Natasha
Marie
Valenzuela

Natalie
Miranda

10.00

400.

Natasha
Marie
Valenzzuela

Natalie
Miranda

Natalie
Miranda

2270

Natalie
Miranda

Natasha
Marie
Valenzuela

Natalie
Miranda

Natasha

Natalie
Miranda

Natasha
Marie
Valenzuela

Natalie
Miranda

Natalie
Miranda

Natalie
Miranda

Natalie

Natalie Miranda

Natalie Miranda

Natalie

Natalie Miranda

Glencoe

Medical Assisting

A Patient-Centered Approach to Administrative and Clinical Competencies

Natalie

Barbara Prickett-Ramutkowski, RN, BSN
Pima Medical Institute, Tucson, Arizona

Abdulai T. Barrie, BS, MS, MD
Business Training Institute, Paramus, New Jersey

Cindy Keller, AAS, CMA
Ivy Tech State College, Lafayette, Indiana

Laurie M. Dazarow, ADN, BS, CMA, MSN, RN, C
Great Lakes Junior College, Saginaw, Michigan

Cindy A. Abel, CMA, PBT (ASCP), BS
Ivy Tech State College, Lafayette, Indiana

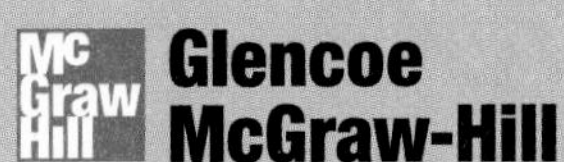

New York, New York
Columbus, Ohio
Woodland Hills, California
Peoria, Illinois

Glencoe/McGraw-Hill 
A Division of The **McGraw-Hill** *Companies*

A Division of the McGraw-Hill Companies

Medical Assisting: A Patient-Centered Approach to Administrative and Clinical Competencies

1 2 3 4 5 6 7 8 9 058 05 04 03 02 01 99 98

Co-developed by
Glencoe/McGraw-Hill
and Visual Education Corporation
Princeton, NJ

WARNING NOTICE: The clinical procedures, medicines, dosages, and other matters described in this publication are based upon research of current literature and consultation with knowledgeable persons in the field. The procedures and matters described in this text reflect currently accepted clinical practice. However, this information cannot and should not be relied upon as necessarily applicable to a given individual's case. Accordingly, each person must be separately diagnosed to discern the patient's unique circumstances. Likewise, the manufacturer's package insert for current drug product information should be consulted before administering any drug. Publisher disclaims all liability for any inaccuracies, omissions, misuse, or misunderstanding of the information contained in this publication. Publisher cautions that this publication is not intended as a substitute for the professional judgment of trained medical personnel.

Library of Congress Cataloging-in-Publication Data

Medical assisting : a patient-centered approach to administrative and clinical competencies / Barbara Prickett-Ramutkowski ... [et al.].
p. cm.
Includes bibliographical references.
ISBN 0–02–802428–1 (student ed.)
ISBN 0–02–802442–7 (student ed. with CD ROM)
1. Medical assistants. I. Prickett-Ramutkowski, Barbara.
[DNLM: 1. Physician Assistants. W 21.5 M4895 1999]
R728.8.M4 1999
610.69'53—dc21
DNLM/DLC
for Library of Congress

97-41917
CIP

Preface

Medical Assisting: A Patient-Centered Approach to Administrative and Clinical Competencies is a comprehensive textbook for the medical assisting student. It acquaints the student with all aspects of the medical assisting profession, both administrative and clinical, from the general to the specific, and it covers key concepts, skills, and tasks that should be familiar to the medical assistant. The book speaks directly to the student, and chapter introductions and conclusions are written to engage the student's attention and to build a sense of positive anticipation about joining the medical assisting profession.

When referring to patients in the third person, we have alternated between passages that describe a male patient and passages that describe a female patient. Thus, the patient will be referred to as "he" half the time and as "she" half the time. The same convention is used to refer to the physician. The medical assistant is consistently addressed as "you."

Patient-Centered Approach

Throughout the book we have taken a patient-centered approach. Wherever tasks involving interaction with patients are described, the focus is on the patient's needs and on the role of the medical assistant in making the patient an active participant in her own care. Several chapters are primarily or exclusively devoted to interaction with patients—such as Chapter 4, on communicating with patients, and Chapter 24, on interviewing the patient.

There is a particular focus on patient education. It is always desirable for patients to be as knowledgeable as possible about their condition. Patients who do not understand what is expected of them may be confused, frightened, angry, and uncooperative; educated patients are better able to understand why compliance is important. Chapter 14 is devoted entirely to patient education. Elsewhere, throughout the book, elements that focus on patient education carry this symbol:

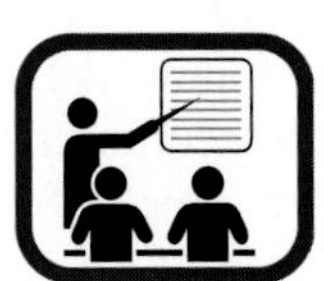

We have also made a consistent effort to discuss patients with special needs. Several chapters in Part II, Administrative Medical Assisting, and half the chapters in Part III, Clinical Medical Assisting, contain special sections of text devoted to the particular concerns of certain patient groups. These groups include the following:

- Pregnant women. Pregnancy has profound effects on every aspect of health, all of which must be taken into account when working with pregnant patients. Where appropriate, we have dealt with special concerns for pregnant patients, such as positioning for an examination, changes in diet, and taking care to avoid harming the fetus with drugs or procedures that would ordinarily pose little or no risk to the patient. Chapter 25, on the general physical examination, includes a separate procedure for meeting the needs of the pregnant patient during an examination.
- Elderly patients. Special care is often required with elderly patients. The body undergoes many changes with age, and patients may have difficulty adjusting to their changing physical needs. Several chapters deal with the special needs of elderly patients, such as Chapter 26, which includes an "Educating the Patient" feature on preventing falls of the elderly.
- Children. The special needs of children are complex, because not only their bodies but their minds and social situations are very different from those of adults. Dealing with children usually means dealing with their parents as well, and medical assistants must hone their communication skills to meet the needs of both patient and parent when working with children. One chapter that focuses on children is Chapter 13, which includes a special text section and a procedure for designing a patient reception area to accommodate children.
- Patients with disabilities. Many different diseases and disabilities require extra effort or consideration on the part of the medical assistant. Patients in wheelchairs and patients with diabetes, hemophilia, or visual or hearing impairments all require specific accommodations. For example, Chapter 22 deals with such patients; it includes a section that discusses the Americans With Disabilities Act and a procedure for making the examination room safe for patients with visual impairments.
- Patients from other cultures. Communicating with patients from other cultures, especially when language barriers are involved, poses a special challenge for the medical assistant. In addition, patients from other cultures may have attitudes about medicine or about social interaction that differ sharply from those of the medical assistant's culture. Chapter 4 is one chapter that deals in depth with patients from other cultures. It contains a text section and a "Caution: Handle With Care" feature about different cultures' attitudes toward medicine.

Because safety is a primary concern for both the patient and the medical assistant, we have emphasized this aspect of the work. Every clinical procedure includes appropriate icons, discussed in Chapter 19, for safety precautions required by the Occupational Safety and Health Administration (OSHA) guidelines. These icons for the OSHA guidelines appear in order of use within each procedure. If hand washing is necessary more than once, the hand washing icon appears twice. If biohazardous waste is generated during the procedure, the biohazardous waste container icon will appear, and so on.

Areas of Competence

A key feature of *Medical Assisting* that will enhance its usefulness to both students and instructors is its reference to the areas of competence defined in the 1997 AAMA Role Delineation Study. The study, which replaces the 1990 DACUM (Developing A CurriculUM) analysis, provides a comprehensive list of duties and skills medical assistants must master at the entry level. The Committee on Accreditation of Allied Health Education Personnel (CAAHEP) requires that all medical assistants be proficient in the 67 entry-level areas of competence when they begin medical assisting work. The opening page of each chapter provides a list of the areas of competence the chapter covers, and the complete Medical Assistant Role Delineation Chart is provided as an appendix. (A correlation chart also appears in the *Instructor's Resource Binder.*) The chapter-by-chapter listing of areas of competence allows instructors to identify skills that have been covered in the course and helps students find the chapters that cover specific skills and duties.

We have been careful to ensure that the text provides ample coverage of topics used to construct the AMT Registered Medical Assistant (RMA) Exam. A correlation chart appears in the *Instructor's Resource Binder.*

Organization of Text

Medical Assisting: A Patient-Centered Approach to Administrative and Clinical Competencies is divided into three parts. Part I provides a basic explanation of the role of the medical assistant in a medical practice. Part II explores the administrative duties of the medical assistant, including basic office work, patient interaction, and financial responsibilities. Part III covers the clinical duties of the medical assistant, from preparing the examination area to assisting with minor surgery.

The ordering of chapters within each part allows the student and the instructor to build a knowledge base starting with the fundamentals and working toward an understanding of highly specialized tasks. Part II introduces the basics of working with office equipment before covering the details of maintaining patient records, scheduling appointments, and processing insurance. Part III begins with a grounding in principles of asepsis, a concept that is crucial to all clinical procedures. Subsequent chapters lead the student through general and specialized physical examinations and eventually into the technical details of laboratory testing, drug administration, electrocardiography, and radiology.

Chapters are also grouped into sections when their subjects relate to a broader topic or area of skills. Each section is set apart, and the general areas of competence covered are included with the list of chapters in that section.

Each chapter opens with a page of material that includes a chapter outline, a list of objectives (skills or knowledge for the student to achieve), a list of key terms, and a list of areas of competence covered in the chapter. The main text of each chapter is organized into topics that move from the general to the specific. Color photographs, anatomical and technical drawings, tables, charts, and in-text features help educate the student about various aspects of medical assisting. The in-text features, set off in boxes within the text, include the following.

- Procedures give step-by-step instructions on how to perform specific administrative or clinical tasks a medical assistant will be required to perform.
- "Tips for the Office" features provide guidelines on keeping the administration of the medical office running smoothly.
- "Educating the Patient" features focus on ways to instruct patients about caring for themselves outside the medical office.
- "Diseases and Disorders" features give detailed information on specific medical conditions—how to recognize, prevent, and treat them.
- "Caution: Handle With Care" features cover precautions to be taken in certain situations or when performing certain tasks.
- "Multiskill Focus" features discuss various specialized medical professions or duties that represent useful additional skills for medical assistants.

Each chapter closes with a summary of the chapter material, focusing on the role of the medical assistant. The summary is followed by end-of-chapter pedagogy, consisting of three types of questions: discussion questions, which involve students in an exploration of issues raised by the chapter material; critical thinking questions, which apply the chapter material to specific, case study-like situations; and application activities, which allow students to practice specific skills in the classroom. End-of-chapter pedagogy is followed by Further Readings—a list of books and articles containing additional information about the subjects presented in the chapter. The instructor may use these further readings to enhance lessons, or the student may use them as references to supplement the text.

The book also includes a glossary and several appendixes for use as reference tools. The Glossary lists all the words presented as key terms in each chapter, along with their definitions, and other terms the student should know. The appendixes include the Medical Assistant Role Delineation Chart and prefixes and suffixes, Latin and Greek terms, abbreviations, and symbols used in medical terminology.

Ancillaries

The *Student Workbook* provides an opportunity for the student to review the material and skills presented in the textbook. On a chapter-by-chapter basis, it provides:

- Vocabulary review exercises, which test knowledge of key terms in the chapter.
- Content review exercises, which test the student's knowledge of key concepts in the chapter.
- Critical thinking exercises, which test the student's understanding of key concepts in the chapter.
- Application exercises, which test mastery of specific skills.
- Case studies, which apply the chapter material to real-life situations or problems.
- Competency checklists for the procedures in the text.

The *Instructor's Resource Binder* provides the instructor with materials to help organize lessons and classroom interactions. It includes:

- A complete lesson plan for each chapter, including an introduction to the lesson, teaching strategies, alternate teaching strategies, case studies, transparency teaching notes, assessment, chapter close, resources, and an answer key to the student textbook.
- Procedure competency checklists, reproduced from the *Student Workbook.*
- An answer key to the *Student Workbook.*
- Charts that show where in the student textbook, the *Student Workbook,* and the *Instructor's Resource Binder,* material is presented that correlates with the 1997 AAMA Role Delineation Study Areas of Competence, the 1990 DACUM Competencies, the SCANS Competencies, the National Health Care Skill Standards, and the AMT Registered Medical Assistant (RMA) Certification Exam Topics.
- Fifty transparencies that reproduce art with captions from the student textbook.

Computer software, including the Glencoe Student Assessment System, the Instructor's Presentation System, and the WCBrown/McGraw-Hill *Dynamic Human* CD-ROM, is also available.

If you have selected the text with CD-ROM, students may study and receive reinforcement on the topics of asepsis; infection control; HIV, hepatitis, and other bloodborne pathogens; minor surgery; and electrocardiography and pulmonary function testing. Also available are CD-ROM packages for classroom use on the topics of infection control and electrocardiography.

Together, the Student Edition, the *Student Workbook,* and the *Instructor's Resource Binder* form a complete teaching and learning package. The *Medical Assisting* course will prepare students to enter the medical assisting field with all the knowledge and skills needed to be a useful resource to patients, a valued asset to employers, and a credit to the medical assisting profession.

Acknowledgments

Many people and organizations provided invaluable assistance in the process of illustrating the highly technical and detailed topics covered in the text. Their contributions helped ensure the accuracy, timeliness, and authenticity of the illustrations in the book.

We would like to thank the following organizations for providing source materials and technical advice: the American Association of Medical Assistants, Chicago, Illinois; Becton Dickinson Microbiology Systems, Inc., Sparks, Maryland; Becton Dickinson VACUTAINER Systems, Inc., Franklin Lakes, New Jersey; Bibbero Systems, Inc., Petaluma, California; Burdick, Inc., Schaumberg, Illinois; the Corel Corporation, Ottawa, Ontario, Canada; Hamilton Media, Hamilton, New Jersey; Nassau Ear, Nose, and Throat, Princeton, New Jersey; Princeton Allergy and Asthma Associates, Princeton, New Jersey; Richmond International, Inc., Boca Raton, Florida; Winfield Medical, Inc., San Diego, California.

We would like to express our appreciation to the following New Jersey physicians and medical facilities for allowing us to photograph a variety of procedures and procedural settings at their facilities: the Eric B. Chandler Medical Center, New Brunswick; Helene Fuld School of Nursing of New Jersey, Trenton; Mercer Medical Center, Trenton; Mercer County Vocational-Technical Health Occupations Center, Trenton; Plainfield Health Center, Plainfield; Princeton Allergy and Asthma Associates, Princeton; the Princeton Medical Group, Princeton; Robert Wood Johnson University Hospital, New Brunswick; Robert Wood Johnson University Hospital at Hamilton, Hamilton; St. Francis Medical Center, Trenton; St. Peter's Medical Center, New Brunswick; Dr. Edward von der Schmidt, neurosurgeon, Princeton; Wound Care Center/Curative Network, New Brunswick.

Reviewers

Every area of the text was reviewed by practitioners and educators in the field. Their insights helped shape the direction of the book.

Janet Aaberg, MS
San Diego Community Colleges
San Diego, CA

Jerri Adler, BA, AA, CMA, CMT
Lane Community College
Eugene, OR

Sr. Patricia Carter, BSN, MS
Stautzenberger College
Findlay, OH

Gwendolyn J. Coleman, RN
Weakley County Vocational Center
Dresden, TN

Lisa Cook, RMA, CMA
Eton Technical Institute
Port Orchard, WA

Barbara Dahl, CMA
Whatcom Community College
Bellingham, WA

Joyce Deutsch, RN, CPC-H, CMA
Indiana Business College
Evansville, IN

Suzanne Ezzo, RN, AST, BS, LVT
Sawyer School
Pittsburgh, PA

Tracie Fuqua, AAS, CMA
Wallace State College
Hanceville, AL

Jeanette Girkin, EdD, CMA
Tulsa Junior College
Tulsa, OK

Glenn Grady, MEd, BSMT (ASCP), CMA
Miller-Motte Business College
Wilmington, NC

Christine E. Hollander, CMA, BS
Denver Institute of Technology
Denver, CO

Sue A. Hunt, MA, RN, CMA
Middlesex Community College
Bedford/Lowell, MA

Chris Kientzle, CMA-C, RMA
Sanford Brown College
Hazelwood, MO

Clare Lewandowski, BS, MA, PhD
Columbus State University College
Columbus, OH

Gwynne Mangiore
Missouri College for Doctors' Assistants
St. Louis, MO

Diane Morlock, CMA
Stautzenberger College
Toledo, OH

Deborah Newton, BS, MA, EMT-I, CMA
Montana State University, College of Technology
Great Falls, MT

Virginia Opitz, RN, BSN, MS, CRRN
North Western Business College
Chicago, IL

Tom Palko, Med, MCS, MT (ASCP)
Arkansas Tech University
Russelville, AR

Hilda Palko, BS, MT (ASCP), CMA
Russelville, AR

Salvatore M. Passanese, AS, BA, MS, PhD
Niagra County Community College
Sanborn, NY

Debra Rosch, CMA
Minnesota School of Business
Brooklyn Center, MN

Jay Shahed, BS, PhD
Robert Morris College
Chicago, IL

Connie W. Stack, BSAH, MLT (ASCP), CMA
Anson Community College
Polkton, NC

Patricia A. Stang, CMA, CPT
Medix School
Baltimore, MD

Geraldine M. Todaro, CMA, CLPLb
Stark State College of Technology
Canton, OH

Kimberly C. Wilson, MT (AMT), CMA
Spencerian College
Louisville, KY

Joan Winters, BS, MS, DLM (ASCP), MT (ASCP)
Wayne Community College
Goldsboro, NC

Brief Contents

Appendixes

Contents

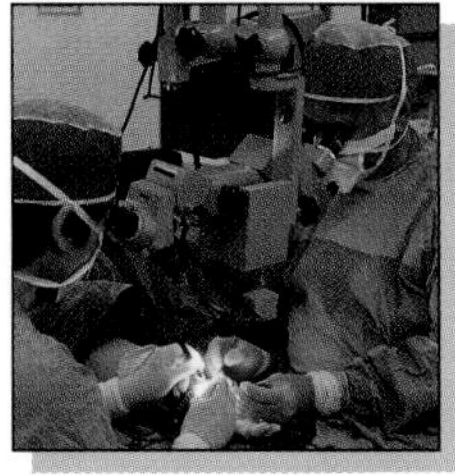

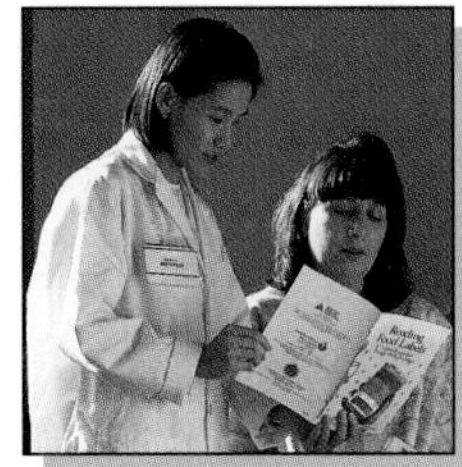

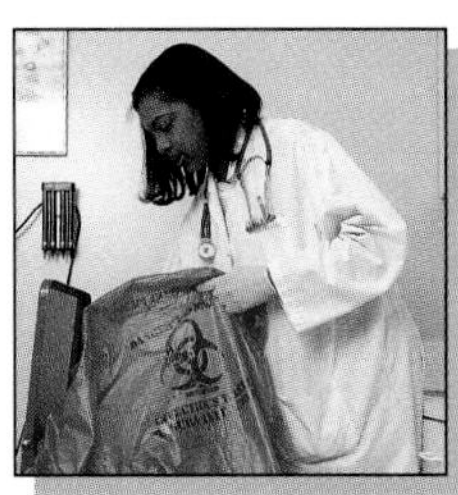

Part One

Introduction to Medical Assisting

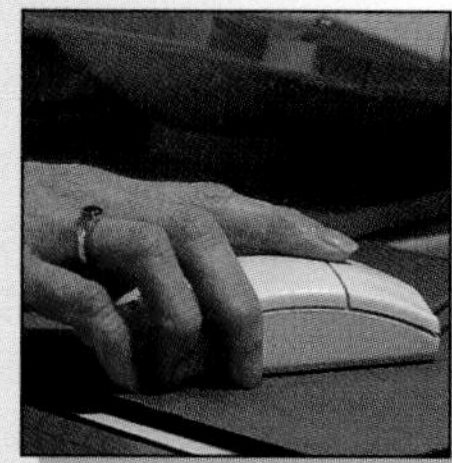

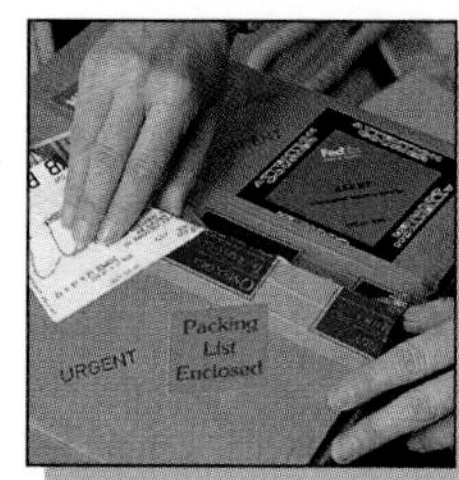
URGENT
Packing
List
Enclosed

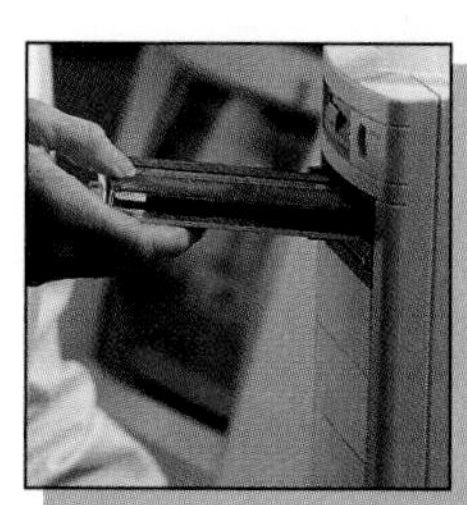

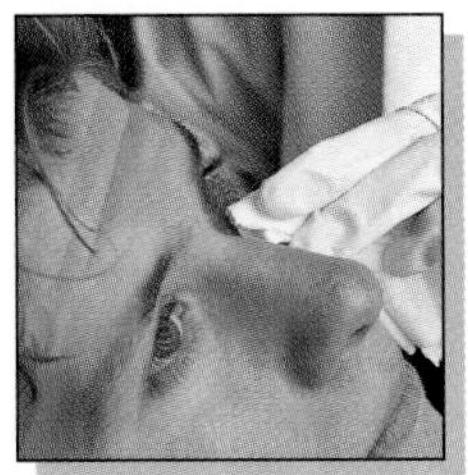
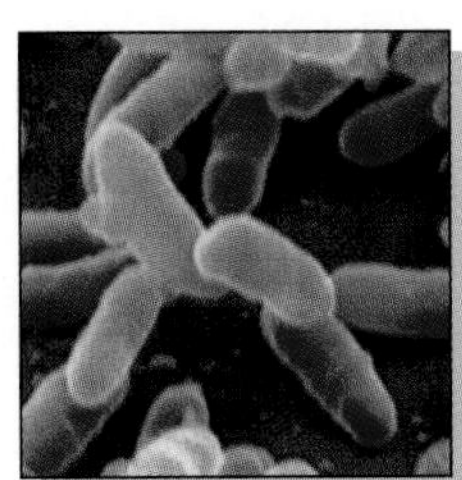
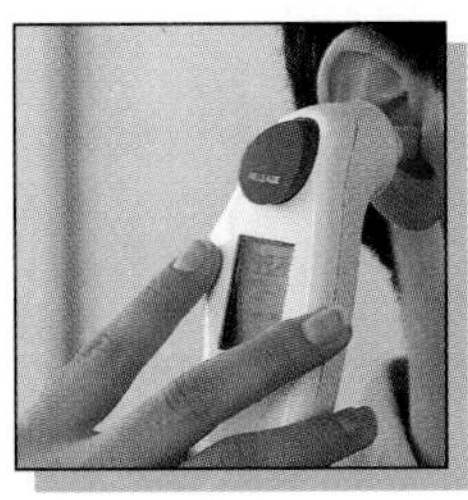

Appendixes

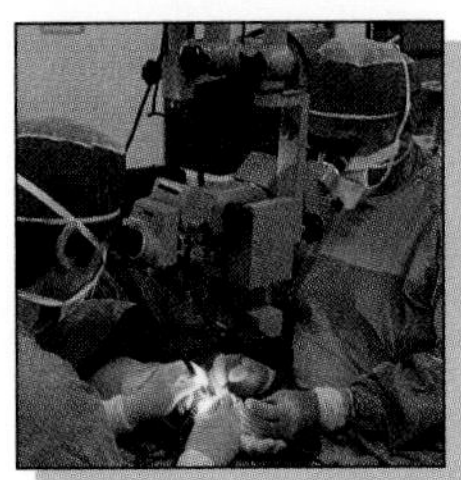
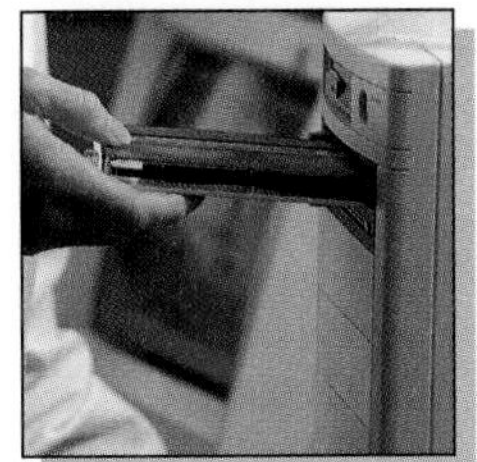
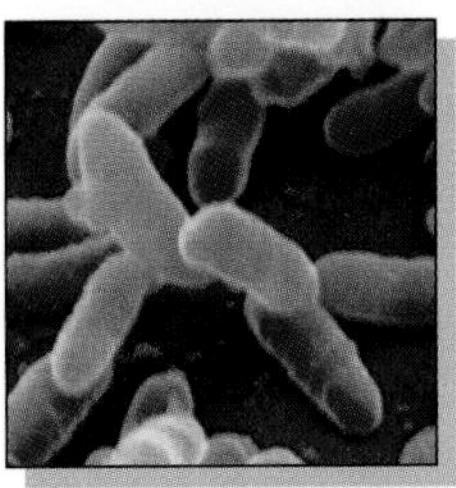

Procedures

Credits and Acknowledgments

Becton Dickinson: 649 *bottom*, 698, 718

Bibbero Systems: 156, 160, 259

Burdick, Inc.: 839 *top left, bottom left, top right*

Center Laboratories: 812

Corbis-Bettmann: 310, 311

David Kelly Crow: xxvi *middle*, 2, 6, 11, 13, 20, 28, 29, 31, 32, 33, 103, 123, 132, 143 *top*, 148, 152, 167, 241, 306 *right*, 308, 318, 326, 327, 378, 386, 387, 424, 425, 436 *bottom*, 490, 494, 496, 499 *bottom*, 559, 561, 594, 637, 673, 760, 780, 790, 843, 855, 856, 857, 873

Difco Laboratories, Detroit, MI: 745 *top*

Tom Dunham: 753 *top*

IVAC Corporation: 436 *top*

Ken Lax: 306 *left*, 467, 472, 475, 476, 499 *top*, 502, 528 *bottom*, 538, 539 *right*, 540, 640, 752 *top*, 753 *bottom*, 758 *bottom*, 759, 761

Lukens Medical Corporation: 653

Robert Matthews: 4, 329, 774

Sara Matthews: 468

MDT Biologic Company: 342

Medical Images, Inc.: 869 *top*
Robert Crandall: 858
C. C. Duncan: 493, 507, 534 *top*, 590
Ken Lax: 221
Leslie O'Shaughnessy: 552
Barry Slaven, MD: 336, 555
Herb Snitzer: 543
Nicholas Thomas: 522, 704

MediSoft: 190

Merrill Property:
Elaine Shay: 754, 758 *top*
Spangler Studio: 752 *bottom*

Lawrence Migdale: 438 *top left*

Courtesy of Mercer Medical Center, Dept. of Radiology, Trenton, NJ: 876 *middle left*, 880 *top*

Cliff Moore: xxvi *right*, 1 *middle*, 44, 45, 56, 58, 61, 62, 68 *middle*, 117, 118, 120, 203, 319, 321, 322, 324, 333, 339 *left*, 341, 379, 380, 389, 487, 519, 563, 564, 565, 568, 570, 571, 615, 635, 641, 642, 643, 649 *top*, 729, 730, 732, 733, 738, 745 *bottom*, 748, 814, 815, 817, 819, 829, 839 *bottom*, 853, 860, 862, 863, 866, 872, 882, 885

Courtesy of MRI Center at Lawrenceville, NJ: 876 *bottom*

Orion Diagnostica Inc., Somerset, NJ: 741 *bottom*

Pelton & Crane: A Siemens Company: 339 *right*, 340

Peter Arnold, Inc.:
Dr. E. Buttane: 744
David Scharf: 727
SIU: 728 *bottom*
Volker Steger: 43, 725 *bottom left*

Photo Researchers, Inc.: 317
Michael Abbey: 396 *bottom left*
Jonathan Ashton/Science Photo Library: 510 *middle right*
Biology Media: 313
Biophoto Associates: 396 *bottom right, top left*, 527 *bottom*, 541
Dr. Tony Brain/Science Photo Library: 728 *middle left*
Scott Camazine: 728 *middle right*, 878 *middle*
CNRI/Science Photo Library: 531
Dickson Despommier: 728 *top right*
John Durham/Science Photo Library: 743
EM Unit, CVL Weybridge/Science Photo Library: 723 *bottom right*
R. J. Erwin: 781 *top left*
Stephen Gerard/Science Source: 878 *top*
GrantPix: 534 *bottom*
James King-Holmes/Science Photo Library: 438 *right*
Andrew McClenaghan/Science Photo Library: 781 *top right*
Will & Deni McIntyre: 1 *left*, 34, 243
Oliver Meckes: 306 *middle*, 725 *top left, top right*
Tom Meyers: 528 *top*
Morendum Animal Health, Ltd./Science Photo Library: 725 *bottom right*, 726
Hank Morgan/Science Source: 138
Professor P. Motta/Univ. "La Sapienza," Rome: 396 *top right*
Larry Mulvehill: 644
NIBSC/Science Photo Library: 723 *left*
NIH/Science Source: 878 *bottom*
John Radcliffe Hospital/Science Photo Library: 518
J. H. Robinson: 728 *top left*
P. Saada/Eurelios/Science Photo Library: 880 *bottom*
Saturn Stills/Science Photo Library: 438 *bottom left*
Science Photo Library: 510 *top left, top right, middle left*, 723 *top right*
Blair Seitz: 521
SIU: 364
Kathy Sloane: xxvi *left*, 27
Garry Watson/Science Photo Library: 359

PhotoEdit: 356
Tony Freeman: 316
Bonnie Kamin: 478
Michael Newman: 625

Phototake:
Ken Sherman: 401

Courtesy of Quakerbridge MRI-CT X-Ray Center, Mercerville, NJ: 876 *top right, middle right*

Courtesy of Radiology Affiliates of Central NJ, PA; Mercerville, NJ: 876 *top left*

Martin M. Rotker: 510 *bottom left*, 527 *top*, 741, 869

Sage Products, Inc.: 323

Kathy Sloane: 1 *right*, 26, 70, 149, 211, 215, 216

The Terry Wild Studio: 68 *left, right*, 72, 76, 78, 79, 80, 86, 89, 97, 98, 99, 143 *bottom*, 155, 162, 166, 169, 172, 180, 195, 199, 200, 201, 204, 206 *left*, 207, 213, 219, 223, 248, 266, 274, 287, 292, 449, 451, 452, 479, 483, 484, 539 *left*, 688, 700, 701, 716, 717, 781 *bottom*

Vistech Consultants: 471 *top right*

Shirley Zeiberg: 182, 206 *right*, 391, 433, 520

Chapter 6, Figure 6-5:
Screen shot reprinted by permission from Microsoft Corporation.

Chapter 6, Figure 6-6:
© I. Hoffmann + Associates Inc. (H + a) Image from the Epilepsy CD-ROM of the H + a Medical Series. All rights reserved.

Chapter 6, Figure 6-7:
Corel WordPerfect is a registered trademark of Corel Corporation or Corel Corporation Limited in Canada, the United States, and/or other countries.

Glencoe

Medical Assisting

A Patient-Centered Approach to Administrative and Clinical Competencies

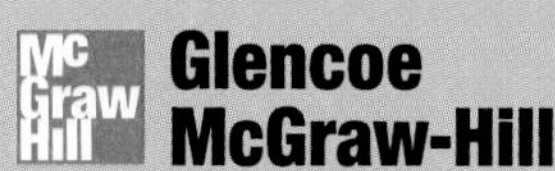

Glencoe McGraw-Hill

New York, New York
Columbus, Ohio
Woodland Hills, California
Peoria, Illinois

Part One

Introduction To Medical Assisting

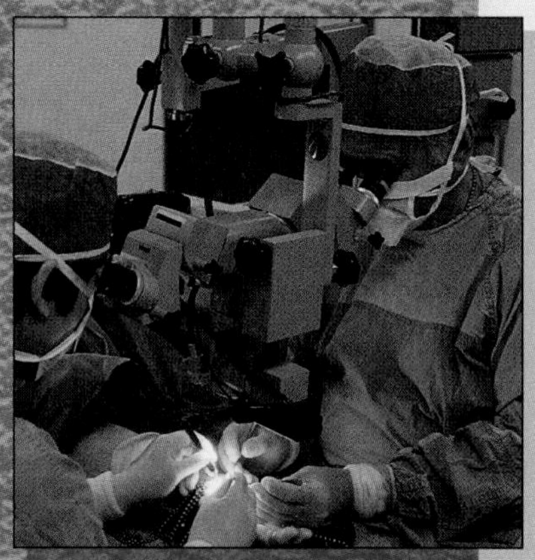

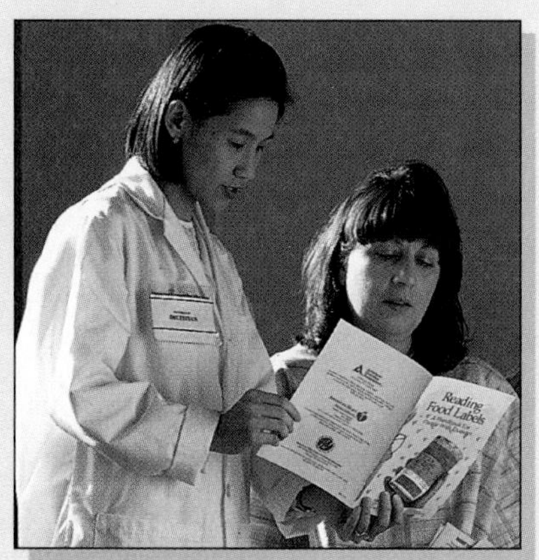

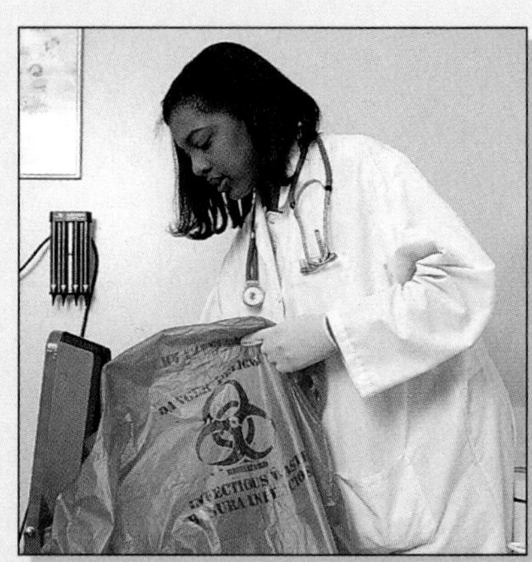

"The medical assisting profession is filled with challenges and rewards every day. Everything is important when you are assisting a patient. You should get to know your patient, and his family, if possible, in order to understand the patient's specific needs. This is especially true with an elderly patient. Treat your patient like a family member. Be considerate and concerned, and always maintain a pleasant attitude.

"It is also essential to know your physician well, and how he or she likes to work. Let the physician know all the information the patient has shared with you, to help him or her make a better diagnosis. Keep informed about what the physician has recommended for treatment. The patient will have questions along the way. It's good medicine to be able to give him solid information about his condition and reinforce the doctor's orders when necessary. A skilled physician and an organized, cooperative, receptive medical assistant promote and maintain exceptional patient care."

Sue Haines,
Medical Assistant, Princeton, New Jersey

Section One

Foundations and Principles

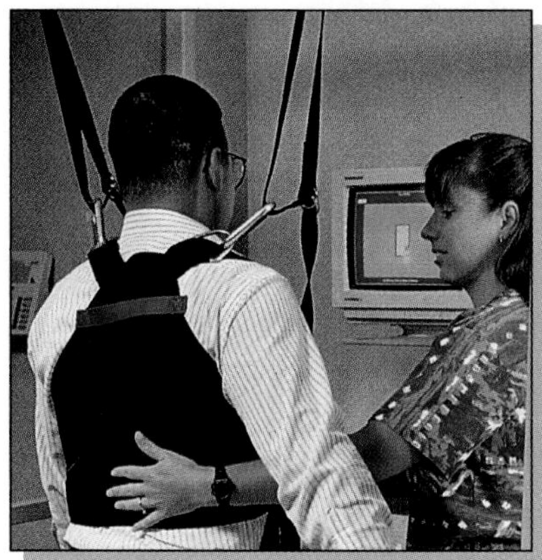

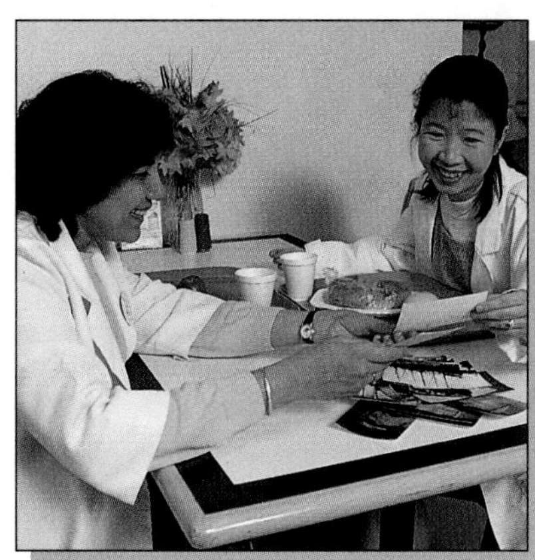

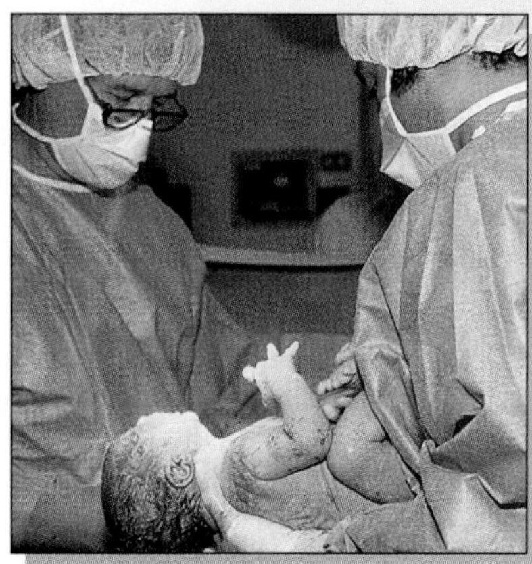

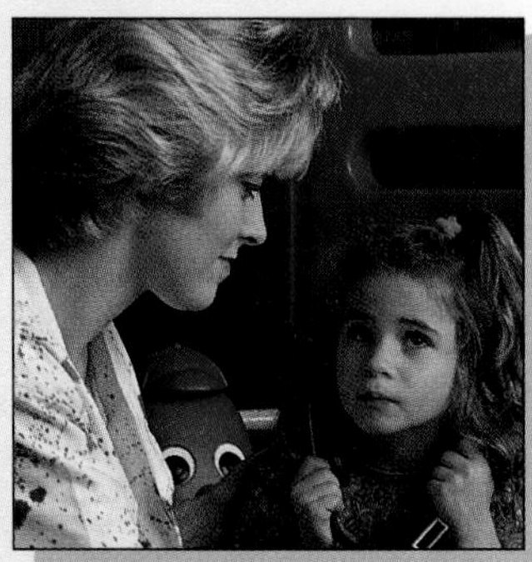

Section One

Foundations and Principles

AREAS OF COMPETENCE

1997 ROLE DELINEATION STUDY

CLINICAL

- Patient Care

GENERAL (Transdisciplinary)

- Professionalism
- Communication Skills
- Legal Concepts

CHAPTER LIST

CHAPTER 1 The Profession of Medical Assisting

CHAPTER OUTLINE

- Growth of the Medical Assisting Profession
- Medical Assistant Credentials
- Membership in a Medical Assisting Association
- Training Programs and Other Learning Opportunities
- Daily Duties of Medical Assistants
- Personal Qualifications of Medical Assistants
- Obtaining a Position
- On the Job
- DACUM Educational Components

Key Terms

accreditation
American Association of Medical Assistants (AAMA)
Certified Medical Assistant (CMA)
contaminated
curriculum vitae
DACUM
externship
portfolio
practitioner
Registered Medical Assistant (RMA)
résumé

OBJECTIVES

After completing Chapter 1, you will be able to:

- Describe the job responsibilities of a medical assistant.
- Discuss the professional training of a medical assistant.
- Identify the personal characteristics a medical assistant needs.
- Define multiskilled health professional.
- Describe how to conduct a job search in the medical assisting profession.
- Explain the importance of continuing education for a medical assistant.
- Describe the process and benefits of certification and registration.
- List the benefits of becoming a member of a professional association.

AREAS OF COMPETENCE

1997 ROLE DELINEATION STUDY

GENERAL (Transdisciplinary)

Professionalism

- Project a professional manner and image
- Demonstrate initiative and responsibility
- Manage time effectively
- Prioritize and perform multiple tasks
- Promote the CMA credential
- Enhance skills through continuing education

Communication Skills

- Use effective and correct verbal and written communications

Legal Concepts

- Practice within the scope of education, training, and personal capabilities

Growth of the Medical Assisting Profession

As a medical assistant you will be an allied health professional trained to work in a variety of health-care settings: medical offices, clinics, and hospitals. Your role, with varied and challenging administrative and clinical duties, will be integral to creating a health-care facility that operates smoothly and provides a patient-centered approach to quality health care. Your specific responsibilities will likely depend on the location and size of the facility as well as its medical specialties.

Medical assisting is now one of the fastest-growing occupations. As the health services industry expands, the U.S. Department of Labor predicts that medical assisting will grow at a much faster rate than the average rate for all occupations through the year 2005. The growth in the number of physicians' group practices and other health-care practices that use support personnel will in turn continue to drive up demand for medical assistants.

According to the U.S. Department of Labor Bureau of Labor Statistics, in 1992 more than 70 percent of medical assistants were employed in physicians' offices. About 12 percent worked in the offices of other health **practitioners** (those who practice a profession), such as chiropractors, optometrists, and podiatrists. Some worked in hospitals, nursing homes, and other health-care facilities.

Modern health insurance, Medicare, and Medicaid now make medical care available to more people, and the number of physicians is increasing. Thus, more medical assistants will be needed to run these physicians' offices.

The following factors will also increase job opportunities for medical assistants: growth of outpatient clinics and health maintenance organizations (HMOs) and the population increase. Specifically, greater numbers of older people now require a relatively high level of medical care (Heyman, 1993). Today more than 20 million persons are over age 65. By the year 2000, approximately 50 percent of the general population will be older than 65. This older population has unique needs and problems (Mitchell and Grippando, 1993).

History of the Medical Assisting Profession

Health professionals served as generalists through the 1950s. During that time nurses performed many basic functions now provided by allied health professionals, including medical laboratory procedures, respiratory therapy, and pulmonary function testing. During the 1960s and 1970s an explosion of knowledge and advances in technology led to specialization. In addition to nurses, nurse practitioners and allied health professionals joined the field of health-care providers. As physicians' needs for office help increased, medical assistants began to receive on-the-job training and to participate in formal academic programs (Bamberg, 1990).

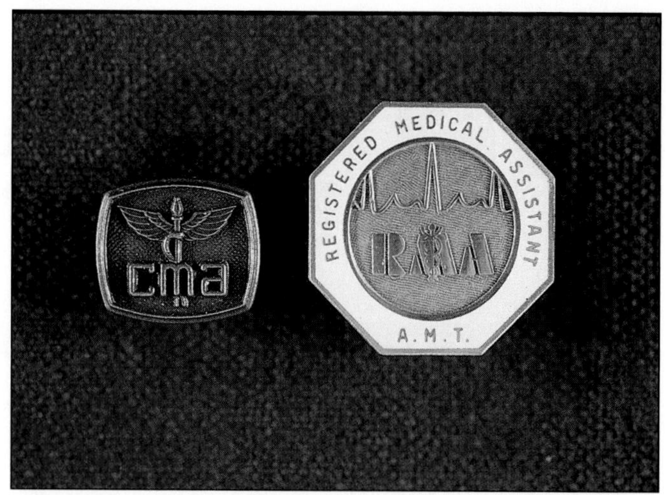

Figure 1-1. The pin on the left is worn by members of the American Association of Medical Assistants. The pin on the right is worn by medical assistants registered by the American Medical Technologists.

Creating the American Association of Medical Assistants

The seed of the idea for a national association of medical assistants—to be called the **American Association of Medical Assistants (AAMA)**—was planted at the 1955 annual state convention of the Kansas Medical Assistants Society. The next year, at an American Medical Association (AMA) meeting, the AAMA was officially created. In 1978 the U.S. Department of Health, Education, and Welfare declared medical assisting an allied health profession. In the early 1970s the American Medical Technologists (which has been a national certifying body for laboratory personnel since 1939) began a program to register medical assistants at accredited schools. You will read more about the benefits of joining one of these organizations later in the chapter. Figure 1-1 shows the pins worn by medical assistants who are certified by the AAMA and by those registered by the American Medical Technologists.

The AAMA's Purpose. The AAMA works to raise standards of medical assisting to a more professional level. It is the only professional association devoted exclusively to the medical assisting profession. Its creator and first president, Maxine Williams, had extensive experience in orchestrating medical assisting projects for the Kansas Medical Assistants Society. She also served as cochair of the planning committee that formed the AAMA.

The AAMA Creed. To maintain the professional standards of the medical assisting profession, the AAMA has developed the following creed, which is reprinted here with the permission of the organization:

> *I believe in the principles and purposes of the profession of medical assisting.*
> *I endeavor to be more effective.*

I aspire to render greater service.
I protect the confidence entrusted to me.
I am dedicated to the care and well-being of all patients.
I am loyal to my physician-employer.
I am true to the ethics of my profession.
I am strengthened by compassion, courage, and faith.

Medical Assistant Credentials

According to Donald A. Balasa, JD, MBA, AAMA executive director and staff legal counsel, "voluntary credentialing . . . is usually national in its scope and most often sponsored by a nongovernmental, private-sector entity" (Balasa, 1994). Many managed care programs (health maintenance organizations), however, want only certified or registered medical assistants on staff. Becoming certified or registered is strongly recommended, as is fulfilling the ongoing requirements to become recertified or reregistered.

RMA Registration

The **Registered Medical Assistant (RMA)** credential is given by the American Medical Technologists (AMT), an organization founded in 1939. RMA credentialing by the AMT ensures that you have taken and passed the AMT certification examination for the Registered Medical Assistant. RMA is a generic term used by the American Registry of Medical Assistants since 1950 and by the AMT since 1984.

The AMT sets forth certain educational and experiential requirements to earn the RMA credential. These include:

- Graduation from an accredited high school or acceptable equivalent.
- Graduation from a medical assistant program or institution accredited by the Accrediting Bureau of Health Education Schools, from a medical assistant program accredited by a regional accrediting commission, or from a formal medical services training program of the U.S. Armed Forces. Alternatively, the applicant can have been employed in the profession of medical assisting for a minimum of 5 years, not more than 2 of which may have been as an instructor in a postsecondary medical assistant program.
- Passing the AMT examination for RMA certification.

CMA Certification

The **Certified Medical Assistant (CMA)** credential is awarded by the Certifying Board of the AAMA. The AAMA's certification examination evaluates mastery of medical assisting competencies based on the 1997 Role Delineation Study, discussed later in this chapter. The National Board of Medical Examiners (NBME) also provides technical assistance in developing the tests.

CMAs must recertify the CMA credential every 5 years. This mandate requires you to learn about new medical developments through education courses or participation in an examination. Hundreds of continuing education courses are sponsored by local, state, and national AAMA groups. The AAMA also offers self-study courses through its Continuing Education Department. As described in the AAMA's publication, *Certified Medical Assistants: Health-Care's Most Versatile Professionals,* the advantages of CMA certification include respect and recognition from peers in the medical assisting profession.

As of June 1998, only applicants of medical assisting programs accredited by the Commission on Accreditation of Allied Health Education Programs (CAAHEP) are eligible to take the certification examination. The examination is administered nationwide every January and June at more than 100 test sites. The AAMA offers the *Candidate's Guide to the Certification Examination* to help applicants prepare for the examination. This guide explains the test format and test-taking strategies. It also includes a sample examination with answers and information about study references.

Major Areas of the RMA/CMA Examinations

The RMA and CMA qualifying examinations are rigorous. Participation in an accredited program, however, will help you learn what you need to know. The examinations cover several distinct areas of knowledge. These include:

- General medical knowledge, including terminology, anatomy, physiology, behavioral science, medical law, and ethics.
- Administrative knowledge, including medical records management, collections, and insurance processing.
- Clinical knowledge, including examination room techniques, medication preparation and administration, pharmacology, and specimen collection.

Membership in a Medical Assisting Association

Professional associations set high standards for quality and performance in a profession. They define the tasks and functions of an occupation. In addition, they provide members with the opportunity to communicate and network with one another. They also present their goals to the profession and to the general public. Becoming a member of a professional association helps you achieve career goals and further the profession of medical assisting.

Professional Support for RMAs

The AMT offers many benefits for RMAs. These include:

- Professional publications.
- Membership in the AMT Institute for Education.

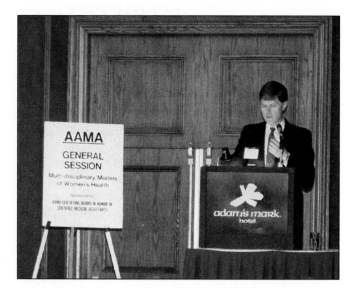

Figure 1-2. Local and state chapters of the AAMA and AMT frequently sponsor seminars and workshops on administrative, clinical, or management topics. In this picture, Donald A. Balasa, executive director and staff legal counsel for the AAMA, addresses a group at the annual AAMA national convention.

- Group insurance programs—liability, health, and life.
- State chapter activities.
- Legal representation in health legislative matters.
- Annual meetings and educational seminars.

Professional Support for CMAs

When you become a member of the AAMA, you will have a large support group of active medical assistants. Membership benefits include:

- Professional publications, such as *The Professional Medical Assistant.*
- A large variety of educational opportunities, such as chapter-sponsored seminars and workshops about the latest administrative, clinical, and management topics (Figure 1-2).
- Group insurance.
- Legal counsel.

Training Programs and Other Learning Opportunities

Formal programs in medical assisting are offered in a variety of educational settings. They include vocational-technical high schools, postsecondary vocational schools, community and junior colleges, and 4-year colleges and universities. Vocational school programs usually last 1 or 2 years and award a certificate or diploma. Community and junior college programs are usually 2-year associate degree programs.

Accreditation

Accreditation is the process by which programs are officially authorized. Two agencies recognized by the U.S. Department of Education accredit programs in medical assisting: CAAHEP and the Accrediting Bureau of Health Education Schools (ABHES).

Accredited programs must cover the following topics: anatomy and physiology; medical terminology; medical law and ethics; psychology; oral and written communications; laboratory, clinical, and administrative procedures; typing; transcription; record keeping; accounting; and insurance processing. High school students may prepare for these courses by studying mathematics, health, biology, typing, office skills, bookkeeping, and computers. You may obtain current information about accreditation standards for medical assisting programs from the AAMA.

Medical assisting programs must also include an externship. An **externship** is practical work experience for a specified time frame in physicians' offices, hospitals, or other health-care facilities.

Additionally, the AAMA lists its minimum standards for accredited programs (called essentials). This list of essentials ensures that all personnel—administrators and faculty—are qualified to perform their jobs.

The AAMA requires that administrative personnel exhibit leadership and management skills. They must also be able to fully perform the functions identified in documented job descriptions. Faculty members must develop and evaluate lesson plans, assess student progress toward the program's objectives, and be knowledgeable regarding course content. They must be qualified through work experience and be able to effectively direct and evaluate student learning and laboratory experiences.

The AAMA also has accreditation requirements for financial and physical resources. Each program's financial resources must meet its obligations to students. Schools must also have adequate physical resources—classrooms, laboratories, clinical and administrative facilities, and equipment and supplies.

The Benefits of Certification/Registration

Certification or registration is not required to practice as a medical assistant. You may practice with a high school diploma or equivalent. Your career options will be greater, however, if you graduate from an accredited school and you become certified or registered.

Graduation from an accredited program helps your career in three ways. First, it shows that you have completed a program that meets nationally accepted standards. Second, it provides recognition of your education by professional peers. Third, it makes you eligible for registration or certification (Heyman, 1993).

A solid medical assisting program provides the following:

- Facilities and equipment that are up to date
- Classes of fewer than 25 students to provide good interaction between instructor and student

- Job placement services
- A cooperative education program and opportunities for continuing education

Externships

In an externship you will obtain work experience while completing a medical assisting program. You will practice skills learned in the classroom in an actual medical office environment.

Externship Requirements. Externships are mandatory in accredited schools. Each program has its own externship requirements. Familiarize yourself with the program requirements as soon as possible. You may be able to obtain an externship site of your choice either at a practice already affiliated with the school or at a practice you find on your own.

The externship is offered in cooperative medical offices or hospitals for a predetermined period (several weeks to several months). Another experienced medical assistant, nurse manager, or licensed nurse practitioner in the externship office often becomes your mentor. This mentor advises and supervises you during the externship.

Externship Duties. Your duties will be planned to meet your program's requirements for real-world work experience. Approach the externship with a positive attitude. Accept any guidance, constructive criticism, or praise as a learning experience.

Obtaining a Reference. Your externship also offers you the opportunity to acquire a good reference. A reference is usually written by your supervisor, who will describe your performance, strengths, and skills. You may use this reference later with prospective employers. As you may be required to provide a list of references when applying for future jobs, ask your externship mentor to prepare a letter of reference for your **portfolio** (a collection of your résumé, reference letters, and other documents of interest, such as awards for volunteer service in a health-related field). Send a thank-you note to your supervisor for allowing you to do an externship and for writing you a reference.

Volunteer Programs

Volunteering is a rewarding experience. Before you even begin a medical assisting program, you can gain experience in a health-care profession through volunteer work. As a volunteer, you will get hands-on training and learn what it is like to assist patients who are ill, disabled, or frightened.

You may volunteer as an aide in a hospital, clinic, nursing home, or doctor's office or as a typist or filing clerk in a medical office or medical record room. Some visiting nurse associations and hospices (homelike medical settings that provide medical care and emotional support to terminally ill patients and their families) also offer volunteer opportunities. These experiences may help you decide if you want to pursue a career as a medical assistant.

The American Red Cross also offers volunteer opportunities for the student medical assistant. The Red Cross needs volunteers for its disaster relief programs locally, statewide, nationally, and abroad.

As part of a disaster relief team at the site of a hurricane, tornado, storm, flood, earthquake, or fire, volunteers learn first-aid and emergency triage skills. Red Cross volunteers gain valuable work experience that may help them obtain a job.

Because volunteers are not paid, it is usually easy to find work opportunities. Just because you are not paid for volunteer work, however, does not mean the experience is not useful for meeting your career goals.

Include information about any volunteer work on your **résumé**—a typewritten document that summarizes your employment and educational history. Be sure to note specific duties, responsibilities, and skills developed during the volunteer experience (Figure 1-3). Résumés are discussed in more detail later in this chapter.

Multiskill Training

Today many hospitals and health-care practices are embracing the idea of a multiskilled health-care professional (MSHP). An MSHP is a cross-trained team member who is able to handle many different duties.

The AAMA includes the word *multiskill* in its definition of the profession of medical assisting:

> *Medical assisting is a multiskilled allied health profession whose practitioners work primarily in ambulatory settings, such as medical offices and clinics. Medical assistants function as members of the healthcare delivery team and perform administrative and clinical procedures. (AAMA, 1991)*

An MSHP may be trained to perform certain clinical procedures. She is not, however, trained to make judgments or interpretations concerning a patient's diagnosis or treatment, as a physician would.

Reducing Health-Care Costs. As a result of health-care reform and downsizing (a reduction in the number of staff members) to control the rising cost of health care, medical practices are eager to reduce personnel costs by hiring multiskilled health professionals. These individuals, who perform the functions of two or more people, are the most cost-efficient employees.

Expanding Your Career Opportunities. Career opportunities are vast if you are self-motivated and willing to learn new skills. If you continue to learn about new administrative and clinical techniques and procedures, you will be an important part of the health-care team.

As you read this book, look for a boxed feature titled Multiskill Focus. This feature highlights additional skills medical assistants can learn and integrate into their jobs

ALICIA HOLT
114 Herald Avenue
Winston, MO 43840
601-444-1216

POSITION:	Full-time medical assistant
EDUCATION:	
June 1996–June 1998	Associate Degree in Science, Mayerville Community College Will take the medical assisting certification examination after graduation
September 1991–June 1995	Winston Central High School
WORK EXPERIENCE:	
May 1998–June 1998	Medical assistant extern Dr. J. D. Perez, pediatrician, Mayerville Pediatrics, Mayerville, MO
September 1994–present	General office clerk Cunningham Medical Supply Company, Winston, MO
June 1994–September 1994	Waitress Bonelli's Italian Restaurant, Winston, MO
VOLUNTEER EXPERIENCE:	
May 1995–present	Recreational aide Watson House for Autistic Children, Mayerville, MO
June 1993–present	Receptionist and information clerk Riverside General Hospital, Atherton, MO
SPECIAL SKILLS:	Typing 55 wpm WordPerfect and Excel Medical Transcription CPR (certified) First Aid (certified)

References available upon request.

Figure 1-3. This medical assistant's résumé includes information about her volunteer work.

to make themselves more marketable as multiskilled health professionals. Following are several examples of positions that are sometimes combined with a medical assistant position:

- Office manager
- Medical laboratory technician
- ECG technician
- Medical transcriptionist
- Medical biller
- Hospital admissions coordinator
- A professional who performs physical exams for applicants to insurance companies
- An administrative assistant at insurance companies (particularly in managed care companies), hospitals, and clinics

If you are multiskilled, you will have an advantage when job hunting. Prospective employers are eager to hire multiskilled medical assistants and may create positions for them.

Daily Duties of Medical Assistants

As a medical assistant you will be the physician's "right arm." Duties include maintaining an efficient office, preparing and maintaining medical records, assisting the physician during examinations, and keeping examining rooms in order. You may also handle the payroll for the office staff (or supervise a payroll service), obtain equipment and supplies, and serve as the link between the physician and representatives of pharmaceutical and medical supply companies. In small practices you will usually handle all duties. In larger practices you may specialize in a particular duty.

Administrative Duties

Your administrative duties may include:

- Greeting patients.
- Handling correspondence.
- Scheduling appointments.
- Answering telephones.
- Creating and maintaining patient medical records.
- Handling billing, bookkeeping, and insurance processing.
- Performing medical transcription.
- Arranging for hospital admissions.
- Scheduling teleconferences for doctors at different locations to discuss cases.
- Supervising personnel.
- Developing and conducting public outreach programs to market the physician's professional services.
- Negotiating leases of equipment and supply contracts.
- Creating a recycling program for the practice. ("Tips for the Office" gives more information on this topic.)
- Serving as liaison between the physician and other individuals, such as pharmaceutical sales representatives and lawyers.

Clinical Duties

Your clinical duties may vary according to state law. They may include:

- Assisting the doctor during examinations.
- Asepsis and infection control.
- Performing diagnostic tests.
- Giving injections, where allowed.
- Performing electrocardiograms (ECGs).
- Drawing blood for testing.
- Disposing of **contaminated** (soiled, or stained) supplies.
- Explaining treatment procedures to patients.
- Performing first aid and cardiopulmonary resuscitation (CPR).
- Patient education.
- Preparing patients for examinations.
- Preparing and administering medications as directed by the physician, and following state laws for invasive procedures.
- Facilitating treatment for patients from diverse cultural backgrounds and for patients with hearing or vision impairments, or physical or mental disabilities.
- Recording vital signs and medical histories.
- Removing sutures or changing dressings on wounds.
- Sterilizing medical instruments.

Other clinical duties may include instructing patients about medication and special diets, authorizing drug refills as directed, and calling pharmacies to order prescriptions. You may also assist with minor surgery or teach patients about special procedures before laboratory tests, surgery, x-rays, or ECGs.

Laboratory Duties

Your laboratory duties may include:

- Performing tests, such as a urine pregnancy test, on the premises.
- Collecting, preparing, and transmitting laboratory specimens.
- Teaching patients to collect specific specimens properly.
- Arranging laboratory services.
- Meeting safety standards and fire protection mandates.

Specialization

You may also choose to specialize in a specific area of health care. For example, podiatric medical assistants make castings of feet, expose and develop x-rays, and assist podiatrists in surgery. Ophthalmic medical

Tips FOR THE OFFICE: Recycling in the Medical Office, Hospital, Laboratory, or Clinic

You may easily incorporate recycling procedures into a medical office, hospital, laboratory, or clinic's daily routine. Medical facilities generate a tremendous amount of recyclable paper material. Recycling may be required by state law. Purchase paper products that can be recycled, or those made of postconsumer recycled materials, and take care in disposing of them (Roseen, 1991).

Some states levy large fines for noncompliance with recycling regulations. It is thus important to have a well-organized office recycling program. There are two essential aspects of recycling: disposal and purchasing. To create a complete recycling program, ensure that materials are disposed of properly and that purchased products have been made from recycled materials.

You may easily call the town's recycling center for guidelines for packaging recycled materials and for a pickup schedule. The recycling center may also provide containers for recyclable materials. You must fulfill all town and state legal recycling requirements.

Most paper products that do not have a glossy coating (like some fax paper) are recyclable. Each recycling center will provide a list of paper materials that can and cannot be recycled.

You must also research disposal techniques for biohazardous materials and follow regulations listed in the office policy manual and the Occupational Safety and Health Administration (OSHA) guidelines. These materials cannot be recycled and must be disposed of properly. They must not be mixed with recyclable waste. You will follow the office policy manual and OSHA guidelines for hazardous medical wastes—including blood products, gloves, cotton swabs, body fluids, and sharps (needles or instruments that puncture the skin). These materials must be disposed of following standard guidelines and in a specially designed protective container.

You must keep recycling issues in mind at all times. Always choose products made from recycled materials—including paper (computer paper and letterhead), printer cartridges, pencils, and many other products.

assistants help ophthalmologists (doctors who provide eye care) by administering diagnostic tests, measuring and recording vision, testing the functioning of eyes and eye muscles, and performing other duties. (Medical specialties and medical assistant specialties are fully discussed in Chapter 2.)

Personal Qualifications of Medical Assistants

There are several personal qualifications that you must have to be an effective and productive medical assistant. You must enjoy working with all types of people, possess good critical thinking skills, and be able to pay attention to detail. Empathy, willingness to learn, flexibility, self-motivation, professionalism, and sound judgment are other important traits. Additionally, you must have a neat, professional appearance, possess good communication skills, and know how to remain calm in a crisis.

Critical Thinking Skills

You will develop critical thinking skills over time, as you apply knowledge about and experience with human nature, medicine, and office administration to new situations. Critical thinking skills include quickly evaluating circumstances, solving problems, and taking action.

Critical thinking skills are used every day. One example is prioritizing your work—deciding which are the most important tasks of the day and which are less important. On a day where everything seems to be "top priority," you must use your professional judgment, knowledge of office policies, and experience with physicians and coworkers to determine what should get done first, second, third, and so on.

You must use critical thinking skills to assess how to react to emergency situations. If you see a patient suddenly pass out in the physician's waiting room, you must quickly see that the patient receives first aid, notify a physician, and alert the patient's family.

Attention to Detail

The profession of medical assisting requires attention to detail. You must check every detail when administering drugs, processing bills and insurance forms, and completing patient charts.

The need for attention to detail is illustrated in the common request to call a patient's pharmacy to order a prescription. You must accurately relay information from the doctor's prescription to the pharmacist. You must ask the pharmacist to read back the information to ensure that he has heard it correctly. Then you must document, in the chart, what has been ordered and when.

Empathy

Empathy is the ability to "put yourself in someone else's shoes" and to identify with and understand another person's feelings. Patients who are ill, frustrated, or frightened appreciate empathic medical personnel.

Many patients require empathy during a medical crisis. For example, a patient with the flu may describe how coughing has prevented him from getting a full night's sleep. You may display empathy by saying, "I know how the flu can disrupt sleep. I just got over it last week myself. It's important to rest in bed, though, even if you can't always sleep."

Willingness to Learn

You must always display a willingness to learn. You will gain new skills more easily and become better acquainted with the administrative and clinical topics and issues related to the practice in which you work if you are willing to learn. Keep an open mind, listen carefully to the professionals with whom you work, observe procedures carefully, listen actively to others, and do your own homework to learn more about medical topics so you can apply new information to your daily activities. For example, if you work in a pediatric practice, you might take a continuing education class on child development at a local community college, at a YWCA, or in a workshop offered by a professional association such as the AAMA or AMT (Figure 1-4).

Flexibility

You will encounter new people and situations every day. An attitude of flexibility will allow you to adapt and to handle them with professionalism.

An example of the need for flexibility occurs when a physician's schedule changes to include evening and weekend hours. The staff may also be asked to change schedules. You must make it a priority to be flexible and to meet the employer's needs.

Self-Motivation

You must be self-motivated and willing to offer assistance with work that needs to be done, even if it is not your assigned job. For example, if you think of a more efficient way to organize patient check-in, discuss it with your supervisor. She may agree and be willing to give your idea a try. If a coworker is on vacation, offer to pitch in and work extra time to keep the office running smoothly.

Professionalism

You should exhibit courtesy, conscientiousness, and a generally businesslike manner at all times on the job. It is important to act professionally with coworkers, patients, doctors, and others in the work setting. You are an agent of your employer—you represent the doctor or doctors in the practice.

One example of professional behavior includes treating all patients with dignity and kindness. Another is making sure that you have completed and documented all your daily duties before leaving work at the end of each day.

You can start acting like a professional even while you are in the classroom studying to become a medical assistant. Presenting a neat appearance, showing courtesy and respect for peers and instructors, having a good attendance record, and arriving on time to class are all important elements that contribute to professionalism in school and in the workplace.

Neat Appearance

A professional always strives to maintain a neat appearance in the workplace. Personal cleanliness is an important part of maintaining a neat appearance. You should take a daily bath or shower, brush your teeth at least twice a day, floss once a day, and use an antiperspirant. You should wear clean, pressed uniforms and clean, white shoes polished on a daily basis. If you are not required to wear a uniform, select appropriate business clothes and clean, polished flat or low-heeled dress shoes. You should not use heavy perfumes or colognes that may irritate others. Fingernails should be clean, trimmed and, for females, polished with a clear or light, natural color. Jewelry should be subtle and tasteful. Wear no more than one ring (or an engagement and wedding ring) for appearance and safety. Body piercing is not acceptable. Women, however, are permitted to have one hole in each ear for pierced earrings. Tattoos, if present, should not show.

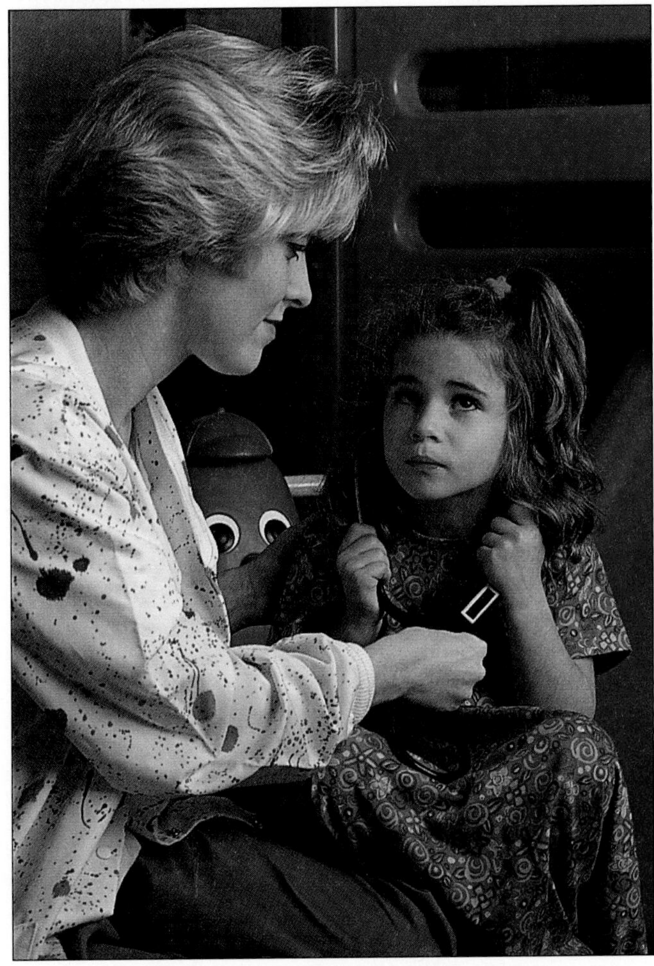

Figure 1-4. A medical assistant who works part-time in a pediatric practice might volunteer one day a week at a preschool to learn more about working with children.

Some activities may make it difficult to maintain a neat appearance—replacing the toner in the copy machine, for example, or filling the developing solution in the x-ray machine. Always store a spare uniform or business outfit at your workplace.

Proper Judgment

You should demonstrate proper judgment in every task. Before making an important decision, you must carefully evaluate each possible outcome.

An example of a situation that requires proper judgment is assessing when an exception should be made in a doctor's schedule of patients. Suppose the next patient on the schedule is in the waiting room. She is having a routine checkup. An unscheduled patient comes in with chest pains. You use proper judgment and allow the patient with chest pains to see the doctor first.

Communication Skills

Effective communication involves careful listening, observing, speaking, and writing. Communication even involves good manners—being polite, tactful, and respectful. You must use good communication skills during every patient discussion and in every interaction you have with physicians, other staff members, and other professionals with whom your practice does business. (Communication skills are discussed in Chapter 4.)

Remaining Calm in a Crisis

There is always the potential for a crisis or emergency in the health-care field. During a crisis you must remain calm and be prepared to handle any situation.

An example of the need for calm and effective action occurs when a patient appears to suffer a stroke while sitting in the waiting room of a busy medical office. You must quickly direct your peers to alert the doctor and remove the other patients from the room while you begin emergency first-aid measures.

Obtaining a Position

If you are well trained, you can usually obtain a position as a medical assistant from an array of opportunities in outpatient and inpatient facilities. Preparation is the key element of any successful job search. Being ready to handle any question that may be asked during the job search gives you the confidence needed for success.

Marketing Your Skills

Prepare academically and psychologically to come out ahead of the competition when you start looking for a job. Medical assisting is one of the fastest-growing professions in the country, yet there is still keen competition for the most desirable jobs. In all stages of your job search, you will need to sell yourself. In other words, you must present yourself to a potential employer as the best person for that job. Work experience (including volunteer work) is often the critical item that will set you apart from other candidates.

Where Are the Job Openings?

The first step in seeking a position as a medical assistant is to look for job openings. Three options with which you should familiarize yourself are advertisements, employment services, and school placement services.

Advertisements. Many prospective employers use classified advertisements in area newspapers to alert potential applicants to a career opportunity within their organization. The advertisement usually describes the duties and responsibilities of the position as well as the type of education and experience required.

A local newspaper's classified advertisements are often a good place to start your search. There is usually a separate section listing health-related jobs.

Employment Services. Employment and temporary agencies provide assistance in locating a specific job. Both types of agencies have a variety of job openings on file. Agencies also place classified ads. You should call to make an appointment with an employment counselor. Appointments at the public employment service may be on a "first-come, first-served" basis.

Agencies usually require you to fill out an application and provide a résumé. If there are positions that match your skills, the service contacts the employer. If there are no appropriate listings, the service places your name on file.

School Placement Services. Many schools offer job placement assistance for students. Typically, employers contact schools to notify them of open positions. Members of the school placement staff then contact students to see if they are interested in interviewing with prospective employers. Many placement offices also post notices on community bulletin boards.

Networking

Networking involves making contacts with relatives, friends, and acquaintances who may have information about how to find a job in your field. People in your network may be able to give you job leads or tell you about openings. This is also called word of mouth—finding job information by talking with other people. They may be able to introduce you to others who work in, or know people who work in, your field. People in your network may help you write, edit, or design your résumé or help you role-play job interviews. Networking is a valuable tool. It can advance your career even while you are employed.

Joining a medical assisting organization and attending conferences are the easiest ways to network. Attend an organization's local chapter meetings and talk with as many people as possible. Remember to bring a pen and notebook. Be prepared to exchange information with

MULTISKILL FOCUS

Ward Secretary

To gain medical assistant credentials, you must fulfill the requirements of either the American Association of Medical Assistants (for a Certified Medical Assistant) or the American Medical Technologists (for a Registered Medical Assistant). After obtaining your medical assistant certification or registration, you may wish to acquire additional skills in specialty areas through course work or on-the-job training. Although this course work or training may not lead to an additional certification or degree, it will enable you to expand your role in the medical office and advance your career as the demand for multiskilled health professionals increases.

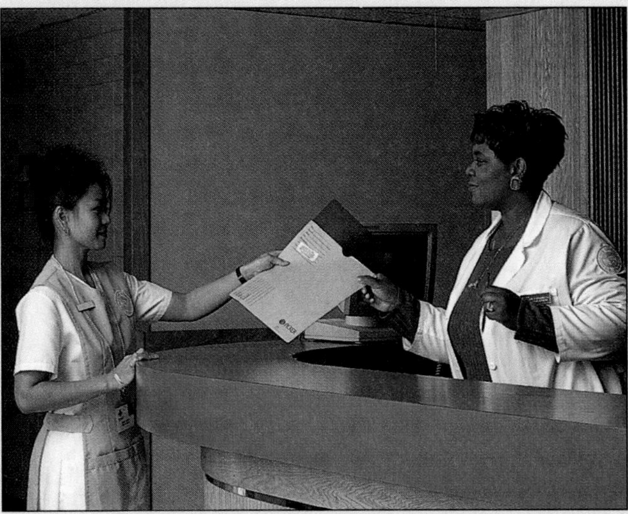

Skills and Duties

Ward secretaries, sometimes called unit secretaries, work in nursing stations or units in a hospital. They keep the nursing station functioning smoothly and free the nursing staff to focus on patient care. A ward secretary usually reports to a head nurse or a unit manager.

The ward secretary has four main areas of responsibility.

1. *Reception.* The ward secretary greets patients and gives them directions. She welcomes visitors and directs them to the rooms of the patients they wish to visit.
2. *Communication.* The ward secretary answers the phone and responds to pages. She addresses patient requests received over the intercom system, such as a request for a nurse or a doctor to come to the patient's room. The ward secretary also delivers mail and messages to patients. Ward secretaries with a command of medical terminology may be involved in coordinating the scheduling of medical personnel for the unit.
3. *Clerical duties.* The ward secretary updates records in patients' charts, transcribes physicians' orders, adds x-rays and laboratory reports to patients' charts, and processes the necessary paperwork for admissions, discharges, transfers, and deaths. In addition, she provides patient information, such as charts and schedules, to doctors and other hospital staff. The ward secretary also schedules patients' visits to other medical units in the hospital, such as laboratories. She keeps track of supply inventories for the unit, places orders for supplies and equipment as needed, and schedules necessary maintenance and repair services.
4. *Safety.* In some hospitals the ward secretary may be responsible for checking each room in the unit to make sure that all equipment—such as lamps, televisions, radios, and furniture—is in good working order. Other safety-related duties include keeping work areas free from clutter and making emergency code calls when necessary.

Workplace Settings

Most ward secretaries work at a nursing station or in a unit or ward in a hospital, but some find work in nursing homes. In some locations the work is divided differently than in a hospital. For example, a clinic might employ one person to handle scheduling and telephone reception and another staff member to greet patients and collect check-in information. Thus the clerical duties of the ward secretary might be separate from those of the receptionist.

Education

Ward secretaries need a high school diploma, and they receive their training on the job, although courses are available that provide valuable background. Sometimes a person who volunteers as a ward secretary in a hospital may be promoted to a paid position.

Where to Go for More Information

American Hospital Association
One North Franklin, Suite 2706
Chicago, IL 60606
(312) 422-3000

National Health Council
1730 M Street, NW, Suite 500
Washington, DC 20036
(202) 785-3910

other attendees. Remember, networking is an exchange of information; it is not one-sided. What you learn through networking may enable you to provide others with information to help their job search or further their career.

Writing a Résumé

One of the most important tools in the job search is a résumé. (You may also be required to submit a résumé when applying for an externship.) A résumé is a concise summary of one's education, skills, and experience. It is sometimes called a **curriculum vitae,** which is Latin for "course of one's life." A résumé tells the employer about the prospective employee's education, work experience, skills, and career goals. It should be limited to one page, although up to two pages is acceptable for someone with several years of work experience.

A résumé is often the first item the employer obtains from a prospective employee. Employers may receive hundreds of résumés from interested applicants. Therefore, your résumé must clearly and accurately summarize your skills and educational achievements.

In short, employers use the résumé to learn about the applicant's skills and to select interview candidates. Remember, you have about 30 seconds to make your point as the employer reads your résumé, so it must be as easy to read as possible.

Information for the Résumé. To begin, write down relevant work, school, and personal information (Procedure 1-1). You won't use all the information, but gathering it helps you become organized. It is important to list:

- Training programs.
- College degree(s).
- Computer knowledge.
- Research projects.
- Foreign languages.
- Part-time and full-time jobs.
- Honors, awards, and scholarships.
- Volunteer, community, and extracurricular activities.
- Paid and unpaid experiences (including externships).
- Participation in special workshops or presentations.
- Professional affiliations and memberships.

Then write down the details. Include dates, functions, activities, results, and achievements. If you are a recent graduate without experience related to the job you want, stress the level of responsibility, achievement, and motivation you have demonstrated in previous jobs.

Next, identify your basic and specific skills. Choose tasks you do well enough to be used profitably by an employer:

- Examples of basic skills: organizing, writing, oral or written communication, analyzing, critical thinking,

PROCEDURE 1-1

Résumé Writing

Objective: To write a résumé that reflects a defined career objective and highlights the applicant's skills

Materials: Paper; pen; dictionary; thesaurus; computer, word processor, or typewriter

Method

1. Write your full name, address (temporary and permanent, if you have both), and telephone number (include the area code).
2. List your general career objective. You may also choose to summarize your skills. If you want to phrase your objective to fit a specific position, you should include that information in a cover letter to accompany the résumé.
3. List the highest level of education or the most recently obtained degree first. Include the school name, degree earned, and date of graduation. Be sure to list any special projects, courses, or participation in overseas study programs.
4. Summarize your work experience. List your most recent or most relevant employment first. Describe your responsibilities, and list job titles, company names, and dates of employment. Summer employment, volunteer work, and student externships may also be included. Use short sentences with strong action words. For example, condense a responsibility into "Handled insurance and billing" or "Drafted correspondence as requested." Use action words like *directed, designed, developed,* and *organized.*
5. List any memberships and affiliations with professional organizations. List them alphabetically or by order of importance.
6. Do not list references on the résumé; just state "References available upon request."
7. Do not list the salary you wish to receive in a medical assisting position. Salary requirements should not be discussed until a job offer is received. If the ad you are answering requests that you include a required salary, it is best to state a range (no broader than $5,000 from lowest to highest point in the range for an annual salary).
8. Type your résumé on an 8½- by 11-inch sheet of high-quality white, off-white, or gray bond paper. Carefully check your résumé for spelling, punctuation, and grammatical errors.

planning, supervising, leading others, computer skills, people skills, creativity, attention to detail, clerical skills, and selling
- Examples of specific skills: processing Medicare and HCFA-1500 insurance forms, obtaining urine specimens, and conducting new patient interviews for patient medical histories

Professional Objective. Once you have identified your accomplishments and skills, you may choose to write a professional objective—a brief statement that demonstrates a career goal. An example of an effective, general objective is, "To work as a medical assistant, applying skills in patient relations and laboratory work while gaining increasing responsibility." If you want to list a specific career objective, such as applying your medical assisting skills in a pediatric medical facility, it would be best to mention it in the cover letter, not on your résumé.

Writing a Cover Letter

Cover letters or letters of application are as important in the job search as a well-written résumé. An effective letter motivates the employer to review the résumé and interview the applicant.

The cover letter should be direct and to the point, no more than a page long, and typed. Figure 1-5 shows an example of a cover letter. Tailor the letter to the individual needs of each position, and address the letter to a specific person in the company.

Check each cover letter for errors in spelling, grammar, and punctuation. It is best to use good-quality bond paper; do not use off-sized or colored paper.

Before you prepare a cover letter, you must research the company or practice. This information will help you tailor your letter to show how your qualifications relate to the company's or practice's needs. Make sure the description of your qualifications and interests directly reflects the words used by the company in the advertisement. Never lie or make up facts about your past in your cover letter. Prospective employers will generally verify all facts presented in your cover letter and résumé.

Sending the Résumé and Cover Letter

When sending the résumé and cover letter, be sure you have the correct address and zip code. Include your return address in the upper left-hand corner of the envelope. Have the envelope weighed at the post office, and use the proper postage.

References

Prospective employers may request reference letters describing the applicant's academic performance and work-related skills. The letters should support the résumé and career objective and fully describe the applicant's skills. Therefore, you should choose reference writers carefully. Faculty members and former employers who can attest to your academic and professional competence are the most appropriate choices. Character references (friends or clergy) are not appropriate unless the application calls for personal as well as professional references. Reference letters should be written only by people who can discuss your work accomplishments, professionalism, leadership, communication, and teamwork abilities.

Preparing a Portfolio

A portfolio, as stated earlier, is a collection of the cover letter, résumé, and list of references. The portfolio represents you, and it should be carefully prepared to make the best possible first impression. If you do not have access to a letter-quality printer, have the portfolio prepared professionally by a service that specializes in this type of work. Professional preparation of the portfolio will enable you to choose matching paper for your cover letters, résumé, and envelopes.

Be sure to get several cost estimates for portfolio preparation. Inquire about the fees for future changes to the portfolio.

Reviewing Your Portfolio

You may also wish to ask a senior member of your local or state medical assistant group to assess your portfolio. A seasoned professional's evaluation can help you create a portfolio that will support a successful job search.

Preparing for an Interview

Preparation for an interview begins long before the interview itself. After you send your cover letters and résumé, you must make sure you have a way to get telephone responses from prospective employers. You must practice how you are going to handle your interview, and you must plan what to wear and how to show yourself in the most positive way.

Telephone Preparation. Before starting your job search, it is wise to invest in an answering machine to receive calls when you are not home. Be sure the outgoing message is clear, concise, and professional. Avoid cute messages or background music. An appropriate message would be, "I'm unable to take your call at the moment, but your call is important to me. Please leave your name, number, the time you called, and a brief message after the tone, and I will call you back as soon as I can. Thank you." Also, make sure all household members who answer the phone (especially children) know proper phone etiquette and how to take a written message. When a prospective employer calls with an interview invitation, write down the interviewer's name, company or practice name, and the day, time, and location of the interview.

Before the Interview. The key to success in an interview is preparation. Ask a friend or family member to pose possible interview questions so you can practice your answers in a comfortable setting. This person may also review your performance.

Your Street Address
City, State, Zip Code

Date

Name of Person to whom you are writing
Title
Company or Organization
Street Address
City, State, Zip Code

Dear Dr., Mr., Mrs., Miss, or Ms. ____________:

1st Paragraph: Tell why you are writing. Name the position or general area of work that interests you. Mention how you learned about the job opening. State why you are interested in the job.

2d Paragraph: Refer to the enclosed résumé and give some background information. Indicate why you should be considered as a candidate, focusing on how your skills can fulfill the needs of the company. Relate your experiences to their needs and mention results/achievements. Do not restate what is said on your résumé—you want to pull together all the information and tell how your background fits the position.

3d Paragraph: Close by making a specific request for an interview. Say that you will follow up with a phone call to arrange a mutually convenient interview time. Offer to provide any additional information that may be needed. Thank the employer for his/her time and consideration.

Sincerely,

(your handwritten signature)

Type your name

Enclosure

Figure 1-5. The object of a cover letter is to convince the recipient to read your résumé.

The research on the practice or hospital you did prior to writing your cover letter will also help you practice for the interview. Identify ways to talk about your background and experience that will match the needs of the practice or hospital. For example, if you are applying to a clinic or office in a neighborhood where the residents speak primarily Spanish and you speak Spanish fluently, look for opportunities during the interview to emphasize this skill. The more information you gather before the interview, the better. Information that should be researched includes:

- The names and specialties of the doctors in the group or hospital department.
- The scope of their practice.

Appropriate Dress. Always prepare the interview outfit at least 1 day before the interview. Dress neatly and conservatively: For men, a simple suit in blue, black, or gray is appropriate. For women, a skirt is usually considered more professional than slacks. The skirt should be about knee-length. Current fad styles may not be appropriate for an interview.

Makeup, including nail polish, should be neutral: avoid bright colors. Use perfumes and colognes sparingly. Keep jewelry to a minimum: earrings, bracelets, and necklaces should be small and conservative and should not make noise. Your hairstyle should also be neat and conservative but flattering, not harsh. Clothes should be cleaned and pressed, and shoes should be polished.

Completing an Application

Some employers request completion of an employment application at an interview even when you provide a résumé. It is still wise to bring extra copies of your résumé to each interview (you may interview with more than one person and each may want to keep a copy). Your résumé may help you fill out the employment application. If the application form is lengthy, ask if you may take it home. You may then carefully type it and send or drop it off the next day. Figure 1-6 shows a sample application form from a national home-care services provider.

Fill out the application neatly. Read and follow the instructions on the form carefully. Your application represents you; it must make a good first impression.

As part of the application process, employers are required by federal law to request documents that prove the applicant's identity and eligibility to work in the United

Date Called	Type of Work Applied For	Appointment Date	Appointment Time	Reschedule Date	Reschedule Time	Availability	No Phone	GR	PC	Credentials	Pay Rate	Surplus Skill

Last Name	First	M.I.	Applicant Profile	Service Code	Pay Rate	Last Hiring Process Step

Address

City | State | Zip Code

Telephone No. | Social Security No. | Today's Date

Please print. Do not complete shaded areas.

EMPLOYMENT APPLICATION
EQUAL OPPORTUNITY EMPLOYER

KELLY Assisted Living®

FOR SUPERVISOR USE ONLY

Are you at least 18? ☐YES ☐NO
Are you familiar with the way a temporary help service works? *(Explain to applicant)* ☐YES ☐NO
Have you ever worked for a temporary help service? ☐YES ☐NO
Did you work for Kelly Assisted Living Services? ☐YES ☐NO
Where? ______
How long ago? ______
When could you start working for us? ______
How long do you plan to work on a temporary basis? ______
Can you work Monday through Friday? ☐YES ☐NO
Can you work Saturday? ☐YES ☐NO
Can you work Sunday? ☐YES ☐NO
Are you available ☐DAYS ☐EVENINGS ☐NIGHTS
Are you available as a Live-in? ☐YES ☐NO
What hours are you available? From______ To______
What form of transportation would you usually use to get to work? *(Car, Public transportation, Other)* ______
Did you bring your professional credentials with you today? ☐YES ☐NO ☐NONE REQUIRED

Check ☑ T if Trained; ☑ E if Experienced; ☑ T and E if Trained and Experienced.

T E
☐ ☐ Home Health Aide
☐ ☐ Homemaker
☐ ☐ Nurse Aide
☐ ☐ Registered Nurse
☐ ☐ Licensed Practical Nurse or Licensed Vocational Nurse

T E
☐ ☐ Other health-related positions
Specify: ______

Do you have experience as a Live-in? ☐YES ☐NO

Check ☑ where work experience was obtained.

☐ Hospital ☐ Home ☐ Industry
☐ Nursing Home ☐ Clinic/Office ☐ Other ______
☐ Community Health

©1990 Kelly Assisted Living Services, Inc. PRINTED IN U.S.A. 816 R9/90

Figure 1-6. Job applicants are often asked to fill out an application form, such as the one shown here. (Reprinted with permission from Kelly Assisted Living Services, Inc.)

States. To maintain the safety and confidentiality of the medical office, hospital, or laboratory, employers may also check a prospective employee's police record, credit rating, and history of chemical or alcohol use or abuse. The applicant may be asked to provide the needed documents or to give the employer authorization to obtain them.

Interviewing Techniques

Plan to arrive early for the interview, and leave time to find the correct location. You should always arrive at least 10 to 15 minutes early. This gives you time to gain your composure and organize your thoughts. Before going to the interviewer's office, use the extra time to go to the rest room to check your appearance and prepare your thoughts for the interview.

What to Bring. As stated earlier, bring extra résumés to the interview, as well as extra copies of recommendation letters. Be prepared for all situations. Also bring a pen and small notepad to write down important information. You can refer to your notes after the interview in a thank-you letter or follow-up phone call.

Appropriate Interview Behavior. Always greet the interviewer with a smile. This is the opportunity to sell yourself to the employer. Offer your hand for a firm, confident handshake, and be alert to the interviewer's body language.

The flow of conversation during an interview should be natural. Maintain eye contact, pay attention to the interviewer, and show interest. Ask intelligent questions that you have prepared before the interview.

Remember, the interview is an opportunity for both the prospective employer and employee to gather information and make a good impression. The résumé describes your skills and experience to a prospective employer. You may already know about the practice, the doctors, and their areas of specialties. The interview does provide an opportunity, however, for the interviewer to ask you specific questions about your professional experience or workplace habits, such as "Can you give me an example of how you worked with others to solve a problem?" Further, you have a chance to ask specific questions of a prospective employer, such as "Will I be able to work directly with patients?"

In addition to reviewing your experience, the interviewer will evaluate your personality and behavior. At the same time, you will be observing the office and learning more about the position. Try to be aware of the office's atmosphere, its equipment and supplies, and the attitudes of the staff. Does it seem like a pleasant, professional place to work? Ask about the office's policies for staff members, and request a tour of the office. Ask yourself if you would be happy in that work environment.

The interviewer will probably have a specific amount of time allotted for the interview. You will be able to anticipate the end of the interview by noting a change in the interviewer's body language. Thank the interviewer for the interview, offer a firm handshake, and express interest in the position.

Questions You Do Not Have to Answer. An interviewer may ask questions that you are not obligated to answer. These questions refer to age, race, sexual orientation, marital status, or number of children. Even if the questions sound harmless or the interviewer seems nonjudgmental, these questions have nothing to do with your skills or abilities. If the interviewer asks even one of these questions, you should reconsider whether you want to work for the organization.

Handling Inappropriate Questions. Be polite and remain professional if you decline to answer a question you feel is inappropriate. You may simply state that you do not believe the requested information is necessary for the employer to evaluate your qualifications for the job. Try to move the discussion onto a more relevant topic.

After the Interview. On the way out of the office, thank all staff members involved in the interview. Ask for a business card from anyone to whom you think you might want to send a thank-you note. After leaving the interview, write down any additional information you want to remember.

Every interview provides the applicant with information about the medical assisting profession. Even if an interview does not result in a job, you will have met new people, developed a larger network of professional contacts, and gained valuable interviewing experience.

Sending a Thank-You Letter. Following an interview it is professional to send a thank-you letter to the person or persons from the company who conducted your interview. You should send this letter within 2 days of the interview. It may be brief, but it should express appreciation for the interview. Mention some key points discussed during the interview, reaffirm your interest in the organization, and state your desire to remain a part of the selection process.

By sending a thank-you letter, you display common business courtesy—this can make a difference in the employer's hiring decision. Even if you are not interested in continuing the interview and selection process, you should thank the employer for holding the interview. Procedure 1-2 explains how to write and send a thank-you letter.

On the Job

Once you have a job you must learn how to be an effective employee. There are many ways that your initiative enables the medical team in the office, hospital, clinic, or laboratory to function effectively. You must identify the important skills in the daily duties, stay competitive and marketable through continuing education, and integrate constructive criticism from your employee evaluations into your daily work and annual goals.

PROCEDURE 1-2

Writing Thank-You Notes

Objective: To write an appropriate, professional thank-you note after an interview or externship

Materials: Paper; pen; dictionary; thesaurus; computer, word processor, or typewriter; #10 business envelope

Method

1. Write the letter within 2 days of the interview or completion of the externship. Begin by writing the date at the top of the letter.
2. Write the name (include credentials and title such as Dr. or Director of Client Services) of the person who interviewed you (or who was your mentor in the externship). Include the complete address of the office or organization.
3. Start the letter with "Dear Dr., Mr., Mrs., Miss, or Ms. ________:"
4. In the first paragraph thank the interviewer for his time and for granting the interview. Discuss some specific impressions: for example, "I found the interview and tour of the facilities an enjoyable experience. I would welcome the opportunity to work in such a state-of-the-art medical setting." If you are writing to thank your mentor for her time during your externship and for allowing you to perform your externship at her office, practice, or clinic, discuss the knowledge and experience you gained during the externship.
5. In the second paragraph mention the aspects of the job or externship that you found most interesting or challenging. For a job interview thank-you note, state how your skills and qualifications will make you an asset to the staff. When preparing an externship thank-you letter, mention interest in any future positions.
6. In the last paragraph thank the interviewer for considering you for the position. Ask to be contacted at his earliest convenience regarding his employment decision.
7. Close the letter with "Sincerely," and type your name. Leave enough space above your typewritten name to sign your name.
8. Type your return address in the upper left-hand corner of the #10 business envelope. Then type the interviewer's name and address in the envelope's center, apply the proper postage, and mail the letter.

Employee Evaluations

Employee evaluations are usually held annually. An initial employment review generally occurs after a probationary period of about 90 days. Evaluations describe an employee's performance. A completed evaluation is placed in an official record of employment. In most situations the employee and employer meet to discuss the employee's performance. The purpose of an annual evaluation should be to check the goals and values of both employer and employee to make sure they support each other (Harlan, 1994).

An employee evaluation form typically outlines the most important qualities and abilities needed for the job. It evaluates the employee's strengths and weaknesses. This form may help determine whether an employee is worthy of a merit raise (a raise based on performance, as opposed to a cost-of-living raise). The quantity and quality of work are assessed on this form, as are initiative, judgment, and cooperation.

Continuing Your Education

You should continue your education after completion of a medical assisting program. You should set specific educational advancement goals on a yearly basis. For example, you may decide to obtain further education to learn more about the medical specialty, such as dermatology, in which you work.

As medical research expands its discoveries and as new technologies emerge, the necessity for self-education increases. You must read to stay abreast of updates in medicine. For example, new advances in heart surgery demand that operating room personnel learn the latest techniques. The need for more highly specialized training presents you with an opportunity for using multiskill training. Medical publications are the best source for the latest medical knowledge. Local and state medical assistant meetings also provide information about advances in the field.

Self-education is an important skill for the medical assistant. Stay up to date in topics about medicine, health care, and wellness, which are frequently covered in the professional and lay media (Figure 1-7). Patients may ask you questions about information they have read or about the effectiveness of certain new treatments. You should alert the physician to patients' concerns or queries.

Advancement Opportunities

Advancement opportunities for medical assistants are plentiful. You may advance to office manager, ward secretary, or medical records clerk. You may become an

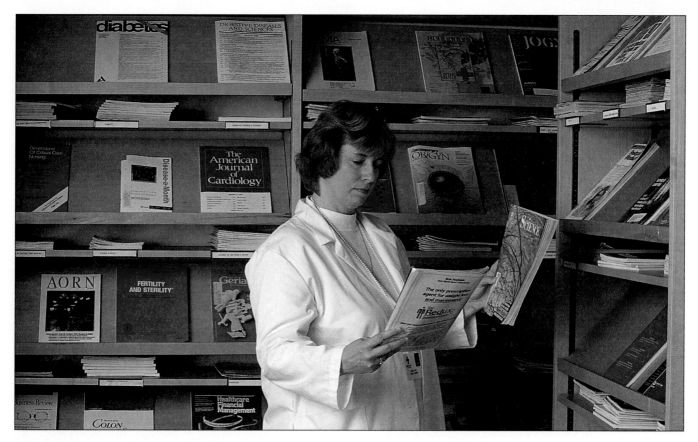

Figure 1-7. Part of self-education involves reading articles in professional and lay magazines about topics that relate to the medical practice in which you work.

ECG technician or phlebotomist (whose duties include collecting blood or administering drugs, blood, and fluids through a vein site). You may also obtain an administrative support position or choose to teach future medical assistants.

Rights of the Medical Assistant

You have the right to be free from any kind of discrimination in the workplace and during the hiring process. These rights are set forth under Title VII of the 1964 Civil Rights Act.

Title VII. The main prohibitions of the civil rights statute are as follows:

> *It shall be unlawful employment practice for an employer to fail or refuse to hire or to discharge any individual, or otherwise to discriminate against any individual with respect to his or her compensation, terms, conditions, or privileges of employment, because of such individual's race, color, religion, sex, or national origin, or to limit, segregate, or classify employees or applicants for employment in any way which would deprive or tend to deprive any individual of employment opportunities or otherwise adversely affect his or her status as an employee, because of such individual's race, color, religion, sex, or national origin. (Lindgren and Taub, 1993)*

This law also protects workers from receiving lower pay than the opposite sex for the same work and from denial of a promotion opportunity because of gender.

Sexual Harassment. Title VII also addresses and defines sexual harassment:

> *Unwelcome sexual advances, requests for sexual favors, and other verbal or physical conduct of a sexual nature . . . when submission to such conduct is made either explicitly or implicitly a term or condition of an individual's employment, submission to or rejection of such conduct by an individual is used as the basis for employment decisions affecting such individual, or such conduct has the purpose or effect of unreasonably interfering with an individual's work performance or creating an intimidating, hostile, or offensive working environment. (Lindgren and Taub, 1993)*

Sexual harassment occurs in a variety of circumstances, and anyone may be sexually harassed. A man or a woman may be the victim or the harasser, and the victim does not have to be of the opposite sex. The victim may be the person being directly harassed or even a coworker who overhears the harassment. The victim has the responsibility to let the harasser know that the conduct is offensive. The victim should also report any instance of sexual harassment to a supervisor or personnel department.

The AAMA Role Delineation Study

In 1996 the AAMA formed a committee whose goal was to revise and update its standards for the accreditation of programs that teach medical assisting. The committee's findings were published in 1997 as the "AAMA Role Delineation Study: Occupational Analysis of the Medical Assisting Profession." The study included a new Role Delineation Chart that outlines the areas of competence you must master as an entry-level medical assistant. This new chart replaces the earlier **DACUM** (Developing A Curriculum) chart, created in 1979 and updated in 1984 and 1990.

Areas of Competence

The Medical Assistant Role Delineation Chart, shown in Appendix I, provides the basis for medical assisting education and evaluation. Mastery of the areas of competence listed in this chart is required for all students in accredited medical assisting programs. The chart shows three general areas of competence: administrative, clinical, and general, or trandisciplinary. Each of these three areas is divided into two or more narrower areas, for a total of ten specific areas of competence. Within each area, a bulleted list of statements descrives the medical assistant's role.

Uses of the Role Delineation Chart

According to the AAMA, the Role Delineation Chart may be used to:

- Describe the field of medical assisting to other health-care professionals.
- Identify entry-level areas of competence for medical assistants.
- Help practitioners assess their own current competence in the field.
- Aid in the development of continuing education programs.
- Prepare appropriate types of materials for home study.

Summary

There are many kinds of on-the-job training, training programs, and careers for medical assistants. As you make the decision to become a medical assistant, you must evaluate your skills and the type of position you would like to obtain. An important goal will be to obtain a real-life view of the medical assistant's daily administrative, clinical, and laboratory duties. These skills and duties are outlined under the areas of competence listed in the AAMA Role Delineation Chart.

You must also research how to obtain on-the-job training or choose a training program that will adequately teach you those skills, how to conduct a job search, and whether or not to become a certified or registered medical assistant. Once you obtain a position you will need information about your on-the-job rights, the information reviewed in an employee evaluation, and the benefits of membership in medical assisting organizations such as the AAMA.

Additionally, you must be aware that the medical assisting profession will continue to change. You will need to stay abreast of changes in technology, procedures, and local, state, and federal regulations governing the way you perform daily duties.

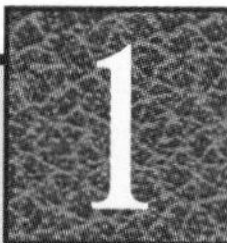

Chapter Review

Discussion Questions

1. How does credentialing help medical assistants obtain broader career advancement opportunities?
2. Name two personal qualifications required of a medical assistant, and explain why each is important for success.
3. What is the purpose of the AAMA Role Delineation Chart?
4. Discuss ways to gain real-world work experience in the field of medical assisting.

Critical Thinking Questions

1. Describe an effective medical assistant, and explain two ways a new medical assistant may learn to be an efficient and effective employee.
2. How will the "aging boom" affect health care and the profession of medical assisting in the future?
3. How can a medical assistant stay up to date about new health-care developments?

Application Activities

1. With a partner, pick one of the following two situations. Without showing your partner, write a description of how you would display the personal attribute stated at the end of the scenario. After you and your partner have written your descriptions, compare them with each other.

   Patient Situation

   Patient says: "I have such a horrible headache. I've been feeling tired lately too."

   Attribute You Wish to Display

   Empathy

   Patient Situation

   Doctor: "I'm really backed up on paperwork. Could you come in an hour early tomorrow morning to help me organize it? You will be paid for the overtime."

   Attribute You Wish to Display

   Flexibility

2. List several challenging but realistic short-term and long-term goals for a medical assistant.
3. Prepare for an upcoming interview by answering the question, "Why do you want to be a medical assistant, and why do you think you will be successful?"

Further Readings

"AAMA Role Delineation Study: Occupational Analysis of the Medical Assisting Profession." Chicago: American Association of Medical Assistants, 1997.

Balasa, Donald A. *Certification and Licensure: Facts You Should Know.* Chicago: American Association of Medical Assistants, 1994.

Bamberg, Richard, Jean Keenon, and Keith D. Blayney. "Multiskilled Medical Assistants in Physician Practices." *The Professional Medical Assistant,* November/December 1990, 14–16.

Caplan, Janice. "Key Steps for a Successful Job Search." *The Professional Medical Assistant,* March/April 1994, 21–22.

Certified Medical Assistants: Health-Care's Most Versatile Professionals. Chicago: American Association of Medical Assistants, 1994.

Essentials and Guidelines for an Accredited Education Program for the Medical Assistant. Chicago: American Association of Medical Assistants, 1991.

Flight, Myrtle R. "Establishing a Standard of Care for MSHPs." *The Professional Medical Assistant,* January/February, 1996, 17–19.

Harlan, Kay. "Conducting an Employee Evaluation: An Opportunity to Nurture Self-Actualization." *The Professional Medical Assistant,* May/June 1994, 4–5.

Heyman, Annette H. "Medical Assistantship: One of America's Fastest-Growing Careers." In *Healthcare Career Directory—Allied Health,* edited by Bradley J. Morgan and Joseph M. Palmisano. Detroit, MI: Gale, 1993.

Ledford, Janice K. "Do's and Don'ts of Résumé Writing." *The Professional Medical Assistant,* March/April 1990, 13–14.

Lindgren, J. Ralph, and Nadine Taub. *The Law of Sex Discrimination.* 2d ed. Minneapolis, MN: West Publishing Company, 1993.

Mitchell, Paula R., and Gloria M. Grippando. *Nursing Perspectives and Issues.* 5th ed. Albany, NY: Delmar, 1993.

Roseen, Stacey J., ed. "The Greening of the Medical Practice." *The Professional Medical Assistant,* March/April 1991, 8–12.

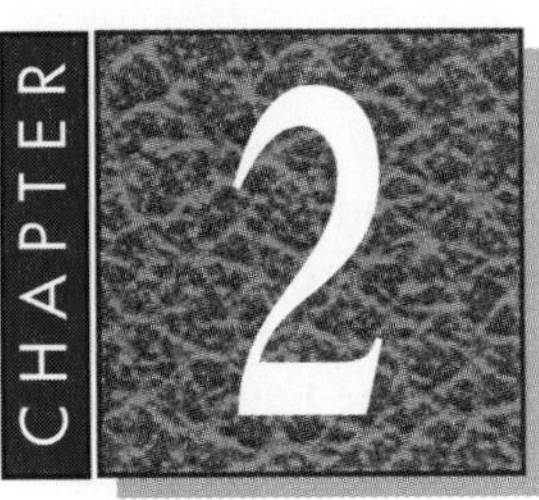

Types of Medical Practice

CHAPTER OUTLINE

- Medical Specialties
- Working With Other Allied Health Professionals
- Specialty Career Options
- Professional Associations

OBJECTIVES

After completing Chapter 2, you will be able to:

- Describe medical specialties and specialists.
- Explain the purpose of the American Board of Medical Specialties.
- Describe the duties of several types of allied health professionals with whom medical assistants may work.
- Name professional associations that may help advance a medical assistant's career.

AREAS OF COMPETENCE

1997 ROLE DELINEATION STUDY

GENERAL (Transdisciplinary)

Professionalism

- Work as a team member
- Promote the CMA credential

Legal Concepts

- Practice within the scope of education, training, and personal capabilities

Key Terms

allergist
anesthetist
cardiologist
dermatologist
doctor of osteopathy
endocrinologist
family practitioner
gastroenterologist
gerontologist
gynecologist
internist
nephrologist
neurologist
oncologist
orthopedist
otorhinolaryngologist
pathologist
pediatrician
physiatrist
plastic surgeon
radiologist
surgeon
triage
urologist

Medical Specialties

Since the beginning of the twentieth century, some physicians have specialized in particular areas of study. There are now approximately 22 major medical specialties. Within each specialty there are several subspecialties. For example, cardiology is a major specialty; pediatric cardiology is a subspecialty. As advances in the diagnosis and treatment of diseases and disorders unfold, the demand for specialized care increases and more medical specialties emerge.

If you graduate from an accredited medical assisting program, you will be well equipped to work with a physician specialist. If you work in the office of a physician specialist, you must continue to learn all the new skills that apply to that specialty. First, however, it is helpful to understand the education and licensing process any medical doctor must undergo to become a board-certified physician.

Physician Education and Licensure

The educational requirements for physicians are rigorous and take several years to complete. To earn the title MD (doctor of medicine), thereby qualifying as a licensed physician, a student must complete a bachelor's degree with a concentration typically in the sciences. Then she must attend a medical school accredited by the Liaison Committee on Medical Education (LCME). Upon completing medical school, she is awarded the degree of MD, but this is not the end of her medical training. She must also pass the U.S. Medical Licensing Examination (USMLE). This examination, commonly known as medical boards, has three parts. Part 1 is usually taken after the second year of medical school, part 2 during the fourth year of medical school, and part 3 during the first or second year of postgraduate medical training.

After medical school an MD begins a residency—a period of practical training in a hospital. The first year of residency is known as an internship. Once it is completed an MD can become certified by the National Board of Medical Examiners (NBME). After completing her internship and passing her medical boards, the MD becomes certified as an NBME Diplomate. If she wishes to specialize in a particular branch of medicine, she must complete an additional 2 to 6 years of residency. She also will apply to the American Board of Medical Specialties (ABMS) to take an examination in her specialty area. After passing the examination, she will be board-certified in her area of specialization. For example, a physician who specializes in pediatrics would receive certification from the American Board of Pediatrics.

The ABMS is an organization of many different medical specialty boards. Its primary purpose is to maintain and improve the quality of medical care and to certify doctors in various specialties. This organization helps the member boards develop professional and educational standards for physician specialists.

Family Practice

Family practitioners (sometimes called general practitioners) are MDs who are generalists and treat all types and ages of patients. They do not specialize in a particular branch of medicine. Many patients seek medical care from a family practitioner and may never have visited a medical specialist. Family practitioners are called primary care physicians by insurance companies. The term refers to individual doctors who oversee patients' long-term health care. Some people, however, have internists as their primary care physicians.

A family practitioner sends a patient to a specialist when she has a specific condition or disease that requires advanced care. For example, a family practitioner refers a patient with a lump in her breast to an **oncologist,** a specialist who treats tumors, or to a general surgeon. Either of these doctors may order a mammogram or perform a needle biopsy of the lump to determine if it is malignant.

If you work in a general practice, you will encounter patients with many different conditions and illnesses. As in any medical setting, you must become knowledgeable about preventing the transmission of viruses. This important topic is discussed in several parts of the book. For more information, see "Caution: Handle With Care."

If you work for a general practitioner, you will often be responsible for arranging patient appointments with specialists. It is important, therefore, for you to know about the duties of each medical specialist. One or more of these specialties may interest you, and you may decide to seek a position as a medical assistant for a physician in that specialty.

Allergy

Allergists diagnose and treat physical reactions to substances, including mold, dust, fur, and pollen from plants or flowers. An individual with allergies is hypersensitive to substances like drugs, chemicals, or elements in nature. An allergic reaction may be minor, such as a rash; serious, such as asthma; or life-threatening, such as swelling of the airways or nasal passages.

Anesthesiology

Anesthetists use medications that cause patients to lose sensation or feeling during surgery. These health-care practitioners administer anesthetics before and during surgery. They also educate patients regarding the anesthetic that will be used and its possible postoperative effects. An anesthesiologist is an MD. A certified registered nurse anesthetist (CRNA) is a registered nurse who has completed an additional program of study recognized by the American Association of Nurse Anesthetists.

Cardiology

Cardiologists diagnose and treat cardiovascular diseases (diseases of the heart and blood vessels). Cardiologists also read electrocardiograms (ECGs) for hospital labora-

CAUTION

HANDLE WITH CARE

Preventing Transmission of Viruses in the Health-Care Setting

Certain procedures are thought to cause the transmission of infection from a medical worker to a patient, and other procedures may also carry that risk. For example, skin-puncture injuries in medical workers are not uncommon. Therefore, many procedures involving needles are considered exposure-prone. If the worker's skin is cut or punctured, the patient could be exposed to the worker's blood.

The risk that a health-care worker will transmit an infection to a patient is small, if proper precautions are taken. Workers participating in high-risk procedures, however, should take extra precautions. Workers with skin conditions characterized by sores that secrete fluid should forgo direct patient care and the handling of equipment used for exposure-prone procedures until the condition has healed. Workers performing high-risk procedures should know their HIV and HBV status. (HIV refers to the virus that causes AIDS; HBV refers to the hepatitis B virus.) HBV vaccination is strongly recommended.

If a health-care worker is infected with HIV or HBV, she should not perform procedures that might result in exposure without the advice of an expert review panel. This panel might include the health-care worker's own physician, someone with expert knowledge about the transmission of infectious disease, a medical professional with expert knowledge about the procedures in question, public health officials, and a member of the infection control committee of the institution.

The panel will advise the worker about when she will be allowed to perform certain procedures. The panel will require her to inform potential patients of the infection before the procedure. The panel must, however, otherwise protect the health-care worker's confidentiality.

Although there has been great controversy on the subject, there are no recommendations in place for required testing of all health-care workers for HIV or HBV because the risk of transmission from worker to patient is not considered great enough to justify the expense. Educational and training activities can help reinforce the extra precautions exposure-prone workers should take.

tories. They educate patients about the positive role healthy diet and regular exercise play in preventing and controlling heart disease.

Dermatology

Dermatologists diagnose and treat diseases of the skin, hair, and nails. Their patients have conditions ranging from warts and acne to skin cancer. Dermatologists treat boils, skin injuries, and infections. They remove growths—such as moles, cysts, and birthmarks—and they treat scars and perform hair transplants.

Doctor of Osteopathy

According to the American Association of Colleges of Osteopathic Medicine (AACOM), **doctors of osteopathy**

> *understand how all the body's systems are interconnected and how each one affects the others. They focus special attention on the musculoskeletal system, which reflects and influences the condition of all other body systems. With osteopathic manipulative treatments, osteopathic physicians use their eyes and hands to identify structural problems and to support the body's natural tendency toward health and self-healing. (AACOM, 1996 Home Page on the Internet)*

Doctors of osteopathy hold the title DO.

Emergency Medicine

Physicians who specialize in emergency medicine work in hospital emergency rooms. They diagnose and treat patients with conditions resulting from an unexpected medical crisis or accident. Common emergencies include trauma, such as gunshot wounds or serious injuries from car accidents; other injuries, such as severe cuts; and sudden illness, such as alcohol or food poisoning.

Endocrinology

Endocrinologists diagnose and treat disorders of the endocrine system. This system regulates many body functions by circulating hormones that are secreted by glands throughout the body. An example of a disorder treated by an endocrinologist is hyperthyroidism, an abnormality of the thyroid gland. Symptoms include weight loss, shakiness, and weakness.

Gastroenterology

Gastroenterologists diagnose and treat disorders of the gastrointestinal tract. These disorders include problems related to the functioning of the stomach, intestines, and associated organs.

Gerontology

Gerontologists study the aging process. Geriatrics is the branch of medicine that deals with the diagnosis and treatment of problems and diseases of the older adult. A specialist in geriatrics may also be called a geriatrician. As the population of older adults continues to increase, there will be greater need for physicians who specialize in diagnosing and treating diseases of the elderly.

Gynecology

Gynecology is the branch of medicine that is concerned with diseases of the female genital tract. **Gynecologists** perform routine physical care and examination of the female reproductive system. Many gynecologists are also obstetricians.

Internal Medicine

Internists specialize in diagnosing and treating problems related to the internal organs. The internal medicine subspecialties include cardiology, critical care medicine, diagnostic laboratory immunology, endocrinology and metabolism, gastroenterology, geriatrics, hematology, infectious diseases, medical oncology, nephrology, pulmonary disease, and rheumatology. Internists must be certified as specialists in these areas.

Nephrology

Nephrologists study, diagnose, and manage diseases of the kidney. They may work in either a clinic or hospital setting. A medical assistant working with a nephrologist may assist in the operation of a dialysis unit for the treatment of patients with kidney disease. In a rural setting a medical assistant might help a doctor operate a mobile dialysis unit that can be taken to the patient's home or to a medical practice that does not have this technology.

Neurology

Neurology is the branch of medical science that deals with the nervous system. **Neurologists** diagnose and treat disorders and diseases of the nervous system, such as strokes. The nervous system is made up of the brain, spinal cord, and nerves that receive, interpret, and transmit messages throughout the body.

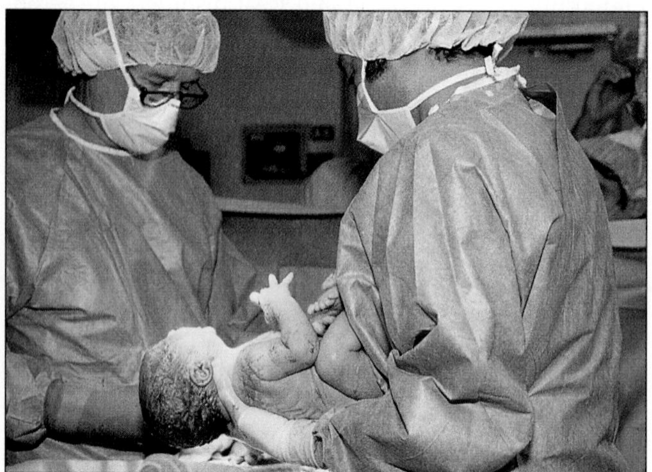

Figure 2-1. Obstetricians who are part of a private practice are usually connected with a specific hospital where they help their patients through labor and delivery.

Obstetrics

Obstetrics involves the study of pregnancy, labor, delivery, and the period following labor called postpartum (Figure 2-1). This field is often combined with gynecology. A physician who practices both specialties is referred to as an obstetrician/gynecologist, or OB/GYN.

Oncology

Oncologists, as stated earlier in the chapter, identify tumors, determine if they are benign or malignant, and treat patients with cancer. Treatment may involve chemotherapy, which is the administration of drugs to destroy cancer cells. Treatment may also involve radiation therapy, which kills cancer cells through the use of x-rays. Oncologists treat both adults and children.

Ophthalmology

An ophthalmologist diagnoses and treats diseases and disorders of the eye. This physician specialist examines patients' eyes for poor vision or disease. Other responsibilities include prescribing corrective lenses or medication, performing surgery, and providing follow-up care after surgery. (Ophthalmologists are sometimes confused with optometrists, but the latter are not MDs. Optometrists, however, perform eye exams to determine the general health of the eye and to prescribe corrective eyeglasses or contact lenses.)

Orthopedics

Orthopedics is a branch of surgery that works to maintain function of the musculoskeletal system and its associated structures. An **orthopedist** diagnoses and treats diseases and disorders of the muscles and bones. Some orthopedists concentrate on treating sports-related injuries, either exclusively for professional athletes or for nonprofessionals of all ages. They are called sports medicine specialists.

Otorhinolaryngology

Otorhinolaryngology involves the study of the ear, nose, and throat. An **otorhinolaryngologist** diagnoses and treats diseases of these body structures. This physician specialist is also referred to as an ear, nose, and throat (ENT) specialist.

Pathology

Pathology is the study of disease. It provides the scientific foundation for all medical practice. The **pathologist** studies the changes a disease produces in the cells, fluids, and processes of the entire body (sometimes by performing autopsies, examinations of the bodies of the deceased) to advance the clinical practice of medicine.

There are two basic types of pathologists. Governments and police departments use forensic pathologists to determine facts about unexplained or violent deaths. Anatomic pathologists often work at hospitals in a research capacity, and they may read biopsies (samplings of cells that could be malignant).

Pediatrics

Pediatrics is concerned with the development and care of children and the diseases of childhood. A **pediatrician** diagnoses and treats childhood diseases and teaches parents skills to keep their children healthy.

Physical Medicine

Physical medicine specialists (**physiatrists**) diagnose and treat diseases and disorders with physical therapy. Physical medicine specialists' patients include both adults and children.

Plastic Surgery

A **plastic surgeon** performs the reconstruction, correction, or improvement of body structures. Patients may be accident victims or disfigured due to disease or abnormal development. Plastic surgery involves facial reconstruction, face-lifts, and skin grafting. Plastic surgery is also used to repair problems like cleft lip and cleft palate.

Radiology

Radiology is the branch of medical science that uses x-rays and radioactive substances to diagnose and treat disease. **Radiologists** specialize in taking and reading x-rays.

Surgery

Surgeons use their hands and medical instruments to diagnose and correct deformities and treat external and internal injuries or disease (Figure 2-2). They work with many different specialists to surgically treat a broad range of disorders. General surgeons may, for example, perform operations as diverse as breast lumpectomy and repair of a pacemaker. There are also subspecialties of surgery, such as neurosurgery, vascular surgery, and orthopedic surgery.

Urology

A **urologist** diagnoses and treats diseases of the kidney, bladder, and urinary system. A urologist's patients include infants, children, and adults of all ages.

Working With Other Allied Health Professionals

You will always work as a member of a health-care team. That health-care team will include doctors, nurses, specialists, and the patients themselves. You must know the duties of the other allied health professionals in your workplace. Even if you do not work with other allied health professionals in the office, you may contact them through correspondence or by telephone. Understanding the duties of other health-care team members will help make you a more effective medical assistant.

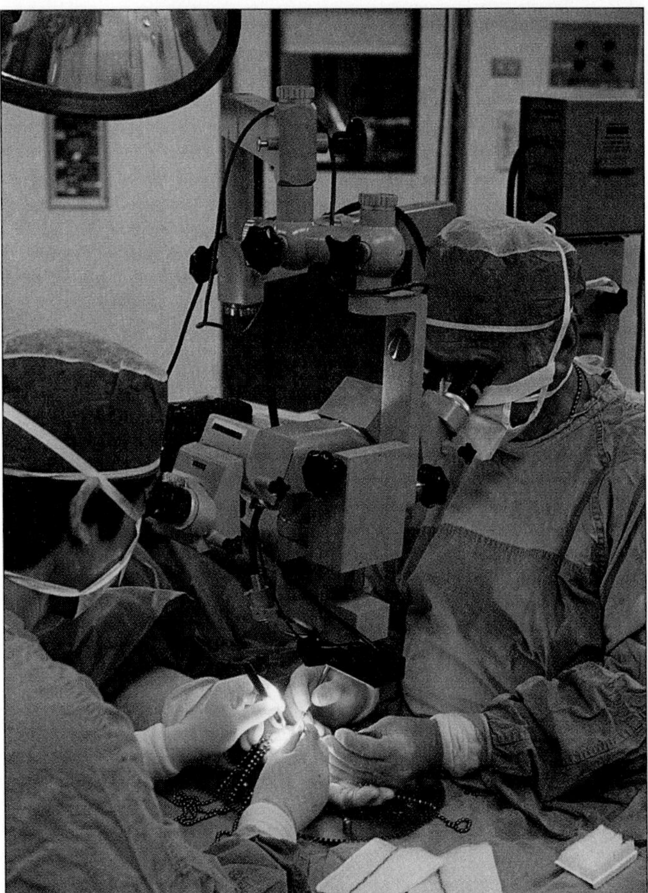

Figure 2-2. Most surgeons specialize in a particular type of surgery, such as heart surgery or hand surgery.

Electroencephalographic Technologist

Electroencephalography (EEG) is the study and recording of the electrical activity of the brain. It is used to diagnose diseases and irregularities of the brain. The EEG technologist (sometimes called a technician) attaches electrodes to the patient's scalp and connects them to a recording instrument. The machine then provides a written record of the electrical activity of the patient's brain. EEG technologists work in hospital EEG laboratories, clinics, and physicians' offices.

Electrocardiograph Technician

The electrocardiograph (ECG) technician is a trained professional who operates an electrocardiograph machine, as pictured in Figure 2-3. An ECG records the electrical impulses reaching the heart muscles. Physicians and cardiologists use the readings from this machine to detect heart abnormalities and to monitor patients with known cardiac problems. Electrocardiograph technicians work in hospitals.

MULTISKILL FOCUS

Medical Office Administrator

To gain medical assistant credentials, you must fulfill the requirements of either the American Association of Medical Assistants (for a Certified Medical Assistant) or the American Medical Technologists (for a Registered Medical Assistant). After obtaining your medical assistant certification, you may wish to acquire additional skills in specialty areas through course work or on-the-job training. Although this course work or training may not lead to an additional certification or degree, it will enable you to expand your role in the medical office and advance your career as the demand for multiskilled health professionals increases.

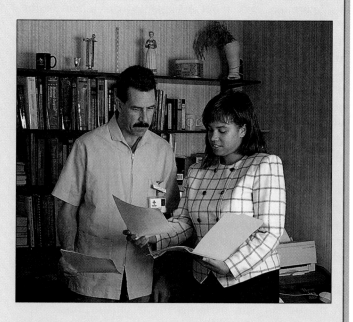

Skills and Duties

A medical office administrator manages the practice of a single physician (solo practice) or of a group practice. His duties are determined, in part, by the size of the practice. If the practice is large, he may have more managerial duties. If it is small, he may act as the receptionist, secretary, and records clerk. (Occasionally, in a solo practice, the practice nurse performs many or all of these functions.) Large group practices with 10 to 15 physicians may have one medical office administrator, while larger group practices with 40 to 50 physicians (such as managed care organizations) may have a highly trained practice administrator who oversees and coordinates the work of several assistant administrators.

The medical office administrator's reception duties begin with greeting and welcoming new patients. He may provide a medical history form for patients and answer any questions they may have. The administrator must have a knowledge of medical terminology in order to answer patients' questions.

This health-care professional coordinates the practice's records and filing. For example, he ensures that x-rays and test results are attached to the appropriate records and that insurance information is up to date. The medical office administrator may also schedule appointments for patients, as well as scheduling referrals with other specialists. He may also keep track of the medical and nursing staff schedule. Sometimes the administrator is the person who calls patients ahead of time to confirm their appointments.

In a solo or small practice, the medical office administrator may perform general secretarial tasks, such as handling the mail and answering the telephone. He must have strong computer and word processing skills, as well as shorthand, typing, and bookkeeping skills. In a large practice the administrator may train and oversee clerical staff and secretaries. He may also interview and evaluate applicants for clerical jobs.

Workplace Settings

Medical office administrators may work in solo practices, group practices, or medical clinics. Specialized health-care facilities, such as nursing homes, may also employ medical office administrators.

Education

Although medical office administrators may learn the medical terminology they need on the job, they usually acquire their secretarial and clerical background through course work, either in a business/vocational school or in a junior or community college. The educational requirements for a medical office administrator vary with the size of the practice and the extent of the administrator's responsibilities. Upper-level positions require a graduate degree.

Where to Go for More Information

American Academy of Medical Administrators
30555 Southfield Road, Suite 150
Southfield, MI 48076
(313) 540-4310

Medical Group Management Association
104 Inverness Terrace East
Englewood Cliffs, CA 80112
(313) 799-1111

National Association of Medical Staff Services
P.O. Box 23590
Knoxville, TN 37933-1590
(615) 531-3571

Medical Technology

Medical technology is an umbrella term that refers to the development and design of clinical laboratory tests (such as diagnostic tests), procedures, and equipment. Two types of allied health professionals that work in medical technology are the medical technologist and the medical laboratory technician.

Medical Technologist. Medical technologists perform laboratory tests and procedures with clinical laboratory equipment. They examine specimens of human body tissues and fluids, analyze blood factors, and culture bacteria to identify disease-causing organisms. They also supervise and train technicians and laboratory aides. Medical technologists have 4-year degrees and may specialize in areas such as blood banking, microbiology, and chemistry. These technologists are employed in clinics, hospitals, private practices, colleges, pharmaceutical companies, government, research, and industry.

Medical Laboratory Technician. Medical laboratory technicians (MLTs) have 1- to 2-year degrees and are responsible for clinical tests performed under the supervision of a physician or medical technologist. They perform tests in the areas of hematology, serology, blood banking, urinalysis, microbiology, and clinical chemistry. Medical laboratory technicians work in hospital laboratories, commercial laboratories, medical clinics, and physicians' offices.

Physician's Assistant

A physician's assistant (PA) is an academically and clinically trained member of the health-care team. The physician's assistant provides direct patient care, but always under the instruction and supervision of a licensed physician. Duties include taking a patient's medical history and performing physical examinations and diagnostic and therapeutic procedures.

Other duties include providing follow-up care and teaching and counseling patients. In some states, physician's assistants can write prescriptions. PAs work in a variety of settings—physicians' private practices, hospitals, clinics, nursing homes, and government and community agencies. They may also teach in physician's assistant programs, after gaining appropriate clinical experience. PAs sometimes work with medical assistants. Training requirements vary, and many states require certification. Most states require registration with the state medical board.

Nuclear Medicine Technologist

A nuclear medicine technologist performs tests to oversee quality control, to prepare and administer radioactive drugs, and to operate radiation detection instruments. This allied health professional is also responsible for correctly positioning the patient, performing imaging procedures, and preparing the information for use by a physician. A nuclear medicine technologist may work in a hospital,

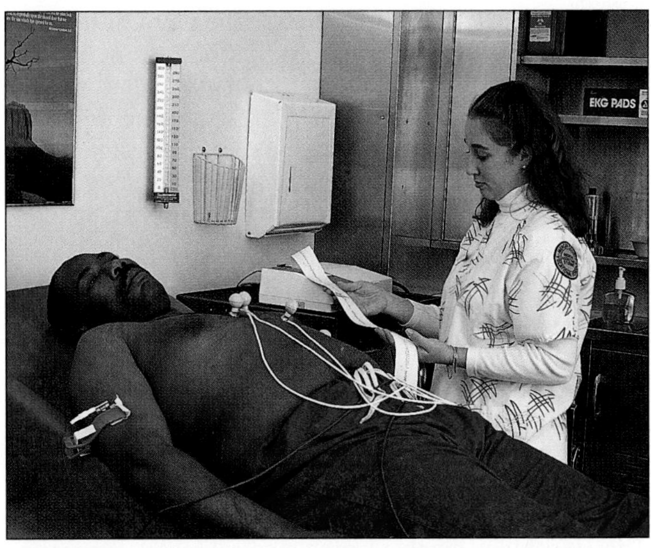

Figure 2-3. The electrocardiograph (ECG) technician is responsible for operating an electrocardiograph machine, which detects heart abnormalities and monitors patients with cardiac problems.

public health institution, or physician's office or—with appropriate clinical experience—in a teaching position at a college or university. There are 2- and 4-year training programs. The registration examination is administered by the American Registry of Radiologic Technologists.

Respiratory Therapist

A respiratory therapist evaluates, treats, and cares for persons with respiratory problems. She works under the supervision of a physician and performs therapeutic procedures based on observation of the patient. Using respiratory equipment, the therapist treats patients with asthma, emphysema, pneumonia, and bronchitis. The respiratory therapist plays an active role in newborn, pediatric, and adult intensive care units. She may work in a hospital, nursing home, physician's office, or commercial company that provides emergency oxygen equipment and services to home-care patients.

Medical Secretary

A medical secretary assists medical, professional, and technical personnel by performing secretarial and clerical support. These functions include taking dictation and typing, as well as composing and preparing letters on a word processor. Other functions include maintaining medical and administrative files. A medical secretary may work in a hospital, nursing home, physician's office, or clinic.

Physical Therapist

A physical therapist (PT) plans and uses physical therapy programs for medically referred patients. The PT helps these patients to restore function, relieve pain, and prevent disability following disease, injury, or loss of body parts. A physical therapist uses various treatment methods, which include therapy with electricity, heat, cold, ultrasound, massage, and exercise. The physical therapist also helps patients accept their disabilities. A physical therapist may work in a hospital, outpatient clinic, rehabilitation center, home-care agency, nursing home, voluntary health agency, private practice, or sports medicine center. A physical therapist must have a bachelor's degree in physical therapy and must pass a state board examination.

Medical Records Technologist

There are two types of medical records technologists: the Registered Records Administrator (RRA) and the Accredited Records Technician (ART). These technologists are responsible for organizing, analyzing, and evaluating medical records. Other responsibilities include compiling administrative and health statistics, coding symptoms, and inputting and retrieving computerized health data. These positions involve typing medical reports, preparing statistical reports on patient treatments, and supervising clerical personnel in the medical records department. Accredited records technicians and registered records administrators work in hospitals, nursing homes, HMOs, physicians' offices, and government agencies.

Phlebotomist

Phlebotomists are allied health professionals trained to draw blood for diagnostic laboratory testing. They work in medical clinics, laboratories, and hospitals. Although medical assistants are also trained to draw blood for standard types of tests, phlebotomists are trained at a more advanced level to be able to draw blood under difficult circumstances or in special situations. For example, if a blood sample is needed for a potassium-level test, it must be drawn in a particular manner that only phlebotomists are trained to do. In most states phlebotomists must be certified by the National Phlebotomy Association or registered by the American Society of Clinical Pathologists.

Radiologic Technologist

A radiologic technologist is a health-care professional who has studied the theory and practice of the technical aspects of the use of x-rays and radioactive materials in the diagnosis and treatment of disease. A radiologic technologist may specialize in radiography, radiation therapy, or nuclear medicine. Radiologic technologists generally work in hospitals; some work in medical laboratories, medical practices, and clinics.

Radiographer

The radiographer (x-ray technician) assists a radiologist in taking x-ray films. These films are used to diagnose broken bones, tumors, ulcers, and disease. A radiographer usually works in the radiology department of a hospital. He may, however, use mobile x-ray equipment in a patient's room or in the operating room. A radiographer may be employed in a hospital, laboratory, clinic, physician's office, government agency, or industry.

Pharmacist

Pharmacists are professionals who have studied the science of drugs and who dispense medication and health supplies to the public. Pharmacists know the chemical and physical qualities of drugs and are knowledgeable about the companies that manufacture drugs.

Pharmacists inform the public about the effects of prescription and nonprescription (over-the-counter) medications. Pharmacists are employed in hospitals, clinics, and nursing homes. They may also work for government agencies, pharmaceutical companies, privately owned pharmacies, or chain store pharmacies. Some pharmacists own their own stores.

There are three levels of pharmacists, each with different training requirements. A pharmacy technician (CPhT) can typically receive on-the-job training. Formal training, although not required by most states, includes certificate programs and 2-year college programs offering associate degrees in science. Voluntary certification is by examination. A registered pharmacist (RPh) requires 5 years of college training with a bachelor's degree in science. Pharmacists must be registered by the state and must pass a state board examination. A doctor of pharmacy (PharmD) requires 6 to 7 years of college training, which may be followed by a residency in a hospital setting.

Registered Dietitian

Registered dietitians help patients and their families make healthful food choices that provide balanced, adequate nutrition (Figure 2-4). Dietitians are sometimes called nutritionists. Dietitians may assist food-service directors at health-care facilities and prepare and serve food to groups. They may also participate in food research and teach nutrition classes. Dietitians work in community health agencies, hospitals, clinics, private practices, and managed care settings. They may also teach at colleges and universities, and they serve as consultants to organizations and individuals.

Nursing Aide/Assistant

Nursing aides assist in the direct care of patients under the supervision of the nursing staff. Typical functions include making beds, bathing patients, taking vital signs, serving meals, and transporting patients to and from treatment areas. Nursing assistants are often employed in psychiatric and acute care hospitals, nursing homes, and home health agencies. On-the-job training can range from 1 week to 3 months.

Practical/Vocational Nurse

Licensed practical nurses (LPNs) and licensed vocational nurses (LVNs) provide nursing care to the sick. Both terms refer to the same type of nurse. Duties involve taking and recording patient temperatures, blood pressure, pulse, and respiration rates. They also include adminis-

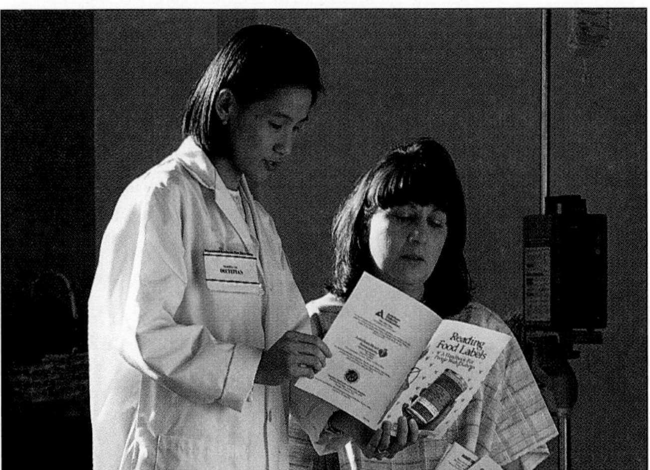

Figure 2-4. Registered dietitians work closely with patients who need to modify their food choices for better health.

tering some medications under supervision, dressing wounds, and applying compresses. LPNs and LVNs are not allowed, however, to perform certain other duties, such as some intravenous (IV) procedures or the administration of certain medications.

Practical/vocational nurses assist registered nurses and physicians by observing patients and reporting changes in their conditions. LPNs/LVNs work in hospitals, nursing homes, clinics, and physicians' offices and in industrial medicine. To meet the needs of the growing aging population in this country, employment opportunities for LPNs and LVNs in long-term care settings have increased.

LPNs/LVNs must graduate from an accredited school of practical (vocational) nursing (usually a 1-year program). They are also required to take a state board examination for licensure as LPNs/LVNs.

Associate Degree Nurse

Associate degrees in nursing (ADNs) are offered at many junior colleges and community colleges and at some universities. These programs combine liberal arts education and nursing education. The length of the ADN program is typically 2 years. ADNs are also considered RNs if they pass the state boards.

Diploma Graduate Nurse

Diploma programs are usually 3-year programs designed as cooperative programs between a community college and a participating hospital. The programs combine course work and clinical experience in the hospital.

Baccalaureate Nurse

A baccalaureate degree refers to a 4-year college or university program. Graduates of a 4-year nursing program are awarded a bachelor of science in nursing (BSN) degree. The curriculum includes courses in liberal arts, general education, and nursing courses. Graduates are prepared to function as nurse generalists and in positions that go beyond the role of hospital staff nurses. BSNs are also considered RNs if they pass the state boards.

Registered Nurse

A nurse who graduates from a nursing program and passes the state board examination for licensure is considered an RN, indicating formal, legal recognition by the state. The RN is a professional who is responsible for planning, giving, and supervising the bedside nursing care of patients. An RN may work in an administrative capacity, assist in daily operations, oversee programs in hospital or institutional settings, or plan community health services.

Registered nurses work in a variety of settings. These settings include hospitals, nursing homes, public health agencies, industry, physicians' offices, government agencies, and educational settings. Some RNs continue their education to earn master's or doctoral degrees.

Nurse Practitioner

A nurse practitioner (NP) is an RN who functions in an expanded nursing role. The NP usually works in an ambulatory patient care setting alongside physicians. An NP may work in an independent nurse practitioner practice with no physicians. An independent nurse practitioner takes health histories, performs physical examinations, conducts screening tests, and educates patients and families about disease prevention.

An NP who works in a physician's practice may perform some duties that a physician would, such as administering physical examinations and treating common illnesses and injuries (Figure 2-5). For example, in an OB/GYN practice the NP can perform a standard annual gynecologic examination, including taking a Pap smear or a culture to test for yeast infection. The nurse practitioner emphasizes preventive health care.

The NP must be an RN with at least a master's degree in nursing, and he must complete 4 to 12 months of an apprenticeship or formal training. With specific formal training the student may become a pediatric nurse practitioner, an obstetric nurse practitioner (midwife), or a psychiatric nurse practitioner. The nurse practitioner works with medical assistants.

Mental Health Technician

A mental health technician, sometimes called a psychiatric aide or counselor, works in a variety of health-care settings with emotionally disturbed and mentally retarded patients. This health professional assists the psychiatric team by observing behavior and providing information to help in the planning of therapy. The mental health technician also participates in supervising group therapy and counseling sessions. This technician may work in a psychiatric clinic, specialized nursing home, psychiatric unit of a hospital, or community health center. Other places of employment include crisis centers and shelters. Training varies widely, from on-the-job

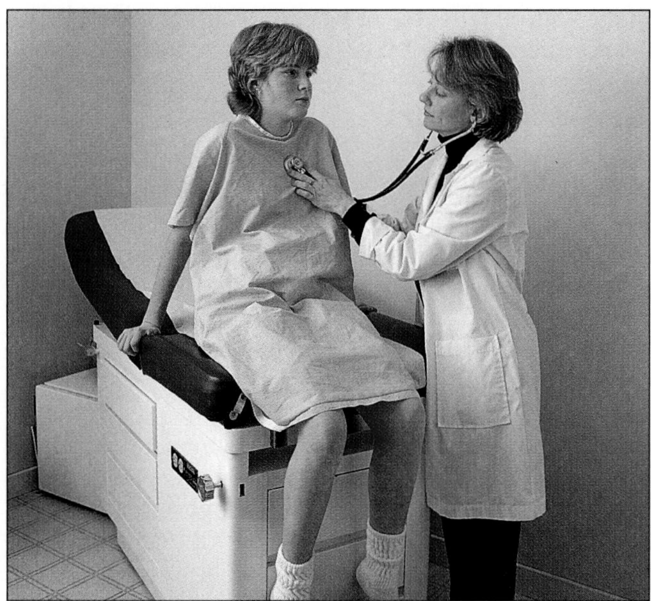

Figure 2-5. Many nurse practitioners work in physicians' offices and are trained to perform routine examinations.

training to advanced degrees, depending on job responsibilities and medical setting.

Occupational Therapist

An occupational therapist works with patients that have physical injuries or illnesses, psychologic or developmental problems, or problems associated with the aging process. This health professional helps patients attain maximum physical and mental health by using educational, vocational, and rehabilitation therapies and activities. The occupational therapist may work in a hospital, clinic, extended care facility, rehabilitation hospital, or government or community agency. To become an occupational therapist, you need a 4-year degree, followed by a 9- to 12-month internship at an accredited hospital. Then you must pass the national board examination, in order to earn the title of OTR—registered occupational therapist.

Medical Transcriptionist

Medical transcriptionists translate a physician's dictation about patient treatments into comprehensive, typed records. Attorneys, insurance companies, and medical specialists need accurate medical records. Medical transcriptionists work in doctors' offices, hospitals, clinics, laboratories, and radiology departments and for medical transcription services and insurance companies. Medical assistants often have medical transcription duties.

Specialty Career Options

The various medical specialties can open up many career possibilities for medical assistants. Deciding to specialize may become one of your career goals 5 or more years from now. Remember that you may need additional training or education for some of these positions. Your hard work will be rewarded, however, as you gain additional job responsibilities.

Choosing an area in which to specialize involves research and careful thought. Local and medical college libraries can supply a great deal of information about the areas in which you may specialize. State employment agencies or schools can help you make career choices.

It is also helpful to check the help-wanted section in local newspapers for information about jobs in specialized areas. Many newspapers separate health-care career opportunities into easy-to-find boxed sections. You may also directly contact companies you would like to work for. Ask about job opportunities, and find out what skills and training the employer requires.

Anesthetist's Assistant

Anesthetist's assistants provide anesthetic care under an anesthetist's direction. Hospitals and high-technology surgical centers frequently employ anesthetist's assistants. These assistants gather patient data and assist in evaluation of patients' physical and mental status. They also record planned surgical procedures, assist with patient monitoring, draw blood samples, perform blood gas analyses, and conduct pulmonary function tests.

Dental Assistant

A dental assistant can practice without formal education or training. In this case, on-the-job training is provided. A dental assistant performs many administrative and laboratory functions that are similar to the duties of a medical assistant. For example, a dental assistant may serve as chair-side assistant, provide instruction in oral hygiene, and prepare and sterilize instruments. To perform expanded clinical and chair-side functions such as those of a hygienist, a dental assistant must have at least 1 year of training in theory and clinical application. This formal education also requires work experience in a dental office.

Dental assistants often work in a private practice. They also work in clinics, dental schools, and local health agencies. Insurance companies hire dental assistants to process dental claims.

Pediatric Medical Assistant

A pediatric medical assistant assists the pediatrician in administrative and clinical duties (Figure 2-6). These duties include obtaining medical histories and preparing patients for examination. Other duties include performing routine tests, sterilizing supplies and equipment, typing, filing, and clerical work. This health professional also educates patients and their parents or guardians about follow-up care and maintains patients' records. A pediatric medical assistant should be able to communicate well with children. Other helpful skills include patience and organizational skills. Pediatric medical assistants work with pediatricians in private practice, hospitals, and clinics.

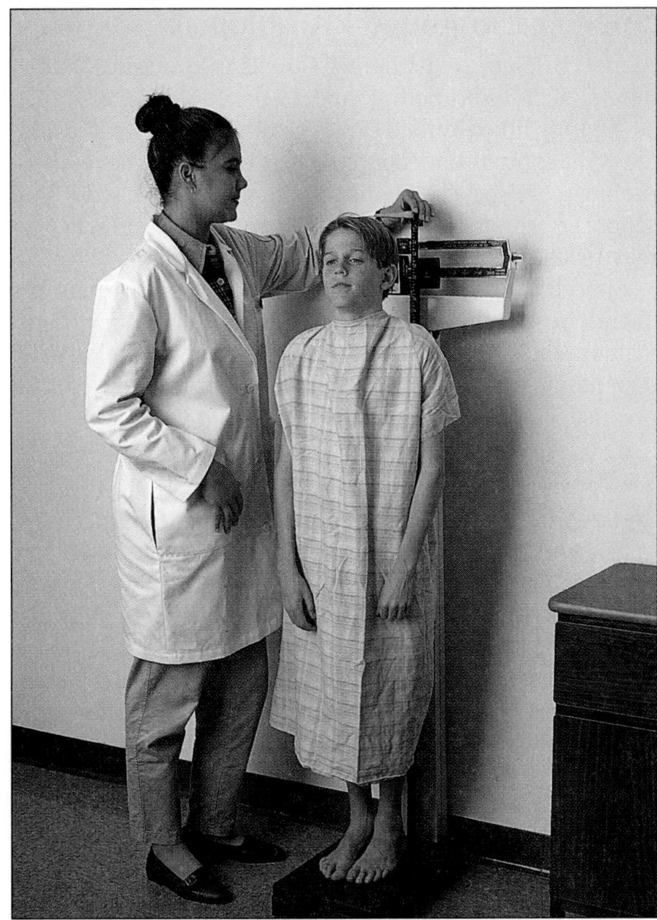

Figure 2-6. If you enjoy working with children, you might consider working as a pediatric medical assistant.

Pharmacy Technician

Pharmacy technicians perform specific routine tasks related to record keeping and preparing and dispensing drugs. Duties include preparing medications for administration and making sure patients receive the correct medication. Pharmacy technicians usually work in hospitals or similar facilities under the supervision of a nurse, pharmacist, or other health-care professional. In a commercial pharmacy they work under the pharmacist's supervision. Opportunities are also available with pharmaceutical firms and wholesale pharmaceutical distributors.

Training can be on-the-job or through certificate programs and 2-year college programs (associate degree). National certification is voluntary by examination and earns the title CPhT (certified pharmacy technician).

Emergency Medical Technician/Paramedic

An emergency medical technician (EMT), sometimes called a paramedic, works under the direction of a physician through a radio communication network. This health professional assesses and manages medical emergencies that occur away from hospitals or other medical settings, such as in private homes, schools, offices, or public areas. An EMT is trained to **triage** patients (to assess the urgency and type of condition presented as well as the immediate medical needs) and to initiate the appropriate treatment for a variety of medical emergencies. While transporting patients to the medical facility, an EMT records, documents, and radios the patient's condition to the physician, describing how the injury occurred. An EMT may work for an ambulance service, fire department, police department, hospital emergency department, private industry, or voluntary care service. Training requirements vary by state but typically require a high school diploma and driver's license, 100 hours of classroom training, and an average of 6 months of practical training on an ambulance squad or in a hospital emergency room.

Surgeon's Assistant

A surgeon's assistant provides patient services under the direction, supervision, and responsibility of a licensed surgeon. This health professional's tasks include obtaining a patient's history and physical data. She then discusses the data with a physician or surgeon to determine what procedures to use to treat the problem. A surgeon's assistant may also assist in performing diagnostic and therapeutic procedures. She must be calm and have good judgment in the high-pressure environment of the operating room. Surgeon's assistants work primarily in hospitals.

Surgeon's assistants are considered a subcategory of physician's assistant. Training programs are usually affiliated with 2- and 4-year colleges and with university schools of medicine and allied health. These programs include practical work in the surgery unit of an affiliated hospital.

Ophthalmic Assistant

An ophthalmic assistant aids ophthalmologists with the routine functions of the practice. This health professional performs simple vision testing, takes medical histories, administers eyedrops, and changes dressings. There are three levels in this category of allied health professional (from most senior to least senior): ophthalmic technologist, ophthalmic technician, and ophthalmic assistant. Duties are determined by the supervising ophthalmologist. No states currently require certification for these positions.

Physical Therapy Assistant

A physical therapy assistant (PTA) works under the direction of a physical therapist to assist with patient treatment. The assistant follows the patient care program created by the physical therapist and physician. This health professional performs tests and treatment procedures, assembles or sets up equipment for therapy sessions, and observes and documents patient behavior and progress (Figure 2-7). A physical therapy assistant may practice in a hospital, nursing home, rehabilitation center, or community or government agency.

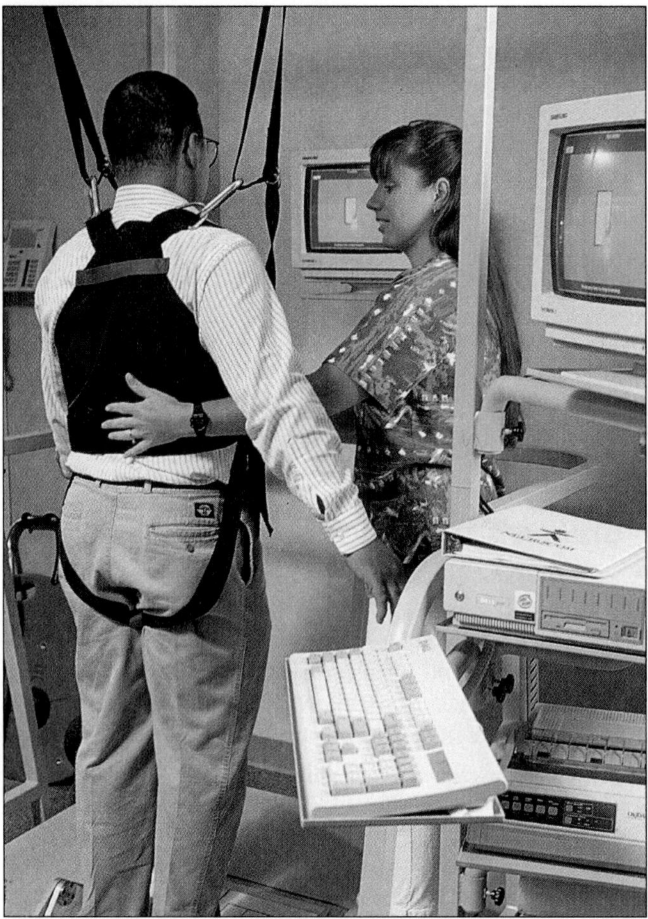

Figure 2-7. Physical therapy assistants provide guidance and support to patients who are recovering from a physical injury or from surgery on a limb or joint.

Radiation Therapy Technologist

A radiation therapy technologist assists the radiologist. He may, for example, assist with administering radiation treatment to patients who have cancer. He may also be responsible for maintaining radiation treatment equipment. The technologist shares responsibility with the radiologist for the accuracy of treatment records. A radiation therapy technologist may work in a hospital, laboratory, clinic, physician's office, or government agency. Training requires a high school diploma and graduation from a 2- or 4-year program in radiography.

Respiratory Therapy Technician

Respiratory therapy technicians work under the supervision of a physician and a respiratory therapist. Respiratory therapists perform procedures such as artificial ventilation. They also clean, sterilize, and maintain the respiratory equipment and document the patient's therapy in the medical record. Respiratory therapy technicians work in hospitals, nursing homes, physicians' offices, and commercial companies that provide emergency oxygen equipment and therapeutic home care.

Speech/Language Pathologist

A speech/language pathologist treats communication disorders, such as stuttering, and associated disorders, such as hearing impairment. This health professional evaluates, diagnoses, and counsels patients who have these problems. A speech/language pathologist may work in a school, hospital, research setting, or private practice or may teach at a college or university.

Speech/language pathologists usually have a master's degree in speech/language pathology or audiology. Certification and licensing requirements vary by state, usually depending on the work setting (public school, private practice, clinic, and so on).

Certified Laboratory Assistant

Certified laboratory assistants perform routine procedures in bacteriology, chemistry, hematology, parasitology, serology, and urinalysis. Laboratory assistants work under the supervision of a medical technologist or hospital anatomic pathologist. They work in laboratories at hospitals, clinics, and physicians' offices and in independent laboratories. One-year training programs are offered by hospitals, vocational schools, and community colleges.

Occupational Therapist Assistant

Occupational therapist assistants work under the supervision of an occupational therapist. They help individuals with mental or physical disabilities reach their highest level of functioning through the teaching of fine motor skills, trades (occupations), and the arts. Duties include preparing materials for activities, maintaining tools and equipment, and documenting the patient's progress. Occupational therapist assistants must earn a 2-year degree (OTA).

Pathologist's Assistant

Pathologist's assistants work under the supervision of a pathologist. Pathologist's assistants sometimes work with forensic pathologists—professionals who study the human body and diseases for legal purposes, in cooperation with government or police investigations. They may prepare frozen sections of dissected body tissue. Assistants working for anatomic pathologists (professionals who study the human body and diseases in a research capacity) may maintain supplies, instruments, and chemicals for the anatomic pathology laboratory. Pathologist's assistants perform laboratory work about 75 percent of the workday. Assistants also perform a variety of administrative duties. They work in community hospitals, university medical centers, and private laboratories.

Professional Associations

Membership in a professional association enables you to become involved in the issues and activities relevant to your field and presents opportunities for continuing education. It is a good idea to become informed about such associations, even those, such as the American Medical Association, that are open to physicians only. The physician you work for may ask you to obtain information about the group's activities and meetings. Table 2-1 summarizes professional associations related to the field of medicine and medical assisting.

American Association of Medical Assistants

The American Association of Medical Assistants (AAMA), as described in Chapter 1, was created to serve the interests of medical assistants and to further the medical assisting profession. The AAMA offers self-paced continuing education classes; workshops and seminars at the local, state, and national levels; and job networking opportunities. Other benefits include legal counsel, group health insurance, professional recognition, and member discounts.

American Association for Medical Transcription

The American Association for Medical Transcription (AAMT) is the professional organization for the advancement of medical transcription. The AAMT also educates medical transcriptionists as medical language specialists. The AAMT offers advice and support to the many medical transcriptionists who are self-employed.

American College of Physicians

Founded in 1915, the American College of Physicians (ACP) is the largest medical specialty organization in the world. It is the only society of internists dedicated to providing education and information resources to the entire field of internal medicine and its subspecialties.

American Hospital Association

The American Hospital Association (AHA) is the nation's largest network of institutional health-care providers. These providers represent every type of hospital: rural and city hospitals, specialty and acute care facilities, freestanding hospitals, academic medical centers, and health systems and networks. The AHA works to support and promote the interests of hospitals and health-care organizations across the country. Organizations as well as individual professionals may join the AHA. Membership benefits include use of the AHA consultant referral service, accessed, for example, by hospitals that need experts in areas not addressed by in-house personnel. Members also have access to AHA's health-care information resources, including teleconferencing and AHA database services.

American Medical Association

The American Medical Association (AMA) was founded in 1847. Its members include 300,000 physicians from every medical specialty. The AMA promotes science and the art of medicine and works to improve public health. The AMA is the world's largest publisher of scientific and medical information and publishes ten monthly medical specialty journals. The AMA also accredits medical programs in the United States and Canada.

The AMA provides an on-line service called AMA/Net for physicians and medical assistants, offering up-to-date information about current medical topics. To use the AMA/Net, the medical office must have a computer, telephone, and modem.

American Medical Technologists

American Medical Technologists (AMT) was established in 1939 as a not-for-profit organization. The AMT offers national certification as a Registered Medical Assistant (RMA) to medical assisting practitioners. It also offers certification to medical technologists, medical laboratory technicians, dental assistants, and phlebotomy technicians. Membership benefits include continuing education classes, workshops and seminars, and job networking opportunities.

American Pharmaceutical Association

The American Pharmaceutical Association (APhA), the national professional society of pharmacists, was founded in 1852. The APhA represents the interests of pharmaceutical professionals, and it strives to help individual members improve their skills. The APhA works to advance the field of pharmacy and the safety of patients. The APhA is active in pharmacy policy development, networking, publishing, research, and public education.

Summary

There are many medical settings in which you can serve as a medical assistant. Some settings will be in specialized branches of medicine. It is important to gain an understanding of the major areas of medicine, as well as the various subspecialties, in order to choose and plan for the type of setting in which you would like to work.

Learning about various allied health professionals—such as pharmacists, nurse practitioners, and medical transcriptionists—will help you interact with others on the job. Learning about specialty career options—such as physical therapy assistants, certified laboratory assistants, and ophthalmic assistants—can give you ideas about integrating new skills into your job as a multiskilled health professional.

Joining a professional organization will enable you to stay informed about issues and activities in the medical assisting field and the specialty or subspecialty in which you work. Professional organizations also provide other benefits to members, such as group health insurance; job networking opportunities; state or chapter meetings, seminars, workshops, and guest presentations; and member discounts. Membership in a professional organization helps you be recognized as a professional. Therefore, it is an important addition to your résumé.

Table 2-1

Professional Medical Organizations

Professional Organization	Membership Requirements	Advantages of Membership
American Association of Medical Assistants (AAMA)	Interested individuals and those who practice medical assisting may join the AAMA.	Offers flexible continuing education programs; publishes bimonthly *The Professional Medical Assistant;* offers legal counsel, professional recognition, various member discounts
American Association for Medical Transcription (AAMT)	Interested individuals and those who practice medical transcription may join the AAMT.	Educates and develops medical transcriptionists as medical language specialists; offers advice and support for self-employed medical transcriptionists
American College of Physicians (ACP)	Physicians and medical students may join.	Provides education and information resources to field of internal medicine and its subspecialties
American Hospital Association (AHA)	Institutional health-care providers and other individuals may join.	Provides consultant referral service and access to health-care information resources
American Medical Association (AMA)	Physicians and medical students may join.	Provides large information source; publishes *Journal of the American Medical Association (JAMA);* offers AMA/Net
American Medical Technologists (AMT)	Medical assistants, medical technologists, medical laboratory technicians, dental assistants, and phlebotomy technicians may join.	Offers national certification as Registered Medical Assistant (RMA); offers certification to other health-care professionals, publications, state chapter activities, continuing education programs
American Pharmaceutical Association (APhA)	Pharmaceutical professionals and physicians may join.	Helps members improve skills; active in pharmacy policy development, networking, publishing, research, public education
American Society of Clinical Pathologists (ASCP)	Any professional involved in laboratory medicine or pathology may join.	Resource for improving the quality of pathology, laboratory medicine; offers educational programs and materials; certifies technologists and technicians

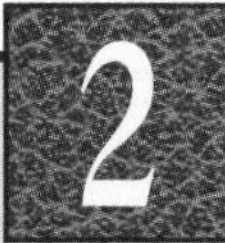

Chapter Review

Discussion Questions

1. Why is geriatrics a growing medical specialty?
2. How might learning about specialty career options help motivate medical assistants in their careers?
3. How do professional organizations help medical assistants perform their job duties?

Critical Thinking Questions

1. How might a medical assistant's experience working with a medical specialist differ from her experience working with a general practitioner, in terms of learning about medicine?
2. If you worked for an obstetrician or OB/GYN, how might you use your spare time to learn more about the specialty and do your job better?
3. Why might a medical assistant be interested in joining a professional association such as the American Hospital Association?

Application Activities

1. Interview a medical assistant, such as a physical therapy assistant, who has chosen a specialty career option. What additional education or training did she need to obtain the position? What are her administrative and clinical duties? What does she like about her job? What does she find most challenging? How did she come to choose the specialty? Report your findings to the class.
2. Create a job-hunting plan for a medical assistant interested in learning about job opportunities in a specialty medical assisting career. Your plan should consist of at least four different ways for the medical assistant to look for jobs.
3. Pick three medical specialties, and identify the skills required for a medical assistant in each specialty.

Further Readings

American Association of Colleges of Osteopathic Medicine. "What Is Osteopathic Medicine?" http://www.aacom.org/what.htm (September 30, 1996).

Balasa, Donald A. "Health System Reform Primer: An Explanation of the Problems and Proposed Solutions." *The Professional Medical Assistant,* January/February 1994, 11–15.

Balasa, Donald A. "How Will Health System Reform Impact the Medical Assisting Profession?" *The Professional Medical Assistant,* July/August 1994, 9–11.

Bezold, Clement. "A Futurist's View of Health Care and Education: Impact on Specialized Accreditation." *Journal of Allied Health,* Winter 1994, 3–9.

Blank, Linda L., ed. *The Role and Education of the Medical Subspecialist in the 21st Century.* Philadelphia: American Board of Internal Medicine, 1994.

Grainger, Ruth Dailey. "Ways to Nurture Your Creativity." *American Journal of Nursing,* January 1991, 14–15.

Harold, Wanda. "The Humanistic Role of the Medical Assistant." *The Professional Medical Assistant,* January/February 1991, 8–10.

Lozada, Marlene. "The Health Occupations Boom." *Vocational Educational Journal,* September 1995, 34–37.

Stanfield, Peggy. *Introduction to the Health Professions.* Boston: Jones and Bartlett, 1990.

Toughill, Eileen H. "Creativity Can Make a Difference." *Geriatric Nursing,* November/December 1990, 276–277.

Wilson, Stephen L., et al. "Utilization of Allied Health Personnel in HMOs." *Journal of Allied Health,* Summer 1989, 361–373.

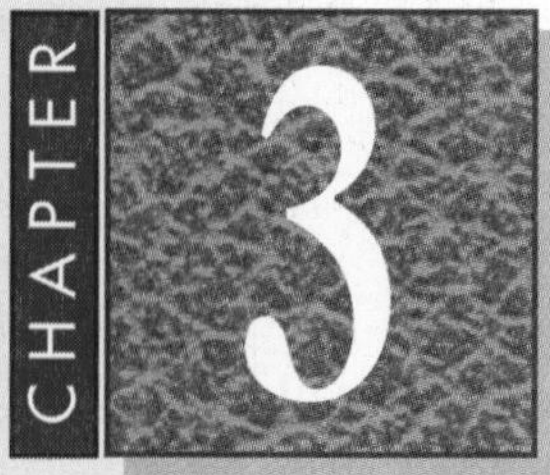

Legal and Ethical Issues in Medical Practice

CHAPTER OUTLINE

- Medical Law
- OSHA Regulations
- Quality Control and Assurance
- Code of Ethics
- Confidentiality Issues and Mandatory Disclosure

OBJECTIVES

After completing Chapter 3, you will be able to:

- Define ethics, bioethics, and law.
- Discuss the measures a medical practice must take to avoid malpractice claims.
- Describe OSHA requirements for a medical office.
- Describe procedures for handling an incident of exposure to hazardous materials.
- Compare and contrast quality control and quality assurance procedures.
- Explain how to protect patient confidentiality.

Key Terms

abandonment
agent
arbitration
bioethics
breach of contract
durable power of attorney
ethics
law
law of agency
liable
living will
malpractice claim
negligence
subpoena
tort
Uniform Donor Card

AREAS OF COMPETENCE

1997 ROLE DELINEATION STUDY

CLINICAL

Fundamental Principles

- Apply principles of aseptic technique and infection control
- Comply with quality assurance practices

Patient Care

- Coordinate patient care information with other health care providers

GENERAL (Transdisciplinary)

Professionalism

- Adhere to ethical principles

Legal Concepts

- Maintain confidentiality
- Practice within the scope of education, training, and personal capabilities
- Use appropriate guidelines when releasing information
- Follow employer's established policies dealing with the health care contract

continued

AREAS OF COMPETENCE *continued*

- Follow federal, state, and local legal guidelines
- Maintain awareness of federal and state health care legislation and regulations
- Comply with established risk management and safety procedures
- Recognize professional credentialing criteria

Medical Law

Medical law plays an important part in medical office procedures. A **law** is a rule of conduct established and enforced by an authority or governing body, such as the federal government. Medical assistants must understand and follow the legal requirements of the practice of medicine with respect to preventing malpractice claims and adhering to standards of care.

Malpractice

Malpractice claims are lawsuits by a patient against a physician for errors in diagnosis or treatment. **Negligence** cases are those in which a person believes that a medical professional did not perform an essential action or performed an improper one, thus harming the patient.

Following are some examples of malpractice:

- Postoperative complications. For example, a patient starts to show signs of internal bleeding in the recovery room. The incision is reopened, and it is discovered that the surgeon did not complete closure of all the severed capillaries at the operation site.
- *Res ipsa loquitur.* This Latin term, which means "The thing speaks for itself," refers to a case in which the doctor's fault is completely obvious. For example, if a lung cancer patient has to have the right lung removed and the surgeon instead removes the left lung, the patient will most likely sue the surgeon for malpractice. Another example is a case in which a surgeon accidentally leaves a surgical instrument inside the patient.

Following are examples of negligence:

- Abandonment. A health-care professional who stops care without providing an equally qualified substitute can be charged with **abandonment.** For example, a labor and delivery nurse is helping a woman in labor. The nurse's shift ends, but all the other nurses are busy and her replacement is late for work. Leaving the woman would constitute abandonment.
- Delayed treatment. A patient shows symptoms of some illness or disorder, but the doctor decides, for whatever reason, to delay treatment. If the patient later learns of the doctor's decision to wait, the patient may believe he has a negligence case.

Negligence cases are sometimes classified using the following legal terms.

1. *Malfeasance* refers to an unlawful act or misconduct.
2. *Misfeasance* refers to a lawful act that is done incorrectly.
3. *Nonfeasance* refers to failure to perform an act that is one's required duty or that is required by law.

The Four Ds of Negligence. The American Medical Association (AMA) lists the following four Ds of negligence:

1. Duty. Patients must show that a physician-patient relationship existed in which the physician owed the patient a duty.
2. Derelict. Patients must show that the physician failed to comply with the standards of the profession. For example, a gynecologist has routinely taken Pap smears of a patient and then, for whatever reason, does not do so. If the patient then shows evidence of cervical cancer, the physician could be said to have been derelict.
3. Direct cause. Patients must show that any damages were a direct cause of a physician's breach of duty. For example, if a patient fell on the sidewalk and damaged her cast, she could not prove that the cast was damaged because it was incorrectly or poorly applied by her physician. It would be clear that the damage to the cast resulted from the fall. If, however, the patient's leg healed incorrectly because of the way the cast had been applied, she might have a case.
4. Damages. Patients must prove that they suffered injury.

To go forward with a malpractice suit, a patient must be prepared to prove all four Ds of negligence.

Malpractice and Civil Law. Malpractice lawsuits are part of civil law. Civil law is concerned with individuals' private rights (as opposed to criminal offenses against public law). Under civil law, a breach of some obligation that causes harm or injury to someone is known as a **tort.** A tort can be intentional or unintentional. Both negligence and breach of contract are considered torts. **Breach of contract** is the failure to adhere to a contract's terms. The implied physician-patient contract includes requirements like maintaining patient confidentiality. (An implied contract is one that is not created by specific, written words, but rather is defined by the conduct of the parties. Usually the parties involved have some special relationship.)

Settling Malpractice Suits. Malpractice suits often require a trial in a court of law. Sometimes, however, they are settled through arbitration. **Arbitration** is a process in which the opposing sides choose a person or persons outside the court system, often with special knowledge in the field, to hear and decide the dispute. (Your local or state medical society has information about your state's policy on arbitration.) If injury, failure to provide reasonable care, or abandonment of the patient is proved to have occurred, the doctor must pay damages (a financial award) to the injured party.

If the doctor you work with becomes involved in a lawsuit, you should be familiar with subpoenas. A **subpoena** is a written court order addressed to a specific person, requiring that person's presence in court on a specific date at a specific time. If you were directly involved in the patient case that precipitated the lawsuit, you might be subpoenaed. Another important term to know is *subpoena duces tecum,* which is a court order to produce documents. If you are in charge of patient records at the practice, you may be required to locate, assemble, photocopy, and arrange for delivery of patient records for this purpose.

Law of Agency. According to the **law of agency,** an employee is considered to be acting as a doctor's **agent** (on the doctor's behalf) while performing professional tasks. The Latin term *respondeat superior,* or "Let the master answer," is sometimes used to refer to this relationship. For example, the employee's word is as binding as if it were the doctor's (so you should never, for example, promise a patient a cure). Therefore, the doctor is responsible, or **liable,** for the negligence of employees. A negligent employee, however, may also be sued directly, because individuals are legally responsible for their own actions. Therefore, a patient can sue both the doctor and the involved employee for negligence. The employer, or the employer's insurance company, can also sue the employee.

The American Association of Medical Assistants (AAMA) recommends that you purchase your own malpractice insurance and have a personal attorney. Most likely, in a case of negligence the doctor would be sued (because you as an employee are acting on the doctor's behalf), and you are usually covered by the doctor's malpractice insurance. Even if you are young and think you do not have many assets, you should still obtain your own insurance.

Terminating Care of a Patient

A physician may wish to terminate care of a patient. Terminating care is sometimes called withdrawing from a case. Following are some typical reasons a physician may choose to withdraw from a case:

- The patient refuses to follow the physician's instructions.
- The patient's family members complain incessantly to or about the physician.
- A personality conflict develops between the physician and patient that cannot be reasonably resolved.
- The patient insists on having pain medication refilled beyond what the physician considers medically necessary.

A physician who terminates care of a patient must do so in a formal, legal manner, following these steps.

1. The physician must write a letter to the patient, expressing the reason for withdrawing from the case and recommending that the patient seek medical care from another physician as soon as possible. Figure 3-1 shows an example of a letter of termination.
2. Send the letter by certified mail with a return receipt requested.
3. Place a copy of the letter (and the return receipt, when received) in the patient's medical record.
4. Summarize in the patient record the physician's reason for terminating care and the actions taken to inform the patient.

LETTER OF WITHDRAWAL FROM CASE

Dear Mr.___________________________:

I find it necessary to inform you that I am withdrawing from further professional attendance upon you for the reason that you have persisted in refusing to follow my medical advice and treatment. Since your condition requires medical attention, I suggest that you place yourself under the care of another physician without delay. If you so desire, I shall be available to attend you for a reasonable time after you have received this letter, but in no event for more than five days.

This should give you ample time to select a physician of your choice from the many competent practitioners in this city. With your approval, I will make available to this physician your case history and information regarding the diagnosis and treatment which you have received from me.

Very truly yours,

___________________________, MD

Figure 3-1. Physicians are required to inform patients in writing if they wish to withdraw from a case. *Source:* Medicolegal Forms With Legal Analysis, American Medical Association, © 1991.

Standard of Care

You are expected to fulfill the standards of the medical assisting profession for applying legal concepts to practice. According to the AAMA, medical assistants should uphold legal concepts in the following ways:

- Maintain confidentiality.
- Practice within the scope of training and capabilities.
- Prepare and maintain medical records.
- Document accurately.
- Use appropriate guidelines when releasing information.
- Follow employer's established policies dealing with the health-care contract.
- Follow legal guidelines and maintain awareness of health-care legislation and regulations.
- Maintain and dispose of regulated substances in compliance with government guidelines.
- Follow established risk-management and safety procedures.
- Recognize professional credentialing criteria.
- Help develop and maintain personnel, policy, and procedure manuals.

Often laws dictate what medical assistants may or may not do. For instance, in some states it is illegal for medical assistants to draw blood. No states consider it legal for medical assistants to diagnose a condition, prescribe a treatment, or let a patient believe that a medical assistant is a nurse or any other type of caregiver. In addition to what is stated by law, you and the physician must establish the procedures that are appropriate for you to perform.

Administrative Duties and the Law

Many of a medical assistant's administrative duties are related to legal requirements. Paperwork for insurance billing, patient consent forms for surgical procedures, and correspondence (such as a physician's letter of withdrawal from a case) must be handled correctly to meet legal standards. Documentation, such as making appropriate and accurate entries in a patient's medical record, is legally important. You may also maintain the physician's appointment book. This book is considered a legal document. It can prove, for instance, that the physician, if unable to see a patient, arranged for the patient to be seen by another physician in the same practice. In other words, the physician provided a qualified substitute as required by law.

You may also be responsible for handling certain state reporting requirements. Items that must be reported include births; certain diseases such as acquired immunodeficiency syndrome (AIDS) and other sexually transmitted diseases; drug abuse; suspected child abuse or abuse of the elderly; injuries caused by violence, such as knife and gunshot wounds; and deaths. Reports are sent to various state departments, depending on the content of the report. For example, suspected child abuse cases are reported to the state department of social services. Addressing these state requirements is called the physician's public duty.

Phone calls must be handled with an awareness of legal issues. For example, if the physician asks you to contact a patient by phone and you call the patient at work, you should not identify yourself or the physician by name to someone else without the patient's permission. You can say, for example, "Please tell Mrs. Arnot that her doctor's office is calling." If you do not take this precaution, the physician can be sued for invasion of privacy. You must abide by similar guidelines if you are responsible for making follow-up calls to a patient after a surgical procedure.

Controlled Substances and the Law

You must also follow the correct procedures for the safekeeping and disposal of controlled substances, such as narcotics, in the medical office. It is important to know the right dosages and potential complications of these drugs, as well as prescription refill rules, in order to understand and interpret the directions of the physician in a legally responsible manner. Prescription pads must be kept secure so that they do not fall into the wrong hands.

Communication and the Law

Communication with the patient and disclosure of information are sensitive legal areas. You are not allowed to decide what information should be given to the patient or by whom. You can, however, provide support and show respect for the patient as a person. In cases involving sexually transmitted diseases (STDs), for example, clear, nonjudgmental communication is of the utmost importance. Sensitivity is also required in dealing with special issues such as illiteracy. For example, a patient may not want to admit being unable to read written instructions. In general, your role in maintaining smooth communication between the patient and the medical office is to help prevent misunderstandings that could lead to legal confrontations.

Legal Documents and the Patient

You need to be aware of two legal documents that are typically completed by a patient prior to major surgery or hospitalization: the living will and the Uniform Donor Card. Traditionally, these documents were completed outside the medical office or in the hospital. The current trend, however, is for medical practice personnel, including medical assistants, to assist patients in developing these important documents.

Living Wills. A **living will,** sometimes called an advance directive, is a legal document addressed to the patient's family and health-care providers. The living will states what type of treatment the patient wishes or does not wish to receive if she becomes terminally ill, unconscious, or permanently comatose (sometimes referred to as being in a persistent vegetative state). For example, a living will typically states whether a patient wishes to be put on life-sustaining equipment should she become permanently comatose. Some living wills contain DNR (do not resuscitate) orders. These orders mean the patient does not wish medical personnel to try to resuscitate her should the heart stop beating. Living wills are a means of helping families of terminally ill patients deal with the inevitable outcome of the illness and may help limit unnecessary medical costs.

The living will is signed when the patient is mentally and physically competent to do so. It must also be signed by two witnesses. Medical practices can help patients develop a living will, sometimes in conjunction with organizations that make available preprinted living will forms. The Society for the Right to Die (based in New York City) and the Association for Freedom to Die (in Columbus, Ohio) are two such organizations.

Patients who have living wills are asked to name, in a document called a **durable power of attorney,** someone who will make decisions regarding medical care on their behalf, if they are unable to do so. Often, a Durable Power of Attorney for Health Care form is completed in conjunction with a living will.

The Uniform Donor Card. In 1968 the Uniform Anatomical Gift Act was passed, setting forth guidelines for all states to follow in complying with a person's wish to make a gift of one or more organs (or the whole body) upon death. An anatomical gift is typically designated for medical research, organ transplants, or placement in a tissue bank. The **Uniform Donor Card** is a legal document that states one's wish to make such a gift. People often carry the Uniform Donor Card in their wallets. Many medical practices offer the service of helping their patients obtain and complete a Uniform Donor Card.

Confidentiality Issues

The physician is legally obligated to keep patient information confidential. Therefore, you must be sure that all patient information is discussed with the patient privately and shared with the staff only when appropriate. For example, the billing department will have to see patient records to code diagnoses and bill appropriately. Also, a staff member who has to make an appointment for a patient to get a herpes test at an outside location will need the patient record to do so.

You must avoid discussing cases with anyone outside the office, even if the patient's name is not mentioned. Only the patient can waive this confidentiality right. All patients' records must be kept out of sight of other patients or visitors, as well as night staff, such as janitorial service employees. Confidentiality also is required in the handling of test results.

OSHA Regulations

The Occupational Safety and Health Administration (OSHA), a division of the U.S. Department of Labor, has created federal laws to protect health-care workers from health hazards on the job. Medical personnel may accidentally contract a dangerous or even fatal disease by coming into contact with a virus a patient is carrying. Medical assistants may also be exposed to toxic substances in the office. OSHA regulations describe the precautions a medical office must take with clothing, housekeeping, record keeping, and training to minimize the risk of disease or injury.

Some of the most important OSHA regulations are those for controlling workers' exposure to infectious disease. These regulations are set forth in the Occupational Safety and Health Administration Bloodborne Pathogens Protection Standard of 1991. A pathogen is any microorganism that causes disease. Microorganisms are microscopic living bodies, such as viruses or bacteria, that may be present in a patient's blood or other body fluids (saliva or semen).

Of particular concern to medical workers are the human immunodeficiency virus (HIV), which causes AIDS, and the hepatitis B virus (HBV). AIDS damages the body's immune system and thus its ability to fight disease. AIDS is always fatal. HBV is a highly contagious disease that is potentially fatal. It causes inflammation of the liver and may cause liver failure. Every year, about 8700 health-care workers become HBV-infected at work, and about 200 die from the disease. (Chapter 21 discusses HIV, hepatitis, and other blood-borne pathogens.)

OSHA requires that medical professionals in medical practices follow what are called Universal Precautions. They were developed by the Centers for Disease Control and Prevention (CDC) to prevent medical professionals from exposing themselves and others to blood-borne pathogens. Exposure can occur, for example, through skin that has been broken from a needle puncture or other wound and through mucous membranes, such as those in the nose and throat. If these areas come into contact with a patient's (or coworker's) blood or body fluids, a virus could be transferred from one person to another. Specific information about Universal Precautions appears in Chapter 19.

Hospitals are required to follow what are called Standard Precautions, also developed by the CDC. Standard Precautions combine Universal Precautions with body substance isolation guidelines. Standard Precautions are also described in Chapter 19.

Protective Gear

The more exposure that is involved, the more protective clothing you need to wear (Figure 3-2). Procedures that usually involve exposure to blood, other body fluids, or broken skin require gloves. There are several kinds of gloves for different situations.

- Disposable gloves are worn only once and then discarded. Do not use a pair that has been torn or damaged.
- Utility gloves are stronger and may be decontaminated. They are used for housecleaning tasks.
- Examination gloves are used for procedures that do not require a sterile environment.
- Sterile gloves are used for sterile procedures such as minor surgery.

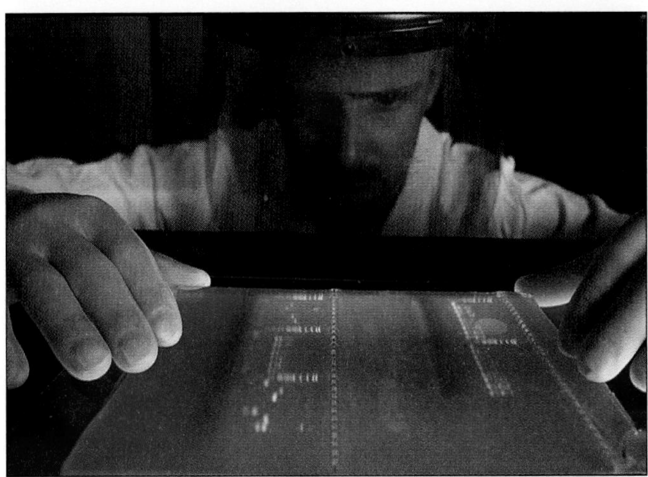

Figure 3-2. Researchers must wear full protective gear in a laboratory that studies infectious diseases. Regulations for such gear are set by OSHA.

Appropriate masks, goggles, or face shields must be used for procedures in which a worker's eyes, nose, or mouth may be exposed. These are procedures that may involve spraying or splashes—for example, examining blood. If potentially infected substances might get onto a worker's clothing, the worker must wear a protective laboratory coat, gown, or apron. Fluid-resistant material is recommended by OSHA.

The law requires that the physician/employer provide all necessary protective clothing to the employee free of charge. The employer also pays for cleaning, maintaining, and replacing the protective items.

Decontamination

After a procedure, you must decontaminate all exposed work surfaces with a 10% bleach solution or with a germ-killing solution containing glutoraldohydes approved by the Environmental Protection Agency (EPA). Replace protective coverings on equipment and surfaces if they have been exposed. Regularly decontaminate receptacles such as bins, pails, and cans as part of routine housekeeping procedures. Never pick up broken glass with your hands. Use tongs, even when wearing gloves, so that the sharp glass does not cut the gloves and expose the skin.

Dispose of any potentially infectious waste materials in special "biohazard bags," which are leakproof and labeled with the biohazard symbol (Figure 3-3). Wastes that fall into this category include blood products, body fluids, human tissues, and vaccines; table paper, linen, towels, and gauze with body fluids on them; and gloves, diapers, sanitary napkins, and cotton swabs. Disposal of sharp instruments ("sharps") is discussed in the next section.

Sharp Equipment

Disposable sharp equipment that has been used must not be bent, broken, recapped, or otherwise tampered with, so as to prevent possible exposure to medical workers. It

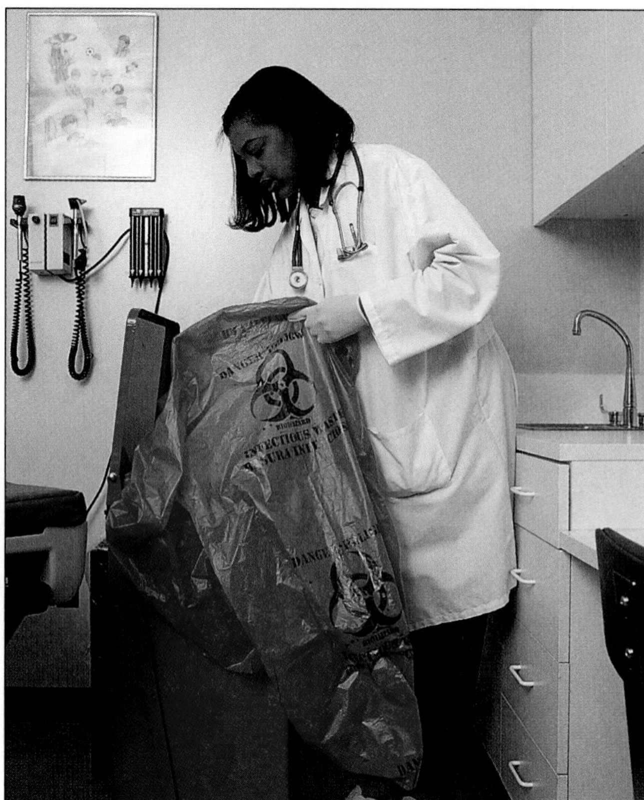

Figure 3-3. The medical assistant may be responsible for disposing of wastes such as gloves, table paper, and gauze with body fluids on them in containers that display the biohazard symbol.

should be placed in a leakproof, puncture-resistant, color-coded, and appropriately labeled container. Reusable sharp equipment must be placed as soon as possible into a puncture-resistant container and taken to a reprocessing area.

Both disposable and reusable instruments are sterilized in their appropriate containers. Sterilizing is usually accomplished by means of an autoclave, a machine that uses pressurized steam. Sterilization of disposable instruments is usually handled by an outside waste management company.

Exposure Incidents

You must give special attention to what to do in case of an exposure incident. This may happen when a medical worker accidentally sticks herself with a used needle. These "puncture exposure incidents" are the most common kind of exposure.

When an exposure incident occurs, the physician/employer must be notified immediately. Quick and proper treatment can help prevent the development of HBV. Timely action can also prevent exposing other people to any infection the worker may have acquired. Reporting the incident to the physician/employer also may encourage him to revise the office's safety procedures in some way to help prevent the same type of incident from happening again.

Postexposure Procedures

OSHA requires specific postexposure evaluation and follow-up procedures. If an exposure incident occurs, the employer must offer the exposed employee a free medical evaluation by a health-care provider of the employer's choice. The employer must refer the employee to a licensed health-care provider who will counsel the employee about what happened and how to prevent the spread of any potential infection. The health-care provider will also take a blood sample and prescribe the appropriate treatment. The employee has the right to refuse both the medical evaluation and the treatment.

When a medical worker starts a job, the physician/employer is required to offer the worker, at no cost, the opportunity to have an HBV vaccination within 10 days. An employee who refuses vaccination must sign a waiver. The employee can change his mind at any time and decide to have the vaccination. If an employee who declined the HBV vaccination is exposed to a patient who is HBV-positive or who is being tested for HBV, it is recommended that the employee be tested for HBV and receive the vaccination if necessary. (The employee may decline to be tested, however.) If the patient is being tested for HBV, the employee is legally required to be informed of the test results. (This is true for HIV as well, and the employee still has the right to refuse testing.) The employee may agree to give blood but not be tested. The blood sample must be kept on hand for 90 days in case the worker later develops symptoms of HBV or HIV infection and then decides to be tested.

The health-care provider that performs the postexposure evaluation must give the employer a written report stating whether HBV vaccination was recommended and received. The report must also state that the employee, if tested, was informed of the blood test results. Any information beyond this must be kept confidential.

If you plan to do an externship in a medical office, the physician does not have to provide you with the HBV vaccine. She may, however, deny you the opportunity to do the externship if you have not received the vaccination elsewhere. Many accredited medical assisting programs offer the vaccine to their students.

Laundry

OSHA has regulations for handling potentially infectious laundry. Hospitals have their own laundry facilities because these facilities are cost-effective. Some larger clinics also have their own laundry facilities. Most doctors' offices, however, send laundry out. Laundry must be bagged and labeled. Any wet laundry to be transported should be packed so that it does not leak. The laundry service the medical office uses should abide by all OSHA regulations. Laundry workers must wear gloves and handle contaminated materials as little as possible. Some doctors' offices use only disposable items, such as paper robes, and do not need laundry service.

Hazardous Materials

You may encounter hazardous equipment and toxic substances in the office. These hazards include vaccines, disinfectants, and laser equipment.

OSHA's Occupational Health and Safety Act of 1970 sets minimum requirements for workplace safety. It also requires employers to keep an inventory of all hazardous materials used in the workplace. Containers of hazardous substances must be labeled in a specific way, listing any potentially harmful ingredients. The employer must post Material Safety Data Sheets (MSDS) about these substances. These sheets specify whether the substance is cancer-causing, list other possible risks, and state OSHA's requirements for controlling exposure. All employees are entitled to be informed about hazardous substances in the workplace and to be trained in how to use them safely.

Training Requirements

Training requirements are part of OSHA's hazardous substance regulations. Every employee who may be exposed to hazardous or infectious substances on the job must be given free information and training during working hours at least once a year. Training must also be held when a new chemical or piece of medical equipment is introduced into the office or when a procedure changes. Training must cover the following topics:

- How to obtain a copy of the OSHA regulations and an explanation of them
- The causes and symptoms of blood-borne diseases
- How blood-borne pathogens are transmitted
- The facility's Exposure Control Plan and how to obtain a copy
- What tasks might result in exposure
- The use and limitations of all the precautions
- All aspects of personal protective equipment
- All aspects of HBV vaccination
- Emergency procedures
- Postexposure procedures
- Warning labels, signs, and color coding

Beyond this federal law, state training requirements vary. The states of Washington and Florida require medical assistants to take a short course specifically covering HIV laws and precautions. Your instructor will familiarize you with your state's policy. OSHA has its own training institute, supports various other training resources, and develops training videotapes and tests for trainees. In some doctors' offices, the laboratory supervisor conducts training for the office staff. Anyone who has gone through a training session can then train others.

General Regulations

General work area laws restrict eating, drinking, smoking, applying cosmetics or lip balm, and handling contact lenses in the work area. These laws also forbid storing food or drinks in refrigerators that are used to store blood or other potentially infectious material. Refrigerators must have working thermometers to ensure proper cooling temperature (see Figure 3-4).

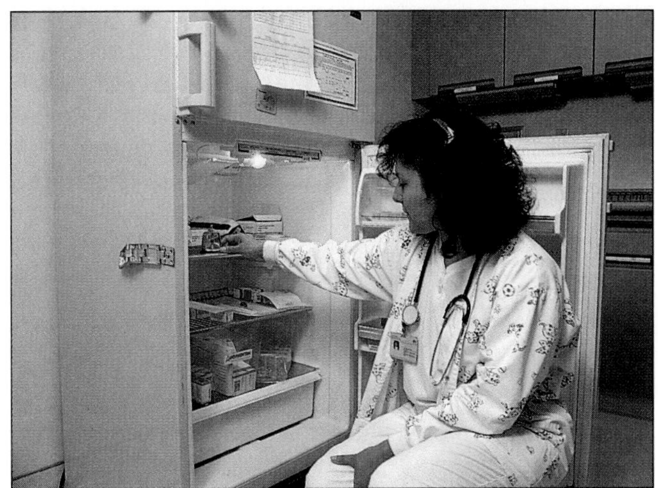

Figure 3-4. OSHA laws require blood or other potentially infectious material to be stored separately from food and drinks. Refrigerators storing such material should have working thermometers to ensure proper cooling temperature.

There are also required procedures for various specific on-the-job injuries. For instance, for eye injuries such as burns and chemical splashes, OSHA requires flushing the eye(s) for 15 minutes with a constant water flow.

Documentation

Lastly, OSHA's record-keeping and documentation requirements are intended to protect the legal rights and safety of everyone in the medical office. The office must have a written Exposure Control Plan describing all precautions against exposure to hazards and blood-borne pathogens and specifying what to do if exposure occurs. Employee medical and exposure records must be kept on file during employment and 30 years afterward. If an employer retires or closes the practice, the employee records are forwarded to the director of OSHA. Also, a log of occupational injuries and illnesses, OSHA Form 200, must be kept for 5 years. The employer must also keep on file for 3 years records documenting an employee's training: dates, topics covered, and names and qualifications of the trainers.

OSHA Inspections

In response to a complaint, or sometimes at random, OSHA may send a compliance officer to inspect a medical office. In 1995 approximately 29,000 inspections were performed. The penalties for not complying with regulations vary according to the severity of the offense. For example, if an inspector finds that the medical assistants have not worn gloves for 2 months because the employer did not make them available, that would entail a severe penalty. If four assistants were wearing gloves but one had forgotten to put them on, there would be a lesser penalty. There are reductions for complying on the spot—perhaps no penalty will be charged. In a serious case, the office could be charged up to $10,000 per broken regulation, multiplied by the number of employees. The penalties are paid directly to OSHA, but the money goes into the federal treasury. If a serious violation occurs in a physicians' office laboratory, the laboratory's payments from Medicare may be suspended.

Quality Control and Assurance

A medical office often has a physicians' office laboratory to perform different types of clinical tests, depending on the physician's specialty and state laws. The Clinical Laboratory Improvement Amendments of 1988 (CLIA '88) lists the regulations for laboratory testing. Physicians must display a certificate from CLIA confirming that their office complies with CLIA regulations. These regulations set standards for the quality of work performed in a laboratory and the accuracy of test results. Congress passed these laws after publicity about deaths caused by errors in the test used to diagnose cancer of the uterus.

According to CLIA '88, there are three categories of laboratory tests: waived tests, moderate-complexity tests, and high-complexity tests. Waived tests, the simplest kind, require the least amount of judgment and pose an insignificant risk to the patient in the event of an error. The laboratory applies for a certificate of waiver from the U.S. Department of Health and Human Services, which grants permission to perform any test on the list of waived tests and to bill it to Medicare or Medicaid. Tests that patients can do at home with kits approved by the department's Food and Drug Administration (FDA), such as the blood glucose test, also fall under this heading.

Most tests are in the moderate-complexity category. Cholesterol testing and checking for the presence or absence of sperm are examples. CLIA lists all waived and moderate-complexity tests and considers all other tests to be of high complexity.

Under CLIA '88, medical assistants are always allowed to perform waived tests. These tests are listed in Figure 3-5. Medical assistants can also perform moderate-complexity tests as long as the physician can ensure that the assistant is appropriately trained and experienced according to federal guidelines. Some state laws may be stricter than the federal laws, so the medical office should check with the state health department to see if there are any local rules about what kinds of tests medical assistants may perform. As you advance in your career, you will most likely be trained to do more and more types of tests, receiving training either by senior staff members or through outside programs.

Waived Tests

- Dipstick or tablet reagent urinalysis (nonautomated) for the following: bilirubin, glucose, hemoglobin, ketone, leukocytes, nitrite, pH, protein, specific gravity, and urobilinogen
- Fecal occult blood
- Ovulation tests—visual color tests for human luteinizing hormone
- Urine pregnancy tests—visual color comparison determination
- Erythrocyte sedimentation rate—nonautomated
- Hemoglobin—(nonautomated) by copper sulfate
- Blood glucose—by glucose monitoring devices cleared by FDA specifically for home use
- Spun microhematocrit
- Hemoglobin—(automated) by single analyte instruments with self-contained or component features to perform specimen-reagent interaction, providing direct measurement and readout

Figure 3-5. Under CLIA '88, medical assistants are always allowed to perform waived tests.

Elements of the Quality Assurance Program

CLIA '88 also requires every medical office to have a quality assurance (QA) program. This program must include a quality control (QC) program specifically for the laboratory. The goal is to track and improve the quality of all aspects of the medical practice—including patient care, laboratory procedures, record keeping, employee evaluations, finances, legal responsibilities, public image, staff morale, insurance issues, and patient education. Documentation is required by QA regulations, to provide evidence that QA procedures are in place in the office. This documentation becomes extremely important if there is an inspection or a legal dispute.

Any QA program must include the following elements:

- Written policies on the standards of patient care and professional behavior
- A QC program
- Training and continuing education programs
- An instrument maintenance program
- Documentation requirements
- Evaluation methods

Software programs are available to help medical offices develop a QA program and procedures manual.

The Laboratory Program

The laboratory QC program must cover testing concerns, such as patient preparation procedures, collection of the specimen (blood, urine, or tissue), labeling, preservation and transportation, test methods, inconsistent results, use and maintenance of equipment, personnel training, complaints and investigations, and corrective actions. (Procedure 3-1 describes the QC procedures for blood

PROCEDURE 3-1

Quality Control Procedures for Blood Specimen Collection

Objective: To follow proper quality control procedures when taking a blood specimen

Materials: Necessary sterile equipment, specimen collection container, and paperwork related to the type of blood test the specimen is being drawn for, requisition form, marker, proper packing materials for transport

Method

1. Review the request form for the test ordered, verify the procedure, prepare the necessary equipment and paperwork, and prepare the work area.
2. Identify the patient and explain the procedure. Confirm the patient's identification. Ask the patient to spell her name. Make sure the patient understands the procedure that is to be performed, even if she has had it done before.
3. Confirm that the patient has followed any pretest preparation requirements such as fasting, taking any necessary medication, or stopping a medication. For example, if a fasting specimen is being taken, the patient should not have eaten anything after midnight of the day before. Some doctors' offices will let the patient drink water or black coffee, however. It often depends on the type of specimen being taken.
4. Collect the specimen properly. Collect it at the right time intervals if that applies. Use sterile equipment and proper technique.
5. Use the correct specimen collection containers and the right preservatives, if required. For example, blood collected into a test tube with additives should be mixed immediately, or it will clot.
6. Immediately label the specimens. The label should include the patient's name, the date and time of collection, the test's name, and the name of the person collecting the specimen. Do not label the containers before collecting the specimen.
7. Follow correct procedures for disposing of hazardous specimen waste and decontaminating the work area. Used needles, for instance, should immediately be placed in a biohazard sharps container.
8. Thank the patient. Keep the patient in the office if any follow-up observation is necessary.
9. If the specimen is to be transported to an outside laboratory, prepare it for transport in the proper container for that type of specimen, according to OSHA regulations. Place the container in a clear plastic bag with a zip closure and dual pockets with the international biohazard label imprinted in red or orange. The requisition form should be placed in the outside pocket of the bag. This ensures protection from contamination if the specimen leaks. Have a courier pick up the specimen and place it in an appropriate carrier (such as an insulated cooler) with the biohazard label. Place specimens to be sent by mail in appropriate plastic containers, and then place the containers inside a heavy-duty plastic container with a screw-down, nonleaking lid. Then place this container in either a heavy-duty cardboard box or nylon bag. The words *Human Specimen* or *Body Fluids* should be imprinted on the box or bag. Seal with a strong tape strip.

specimen collection.) The accuracy of the tests, and the instruments and chemicals that are used, must be monitored through QC procedures and documented. (Laboratory QC programs are discussed in more detail in Chapter 32.)

Code of Ethics

Medical ethics is a vital part of medical practice, and following an ethical code is an important part of your job. **Ethics** deals with general principles of right and wrong, as opposed to requirements of law. A professional is expected to act in ways that reflect society's ideas of right and wrong, even if such behavior is not enforced by law. Often, however, the law is based on ethical considerations.

Bioethics deals with issues that arise related to medical advances. Here are two examples of bioethical issues.

1. A treatment for Parkinson's disease was developed that uses fetal tissue. Some women, upon learning about this treatment, might get pregnant just to have an abortion and sell the fetal tissue. Is this ethical?
2. If a couple cannot have a baby because of a medical condition of the mother, using a surrogate mother is an option some couples choose. The surrogate mother is artificially inseminated with the sperm of the husband and carries the baby to term. The couple then raises the child. Ethically speaking, who is the real mother, the woman who bears the child or the woman who raises the child? If the surrogate mother wants to keep the baby after it is born, does she have a right to do so?

Practicing appropriate professional ethics has a positive impact on your reputation and the success of your employer's business. Many medical organizations, therefore, have created guidelines for the acceptable and preferred manners and behaviors, or etiquette, of medical assistants and physicians.

The principles of medical ethics have developed over time. The Hippocratic oath, in which medical students pledge to practice medicine ethically, was developed in ancient Greece. It is still used today and is one of the original bases of modern medical ethics. Hippocrates, the fourth-century-B.C. Greek physician commonly called the "father of medicine," is traditionally considered the author of this oath, but its authorship is actually unknown.

Among the promises of the Hippocratic oath are to use the form of treatment believed to be best for the patient, to refrain from harmful actions, and to keep a patient's private information confidential.

The AMA defines ethical behavior for doctors in *Code of Medical Ethics: Current Opinions with Annotations* (1996). Medical assistants, as well as doctors, need to be aware of these principles.

> *A physician shall be dedicated to providing competent medical service with compassion and respect for human dignity.*

This concept means that medical professionals will respect all aspects of the patient as a person, including intellect and emotions. The doctor must decide what treatment would result in the best, most dignified quality of life for the patient, and the doctor must respect a patient's choice to forgo treatment.

> *A physician shall deal honestly with patients and colleagues and strive to expose those physicians deficient in character or competence or who engage in fraud or deception.*

Medical professionals, including medical assistants, should respect colleagues, but they must also respect and protect the profession and public welfare enough to report colleagues who are breaking the law, acting unethically, or unable to perform competently. Dilemmas may arise where one suspects, but is not able to prove, for instance, that a coworker has a substance abuse problem or another problem that is affecting performance. Ignoring such a situation in medical practice could cost someone's life as well as lead to lawsuits.

In terms of billing, a doctor should bill only for direct services, not for indirect ones, such as referrals. The doctor also should not bill for services that do not really pertain to the practice of medicine, such as dispensing drugs.

It is also unethical for the doctor to influence the patient about where to fill prescriptions or obtain other medical services when the doctor has a personal financial interest in any of the choices.

> *A physician shall respect the law and also recognize a responsibility to seek changes in requirements that are contrary to the patient's best interests.*

Several legal or employer requirements have come under scrutiny as being contrary to a patient's best interests. Among them are discharging patients from the hospital after a certain time limit for certain procedures, which may be too soon for many patients. Insurance company payment policies have sometimes been criticized as unfair. So have health maintenance organization (HMO) financial policies that may conflict with a doctor's preference in treatment.

> *A physician shall respect the rights of patients, of colleagues, and of other health professionals and shall safeguard patient confidences within the constraints of law.*

A document called the Patient's Bill of Rights, established by the American Hospital Association in 1973 and revised in 1992, lists ethical principles protecting the patient. (The text of the Patient's Bill of Rights appears in Chapter 24.) Some states have even passed this code of ethics into law. Among a patient's rights are the right to information about alternative treatments, the right to refuse to participate in research projects, and the right to privacy.

> *A physician shall continue to study; apply and advance scientific knowledge; make relevant information available to patients, colleagues, and the public; obtain consultation; and use the talents of other health professionals when indicated.*

Keeping up with the latest advancements in medicine is crucial for providing high-quality, ethical care. Most states require doctors to accumulate "continuing education units" to maintain a license to practice. These units are earned by means of educational activities such as courses and scientific meetings. The AAMA requires medical assistants to renew their certification every 5 years, by either accumulating continuing education credits through the AAMA or retaking the certification examination.

> *A physician shall, in the provision of appropriate patient care, except in emergencies, be free to choose whom to serve, with whom to associate, and the environment in which to provide medical services.*

Ethically, doctors can set their hours, decide what kind of medicine to practice and where, decide whom to accept as a patient, and take time off as long as a qualified substitute performs their duties. Doctors may decline to accept new patients because of a full workload. In an emergency, however, a doctor may be ethically obligated to care for a patient, even if the patient is not of the doctor's choosing. The doctor should not abandon that patient until another physician is available.

> *A physician shall recognize a responsibility to participate in activities contributing to an improved community. This ethical obligation holds true for the allied health professions as well.*

In addition to knowing the physician's codes of ethics, medical assistants should follow the AAMA's Code of Ethics, which appears in Figure 3-6.

CODE OF ETHICS

The Code of Ethics of the AAMA shall set forth principles of ethical and moral conduct as they relate to the medical profession and the particular practice of medical assisting.

Members of the AAMA dedicated to the conscientious pursuit of their profession, and thus desiring to merit the high regard of the entire medical profession and the respect of the general public which they serve, do pledge themselves to strive always to:

A. render service with full respect for the dignity of humanity;

B. respect confidential information obtained through employment unless legally authorized or required by responsible performance of duty to divulge such information;

C. uphold the honor and high principles of the profession and accept its disciplines;

D. seek to continually improve the knowledge and skills of medical assistants for the benefit of patients and professional colleagues;

E. participate in additional service activities aimed toward improving the health and well-being of the community.

Figure 3-6. The AAMA's Code of Ethics sets the ethical standard for the profession of medical assisting. (Reprinted with permission of the American Association of Medical Assistants.)

Confidentiality Issues and Mandatory Disclosure

Related to law, ethics, and quality care is the issue of when the medical assistant can disclose information and when it must be kept confidential. The incidents doctors are legally required to report to the state were outlined earlier in the chapter. A doctor can be charged with criminal action for not following state and federal laws.

Ethics and professional judgment are always important. Consider the question of whether to contact the partners of a patient who has a sexually transmitted disease and whether to keep the patient's name from those people. The law says that the physician must instruct patients on how to notify possibly affected third parties and give them referrals to get the proper assistance. If the patient refuses to inform involved outside parties, then the doctor's office may offer to notify current and former partners. "Caution: Handle With Care" addresses this issue.

In general, the patient's ethical right to confidentiality and privacy is protected by law. Only the patient can waive the right to confidentiality. A physician cannot publicize a patient case in journal articles or invite other health professionals to observe a case without the patient's written consent. Most states also prohibit a doctor from testifying in court about a patient without the patient's approval. When a patient sues a physician, however, the patient automatically gives up the right to confidentiality.

In terms of rights to the patient's chart, the physician owns the chart, but the patient owns the information. The patient has a right to a copy of the chart for a reasonable fee. (It is illegal for the patient to be denied a copy of his chart if he is unable to pay the fee.)

Following are six principles for preventing improper release of information from the medical office.

1. When in doubt about whether to release information, it is better not to release it.
2. It is the patient's, not the doctor's, right to keep patient information confidential. If the patient wants to disclose the information, it is unethical for the physician not to do so.
3. All patients should be treated with the same degree of confidentiality, whatever the health-care professional's personal opinion of the patient might be.
4. You should be aware of all applicable laws and of the regulations of agencies such as public health departments.

CAUTION
HANDLE WITH CARE

Notifying Those at Risk for Sexually Transmitted Disease

There are few things more difficult for a patient with a sexually transmitted disease (STD) than telling current and former partners about the diagnosis. In fact, some patients elect not to do so. When patients refuse to alert their partners, the medical office can offer to make those contacts. Often that responsibility lies with the medical assistant.

You are most likely to encounter such a situation if you are a medical assistant working in a family practice, an obstetrics/gynecology practice, or a clinic. Becoming familiar with all facets of the situation—from ensuring patient confidentiality to handling potentially difficult confrontations—will help you best serve the patient.

The first step is to get the appropriate information from the patient who has contracted the STD. Because the patient may be sensitive about revealing former and current partners, help him or her feel more comfortable. First, spend some time talking about the STD. How much does the patient know about it? Educate the patient about implications, including the probable short- and long-term effects of the disease. Explain how the STD is transmitted. Alert the patient to precautions to take so he or she will not continue to transmit the disease to others. Help the patient understand why it is important for people who may have contracted the disease from him or her to know they may have it.

Then, offer to contact the patient's former and current partners. Fully explain each step in the notification process, assuring the patient that his or her name will not be revealed under any circumstances. Answer any questions and address any concerns about the notification process. If the patient is still reluctant to provide information, give him or her some time to think about it away from the office, and follow up periodically with a phone call.

Once the patient agrees to reveal names, write down the names and other information, preferably phone numbers. To make sure you have correct information, read it back to the patient, spelling each person's name in turn and reciting the phone number or address. Write down the phonetic pronunciations of any difficult names. Tell the patient when you will make the notifications.

You now are ready to contact these individuals. Professionals who work with STD patients recommend guidelines for contacting current and former partners to alert them about potential exposure to an STD. Note that these guidelines are applicable only to STDs other than AIDS.

Determine how you will contact each individual: in writing, in person, or by phone.

1. If you use U.S. mail, mark the outside of the addressed envelope "Personal." On a note inside, simply ask the person to call you at the medical office. Do not put the topic of the call in writing.
2. If you make the contact in person, ask where you can talk privately. Even if the person appears to be alone, others may still be able to overhear the conversation.
3. If you use the phone, identify yourself and your office, and ask for the specific individual. Do not reveal the nature of your call to anyone but that person. If pressed, tell the person who answers the phone that you are calling regarding a personal matter.

Once on the phone or alone with the person, confirm that you are talking to the correct person. Mention that you wish to talk about a highly personal matter, and ask if it is a good time to continue the discussion. If not, arrange for a more appropriate time.

Inform the individual that he or she has come in contact with someone who has a sexually transmitted disease. Recommend that the person visit a doctor's office or clinic to be tested for the disease.

Be prepared for a variety of reactions, from surprise to anger. Respond calmly and coolly. Expect to respond to questions and statements such as:

- Who gave you my name?
- Do I have the disease?
- Am I really at risk? I haven't had intercourse recently (or) I've only had intercourse with my spouse.
- I feel fine. I just went to my doctor recently.

Let the person know that you cannot reveal the name of the partner because the information is strictly confidential. Assure the person that you will not reveal his or her name to anyone either.

Explain that exposure to the disease does not mean a person has contracted it. Encourage the person to get tested to know for sure.

Tell the person that he or she is still at risk, even if the person hasn't had intercourse recently or has had it only with a spouse. Let the person know that someone with whom he or she came in close contact at some point has contracted the disease.

Even if the person says, "I feel fine," he or she may still have the disease. Again, stress the importance of getting tested.

Provide your name and phone number for contact about further questions. Recommend local offices and clinics for testing, and provide phone numbers. If the person will come to your office, offer to make the appointment.

Finally, document the results of your call. Log in the original patient's file the date that you completed notification. Include any pertinent details about the notification. Alert the patient when all people on the list have been notified.

5. When it is necessary to break confidentiality and when there is a conflict between ethics and confidentiality, discuss it with the patient. If the law does not dictate what to do in the situation, the attending physician should make the judgment based on the urgency of the situation and any danger that might be posed to the patient or others.
6. Get written approval from the patient before releasing information. For common situations, the patient should sign a standard release-of-records form.

The AMA has several standard forms for authorization of disclosure and includes disclosure clauses in many other forms. For example, the consent-to-surgery form includes a clause about consenting to picture taking and observation during the surgery. When using a standard form, cross out anything that does not apply in that particular situation. Medical practices often develop their own customized forms.

Summary

You must carefully follow all state, federal, and individual practice rules and laws while performing your daily duties. You must also follow the AAMA Code of Ethics for medical assistants. It is an important part of your duties to help the doctor avoid malpractice claims—lawsuits by the patient against the physician for errors in diagnosis or treatment.

To perform effectively as a medical assistant, you must maintain an office that follows all OSHA regulations for safety, hazardous equipment, and toxic substances. The office also must meet QC and QA guidelines for all tests, specimens, and treatments. It is your responsibility to ensure patient privacy and confidentiality of patient records, to fully document patient treatment, and to maintain patient records in an orderly and readily accessible fashion.

3 Chapter Review

Discussion Questions

1. How does the law of agency make it possible for a patient to sue both the medical assistant and the physician for an act of negligence committed by the medical assistant?
2. What rights do patients have regarding confidentiality and ownership of their medical records? When does a patient give up the right to confidentiality?
3. What is the purpose of quality control and quality assurance programs?

Critical Thinking Questions

1. What is an example of a bioethical issue? Give two opposing views of the issue.
2. What are two different situations that could turn into a malpractice or abandonment suit if committed by physicians or their medical staff members?
3. What should a medical assistant do who may have been exposed to HIV or HBV outside of work?

Application Activities

1. Imagine that a patient who may need a blood transfusion tells you that his religious beliefs do not permit that type of medical intervention. What course of action would you take?
2. In a medical law textbook or journal, research a malpractice case. Prepare a 10-minute presentation for the class in which you summarize both sides of the case (patient and caregiver). Include when and where the case took place. Explain how the case was settled and whether the settlement took place in a court of law or through arbitration. Close with your opinion about whether the case was settled fairly.
3. Research a piece of legislation on a health-care issue or practice, either a bill passed in the last 5 years or a bill currently being considered in Washington. What impact has this bill had or might this bill have on the medical assisting profession? Summarize your findings in a one- to two-page report.

Further Readings

Balasa, Donald A. “Federal Lab Regulations Seem Favorable for Medical Assistants.” *The Professional Medical Assistant,* January/February 1992, 22–23.

Code of Medical Ethics: Current Opinions with Annotations. Chicago: American Medical Association, 1996.

“Lab Regulators Gain Penalty Options Under CLIA Sanctions.” *Medical Laboratory Observer* 23, no. 2 (June 1991).

Opoien, J. W., and Donald Balasa. “Physician Liability and the Medical Assistant.” *Iowa Medicine,* August 1991, 334–335.

Renfro, Joy. “Quality Assurance: A Useful Tool for the Physician’s Office.” *The Professional Medical Assistant,* November/December 1990, 6–8.

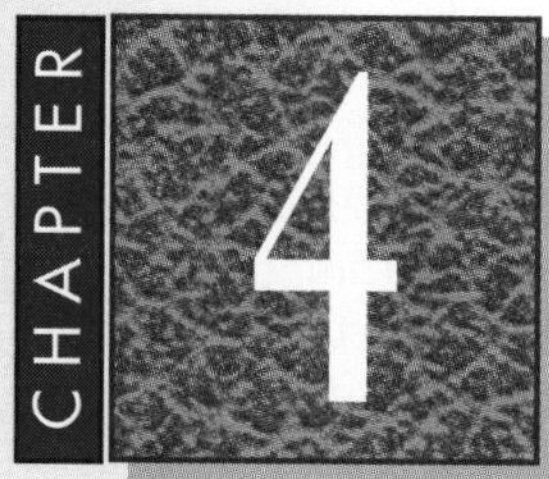

Communication With Patients, Families, and Coworkers

CHAPTER OUTLINE

- Communicating With Patients and Families
- The Communication Circle
- Types of Communication
- Improving Your Communication Skills
- Communicating in Special Circumstances
- Communicating With Coworkers
- Managing Stress
- The Policy and Procedures Manual

Key Terms

active listening
aggressive
assertive
body language
closed posture
conflict
empathy
feedback
interpersonal skill
open posture
passive listening
personal space
rapport

OBJECTIVES

After completing Chapter 4, you will be able to:

- Identify elements of the communication circle.
- Give examples of positive and negative communication.
- List ways to improve listening and interpersonal skills.
- Explain the difference between assertiveness and aggressiveness.
- Give examples of effective communication strategies with patients in special circumstances.
- Discuss ways to establish positive communication with coworkers and superiors.
- Explain how stress relates to communication and identify strategies to reduce stress.
- Describe how the office policy and procedures manual is used as a communication tool in the medical office.

AREAS OF COMPETENCE

1997 ROLE DELINEATION STUDY

GENERAL (Transdisciplinary)

Professionalism

- Project a professional manner and image
- Demonstrate initiative and responsibility
- Work as a team member
- Adapt to change

Communication Skills

- Treat all patients with compassion and empathy
- Recognize and respect cultural diversity

continued

AREAS OF COMPETENCE continued

- Adapt communications to individual's ability to understand
- Use effective and correct verbal and written communications
- Recognize and respond to verbal and nonverbal communications
- Serve as liaison
- Promote the practice through positive public relations

Legal Concepts

- Participate in the development and maintenance of personnel, policy, and procedure manuals

Communicating With Patients and Families

Think about the last time you had a doctor's appointment. How well did the staff and physicians communicate with you? Were you greeted cordially and pleasantly invited to take a seat, or did someone thrust a clipboard at you and say "Fill this out"? If you had a long wait in the waiting room or examination room, did someone come in to explain the delay? Did you become frustrated and angry because nobody told you what was happening?

As a medical assistant, you are a key communicator between the office and patients and families. The way you greet patients, explain procedures, ask and answer questions, and attend to the individual needs of patients forms your communication style. Your interaction with the patient sets the tone for the office visit and can significantly influence how comfortable the patient feels in your practice. Developing strong communication skills in the medical office is just as important as mastering administrative and clinical tasks.

The Communication Circle

As you interact with patients and their families, you will be responsible for giving information and ensuring that the patient understands what you, the doctor, and other members of the staff have communicated. You will also be responsible for receiving information from the patient. For example, patients will describe their symptoms. They may also discuss their feelings or ask questions about a treatment or procedure. The giving and receiving of information forms the communication circle.

Elements of the Communication Circle

The communication circle involves three elements: a message, a source, and a receiver. Messages are usually verbal or written. (As you will see later in the chapter, some messages are nonverbal.) The source sends the message, and the receiver receives it. The communication circle is formed as the source sends a message to the receiver and the receiver responds (Figure 4-1).

Consider this example, in which Simone, a medical assistant who works in a physical therapy office, is speaking with Mrs. Sommer, a patient who is having therapy for a back injury. Watch the communication circle at work.

Simone: The physical therapist says you're making great progress and that you can start on some simple back exercises at home. I'd like to go over them with you. Then I'll give you a sheet that illustrates the exercises. How does that sound to you?

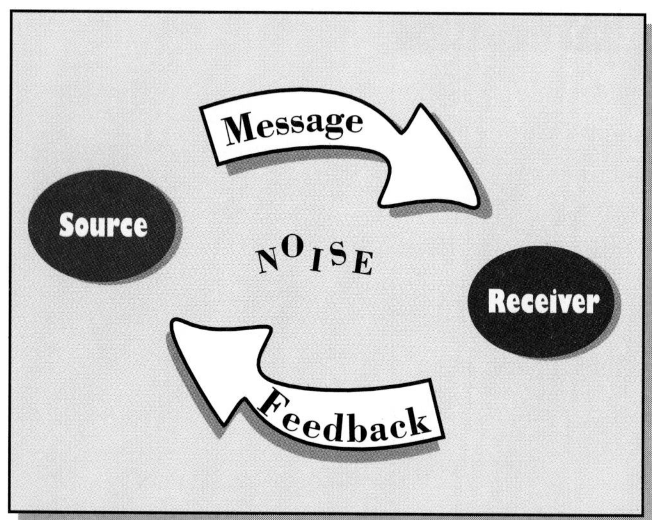

Figure 4-1. The process of communication involves an exchange of messages through verbal and nonverbal means.

Mrs. Sommer: I'm a little nervous about doing exercises. I still have some pain when I bend over.

Simone: I understand. It's important, though, to start using those muscles again. Why don't you show me exactly where it hurts. Then we can go over proper body mechanics, such as bending down to pick something up and getting in and out of chairs, the car, and bed. Then we'll just start with one or two of the exercises and save the rest for next time, when you're feeling more ready.

Mrs. Sommer: Yes, I only feel up to doing a little bit today.

The medical assistant (the source) gives a verbal message (about back exercises) to the patient (the receiver). The patient responds by drawing attention to her pain and uneasiness about certain movements. The patient's response is also a message to the medical assistant, who responds in turn. The giving and receiving of information continues within the communication circle until the exchange is finished.

Feedback. Another word for response is **feedback,** which is verbal or nonverbal evidence that the receiver got and understood the message. When you communicate information to a patient or ask a patient a question, always look for feedback. For example, if you calculate a pregnant patient's due date and tell her she's 12 weeks pregnant, look for a response. If she responds, "Oh, good, that means I'm out of danger of having a miscarriage," you would respond that whereas most miscarriages occur in the first 12 weeks, some risk of miscarriage remains throughout the pregnancy. If she responds, "I thought I was 14 weeks pregnant," you would need to clarify how you worked out your calculation and compare it with hers, to uncover any discrepancy. Good communication in the medical office requires patient feedback at every step.

Noise. Anything that distorts the message in any way or interferes with the communication process can be referred to as noise. Noise refers not only to sounds, such as a siren or jackhammer on the street below the medical office suite. It also refers to room temperature and other types of physical comfort or discomfort, such as pain, and to emotions, such as fear or sadness. If patients are feeling uncomfortable in a chilly or hot room, upset about their illness, or in great pain, they may not pay close attention to what you are saying. Conversely, if you are feeling upset about a personal problem outside work or if you are unwell or preoccupied with all the things you have on your to-do list, you may not communicate well.

As you deal with each patient, try to screen out or eliminate both literal and figurative noise. For example, before you start a conversation with a patient in an examination room, you might ask, "Are you too chilly or too hot? Is the temperature in here comfortable for you?" If there is construction going on outside the building, see if there is a less noisy inner room or office that you might be able to use. If a patient seems nervous or upset, address those feelings before you launch into a factual discussion.

If you are feeling stressed or out of sorts, that feeling constitutes a type of noise. Try to take a "breather" between patients or a break from desk work—walk downstairs, get some fresh air, stretch your legs. Feeling dehydrated or hungry affects your communication efforts too. Limit your caffeine and sugar intake. Drink plenty of water and juice throughout the day. Eat a good lunch and healthful snacks. Leave your personal problems at home.

Humanizing the Communication Process in the Medical Office

As highly structured managed care organizations and technological advances rapidly change the face of health care, many patients feel that health care is becoming impersonal. Every time you communicate with patients, you can counteract this perception by playing a humanistic role in the health-care process. Being humanistic means that you work to help patients feel attended to and respected as individuals, not just as descriptions on a chart. Good communication supports this patient-centered approach.

Make a point of developing and using strong communication skills to show patients that you, the doctors, and other staff members care about them and their feelings. Taking care to treat patients as people helps humanize the communication process in the medical office.

Types of Communication

Communication can be positive or negative. It can also be verbal, nonverbal, or written. To help ensure effective communication with patients, familiarize yourself with these different types of communication. (Written communication is discussed in Chapter 7.)

Positive Communication

In the medical office, communication that promotes patients' comfort and well-being is essential. Treating patients brusquely or rudely is unacceptable in the health-care setting. It is your responsibility—not the patient's—to set the stage for positive communication.

When information—even bad news—is communicated with some positive aspect, patients are more likely to listen attentively and respond positively themselves. For example, you might explain to a patient who is about to get an injection, "This will sting, but only for a couple of seconds. When we're through, you're free to go." You would not just say, "This is going to hurt."

Other examples of positive communication are:

- Being friendly, warm, and attentive ("It's good to see you again, Mrs. Armstrong. I know you're on your lunch hour, so let's get started right away.")
- Verbalizing concern for patients ("Are you comfortable?" "I understand it hurts when I do this; I'll be gentle." "This paperwork won't take long at all.")
- Encouraging patients to ask questions ("I hope I've explained the procedure well. Do you have any questions, or are there any parts you would like to go over again?")
- Asking patients to repeat your instructions to make sure they understand
- Looking directly at patients when you speak to them
- Smiling (naturally, not in a forced way)
- Speaking slowly and clearly
- Listening carefully

Negative Communication

Most people do not purposely try to communicate negatively. Some people, however, may not realize that their communication style has a negative impact on others. Look for and ask for feedback to help you curb negative communication habits. Ask yourself, "Do the physicians and my other coworkers seem glad to speak with me? Are they open and responsive to me?" "Do patients seem at ease with me, or are they very quiet, turned off, or distant?" (Note that some patients may respond this way because of the way they feel, not because of the way you are communicating with them.) Here are some examples of negative communication:

- Mumbling
- Speaking brusquely or sharply
- Avoiding eye contact
- Interrupting patients as they are speaking
- Rushing through explanations or instructions
- Treating patients impersonally
- Making patients feel they are taking up too much of your time or asking too many questions
- Forgetting common courtesies, such as saying please and thank you
- Showing boredom

A good way to avoid negative communication is to open your eyes and ears to others in service-oriented workplace settings. The next time you buy something at a store, call a company for information over the phone, or eat out at a restaurant, take note of the way the staff treats you. Do they answer your questions courteously? Do they give you the information you ask for? Do they make you feel welcome? What specifically makes their communication style positive or negative? Remember, you can always improve your communication skills.

Body Language

Verbal communication refers to communication that is spoken. Nonverbal communication is also known as **body language.** Body language includes facial expressions, eye contact, posture, touch, and attention to personal space. In many instances, people's body language conveys their true feelings, even when their words may say otherwise. A patient might say "I'm OK about that," but if she is sitting with her arms folded tightly across her chest and avoids looking at you, she may not mean what she says.

Facial Expression. Your face is the most expressive part of your body. You can often tell whether someone has understood your message simply by his facial expression. For example, when you are explaining a procedure to a patient, look at his expression. Does it seem puzzled? Is his brow wrinkled? Does he look surprised? Facial expressions can give you clues about how to tailor your communication efforts. They also serve as a form of feedback.

Eye Contact. Eye contact is an important part of positive communication. Look directly at patients when speaking to them. Looking away or down communicates that you are not interested in the person or that you are avoiding her for some reason.

There may be cultural differences in the ways patients react to eye contact. In some cultures, for example, it is common to avoid eye contact out of respect for someone who is considered a superior. Thus, children may be taught not to look adults in the eye.

Posture. The way you hold or move your head, arms, hands, and the rest of your body can project strong nonverbal messages. During communication, posture can usually be described as open or closed.

Open Posture. A feeling of receptiveness and friendliness can be conveyed with an **open posture.** In this position, your arms lie comfortably at your sides or in your lap. You face the other person, and you may lean forward in your chair. This demonstrates that you are listening and are interested in what the other person has to say. Open posture is a form of positive communication.

Closed Posture. A **closed posture** conveys the opposite, a feeling of not being totally receptive to what is being said. It can also signal that someone is angry or upset. A person in a closed posture may hold his arms rigidly or fold them across his chest. He may lean back in his chair, away from the other person. He may turn away to avoid eye contact. Slouching is a kind of closed posture that can convey fatigue or lack of caring. Watch for patients with closed postures that may indicate tension or pain. Avoid closed postures yourself—they have a negative effect on your communication efforts.

Touch. Touch is a powerful form of nonverbal communication. A touch on the arm or a hug can be a means of saying hello, sharing condolences, or expressing congratulations. Family background, culture, age, and gender all influence people's perception of touch. Some people may welcome a touch or think nothing of it. Others may view touching as an invasion of their privacy. In general, in the medical setting, a touch on the shoulder, forearm, or back of the hand to express interest or concern is acceptable.

Personal Space. When communicating with others, it is important to be aware of the concept of personal space. **Personal space** is an area that surrounds an individual. By not intruding on a patient's personal space, you show respect for his feelings of privacy.

In most social situations, it is common for people to stand 4 to 12 ft away from each other. For personal conversation, you would typically stand between 1½ and 4 ft away from a person. Some patients may feel uncomfortable—and may become anxious—when you stand or sit close to them. Others prefer the reassurance of having people close to them when they speak. Watch patients carefully. If they lean back when you lean forward or if they fold their arms or turn their head away, you may be invading their personal space. If they lean or step toward you, they may be seeking to close up the personal space.

Improving Your Communication Skills

Sharpening your communication skills should be an ongoing effort and will help you become a more effective communicator. Good communication skills can enhance the quality of your interaction with patients and coworkers alike. Among the skills involved in communication are listening skills, interpersonal skills, and assertiveness skills.

Listening Skills

Listening involves both hearing and interpreting a message. Listening requires you to pay close attention not only to what is being said but also to nonverbal cues, such as those communicated through body language.

Listening can be passive or active. **Passive listening** is simply hearing what someone has to say without the need for a reply. An example is listening to a news program on the radio; the communication is mainly one-way. **Active listening** involves two-way communication. You are actively involved in the process, offering feedback or asking questions. Active listening takes place, for example, when you interview a patient for her medical history. Active listening is an essential skill in the medical office.

There are several ways to improve your listening skills:

- Prepare to listen. Position yourself at the same level (sitting, standing) as the person who is speaking, and assume an open posture (Figure 4-2).
- Relax and listen attentively. Do not simply pretend to listen to what is being said.
- Maintain eye contact.
- Maintain appropriate personal space.
- Think before you respond.
- Provide feedback. Restate the speaker's message in your own words to show that you understand.
- If you do not understand something that was said, ask the person to repeat it.

Interpersonal Skills

When you interact with people, you use **interpersonal skills.** When you make a patient feel at ease by being warm and friendly, you are demonstrating good interpersonal skills. In addition to warmth and friendliness, valuable interpersonal skills include empathy, respect, genuineness, openness, and consideration and sensitivity.

Warmth and Friendliness. A friendly but professional approach, a pleasant greeting, and a smile get you off to a good start when communicating with patients. When your approach is sincere, patients will be more relaxed and open.

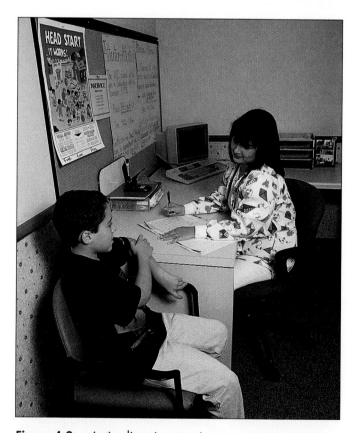

Figure 4-2. Active listening requires two-way communication and positive body language.

Empathy. The process of identifying with someone else's feelings is **empathy**. When you are empathetic, you are sensitive to the other person's feelings and problems. For example, if a patient is experiencing a migraine headache and you have never had one, you can still let her know you are trying to imagine, or relate to, her situation. In other words, you can acknowledge the severity of her pain and show support and care. You must, however, always remain objective in your interaction with patients.

Respect. Showing respect can mean using a title of courtesy, such as "Mr." or "Mrs.," when communicating with patients. It can also mean acknowledging a patient's wishes or choices without passing judgment.

Genuineness. Being genuine in your interactions with patients means that you refrain from "putting on an act" or just going through the motions of your job. Patients like to know that their health-care providers are real people. In a medical setting, being genuine means caring for each patient on an individual basis, giving patients the full attention they deserve, and showing respect for them. Being genuine in your communication with patients encourages them to place trust in you and in what you say.

Openness. Openness means being willing to listen to and consider others' viewpoints and concerns and being receptive to their needs. An open individual is accepting of others and not biased for or against them.

Consideration and Sensitivity. You should always try to show consideration toward patients and act in a thoughtful, kind way. You must be sensitive to their individual concerns, fears, and needs.

Assertiveness Skills

As a professional, you need to be **assertive;** that is, to be firm and to stand up for yourself while still showing respect for others. Being assertive means trusting your instincts, feelings, and opinions (not in terms of diagnosing, which only the doctor can do, but in terms of basic communication with patients), and acting on them. For example, when you see that a patient looks uneasy, speak up. You might say, "You look concerned. How can I help you feel more comfortable?"

Being assertive is different from being aggressive. When people are **aggressive,** they try to impose their position on others or try to manipulate them. Aggressive people are bossy and can be quarrelsome. They do not appear to take into consideration others' feelings, needs, thoughts, ideas, and opinions before they act or speak.

To be assertive, you must be open, honest, and direct. Be aware of your body position: an open posture conveys the proper message. When you communicate, speak confidently and use "I" statements such as "I feel . . ." or "I think. . . ." (Assertiveness is also discussed later in the chapter in the section on communicating with coworkers.)

Developing your assertiveness skills increases your sense of self-worth and your confidence as a professional. Being assertive will also help you prevent or resolve conflicts more peacefully and increase your leadership ability. People look up to and respect professionals who are assertive in the workplace.

Communicating in Special Circumstances

If you make an effort to develop good interpersonal skills, most patients will not be difficult to communicate with. You will, however, encounter patients in special circumstances, when they may be anxious or angry. These situations sometimes inhibit communication. Patients from different cultures may pose challenges to communication. Others may have some type of impairment or disability that makes communication difficult. Similarly, young patients, parents with children who are ill or injured, and patients with terminal illnesses may present communication difficulties. Learning about the special needs of these patients and polishing your own communication skills will help you become an effective communicator in any number of situations.

The Anxious Patient

It is common for patients to be anxious in a doctor's office or other health-care setting. This reaction is commonly known as the "white-coat syndrome." There can be many reasons for anxiety. A patient can become anxious because she is ill and does not know what is wrong with her—she may fear the worst. A patient may have recently been diagnosed with an illness that he knows nothing about, which may necessitate a severe lifestyle change. Fear of bad news or fear that some procedure is going to be painful can create anxiety. Anxiety can interfere with the communication process. For example, because of anxiety a patient may not listen well or pay attention to what you are saying.

Some patients—particularly children—may be unable to verbalize their feelings of fear and anxiety. Watch for signs of anxiety. They may include a tense appearance, increased blood pressure and rates of breathing and pulse, sweaty palms, reported problems with sleep or appetite, irritability, and agitation. Procedure 4-1 will help you communicate with patients who are anxious.

The Angry Patient

In a medical setting, anger may occur for many reasons. Anger may be a mask for fear about an illness or the outcome of surgery. Anger may come from a patient's feeling of being treated unfairly or without compassion. Anger may stem from a patient's resentment about being ill or injured. Anger may be a reaction to frustration, rejection, disappointment, feelings of loss of control or self-esteem, or invasion of privacy.

As a medical assistant, you will encounter angry patients and will need to help them express their anger constructively, for the sake of their health. At the same time,

PROCEDURE 4-1

Communicating With the Anxious Patient

Objective: To use communication and interpersonal skills to calm an anxious patient

Materials: None

Method

1. Identify signs of anxiety in the patient.
2. Acknowledge the patient's anxiety. (Ignoring a patient's anxiety often makes it worse.)
3. Identify possible sources of anxiety, such as fear of a procedure or test result, along with supportive resources available to the patient, such as family members and friends. Understanding the source of anxiety in a patient and identifying the supportive resources available can help you communicate with the patient more effectively.
4. Do what you can to alleviate the patient's physical discomfort. For example, find a calm, quiet place for the patient to wait, a comfortable chair, a drink of water, or access to the bathroom (Figure 4-3).
5. Allow ample personal space for conversation. Note: You would normally allow a 1½- to 4-ft distance between yourself and the patient. Adjust this space as necessary.
6. Create a climate of warmth, acceptance, and trust.
   a. Recognize and control your own anxiety. Your air of calm can decrease the patient's anxiety.
   b. Provide reassurance by demonstrating genuine care, respect, and empathy.
   c. Act confidently and dependably, maintaining truthfulness and confidentiality at all times.
7. Using the appropriate communication skills, have the patient describe the experience that is causing anxiety, her thoughts about it, and her feelings. Proceeding in this order allows the patient to describe what is causing the anxiety and to clarify her thoughts and feelings about it.
   a. Maintain an open posture.
   b. Maintain eye contact, if culturally appropriate.
   c. Use active listening skills.
   d. Listen without interrupting.
8. Do not belittle the patient's thoughts and feelings. This can cause a breakdown in communication, increase anxiety, and make the patient feel isolated.
9. Be empathic to the patient's concerns.
10. Help the patient recognize and cope with the anxiety.
    a. Provide information to the patient. Patients are often fearful of the unknown. Helping them understand their disease or the procedure they are about to undergo will help decrease their anxiety.
    b. Suggest coping behaviors, such as deep breathing or other relaxation exercises.
11. Notify the doctor of the patient's concerns.

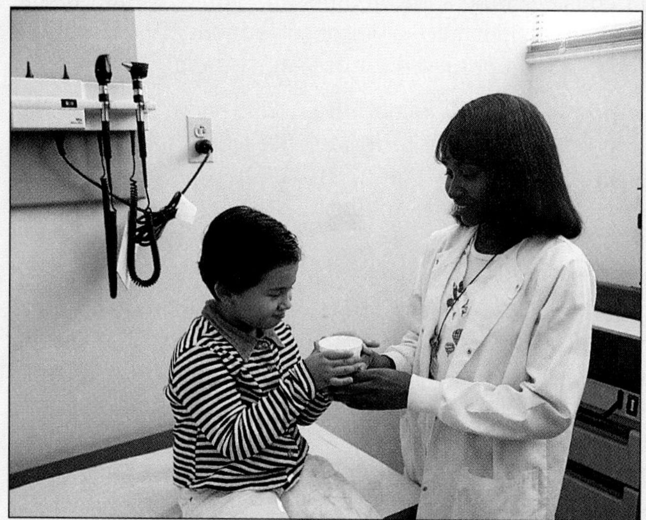

Figure 4-3. You can calm children's anxiety by spending time talking with them, playing a game, reading a story, or just offering a glass of water.

you must learn not to take expressions of anger personally; you may just be the unlucky target. A goal with angry patients is to help them refocus emotional energy toward solving the problem. Study the following tips for communicating with an angry patient.

1. Learn to recognize anger and its causes. Anger is easy to recognize in most people, but it can be subtle in others. Patients who speak in a tense tone, are stubborn, or appear to ignore your attempts at communication may be angry.
2. Remain calm and continue to demonstrate genuineness and respect. Communicate that you respect and care about the patient's feelings.
3. Focus on the patient's physical and medical needs.
4. Maintain adequate personal space. Place yourself on the same level as the patient. If the patient is standing, encourage him to sit down. Maintain an open posture to show that you are receptive to listening. Maintain eye contact, but avoid staring at the patient, which can make the person angrier.

5. Avoid the feeling that you need to defend yourself or to give reasons why the patient should not be angry. Instead, listen attentively and with an open mind to what the patient is saying. Most patients' anger will lessen if they know someone is really listening to them and showing an interest in their emotions and needs.
6. Encourage patients to be specific in describing the cause of their anger, their thoughts about it, and their feelings. Be empathic and acknowledge the patient's feelings and perceptions. Follow through with any promises you might make concerning correction of a problem, but avoid totally agreeing or disagreeing with the patient. State what you can and cannot do for the patient.
7. Present your point of view calmly and firmly to help the patient better understand the situation. If patients are receptive to your viewpoint, their perspective may change for the better.
8. Avoid a breakdown in communication. Allow the patient to voice anger. Trying to outtalk the patient or overexplain will only annoy and irritate him. You might also suggest that the patient spend a few moments alone to gather his thoughts or to cool off before continuing any type of communication.
9. If you feel threatened by a patient's anger or if it looks as if the patient's anger may become violent, leave the room and seek assistance from one of the physicians or other members of the office staff. Document any threats in the patient's chart.

Patients of Other Cultures

Our beliefs, attitudes, values, use of language, and views of the world are unique to us, but they are also shaped by our cultural background. In any health-care setting, you will most likely have contact with patients of diverse cultures and ethnic groups. Each culture and ethnic group has its own behaviors, traditions, and values. Rather than viewing these differences as barriers to communication, strive to understand and be tolerant of them.

Remember that these beliefs are neither superior nor inferior to your own. They are simply different. Never allow yourself to make value judgments or to stereotype a patient, a culture, or an ethnic group. Each patient is an individual in her own right.

Different Views and Perceptions. It is common for patients in many cultures to view health-care professionals as superior to themselves intellectually, socially, and economically. Patients from minority ethnic groups may feel that health-care professionals of the majority ethnic group cannot understand them or identify with them. In some cases, unfortunately, they may be right. The professional's attitude of superiority may stem from the feeling that because she knows more about medical issues than the patient does, she is somehow more important than the patient.

Do your best to treat patients of all cultures and ethnic groups with equal respect. Effective communication cannot take place unless you respect the patient's dignity and maintain the patient's sense of self-worth.

Maintaining an open mind will help you see and understand differences in cultural perceptions to which you must be sensitive. For example, patients may have different views of their role and the role of their families in the health-care process. They may view the roles of men and women differently than you do. Patients may also have different views of the cause of their illness and how it should be treated. "Caution: Handle With Care" discusses different cultural views of health care.

The Language Barrier. Patients who cannot speak or understand English may have difficulty expressing their needs or feelings effectively. You may need to speak through an interpreter to gather and convey information or to discuss sensitive issues with a patient. Instead of using medical terms, which can be difficult to translate, try to say the same thing using basic, familiar words and simple phrases.

If the patient comes to the office often, take the time to learn some basic phrases in the patient's native language, such as "How are you feeling today?" and "Is there anything I can get you?" Even if the rest of your conversation must take place in English, your small efforts will be much appreciated.

The Patient With a Visual Impairment

When communicating with a patient who has a visual impairment, be aware of what you say and how you say it. Since people with visual impairments cannot usually rely on nonverbal clues, your tone of voice, inflection, and speech volume take on greater importance.

Following are some suggestions for communicating with a patient who has a visual impairment.

- Use large-print materials whenever possible.
- Make sure there is adequate lighting in all patient areas.
- Use a normal speaking voice.
- Talk directly and honestly. Explain instructions thoroughly.
- Do not talk down to the patient; preserve the patient's dignity.

The Patient With a Hearing Impairment

Hearing loss can range from mild to severe. How you communicate depends on the degree of impairment and on whether the patient has effective use of a hearing aid.

Following are some tips to help you communicate effectively with a hearing-impaired patient.

- Find a quiet area to talk, and try to minimize background noise.
- Position yourself close to and facing the patient. The patient will rely on visual clues such as the movement of your lips and mouth, your facial expression, and your body language (Figure 4-4).

CAUTION HANDLE WITH CARE

Multicultural Attitudes About Modern Medicine

Patients' cultural backgrounds have a great effect on their attitudes toward health and illness. Patients from different cultural backgrounds often have beliefs about the causes of illness, what symptoms mean, and what to expect from health-care professionals that are often different from those of modern medicine (Buchwald et al., 1994). Understanding some of these perceptions, behaviors, and expectations will help you communicate effectively with patients of different cultures.

Beliefs About Causes of Illness

Some cultures have beliefs about the causes of illness that differ sharply from accepted notions in the mainstream culture. As an example, many cultures believe that some illnesses are caused by hot or cold forces in the body. Some believe that winds and drafts cause illness or that illness can be caused by blood that is too thick or too thin. Others believe that having bad feelings toward others can create ill health.

Because of such beliefs, it may be hard to obtain information from patients about possible reasons for their medical problems. It may also be hard for some patients to realize the importance of taking medication to treat certain illnesses. In this case, you may have to be very persuasive and firm when giving the patient instructions for medication usage. It may be helpful or necessary to involve other family members in persuading the patient.

How Symptoms Are Presented and What They Mean

People from different cultures may differ in the way they perceive and report symptoms. Some may express pain very emotionally because their culture may feel that suppressing pain is harmful. In contrast, people from other cultures may not admit that they are in pain, thinking that acknowledging pain is a sign of weakness. People of all cultures may be more likely to report physical symptoms of illness than they are to report psychologic symptoms. Be aware of nonverbal indications of pain or other symptoms.

Treatment Expectations

Patients from other cultures may be totally unaccustomed to some of the practices of modern medicine. Patients of certain ethnic or cultural groups often consult other types of healers before seeing a doctor. They are likely to have different expectations of treatment from each.

Patients from other cultures may be wary of certain treatments because these treatments are so different from what they are accustomed to. This is especially true of some of the medical procedures and interventions considered to be state of the art, such as laser surgery or diabetes management.

When dealing with patients of other cultures, keep in mind their perspectives on health care. Try to avoid generalizations and cultural stereotyping, however, because there can be a variation of attitudes within ethnic groups. Treat each patient as an individual, and you will be providing the best care possible.

- Speak slowly, so the patient can follow what you are saying.
- Remember that elderly patients lose the ability to hear high-pitched sounds first. Try speaking in lower tones.
- Speak in a clear, firm voice, but do not shout, especially if the patient wears a hearing aid.
- To verify understanding, ask questions that will encourage the patient to repeat what you said.
- Whenever possible, use written materials to reinforce verbal information.

The Patient Who Is Mentally or Emotionally Disturbed

There may be times when you will need to communicate with patients who are mentally or emotionally disturbed. When dealing with this type of patient, you need to determine what level of communication the patient can understand. Keep these suggestions in mind to improve communication.

- It is important to remain calm if the patient becomes agitated or confused.
- Avoid raising your voice or appearing impatient.
- If you do not understand, ask the patient to repeat what he said.

The Elderly Patient

Medical assistants now spend at least 50% of their time caring for older patients. Be aware of the vast differences in the capabilities of people of this age group. Do not stereotype all elderly patients as frail or confused. Most are not, and each patient deserves to be treated according to her own individual abilities.

Always treat elderly patients with respect. Regardless of their physical or mental state, elderly patients are adults. Do not talk down to them. Use the title "Mrs." or "Mr." to address older people unless they ask you to call them by their first name.

Denial or Confusion. Some elderly patients deny that they are ill. For example, in a survey of elderly people, the majority of whom had at least one chronic condition, 85% reported that they were in good or excellent health

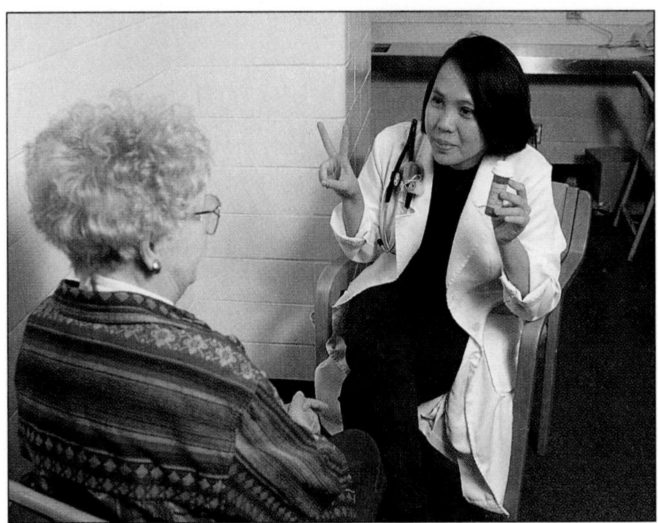

Figure 4-4. When communicating with a patient who has a hearing impairment, position yourself close to the patient and use gestures and effective body language.

(Bradley and Edinberg, 1990). Patients' perception of how they feel may be quite different from their actual state of health.

The reverse situation can also occur. Elderly patients may overreact to a problem and consider themselves sicker than they really are. They may become dependent, passive, or anxious. Elderly patients may also over- or underestimate their ability to perform certain tasks or to deal with certain limitations.

Elderly patients may be confused if they have some impairment in memory, judgment, or other mental abilities. Signs of confusion can occur with Alzheimer's disease, senility, depression, head injury, or misuse of medications or alcohol. Elderly patients may or may not be aware of their condition. They may have difficulty understanding instructions.

The following tips can help you communicate with elderly patients.

- Act as if you expect the patient to understand.
- Respond calmly to any confusion on the patient's part. Tell the truth. Use facts. Do not go along with misconceptions or make up explanations.
- Use simple questions and terms, but avoid using baby talk or speaking to the patient as if he were a child.
- Explain points slowly and clearly, using concrete terms rather than abstract expressions. Say, for example, "You may feel a pinprick and a sting when I put the needle in" instead of "You may feel some discomfort in your arm."
- Ask the patient to relax and speak slowly.
- If you do not understand the patient, simply say that you cannot understand her well and ask her to repeat what she said. Do not say you understand when in fact you do not. It is important not to belittle the patient. It is equally important to inform yourself about what could be very important information.

The Importance of Touch. Because they often live alone, many elderly patients experience a lack of physical touch. Using touch—offering to hold a patient's hand or placing an arm around his shoulder—communicates that you care about the patient's well-being.

The Young Patient

A doctor's office can be a frightening place for children. They often associate the doctor's office with getting a shot or being sick. Sometimes parents have misled their children about what to expect from a visit to the doctor. When dealing with children, it is better to recognize and accept their fear and anxiety than to dismiss these emotions. When children realize that you take their feelings seriously, they are more apt to be receptive to your requests and suggestions.

Explain any procedure, no matter how basic (such as testing a reflex with a reflex hammer), in very simple terms. Let the child examine the instrument.

Other suggestions include using praise ("You were very brave") and always being truthful. Do not tell children that a procedure will not hurt if it will, or you will lose their trust.

As children get older, you can use more detailed descriptions when explaining procedures. Remember that after the age of 7 or 8, children can tell if they are being talked down to or treated like babies. Encourage them to participate actively in their care, and direct any questions or instructions to them, when appropriate. You should also respect the adolescent's request not to have a parent present during private conversations.

Parents

Parents are naturally concerned about their children and are likely to be worried or anxious when a child is ill. Children often react to a situation based on how they see their parents react. Reassuring parents and keeping them calm can also help children relax.

The Patient With AIDS and the Patient Who Is HIV-Positive

Patients with acquired immunodeficiency syndrome (AIDS) and patients who have the human immunodeficiency virus (HIV), the virus that causes AIDS, have a grave illness to deal with. They also face a society that often stigmatizes them, saying they have only themselves to blame. These patients often feel guilty, angry, and depressed. Many literally hate themselves.

To communicate effectively with these patients, you need accurate information about the disease and the risks involved. Take the initiative to educate yourself about AIDS and HIV. Patients will have many questions. Part of your role as a good communicator will be to answer as many questions as you can. If a patient asks a question you cannot answer, tell the physician, so he can respond quickly.

Above all, remember that HIV is not transmitted through casual or common physical contact, such as brushing by a person in a crowded hall or shaking hands. It is transferred only through bodily fluids. Patients with AIDS and those who are HIV-positive need to know you are not afraid to be near them, to touch them, or to talk to them. Like any patient whose body is being ravaged by a serious illness, these patients need human contact (verbal and physical), and they need to be treated with dignity.

Patients' Families and Friends

Family members or friends sometimes accompany a patient to the office. These individuals can provide important emotional support to the patient. Always ask patients if they want a family member or friend to accompany them to the examination room, however. Do not just assume their preference. Acknowledge family members and friends, and communicate with them as you do with patients. They should be kept informed of the patient's progress, whenever possible, to avoid unnecessary anxiety on their part. You must always protect patient confidentiality, however. Too often, health-care workers think that it is acceptable to discuss patient cases in detail with family members, even without the consent of the patient.

Communicating With Coworkers

The quality of the communication you have with coworkers greatly influences the development of a positive or negative work climate and a team approach to patient care. In turn, the workplace atmosphere ultimately affects your communication with patients.

Positive Communication With Coworkers

In your interactions with coworkers, use the same skills and qualities that you use to communicate with patients. Have respect and empathy; be caring, thoughtful, and genuine; and use active listening skills. These skills will help you develop **rapport,** which is a harmonious, positive relationship, with your coworkers (Figure 4-5).

Following are some rules for communication in the medical office.

1. Use proper channels of communication. For example, if you are having problems getting along with a coworker, try first to work it out with her. Do not go over her head and complain to her supervisor. Your coworker may not have realized the effect of her behavior and may wish to correct it without involving her supervisor. If you go to the supervisor right away, working relationships can become even more strained.
2. Have the proper attitude. You can avoid conflict and resolve most problems if you maintain a positive attitude. A friendly approach is much more effective than a hostile approach. Remember that many problems are simply the result of misinformation or lack of communication.
3. Plan an appropriate time for communication. If you have something important to discuss, schedule a time to do so. For example, if you want to talk with the office manager about renewing the lease of a piece of office equipment, tell him you would like to discuss that topic and ask him to let you know a time that is convenient.

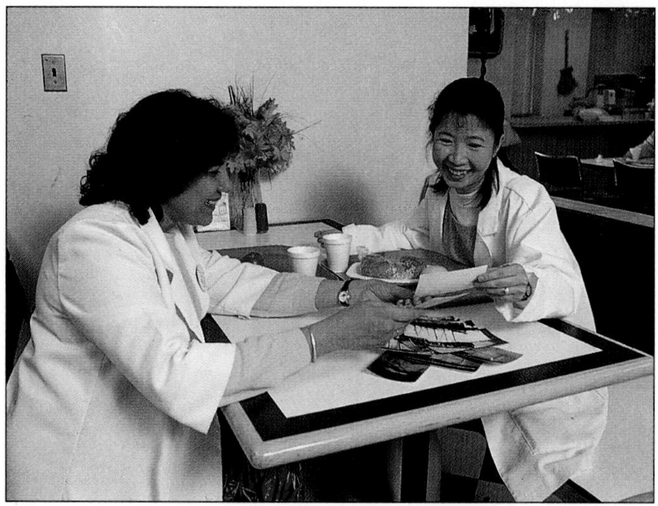

Figure 4-5. Rapport with coworkers is easy to build when you are open, friendly, and thoughtful.

As an example of good communication with coworkers, consider this exchange between Mai Lee, a medical assistant, and Margot, a coworker in a pediatric practice. Note the way Mai Lee demonstrates assertiveness.

Mai Lee: I know you spent a lot of time choosing the new toys for the reception area. I love the wooden safari animal puzzles.

Margot: Thanks. I think the children really enjoy themselves now.

Mai Lee: I wanted to mention to you, though, that I'm concerned about the toy tea set with miniature cupcakes and sandwiches. Anything that's smaller than a golf ball is a choking hazard to infants and toddlers.

Margot: I don't think the little ones pay much attention to the tea set. It's mostly for older kids.

Mai Lee: Yes, but I'm still afraid that a baby could put one of those pieces in his mouth. What if we put up a little shelf in the play area that is low enough for kids 4 years old or more to reach but high enough to be out of reach of the babies. We could put the tea set on it in a clear plastic box and any other toys with small parts.

Margot: I see your point. Sounds like a good idea to me.

Mai Lee started with a statement that acknowledged the coworker's situation and feelings. Then she stated her own opinion. When her coworker disagreed, she repeated her concern, describing what might happen if the situation remained unchanged. Then she made a constructive suggestion for solving the problem without hurting the coworker's feelings. As you interact with coworkers, be sensitive to the timing of your conversations, the manner in which you present your ideas and thoughts, and your coworkers' feelings.

Communicating With Superiors

Positive or negative communication can affect the quality of your relationships with superiors. For example, problems arise when communication about job responsibilities is unclear or when you feel that one of your superiors does not trust or respect you, or vice versa.

Consider these suggestions when communicating with superiors.

1. Keep superiors informed. If the office copier is not working properly, talk to your supervisor about it before a breakdown occurs that will hold everyone up. If several patients express the same types of complaint about the examination rooms, make sure the right people are told. If the doctor asks you to call a patient and you reach the patient, tell the doctor.
2. Ask questions. If you are unsure about an administrative task or the meaning of a medical term, for example, do not hesitate to ask a superior. It is better to ask a question before acting than to make a mistake. It is also better to ask than to risk annoying someone because you carried out a task or wrote a term incorrectly. Asking questions of superiors means that you respect them professionally.
3. Minimize interruptions. For example, before launching into a discussion, make sure the superior you are talking to has time to talk. Opening with "Can I interrupt you for a moment, or should I come back?" or "Do you have a minute to talk?" goes a long way toward establishing good communication. It is also better to go to your supervisor when you have several questions to ask rather than to interrupt her repeatedly.
4. Show initiative. Any superior will greatly appreciate this quality. For example, if you think you can come up with a more efficient way to get the office newsletter written and distributed, write out a plan and show it to your supervisor. He is likely to welcome any ideas that improve office efficiency or patient satisfaction.

Dealing With Conflict

Conflict, or friction, in the workplace can result from opposition of opinions or ideas or even from a difference in personalities. Conflict can arise when the lines of communication break down or when a misunderstanding occurs. Conflict can also result from prejudices or preconceived notions about people or from lack of mutual respect or trust between a staff member and a superior. Whatever the cause, conflict is counterproductive to the efficiency of an office.

Following these suggestions can help prevent conflict in the office and improve communication among coworkers.

1. Do not "feed into" other people's negative attitudes. For example, if a coworker is criticizing one of the doctors, change the subject.
2. Try your best at all times to be personable and supportive of coworkers. For example, everyone has bad days. If a coworker is having a bad day, offer to pitch in and help or to run out and get her lunch if she is too busy to go out.
3. Refrain from passing judgment on others or stereotyping them (women are bad at math, men don't know how to communicate, and so on). Coworkers should show respect for one another and try to be tolerant and nonjudgmental.
4. Do not gossip. You are there to work. Act professionally at all times.
5. Do not jump to conclusions. For example, if you get a memo about a change in your schedule that disturbs you, bring your concern to your supervisor. She may be able to be flexible on certain points. You do not know until you ask.

Managing Stress

Stress can be a barrier to communication. For example, if you are feeling very pressured at work, you might snap at a coworker or patient, or you might forget to give the physician an important message.

Professionals in the health-care field may experience high levels of stress in their daily work environment. Stress can result from a feeling of being under pressure, or it can be a reaction to anger, frustration, or a change in your routine. Stress can increase your blood pressure, speed up your breathing and heart rate, and cause muscle tension. To minimize stress—for the sake of your health as well as for good communication in the office—it is helpful to understand some basic information about stress.

Stress—Good or Bad?

A certain amount of stress is normal. A little bit of stress—the kind that makes you feel excited or challenged by the task at hand—can motivate you to get things done and push you toward a higher level of productivity. Ongoing stress, however, can be overwhelming and affect you physically. For example, it can lower your resistance to colds and increase your risk for developing heart disease, diabetes, high blood pressure, ulcers, allergies, asthma, colitis, cancer, and certain autoimmune diseases, which cause the body's immune

Potential Causes of Stress

- Death of a spouse or family member
- Divorce or separation
- Hospitalization (yours or a family member's) due to injury or illness
- Marriage or reconciliation from a separation
- Loss of a job or retirement
- Sexual problems
- Having a new baby
- Significant change in your financial status (for better or worse)
- Job change
- Children leaving or returning home
- Significant personal success, such as a promotion at work
- Moving or remodeling your home
- Problems at work, such as your boss's retiring, that may put your job at risk
- Substantial debt, such as a mortgage or overspending on credit cards

Figure 4-6. Be aware of the common causes of stress. Find stress-reducing techniques that work for you.

system to attack normal tissue. Figure 4-6 shows the potential causes of stress.

Reducing Stress

Some stress at work is inevitable. An important goal is to learn how to manage or reduce stress. Take into account your strengths and limitations, and be realistic about how much you can handle at work and in your life outside work. Pushing yourself a certain amount can be motivating. Pushing yourself too much is dangerous. Review Figure 4-7 for tips on reducing stress.

The Policy and Procedures Manual

The policy and procedures manual is a key written communication tool in the medical office. No discussion of communication in the medical office would be complete without a description of this important document. The manual is used by permanent employees as well as by temporary employees who may be hired when others are ill or on vacation or when there is an unusually heavy

Tips for Reducing Stress

- Maintain a healthy balance in your life among work, family, and leisure activities.
- Exercise regularly.
- Eat balanced, nutritious meals and healthful snacks. Avoid foods high in caffeine, salt, sugar, and fat.
- Get enough sleep.
- Allow time for yourself, and plan time to relax.
- Rely on the support that family, friends, and coworkers have to offer. Don't be afraid to share your feelings.
- Try to be realistic about what you can and cannot do. Do not be afraid to admit that you cannot take on another responsibility.
- Try to set realistic goals for yourself.
- Remember that there are always choices, even when there appear to be none.
- Be organized. Good planning can help you manage your workload.
- Redirect excess energy constructively—clean your closet, work in the garden, do volunteer work, have friends over for dinner, exercise.
- Change some of the things you have control over.
- Keep yourself focused. Focus your full energy on one thing at a time, and finish one project before starting another.
- Identify sources of conflict, and try to resolve them.
- Learn and use relaxation techniques, such as deep breathing, meditation, or imagining yourself in a quiet, peaceful place. Choose what works for you.
- Maintain a healthy sense of humor. Laughter can help relieve stress. Joke with friends after work. Go see a funny movie.
- Try not to overreact. Ask yourself if a situation is really worth getting upset or worried about.
- Seek help from social or professional support groups, if necessary.

Figure 4-7. These tips will help you avoid and reduce stress in your professional and personal life.

workload. The manual covers all office policies and clinical procedures. It is usually developed as a joint effort by the physician (or physicians) and the staff (often the medical assistant).

Policies

Policies are rules or guidelines that dictate the day-to-day workings of an office. Although individual policies vary from office to office, most medical office manuals describe the following policy areas:

- Office purposes, objectives, and goals as set down by the physician(s)
- Rules and regulations
- Job descriptions and duties of staff personnel
- Office hours
- Dress code
- Insurance and other benefits
- Vacation, sick leave, and other time away from the office
- Salary and performance evaluations
- Maintenance of equipment and supplies
- Mailings
- Bookkeeping
- Scheduling appointments and maintaining patient records
- Occupational Safety and Health Administration (OSHA) guidelines

The policy section of the manual also typically describes the chain of command for the office, or the person to whom each employee reports. This information is sometimes presented in chart form and called an organizational chart. For example, the receptionist, secretary, medical assistant, and billing person might report to the office manager. The office manager, in turn, might report directly to the physician or physicians. This chain of command varies from office to office, depending on the size and needs of the practice.

Procedures

Detailed instructions for specific procedures are covered in the procedures section of the manual. The areas discussed include clinical procedures and quality assurance programs.

Each clinical procedure should include instructions about the following:

- Purpose of the test, clinical application, and usefulness
- Specimen required and collection method; special patient preparation or restrictions
- Reagents, standards, controls, and media used; special supplies
- Instrumentation, including calibration and schedules
- Step-by-step directions
- Calculations
- Frequency and tolerance of controls; corrective action to be taken if tolerances are exceeded
- Expected values; values requiring special notification; interpretation of values
- Procedure notes (e.g., linearity or detection limits)
- Limitations of method (e.g., interfering substances and/or pitfalls and precautions)
- Method validation
- References
- Effective date and schedule for review
- Distribution

Developing a Manual

Although it is likely that your office will already have a manual, you may be involved in reorganizing, producing, or updating the manual. In any event, it is important to understand how a manual is developed.

Planning. To begin planning a manual, first determine a format, or how you will organize the information. The format depends on the office's needs and organization. Many offices prefer a loose-leaf notebook in which pages can easily be replaced when changes or updates are necessary. Figure 4-8 shows a sample page from a manual.

After determining a format, create an outline, organizing the topics and subtopics. Have it approved by the office manager and physician or physicians. In the procedures section, begin each procedure sheet on a new page. Include the following for each procedure page:

- The style to be used for each procedure, whether quantitative or qualitative
- The month and year the procedure was adopted
- The page number and total number of pages for that procedure
- A cover sheet for noting changes, additions, or corrections to the procedure, including whether the procedure replaces an earlier one
- The name of the writer and the name of the physician who approved the text of the procedure

Developing and Updating Material. Sources you may refer to for developing or updating the manual might include scientific or medical journals, manufacturer product literature, textbooks, standards publications, research and validation data, and written personal communications.

For more information on the design, development, and use of technical procedure manuals, contact the National Committee for Clinical Laboratory Standards (NCCLS) in Wayne, Pennsylvania.

MILLSTONE MEDICAL ASSOCIATES

Policy and Procedures Manual

Procedure for Creating a Medical File for a New Patient

GOAL: To create a complete medical record for each new patient containing all necessary personal and medical information

PROCEDURE:

1. Establish that the patient is new to the doctor's office.
2. Ask the patient for all necessary insurance information. If the patient has an insurance card, make a photocopy of it for his file.
3. Ask the patient to fill out the patient information form. Keyboard the information onto a new patient information form, for legibility.
4. Review all information with the patient, to check for accuracy.
5. Label the new patient's folder, according to office procedure. Type either the patient's name (for an alphabetic file) or the correct number (for a numerical file).
6. If filing is done numerically, fill out a cross-reference form on the computer, along with a patient ID card to be stored in a secure location.
7. Add the patient's name to the necessary financial records, including the office ledger, whether on paper or on the computer.
8. After completing the folder label information, place the new patient information form inside the folder, along with any other personal or medical information that pertains to the patient.
9. On the outside of the patient's folder, clip a routing slip.

Figure 4-8. This page from a policy and procedures manual provides the office staff with information about creating a medical file for a new patient.

Summary

As a medical assistant, you are a key communicator between the office and patients and families. The way you greet patients, the way you explain procedures, the manner in which you ask and answer questions, and your attentiveness to patients' individual needs combine to form your communication style. Effective communication skills—which include listening, interpersonal, and assertiveness skills—will help you improve your communication style. These skills will also enable you to develop good communication with patients under special circumstances. Patients with special needs include those who are anxious or angry, elderly, or from other cultures and those who have hearing or visual impairments.

Good communication skills also enable you to develop satisfying and professional working relationships with coworkers and superiors. Effective communication helps the office function smoothly, helps reduce conflicts and stress, and helps motivate individuals to achieve personal and professional goals.

An important communication document in the medical office is the policy and procedures manual. This manual covers all office policies and clinical procedures and is usually developed as a joint effort by the doctor (or doctors) and the staff (often the medical assistant).

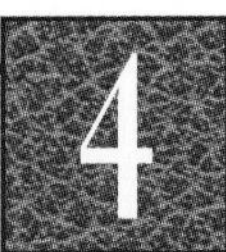

4 Chapter Review

Discussion Questions

1. Discuss the difference between verbal and nonverbal communication. Give examples of each.
2. Name two interpersonal skills. Give an example of how you can demonstrate each skill.
3. Suggest some of the communication problems that can arise with patients from other cultures. How might you deal with these problems?

Critical Thinking Questions

1. You are with a patient who is anxious about having her blood drawn. What specific steps would you take to address her anxiety, and what would you say to her at each step to prepare her for the procedure?
2. You are having difficulty with one of your coworkers who is constantly late returning from lunch, leaving you to handle his patients. How might you assertively discuss the situation with him to resolve the conflict?
3. You notice that one of your coworkers appears to be under a lot of stress. What steps could you take to help her?

Application Activities

1. With a partner, practice your communication skills by assuming the roles of a medical assistant and a patient who is angry after having to wait for an hour in the office waiting room.
2. With a partner or group, take turns using body language to indicate a variety of emotions, and see if the others can correctly guess what message you are sending.
3. With a group of classmates, create an outline for an office policy and procedures manual. Identify sections that might need updating on an ongoing basis and why the updating might be necessary.

Further Readings

Balzer-Riley, Julia W. *Communications in Nursing: Communicating Assertively and Responsibly in Nursing: A Guidebook.* 3d ed. St. Louis, MO: Mosby–Year Book, 1996.

Bradley, Jean C., and Mark A. Edinberg. *Communication in the Nursing Context.* 3d ed. Norwalk, CT: Appleton & Lange, 1990.

Buchwald, Dedra, et al. "Caring for Patients in a Multicultural Society." *Patient Care,* June 15, 1994, 105–109, 113–114, 116, 119–120.

Harold, Wanda. "The Humanistic Role of the Medical Assistant." *The Professional Medical Assistant,* January/February 1991, 8–10.

Marszal, Celia. "The Patient Is a Person." *The Professional Medical Assistant,* March/April 1996, 21–22.

Myerscough, Philip R. *Talking With Patients: A Basic Clinical Skill.* 2d ed. New York: Oxford University Press, 1992.

Northouse, Peter G., and Laurel L. Northouse. *Health Communication Strategies for Health Professionals.* 2d ed. Norwalk, CT: Appleton & Lange, 1992.

Part Two

Administrative Medical Assisting

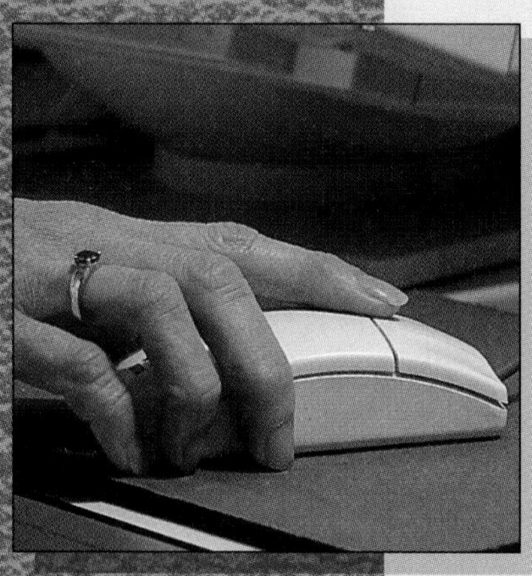

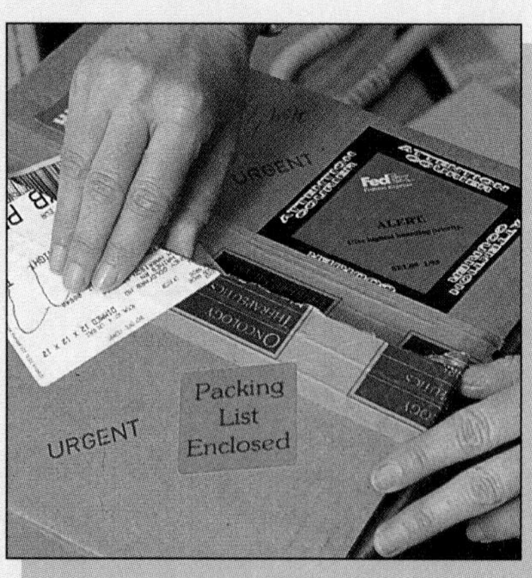

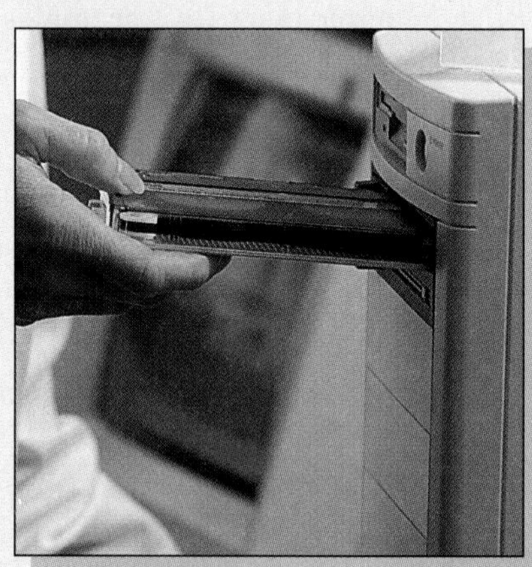

"In my 15 years as a medical assistant and transcriptionist in a large cardiology practice, I have gained invaluable experience that enhances the care of our patients. Cardiology patients require complex care. State-of-the-art equipment, pleasant office surroundings, and a well-educated, warm, and caring staff are key elements in helping patients feel at ease. As I work with patients, I do everything I can to help them feel comfortable in the office. Using reassuring words and good listening skills helps them overcome the anxieties they may have about their illness or a test they are about to have performed.

"Administrative duties are as important as clinical duties. For example, make sure the medical transcription work space is quiet and comfortable. Transcription requires intense concentration to ensure accuracy. Accuracy in all administrative tasks contributes to the success of each patient's treatment plan."

Kaye H. Listug,
Medical Assistant, La Mesa, California

Section One

Office Work

Chapter 5: Using and Maintaining Office Equipment
Chapter 6: Using Computers in the Office
Chapter 7: Managing Correspondence and Mail
Chapter 8: Managing Office Supplies
Chapter 9: Maintaining Patient Records
Chapter 10: Managing the Office Medical Records

Section Two

Interacting With Patients

Chapter 11: Telephone Techniques
Chapter 12: Scheduling Appointments and Maintaining the Physician's Schedule
Chapter 13: Patient Reception Area
Chapter 14: Patient Education

Section Three

Financial Responsibilities

Chapter 15: Processing Insurance Claims
Chapter 16: Bookkeeping and Banking
Chapter 17: Billing and Collections
Chapter 18: Accounts Payable, Payroll, and Contracts

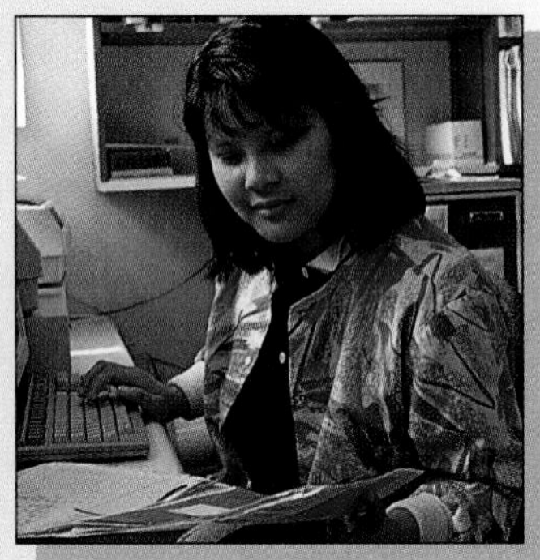

Section One

Office Work

AREAS OF COMPETENCE

1997 ROLE DELINEATION STUDY

ADMINISTRATIVE

- **Administrative Procedures**

CLINICAL

- **Patient Care**

GENERAL (Transdisciplinary)

- **Communication Skills**
- **Legal Concepts**
- **Operational Functions**

CHAPTER LIST

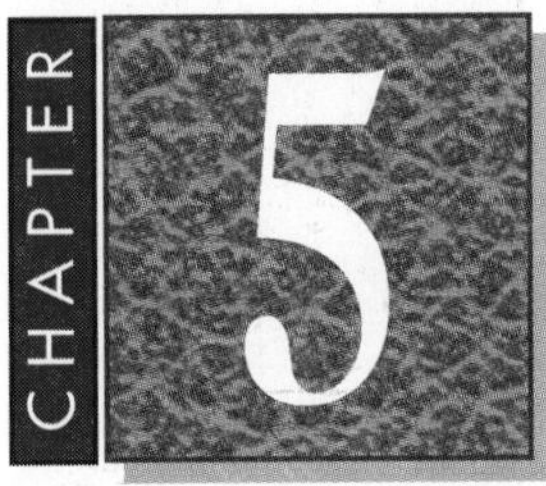

Using and Maintaining Office Equipment

CHAPTER OUTLINE

- Office Communication Equipment
- Office Automation Equipment
- Purchasing Decisions
- Maintaining Office Equipment

OBJECTIVES

After completing Chapter 5, you will be able to:

- Describe the types of office equipment used in a medical practice.
- Explain how each piece of office equipment is used.
- List the steps in making purchasing decisions for office equipment.
- Compare and contrast leasing and buying.
- Describe a warranty, a maintenance contract, and a service contract, and discuss the importance of each.
- Identify when troubleshooting is appropriate and what actions may be taken.
- List the information included in an equipment inventory.

Key Terms

cover sheet
lease
maintenance contract
microfiche
microfilm
service contract
troubleshooting
voice mail
warranty

AREAS OF COMPETENCE

1997 ROLE DELINEATION STUDY

ADMINISTRATIVE

Administrative Procedures

- Perform basic clerical functions
- Perform medical transcription

GENERAL (Transdisciplinary)

Operational Functions

- Maintain supply inventory
- Evaluate and recommend equipment and supplies

Office Communication Equipment

When you think of equipment for a medical office, you probably imagine x-ray machines, blood pressure monitors, and stethoscopes. You will, however, find many other kinds of equipment in a medical practice. Medical offices also use business communication equipment, which includes telephones, facsimile machines, computers, and photocopiers. One of your duties as a medical assistant may be to operate the medical office's communication equipment.

Just as medical equipment has evolved over the years, so has office equipment. The office communication equipment available years ago handled only the most basic tasks. Medical practices may have had a single telephone and a typewriter. If copies of patient records were required, medical assistants handwrote a duplicate set or used carbon paper to make additional copies.

Today technology allows almost instantaneous communication of information throughout the world. This instant communication can be critical for the fast-paced medical profession, where information often translates to the need for immediate treatment, sometimes in life-threatening situations. Communicating effectively within a medical office can be as vital as providing the correct treatment to patients—and often ensures that they receive such treatment (Figure 5-1).

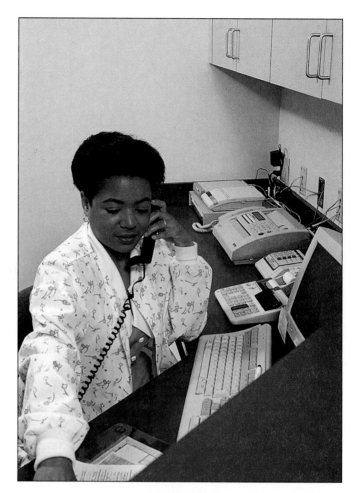

Figure 5-1. Most medical offices today rely on many up-to-date pieces of communication equipment.

Telephone Systems

Although the telephone is a common item in offices, it is one of the most important pieces of communication equipment in a medical practice. Not only is it the instrument patients use to communicate with the office; it is also the main means of communication with other doctors, hospitals, laboratories, and other businesses important to the practice.

Multiple Lines. Few practices can function with just one telephone line because if that line is in use, no other calls can come in or go out. Most medical offices have a telephone system that includes two or more telephones and several telephone lines. The six-button telephone is a popular choice in medical practices. This system has four lines for incoming or outgoing calls, an intercom line, and a button for putting a call on hold.

A telephone system can be set up so that incoming calls ring on all the telephones in the office. A more common setup in busy practices is to use a switchboard, a device that receives all calls. The receptionist then routes calls to the appropriate telephone extensions.

Automated Menu. Instead of using a switchboard, some medical practices route calls by means of an automated menu. Callers listen to the recorded menu and, in response, press a number on their telephone keypad. For example, the menu will say, "Press 2 to speak to Dr. Lowell." The caller presses 2, and the phone rings in Dr. Lowell's office. "Tips for the Office" provides more information on routing calls through an automated menu. If your office uses such a menu, make sure the voice prompts are clear and understandable.

Voice Mail. An automated menu is often used in conjunction with **voice mail,** which is an advanced form of answering machine. If a doctor is out of her office or taking another telephone call, the call is answered by voice mail, and the caller can leave a message. One of the benefits of a voice mail system is that callers never receive a busy signal.

Answering Machine. Many offices use a telephone answering machine to answer calls after office hours, on weekends and holidays, and when the office is closed for any reason. A typical recorded message announces that the office is closed and states when it will reopen. The message must always indicate how the caller can reach the doctor or the answering service in an emergency.

An answering machine may be programmed simply to play a taped message from the office, or it may also record messages from callers. If callers can leave messages, you should check the answering machine to retrieve them at the start of each day.

Answering Service. Instead of or in addition to an answering machine, most medical offices use an answering service. Unlike answering machines, answering services provide people to answer the telephone. They take messages and communicate them to the doctor on call. The doctor on call is responsible for handling emergencies that may occur when the office is closed, such as at night or on weekends or holidays.

Upon receiving a call from the answering service, the doctor calls the patient. For example, the doctor may recommend ways for the patient to alleviate her pain and ask her to come into the office the next morning.

Answering services can be used in two ways. The doctor's office may have an answering machine to record calls of a routine nature and give the number of the answering service to call in emergencies. Alternatively, the answering service may have a direct connection to the doctor's office, picking up calls after a certain number of rings day or night or during specific hours.

Although most answering services provide satisfactory, sometimes even outstanding, service, it is good practice to check up on the service every so often by calling it during its coverage hours. This quality check ensures that the service meets office standards and expectations.

Pagers

Physicians often need to be reached when they are out of the office, so many carry pagers. Pagers are small electronic devices that give a signal to indicate that someone is trying to reach the physician.

Technology of Paging. Each paging device is assigned a telephone number. When someone calls that number, the pager picks up the signal and beeps, buzzes, or vibrates to indicate that a call has been made. Most pagers have a window that displays the caller's telephone number so that the person who has been paged can return the call promptly. Certain models display a short message. Some pagers store telephone numbers so that the receiver can return several calls without having to write down the numbers.

Paging a Physician. Many telephone messages can wait until the physician returns to the office or calls in for messages. When a message needs to be delivered immediately, however, paging is an efficient response. The paging process is as simple as making a telephone call.

1. A list of pager numbers for each physician in the practice should be kept in a prominent place in the office, such as by the main switchboard. Make sure you know where these numbers are kept. Look up the telephone number for the pager of the physician you need to contact.
2. Dial the telephone number for the pager.
3. You will hear the telephone ringing and the call picked up. Listen for a high-pitched tone, which signals the connection between the telephone and the pager.
4. To operate most pagers, you need to dial the telephone number you wish the physician to call, followed by the pound sign (#), located below the number 9 on a push-button telephone. (Some pager services have an operator and work much like an an-

Tips FOR THE OFFICE

Routing Calls Through an Automated Menu

An automated menu system answers calls for you and separates requests into categories so that you can deal with them efficiently. You may already be familiar with automated menus, which are widely used by many large businesses. Someone who calls an automated system hears a recorded message identifying the business. The message gives the caller a list of options from which to choose to identify the purpose of the call. The caller selects an option by pressing the corresponding button on her push-button telephone. If she does not have a push-button telephone, her call is automatically routed so that she can talk to a person or leave a voice mail message.

How does an automated menu system save time and effort in a medical office? You don't have to answer calls as they come in but can instead reserve a block of time in which to listen and respond to messages. This system allows you to complete other work without interruption.

To set up an automated system, you need to plan specific categories from which patients can choose. Categories may include (1) making and changing appointments, (2) asking billing questions, (3) asking medical questions of the doctors or nurses, and (4) reporting patient emergencies.

When the caller presses the code for a patient emergency, the call rings in the office because it needs to be answered immediately. You or other staff members can respond to calls in the other categories in a timely fashion. Questions for doctors or nurses can be routed immediately to the appropriate voice mail, bypassing you and the office receptionist.

Automated menu systems can be set up by telephone vendors listed in the yellow pages. When choosing an automated telephone system, be careful that callers do not become lost in the process. It is a good idea to set up a system that allows callers to return easily to the main menu. Following up on messages promptly will also help callers feel comfortable with your voice mail system, so you should check for messages at least once every hour.

swering service. Give the operator a message, and the operator will contact the physician.)

5. Listen for a beep or a series of beeps signaling that the page has been transmitted. Then hang up the phone. The physician will call the number at his earliest convenience.

Facsimile Machines

Critical documents, such as laboratory reports or patient records, often need to be sent immediately to locations outside the office. Documents can be sent by means of a facsimile machine, or fax machine. A fax machine scans each page, translates it into electronic impulses, and transmits those impulses over the telephone line. When they are received by another fax machine, they are converted into an exact copy of the original document.

A fax machine in a medical office should have its own telephone line. A separate line ensures that transmission of incoming and outgoing faxes will not be interrupted and that the machine will not tie up a needed telephone line when sending or receiving information.

Benefits of Faxing. A fax machine can send an exact copy of a document within minutes. The cost for sending a fax is the same as for making a telephone call to that location. For a short document, this is usually less expensive than an overnight mail service.

Many fax machines have a copier function and can be used as an extra copy machine. This function may only be useful, however, if the machine uses plain paper. The telephone for the fax may also be used as an extra extension for outgoing calls, if needed.

Thermal Paper vs Plain Paper. Some fax machines print on rolls of specially treated paper called electrothermal, or thermal, paper, which reacts to heat and electricity. Thermal paper tends to fade over time, so documents received on this type of paper may need to be photocopied. Many new models of fax machines use plain paper instead of thermal paper, avoiding the need for making copies. Information is transferred to the plain paper by either a carbon ribbon or a laser beam.

Sending a Fax. Sending a fax is a simple process. One or more pages of a document can be sent at any given time.

1. Prepare a **cover sheet,** which provides information about the transmission. Cover sheets can vary in appearance but usually include the name, telephone number, and fax number of the sender and the receiver; the number of pages being transmitted; the date; and whether the information is confidential.

City Medical Associates

555 London Street Strathspey, PA 19919

Janet Michaels, MD — INTERNAL MEDICINE — Scott J. Michaels, MD

FACSIMILE COVER SHEET

Date: ______________________

To: ______________________ From: ______________________

Fax #: ______________________ Fax #: ______________________

# of pages (including this cover sheet): ________

Message: ____

____

Figure 5-2. Every document that is sent by fax transmission should include a cover sheet, which provides details about the transmission.

Often medical practices use preprinted cover sheets, with blanks that can be filled in for each transmission. (A sample cover sheet is shown in Figure 5-2.)

2. Place all pages face down in the fax machine's sending tray or area. Dial the telephone number of the receiving fax machine, using either the telephone attached to the fax machine or the numbers on the fax keyboard.
3. If you use the fax telephone, listen for a high-pitched tone. Then press the "Send" or "Start" button, and hang up the telephone. Your fax is now being sent.
4. If you use the fax keyboard, press the "Send" or "Start" button after dialing the telephone number. This button will start the call.
5. Watch for the fax machine to make a connection. Often a green light appears as the document feeds through the machine.
6. If the fax machine is not able to make a connection, as when the receiving fax line is busy, it may have a feature that automatically redials the number every few minutes for a specified number of attempts.
7. When a fax has been successfully sent, most fax machines print a confirmation message. When a fax has not been sent, the machine either prints an error message or indicates on the screen that the transmission was unsuccessful.

Receiving a Fax. Faxes can be received 24 hours a day if the fax machine is turned on and has an adequate supply of paper. If the fax machine is not already sending or receiving a fax, the fax telephone rings briefly, signaling the start of a transmission. The transmission begins shortly thereafter, with the machine printing out the document as it is sent. When completed, the machine usually prints a transmission report, with the number of pages, the date and time, and the originating fax number.

Typewriters

Typewriters can be used to create correspondence, interoffice documents, and patient bills. Typewritten documents are easier to read than handwritten ones and project a more businesslike appearance.

Models and Features. Although typewriter models differ in features, all use a standard keyboard. Placement of the keys is identical on each typewriter. The arrangement is not alphabetic. Rather, the most frequently used keys are near the middle, where your fingers can most easily reach them, and the least used keys are toward the outside.

A wide variety of typewriter models are available. Most offices use electric or electronic models. Although both are powered by electricity, they differ in their ability to perform certain functions. For example, electronic typewriters can store limited amounts of information for further use, but electric typewriters cannot. Both electric and electronic typewriters provide a wide selection of features, including, but not limited to, automatic carriage return, automatic centering, self-correction, and changeable typefaces or fonts.

Typewriters vs Word Processors. Typewriters should not be confused with word processors, which perform a similar function but are more sophisticated. Word processors can store entire documents in memory, thereby allowing much greater flexibility in manipulating material than do typewriters. Word processors display documents on a screen, and these documents can be revised as often as needed before being printed out. Word processors are typically more expensive than typewriters, but they are less expensive than computers and make it easy to generate perfect documents.

Today many medical practices use computers with word processing software. (Chapter 6 discusses the use of computers in a medical office.)

Office Automation Equipment

Using automated equipment enables you to perform a task more easily and quickly than doing it manually. For example, adding numbers on a calculator is a much faster process than doing it on paper. Many of the administrative tasks in a medical practice can be accomplished with automated equipment, giving you more time to perform other procedures.

Photocopiers

A photocopier, also called a copier or copy machine, instantly reproduces office correspondence, forms, bills, patient records, and other documents. Before photocopiers were available, offices used carbon paper to reproduce documents as they were being typed. The number of copies that could be made was limited.

A photocopier takes a picture of the document it is to reproduce and prints it on plain paper using a heat process. Photocopiers use either liquid or dry toner, a form of ink. They can make an unlimited number of copies. Photocopiers do not require treated or otherwise special paper. Various kinds of paper can be used in the machine, including office stationery and colored paper. Many photocopiers accept different sizes of paper, from the standard 8½- by 11-inch paper to 8½- by 14-inch legal paper and even larger.

Photocopiers come in many models, from desktop machines for limited use to industrial models for continual heavy use. The machines vary in features and speed.

Special Features. Copiers offer a wide range of special features. They may collate (assemble sets of multiple pages in order) and staple pages, enlarge or reduce images, and produce double-sided copies (print on both sides of the page). Some can also adjust contrast and even track the cost of a job via a specific code input into the machine. Although the majority of photocopiers used in medical offices produce black-and-white copies, photocopiers are available that make color copies. Some copiers can make transparencies (text and images printed on clear acetate), which physicians often use for presentations.

One of the more useful features of photocopiers is the "Help" function. Selecting this function displays directions in plain English that explain how to fix a paper jam or deal with other routine copier problems. Some copiers are even programmed to indicate that service is needed.

Making Copies. Although the procedure for making copies differs slightly from machine to machine, most machines can be operated by following these basic steps.

1. Make sure the machine is turned on and warmed up. It will display a signal when it is ready for copying.
2. Prepare your materials, removing paper clips, staples, and self-adhesive flags.
3. Place the document to be copied in the automatic feeder tray or upside down directly on the glass. The feeder tray can accommodate many pages; you may place only one page at a time on the glass. Automatic feeding is a faster process, and you should use it when you wish to collate or staple packets. Page-by-page copying is advantageous if you need to copy a single sheet or to enlarge or reduce the image. To use any special features, such as making double-sided copies or stapling the copies, you have to press a button on the machine.
4. Set the machine for the desired paper size.
5. Key in the number of copies you want to make, and press the "Start" button. The copies are made automatically.
6. If necessary, press the "Clear" or "Reset" button when your job is finished to prepare the machine for the next user.

Adding Machines and Calculators

For handling tasks such as patient billing, bank deposits, and payroll, medical practices depend on adding machines and calculators. The difference between the two types of machines is minimal. Adding machines typically plug into an outlet and produce a paper tape on which calculations are printed. Calculators are more often battery- or solar-powered, with memory to store figures. Calculators are portable and usually do not produce a paper tape.

Routine Calculations. Both adding machines and calculators are sufficient for routine office calculations. These machines perform basic arithmetic functions, such as addition, subtraction, multiplication, and division. Many of today's models perform such specialized functions as computing percentages and storing data. Some are even computerized.

Checking Your Work. It is easy to hit an incorrect key or to key in a number twice when using an adding machine or a calculator. Therefore, check all mathematical computations. An error on a bill causes problems for both the patient and the office.

If the machine produces a paper tape, check the numbers on the tape against the numbers you are adding. The paper tape is especially useful when adding a long series of numbers. Without a printed record, you must perform the same calculations again to make sure the total is correct.

Postage Meters

Every medical office uses the U.S. Postal Service. Patient bills, routine correspondence, purchase orders, and payments are just some of the items typically sent by mail. (See Chapter 7 for additional information on mailing correspondence.)

Although some medical offices use stamps, most use a postage meter. A postage meter is a machine that applies postage to an envelope or package, eliminating the need for postage stamps (Figure 5-3). There are often two parts to a postage meter: the meter, which belongs to the post office, and the mailing machine, which the practice can own. The meter actually applies the postage, and the mailing machine does the rest, such as sealing the envelope.

Benefits of Using a Postage Meter. There are several advantages to using a postage meter instead of purchasing stamps. It saves frequent trips to the post office. It also saves money for the office by providing the exact amount of postage needed for each item. When you have to use a combination of stamps, you may exceed the required postage. It is unlikely as well as impractical for a practice to keep every denomination of stamps on hand.

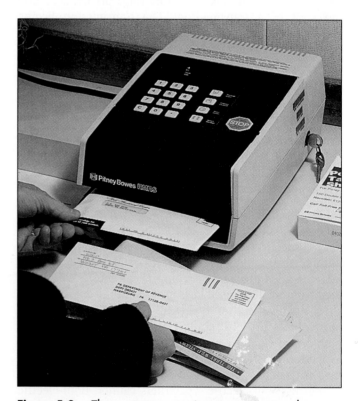

Figure 5-3. The postage meter is a convenient and cost-effective way to apply postage to office correspondence and packages.

Some postage meters can imprint envelopes with the name of your medical practice or with a message at the same time postage is applied. The message appears immediately to the left of the postal mark, at the top of the envelope.

Many types of postage meters are available, from basic models for a small office to advanced models for large businesses. The latest machines include automatic date setting, memory to program a large mailing, and display alerts for low postage or the need for ribbon replacement. Some models can apply postage to parcels without the use of labels or tape. Procedure 5-1 shows you how to use a postage meter.

Prepaying for Postage. To use a postage meter, you must prepay the postage. You can take your meter to the post office to add postage, or you can use a postage meter service. A service maintains the postal account for you. Although the money in each account is the property of the U.S. Postal Service, the provider manages the account and adds postage to the meter. Postage can also be added to the meter by telephone or by modem, with data sent directly to the meter over the telephone line. The process takes only a few minutes, and the call is often toll-free. Before postage can be added, however, money must be deposited into an account. Keeping the postage account current ensures that all mail is sent on a timely basis. This task may be one of your responsibilities.

On any meter, you can check the amount of postage used and the amount remaining with the touch of a button. On some models, the meter must have $10 or more for the machine to apply postage to an envelope or package.

Postage Scales

Besides the postage meter, you also need a scale. Postal scales are a good investment because they show both the weight and the amount of postage required. Some postage

PROCEDURE 5-1

How to Use a Postage Meter

Objective: To correctly apply postage to an envelope or package for mailing, according to U.S. Postal Service guidelines

Materials: Postage meter, addressed envelope or package, postal scale

Method

1. For the postage meter to function, there must be money in your postal account. Contact the company that is managing your account or your local post office for more information.
2. Verify the day's date. U.S. Postal Service guidelines prohibit mailing envelopes and packages that are postmarked with an incorrect date. Check that the postage meter is plugged in and switched on before you proceed.
3. Locate the area where the meter registers the date. Many machines have a lid that can be flipped up, with rows of numbers underneath. Months are represented numerically, with 1 symbolizing January, 2 symbolizing February, and so on. Check that the date is correct. If it is not, change the numbers to the correct date.
4. Make sure that all materials have been included in the envelope or package. Weigh the envelope or package on a postal scale. Standard business envelopes weighing up to 1 oz require the minimum postage (the equivalent of one first-class stamp). Oversize envelopes and packages require additional postage. A postal scale will indicate the amount of postage required.
5. Key in the postage amount on the meter, and press the button that enters the amount. For amounts over $1, you may have to press a "$" button or the "Enter" button twice. This feature verifies large amounts, catching errors in case you mistakenly press too many keys.
6. Check that the amount you typed is the correct amount. Envelopes and packages with too little postage will be returned by the U.S. Postal Service. If you send an envelope or package with too much postage, the practice will not be reimbursed.
7. If you are applying postage to an envelope, hold it flat and right-side up (so that you can read the address). Seal the envelope (unless the meter seals it for you). As you face the postage meter, locate the plate or area where the envelope can slide through. This feature is usually near the bottom of the meter. Place the envelope on the left side, and give it a gentle push toward the right. Some models hold the envelope in a stationary position. (If the meter seals the envelope for you, be sure to place it correctly to allow for sealing. The meter will grab the envelope and pull it through quickly.)
8. For packages, you need to create a postage label to affix to the package. Follow the same procedure for a label as for an envelope. Affix the postmarked label on the package in the upper right-hand corner.
9. Check that the printed postmark has the correct date and amount and that it is legible.

meters include a scale. If you need a postal scale but one is not available, you can use any scale that weighs in ounces. You can then translate the weight into the correct postage by using a current postal rate chart, available from the U.S. Postal Service.

Posting Mail

Before you begin posting mail, make sure the envelope or package is complete, with all materials included. After applying the postage, place the postmarked envelope or package in the area of your office designated for mail pickup.

Dictation-Transcription Equipment

Physicians usually do not type their own correspondence, patient records, or other documents. Medical assistants, although not professional medical transcriptionists, may be asked to transcribe recorded words into written text. Using dictation-transcription equipment is the most efficient way to complete this task. *Dictation* is another word for speaking; *transcription* is another word for writing. Together they mean to transform spoken words into written form.

Medical assistants performing transcription often use a desktop dictation-transcription machine, a unit similar in size and appearance to a telephone. A smaller attachment resembles a handheld tape recorder. The machine includes special controls to record and play tapes.

Dictating and Transcribing. Before a tape can be transcribed, it must be recorded. A doctor can take several steps during the recording process to make the job of transcribing the tape as easy as possible.

1. The doctor should indicate the date and the type of document being dictated and provide explicit instruc-

PROCEDURE 5-2

How to Use a Dictation-Transcription Machine

Objective: To correctly use a dictation-transcription machine to convert verbal communication into the written word

Materials: Dictation-transcription machine; audiocassette or magnetic tape or disk with the recorded dictation; typewriter, word processor, or computer; blank paper or stationery; medical dictionary; regular dictionary; pen; correction fluid or tape (for the typewriter)

Method

1. Insert the tape into the dictation-transcription machine (Figure 5-4). In front of you, next to the machine, will be a typewriter, word processor, or computer, on which you will type the information. Turn on the typewriter, word processor, or computer if it is not on already.
2. Place all materials, including a regular dictionary and a medical dictionary, within easy reach, and clear the area of items you will not use.
3. Choose the paper you will use, and insert it. Set the margins and line spacing. You can estimate the length of the document by using the scanning control.
4. Dictation-transcription machines use foot pedals to allow your fingers to remain on the keyboard. Press down the foot pedal to start and stop the dictation-transcription machine.
5. To rewind the tape, use the reverse foot pedal.
6. Pause the recording with the pause foot pedal, if your machine has one, or stop it with the stop/start pedal.
7. Adjust the speed and volume controls to help you work most efficiently.
8. Proofread the final document, and make any corrections directly on the document. Use correction fluid or correction tape as necessary. Make sure that the corrected document looks professional and businesslike. Retype it if necessary. Proofread the final copy once again. If possible, ask someone else to proofread it also.
9. Turn off all equipment that should not be left on.

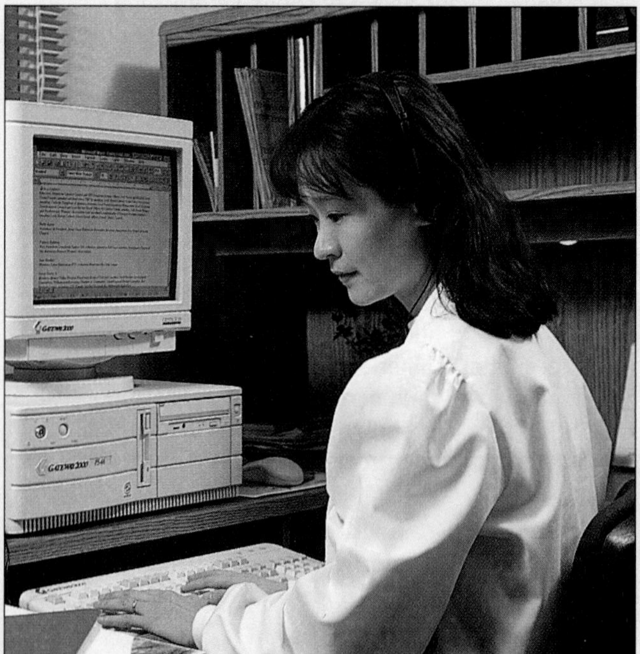

Figure 5-4. One of your responsibilities as a medical assistant may be to use dictation-transcription equipment.

tions about the document. For example, the doctor should indicate that a particular document is a letter and that it is to be produced on office stationery and mailed to a patient.

2. The doctor should spell out all names and addresses as well as any unfamiliar terms.
3. Where possible, the doctor should dictate punctuation, by saying, for example, "comma" or "Begin new paragraph."
4. The doctor should speak clearly and slowly. The doctor should neither eat while dictating nor record in a noisy environment, such as the emergency room of a hospital, if at all possible.

Procedure 5-2 shows you how to operate a dictation-transcription machine. Chapter 9 explains how to create accurate, complete transcriptions.

Special Controls. Dictation-transcription machines often have special controls to streamline the transcription process. Volume and tone controls make dictation clearer, and speed controls separate words. Setting the speed to the rate at which you are comfortable typing also makes the transcription process more efficient. In addition, headphones allow you to concentrate on the recording, shutting out distracting office noise.

More specialized controls include scanning, which allows you to review a tape's contents quickly, and indicator strips, which mark important material. Some machines are also equipped with an automatic backspace control, which rewinds the tape slightly each time it is stopped, so that no words are missed. For the recording process, the machine may be equipped with an insert control, to allow someone to place additional dictation in the middle of existing dictation. The machine may also include a voice-activated sensor for hands-free recording. After a transcribed document has been approved, you may wish to use the machine's erase function to create a clean tape.

Check Writers

Medical practice personnel need to write checks to pay for equipment, supplies, and payroll. This common office procedure can be automated by using a check writer, which is a machine that imprints checks. The safety advantage of using such a machine is that the name of the payee (the person receiving the check) and the amount of the check, once imprinted, cannot be altered.

Producing a Check. To produce a check using a check writer, you first put in a blank check or a sheet of blank checks. Then you key in the date, payee's name, and payment amount. The check writer imprints the check with this information and perforates it with the payee's name. The perforations are actual little holes in the paper, which prevent anyone from changing the name on the check. A doctor or another authorized person then signs the check. To complete the process, record the check in the office checkbook.

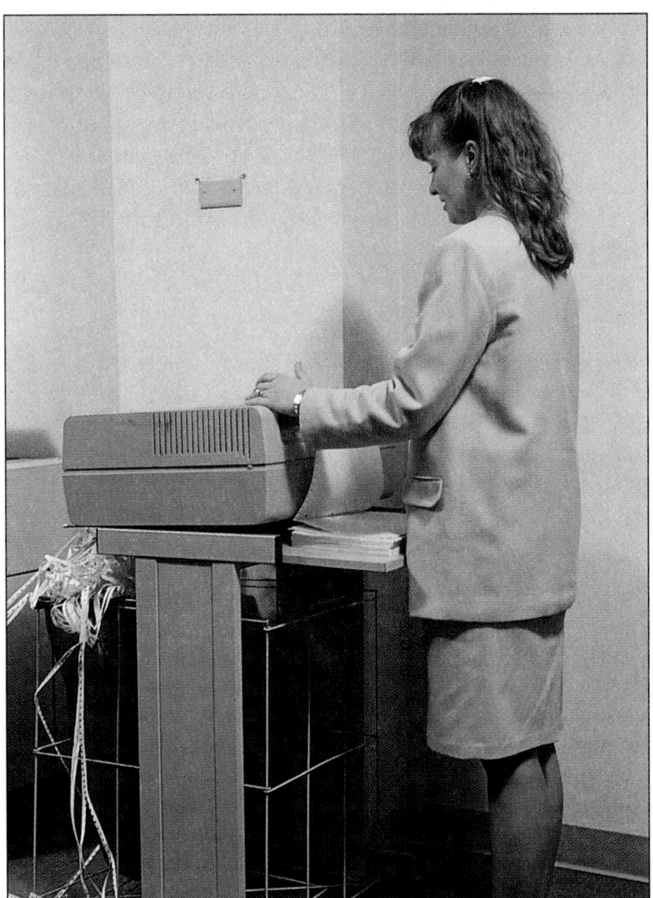

Figure 5-5. As a medical assistant, you may be asked to use a paper shredder to destroy confidential documents that are no longer needed by the practice.

Voiding a Check. If the information on an imprinted check is incorrect, it cannot be changed. Therefore, you must issue a new check and void the previous one. To void the check, write VOID in clear letters across it, or use a VOID stamp with red ink. Then file the check with the office bank records so that the practice's money manager is aware that it has been voided.

Paper Shredders

Paper shredders are usually associated with government offices but are also quite common in medical practices. A paper shredder, such as the one shown in Figure 5-5, is often used when confidential documents, such as patient records, need to be destroyed. Paper shredders cut documents into tiny pieces to make them unreadable.

The most common type of shredder cuts paper into ribbonlike strips, which differ in width, depending on the model. Other shredders cut the paper in two directions, forming small pieces. Some paper shredders offer additional options, such as an electronic eye that automatically starts the machine when paper is inserted and stops when it is done. Other features available are paper jam detection, automatic reverse, and automatic shutdown when the machine gets too hot.

How to Shred Materials. A paper shredder is ready to use when it is turned on. To shred a document, insert it into the feed tray at the top of the shredder. The machine feeds the paper through hundreds of knifelike cutters, instantaneously shredding the paper. A basket attached beneath the shredder catches the bits of paper. Different models can accommodate different amounts of paper through the cutters. Shredder baskets must be emptied periodically to allow room for additional shredded paper. Some shredders signal when the basket is full.

When to Shred Materials. Medical practices often need to eliminate old patient records or other sensitive materials. These items cannot simply be thrown into the trash because of confidentiality problems. The shredder is an effective disposal solution. If records have incorrect information that has been corrected on subsequent documents, the old records are shredded so that the incorrect information is not mistakenly placed in the patient's folder.

A document that has been shredded cannot be put back together. Therefore, do not decide on your own to shred a document. The physician usually tells you when a document should be shredded. If you are not sure whether to shred a document, check with a senior staff member before beginning the process.

Microfilm and Microfiche Readers

If all information were stored on paper in file folders, medical offices would need additional rooms to hold it all. Therefore, some medical offices store information on microfilm or microfiche. **Microfilm** is a roll of film imprinted with information and stored on a reel. Film can also be stored in cartridges, to protect the film from being touched. **Microfiche** is film imprinted with information and stored in rectangular sheets.

Information stored on microfilm and microfiche is dramatically reduced in size. Because each roll or sheet can hold a large amount of material, less storage space is required than for comparable paper files. Because the information is so tiny, however, reading it requires special machines, such as those shown in Figures 5-6 and 5-7.

Even if your office does not store records on microfilm or microfiche, you may still need to have a reader because back issues of medical journals and other publications are often available only in these formats.

Models and Features. Microfilm and microfiche machines come in many different sizes. Most medical offices use a desktop model to conserve space. The main difference between a desktop model and other models is size. The features and controls are similar.

Basic controls on microfilm and microfiche readers allow adjustment of the image—zooming into an area, focusing, and rotating it—and fast-forwarding to other parts of the film. Advanced controls include image editing, an odometer that measures the amount of film scanned, and search functions that can be connected to a computer to locate specific items.

Reading and Printing. For ease of use, you should label and date each roll of microfilm or each microfiche sheet with the information it contains. Then you will be able to locate information easily when you need it.

Because the film is stored in different formats, microfilm and microfiche require different mechanisms to read

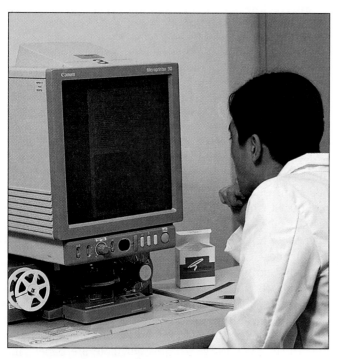

Figure 5-6. Storing information on microfilm helps reduce the amount of storage space needed by the practice.

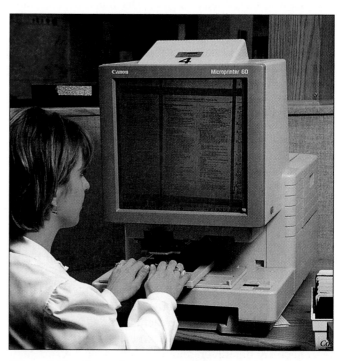

Figure 5-7. Special equipment must be used to read text that has been converted to microfiche.

them. For example, microfilm requires a roller attachment; microfiche requires a flat surface. Newer models can accommodate different formats with the use of detachable, interchangeable reading mechanisms.

Microfilm is inserted onto a rod and threaded onto the microfilm reader. Microfiche is placed directly on the glass tray of a microfiche reader. If you are unsure, check the directions in the manual for your reader.

The reading process is similar for all machines, with information displayed on a large screen. The screen displays only a small portion of the information stored on the film. You can fast-forward through the film to read additional information. Most machines allow you to print out the image on the screen.

Purchasing Decisions

As a medical assistant, you may be involved in making purchasing decisions for office equipment. For example, the physician or office manager may ask you to investigate whether the practice needs a certain piece of equipment, such as a new photocopier or microfiche reader. To make a sound decision about whether the office will benefit from such a purchase, you will need to conduct thorough research.

Evaluating Office Needs

The first step in the research process is to document the tasks that a piece of equipment can complete. In the case of a typewriter, for example, tasks include writing letters and bills, recording the staff's schedule, and preparing a fax cover sheet, as well as producing other office documents. To obtain a complete list of office needs, consult other staff members for their ideas.

If you are replacing an old piece of equipment, you will want to know what advantages the new piece of equipment offers over the current one. Next to each task on your list, indicate the benefits offered by the new product. For example, next to typing office correspondence, you might list several benefits of an electronic typewriter or a computer over a manual typewriter. Both the electronic typewriter and the computer are easy to use; they self-correct, making correction fluid or tape unnecessary; and they store information, thus saving typing time. Some medical magazines, such as *Medical Economics* and *The Professional Medical Assistant,* review medical office equipment periodically and are good resources to consult in making your purchasing decisions.

Contacting Suppliers. Put together a list of the features you would like in your machine. Then contact suppliers who sell models that offer those features. You can call the manufacturer directly to find out the name of a local vendor. Many manufacturers prepare brochures giving information about their products. If time allows, you can request that these be sent to you.

Look in the yellow pages for office supply stores and other companies that sell office equipment. Obtain product and pricing information on each model. For certain equipment, such as photocopiers, a sales representative will come to your office to demonstrate and discuss the product.

Evaluating Warranty Options. Most products come with a warranty. A **warranty** is a contract that guarantees free service and replacement of parts for a certain period, usually 1 year. Warranties are valid only for specified service and repairs. They usually do not cover accidents, vandalism, acts of God (such as damage caused by floods or earthquakes), or mistreatment of the machine. In most cases, warranty repairs must be made at an authorized service center.

If you want more coverage than the warranty allows, you can buy an extended warranty. Extended warranties increase the amount of time that equipment is covered. For expensive pieces of equipment or parts, the additional cost of an extended warranty may be justified.

After you purchase a product, you should fill out the warranty card and mail it to the manufacturer. File the receipt in a safe place in the office where it can easily be retrieved.

Preparing a Recommendation. After you have obtained all the information, you are ready to evaluate it. To compare and contrast the different models, construct a chart. Place the product model names in columns across the top. Down the left side, list factors that will influence the purchase decision: cost, warranty options (including the length of the warranty and the price of an extended warranty), special features, and delivery time. Then fill in the information. This chart will provide an easy-to-use summary of your research.

Analyze the list, and choose the product you think will best meet the needs of the office. Then meet with the physician or office manager to discuss your recommendation.

Leasing vs Buying Equipment

Once the product has been selected, there is one more decision to make: whether to lease or to buy the item. When buying a product, the purchaser becomes the owner of the product. Owners are free to do with the product anything they choose, which may include selling it to someone else.

For most large pieces of office equipment, such as photocopiers, there is also an option to **lease** the equipment. Leasing, or renting, usually involves an initial charge and a monthly fee. On average, the initial charge is equal to about two monthly payments.

Lease Agreement. A lease is for a specified time, after which time the equipment is returned to the seller (Figure 5-8). Some leases allow purchase of the equipment at the end of the rental period for an additional payment.

Metropolitan Office Systems

Lease Agreement

Customer (Location)

Standard Education Corporation
Full Legal Name (Please Print)

119 Washington Blvd.
Address

Spokane, WA 98548
City County State Zip

Customer (Billing address, if different)

Full Legal Name (Please Print)

Address

City County State Zip

Billing Contact

Phone

Dealer:

Quantity	Description: Make, Model, and Serial Number	Quantity	Description: Make, Model, and Serial Number
1	FT 6655 Copier AA3365430358		
1	Sorter A337502010902		
1	Document Feeder A338506		
1	RT314 Large-capacity Tray		

Minimum Lease Term:	Payment Due:	Amount of Monthly Payment With Sales, Use, and Property Tax:	Advance Payment of $965.56 (Tax Included) by Check #	Documentation Fee
60 Months	X Monthly ___ Quarterly ___ Annually ___ Other: $455.46	$482.78	___ First Month's Rent X First and Last ___ Security Deposit (Without Tax) ___ Other ___	$ -0-

Figure 5-8. Read lease agreements carefully.

The details of the purchase option are covered in the lease agreement.

Advantages of Leasing. When you lease a product, your office does not own it, but you have several advantages. Leasing allows purchasers to keep more of their money. The initial cost of obtaining the machine is a fraction of the full cost of purchasing it. Therefore, the remainder of the money can earn interest in the bank or be used for other expenses. Leasing is advantageous when you do not have enough money to buy the equipment but need the services it provides. In addition, leasing allows businesses to update equipment every few years at the end of each lease period. Updating may not be as affordable if you buy equipment. Often the company that leases the product is also responsible for servicing it. Finally, in most cases, businesses are able to take lease payments as a tax deduction each year.

Leasing is not the best solution for everyone. It is important to weigh the advantages of leasing against the advantages of buying equipment for your medical practice.

Negotiating. Whether you decide to lease or buy equipment, always ask whether the price is firm or if there is room for negotiation. Although most equipment prices are set, terms can sometimes be negotiated on more expensive pieces of equipment. Companies that lease office equipment are often flexible in determining the monthly payment. For example, many companies accept smaller payments to start out, with larger payments near the end, or vice versa.

Some suppliers will match their competitors' prices. Also, if you are purchasing several pieces of equipment at the same time, a supplier may be able to offer some savings on the total cost of the purchase or provide some service, such as delivery, free of charge.

Maintaining Office Equipment

Office equipment must be regularly maintained to provide high-quality service. Daily or weekly maintenance, such as cleaning the glass on the photocopier or replacing toner, can be performed by the office staff. However, more extensive maintenance should be done by the equipment supplier.

Equipment Manuals

The best source of information about maintaining a piece of equipment is the manual that comes with it. This booklet gives basic information about the equipment, including how to set it up, how it works, special features, and problems you may encounter. The information in an equipment manual is extremely valuable. If the manual is lost, call the manufacturer to obtain another one. Equipment manuals should be filed where they can be retrieved easily.

Maintenance and Service Contracts

Equipment suppliers provide standard maintenance contracts when office equipment is purchased. A **maintenance contract** specifies when the equipment will be cleaned, checked for worn parts, and repaired. A standard maintenance contract may include regular checkups as well as emergency repairs.

In addition, some suppliers offer a **service contract,** which covers services that are not included under the standard maintenance agreement. For example, a service contract may cover emergency repairs if they are not covered under standard maintenance. In some cases, service contracts are combined with maintenance contracts in one document.

It is important to keep track of all maintenance performed on your equipment. Many offices keep a maintenance log, where staff members record the date and purpose of each service call. This log is helpful in identifying whether equipment should be replaced because of its need for frequent servicing.

Troubleshooting

You can call a service supplier the minute a piece of equipment stops functioning properly, but you can also take steps to see whether you can determine and correct the problem yourself. This process is called **troubleshooting.** Resolving the problem can save you the cost of a service call that may not be covered by your standard agreement.

The first step in troubleshooting is to eliminate possible simple causes of a problem. For example, if the machine is powered by electricity, make sure that it is plugged into a functioning outlet and that it is turned on. Are all doors and other openings in their correct positions? Are all machine connections firmly in place?

If you cannot discover a simple cause for the problem, it is time to test the machine to determine what it is failing to do. In the case of a malfunctioning photocopier, for example, try making a copy, and note the response. Write down any error messages the machine provides.

Next consult the equipment manual. Many manuals devote a section to troubleshooting. If you cannot find the solution after reading the manual, call the manufacturer or the place of purchase for additional assistance. Be prepared to explain the steps you have already taken toward resolving the problem.

Equipment Inventory

Each piece of equipment is an asset of a business. It is part of the business's net worth and should be listed on the medical practice's balance sheet. Therefore, taking inventory of office equipment provides relevant information for the practice's money manager. It may also indicate whether old machinery is due for replacement.

There is no set format for taking an office equipment inventory. Figure 5-9 shows one example. Many offices use a master inventory sheet to survey all equipment at a glance. The master sheet usually includes such general information as equipment names and the quantity of each type of equipment.

Many offices also keep more detailed information about each individual piece of equipment in files or on a single sheet of paper. Detailed information may include the following:

- Name of the equipment, including the brand name
- Brief description of the equipment
- Model number and registration number
- Date of purchase

EQUIPMENT INVENTORY

ITEM	PURCHASE DATE	PURCHASE PRICE
1. TotalOffice oak desk	10/15/94	$295.00
2. TotalOffice rolling desk chair	10/15/94	$119.00
3. TotalOffice 4-drawer file cabinet	1/28/95	$150.00
4. TotalOffice 2-drawer file cabinet	1/28/95	$100.00
5. HYtech Pentium 100 computer	5/29/96	$1150.00
6. HYtech 14-inch monitor	5/29/96	$200.00

Figure 5-9. An equipment inventory sheet includes equipment names and the quantity of each type of equipment.

- Place of purchase, including contact information
- Estimated life of the product
- Product warranty
- Maintenance and service contracts

All equipment inventories should be updated periodically.

Summary

In many ways, state-of-the-art office equipment is as important for a medical office as its medical equipment. Although every office does not have the same equipment, common machines include telephones, computers, pagers, fax machines, dictation-transcription equipment, photocopiers, adding machines and calculators, postage meters, check writers, paper shredders, and microfilm or microfiche readers.

As a medical assistant, you may be expected not only to operate this equipment but also to help make purchasing decisions by researching various options. This research includes obtaining information about product features, warranties, and maintenance. Yet another decision is whether to lease or buy the equipment.

Equipment is an asset for a medical office. The office staff needs to maintain a comprehensive inventory of the products leased and purchased. It is important to keep up to date with new technologies that will help the administrative office function smoothly and efficiently.

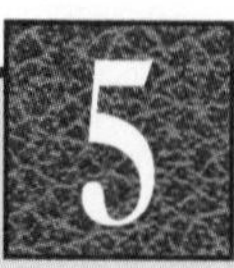

Chapter Review

Discussion Questions

1. How does office equipment help today's medical practice function efficiently? Provide several examples.
2. Compare and contrast leasing and buying a new piece of office equipment. When does it make sense to lease rather than buy?
3. What are some features of a standard product warranty?

Critical Thinking Questions

1. Summarize the skills a medical assistant needs to oversee staff training on all office equipment.
2. Explain how you would justify the purchase of a new photocopier to your office manager.
3. Explain how you would troubleshoot an electronic typewriter that seems not to be working.

Application Activities

1. Your office frequently uses temporary employees to help with copying. The office manager has asked you to prepare written directions to post by the photocopier as a reference for these employees. Write the directions on a sheet of paper. Assume that the person reading the directions has never used a photocopier. Include somewhere in the directions how to handle paper clips and staples.
2. Develop a script for the automated menu that will be used with your medical practice's new voice mail system. Remember to include the name of your practice and the different choices for callers, including an emergency response option.
3. Assume that you work in a busy internal medicine group practice with four doctors. Your supervisor has asked you to look into purchasing a new fax machine for the office. Using office supply catalogs, compare and contrast three models of fax machines. Make a chart outlining the features of each and giving a short explanation of how each feature would or would not benefit the practice. Write a paragraph explaining which of the three models you would recommend and why.

Further Readings

LeGallee, Julie. "Typewriters: Are Computers Driving Them to Pasture?" *The Office,* August 1993, 16.

Maynard, Roberta. "The Facts About Your Fax Costs." *Nation's Business,* August 1995, 10.

McCabe, Susan. "Office Equipment: Making Your Dealer Your Ally." *Managing Office Technology,* December 1995, 18.

Romei, Laura K. "Shredders: The Other Cutting-Edge Technology." *Managing Office Technology,* November 1995, 66.

Sheehan, Christopher. "Cutting Cost With Copier Controls." *The Office,* February 1993, 22.

Trembly, Ara C. "Multifunction Market Set to Explode." *Managing Office Technology,* June 1994, 15.

Willen, Janet L. "Should You Lease Office Equipment?" *Nation's Business,* May 1995, 59.

Using Computers in the Office

CHAPTER OUTLINE

- The Computer Revolution
- Types of Computers
- Components of the Computer
- Using Computer Software
- Selecting Computer Equipment
- Security in the Computerized Office
- Computer System Care and Maintenance
- Computers of the Future

OBJECTIVES

After completing Chapter 6, you will be able to:

- List and describe common types of computers.
- Identify computer hardware and software components and explain the functions of each.
- Describe the types of computer software commonly used in the medical office.
- Discuss how to select computer equipment for the medical office.
- Explain the importance of security measures for computerized medical records.
- Describe the basic care and maintenance of computer equipment.
- Identify new advances in computer technology and explain their importance to the medical office.

AREAS OF COMPETENCE

1997 ROLE DELINEATION STUDY

GENERAL (Transdisciplinary)

Operational Functions

- Evaluate and recommend equipment and supplies
- Apply computer techniques to support office operations

Key Terms

CD-ROM
central processing unit (CPU)
cursor
database
dot matrix printer
electronic mail
hard copy
hardware
icon
ink-jet printer
Internet
laser printer
modem
motherboard
multimedia
multitasking
network
random-access memory (RAM)
read-only memory (ROM)
scanner
screen saver
software
tower case
tutorial

The Computer Revolution

Over the past decade computers have revolutionized the way we live and work. Computers make many tasks easier because they process information with great speed and accuracy. They are also capable of storing vast amounts of information in a small space.

In today's world computer skills are essential for most career choices, and medical assisting is no exception. Medical practices that have not yet made the switch to a computerized practice will most likely do so in the near future. As a medical assistant, you need to understand the fundamentals of computers and their uses. This knowledge will enable you to perform many office tasks with ease. In addition, the more you know about computers, the more likely you will be able to solve or avoid computer problems.

Types of Computers

Three basic types of computers are used today: mainframe computers, minicomputers, and personal computers. Each type of computer is suitable for a certain type of work in a particular kind of workplace.

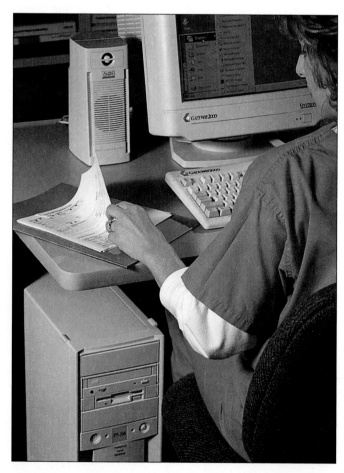

Figure 6-1. Offices can free up much-needed desktop space by using computers in tower cases, which can be kept on the floor.

Mainframe Computers

Mainframes are the largest and most expensive of the three types of computers. Often used by government facilities and large institutions, including universities and hospitals, mainframes can process and store huge quantities of information.

Minicomputers

Minicomputers are smaller than mainframes but larger than personal computers. Minicomputers have traditionally been used in network settings. A **network** is a system that links several computers together. In this environment a minicomputer typically functions as a server, which is a computer used as a centralized storage location for shared information. Today, however, personal computers are becoming as powerful as minicomputers and may eventually replace them.

Personal Computers

Also called microcomputers, personal computers can be found in homes, offices, and schools. They are ideal for these settings because they are small, self-contained units. Because users have different needs, personal computers are available in three different types: desktop, notebook, and palmtop.

Desktop. The most common type of personal computer, a desktop model fits easily on a desk or other flat surface. The system unit of many newer desktop models is housed in a **tower case,** which extends vertically instead of horizontally. A tower case—often placed on the floor next to the desk—allows more surface area at the workstation (see Figure 6-1). Both large and small medical offices commonly use desktop computers.

Notebook. A notebook computer (also called a laptop) is small—about the size of a thick magazine—and weighs only a few pounds. Notebooks operate either on battery power or on an AC adapter. As advances in technology make notebooks smaller, more powerful, and less expensive, they are expected to become more popular. Their portability makes them especially convenient for people who travel on business. Using notebook computers, physicians and other health-care professionals can communicate with the medical office computer from their homes or any other location.

Palmtop. As the name suggests, a palmtop computer is about the size of your palm and is extremely light. Because they are so small, palmtops generally cannot perform all the functions of desktop or even notebook computers. The keyboard of a palmtop does not contain all the extra function keys found on a standard keyboard, and the keys themselves are quite small. For these reasons, palmtops are usually not used for such tasks as word processing. They may, however, be useful for health-care professionals who need to enter patient data from locations outside the medical office.

Components of the Computer

Computer components are divided into hardware and software. **Hardware** comprises the physical components of a computer system, including the monitor, keyboard, and printer. **Software** is a set of instructions, or a program, that tells the computer what to do. Software includes both the operating system and applications that run on the operating system.

Hardware

The computer's hardware serves four main functions: inputting data, processing data, storing data, and outputting data. Various hardware components are needed to perform each of these functions.

Input Devices. For a computer to handle information, such as patient records, the data must first be entered, or input. Several types of input devices may be used to enter data into the computer. Keyboards, pointing devices, modems, and scanners are input devices. After information is entered into the computer, it can be displayed on the monitor, processed, or stored.

Keyboard. The keyboard is the most common input device. The main part of a keyboard resembles a typewriter. Most keyboards have several additional keys, however. A typical keyboard contains the following:

- Standard typewriter keys to enter letters, numbers, symbols, and punctuation marks
- Separate numerical keypad for entering numbers faster and more easily
- Arrow keys to move the **cursor,** a blinking line or cube on the computer screen showing where the next character that is keyed will appear
- Function keys to perform such tasks as saving and printing files

When you use the keyboard, it is important to position your hands properly to avoid injury. "Diseases and Disorders" provides tips for preventing and coping with carpal tunnel syndrome, a condition resulting from repetitive motion.

Pointing Device. Many of today's sophisticated software programs need not only a keyboard but also a pointing device to enter information into the computer. When you move the pointing device, an arrow appears. You can point and click the arrow on various buttons that appear on the screen. The three types of pointing devices are the mouse, the trackball, and the touch pad.

1. A mouse, the most common pointing device, has two or three buttons on top and a rolling ball on the bottom. You move the mouse across a mouse pad until the arrow points at the desired button or object on the screen. Then, as shown in Figure 6-3, you push one of the buttons on the mouse to access a function, such as opening a file.
2. A trackball is similar to a mouse except that the rolling ball is on the top of the device instead of on the bottom. Rather than pushing a trackball across a pad, you roll the ball with your fingers while the trackball remains stationary.
3. A touch pad is the newest type of pointing device and is becoming popular, especially on notebook computers. It is a small, flat device that is highly sensitive to the touch. To move the arrow on the screen, you simply slide your finger across the touch pad. To click on an item, you push a button similar to that on a mouse or trackball, or you tap your finger on the touch pad.

Modem. This term is a shortened form of the words *modulator-demodulator.* A **modem** is a device used to transfer information from one computer to another over telephone lines. Because modems allow information to be transferred both to and from a computer, they are considered input/output devices. The speed at which a modem transfers data is called the baud rate. Although the current standard modem speed is 28,800 baud, modem speeds are continually being improved. Modems are essential for any medical office that needs to transfer files electronically, as when submitting insurance claim forms.

An advanced type of modem is a fax modem. This device allows the computer to send and receive files much as a fax machine does. A fax modem is not quite as versatile as a regular fax machine, however. The information being sent must first be input into the computer. You could not, for example, use a fax modem to send a patient record with handwritten notes on it.

Scanner. A **scanner** is a device used to input printed matter and convert it into a format that can be read by the computer. Scanners are useful in the medical office because patient reports from another doctor, a hospital, or another outside source can be easily entered into the computer. Using a scanner is much faster than keyboarding, or inputting the information with a keyboard. Following are three types of scanners that are available.

- Handheld scanners are generally the least expensive but are more difficult to use and produce lower-quality results than the other two types.
- A single-sheet scanner feeds one sheet of paper through at a time and looks similar to a single-sheet printer.
- A flatbed scanner is the most expensive type of scanner but is the easiest to use and produces the highest-quality input. It works much like a small photocopier: the paper lies flat and still on a glass surface while the machine scans it.

Processing Devices. There are two major processing components inside the system unit, or computer cabinet. The **motherboard** is the main circuit board that controls the other components in the system. The **central processing unit (CPU),** or microprocessor, is the primary computer chip responsible for interpreting and executing programs.

DISEASES AND DISORDERS

Carpal Tunnel Syndrome

As the number of computers used in the home and workplace has escalated in recent years, the number of cases of carpal tunnel syndrome has also risen dramatically. Carpal tunnel syndrome is a hand disorder that is often associated with computer use. The term for this condition comes from the name for a canal (the carpal tunnel) located in the wrist. Several tendons pass through this tunnel, allowing the hand to open and close.

Carpal tunnel syndrome results from repetitive motion, such as keyboarding, for hours at a time. This motion may cause swelling to develop around the tendons and carpal tunnel. The swelling compresses the nerve. The people most likely to develop carpal tunnel syndrome are workers whose jobs require them to perform repetitive hand and finger motions.

Symptoms

The symptoms associated with carpal tunnel syndrome include the following:

- Tingling or burning in the hands or fingers
- Weakness or numbness in the hands or fingers
- Difficulty opening or closing the hands
- Pain that stems from the wrist and travels up the arm

Tips for Prevention

If you use a keyboard for extended periods, you should practice proper techniques to prevent carpal tunnel syndrome.

1. While seated, hold your arms relaxed at your sides, and check to make sure that your keyboard is positioned slightly higher than your elbows. As you input, keep your elbows at your sides, and relax your shoulders (see Figure 6-2).
2. Use only your fingers to press keys, and do not use more pressure than necessary. Use a wrist rest, and keep your wrists relaxed and straight.
3. When you need to strike difficult-to-reach keys, move your whole hand rather than stretching your fingers. When you need to press two keys at the same time, such as "Control" and "F1," use two hands.
4. Try to break up long periods of keyboard work with other tasks that do not require computer use.

Tips for Relieving Symptoms

If you have symptoms of carpal tunnel syndrome, try these suggestions for relief.

- Elevate your arms.
- Wear a splint on the hand and forearm.
- Discuss your symptoms with a physician, who may prescribe medication.

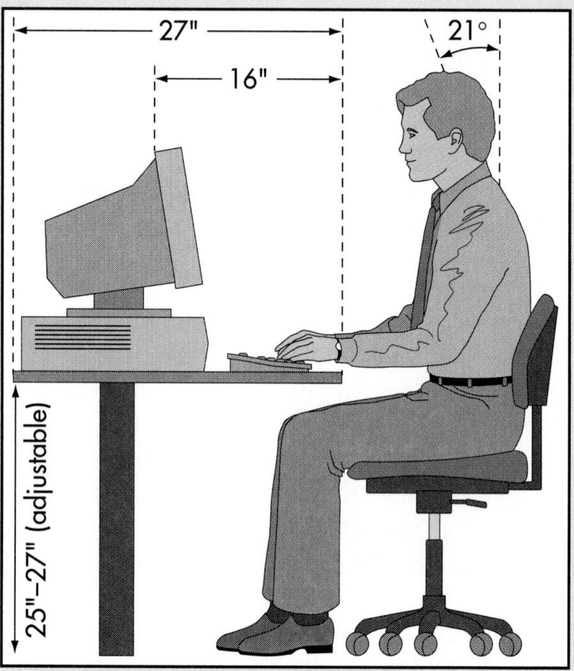

Figure 6-2. Maintaining proper posture and hand positions helps to avoid injury when keyboarding.

How quickly the computer processes information depends on the type of microprocessor and its speed, which is measured in megahertz (MHz). Most microprocessors are known by a number, such as 486. A popular microprocessor is the Intel Pentium. Pentium microprocessors come in many common speeds, including 133, 150, and 166 MHz.

Storage Devices. One of the main tasks of a computer is to store information for later retrieval. The computer uses memory to store information either temporarily or permanently. Several types of drives are used for permanent information storage.

Memory. Computers use two types of memory to store data: **random-access memory (RAM)** and read-only memory (ROM). RAM is temporary, or programmable, memory. While you are working on a software program, the computer is accessing RAM. In general, the more RAM that is available, the faster the computer will perform. As software programs become more sophisticated, they require more RAM. Only a few years ago, 4 megabytes (MB) of RAM was the minimum amount needed to run most programs. (Megabytes are a measurement of memory space.) Today, however, many applications require much more RAM.

Read-only memory (ROM) is permanent memory. The computer can read it, but you cannot make changes to it. The purpose of ROM is to provide the basic operating instructions the computer needs to function.

Hard Disk Drive. The hard disk drive is where informa-

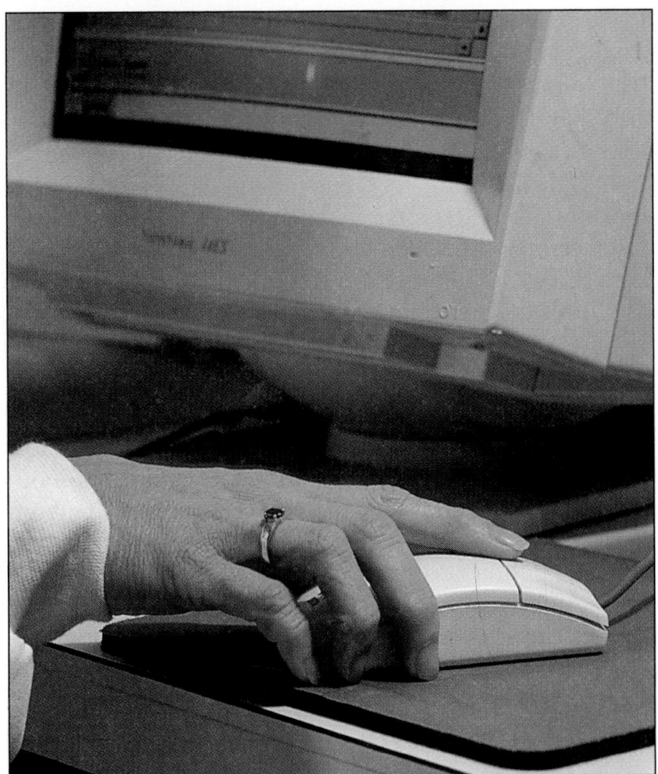

Figure 6-3. Using a mouse, you can point and click to access a variety of functions.

tion is stored permanently for later retrieval. Software programs and important data are usually stored on the hard disk for quick and easy access. The amount of hard disk space needed to store software programs is increasing rapidly. The more software programs you want to store, the larger the hard disk you will need. Some computers have a 500- or 850-MB hard disk. Many computers have hard disk capacity of 1.6 gigabytes (GB), 2.0 GB, or more. (One gigabyte equals 1000 megabytes.)

Diskette Drive. This device can read from and write to diskettes (also called disks). The two standard diskette formats are 5¼-inch disks, which are flexible, and 3½-inch disks, which are rigid. Because the 3½-inch disks are more compact, can store more information, and are sturdier than the 5¼-inch disks, they have become more popular.

CD-ROM Drive. CD-ROMs look just like audio compact discs, but they contain software programs. The term **CD-ROM** stands for "compact disc—read-only memory." The main advantage of a CD-ROM over a diskette is its ability to store huge amounts of data.

CD-ROM drives have become standard equipment on most personal computers. Although many software packages are available on both CD-ROM and diskettes, some large programs are available only on CD-ROM. These programs include multimedia applications such as medical encyclopedias. **Multimedia** refers to software that uses more than one medium—such as graphics, sound, and text—to convey information.

Tape Drive. This storage device is used to back up (make a copy of) the files on the hard disk. The information is copied onto magnetic tapes that look similar to audiotapes. If the hard drive malfunctions, you will have a copy of the information on these tapes. It is possible to back up the information onto diskettes. Most hard disks, however, contain so much information that a large number of diskettes would be required to back up all the data. With most tape drives, the entire contents of the hard disk can be stored on one or two tapes. Store these tapes at night in a fireproof container.

Output Devices. Output devices are used to display information after it has been processed. A monitor and a printer are two output devices needed in the medical office.

Monitor. A computer monitor looks like a television screen. It displays the information that is currently active, such as a word processing document. Monitors are available in both color and monochrome (amber, green, or white against a black background). A color monitor is required to run many software programs, including multimedia applications.

Color monitors vary in the number of colors they can display and in the resolution of the images. *Resolution* refers to the crispness of the images and is measured in dot pitch. The lower the dot pitch, the higher the resolution. For example, a monitor with a 0.26 dot pitch displays sharper images than a monitor with a 0.39 dot pitch. Using a high-resolution monitor can help you avoid eye strain.

Printer. A printer is required to produce a **hard copy,** which is a readable paper copy or printout of information (see Figure 6-4). You will need a printer to print out correspondence, patient reports, bills, insurance claims, and other documents. Printer resolution is noted in terms of dots per inch (dpi). The higher the dpi, the better the

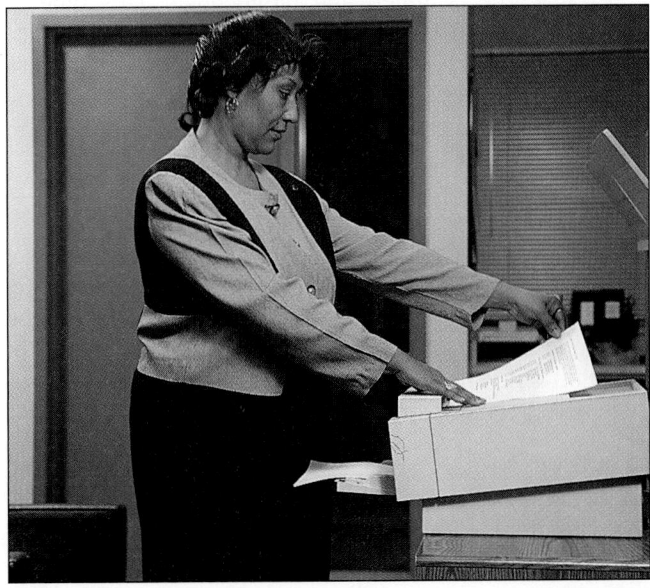

Figure 6-4. You may need to print out hard copies of documents to send to patients, vendors, insurance companies, or other doctors' offices.

print quality. Printer output varies, depending on the type of printer and the model. The three most commonly used printers are dot matrix, ink-jet, and laser.

1. **Dot matrix printers** create characters by placing a series of tiny dots next to one another. The dot matrix printer is the only type that is an impact printer, which means that it makes an impression on the paper as it prints. Although it is the least expensive of the three types, the dot matrix printer is slower and noisier and produces a lower-quality output than the other types. Because it is an impact printer, however, it is the only type that is capable of producing multiple copies with carbon paper or other multicopy forms.
2. **Ink-jet printers** also form characters using a series of dots, but they are nonimpact printers in which the dots are created by tiny drops of ink. Many ink-jet printers are capable of printing in both black and color. Because of their high-quality output and affordable prices, ink-jet printers are popular for home and small-office use.
3. **Laser printers** are high-resolution printers that use a technology similar to that of photocopiers. Of the three printer types, laser printers are the fastest and produce the highest-quality output. Laser printers are more expensive than dot matrix or ink-jet printers. Prices have dropped significantly over the years, however, so laser printers may be affordable even for small medical offices.

Because each type of printer has advantages and disadvantages, some medical offices may purchase more than one type. For example, a medical office may have a dot matrix printer for creating internal memos and multipage insurance forms and a laser printer for creating documents whose quality resembles that of typeset documents.

A current trend in printers is the "all-in-one" model, which functions not only as an ink-jet printer but also as a fax machine, scanner, and photocopier. This type of machine may be convenient for a small medical office that requires each of these functions but does not have space for four separate devices. In addition, purchasing an all-in-one unit is usually more economical than purchasing the machines separately.

Software

Computer software is generally divided into two categories: operating system and application software. The operating system controls the computer's operation. Application software allows you to perform specific tasks, such as scheduling appointments.

Operating System. When you turn on a computer, the operating system starts working, providing instructions the computer needs to function. Because most medical practices use IBM-compatible personal computers, the operating systems discussed here are DOS (disk operating system) and Microsoft Windows and Windows 95. IBM-compatible computers are most suitable for businesses that use computers primarily to manipulate words. Apple computers are used by businesses, such as advertising agencies or design firms, that are extensively involved in graphics, visual images, or desktop publishing.

DOS. DOS is the original operating system created for IBM and IBM-compatible computers. It uses a command line interface—you must learn and use commands to perform certain tasks. For example, to copy a file from a hard drive to a diskette drive, you must type a command that instructs the computer to copy the file.

Windows. This operating system employs a graphical user interface (GUI) instead of a command line interface. With a GUI, menu choices are identified by **icons,** or graphic symbols. For example, the "Print" command is usually identified by a button with a tiny illustration of a printer on it. To print a document, you move the pointing device until the arrow is on the printer icon and then click the button.

An important advantage of the Windows operating system over DOS is that it is easier to learn because you do not have to remember commands. Another benefit of Windows is that it is a **multitasking** system—users can run two or more software programs simultaneously. You could, for example, enter patient information into a **database,** a collection of records created and stored on the computer, while a word processing program is running in the background. DOS is not a multitasking system; you can run only one application at a time.

Windows 95. This operating system, introduced in 1995, is similar to Windows but has many additional features (see Figure 6-5). In most businesses, Windows 95 is quickly becoming the standard operating system for IBM and IBM-compatible computers. Most new computers are shipped with Windows 95 preinstalled, and many software programs are being written to run exclusively under this operating system.

Applications. Most of the software sold in stores is application software. It is used for a specific purpose, or application. Word processing, database, and accounting software are just a few examples of the wide variety of applications available.

Using Computer Software

Computer software has been developed for nearly every office function imaginable. Using software, you can complete tasks with greater speed, accuracy, and ease than with a manual system. Learning how to use the software correctly, however, is the key to getting the most out of your computer system.

Word Processing

As in any office, word processing is a common computer application in the medical office. It has replaced the typewriter for writing correspondence and reports,

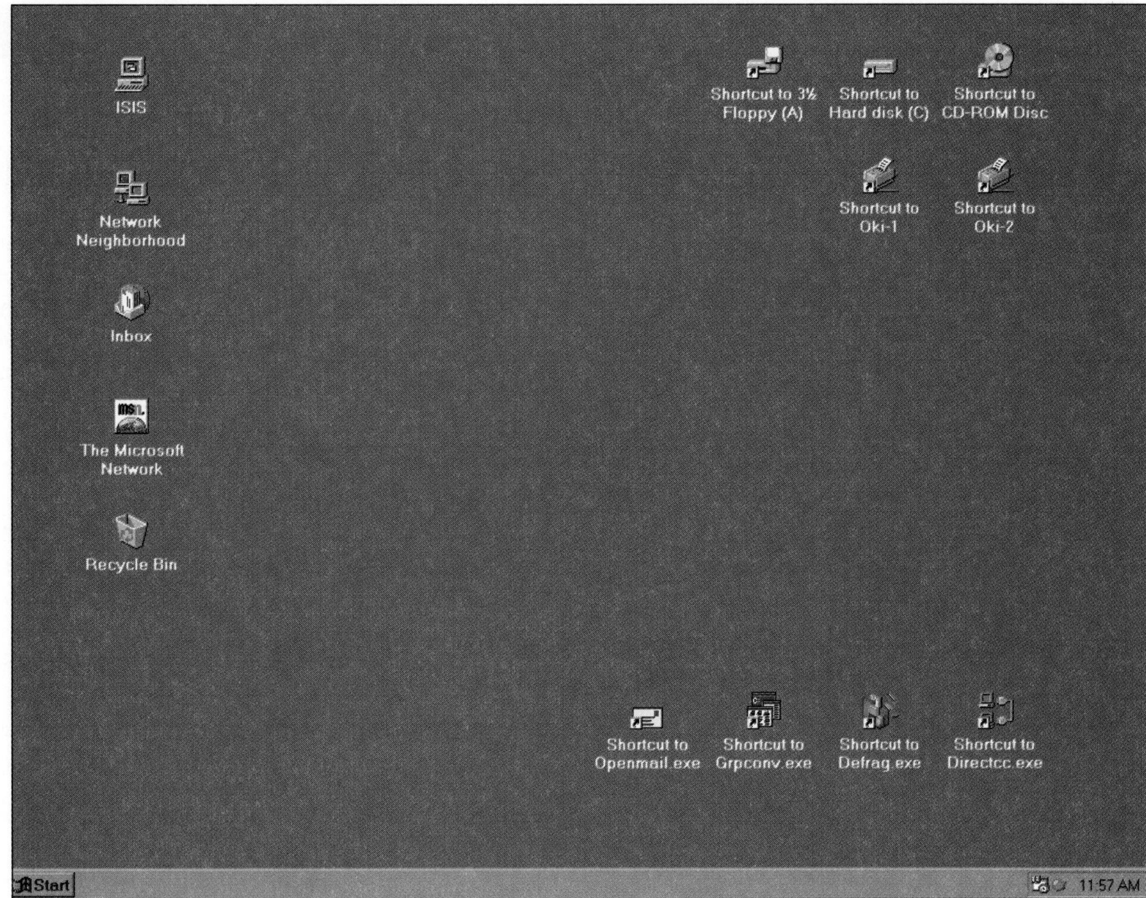

Figure 6-5. The Windows 95 operating system employs a graphical user interface. Icons identify programs or other menu choices.

transcribing physicians' notes, and performing many other functions. Correcting errors is easy on a word processor, and you can save documents for later retrieval and modification. Procedure 6-1 shows you how to use a word processing program to create a form letter. A form letter can be merged with a patient mailing list to create letters that are personalized with patients' names.

Database Management

As mentioned earlier, a database is a collection of records created and stored on a computer. In a medical office, databases are used to store patient records, such as billing information, medical chart data, and insurance company facts. These records can be sorted and retrieved in many ways and for a variety of purposes. You may be asked to find, add to, or modify information in a database. For example, you might use a database to determine all the patients covered by a particular insurance company.

Accounting and Billing

Accounting and billing software is extremely useful in an office environment. It enables you to perform many tasks, including keeping track of patients' accounts, creating billing statements, preparing financial reports, and maintaining tax records. (You will learn more about accounting and billing functions in Chapters 17 and 18.)

Appointment Scheduling

Instead of writing in an appointment book, you can use software to schedule appointments. Some scheduling packages allow you to enter patient preferences, such as day of the week and time, and then to list available appointments based on that information. If the office system is on a network, scheduling software is particularly valuable, because more than one user can access the appointment schedule at a time.

Electronic Transactions

Using a computer equipped with a modem and communications software, you can perform several types of electronic transactions. This technology enables you to send and receive information instantaneously rather than waiting the days or weeks required for regular mail. Common electronic transactions include sending insurance claims and communicating with other computer users.

Sending Insurance Claims. Insurance claims can be submitted directly from the medical office to an insur-

PROCEDURE 6-1

Creating a Form Letter

Objective: To use a word processing program to create a form letter

Materials: Computer equipped with a word processing program, printer, form letter to be input

Method

1. Turn on the computer. Select the word processing program you want to use.
2. Use the keyboard to begin entering text into a new document.
3. To edit text, press the arrow keys to move the cursor to the position at which you want to insert or delete characters, and enter the text. Use the "Insert" mode to add characters or the "Typeover" mode to type over and replace existing text.
4. To delete text, position the cursor to the left of the characters to be deleted and press the "Delete" key. Alternatively, you can place the cursor to the right of the characters to be deleted and press the "Backspace" key (the left-pointing arrow usually found at the top right corner of the keyboard).
5. If you need to move an entire block of text, you must begin by highlighting it. In most Windows-based programs, you first click the mouse at the beginning of the text to be highlighted. Then you hold down the left mouse button, drag the mouse to the end of the block of text, and release your finger from the mouse. The text should now be highlighted. Choose the button or command for cutting text. Then move the cursor to the place where you want to move the text, and select the button or command for retrieving or pasting text.
6. As you input the letter, it is important to save your work every 15 minutes or so. Some programs do this automatically. If yours does not, use the "Save" command or button to save the file. Be sure to save the file again when you have completed the letter.
7. Print the letter using the "Print" command or button.

ance company. This procedure enables claims to be processed quickly and efficiently. (Processing insurance claims is discussed in Chapter 15.)

Communicating. The ability to communicate and share information with other computer users and systems is important in many medical offices. This communication may take place through electronic mail, on-line services, and the Internet. "Tips for the Office" gives ideas for saving time and money while you are on-line.

Electronic Mail. Commonly known as E-mail, **electronic mail** is a method of sending and receiving messages through a network. With E-mail, you can communicate with computer users in your own office, across town, or on the other side of the world.

On-Line Services. These services, such as America Online and CompuServe, provide a means for health-care professionals to communicate with one another. Most on-line services contain forums that offer information and discussion groups focusing on a wide range of medical topics. Health-care workers can learn about the latest medical research and technology or exchange ideas with others in their field. In addition, some on-line services provide access to medical databases such as MEDLINE, created by the National Library of Medicine. Users can search MEDLINE for records and abstracts from thousands of medical journals from around the world. Most on-line services also offer access to the Internet.

Internet. The **Internet** is a global network of computers. Through the Internet, you can communicate with millions of computer users around the world. In addition, many large medical facilities, universities, and other organizations—such as the National Institutes of Health and the Centers for Disease Control and Prevention—provide medical resources, databases, and other information on the Internet. Users can visit such Internet sites as the Virtual Hospital, sponsored by the University of Iowa, and the Cyberspace Hospital, sponsored by the National University of Singapore. At these sites you may find multimedia textbooks, presentations, and links to other related sites on the Internet. Table 6-1 describes these and other popular medical resources available on the Internet.

Research

The advent of CD-ROM technology has revolutionized the world of research. Not only can an immense amount of information be contained on one compact disc, but the CD-ROM usually provides additional information in the form of videos and sound (see Figure 6-6). A CD-ROM encyclopedia, for example, might also provide spoken pronunciations of medical terms. This type of software may help patients—especially children—understand the human body as well as various medical conditions.

Software Training

Software programs are often quite complex. Most people need a period of training before they feel comfortable using the application. Several methods of training—some from outside sources and some provided by the software manufacturer—are available.

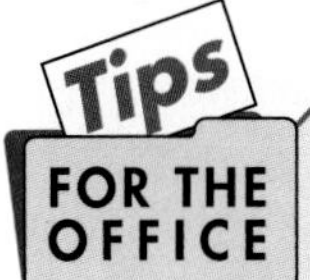

Saving Time and Money On-Line

If the medical office where you work is computerized, the system most likely has a modem for sending E-mail and transferring files electronically. The modem may also be used to access various on-line services and the Internet, a global network of computers. If this access is not currently available in the medical office, it probably will be in the near future. You may even be asked to help choose an on-line service or Internet provider for the office.

Having access to an on-line service and the Internet is worthwhile for many medical offices. Unless the people using these services are careful, however, this access can be very costly. In general, the more time you spend on-line, the more expensive the service becomes. For this reason, knowing how to use these communications systems wisely is a valuable asset.

Choosing an On-Line Service

If you have the opportunity to help select an on-line service for the office, compare several services for the following:

1. Free trial membership. Many services offer a free 1-month membership during which you can try out the service. The trial periods enable office staff members to test several services to determine which one best suits their needs.
2. Local access telephone number. Make sure the service provides an access number within the local dialing area of the office. If it does not, the office will be charged long-distance telephone rates each time someone goes on-line. These fees are separate from the on-line service's rates and can add up quickly.
3. Volume discount plan. If the office will be using the on-line service often, it is a good idea to find a provider that offers a discount for frequent usage. Rather than charging a per-hour rate over the first 5 hours of use, for example, these services charge a flat rate for 20 or 30 hours of use per month. Some even offer unlimited use for a flat rate.
4. Extra fees. Although access to most of the information found in on-line services is included in the membership fee, some providers charge extra for premium or extended services. If you want to read or print out the full text of an article in a medical journal, for example, some providers charge an additional fee. Make sure you consider these extra fees when comparing costs of on-line services.
5. Availability of health-care information. Some on-line services provide discussion groups (commonly known as chat rooms) and resources that would be useful to the medical office. Other services may not offer as much relevant information. By comparing several services, you can determine which one provides the resources your office needs most.

Sending and Receiving E-Mail

When using E-mail, follow these guidelines to use your on-line time efficiently.

1. Compose messages off-line. Most services allow you to write E-mail messages before you actually go on-line. When you have finished writing the message, you simply log onto the service and click a button to send the E-mail. This technique will save a great deal of on-line time, especially if you must frequently send lengthy messages.
2. Read messages off-line. When you receive an E-mail message, you do not have to read it immediately. You will spend less time on-line if you save the message on the hard disk to read or print out later.
3. Use computerized address books. As part of the E-mail system, most services provide an on-line address book in which you can store frequently used E-mail addresses. Instead of wasting time searching for an E-mail address in a standard card file, you simply click on the person's name in the address book, and the mail is automatically sent to that person. You can also use the address book to send the same E-mail message to several people at once.

Doing Research

Although a great deal of valuable information can be found through on-line services and the Internet, searching for this information can be time-consuming. Here are some tips to make the most of your on-line time.

1. Use favorite places. Most on-line services allow you to keep a list of favorite places, or sites that you visit frequently. Instead of trying to remember a long Internet address or searching for the location of information you found last week, you simply add these sites to your favorite places and click on the name to visit them.
2. Refine your searches. Searching for *arthritis,* for example, might produce hundreds of references that you would have to read through to determine their relevance. Narrowing your search to *juvenile rheumatoid arthritis,* on the other hand, would produce fewer references but would provide more exact matches.
3. Download files. *Download* means to transfer a file to the hard disk. Instead of reading through information while you are on-line, you can usually save on-line time by downloading the files and retrieving them later (after you have logged off the on-line service).

Table 6-1

Medical Resources on the Internet

Organization	Web Address	Description
American Medical Association	http://www.ama-assn.org	News announcements and press releases; articles from *JAMA* and other AMA journals; links to other medicine-related Internet sites
Cyberspace Hospital	http://ch.nus.sg	Various departments and services, organized like a real hospital; medical bulletins; capability for users to search for information on medical topics
HealthWeb	http://hsinfo.ghsl.nwu.edu/healthweb/index.html	Starting point for searching the Internet because it contains links to a wide variety of medical resources
National Institutes of Health	http://www.nih.gov	Medical news and current events; press releases; biomedical information about health issues; scientific resources; links to Internet sites of related government agencies
National Library of Medicine	http://www.nlm.nih.gov	Internet site for world's largest biomedical library; research and development activities; connections to on-line medical information services
New England Journal of Medicine	http://www.nejm.org	Articles and abstracts; archives of past issues
U.S. Department of Health and Human Services	http://www.os.dhhs.gov	Programs and activities of this agency; links to divisions of agency, including Centers for Disease Control and Prevention, Food and Drug Administration, and National Institutes of Health
Virtual Hospital	http://vh.radiology.uiowa.edu	Information on a variety of health issues, medical resources, tutorials, and multimedia textbooks

Classes. Many computer vendors offer training classes for the software packages they sell. In addition, community colleges and high schools sometimes offer adult education classes for a variety of applications, including word processing and communications. These classes are usually at the beginner or intermediate level.

Tutorials. Many software packages come with a **tutorial,** which is a small program designed to give users an overall picture of the product and its functions. The tutorial usually provides a step-by-step walk-through and exercises in which you can try out your newly acquired knowledge.

Documentation. Nearly all software manufacturers provide some type of documentation with their programs. Documentation is usually in the form of written instruction manuals or on-line help that is accessed from within the program.

Manuals. Some manuals provide detailed information on how the software operates and may include an index and sections on troubleshooting and commonly asked questions. Other manuals may simply give installation instructions and brief information on program basics. This type of manual then refers users to the software's on-line help.

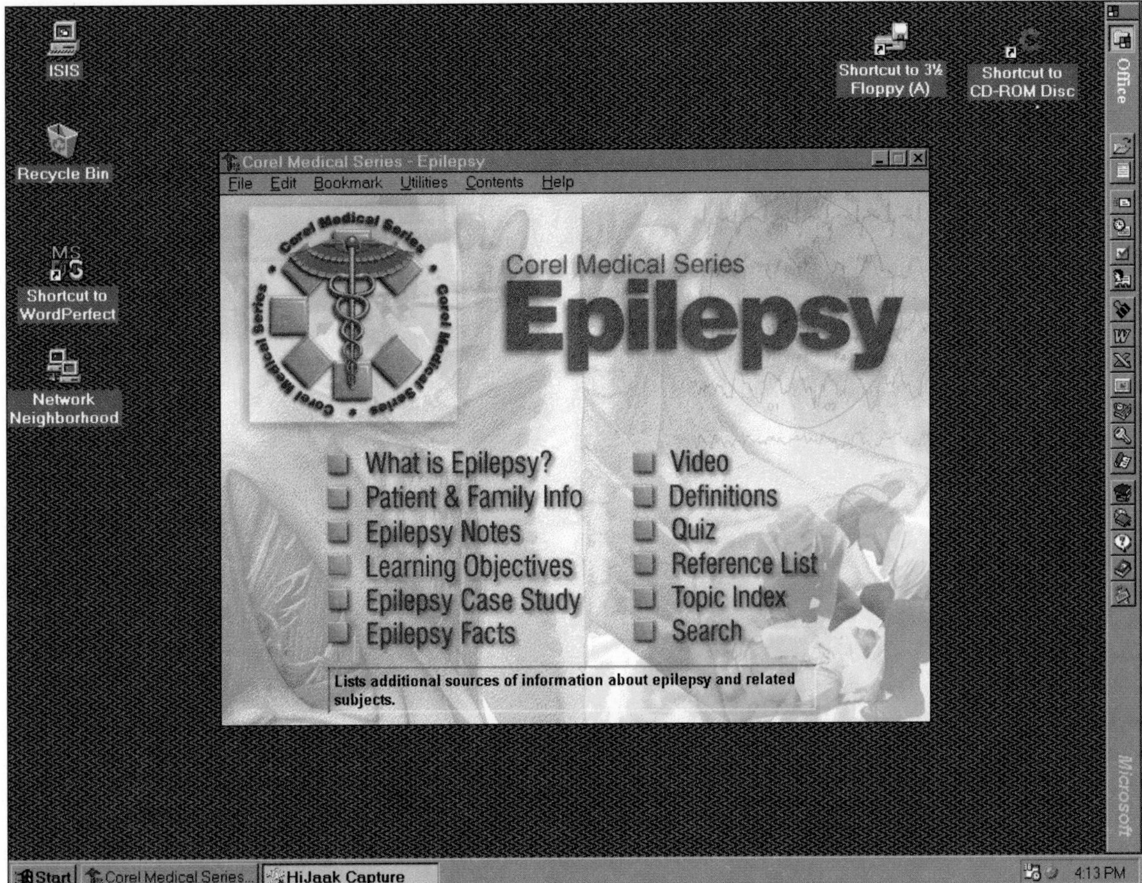

Figure 6-6. A CD-ROM provides features, such as video and sound, that are not possible in a standard printed book.

On-Line Help. In most software applications, users access the on-line help screen by clicking on a "Help" button or by pressing a certain function key, such as "F1." The on-line help usually provides a "Contents" section (shown in Figure 6-7), in which you can browse for topics. An Index, in which you can search for key words, is also provided.

Technical Support. More likely than not, you will eventually encounter a software problem that you cannot solve on your own. If you have had no luck searching through the software documentation, you probably need to call the technical support phone number (a toll-free number usually listed in the documentation). Most software companies provide a team of knowledgeable individuals who will try to solve your problem over the telephone. Before you call for technical support, make sure you have the software registration number handy. Also, you should be sitting at the computer and have it turned on so that you can follow the suggested steps.

Another instance in which you might use technical support is when you upgrade your software to a newer version. Many software companies automatically notify you about upgrades that become available. If you choose to upgrade your software, you may have questions about new functions, price, or installation procedures. A software company's technical support staff can help you.

Selecting Computer Equipment

Perhaps you are working in a medical office that is not yet computerized. If the decision is made to convert to a computerized system, you may be asked to help select equipment. Even if your office already uses computers, the system will probably need to be upgraded at some point to provide more functions. In either situation, you may be asked for your input in selecting software, adding a network, or choosing a vendor.

The first step for helping in the selection process is to learn as much as you can about hardware and software. You can get information by taking an introductory computer class at an adult school or community college; by reading computer magazines or books; or by talking to friends, relatives, or coworkers who use computers.

Converting to a Computerized Office

When an office converts from a manual system to computers, staff members should determine how the new computer system will be used. The objective is to obtain a system which not only meets current office needs but which can also be expanded and upgraded to meet future needs. To get the longest use from a computer system, a good general guideline is to buy the most advanced system possible within the allowed budget.

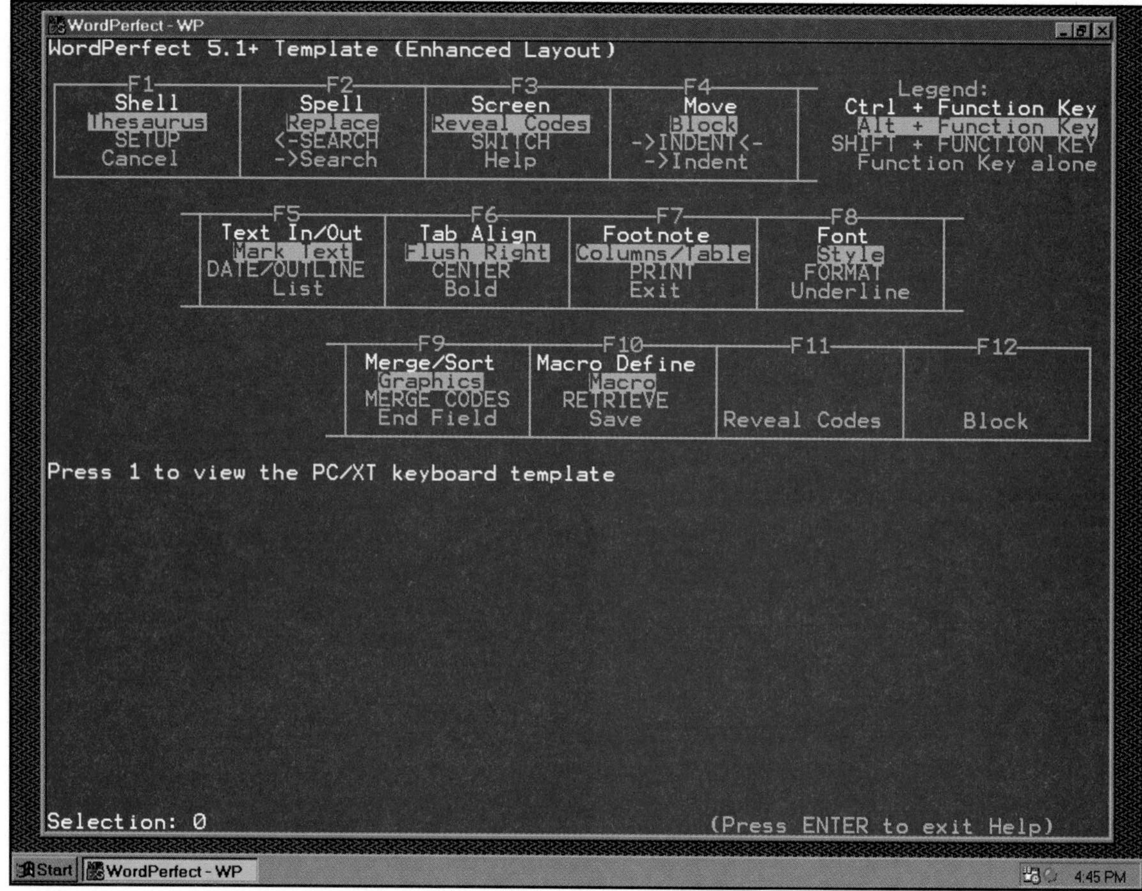

Figure 6-7. An on-line help system allows you to access helpful information when you are using a software program.

Upgrading the Office System

Computer hardware is changing and improving at such a rapid pace that a new system seems to become outdated almost as soon as it is purchased. In addition, more-advanced software is introduced every day, and this software requires more-advanced hardware to run. Consequently, an office system purchased only a year or two ago may need to be upgraded. Sometimes an upgrade simply requires replacement or addition of certain components. For instance, a laser printer can take the place of a dot matrix printer, or a CD-ROM drive can be added. In other cases, such a solution is not possible or cost-effective, so an entirely new system must be purchased.

Selecting Software

After a decision is made regarding the type of software needed, such as an accounting program, a specific product must be chosen. To make an informed decision, you can read software reviews in computer magazines or trade publications. You might also check with other medical offices to get opinions on software packages. A crucial step in selecting software is to make sure the office computer system meets the minimum system requirements listed on the software box. For example, a medical encyclopedia may require a 486 processor, Windows 95, 8 MB of RAM, 10 MB of available hard disk space, and a CD-ROM drive.

Adding a Network

There are several advantages to adding a network to the computer system in a medical office. A computer network enables users to share software programs and files and allows more than one person to work on the same patient's information at one time. While you are working on a patient's insurance claim, for example, another assistant might be inputting billing information. Some medical offices are virtually paperless. They use a highly sophisticated network with a notebook or desktop computer in every examination room (Figure 6-8). Doctors input information into patients' computerized charts. If a doctor is in her office and a patient is waiting, a staff member at the front desk sends an E-mail message to the doctor's desktop computer, and a beep sounds as an alert. Networks also allow large medical facilities to communicate with employees via E-mail. For instance, an internal memo about changes in office policies may be sent by E-mail to all employees.

Choosing a Vendor

When purchasing computer equipment, you should look for a reputable vendor who not only offers a reasonable price but also provides training, service, and technical support. A first step might be to check with personnel in other medical offices that use a computer system. Find

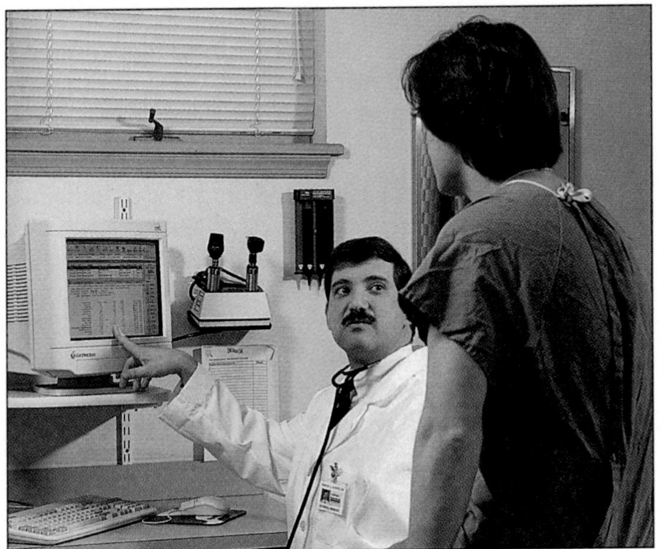

Figure 6-8. Some medical offices use highly sophisticated computer networks.

out which dealer they use and if they are satisfied with the system, salespeople, and support. You can also ask dealers for names of references—medical offices that have purchased systems from them. It is a good idea to get cost estimates from at least three vendors, and it is preferable to buy all hardware components from the same vendor.

Security in the Computerized Office

Although security measures are important in any office, they are especially important in a computerized medical office. Great care must be taken to safeguard confidential files, make backup copies on a regular basis, and prevent system contamination.

Safeguarding Confidential Files

Much of the information collected in a medical office is confidential. Just as with paper records, confidential information stored on the computer should be accessible only to authorized personnel. Two common ways to provide security in a computerized office are to employ passwords and to install an activity-monitoring system.

Passwords. In many hospitals and physicians' offices, each employee who is allowed access to computerized patient files is given a password. The employee must enter the password into the computer when using the files. If you are given a password, do not divulge it to anyone else unless your office manager asks you to do so. If an employee leaves or is fired, that person's password should be immediately erased from the system.

Activity-Monitoring Systems. In conjunction with passwords, some health-care facilities use a computer system that monitors user activity. Whenever someone accesses computer records, the system automatically keeps track of the user's name and the files that have been viewed or modified. In this way, problems or security breaches can be traced back to specific employees.

Making and Storing Backup Files

For securing important computer files, it is essential to routinely make diskette or tape backups of them (see Figure 6-9). How often backups are made varies among medical offices; your supervisor will tell you the policy for your office. Just as important as making the backups is storing them properly. Backup files should not be stored near the original files. Ideally, they should be kept outside the medical office—perhaps at the physician's home—so that they will be secure in case of fire, burglary, or other catastrophe at the office.

Preventing System Contamination

Another important security issue in the computerized medical office is computer viruses. Computer viruses are programs written specifically to contaminate the hard disk by damaging or destroying data.

One way that viruses can be passed from computer to computer is through shared diskettes that have been infected. Another way is through infected files retrieved from on-line services, the Internet, and electronic bulletin boards. Several software programs are available to detect

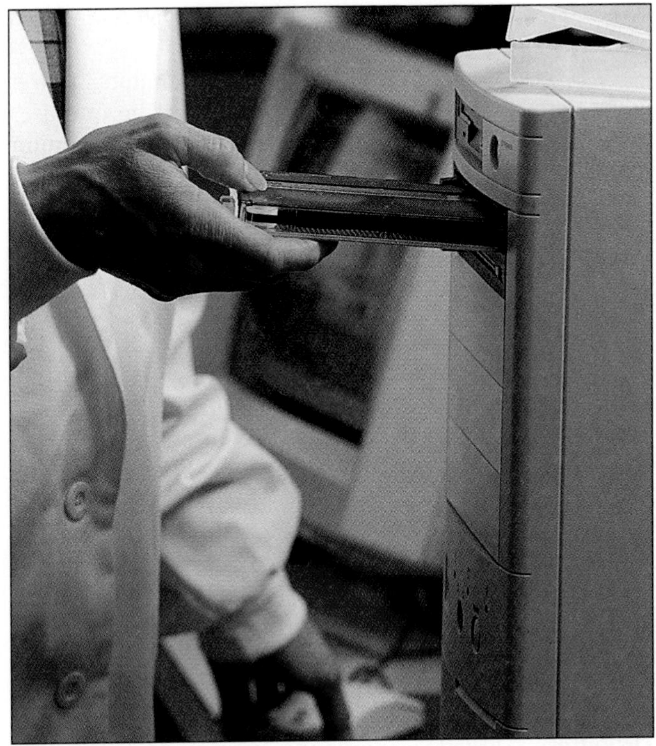

Figure 6-9. It is important to back up computer files and store them properly.

and correct computer viruses. Most are fairly inexpensive but provide an invaluable service.

Computer System Care and Maintenance

Like a car, a computer needs routine care and maintenance to stay in sound condition. The computer user's manual outlines the steps required. Also, a good general rule is not to eat or drink near the computer. Crumbs and spilled liquids can damage the system components and storage devices.

System Unit

The system unit should be placed in a well-ventilated location, with nothing blocking the fan in the back of the cabinet. To keep the system's delicate circuitry from being damaged by an electrical power surge, you should use a power strip with a surge protector. You plug the computer into the power strip, and then plug the power strip into the electrical outlet.

Monitor

The computer monitor needs to be protected from screen burn-in, which may happen if the same image stays on the computer screen for an extended time. To prevent burn-in, you can use a **screen saver,** which automatically changes the monitor display at short intervals or constantly shows moving images. Both the Windows and Windows 95 operating systems come equipped with screen savers. A wide variety of screen savers are also available as separate software packages.

To protect their screens, many newer monitors "power down" after a certain period of inactivity. If no one uses the computer for 30 minutes, for example, the monitor screen goes blank. To resume using the computer after the screen saver has been activated or the monitor has powered down, you simply touch any key or move the mouse.

Printer

Maintenance of a printer generally consists of replacing the ribbon, ink cartridge, or toner cartridge. You can tell when the ribbon or cartridge needs to be changed because the ink on your printouts becomes very light. Replacement is usually a simple process, described in the printer manual.

Information Storage Devices

Diskettes, CD-ROMs, and magnetic tapes are highly sensitive devices. Even a small scratch may cause permanent damage or make it impossible to retrieve data. To avoid problems, handle and store disks and tapes properly.

Diskettes. Diskettes should be kept away from magnetic fields, such as a paper clip holder that has a magnet in it. They should also be kept out of direct sunlight and away from extreme temperatures. In addition, store 5¼-inch disks in their sleeves, and never bend them or touch the exposed part of the disk. Although 3½-inch disks are sturdier than 5¼-inch disks, they should still be handled with care.

CD-ROMs. Figure 6-10 shows the proper way to handle a CD-ROM. When you pick it up, touch only the edges or the edge and the hole in the center. CD-ROMs should be stored in the clear plastic case in which they are packaged, sometimes called a jewel case. If a CD-ROM becomes dusty or smudged with fingerprints, you can clean it by rubbing it gently with a soft cloth. Always rub from the center to the outside. *Never* rub in a circular motion.

Magnetic Tapes. These tapes should be treated much as you would treat audiotapes. They should be stored in a relatively cool, dry place, away from magnetic fields.

Computers of the Future

Computers are evolving at such a rapid pace that it is virtually impossible to predict the changes that will take place even in the next few years. Some important new technologies, however, have already been introduced in

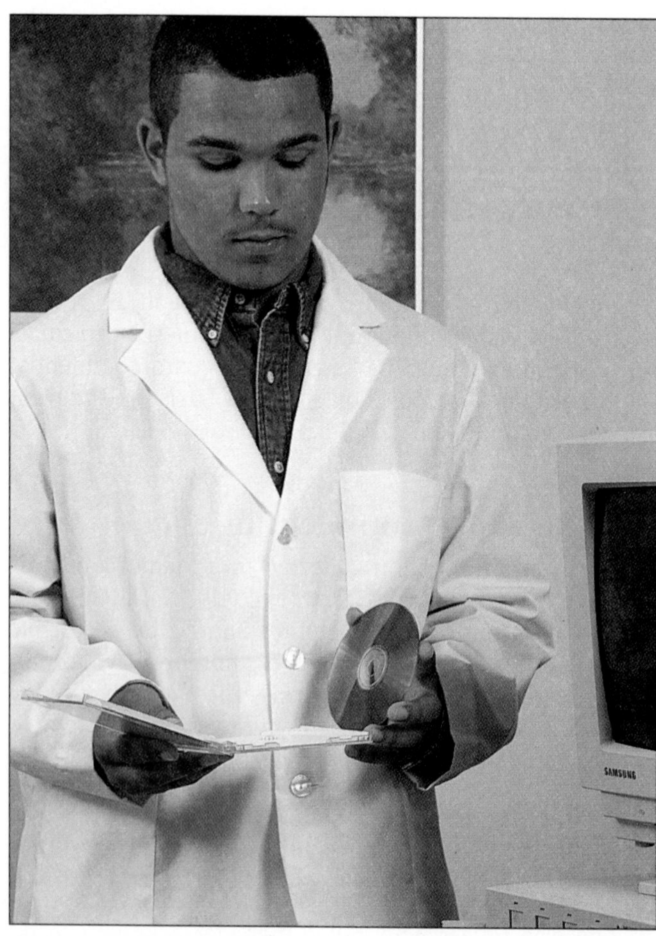

Figure 6-10. When handling a CD-ROM, be careful not to touch the flat surface of the disc.

MULTISKILL FOCUS

Dental Office Administrator

To gain medical assistant credentials, you must fulfill the requirements of either the American Association of Medical Assistants (for a Certified Medical Assistant) or the American Medical Technologists (for a Registered Medical Assistant). After obtaining your medical assistant certification or registration, you may wish to acquire additional skills in specialty areas through course work or on-the-job training. Although this course work or training may not lead to an additional certification or degree, it will enable you to expand your role in the medical office and advance your career as the demand for multiskilled health professionals increases.

Skills and Duties

A dental office administrator carries out clerical and administrative duties for a dentist or a dental group. His duties may vary with the size of the practice. In a large practice he may oversee the clerical staff. In a small practice he may have more varied tasks, including staffing the reception desk, maintaining records, and performing other secretarial duties.

The duties of a dental office administrator mostly fall into the following categories:

1. *Communication.* In many offices, this task is the administrator's main responsibility. He answers the telephones and manages the correspondence for the practice, which may include billing.
2. *Reception.* The office administrator greets and welcomes patients. He must have a knowledge of dental terminology in order to assist patients with dental paperwork.
3. *Scheduling.* The dental office administrator coordinates patient appointments and may schedule referrals with other specialists, such as orthodontists. He may also maintain the schedules of the dental hygienists and other office staff. Sometimes the administrator is responsible for calling patients to confirm appointments ahead of time.
4. *Records and filing.* The administrator may manage the patient records and other files. He attaches dental x-rays to the appropriate records and maintains up-to-date insurance information to ensure accurate billing.
5. *Secretarial duties.* The dental office administrator has a range of other duties that vary from practice to practice. Typically, he is responsible for managing office supplies. He often needs to type or take shorthand. He also uses computer and word processing skills. Specialized skills, such as bookkeeping, may also be helpful.
6. *Supervision.* In a large dental practice, the administrator trains and oversees clerical staff and secretaries.

Workplace Settings

Dental office administrators may work in a private practice, a group practice, or a dental clinic.

Education

Dental office administrators often learn the dental and medical terminology they need on the job. They may acquire secretarial training by taking courses, either in a business/vocational school or in a junior or community college. A high school diploma is usually required. Further education may be necessary in a practice where the administrator must supervise other staff members.

Where to Go for More Information

American Academy of Dental Practice Administrators
1063 Whippoorwill Lane
Palatine, IL 60067
(312) 934-4404

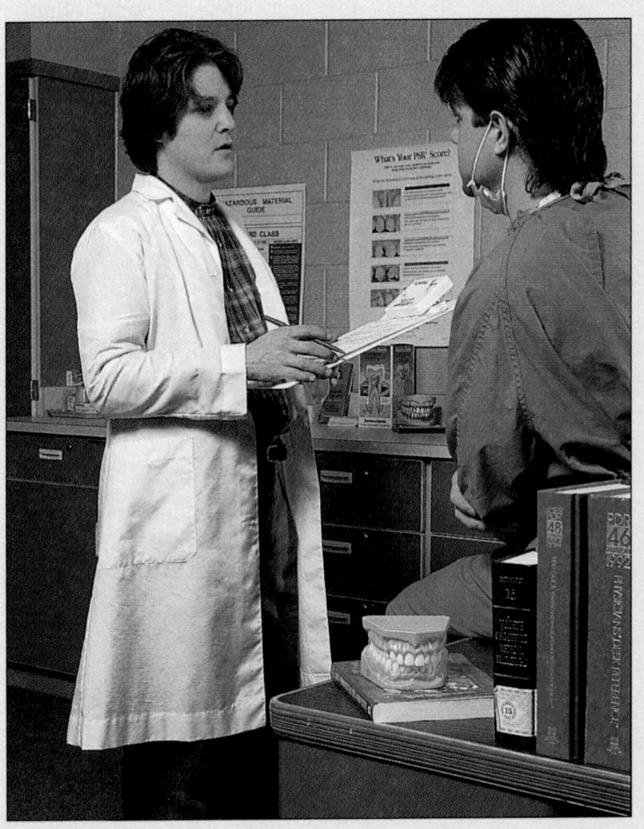

the medical office and will be improved in the near future. Telemedicine, CD-R technology, and speech recognition technology are only three examples of new computer technologies. Undoubtedly, more will be explored and developed every year.

Telemedicine

Telemedicine refers to the use of telecommunications to transmit video images of patient information. These images are already used to provide medical support to physicians caring for patients in rural areas. Some experts feel that telemedicine has great potential and that advancements in computer technology will make telemedicine more popular in the future.

CD-R Technology

While CD-ROMs can only be *read* by the computer, CD-R (compact disc-recordable) media can be read *and* written to. CD-R technology allows you to use compact discs like diskettes—to store data and information. Recordable CDs, however, can store much more information than diskettes can. Although CD-R technology is currently available, it is not yet widely used because it is still fairly expensive.

Speech Recognition Technology

This technology enables the computer to comprehend and interpret spoken words. The user simply speaks into a microphone instead of inputting information with a keyboard or a scanner. Because every human voice is different, however, and the English language is vast and complex, this technology is difficult to perfect. As speech recognition technology becomes more advanced, more accurate, and less expensive, it will most likely gain widespread acceptance. It has a great deal of potential, including the ability to virtually eliminate the need for medical assistants to transcribe physicians' notes.

Summary

Many medical offices have already converted from a paper-based system of record keeping to a computer-based one. You should familiarize yourself with the types of computers available and the hardware and software components that make up a computer system. A variety of software programs are used in the medical office, including word processing, database management, accounting and billing, appointment scheduling, and electronic transactions, such as submitting insurance claims. Other computer technology you need to know about includes modems, scanners, and CD-ROM software.

Whether you are converting to a computerized office or simply upgrading an existing system, learn the guidelines for selecting computer hardware and software. In a computerized office it is also important to know how to secure computerized files and to care for and maintain computer equipment.

6 Chapter Review

Discussion Questions

1. Compare and contrast the three types of printers. What are the advantages and disadvantages of each?
2. Why, do you think, has the Internet become such a popular method of communication? In what ways does it benefit the medical community?
3. Do you think that computerized patient records are more or less secure than paper records? Explain your answer.

Critical Thinking Questions

1. Describe how you would train yourself to use a new software program, and outline the steps you would take to solve a problem with the software.
2. Analyze how you would handle a situation in which a new coworker asks to borrow your password so she can learn how to use the computer.
3. Summarize the proper care and maintenance of computer diskettes. Evaluate how these procedures can prevent problems from occurring.

Application Activities

1. Look through computer magazines or trade journals for descriptions or reviews of software in each of the following categories: word processing, database management, accounting and billing, appointment scheduling, electronic transactions, and medical research. Make a chart comparing two or three software packages in each category. For each software title, include a brief description or evaluation, the manufacturer's name, and the price. Based on your research, choose one software package that you think is the best product in each category. Briefly explain each of your choices.
2. The medical office manager where you work has decided to upgrade the computer system. She has asked you to choose three vendors from which to

continued

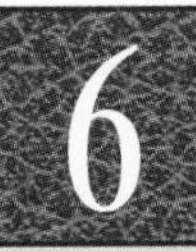

Chapter Review continued

get information and cost estimates for a new system. Describe the process by which you would select the vendors, and make a list of questions you would ask salespersons to evaluate the services.

3. Research one of the technological advances mentioned in this chapter—telemedicine, CD-R technology, or speech recognition technology—to learn more about it. Find out how the technology benefits the medical office. Write a one-page report on your findings.

Further Readings

Ball, M. H., et al., eds. *Aspects of the Computer-Based Patient Record.* New York: Springer-Verlag, 1995.

Baptist, Claire, et al. *Computers in the Medical Office: Using Medisoft.* New York: Glencoe, 1995.

Bjelland, Harley. *On-line Systems for Medical Professionals: How to Use and Access Databases.* Los Angeles: Practice Management Information Corp., 1992.

Glowniak, Jerry V. "Medical Resources on the Internet." *Annals of Internal Medicine,* 15 July 1995, 123–131.

Lindberg, Donald A. B., and Betsy L. Humphreys. "Computers in Medicine." *JAMA, The Journal of the American Medical Association,* 7 June 1995, 1667–1668.

Renfro, Joy. "Using Information Technology to Improve America's Health Care Delivery System." *The Professional Medical Assistant,* May/June 1996, 21–24.

Tietze, M. F., and J. T. Huber. "Electronic Information Retrieval in Nursing." *Nursing Management,* July 1995, 36–37, 41–42.

Xiradis-Aberle, Lori, and Craig L. Aberle. *How to Computerize Your Small Business.* New York: John Wiley, 1995.

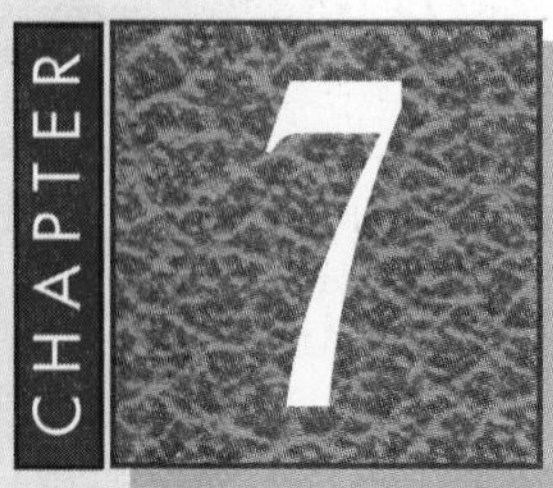

Managing Correspondence and Mail

CHAPTER OUTLINE

- Correspondence and Professionalism
- Choosing Correspondence Supplies
- Written Correspondence
- Effective Writing
- Editing and Proofreading
- Preparing Outgoing Mail
- Mailing Equipment and Supplies
- U.S. Postal Service Delivery
- Other Delivery Services
- Processing Incoming Mail

OBJECTIVES

After completing Chapter 7, you will be able to:

- List the supplies necessary for creating and mailing professional-looking correspondence.
- Identify the types of correspondence used in medical office communications.
- Describe the parts of a letter and the different letter and punctuation styles.
- Compose a business letter.
- Explain the tasks involved in editing and proofreading.
- Describe the process of handling incoming and outgoing mail.
- Compare and contrast the services provided by the U.S. Postal Service and other delivery services.

AREAS OF COMPETENCE

1997 ROLE DELINEATION STUDY

ADMINISTRATIVE

Administrative Procedures

- Perform basic clerical functions

GENERAL (Transdisciplinary)

Communication Skills

- Use effective and correct verbal and written communications
- Receive, organize, prioritize, and transmit information

Key Terms

annotate
clarity
concise
courtesy title
dateline
editing
full-block letter style
identification line
letterhead
modified-block letter style
proofreading
salutation
simplified letter style

Correspondence and Professionalism

As in any business, correspondence from health-care professionals to patients and colleagues must be handled carefully, with appropriate attention to content and presentation. By learning how to create, send, and receive correspondence and other types of mail, you can ensure positive, effective communication between your office and others. Well-written, neatly prepared correspondence is one of the most important means of communicating a professional image for the medical office (Figure 7-1).

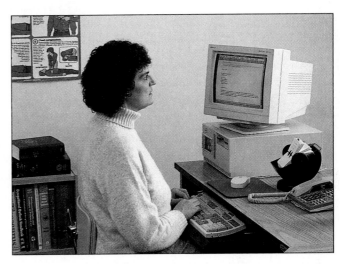

Figure 7-1. The correspondence that goes out of and comes into a medical office is vital to a well-run practice.

Choosing Correspondence Supplies

The first step in preparing professional-looking correspondence is choosing the right supplies. Many offices already have most of these supplies on hand. However, you may be responsible for choosing and ordering such supplies. You may need to make decisions about letterhead paper, envelopes, labels, invoices, and statements.

Letterhead Paper

Letterhead refers to formal business stationery on which the doctor's (or office's) name and address are printed at the top. In most cases, the office phone number is listed, along with the names of all the associates in the practice. Letterhead is used for correspondence with patients, colleagues, and vendors.

The fiber content of paper is the amount of wood pulp in the paper. Letterhead paper can be cotton fiber bond (sometimes called rag bond) or sulfite bond. Cotton fiber bond contains cotton pulp along with chemically treated wood pulp. It is usually more expensive than other types of paper. Cotton bond contains a watermark, which is an impression or pattern that can be seen when the paper is held up to the light. A watermark indicates that the paper is of high quality. The most popular cotton bond used for letterhead is 25% cotton because it is economical, but all higher grades can be used.

Sulfite bond is made from chemically treated wood pulp. It is smoother than cotton bond and less expensive. Sulfite bond comes in five grades, numbered one through five. Grade one is a cost-effective bond for letterhead. This grade of sulfite bond also has a watermark. You often cannot tell the difference between this grade of sulfite bond and cotton bond.

The finish of a paper refers to the paper's look and feel. Papers with a smooth finish are the most popular type for letterheads. They are less expensive and work well with most printers. Another type of finish used in high-quality letterhead is linen laid. This type has a rougher feel because it is embossed with a design, much like linen fabric.

Envelopes

Envelopes are used for correspondence, invoices, and statements. Typically, business letterhead, matching envelopes, and sometimes invoice and statement letterhead are printed together.

Familiarize yourself with the several types of envelopes used in the medical office.

1. The most common envelope size used for correspondence is the No. 10 envelope (also called business size). It measures 4⅛ by 9½ inches.
2. Envelopes used for invoices and statements can range from No. 6 (3⅝ by 6½ inches) to No. 10. These envelopes commonly have a transparent window that allows the address on the invoice or statement to show through, saving time and reducing the potential for errors involved in retyping the address.
3. Smaller payment-return envelopes—preaddressed to the doctor's office—are often included along with a bill, for the patient's convenience.
4. Tan kraft envelopes, also called clasp envelopes, are used to send large or bulky documents.
5. Padded envelopes are used to send documents or materials, such as slides, that may be damaged in the normal course of mail handling.

Labels

Address labels, printed from a computerized mailing list, can greatly speed the process of addressing envelopes for bulk mailings. For example, you may have to send a notice of a change in office hours or a quarterly office newsletter to a large number of patients in a practice.

Invoices and Statements

There are several different types of invoices and statements in use today. They include:

- Preprinted invoices (used to send an original bill).
- Preprinted statements (used to send a reminder when an account is 30 or more days past due).
- Computer-generated invoices and statements.
- Superbills (discussed in Chapter 17).
- Data mailers.

Written Correspondence

A letter is a form of communication—much like holding a conversation in person. The recipient will form an impression of the physician or the office based upon the letter. Therefore, letters must be clear and well written and must politely convey the appropriate information.

Types of Correspondence in the Medical Office

As a medical assistant, you will be responsible for preparing routine letters at the physician's request. You may transcribe some letters from the physician's dictation and compose others from notes.

The purpose of most letters is to explain, clarify, or give instructions or other information. Correspondence includes letters of referral; letters about scheduling, canceling, or rescheduling appointments; patient reports for insurance companies; instructions for examinations or laboratory tests; answers to insurance or billing questions; and cover letters or form letters to order supplies, equipment, or magazine subscriptions.

Parts of a Business Letter

Figure 7-2 illustrates the parts of a typical business letter. Details about format may vary from office to office.

Dateline. The dateline consists of the month, day, and year. It should begin about three lines below the preprinted letterhead text. The month should always be spelled out, and there should be a comma after the day.

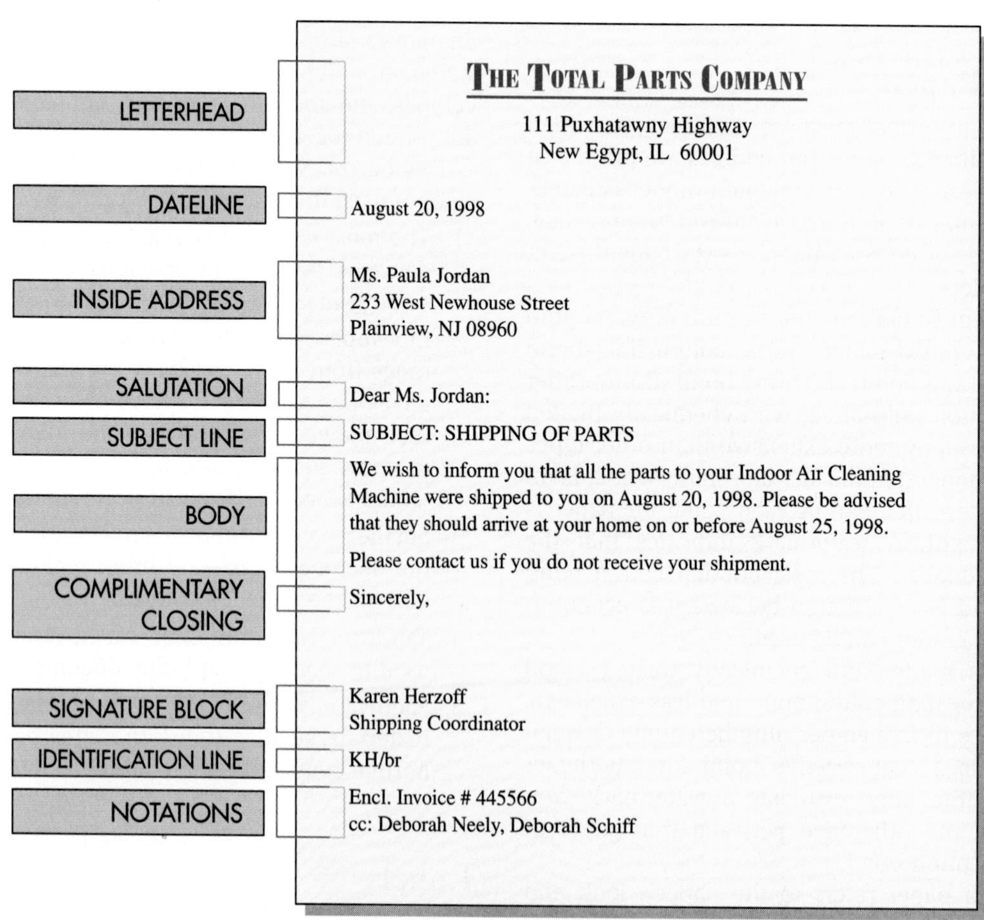

LETTERHEAD
DATELINE
INSIDE ADDRESS
SALUTATION
SUBJECT LINE
BODY
COMPLIMENTARY CLOSING
SIGNATURE BLOCK
IDENTIFICATION LINE
NOTATIONS
THE TOTAL PARTS COMPANY
111 Puxhatawny Highway
New Egypt, IL 60001
August 20, 1998
Ms. Paula Jordan
233 West Newhouse Street
Plainview, NJ 08960
Dear Ms. Jordan:
SUBJECT: SHIPPING OF PARTS
We wish to inform you that all the parts to your Indoor Air Cleaning Machine were shipped to you on August 20, 1998. Please be advised that they should arrive at your home on or before August 25, 1998.
Please contact us if you do not receive your shipment.
Sincerely,
Karen Herzoff
Shipping Coordinator
KH/br
Encl. Invoice # 445566
cc: Deborah Neely, Deborah Schiff

Figure 7-2. Knowing the parts of a typical business letter enables medical assistants to create written communications that reflect well on the office.

Inside Address. The inside address contains all the necessary information for correct delivery of the letter. In general, you should:

- Include a **courtesy title** (Dr., Mr., Mrs., and so on) and the intended receiver's full name. Note: If Dr. is used, it is not followed by MD after the name. For example, either of these forms is acceptable: Dr. John Smith; John Smith, MD. This form is not acceptable: Dr. John Smith, MD.
- Include the intended receiver's title on the same line with the name, separated by a comma, or on the line below it.
- Include the company name, if applicable.
- Use numerals for the street address, except the single numbers one through nine, which should be spelled out—for example, Two Markham Place.
- Spell out numerical names of streets if they are numbers less than ten.
- Spell out the words *Street, Drive,* and so on.
- Include the full city name; do not abbreviate.
- Use the two-letter state abbreviation recommended by the U.S. Postal Service (USPS) (Table 7-1).
- Leave one space between the state and the zip code; include the zip + 4 code, if known.

Attention Line. An attention line is used when a letter is addressed to a company but sent to the attention of a particular individual. If you do not know the name of the individual, call the company directly to inquire the name of the appropriate contact person. A colon between the word *Attention* and the person's name is optional.

Salutation. When addressing a person by name, use a salutation, a written greeting such as *Dear*, followed by Mr., Mrs., or Ms., and the person's last name. When you do not know the name, it is becoming common practice to use the business title or department in the salutation, as in "Dear Laboratory Director" or "Dear Claims Department." This also avoids confusion if you do not know the gender of a person with a name such as Pat or Chris.

Subject Line. A subject line is sometimes used to bring the subject of the letter to the reader's attention. It is typed two lines below the salutation and two lines above the body of the letter.

Table 7-1

USPS State Abbreviations

State	Abbreviation	State	Abbreviation
Alabama	AL	Indiana	IN
Alaska	AK	Iowa	IA
Arizona	AZ	Kansas	KS
Arkansas	AR	Kentucky	KY
California	CA	Louisiana	LA
Colorado	CO	Maine	ME
Connecticut	CT	Maryland	MD
Delaware	DE	Massachusetts	MA
District of Columbia	DC	Michigan	MI
Florida	FL	Minnesota	MN
Georgia	GA	Mississippi	MS
Hawaii	HI	Missouri	MO
Idaho	ID	Montana	MT
Illinois	IL	Nebraska	NE

continued

Table 7-1 continued

USPS State Abbreviations

State	Abbreviation	State	Abbreviation
Nevada	NV	Rhode Island	RI
New Hampshire	NH	South Carolina	SC
New Jersey	NJ	South Dakota	SD
New Mexico	NM	Tennesee	TN
New York	NY	Texas	TX
North Carolina	NC	Utah	UT
North Dakota	ND	Vermont	VT
Ohio	OH	Virginia	VA
Oklahoma	OK	Washington	WA
Oregon	OR	West Virginia	WV
Pennsylvania	PA	Wisconsin	WI
Puerto Rico	PR	Wyoming	WY

Body. The body of the letter begins two lines below the salutation or subject line. The text is single-spaced with double-spacing between paragraphs.

If the body contains a list, set the list apart from the rest of the text. Leave an extra line of space above and below the list. For each item in the list, indent five to ten spaces from each margin. Single-space within items, but leave an extra line between items. A bulleted list has a small, solid, round circle before each item.

Complimentary Closing. The closing is placed two lines below the last line of the body. "Sincerely" is a common closing. "Very truly yours" and "Best regards" are also acceptable closings in business correspondence.

Signature Block. The signature block contains the writer's name on the first line and the writer's business title on the second line. The block is aligned with the complimentary closing and typed four lines below it, to allow space for the signature.

Identification Line. The letter writer's initials followed by a colon or slash and the typist's initials are sometimes included in the letter. These initials are called the identification line. This line is typed flush left, two lines below the signature block.

Notations. Notations include information such as the number of enclosures that are included with the letter and the names of other people who will be receiving copies of the letter (sometimes referred to as cc's, or carbon copies). If there are enclosures, a notation should appear flush left, one or two lines below the identification line (or one or two lines below the signature block, if no identification line is present). You may abbreviate the word *Enclosure* by typing *Enc, Encl,* or *Encs* (with or without punctuation, depending on the style of the letter you are writing). The copy notation, *cc,* appears after the enclosure notation and includes one or more names or initials.

Punctuation Styles

Two different styles of punctuation are used in correspondence: open punctuation and mixed punctuation. A writer should use one punctuation style consistently throughout a letter.

Open Punctuation. This style uses no punctuation after the following items when they appear in a letter:

- The word *Attention* in the attention line
- The salutation
- The complimentary closing
- The signature block
- The enclosure and copy notations

Mixed Punctuation. This style includes the following punctuation marks used in specific instances:

- A colon after *Attention* in the attention line
- A colon after the salutation
- A comma after the complimentary closing
- A colon or period after the enclosure notation
- A colon after the copy notation

Letter Format

Follow these general formatting guidelines for all letters.

1. With paper 8½ inches wide, it is common to use 1-inch margins on the left and right.
2. Roughly center the letter on the page according to the length of the letter. (Most word processing programs can do this centering automatically.) For shorter letters, you can use wider margins and start the address farther down the page. For longer letters, use standard margins but start higher up on the page.
3. Single-space the body of the letter. Double-space between paragraphs or parts of the letter.
4. Use short sentences (no more than 20 words on average).
5. Have at least two sentences in each paragraph.
6. Divide long paragraphs—more than 10 lines of type—into shorter ones.

For multipage letters, use letterhead for the first page and blank paper for the subsequent pages. (When you order letterhead, be sure to order blank paper of the same type as the letterhead for subsequent sheets.)

Using a 1-inch margin at the top, include a heading with the addressee, date, and page number on all pages following the first one. Resume typing or printing the text about three lines below the heading.

Letter Styles

Different letter styles are used for different purposes. Your office is likely to have a preferred style in place. The four most common letter styles are full-block, modified-block, modified-block with indented paragraphs, and simplified.

Full-Block Style. The full-block letter style, also called block style, is typed with all lines flush left. Figure 7-3 shows an example of the block letter style. This style may include a subject line two lines below the salutation. Block-style letters are quick and easy to write because there are no indented paragraphs to slow the typist. Block style is one of the most common formats used in the medical office.

Modified-Block Style. The modified-block letter style is similar to full block but differs in that the dateline, complimentary closing, signature block, and notations are aligned and begin at the center of the page or slightly to the right. This type of letter has a traditional, balanced appearance.

Modified-Block Style With Indented Paragraphs. This style is identical to the modified-block style except that the paragraphs are indented.

Simplified Style. The simplified letter style is a modification of the full-block style and is the most modern letter style. Figure 7-4 shows an example of the simplified letter style. The salutation is omitted, eliminating the need for a courtesy title. A subject line in all-capital letters is placed between the address and the body of the letter. The subject line summarizes the main point of the letter, but does not actually use the word *subject.* All text is typed flush left. The complimentary closing is omitted, and the sender's name and title are typed in capital letters in a single line at the end of the letter. Note that this letter style always uses open punctuation, so it is both easy to read and quick to type. In most situations in a medical office, however, the simplified letter style may be too informal.

Effective Writing

To create effective, professional correspondence that reflects well on the practice, be sure that you use an appropriate style, clear and concise language, and the active voice. Following are some general tips to help you write effective letters.

1. Before you write, know the type of person to whom you are writing. Is the letter to a physician, a patient, a vendor, or fellow staff members? Decide if the tone should be formal or more relaxed.
2. Know the purpose of the letter before you begin, and make sure your letter accurately conveys that purpose.
3. Be **concise**—that is, say what you mean as briefly as possible. Be specific, and do not use unnecessary words.
4. Show **clarity** in your writing; state your message so that it can be understood easily.
5. Use the active voice whenever possible. Voice shows whether the subject of a sentence is acting or is being acted upon. Here is an example of the active voice:

   "Dr. Huang is seeing 18 patients today."

   Here is an example of the same sentence, written in the passive voice:

   "Eighteen patients will be seen by Dr. Huang today."

   Note that the active voice is more direct and livelier to read.
6. Use the passive voice, however, to soften the impact of negative news:

   "Your account will be turned over to a collection agency if we do not receive payment promptly."

ABC PUBLISHERS, INC.

July 10, 1998

Ms. Lara Erickson
2594 Hughes Boulevard
Hamilton City, NJ 08999

Dear Ms. Erickson:

SUBJECT: SHIPMENT DELAY

Thank you for contacting us regarding your order for *Smith and Doe's New Medical Dictionary*. Due to an unexpectedly heavy demand for the book, we are experiencing delays in processing and shipping orders.

We expect to ship your book in four weeks, around August 15. Because of this delay, we offer you the option of canceling your order with a full refund. If you would like to cancel at this point, please fill out and return the enclosed postcard. If we do not hear from you, your order will be shipped when ready.

We are sorry for any inconvenience this delay may cause you. Please be assured that ABC Publishers values its customers and always endeavors to fulfill orders in a timely fashion.

Sincerely yours,

Andrew Williams

Andrew Williams
Customer Service Manager

AW/cjc
Enclosure

117 New Avenue New York, NY 10000

Figure 7-3. The full-block letter style is quicker and easier to type than other styles.

ABC PUBLISHERS, INC.

July 10, 1998

Ms. Lara Erickson
2594 Hughes Boulevard
Hamilton City, NJ 08999

SHIPMENT DELAY

Thank you for contacting us regarding your order for *Smith and Doe's New Medical Dictionary*. Due to an unexpectedly heavy demand for the book, we are experiencing delays in processing and shipping orders.

We expect to ship your book in four weeks, around August 15. Because of this delay, we offer you the option of canceling your order with a full refund. If you would like to cancel at this point, please fill out and return the enclosed postcard. If we do not hear from you, your order will be shipped when ready.

We are sorry for any inconvenience this delay may cause you. Please be assured that ABC Publishers values its customers and always endeavors to fulfill orders in a timely fashion.

Andrew Williams

ANDREW WILLIAMS, CUSTOMER SERVICE MANAGER

AW/cjc
Enclosure

117 New Avenue New York, NY 10000

Figure 7-4. The simplified letter style is considered by some executives to be the most readable style for correspondence.

It would sound harsher to say:

"We will turn over your account to a collection agency if we do not receive payment promptly."

7. Always be polite and courteous.
8. Always check spelling and the accuracy of dates and monetary figures.

Editing and Proofreading

Editing and proofreading take place after you create the first draft of a letter. Editing involves checking a document for factual accuracy, logical flow, conciseness, clarity, and tone. Proofreading involves checking a document for grammatical, spelling, and format errors. Be sure to edit and proofread all correspondence before mailing.

Tools for Editing and Proofreading

Reference books can help you prepare letters that appear professional. Keep the following tools available.

Dictionary. An up-to-date dictionary gives you more than definitions of words. A dictionary tells you how to spell, divide, and pronounce a word and what part of speech it is, such as a noun or adjective.

Medical Dictionary. It is nearly impossible for even the most experienced health-care professional to be familiar with every medical term. A medical dictionary will serve as a handy reference for terms with which you are unfamiliar or about which you would like more information.

Becoming familiar with some of the prefixes and suffixes commonly used in medical terms can help you understand the meanings of many words. Appendix B lists some common medical prefixes and suffixes.

Physicians' Desk Reference (PDR). The *PDR* may be thought of as a dictionary of medications. Published yearly, it provides up-to-date information on both prescription and nonprescription drugs. You can consult the *PDR* for the correct spelling of a particular drug or for other information about its usage, side effects, contraindications, and so on.

English Grammar and Usage Manuals. These manuals answer questions concerning grammar and word usage. They usually contain sections on punctuation, capitalization, and other details of written communication.

Word Processing Spelling Checkers. Most word processing programs used in medical offices have built-in spelling checkers. There are also programs designed specifically to check spelling in medical documents. These spelling checkers include most common medical terms that would not be found in a regular software program.

Spelling checkers pick up many spelling errors and often give you suggestions for correct spellings. If you indicate the choice you meant to input, the program automatically replaces the misspelled word. These programs may not detect all spelling errors, however. They should not be relied on as the only means of checking a document. For example, spelling checkers cannot tell you that you used the wrong word if you type the word *form* instead of *from,* because *form* is also a correctly spelled word.

Some software packages offer grammar-checking and style-checking features. These programs can identify certain problems, but the person using them still needs to know basic rules of grammar and style to correct errors.

Editing

The **editing** process ensures that a document is accurate, clear, and complete; free of grammatical errors; organized logically; and written in an appropriate style. It is a good idea to leave some time between the writing and editing stages so that you can look at the document in a fresh light. As you edit, you must examine language usage, content, and style.

Language Usage. Learn basic grammar rules. When in doubt, refer to a grammar handbook or reference manual. Make sure all sentences are complete. Ask yourself, Is this the best way to convey what I want to say? Do my word choices reflect the overall tone of the document? For example, in a business letter, you would avoid choosing phrases that are too colloquial or cute, such as "Thanks a million" or "Take it easy."

Content. A letter should contain all the necessary information the writer intends to convey. If you are editing someone else's letter and something appears to be missing, check with the writer. She may have omitted information by mistake.

The content of a letter should follow a logical thought pattern. Discuss one topic at a time. Do not jump back and forth between topics. Here are two other suggestions to help you stay organized.

- Make sure the purpose of the letter is stated directly at the beginning.
- When introducing a new idea or topic, begin a new paragraph.

Style. Use a writing style that is appropriate to the reader. A letter written to a patient is likely to require a different style from one written to a physician.

Proofreading

Proofreading means checking a document for errors. After you edit a document, put it aside for a short time before proofreading it. Ideally, have a coworker proofread your work. There are three types of errors that can occur when preparing a document: formatting, data, and mechanical.

Formatting Errors. These errors involve the positioning of the various parts of a letter. They may include errors in indenting, line length, or line spacing. To avoid these errors:

- Scan the letter to make sure that the indentions are consistent, that the spacing is correct, and that the text is centered from left to right and top to bottom.
- Make sure you have followed the office style.

Data Errors. These errors involve typing monetary figures, such as a balance on a patient statement. Verify the accuracy of all figures by checking them twice or by having one or two coworkers check them.

Mechanical Errors. These errors involve spelling, punctuation, spacing between words, and division of words. Mechanical errors also include reversing words or characters, typing them twice, or omitting them altogether. Here are some tips to help you avoid mechanical errors.

1. Learn basic spelling, punctuation, and word division rules. When in doubt, be sure to check a manual on English usage. Table 7-2 presents some basic rules concerning the mechanics of writing. Figure 7-5 lists some of the most commonly misspelled medical terms and other words.
2. Check carefully for transposed characters or words.
3. Avoid dividing words at the end of a line. Most word processing programs automatically "wrap" words to the next line, so if you are writing on a computer, dividing words should not present a problem.

Table 7-2

Basic Rules of Writing

Word Division	Divide: • According to pronunciation. • Compound words between the two words from which they derive. • Hyphenated compound words at the hyphen. • After a prefix. • Before a suffix. • Between two consonants that appear between vowels. • Before *-ing* unless the last consonant is doubled; in that case, divide before the second consonant. Do not divide: • Such suffixes as *-sion, -tial,* and *-gion.* • A word so that only one letter is left on a line.
Capitalization	Capitalize: • All proper names. • All titles, positions, or indications of family relation when preceding a proper name or in place of a proper noun (not when used alone or with possessive pronouns or articles). • Days of the week, months, and holidays. • Names of organizations and membership designations. • Racial, religious, and political designations. • Adjectives, nouns, and verbs that are derived from proper nouns (including currently copyrighted trade names). • Specific addresses and geographic locations. • Sums of money written in legal or business documents. • Titles, headings of books, magazines, and newspapers.

continued

Table 7-2 continued	
Basic Rules of Writing	
Plurals	• Add *s* or *es* to most singular nouns. (Plural forms of most medical terms do not follow this rule.) • With medical terms ending in *is,* drop the *is* and add *es:* metastasis/metastases epiphysis/epiphyses • With terms ending in *um,* drop the *um* and add *a:* diverticulum/diverticula atrium/atria • With terms ending in *us,* drop the *us* and add *i:* calculus/calculi bronchus/bronchi (Two exceptions to this are virus/viruses and sinus/sinuses.) • With terms ending in *a,* keep the *a* and add *e:* vertebra/vertebrae
Possessives	To show ownership or relation to another noun: • For singular nouns, add an apostrophe and an *s.* • For plural nouns that do not end in an *s,* add an apostrophe and an *s.* • For plural nouns that end in an *s,* just add an apostrophe.
Numbers	Use numerals: • In general writing, when the number is 11 or greater. • With abbreviations and symbols. • When discussing laboratory results or statistics. • When referring to specific sums of money. • When using a series of numbers in a sentence. Tips: • Use commas when numerals have more than three digits. • Do not use commas when referring to account numbers, page numbers, or policy numbers. • Use a hyphen with numerals to indicate a range.

As you can see, creating a business letter involves many steps. Procedure 7-1 organizes these steps for you.

Preparing Outgoing Mail

After you have created, edited, and proofread a letter, you need to prepare it for mailing. This preparation includes having the letter signed, preparing the envelope, and folding and inserting the letter into the envelope. It will then be ready for postage to be calculated and affixed.

Signing Letters

After the letter is complete—it has been proofread and the envelope and enclosures have been prepared—it is ready for signing. Some doctors authorize other staff members to sign for them. If you have been authorized to sign letters, you should sign the doctor's name and place your initials after the doctor's signature.

If the doctor prefers to sign all letters, you should place the letter on the doctor's desk in a file folder marked "For Your Signature." If the letter is of an urgent nature, give it to the doctor as soon as possible. Otherwise, you can collect several letters in the folder and present the entire group for signing at one time.

Preparing the Envelope

To ensure the quickest delivery of mail, the USPS has issued several guidelines for preparing envelopes. The USPS uses electronic optical character readers (OCRs) to help speed mail processing. OCRs read the last two lines of an address and sort the mail accordingly. To take advantage of this technology, envelopes must be no smaller than 3½ by 5 inches and no larger than 6⅛ by 11½ inches. They must be addressed in a specific format that can be read by the OCR. Use USPS guidelines for addressing envelopes.

Address Placement. The address must be placed in a certain location on the envelope for reading by the OCR (Figure 7-6). The area the OCR can read has the following characteristics.

1. It is bordered by a 1-inch margin on both the left and right sides of the envelope.

Commonly Misspelled Medical Terms and Other Words

Medical Terms

abscess	diluent	larynx	pleurisy
aerobic	dissect	leukemia	pneumonia
anergic	eosinophil	leukocyte	polyp
anesthetic	epididymis	malaise	prescription
aneurysm	epistaxis	menstruation	prophylaxis
anteflexion	erythema	metastasis	prostate
arrhythmia	eustachian	muscle	prosthesis
asepsis	fissure	neuron	pruritus
asthma	flexure	nosocomial	psoriasis
auricle	fomites	occlusion	pyrexia
benign	glaucoma	oscilloscope	respiration
bilirubin	glomerular	osseous	rheumatism
bronchial	gonorrhea	palliative	scirrhous
capillary	hemocytometer	parasite	serous
cervical	hemorrhage	parenteral	specimen
chancre	hemorrhoids	parietal	sphincter
choroid	homeostasis	paroxysm	sphygmomanometer
chromosome	humerus	pericardium	squamous
cirrhosis	ileum	perineum	staphylococcus
clavicle	ilium	peristalsis	surgeon
curettage	infarction	peritoneum	vaccine
cyanosis	inoculate	pharynx	vein
defibrillator	intussusception	pituitary	venous
desiccation	ischium	plantar	wheal

Other Words

absence	aggravate	appropriate	brochure
accept	all right	approximate	bulletin
accessible	a lot	argument	business
accommodate	already	assistance	category
accumulate	altogether	associate	changeable
achieve	analysis	auxiliary	characteristic
acquire	analyze	balloon	cigarette
adequate	apparatus	bankruptcy	circumstance
advantageous	apparent	believe	clientele
affect	appearance	benefited	committee

continued

Figure 7-5. Familiarize yourself with these commonly misspelled words, and check their spelling carefully whenever you use them.

Commonly Misspelled Medical Terms and Other Words continued

Other Words

comparative
complement
compliment
concede
conscientious
conscious
controversy
corroborate
counsel
courtesy
defendant
definite
dependent
description
desirable
development
dilemma
disappear
disappoint
disapprove
disastrous
discreet
discrete
discrimination
dissatisfied
dissipate
earnest
ecstasy
effect
eligible
embarrass
emphasis
entrepreneur
envelope
environment
exceed
except
exercise
exhibit
exhilaration

existence
fantasy
fascinate
February
fluorescent
forty
grammar
grievance
guarantee
handkerchief
height
humorous
hygiene
incidentally
indispensable
inimitable
insistent
irrelevant
irresistible
irritable
its
it's
labeled
laboratory
led
leisure
liable
liaison
license
liquefy
maintenance
maneuver
miscellaneous
misspelled
necessary
noticeable
occasion
occurrence
offense

oscillate
paid
pamphlet
panicky
paradigm
parallel
paralyze
pastime
persevere
persistent
personal
personnel
persuade
phenomenon
plagiarism
pleasant
possession
precede
precedent
predictable
predominant
prejudice
preparation
prerogative
prevalent
principal
principle
privilege
procedure
proceed
professor
pronunciation
psychiatry
psychology
pursue
questionnaire
rearrange
recede
receive

recommend
referral
relieve
repetition
rescind
résumé
rhythm
ridiculous
schedule
secretary
seize
separate
similar
sizable
stationary
stationery
stomach
subpoena
succeed
suddenness
supersede
surprise
tariff
technique
temperament
temperature
thorough
transferred
truly
tyrannize
unnecessary
until
vacillate
vacuum
vegetable
vicious
warrant
Wednesday
weird

2. It has a $\frac{5}{8}$-inch margin on the bottom. The top of the city/state/zip code line (the last line in the address block) must be no higher than $2\frac{1}{4}$ inches from the bottom edge of the envelope.
3. An area $4\frac{1}{2}$ inches wide in the bottom right-hand corner of the envelope should be left clear. The OCR reads the address and prints a bar code that corresponds to the zip code in this area.

Address Format. When you type an address, follow these format guidelines.

1. Type or machine-print (for example, by computer) the address. (The OCR cannot read handwriting.) Avoid fancy script fonts.
2. Use all-capital letters, and single-space the lines. Use only one or two spaces between numbers and words in the address.
3. Use only USPS-approved abbreviations for location designations, as presented in Table 7-3.
4. Put the addressee's name on the first line of the address block, the department (if any) on the second

PROCEDURE 7-1

Creating a Letter

Objective: To follow standard procedure for constructing a business letter

Materials: Word processor or personal computer, letterhead paper, dictionaries or other sources

Method

1. Format the letter according to the office's standard procedure. Use the same punctuation style throughout.
2. Start the dateline three lines below the last line of the printed letterhead.
   (Note: Depending upon the length of the letter, it is acceptable to start between two and six lines below the letterhead.)
3. Two lines below the dateline, type in any special mailing instructions (such as REGISTERED MAIL, CERTIFIED MAIL, and so on).
4. Three lines below any special instructions, begin the inside address.
   (Note: It is acceptable to start the inside address anywhere from 3 to 12 lines below the dateline, depending upon the length of the letter.)
   - Type the addressee's courtesy title (Mr., Mrs., Dr., and so on) and full name on the first line.
   - Type the addressee's business title on the second line.
   - Type the company name on the third line.
   - Type the street address on the fourth line, including the apartment or suite number.
   - Type the city, state, and zip code on the fifth line. Use the standard two-letter abbreviation for the state, followed by one space and the zip code.
5. Two lines below the inside address, type the salutation.
6. Two lines below the salutation, type the subject line, if applicable.
7. Two lines below the subject line, begin the body of the letter.
   - Single-space between lines.
   - Double-space between paragraphs.
8. Two lines below the body of the letter, type the complimentary closing.
9. Leave three blank lines (return four times), and begin the signature block. (Enough space must be left to allow for the signature.)
   - Type the sender's name on the first line.
   - Type the sender's title on the second line.
10. Two lines below the sender's title, type the identification line. Type the sender's initials in all capitals and your initials in lowercase letters, separating the two sets of initials with a colon or a slash.
11. One or two lines below the identification line, type the enclosure notation, if applicable.
12. Two lines below the enclosure notation, type the copy notation, if applicable.
13. Edit the letter.
14. Proofread the letter.

line, and the company name on the third line. If the letter is to go to someone's attention at a company, put the company name on the first line and "Attention: [Name]" on the second line.

5. The line above the city, state, and zip code should contain the street address or post office box number. Include suite or apartment numbers on the same line as the street address.
6. The last line of the address must include the city, state, and zip code. Use the zip + 4 code whenever possible.
7. Include the hyphen in the zip + 4 code, for example, 08520-6142.
8. Type any special notations (such as SPECIAL DELIVERY, CERTIFIED, or REGISTERED) two lines below the postage in all-capital letters. This information should appear outside the area the OCR can read.
9. Type any handling instructions (such as *Personal* or *Confidential*) three lines below the return address. This information should also be outside the area the OCR can read.
10. Letters going to foreign countries should have the name of the country on the last line of the address block in all-capital letters.

Folding and Inserting Mail

Letters and invoices must be folded neatly before they are inserted into the envelopes. The proper way to fold a letter depends on the type of envelope into which the letter will fit.

- With a small envelope, fold the enclosure in half lengthwise, and insert it.
- With a regular business-size envelope, fold the letter in thirds. Fold the bottom third up first, then the top third down, and insert the letter.

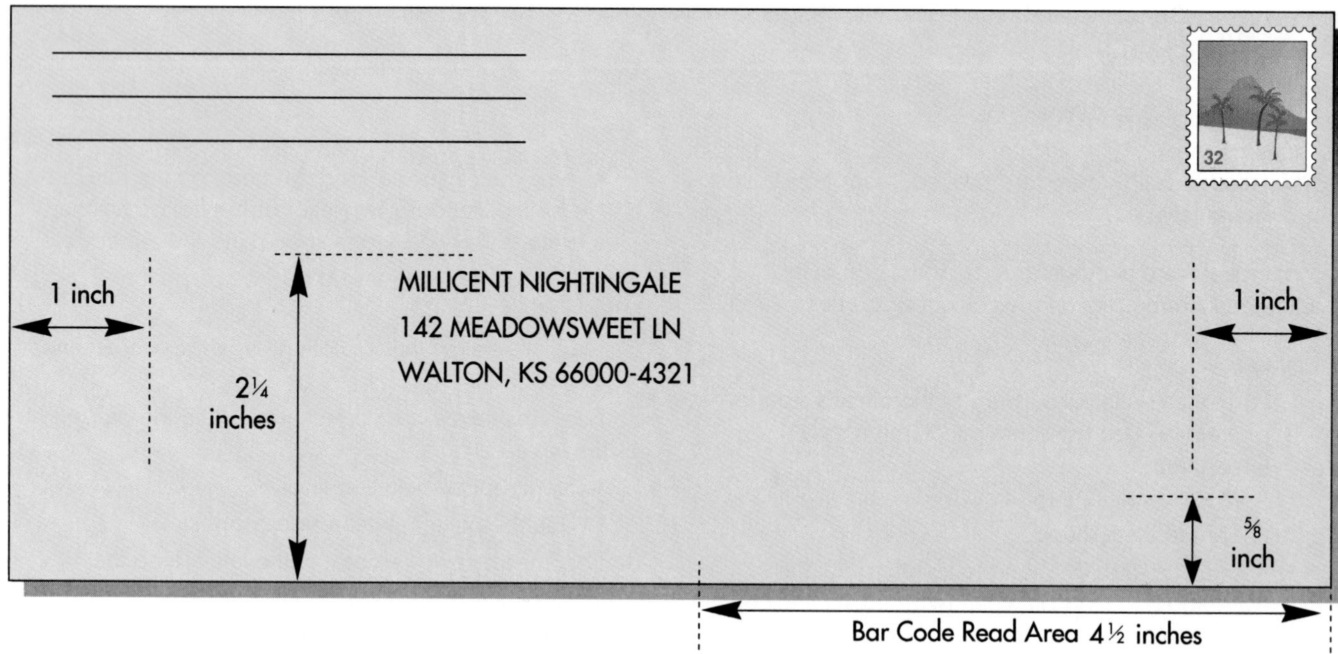

Figure 7-6. Following this format for typing an envelope assures that it can be processed by USPS electronic equipment.

- With a window envelope, use an "accordion fold." Fold the bottom third up. Then, fold the top third back so that the address appears in the window, and insert the enclosure.

Before folding the letter, double-check that it has been signed, that all enclosures are included, and that the address on the letter matches the one on the envelope. Any enclosures that are not attached to the letter should be placed inside the folds so that they will be removed from the envelope along with the letter.

Mailing Equipment and Supplies

The proper equipment and supplies will help you handle the mail efficiently and cost-effectively. In addition to letterhead, blank stationery for multipage letters, and envelopes, you will need some standard supplies. The USPS provides forms, labels, and packaging for items that need special attention, such as airmail, Priority Mail, Express Mail, certified mail, or registered mail. Private delivery

Table 7-3

USPS Abbreviations

Word	Abbreviation	Word	Abbreviation
Avenue	AVE	Highway	HWY
Boulevard	BLVD	Junction	JCT
Center	CTR	Lane	LN
Circle	CIR	North	N
Corner	COR	Parkway	PKY
Court	CT	Place	PL
Drive	DR	Plaza	PLZ
East	E	South	S
Expressway	EXPY	West	W

companies, such as United Parcel Service (UPS), also provide shipping supplies to their customers.

Airmail Supplies

In the past, any piece of mail that was transported by air was designated as airmail. Today nearly all first-class mail outside a local area is routinely sent by air. However, airmail services are still available for some packages and for most mail going to foreign countries.

If you are sending an item by airmail, attach special airmail stickers, available from the post office, on all sides. (The word *AIRMAIL* can also be neatly written on all sides.) Special airmail envelopes for letters can be purchased from the USPS.

Envelopes for Overnight Delivery Services

For correspondence or packages that must be delivered by the next day, a number of overnight delivery services are available through the USPS and private companies. Most companies require the use of their own envelopes and mailing materials. Make sure you keep adequate supplies on hand so that you do not run out at the last minute.

Postal Rates, Scales, and Meters

Postal rates and regulations change periodically, and every medical office should have a copy of the latest guidelines. These guidelines are available from the USPS. Postal scales and meters are described in Chapter 5.

U.S. Postal Service Delivery

The USPS offers a variety of domestic and international delivery services for letters and packages. Following are some of the services you will be most likely to use in a medical office setting.

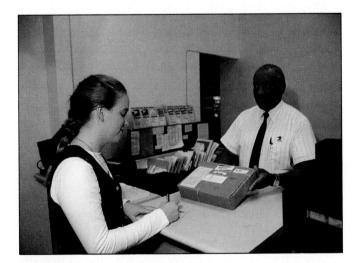

Figure 7-7. If no one is in the office when the mail is delivered, the medical assistant may need to go to the post office to sign for a certified letter or package.

Regular Mail Service

Regular mail delivery includes several classes of mail, as well as other designations such as Priority Mail and Express Mail. The class or designation determines how quickly a piece of mail is delivered.

First-Class Mail. Most correspondence generated in a medical office—letters, postcards, and invoices—is sent by first-class mail. Items must weigh 11 oz or less to be considered first-class. (An item over 11 oz that requires quick delivery must be sent by Priority Mail, which is discussed later in the chapter.) The cost of mailing a first-class item is based on its weight. The standard rate is for items 1 oz or less that are not larger than 6⅛ inches high and 11½ inches wide. Additional postage is required for items that are heavier or larger. Postage for postcards is less than the letter rate.

Fourth-Class Mail. This class is also called parcel post. It is used for items weighing 1 lb or more that do not require speedy delivery. Rates are based upon weight and distance. There is a special fourth-class rate for mailing books, manuscripts, and some types of medical information.

Priority Mail. Priority class is useful for heavier items that require quicker delivery than is available for fourth-class mail. Any first-class item that weighs between 11 oz and 70 lb requires Priority Mail service. Although the rate for Priority Mail varies with the weight of the item and the distance it must travel, the USPS offers a flat rate for all material that can fit into its special Priority Mail envelope. The USPS guarantees delivery of Priority Mail items in 2 to 3 days.

Express Mail. Express Mail is the quickest USPS service. Different types are available, including next-day and second-day delivery. Express Mail deliveries are made 365 days a year. Rates vary, depending upon the weight and the specific service. A special flat-rate envelope is also available. Items sent by Express Mail are automatically insured against loss or damage. You can drop off packages at the post office or arrange for pickup service.

Special Postal Services

The USPS offers a variety of special mail delivery services in addition to the regular classes of mail. These services may require an additional fee above and beyond the cost of postage.

Special Delivery. Use special delivery if you want an item delivered as soon as it reaches the recipient's post office. Delivery of the item is typically made before the regularly scheduled mail delivery. Special delivery service is available within certain distance limits and during certain hours.

Certified Mail. Certified mail offers a guarantee that the item has been sent to the proper place. The item is marked as certified mail and requires the postal carrier to obtain a signature upon delivery (Figure 7-7). The sender may purchase a receipt showing that the item was received.

Return Receipt Requested. You may request a return receipt to obtain proof that an item was delivered. The receipt indicates who received the item and when. You can obtain a return receipt for various types of mail.

Registered Mail. Use registered mail to send items that are valuable, irreplaceable, or otherwise important. Registered mail provides the sender with evidence of mailing and delivery. It also provides the security that an item is being tracked as it is transported through the postal system. Because of this tracking process, delivery may be slightly delayed.

To register a piece of mail, take it to the post office, and indicate the full value of the item. Both first-class mail and Priority Mail can be registered.

International Mail

The USPS offers both surface (via ship) and airmail service to most foreign countries. Information on rates and fees is available from the post office.

There are various types of international mail, which are similar to the domestic classes. The USPS also provides international Express Mail and Priority Mail services, along with special mail delivery services such as registered mail, certified mail, and special delivery.

Tracing Mail

If a piece of registered or certified mail does not reach its destination by the expected time, you can ask the post office to trace it (Figure 7-8). You will need to present your original receipt for the item.

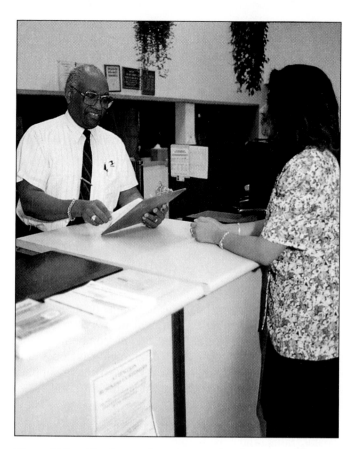

Figure 7-8. Tracing an item is a service that post offices perform when important items are delayed or do not reach their destinations.

Messengers

When items must be delivered within the local area on the same day, local messenger services are an option. Many messenger companies are listed in the yellow pages of the telephone book.

Other Delivery Services

In addition to the USPS, other companies provide mail and package delivery services. The costs and types of services vary.

United Parcel Service (UPS)

UPS delivers packages and provides overnight letter and express services. You can either drop off packages at a UPS location or have them picked up at your office. Fees vary with the services provided such as ground or air. Packages are automatically insured against theft or damage.

Express Delivery Services

Companies such as Federal Express and Airborne Express provide several types of quick delivery services for letters and packages. Rates vary according to the weight, time of delivery, and, in some cases, whether you have the package picked up at your office or drop it off at one of the company's local branches.

Processing Incoming Mail

Mail is an important connection between the office and other professionals and patients. Often an office has an established procedure for handling the mail. It is best to set aside a specific time of the day to process all the incoming mail at once rather than trying to do a little bit at a time.

Although it sounds simple, processing mail involves more than merely opening envelopes. In general, it involves the following steps: sorting, opening, recording, annotating, and distributing.

Sorting and Opening

The first step in processing mail is to sort it. Mail is typically sorted according to its priority. Sort mail in an uncluttered area to avoid mixing it with other paperwork. Follow a regular sorting procedure each time so that you do not miss any steps. Procedure 7-2 outlines suggested steps for sorting and opening the mail. "Tips for the Office" discusses how to recognize urgent incoming mail.

PROCEDURE 7-2

Sorting and Opening Mail

Objective: To follow a standard procedure for sorting, opening, and processing incoming office mail

Materials: Letter opener, date and time stamp (manual or automatic), stapler, paper clips, adhesive notes

Method

1. Check the address on each letter or package to be sure that it has been delivered to the correct location.
2. Sort the mail into piles according to priority and type of mail. Your system may include the following:
   - Top priority. This pile will contain any items that were sent by overnight mail delivery, in addition to items sent by registered mail, certified mail, or special delivery. (Faxes and E-mail messages are also top priority.)
   - Second priority. This pile will include personal or confidential mail.
   - Third priority. This pile will contain all first-class mail, airmail, and Priority Mail items. These items should be divided into payments received, insurance forms, reports, and other correspondence.
   - Fourth priority. This pile will consist of packages.
   - Fifth priority. This pile will contain magazines and newspapers.
   - Sixth priority. This last pile will include advertisements and catalogs.
3. Set aside all letters labeled "Personal" or "Confidential." Unless you have permission to open these letters, only the addressee should open them.
4. Arrange all the envelopes with the flaps facing up and away from you.
5. Tap the lower edge of the envelope to shift the contents to the bottom. This step helps to prevent cutting any of the contents when you open the envelope.
6. Open all the envelopes. (It is more efficient to open all the envelopes first and then to remove the contents.)
7. Remove and unfold the contents, making sure that nothing remains in the envelope.
8. Review each document, and check the sender's name and address.
   - If the letter has no return address, save the envelope, or cut the address off the envelope, and tape it to the letter.
   - Check to see if the address matches the one on the envelope. If there is a difference, staple the envelope to the letter, and make a note to verify the correct address with the sender.
9. Compare the enclosure notation on the letter with the actual enclosures to make sure that all items are included. Make a note to contact the sender if anything is missing.
10. Clip together each letter and its enclosures.
11. Check the date of the letter. If there is a significant delay between the date of the letter and the postmark, keep the envelope. (It may be necessary to refer to the postmark in legal matters or cases of collection.)
12. If all contents appear to be in order, you can discard the envelope.
13. Review all bills and statements.
    - Make sure the amount enclosed is the same as the amount listed on the statement.
    - Make a note of any discrepancies.
14. Stamp each piece of correspondence with the date (and sometimes the time) to record its receipt. If possible, stamp each item in the same location—such as the upper right-hand corner. (It may be necessary to refer to the date in legal matters or in cases of collection.)

Recording

It is a good idea to keep a log of each day's mail. This daily record lists the mail received and indicates follow-up correspondence and the date it is completed. This method helps in tracing items and keeping track of correspondence.

Annotating

Because you will be reading much of the incoming mail, you may also be encouraged to annotate it. To **annotate** means to underline or highlight key points of the letter or to write reminders, comments, or suggested actions in the margins or on self-adhesive notes. Annotating may involve pulling a patient's chart or any previous related correspondence from a file and attaching it to the letter.

Distributing

The next step is to sort letters into separate batches for distribution. These batches might include correspondence that requires the physician's attention, payments to be directed to the person in charge of billing, and correspondence that requires your attention. Each batch

Tips FOR THE OFFICE

How to Spot Urgent Incoming Mail

How can you tell if a piece of incoming mail is urgent? First-class mail marked "Urgent" tells you that it requires immediate attention. Here are some other signals to look for.

Overnight Mail
Any package that has been sent by an overnight carrier or by USPS Express Mail should be considered urgent and should be opened immediately.

Certified Mail
Certified mail requires your signature upon delivery. The sender used certified mail to be sure that the item would be sent to the proper person.

Registered Mail
Items sent by registered mail typically are valuable, irreplaceable, or otherwise important. Registered mail provides the sender with evidence of mailing and delivery.

Special Delivery
An item sent by special delivery is likely to be delivered sometime before the normal mail delivery—possibly even on a Sunday or holiday. The sender requested special delivery to ensure that the item would be delivered promptly after it was received at the addressee's post office.

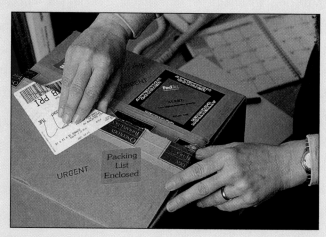

Figure 7-9. Urgent materials receive top priority upon arrival at an office.

should be presented to the appropriate person in a file folder or arranged with the highest-priority items on top. You may be given specific instructions on how to distribute magazines, newspapers, and advertising circulars.

Handling Drug and Product Samples

Many physicians receive a number of drug and product samples in the mail. Handling procedures vary from office to office. Samples of nonprescription products, such as hand creams or cough drops, may be displayed in the patient treatment area for patients to take.

The physician may ask that you put samples of any new prescription drugs in the consultation room for him to evaluate. Store other drug samples in a locked cabinet reserved solely for such samples. Sort and label the samples by category, such as antibiotics, sedatives, painkillers, and so on. Never give samples to patients unless specified by the physician. If the physician directs you to give samples to a patient, make sure to write this information in the patient's chart and date the entry.

When a box of samples is half empty, it is common practice to destroy half of the remaining samples by pouring liquids down the drain and putting pills in a garbage disposal. Samples should not be put in the trash. (The remaining samples that have not been destroyed may be used at the physician's direction.) Once a month, any samples that are past their expiration date should be destroyed (Figure 7-10).

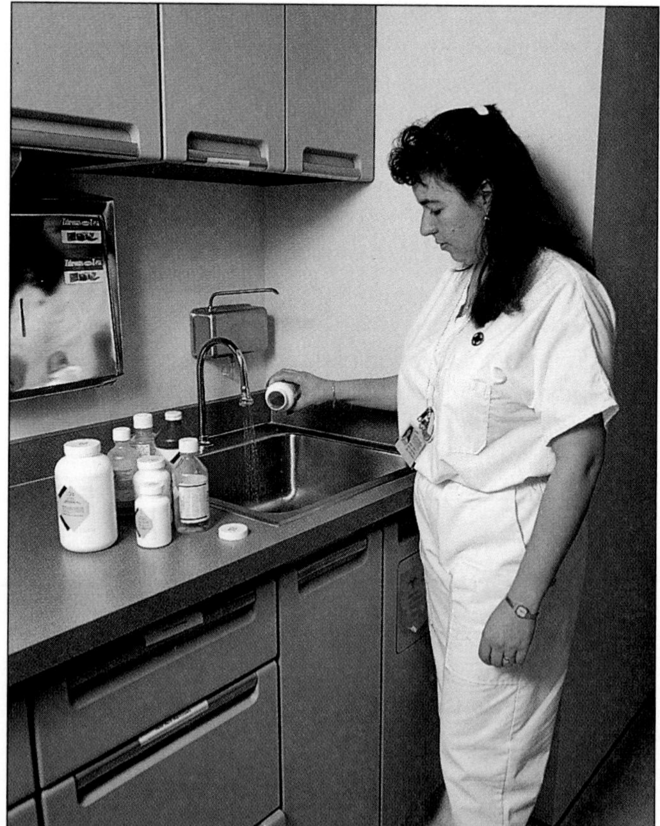

Figure 7-10. Certain nontoxic medical supplies must be carefully disposed of according to medical office policy.

Summary

As a medical assistant, you are responsible for many of the tasks involved in writing correspondence and processing outgoing and incoming mail in the medical office. Proper and efficient management of correspondence and mail is essential to promoting a positive, professional office image.

Choosing the proper letterhead and envelopes helps to ensure professional-looking correspondence. Knowing the parts of a letter and the various letter styles and formats used in the business environment today helps you create effective correspondence. Knowing how to edit and proofread and how to use writing reference books helps ensure that your letters are understandable and well written.

Familiarity with the types of mail services available enables you to choose the proper services to meet the office's mailing needs. Following proper procedures and recommended USPS guidelines ensures that office mail will be received in the most timely manner.

Handling incoming mail is also an important responsibility. Following an established procedure allows you to process and route the mail efficiently.

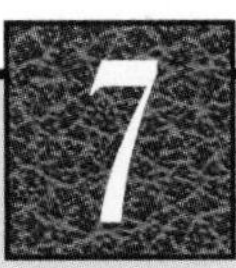

Chapter Review

Discussion Questions

1. Give three examples of types of correspondence commonly found in a medical practice.
2. Describe the five steps involved in processing incoming mail.
3. Explain the differences between certified mail, return receipt requested, and registered mail.

Critical Thinking Questions

1. How might you improve your skills in writing business letters both in the office and outside work?
2. Imagine that the waiting room is packed with people, and your coworker is out sick. You have received a large amount of mail today, and you can tell that the doctor will consider much of it important or even urgent. How would you deal with the mail?
3. Imagine that you need to send several bills to patients for delivery tomorrow. For some, you need proof that the patient received the delivery. How would you mail them?

Application Activities

1. You are employed in Dr. Angelo Carillo's office. A young patient of yours, Rodney Sills, has broken his wrist, and Dr. Carillo says that Rodney will be unable to participate in gym class for 10 weeks. Create a letter notifying his gym instructor of the situation.
2. Prepare a No. 10 business envelope using the USPS guidelines for addressing envelopes. Include the following information.

   Return address:

   Dr. Angelo Carillo, 123 Winding Way, Suite 2, Rockland, NJ 09876

   Mailing address:

   ABC Insurance, 987 Hill Street, Marrakesh, CA 01234

   Attention:

   Susan Jones, Claims Department

   Special Instructions:

   Certified Mail
3. Using proper letter formatting technique and the basic rules of writing reviewed in this chapter, correct the following letter:

   September 18th, 1997

   Mountainside Hospital
Samuel Adams, Educational Coordinator
1 Mountainside Lane
San Francisco, California, 94112

   Dear mr. Adams:

   I am writing in response to your letter of the 10th. I am very interested in presenting a talk at your Health Fare in February. I am avialable to speak on either the 20th or the 21st.

   If there is any flexibility in scheduling, I would prefer to present my talk in the afternoon. Also, please let me know how long I should prepare to speak. I am including a copy of an article I recently wrote on the same subject for the local paper.

   I am looking forward to hearing from you.

   Sincerly,

   Enclosure

   Dr. Angelo Carillo

   AC/SCB

Further Readings

Becklin, Karonne J., and Edith M. Sunnarborg. *Medical Office Procedures.* 4th ed. Westerville, OH: Glencoe, 1996.

Bureau of Business Practice Editorial Staff. *The Secretary's Complete Self-Training Manual.* Waterford, CT: Prentice Hall, 1992.

Jaderstrom, Susan, Leonard Kruk, and Joanne Miller. *Professional Secretaries International® Complete Office Handbook: The Secretary's Guide to Today's Electronic Office.* New York: Random House, 1992.

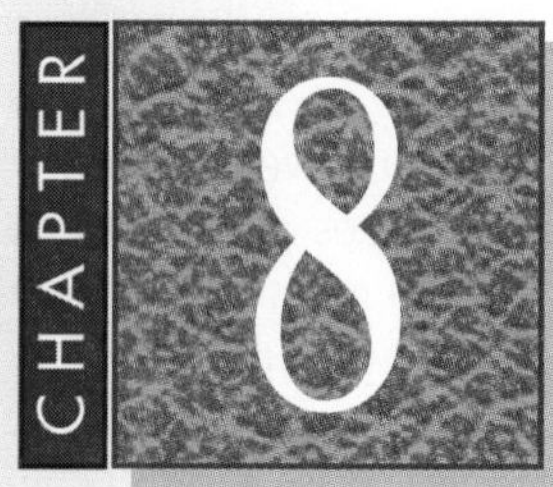

Managing Office Supplies

CHAPTER OUTLINE

- Organizing Medical Office Supplies
- Taking Inventory of Medical Office Supplies
- Ordering Supplies

OBJECTIVES

After completing Chapter 8, you will be able to:

- Give examples of vital, incidental, and periodic supplies used in a typical medical office.
- Describe how to store administrative and clinical supplies.
- Implement a system for tracking the inventory of supplies.
- Schedule inventories and ordering times to maximize office efficiency.
- Locate and evaluate supply sources.
- Use strategies to obtain the best-quality supplies while controlling cost.
- Follow procedures for ordering supplies.
- Check a supply order and pay for the supplies.

AREAS OF COMPETENCE

1997 ROLE DELINEATION STUDY

GENERAL (Transdisciplinary)

Operational Functions

- Maintain supply inventory
- Evaluate and recommend equipment and supplies

Key Terms

disbursement
durable item
efficiency
expendable item
inventory
invoice
purchase order
purchasing group
requisition
reputable
unit price

Organizing Medical Office Supplies

Purchasing and maintaining administrative and medical supplies are essential skills that you will use in managing the office. You will be responsible for taking inventory of equipment and supplies, evaluating and recommending equipment and supplies, and negotiating prices with suppliers. When managing office supplies, your goal is to achieve **efficiency,** which is the ability to produce the desired result with the least effort, expense, and waste.

The word *supplies* refers to **expendable items,** or items that are used and then must be restocked, such as prescription pads (Figure 8-1). More **durable items,** or pieces of equipment that are used indefinitely—such as telephones, computers, and examination tables—are not considered supplies. Also in the category of durable items is medical equipment, such as stethoscopes and reflex hammers. Ordering durable administrative items is discussed in Chapter 5.

Determining Responsibility for Organizing Supplies

It is recommended that the responsibility for organizing office supplies lie with at most one or two individuals. Often this responsibility is given to the medical assistant. In a small practice, one medical assistant may be able to handle this responsibility. A practice with several physicians may require two or three medical assistants to take care of supplies. When two medical assistants handle this responsibility, one is often assigned to handle administrative items and the other to handle clinical (medical) supplies. In a large practice, a third assistant might handle computer, copier, and fax supplies.

Categorizing Supplies

Most supplies in the medical office fall into two main categories: administrative and clinical. Examples of administrative supplies are those that keep the office running, such as stationery, insurance forms, pens, pencils, and clipboards. Clinical supplies are medically related and include alcohol swabs, tongue depressors, disposable tips for otoscopes, and disposable sheaths for thermometers.

There are also general supplies, which are used by both patients and staff. Examples of general supplies are paper towels, liquid hypoallergenic soap, and facial and toilet tissue.

The Supply List. You will need to determine what items in your office are used routinely and reordered systematically. Keep a list of these items, and update it as needed. This supply list is usually kept in the office procedures manual. Appropriate sections of the list may be posted on the cabinets where those items are stored.

To help keep track of supplies, categorize them according to the urgency of need. Although all supplies in your office are necessary, some supplies are more important than others. Figure 8-2 can help you determine vital, incidental, and periodic supplies for your office.

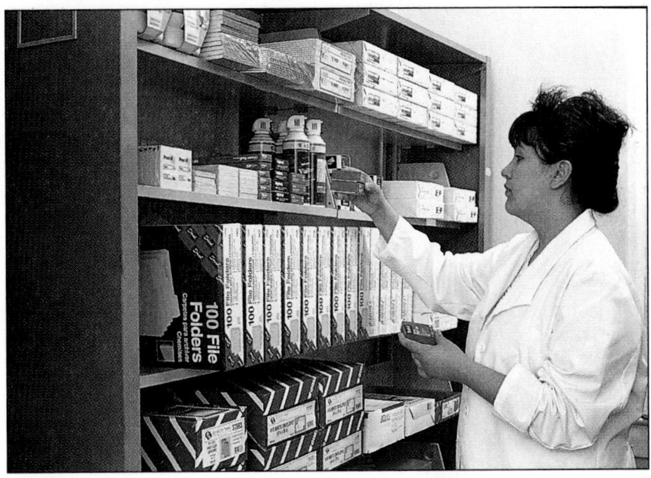

Figure 8-1. Making sure that supplies are in order is a continuous process that assures an efficient, well-prepared office.

Vital Supplies. These items are absolutely necessary to ensure the smooth running of the practice. They include paper examination table covers and prescription pads. Without these items, the physician would be unable to work in a clean examination environment or to readily prescribe medication for patients during office visits. Another type of vital supply is an item that requires a special order, such as a printed form. Special orders take time to obtain, so they must be ordered well before supplies run low.

Incidental Supplies. These supplies are needed in the office but do not threaten the efficiency of the office if the supply runs low. Incidental supplies include staples and rubber bands, which can be purchased quickly and easily at a local stationery store.

Periodic Supplies. These supplies require ordering only occasionally. For example, you will order appointment books only once or twice a year, probably in small numbers. The urgency of ordering some periodic items can depend on the size of the office. A multiphysician office, for example, would require more appointment books than a single-physician office. Another example of a periodic item might be holiday cards to send to the physician's colleagues and patients.

Storing Office Supplies

Storing office supplies requires good organizational skills and attention to detail. Many people in an office use these supplies, so the items should be stored neatly and in an orderly way. In addition, it is important to store supplies safely to prevent loss or theft, damage, or deterioration.

Typical Supplies in a Medical Office

Administrative Supplies

Appointment books, daybooks
Back-to-school/back-to-work slips
Clipboards
Computer supplies
Copy and facsimile (fax) machine paper
File folders, coding tabs
History and physical examination sheets/cards
Insurance forms: disability, HMO and other third party payers, life insurance examinations, Veterans Administration, workers' compensation
Insurance manuals
Local welfare department forms
Patient education materials
Pens, pencils, erasers
Rubber bands, paper clips
Social Security forms
Stamps
Stationery: appointment cards, bookkeeping supplies (ledgers, statements, billing forms), letterhead, second sheets, envelopes, business cards, prescription pads, notebooks, notepads, telephone memo pads

Clinical Supplies

Alcohol swabs
Applicators
Bandaging materials: adhesive tape, gauze pads, gauze sponges, elastic bandages, adhesive bandages, roller bandages (gauze and elastic)
Cloth or paper gowns
Cotton, cotton swabs
Culture tubes
50% dextrose solution
Disposable sheaths for thermometers

continued

Figure 8-2. Familiarize yourself with the typical supplies in a medical office.

Location. In a small medical office, supplies are generally kept near the areas of the office where they are used. Administrative supplies are usually stored behind or adjacent to the reception area, with clinical supplies stored near the examination rooms. If the practice has a laboratory, pertinent supplies are stored in or near the laboratory. Offices that have separate supply rooms offer more storage space.

Storage Cabinets. Each storage cabinet should be labeled with a list of its contents. Keep all stock of one item together. Store small items together according to type.

Finding supplies is easier if you keep small items at eye level. Put large, bulky goods, such as reams of stationery, on lower shelves. Label boxes and containers clearly so that all employees can readily find what they need and to make the inventory process easier.

To reduce the risk of errors on reorders, keep each item's original label attached to it. Cover the label with clear tape, if necessary. If you must replace a worn label, do it immediately when needed, making sure the new label has the same detailed information as the old one. Bottles with pouring spouts should be labeled on the side opposite the spout to prevent the liquid from dripping onto the label. Use a laundry marking pen to label linens with the name of your office. Linen services usually premark linens with the name of the company or the practice.

Many items have a shelf life after which they are not usable. By not overordering and by rotating supplies—using older ones first—your office will be able to use items during their shelf life. This is true not only for perishable items such as medications, but also for linens and paper, which can deteriorate. Keep in mind when stocking medications or chemicals that a more recent shipment may have an earlier expiration date than a previous shipment. Always check expiration dates when storing supplies. Be careful to arrange them so that items with earlier expiration dates are in front of those with later dates.

Administrative Supplies. In addition to such expendable items as pens, pencils, and paper clips, paper products are important to a medical office. In general, paper products should be stored flat in their original boxes or wrappings to prevent pages from bending or curling. However, information booklets may be stored upright to save space. Envelopes and other paper goods with gummed surfaces must be kept dry to prevent them from sticking together.

Clinical Supplies. The rules of good housekeeping and asepsis (see Chapter 19) apply to storage areas for clinical supplies. These areas must be kept clean and protected from damage and exposure to the elements.

All dressings and most bandaging materials must be kept sterile. For example, gauze that may be used to bandage an open wound must be sterile. Elastic rolled bandages, which do not touch open wounds, must be clean but not necessarily sterile.

Chemicals, drugs, and solutions should be kept in a cool, dark place because light causes some substances to deteriorate. Store all liquids in their original containers. Line cabinets with plastic-coated shelf paper, and wipe it frequently with a damp cloth.

Typical Supplies in a Medical Office continued

Clinical Supplies

Disposable tips for otoscopes
Gloves: sterile, examination
Hemoccult test kits
Iodine or Betadine pads
Lancets
Lubricating jelly
Microscopic slides and fixative
Needles, syringes
Nitroglycerin tablets
Safety pins
Silver nitrate sticks
Suture removal kits
Sutures
Thermometer covers
Tongue depressors
Topical skin freeze
Urinalysis test sticks
Urine containers
Injectable medications: diazepam (Valium), diphenhydramine hydrochloride (Benadryl), epinephrine (Adrenalin), furosemide (Lasix), isoproterenol (Isuprel), lidocaine (Xylocaine: 1%, 2%, and plain), meperidine hydrochloride (Demerol), morphine, phenobarbital, sodium bicarbonate, sterile saline, sterile water
Other medicines, chemicals, solutions, ointments, lotions, and disinfectants, as needed

General Supplies

Liquid hypoallergenic soap
Paper cups
Paper towels
Tampons
Tissues: facial, toilet

Store poisons and narcotics separately from other products. Narcotics must be stored securely out of sight in a locked cabinet. Never store strong acids near alkaline solutions or flammable items near sources of heat. Solutions that will be stored for a considerable length of time should have a small amount of space at the top of the bottle to allow for heat expansion.

Some liquids should be stored in the refrigerator. Check each item for specific storage instructions. If storage space is limited, consider eliminating some items—especially bulky ones that are rarely used or items that patients can purchase at surgical supply stores.

Taking Inventory of Medical Office Supplies

The list of supplies your office uses regularly and the quantities you have in storage constitute the office **inventory.** Keeping track of the office's inventory is a job that requires careful planning, attention to detail, and basic math skills. Accurate inventory activity ensures that the office never runs out of much-needed supplies.

Understanding Your Responsibilities

It is important to have an understanding with the doctor or doctors in the practice about the extent of your responsibilities for maintaining supplies. Some doctors are more involved with the details of running an office than others. Your responsibilities may grow as you become more experienced. The doctor, however, usually takes care of certain duties, such as meeting with drug company representatives or authorizing large purchases.

Generally you will be responsible for overseeing the flow of supplies bought and used, calculating the budget for supplies, selecting supplies and vendors, following correct purchasing and payment procedures, and storing the goods properly.

The Inventory Filing System. To oversee the flow of inventory efficiently, you will need a filing system. (See Procedure 8-1.) This system consists of several elements:

- The list of supplies (discussed earlier in the chapter)
- An itemized inventory
- An inventory card or record page for each item
- A list of the names and addresses of current vendors
- A file of current catalogs from vendors (including some vendors not currently used, for comparison shopping)
- A want list of brands or items that the office does not currently use but may want to try in the future
- Files for **invoices,** or bills from vendors, and completed order forms
- Reorder reminder cards to indicate when an in-stock item should be reordered
- Color-coded, removable self-adhesive flags to indicate "Need to Order" or "On Order"
- An inventory and ordering schedule
- Order forms for each vendor (may be multiple-copy forms, fax forms, electronic forms, or E-mail forms)

The Inventory Card or Record Page. The inventory card or record page for each item or category of items may be a 4- by 6-inch index card or a page in a loose-leaf

PROCEDURE 8-1

Step-by-Step Overview of Inventory Procedures

Objective: To set up an effective inventory program for a medical office

Materials: Pen, paper, file folders, vendor catalogs, index cards or loose-leaf binder and blank pages, reorder reminder cards, vendor order forms

Method

1. Define with your physician/employer the extent of your responsibility in managing supplies. Know whether the physician's approval or supervision is required for certain procedures, whether any systems have already been established, and if the physician has any preference for a particular vendor or trade-name item. If your medical practice is large, determine which medical assistant is responsible for each aspect of supply management.
2. Know what administrative and clinical supplies should be stocked in your office. Create a formal supply list of vital, incidental, and periodic items, and keep a copy in the office's procedures manual.
3. Start a file containing a list of current vendors with copies of their catalogs.
4. Create a want list of brands or products the office does not currently use but might like to try. Inform other staff members of the list so that they can make entries.
5. Make a file for supply invoices and completed order forms. (Keep these documents on file for at least 3 years.)
6. Devise an inventory system of index cards or loose-leaf pages for each item. List the following data for each item on its card:
   - Date and quantity of each order
   - Name and contact information for the vendor and sales representative
   - Date each shipment was received
   - Total cost and unit cost, or price per piece for the item
   - Payment method used
   - Results of periodic counts of the item
   - Quantity expected to cover the office for a given period of time
   - Reorder quantity (the quantity remaining on the shelf that indicates when reorder should be made)
7. Have a system for flagging items that need to be ordered and those that are already on order. For example, mark their cards or pages with a self-adhesive tab or note. Make or buy reorder reminder cards to put into the stock of each item at the reorder quantity level.
8. Establish with the physician a regular schedule for taking inventory. Every 1 to 2 weeks is usually sufficient. As a backup system for remembering to check stock and reorder, estimate the times for these activities. Mark them on your calendar, or create a tickler file on your computer.
9. Order at the same times each week or month, after inventory is taken. However, if there is an unexpected shortage of an item, and there is still more than a week or so before the regular ordering time, place the order immediately.
10. Fill in the vendor's order form (or type a letter of request). Order by telephone, fax, or E-mail, if possible, to expedite the order. Be sure to follow procedures that have been approved by the physician or office manager. When placing an order, have all the necessary information at hand, including the correct name of the item and the order and account numbers. Record the order information in the inventory file for that item. Be sure to obtain from the vendor an estimated arrival time for the order, and mark that date and order number on your calendar.
11. When you receive the shipment, record the date and the amount received on the item's inventory card or record page. Check the shipment against the original order and the packing slip inside the package to ensure that the right items, sizes, styles, packaging, and amounts have arrived. If there is any error, immediately call the vendor, with the catalog page and the inventory card or record page at hand.
12. Check the invoice carefully against the original order and the packing slip, making sure that the bill has not already been paid. Sign or stamp the invoice to show that the order was received.
13. Write a check to the vendor to be signed by the physician. Be sure to show the physician the original order, packing slip, and invoice. Record the check number, date, and amount of payment on the invoice, and initial it or have the physician do so. Write the invoice number on the front of the check.
14. Mail the check and the vendor's copy of the invoice to the vendor in a reasonable amount of time, and file the office copy of the invoice with the original order and packing slip.

binder (Figure 8-3). These separate cards or pages make it easy to group together the items that need to be ordered at any given time. Records kept on the card or page help you monitor how quickly items are used and how much should be ordered each time.

Some information may change. As you become more proficient at monitoring inventory or as the practice grows or diminishes in size, you may find that quantities, vendors, or reorder quantities need to be adjusted. Along with the doctor, you will be able to determine the ideal quantity of each item to have on hand, depending on the size of the practice, the available storage space, and the ordering schedule.

It is important to check the storage areas regularly, preferably at specific times, and to count the items on hand. When the supply of an item begins to run low, you (or another staff member) should flag the inventory card or record page to indicate the need to reorder it at the next regular ordering time.

Color-coded, removable self-adhesive flags on the inventory card or record page are an efficient way to track inventory. A red flag, for example, might indicate that a supply needs to be ordered. A yellow flag might be substituted when the item has been ordered.

Reorder Reminder Cards. Reorder reminder cards (Figure 8-4) are usually brightly colored cards inserted directly into stock on the supply shelf to indicate when it is time to reorder an item. For example, if you have determined that four boxes of staples is a sufficient quantity to keep on hand and your office supply orders are filled in 2 business days, you might place the reorder reminder card between the third and fourth boxes of staples. The reorder quantity on the inventory card or record page for staples would indicate "four boxes."

The reorder reminder cards also remind other staff members to tell you when an item is in short supply. In some offices, the medical assistant labels the reminder card with the name of the supply item, such as "staples." This method allows any staff member to pull the card when the last box of staples before the reminder card is taken from the supply shelf. The staff member can then place the card in a "To Be Ordered" envelope. Staff members in some offices request supplies by writing them in a want book or on a want list.

Inventory Reminder Kits. Some mail-order supply vendors sell inventory kits, complete with cards and tabs or flags. Computerized inventory systems are also available. Shelves still need to be checked and counts logged on to the computer, however. Therefore, smaller offices generally do not benefit as much as larger ones from a computerized inventory system.

(ITEM NAME) *Exam Table Paper 21"*

ORDER QUANTITY *12* REORDER POINT *4*

ORDER	QTY	REC'D	UNIT COST	PRICE	PREPAID	ON ACCT.	ORDER	QTY	REC'D	UNIT COST	PRICE	PREPAID	ON ACCT.
1/4	12	1/8	$12.25	$147.00	Check 1214	X							
2/5	12	2/9	$12.25	$147.00	Check 2110	X							

INVENTORY COUNT

	JAN.	FEB.	MAR.	APR.	MAY	JUNE	JULY	AUG.	SEPT.	OCT.	NOV.	DEC.
DATE ____	7	10										
DATE ____												

ORDER SOURCE

Smith Physician's Supply Co.
493 Carlton Avenue
South Union, NJ 07422
908-899-6123 Contact: Martin Kohn

UNIT PRICE

12 - $147.00
36 - $441.00

Figure 8-3. The inventory card or record page is the primary inventory-tracking tool in managing medical office supplies.

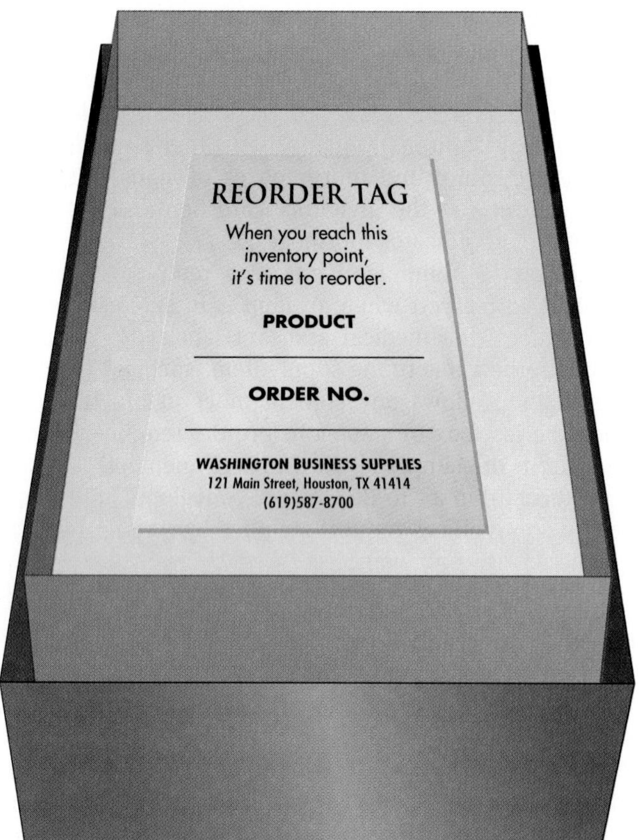

Figure 8-4. Reorder reminder cards are usually brightly colored cards inserted directly into the spare stock of an item on the supply shelf to indicate when it is time to reorder the item.

Scheduling Inventory and Ordering

Establish a regular schedule for counting the supplies in the office. Taking inventory every 1 or 2 weeks is usually sufficient. Estimating when you will probably need to reorder a particular item—and putting that date on your calendar or in your appointment book—is also helpful. You and the physician can determine how often storage areas should be checked.

Established Ordering Times. There should be established ordering times, such as the same day each week or month, after inventory is taken. For example, you might take inventory the first Tuesday of every month and order supplies the first Thursday of every month.

A regular schedule for taking inventory and ordering helps all staff members remember when they must give their requests to you. Although you may need to adjust the ordering time occasionally, try to adhere to the schedule to avoid the expense and inconvenience of rush orders.

When to Order Ahead of Schedule. When you take inventory, and the spare supply of an item has not reached but is close to the placement of the reorder reminder card, you must decide whether you should reorder then or wait until the next regular ordering time. You will probably find it is more efficient to go ahead and order rather than wait. Ordering early assures you that the supply will not be depleted before the next regular ordering time.

Ordering ahead of schedule can be especially important if there is a large demand for a particular product and manufacturers' production levels have not caught up with that demand. This situation can occur if there has been an outbreak of a particular flu or virus, or if the Food and Drug Administration has determined that a certain product is harmful, resulting in higher demand for an alternative product.

Unanticipated Shortage of a Supply Item. If the supply of an item reaches the reorder reminder card, and there is still a long time before the next regular ordering time, place the order immediately so that you do not risk running out of the item.

To help you oversee inventory effectively, request that your coworkers finish one container before opening a new one, and keep all stock of the same item in one place. The need to count inventory of an item in more than one location or container increases the likelihood of errors.

As a medical assistant, you want to be sure that there are always sufficient quantities of supplies to keep the office running efficiently. It is unwise to stock spare supplies in too great a quantity, however, because the administrative budget is not likely to support such expenditures. In addition, spare quantities of supplies can be a storage problem.

Ordering Supplies

Ordering supplies requires a procedure to deal with vendors and to order and check supplies. You can avoid common purchasing mistakes by understanding the most efficient way to order supplies for your office.

Locating and Evaluating Supply Vendors

A vendor will most likely already be in place when you join a practice. You should, however, be aware of competitors' prices, services, and other incentives intended to attract your office as a customer. Sometimes the incentives—such as bonus supplies with certain purchases—can represent sizable savings. Remember also that your time has a dollar value to the practice, and services that save you time are worth comparing when evaluating vendors.

Obtaining recommendations from other medical offices is a good way to locate office-supply dealers who sell items at reasonable prices and are also reputable. **Reputable** vendors fulfill orders accurately with quality items, deliver products in good condition, and charge fair prices. Keep in mind when evaluating vendors that the physician may have preferences for certain trade names or vendors.

Gathering Competitive Prices. The costs of maintaining a medical practice are continually rising. Saving money on supplies through careful purchasing strategies is one way to help your physician/employer reduce spending. The medical assistant is often largely responsible for comparison pricing, ordering, and establishing and maintaining relationships with vendors. Your awareness of the most up-to-date information about vendors and supplies is valuable to your physician/employer. Discuss prices with the physician, who in turn may want to discuss them with an accountant.

Setting Up a Supply Budget. The average medical practice spends 4% to 6% of its annual gross income on administrative, clinical, and general supplies. If an office is spending more than 6%, it may be time to reevaluate the office's spending practices. Remember, though, that any budget is only a guide. A budget is meant to serve your office, not the reverse. You and your physician/employer may need to adjust the supply budget based on prices and discounts available from vendors.

Comparing Vendors. To collect competitive data from vendors, contact them by telephone or in writing to request catalogs and other forms of product information. If you are not in charge of routing mail, make sure that supply-related mail, such as product catalogs and sale notices, is routed to you. Catalogs usually include basic information, such as the dealer's name, address, and telephone number, order numbers for items, and vendor policy (Figure 8-5). When investigating a vendor, obtain the following information:

- Prices—costs for supplies, delivery, and any other services; special discounts; minimum quantities applicable; bonus supplies with purchases
- Quality—product descriptions, illustrations, trade names, recommendations for use, durability, guarantees
- Service—availability of products, delivery time and procedures, sales representative availability, damaged-goods policy
- Payment policies

Competitive Pricing and Quality

Part of your responsibility in managing office supplies is to stay informed about the pricing and quality of competitors to your vendors. Savings can add up quickly, and ongoing comparison pricing can save the practice hundreds of dollars a year.

Unit Pricing. Because many medical items come in a variety of package sizes, you need to be aware of how much the office is actually paying per item. To calculate an item's **unit price,** divide the total price of the package by the quantity, or number of items. For example, if a package of 12 pens costs $12, the unit price, or price per pen, is $1 ($12 divided by 12 pens). If another vendor provides the same type of pen in a package of 18 for $17.10, the unit price is 95 cents ($17.10 divided by 18 pens). The second set of pens is the better buy.

Unit prices are generally lower at larger quantities. Therefore, it makes sense to place one large order for a nonperishable item to cover the office until the next ordering time. Generally, however, you should not order more than a year's supply of any one item, particularly if the item is custom-printed. Addresses, insurance codes, or additions to medical staff can change. When placing quantity discount orders, always consider the following factors: whether the supply can be used within a reasonable time, the possibility of spoilage or deterioration, the amount of storage space in the office, and whether the doctor will continue to use the item. Avoid overspending by not ordering more of an item than is reasonable or necessary.

Rush Orders. As stated earlier in the chapter, unexpected rush orders usually cost the office more money than regularly scheduled orders. (In some cases, a vendor may not charge extra to a steady customer, but these cases would be exceptions.) To avoid rush orders, be aware of approximately how long the vendor takes to deliver an order. You can obtain this information from the vendor policy and by keeping accurate records of your own experience with deliveries.

Mail-Order Companies. Using large, established mail-order companies often saves money for the medical office, but there may be less control over orders and a greater potential for hidden costs. The neighborhood pharmacy may also offer discounts, but ordering from wholesalers or directly from the manufacturer is usually more economical. "Tips for the Office" provides helpful information about cost-efficient ordering by telephone or fax or through an on-line service.

Purchasing Groups. Purchasing groups are groups of physicians that order supplies together to obtain a quantity discount. For example, several medical offices associated with a nearby hospital may order through the hospital. In return for this convenience, the physicians pay dues and guarantee the vendors a certain amount of business. Some programs require members to spend a certain percentage of their supply budget through the group. Groups may also require that members not disclose the group's prices to other physicians. The larger medical practices that participate in these groups save an average of 20% on supplies. The savings are not usually significant for small offices.

Group Buying Pools. If a medical office wants to use local vendors instead of, or in addition to, a purchasing group or if it is too small to benefit from a purchasing group, it can still pool resources with other area offices to

BY PHONE

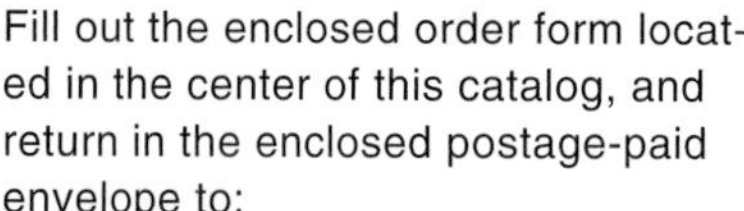

Call our toll-free number:
(800) BIBBERO
(800-242-2376)
Monday thru Friday,
6:00 A.M. – 5:00 P.M. (PST)

BY MAIL

Complete order form and mail to:
Bibbero Systems, Inc.
1300 N. McDowell Blvd.
Petaluma, CA 94954-1180

BY FAX

Complete order form and transmit via
FAX to : 800-242-9330
Our FAX line is open 24 hours daily.

Fill out the enclosed order form located in the center of this catalog, and return in the enclosed postage-paid envelope to:

Bibbero Systems, Inc.
1300 N. McDowell Blvd.
Petaluma, CA 94954-1180

If you are in a hurry, call us toll free at: 800-242-2376 or FAX us at 800-242-9330. Our Customer Service Department will be happy to assist you.

For items requiring custom imprinting, please enclose with your order the following information, either typed or printed: Name, Specialty, Address, City/State & Zip Code, Telephone Number and State License Number.

Send us your specifications for any type of special form - Patient Registration, History Forms, Dividers, Charts, etc. – and we will furnish quotes at no charge. We can print single page or multiple part forms.

Please Note: All custom printed orders are subject to an overrun or underrun variance of 10%.

TERMS

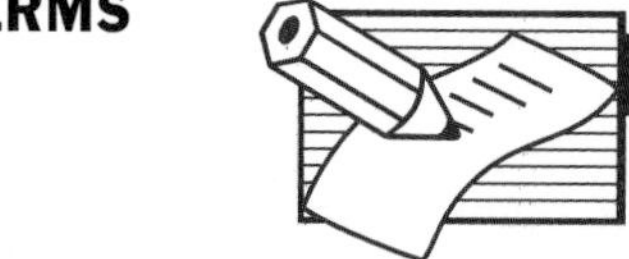

Full payment is due upon receipt of merchandise. Accounts are considered overdue after thirty (30) days and will be subject to a 1% monthly service charge. A service charge of $10.00 will be applied to all returned checks. For information regarding special financial arrangements, please contact our Credit Department at 800-242-2376.

GUARANTEE!

Your Satisfaction Guaranteed!

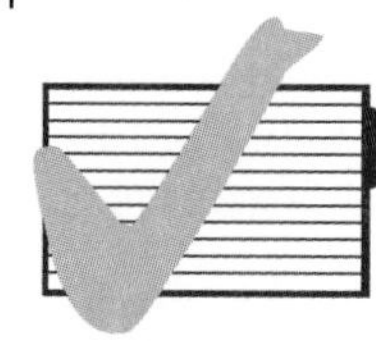

We guarantee our stock products. Return any of our stock products within 60 days of purchase for full credit, exchange or refund of your purchase price. After 60 days, your return will be subject to prior approval and a 15% restocking charge. All returns must have an authorization number. Call our Customer Service Department at 800-242-2376 for your authorization number and enclose it with your return. Opened and/or partially used packages cannot be returned. Personalized items, made to order, special orders and unlocked or opened software cannot be returned.

SHIPPING POLICY

Stock items are normally shipped the same day.

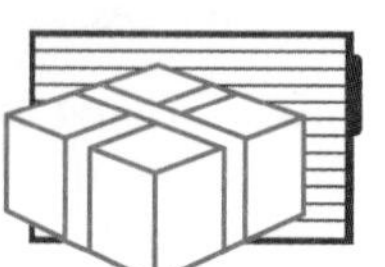

Stock orders received by 11:00 A.M. are normally shipped the same day. Out-of-stock items are automatically back ordered. Custom printed orders normally leave our plant within 10-15 working days after proof approval.

Combined stock and custom printed orders are shipped together, if requested. All orders are shipped via the best method available to your location. Common carriers are used for large volume orders. Overnight air and 2nd day delivery services are available on request.

FREE DELIVERY

Free delivery on pre-paid orders totaling $300.00 or more.

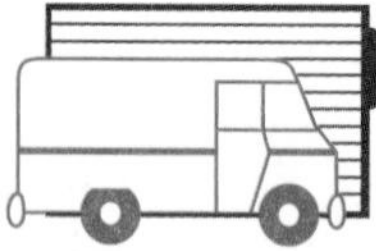

All orders prepaid by check, Visa, MasterCard or American Express totaling $300.00 or more will be shipped freight free within the continental U.S. This offer excludes furniture, cabinets, and special order items. We regret that the high cost of shipping outside the 48 contiguous states prohibits us from extending this service; we will use the most economical shipping method available to your location.

We accept Visa, MasterCard, & American Express for all your purchases.

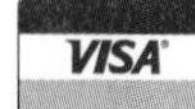

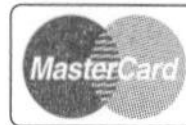

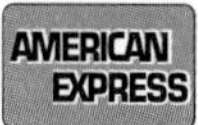

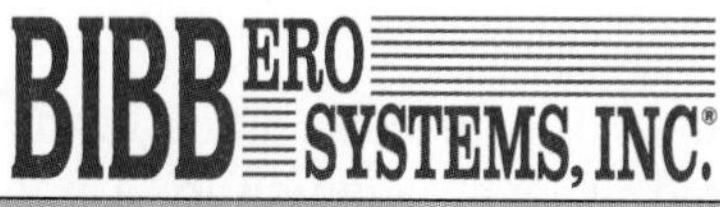

Figure 8-5. Examine supply catalogs carefully to find out vendors' company policies.

qualify for quantity discounts. Even if the offices are ordering different items, discounts are based on the total order, and savings can range from 10% to 20%. Under this arrangement the offices must usually take responsibility for distributing the items among themselves. A buying pool is convenient for medical practices that are in the same building or office complex (Figure 8-6).

Benefits of Using Local Vendors

There are many potential vendors, including local dealers, mail-order companies, and nearby pharmacies. Try to establish good credit and business relationships with reputable local vendors. These companies often charge a little more than mail-order companies. Still, spending most of the office's supply budget through one favored local

Tips FOR THE OFFICE

Ordering by Telephone or Fax or On-Line

You may occasionally purchase office supplies at a local retail outlet, but most often you will order them without leaving your office. Three common ways to do so are by telephone, by facsimile (or fax) machine, and through an on-line service. Here are tips to help make sure every order—no matter which option you choose—is successfully placed.

Ordering by Telephone

1. Clear communication is a must when ordering by telephone. Speak slowly, and enunciate your words carefully to make sure you are understood. It is also a good idea to spell each word of the practice's name and the address to ensure proper delivery. Use expressions like "S as in Sam, P as in people" to clarify your spelling.
2. Ask the representative taking your order to repeat the order. Check that every item is included with the appropriate price, quantity, style, and color.
3. Confirm the expected delivery date so that you will know if something is late. Also confirm how payment will be made, to prevent unexpected delays.
4. Record the name and telephone number of the person who takes the order in case there is a problem with the order. Get an order number (sometimes called a confirmation number) in case you have to call back with a question or a change in your order.
5. If possible, avoid placing telephone orders on Mondays and Fridays, when call volume is typically high.

Ordering by Fax

1. When ordering by fax, use the form provided by the vendor if one is available. This form uses the format to which the supply company is accustomed and will speed the processing of your order.
2. Type your order, or write it neatly and legibly, to prevent miscommunication. Fill out the form completely. Make sure you indicate quantities, descriptions, and prices (including shipping) for each item you order.
3. Proofread your order before you send it. Checking the accuracy of the order now will save time later.
4. Follow up by telephone to make sure your order was received and understood and to confirm the delivery date and payment requirements.

Ordering On-Line

1. Ordering on-line requires a computer and a modem connection to the Internet or to an on-line service. Before ordering on-line, make sure you are fully familiar with the equipment and the process, or have your supervisor or the supply company's sales representative oversee your initial orders.
2. Type your name and address accurately.
3. If pictures of supplies are not available on-line, consult the company's printed catalog or CD-ROM catalog. If you do not have access to a catalog, read the on-line text descriptions carefully, checking trade names and specifications, to select the appropriate merchandise. If you have questions, consult the supply company by telephone.
4. When you have completed the selections, the on-line service will display your order so that you can confirm it. Check that all the information is accurate, including your name, address, and telephone number.
5. If you have an account with the company, you may type in your account number to place the order. Otherwise, you may wish to arrange to make payment upon delivery. If you prefer to pay by credit card, first make sure that the company is reputable and that it uses a security system that prevents your number from being read by anyone unauthorized to do so.

If, despite your best efforts, your order is [illegible]cessed incorrectly, take appropriate action immed[illegible] [illegible]though ordering by telephone or fax or [illegible] [illegible]nient, it still requires additional time t[illegible] that must be returned.

By law, orders that you place [illegible] a reasonable time. The Feder[illegible] monitors purchases by telep[illegible] vices to protect consumer[illegible] panies to provide merc[illegible] you the option of ca[illegible] full refund.

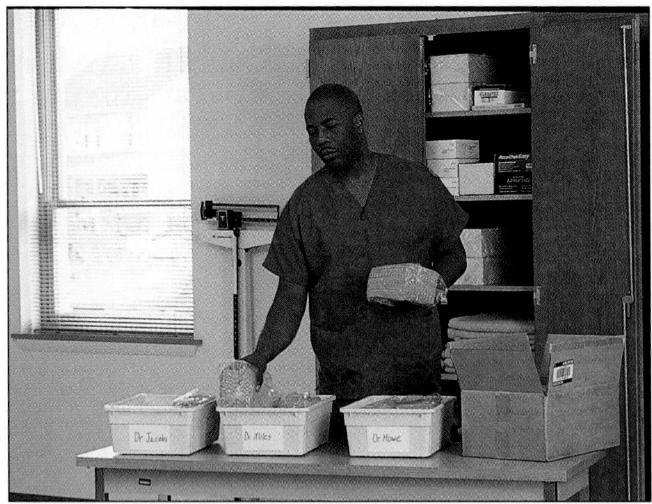

Figure 8-6. Ordering jointly with other offices can cut expenses for everyone.

dealer often results in discounts, special service in the event of an emergency, and information about upcoming sales and specials. Local dealers may also offer more personal assistance, perhaps even a salesperson's help with taking inventory, to compete with larger vendors whose business is based primarily on catalog sales. The extra service may be worth the higher cost.

Buying from local vendors can also provide a public relations benefit for physicians; it means keeping business in the community. However, specialty items may need to be ordered from other vendors. For example, letterhead should be ordered from a reliable printer, whether that printer is located in the community or out of state.

Payment Schedules

Another factor that affects the cost of supplies is the payment schedule. Many vendors do not charge for handling if an order is prepaid. Others offer a discount for enclosing a check with an order. Some delay billing for 30 to 90 days, allowing the physician to keep the money in the bank, collecting interest for a longer period.

The vendor's invoice usually describes payment terms. Two examples of payment terms follow.

- If the invoice says "Net 30," you have 30 days in which to pay the total amount.
- "1% 10 Days Net 30" means that you will get a savings of 1% of the total price by paying within 10 days.

Copies of all bills and order forms for supplies should be kept on file for at least 5 years in case the practice is audited by the Internal Revenue Service (IRS).

...ge Space as a Cost Factor

...n purchases, you need to consider the ...ce. Ideally, there should be enough ... occasional large purchases for

quantity discounts. If there is not, a vendor might allow you to take partial shipments on a large order. The vendor might also allow you to pay for the partial shipments with partial payments, but you will probably have to request this plan.

Ordering Procedures

Ordering procedures for supplies vary from office to office but always involve these tasks: completing paperwork, checking orders received, correcting errors in shipments, and making payment.

Order Forms. Before ordering merchandise, you should inquire about a vendor's ordering options, discuss them with the physician, and determine which method is best for the office. Many vendors now accept telephone, fax, and E-mail as well as traditional written order forms. Many vendors will also send a sales representative to your office to help you decide which items to purchase and to show you how to complete an order form accurately. Sometimes the sales representative can give you better deals than those described in the catalog. Whatever form you use, be sure to keep a copy of each order you submit.

Before you place an order, gather all the necessary information, such as correct names of items, item numbers, and order and account numbers. This information helps ensure the accuracy of the order. Immediately after placing the order, note all order information on the inventory card or record page for that item.

Purchase Requisitions. You will need to follow any special ordering procedures established in your medical office. The specific procedures and the level of authority a medical assistant has vary from one office to another. Sometimes placing an order requires a **requisition** (a formal request from a staff member or doctor), which is given to the medical assistant who does the actual ordering. The doctor's approval may be necessary for large purchases—for example, for orders that total more than $300. Recurring orders may not require the doctor's approval, but you may need to get approval before ordering a new brand or quantities of a particular item over a certain amount.

In a group practice where doctors order different items and several staffers are in charge of ordering, procedures for ordering can be complicated. One common way to simplify matters is to use **purchase orders,** forms that authorize a purchase for the practice. Figure 8-7 shows a sample purchase order. Purchase orders are usually preprinted with consecutive numbers. The medical assistant submits approved purchase orders to the vendor for fulfillment. This method is most often used for expensive items, such as office equipment, but some large practices also use purchase orders for supplies.

Checking Orders Received. When the shipment of supplies arrives, record the date received on the inventory card or record page, as well as the quantity of each item. Check the shipment against the order form to make sure the correct items—in the correct sizes, styles, packaging, and quantity—have been delivered.

Then check the contents against the packing slip (a description of the package contents) enclosed in the package. This checking takes time, but catching even one error is worth the time taken. If several people on a staff have ordering responsibility, they can share the task.

Correcting Errors. If you find an error in a shipment, contact the vendor immediately so that the records can be corrected and missing supplies can be delivered immediately. When you call to report errors, be sure you have all the paperwork in front of you. You will need the invoice number, order date, name of the person who placed the order, name of the person who took the order, and a list of questions or a description of the complaint. If a catalog was used in ordering, have it open to the appropriate page.

Invoices. Typically the vendor sends an invoice to the medical office, either accompanying the merchandise or separately. This invoice also should be checked carefully against the original order and the packing slip. Be sure to check the arithmetic as well. Then sign or stamp the invoice to confirm that the order was received. If an item you order is temporarily out of stock, the vendor usually sends an invoice stamped "Back Ordered." Later, when the item is back in stock, the vendor will ship it to your office.

Make sure the invoice has not already been paid. It is a good habit to record the check number, date, and amount of payment on the invoice. You may initial it or have the doctor initial it.

Disbursements. An invoice is paid with a **disbursement** (payment of funds) to a vendor. Disbursements may be made in cash or by check or money order. Usually you will write a check to the vendor and have the physician sign it. Be sure to show the physician the original order, packing slip, and invoice. On the front of the check, record the invoice number. Finally, mail the check to the vendor with the vendor's copy of the invoice. File the office copy of the invoice, along with the original order and the packing slip, according to your inventory filing system (Figure 8-8).

If you make a cash disbursement, obtain a receipt to keep on file. If you are the one responsible for maintaining the practice's financial records and presenting them to the accountant, you may also be responsible for recording the payment information in the office's accounting books.

PURCHASE ORDER

Submitted by: ______________________
Order Number: ______________________
Date Ordered: ______________________
Date Required: ______________________

SHIP TO: Dr. Carlotta Montoni
201 Oak Walk, Suite 32
Gilead, PA 19034

PHONE: 215-610-4120

	ITEM	DESCRIPTION/MODEL	COLOR	SIZE	QUANTITY	PRICE EACH	TOTAL
1.							
2.							
3.							
4.							
5.							
6.							
7.							
8.							
						TOTAL	

Approved: ______________________ Date: ______________________

Figure 8-7. A purchase order, when approved by the physician or office manager, is an authorization from the practice for a purchase.

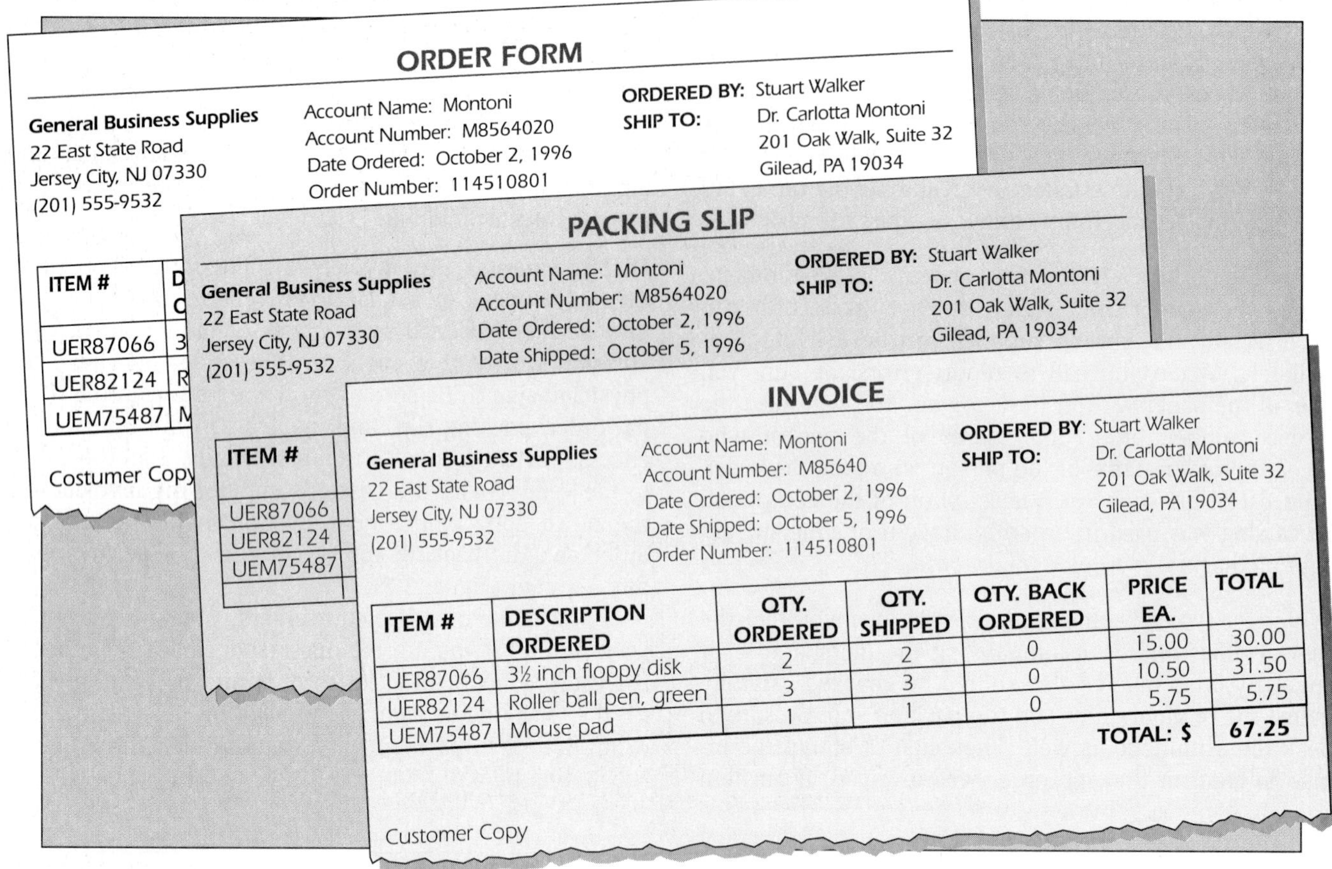

ORDER FORM

General Business Supplies
22 East State Road
Jersey City, NJ 07330
(201) 555-9532

Account Name: Montoni
Account Number: M8564020
Date Ordered: October 2, 1996
Order Number: 114510801

ORDERED BY: Stuart Walker
SHIP TO: Dr. Carlotta Montoni
201 Oak Walk, Suite 32
Gilead, PA 19034

ITEM #
UER87066
UER82124
UEM75487

PACKING SLIP

General Business Supplies
22 East State Road
Jersey City, NJ 07330
(201) 555-9532

Account Name: Montoni
Account Number: M8564020
Date Ordered: October 2, 1996
Date Shipped: October 5, 1996

ORDERED BY: Stuart Walker
SHIP TO: Dr. Carlotta Montoni
201 Oak Walk, Suite 32
Gilead, PA 19034

ITEM #
UER87066
UER82124
UEM75487

INVOICE

General Business Supplies
22 East State Road
Jersey City, NJ 07330
(201) 555-9532

Account Name: Montoni
Account Number: M85640
Date Ordered: October 2, 1996
Date Shipped: October 5, 1996
Order Number: 114510801

ORDERED BY: Stuart Walker
SHIP TO: Dr. Carlotta Montoni
201 Oak Walk, Suite 32
Gilead, PA 19034

ITEM #	DESCRIPTION ORDERED	QTY. ORDERED	QTY. SHIPPED	QTY. BACK ORDERED	PRICE EA.	TOTAL
UER87066	3½ inch floppy disk	2	2	0	15.00	30.00
UER82124	Roller ball pen, green	3	3	0	10.50	31.50
UEM75487	Mouse pad	1	1	0	5.75	5.75
					TOTAL: $	67.25

Customer Copy

Figure 8-8. Check the information on the vendor invoice against the original order and the packing slip to make sure there are no errors.

Avoiding Common Purchasing Mistakes

Even the most watchful professional can make purchasing mistakes. The best you can do is to educate yourself about common mistakes and try to avoid them. For example, be aware of the possibility of dishonest telephone solicitations. A caller may claim to be a sales representative for the manufacturer of the office photocopier, offering bargains on paper or toner. The caller may require advance payment to be sent to a post office box. The bargains may never arrive.

The best way to deal with these solicitations is to tell the caller that your office does not purchase supplies by telephone. If a telephone offer appears to be legitimate and to offer substantial savings, ask for the name and telephone number of the firm so that you can return the call at a more convenient time. Then you can verify the number with the telephone company and check the firm's name with the Better Business Bureau.

Another disreputable tactic some vendors use is bait and switch: the price of one item is lowered to attract the customer, but that item is always "sold out" and the customer is encouraged to buy a more expensive one. A vendor may also mislead you by raising the price of an item you have been ordering without informing you. Always confirm the current price, check invoices as they come in, and record everything in the item's file. Having your inventory card or record page open while ordering will prompt you to notice and question price changes. If there is an honest error, a reputable firm will readily and courteously correct it.

Problems can also be avoided by carefully supervising a new vendor's sales representative until a comfortable, professional rapport has been established. Discuss your inventory system with representatives, and ask them questions about their procedures.

Summary

A typical medical practice uses both administrative and clinical office supplies. Supplies can be categorized as vital, incidental, and periodic.

Keeping track of supplies involves creating supply lists and taking inventory. You must know the storage requirements for various kinds of supplies. An inventory filing system can help you organize office supply tasks. Maintaining adequate supplies and well-organized storage space contributes to the smooth running of the office.

You will also locate, evaluate, and establish and maintain working relationships with vendors. It is important to be adept at comparison pricing and to stay abreast of competitors' product quality, pricing policies, and services.

Just as cost-effectiveness is stressed in medical care, it is important to look for ways to control costs when ordering supplies. Checking orders carefully and avoiding dishonest telephone solicitations are two examples of ways to control costs.

8 Chapter Review

Discussion Questions

1. When starting a new job with a practice, what are three specific inquiries you might make about maintaining office supplies?
2. Discuss how procedures for maintaining office supplies in a multiphysician practice might differ from those in a solo medical practice.
3. Name two ways you might adjust the inventory system after the office unexpectedly runs out of letterhead.

Critical Thinking Questions

1. You just learned that Superior Office Supplies, one of your main vendors, is going out of business soon. How can you prepare for the change?
2. You are surprised to notice that the supply of prescription pads is at an extremely low level for typical office usage. What step could you take to replace the item that would be both quick and cost-effective?
3. While taking the biweekly supply inventory, you notice that the number of self-adhesive flags remaining on the shelf is much lower than usual. How would you investigate why this shortage happened, and how might you prevent a repeat occurrence?

Application Activities

1. Using vendor catalogs, make a list of ten typical office supply items for a medical practice. Create a fictional office supply list and ordering schedule (including quantities and prices) for the practice.
2. Select a supply company catalog, and become familiar with it. Imagine that you are a sales representative for that company, and make a presentation to your class as if it were a typical medical practice. Your goal is to have the medical office choose your company as its vendor. Be prepared to answer questions about how your company handles various customer concerns.
3. Make a diagram of an office supply cabinet, indicating how you would label and store items for maximum efficiency. Try to use several of the inventory elements discussed in the chapter.

Further Readings

Carpenter, David C. "How to Get the Best All-Around Deals on Supplies: Quality and Customer Service Are as Important as Low Prices." *Medical Economics,* 18 March 1991, 86.

Murray, Dennis. "Save Big on Equipment and Supplies: Medical Office Equipment Purchasing." *Medical Economics,* 13 September 1993, 55.

Sweeney, Dorothy R. "Keeping a Lid on Supply Costs." *Medical Economics,* 16 March 1992, 195.

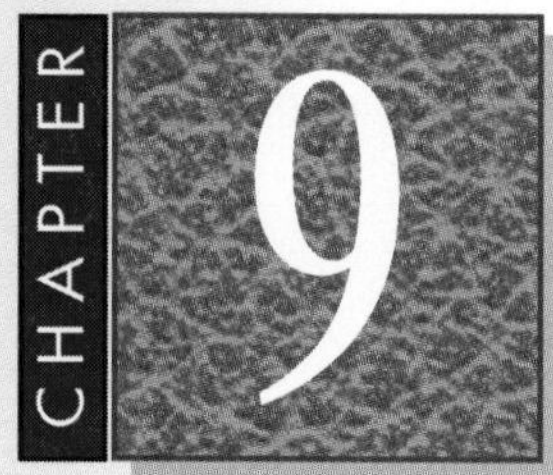

Maintaining Patient Records

CHAPTER OUTLINE

- Importance of Patient Records
- Contents of Patient Charts
- Initiating and Maintaining Patient Records
- The Six Cs of Charting
- Types of Medical Records
- Appearance, Timeliness, and Accuracy of Records
- Medical Transcription
- Correcting and Updating Patient Records
- Release of Records

Key Terms

documentation
informed consent form
patient record/chart
POMR
sign
SOAP
symptom
transcription
transfer

OBJECTIVES

After completing Chapter 9, you will be able to:

- Explain the purpose of compiling patient medical records.
- Describe the contents of patient record forms.
- Describe how to create and maintain a patient record.
- Identify and describe common approaches to documenting information in medical records.
- Discuss the need for neatness, timeliness, accuracy, and professional tone in patient records.
- Discuss tips for performing accurate transcription.
- Explain how to correct a medical record.
- Explain how to update a medical record.
- Identify when and how a medical record may be released.

AREAS OF COMPETENCE

1997 ROLE DELINEATION STUDY

ADMINISTRATIVE

Administrative Procedures

- Perform medical transcription

CLINICAL

Patient Care

- Obtain patient history and vital signs
- Coordinate patient care information with other health care providers

GENERAL (Transdisciplinary)

Communication Skills

- Receive, organize, prioritize, and transmit information

continued

AREAS OF COMPETENCE continued

Legal Concepts

- Prepare and maintain medical records
- Document accurately
- Use appropriate guidelines when releasing information
- Follow federal, state, and local legal guidelines

Importance of Patient Records

One of your most important duties as a medical assistant will be filling out and maintaining accurate and thorough patient records. **Patient records,** also known as **charts,** contain important information about a patient's medical history and present condition. Patient records serve as communication tools as well as legal documents. They also play a role in patient and staff education and may be used for quality control and research.

These records provide physicians with all the important information, observations, and opinions that have been recorded about a patient. The health-care professional can read the complete patient medical history and information about treatment and outcomes. The information in the records can also be sent to other physicians or health-care specialists if the patient needs further treatment, changes physicians, or moves to a new location. Medical records include the following information about the patient:

- Address and phone number
- Insurance coverage
- Name of the person responsible for payment
- Occupation
- Medical history
- Current complaint or condition
- Health-care needs
- Medical treatment plan or services received
- Radiology and laboratory reports (sometimes)
- Response to care

Legal Guidelines for Patient Records

Patient records are important for legal reasons. As a general rule, if information is not documented, no one can prove that an event or procedure took place. Medical records are used in lawsuits and malpractice cases to support a patient's claim of malpractice against a doctor and to support the doctor in defense against a claim.

Standards for Records

Records that are complete, accurate, and well documented can be convincing evidence that a doctor provided appropriate care. On the other hand, altered, incomplete, inaccurate, or illegible records may imply that a doctor's entire medical practice is below standard.

Additional Uses of Patient Records

Patient records serve as ongoing references about individual patients' medical care. They are also valuable for patient education, quality of treatment, and research.

Patient Education. Patient records can be used to educate patients about their own conditions and treatment plans. The physician can point out how test results have changed or how the patient's general health has improved or lessened. She can also emphasize the importance of following treatment instructions. The medical assistant in turn may use some of this information in educating the patient about his condition or its management. Records can also be used to educate the health-care staff about unusual medical conditions, patient progress, or results of treatment plans.

Quality of Treatment. Patient records may be used to evaluate the quality of treatment a facility or doctor's office provides. Auditing groups, such as peer review organizations or the Joint Commission on Accreditation of Healthcare Organizations (JCAHO), may review the charts to monitor whether the care provided and the fees charged meet accepted standards. Records also provide statistics for health-care analysis and future health-care plans and policy decisions.

Research. Patient records also play an important role in medical research. For example, a medical research team may be testing a new hypertension drug with volunteers who fit a certain medical category—perhaps men between the ages of 45 and 54 who have high blood pressure. Carefully kept records are valuable sources of data about patient responses, behavior, symptoms, side effects, and outcomes (see Figure 9-1).

On the other hand, information in charts may spur researchers to begin a study. For example, the records may show that 80% of all patients taking a particular heart medication experience dizziness. Researchers can investigate why this reaction might be happening.

Contents of Patient Charts

You will fill out a record for each new patient who comes to the office. Although each physician's office has its own forms and medical charts, in general, all records must contain certain standard information.

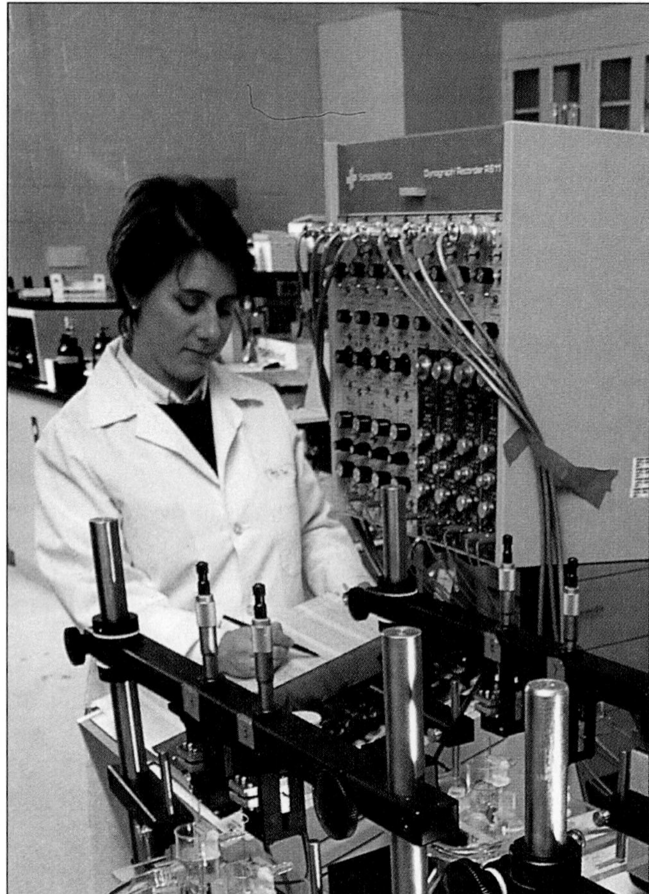

Figure 9-1. Medical researchers may rely on data gathered from patient records.

Standard Chart Information

Standard chart information covers a spectrum of different, carefully detailed notes and facts about a patient, from his medical history to the doctor's diagnosis and comments on follow-up care. You must have an understanding of what each part means.

Patient Registration Form. This part of the record should list the date of the patient's current visit, the patient's age, address, Social Security number, medical insurance, occupation, marital status, and number of children, and the name of the person to contact in an emergency. Some patient registration forms include family medical history and a list of medical problems. This information is usually placed at the front or top half of the chart for easy reference. Figure 9-2 is an example of a patient registration form.

Patient Medical History. This section includes the patient's past medical history (including illnesses, surgeries, known allergies, or current medications), family medical history, and social and occupational history (including diet, exercise, smoking, and use of alcohol or drugs). Usually, the history form ends with a section for the patient to describe the condition or complaint that is the reason for her visit. Medicare and managed care insurance now require that the patient's complaint be entered into the medical record. Preferably this complaint should be recorded in the patient's own words.

Physical Examination Results. Sometimes a form is used to record the results of a general physical examination. Figure 9-3 shows a combination medical history and physical examination form.

Results of Laboratory and Other Tests. Test results include findings from tests performed in the office and those received from other doctors, hospitals, or independent laboratories. Some offices use a laboratory summary sheet to help the doctor detect significant changes more easily.

Records From Other Physicians or Hospitals. These records should be entered into the patient's chart. A copy of the patient's written request authorizing release of the records from the other sources should also be included.

Doctor's Diagnosis and Treatment Plan. The doctor's diagnosis must be recorded, along with the treatment plan, which may consist of treatment options, the final treatment list, instructions to the patient, and any medications prescribed. The doctor may also put specific comments or impressions on record.

Operative Reports, Follow-Up Visits, and Telephone Calls. Continuation of the record lasts as long as the patient is under the doctor's care. You should record and date all procedures, surgeries, follow-up care, and additional notes the doctor makes regarding the patient's case. You can use continuation forms to add more pages. In addition, you may keep a separate log of telephone calls to and from the patient.

Informed Consent Forms. **Informed consent forms,** such as the one shown in Figure 9-4, verify that a patient understands the treatment offered and the possible outcomes or side effects of the treatment. Consent forms may specify what the outcome might be if the patient receives no treatment. They may also describe alternative treatments and possible risks. The patient signs the consent form but may withdraw consent if she changes her mind.

Discharge Summary Forms. The discharge summary form generally includes information that summarizes the reason the patient entered the hospital; tests, procedures, or operations performed in the hospital; medications administered in the hospital; and the disposition, or outcome, of the case. A medical assistant working in a hospital (not a doctor's office) would complete this form. Elements of the form may include the following:

- Date of admission
- Brief history
- Date of discharge
- Admitting diagnosis
- Operations and procedures or hospital course (course of action taken in the hospital)
- Complications

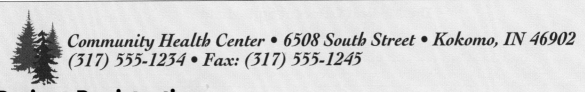

Patient Registration
Patient Information

Name: ________________ Today's Date: ________

Address: ________________

City: ________ State: ________ Zip Code: ________

Telephone (Home): ________ (Work): ________

Birthdate: ________ Age: ____ Sex: M F No. of Children ____ Marital Status: M S W D

Social Security Number: ________ Employer: ________ Occupation: ________

Primary Physician: ________________

Referred by: ________________

Person to Contact in Emergency: ________________

Emergency Telephone: ________________

Special Needs: ________________

Responsible Party

Party Responsible for Payment: Self Spouse Parent Other

Name (If Other Than Self): ________________

Address: ________________

City: ________ State: ________ Zip Code: ________

Primary Insurance

Primary Medical Insurance: ________________

Insured party: Self Spouse Parent Other

ID#/Social Security No.: ________ Group/Plan No.: ________

Name (If Other Than Self): ________________

Address: ________________

City: ________ State: ________ Zip Code: ________

Secondary Insurance

Secondary Medical Insurance: ________________

Insured party: Self Spouse Parent Other

ID#/Social Security No.: ________ Group/Plan No.: ________

Name (If Other Than Self): ________________

Address: ________________

City: ________ State: ________ Zip Code: ________

Figure 9-2. The patient registration form is often the first document used in initiating a patient record.

The Medical Center at Springfield

Medical History

Name Age Sex S M W D

Address Phone Date

Occupation Ref. by

Chief Complaint

Present Illness

History —Military

—Social

—Family

—Marital

—Menstrual Menarche Para. LMP

—Illness Measles Pert. Var. Pneu. Pleur. Typh. Mal. Rh. Fev. Sc. Fev. Diphth. Other

—Surgery

—Allergies

—Current Medications

Physical Examination

Temp. Pulse Resp. BP Ht. Wt.

General Appearance Skin Mucous Membrane

Eyes: Vision Pupil Fundus

Ears:

Nose:

Throat: Pharynx Tonsils

Chest: Breasts

Heart:

Lungs:

Abdomen:

Genitalia:

Rectum:

Pelvic:

Extremities: Pulses:

Lymph Nodes: Neck Axilla Inguinal Abdominal

Neurological:

Diagnosis:

Treatment:

Laboratory Findings:

Date Blood

Date Urine

Figure 9-3. In some doctors' offices, the medical history form and the physical examination form are combined.

THE OAK HILLS MEDICAL CENTER
Oak Hills, MA

CONSENT TO OPERATION, ADMINISTRATION OF ANESTHETICS, AND RENDERING OF OTHER MEDICAL SERVICE

Patient: ______________________________ Age: __________
Date: ______________________ Time: ______________________

1. I AUTHORIZE AND DIRECT ______________________, with the associates and assistants of his/her choice, to perform upon myself the following operation
____
____
____

If any unforeseen conditions arise in the course of the operation or in the postoperative period, calling in their judgment for other operations or procedures, I further request and authorize them to do whatever is deemed advisable for my health and well-being.

2. The positive and negative aspects of autologous blood transfusions (receiving my own blood donated prior to surgery), designated blood transfusions (donated in advance by family/friends for my use), or homologous blood transfusions (from general donor population) have been explained to me. I understand autologous and designated transfusions can be accommodated only for nonemergency surgery.

6. I certify that I understand the above consent to operation and that the explanations referred to have been made.

______________________ ______________________
Witness (of signature only) Signature

Figure 9-4. Patients are asked to sign informed consent forms to confirm that they understand the treatment offered.

- Instructions to the patient for follow-up care after discharge from the hospital
- Physician's signature

Correspondence With or About the Patient. All written correspondence from the patient or from other doctors, laboratories, or independent health-care agencies should be kept in the patient's chart. Make sure that each piece of correspondence is marked or stamped with the date the doctor's office received the document.

Information Received by Fax

Some information—such as laboratory results, physician comments, or correspondence—may be received by fax transmission. Always request that the original be mailed if possible. If the original is not available, make a photocopy of the fax. Fax copies made on thermal paper, as opposed to those made from a plain-paper fax, fade over time and may become unreadable.

Dating and Initialing

You must be careful not only to date everything you put into the patient chart but also to initial the entry. This system makes it easy to tell which items the assistant enters into the chart and which items others enter. In many practices the physician initials reports before they are filed to prove that he saw them.

Initiating and Maintaining Patient Records

Besides the receptionist, you will often be the first health-care professional that new patients talk with when they visit a doctor's office. During your first contact with a patient, you will initiate a patient record. Recording information in the medical record is called **documentation.** Complete, thorough documentation ensures that the doc-

Tips FOR THE OFFICE

Talking With the Older Patient

If you work in a practice that specializes in geriatrics or in any practice with older patients, certain communication skills will help you in your job. You may find yourself in various situations in which knowing how to talk with the older patient will be a necessary skill. Taking a medical history or helping a patient describe her symptoms are two such situations. The following tips will help you and the patient communicate with each other more effectively.

1. Many older patients are hard of hearing, but *not deaf*. Speak slightly more slowly than you normally would. Speak clearly and loudly (but do not shout—shouting will insult and anger an older patient who does hear well). Enunciate well, and use a lower tone of voice (elderly people lose the ability to hear high-frequency sounds first). If the patient asks you to repeat a question, rephrase it instead of repeating it verbatim.
2. Look at the patient directly so that she knows you care about what she has to say and so that you can make sure she understands what you tell or ask her.
3. You can show respect for the patient's age by addressing the patient with Mr., Mrs., Ms., or Miss, unless he or she asks to be called by his or her first name.
4. Be patient. Some older patients live alone or in relative isolation and may be out of practice with the two-way communication skills that make a conversation or interview go smoothly. The simple act of being interviewed, even for what may seem to you a straightforward medical history, may unsettle the older patient. For example, he may need to stop and think of a word here and there. Do not supply the word. Wait—let the patient think of it on his own. Also, do not rush through your questions. Rushing will only make the patient feel anxious and incompetent if she feels she cannot keep up with you.
5. Practice active listening skills. Pay attention to the patient's verbal and nonverbal cues. Do not interrupt the patient. After the patient finishes giving each answer, repeat it, to give him a chance to correct you if you misheard or misunderstood.
6. If you are interviewing the patient to obtain a medical history, explain before you begin the type of questions you will ask and how the information will be used.
7. If you need to use medical terminology, try also to express the same information in lay terms. For example, you might ask, "Do you use a diuretic or pill to help you eliminate fluids?"
8. Be cheerful and friendly but not sugary-sweet. Do not talk down to older patients; they are not stupid.
9. Avoid sounding surprised or excited by any answer to a question or to any information the patient gives.
10. Under no circumstances use endearments such as dear, honey, or sweetie.
11. Look for ways to make a connection so that the patient feels relaxed and comfortable. In the course of taking a patient's history, you might find out that he enjoys swimming. Maybe you do, too—and you can describe a beautiful lake you once went swimming in.
12. Show an interest in the patient as a person. Ask about something she is interested in. For example, a patient might be wearing a piece of handmade jewelry. Ask where it came from. She might have a wonderful story to tell.

tor will have detailed notes about each of her contacts with the patient and about the treatment plan, patient responses and progress, and treatment outcomes.

Initial Interview

You usually perform the following tasks on your own, depending on the doctor's practice and your experience and background. Familiarize yourself with each task.

Completing Medical History Forms. You will help new patients fill out medical history forms or questionnaires. You may retrieve current patients' records from the files to update them. Type the patient's name and other identifying information on the first page and on all subsequent pages of the form.

You may interview patients to fill in some of the remaining blanks about medical history. Some doctors prefer to ask patients questions themselves. Others believe that people sometimes talk more freely with an assistant than they do with the doctor.

Documenting Patient Statements. You will record any signs, symptoms, or other information the patient wishes to share. Document this information in the patient's words, not your interpretation of the words. Record these data in specific detail. For example, if the patient drinks alcohol, you should record the number of drinks per week, the type of liquor consumed, and whether the drinking has affected the patient's behavior and health.

Conduct the interview in a private room or in a semiprivate office away from the reception area, as shown in Figure 9-5. Patients usually do not like to discuss their medical or personal problems in front of others. Your opinion of the patient, such as "the patient seems mentally unstable," is your own and should not be discussed or documented. "Tips for the Office" will help you take information from elderly patients.

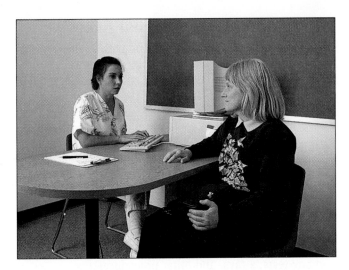

Figure 9-5. Conduct interviews with patients in a private or semiprivate room to make them feel more comfortable.

Documenting Test Results. Put a copy in the chart of any test results, x-ray reports, or other diagnostic results that the patient has brought with him. You may also record this information on a separate test summary sheet in the chart.

Examination Preparation and Vital Signs. In many instances, you will prepare patients for examination. You will record vital signs, medication the patient is currently taking, and any responses to treatment. Before you leave a patient, ask, "Is there anything else you would like the doctor to know?" The patient may be more comfortable sharing further information with you than with the doctor.

Follow-Up

After you record the initial interview and background information, the doctor decides what entries will be made regarding examinations, diagnosis, treatment options and plans, and comments or observations about each case. You then maintain the patient record by performing the following duties.

1. Transcribe notes the doctor dictates about the patient's progress, follow-up visits, procedures, current status, and other necessary information.
2. Post laboratory test results or results of examinations in the record or on the summary sheet.
3. Record telephone calls from the patient and calls that the doctor or other office staff members make to the patient (Figure 9-6). Telephone calls can be an important part of good follow-up care. Calls must be dated, and the content of the conversations must be documented. You must initial the entry. Even if the doctor did not reach the patient, the call should be recorded and dated. State whether the doctor got an answer, left a message on an answering machine or with a person, and so on. Legally, if an item is not in the record, it did not happen.
4. Record medical instructions or discharge instructions the doctor gives. At the doctor's request, you may counsel or educate the patient regarding treatment regimen or home-care procedures the patient must follow. This information must be entered into the record, dated, and initialed. Some offices make carbon copies or photocopies of patient instructions.

The Six Cs of Charting

To maintain accurate patient records, always keep these six Cs in mind when filling out and maintaining charts: Client's (patient's) words, Clarity, Completeness, Conciseness, Chronological order, and Confidentiality.

1. *Client's words.* Be careful to record the patient's exact words rather than your interpretation of them. For instance, if a client says, "My right knee feels like it's thick or full of fluid," write that down. Do not rephrase the sentence to say, "Client says he's got fluid on the knee." Often the patient's exact words, no matter how odd they may sound, provide important clues for the physician in making a diagnosis.
2. *Clarity.* Use precise descriptions and accepted medical terminology when describing a patient's condition. For instance, "Patient got out of bed and walked 20 feet

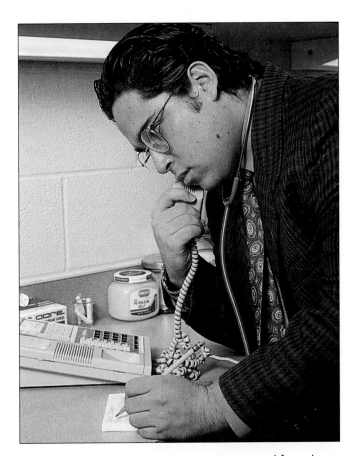

Figure 9-6. All telephone conversations to and from the patient must be logged in the patient record.

without shortness of breath" is much clearer than "Patient got out of bed and felt fine."

3. *Completeness.* Fill out completely all the forms used in the patient record. Provide complete information that is readily understandable to others whenever you make any notation in the patient chart.
4. *Conciseness.* While striving for clarity, also be concise, or brief and to the point. Abbreviations and specific medical terminology can often save time and space when recording information. For instance, you can write "Patient got OOB and walked 20 ft w/o SOB." OOB and SOB are standard abbreviations for "out of bed" and "shortness of breath," respectively. Every member of the office staff should use the same abbreviations to avoid misunderstandings. Table 9-1 lists some common medical abbreviations.
5. *Chronological order.* All entries in patient records must be dated to show the order in which they are made. This factor is critical, not only for documenting patient care but also in case there is a legal question about the type and date of medical services.
6. *Confidentiality.* All the information in patient records and forms is confidential, to protect the patient's privacy. Only the patient, attending physicians, and the medical assistant (who needs the record to tend to the patient and/or to make entries into the record) are allowed to see the charts without the patient's written consent. Never discuss a patient's records, forward them to another office, fax them, or show them to anyone but the physician unless you have the patient's written permission to do so.

Types of Medical Records

You should be familiar with the different approaches to documenting patient information. The most common methods are conventional/source-oriented and problem-oriented medical records.

Conventional, or Source-Oriented, Records

In the conventional, or source-oriented, approach, patient information is arranged according to who supplied the data—the patient, doctor, specialist, or someone else. The medical form may have a space for patient remarks, followed by a section for the doctor's comments.

These records describe all problems and treatments on the same form in simple chronological order. For example, a patient's broken wrist would be recorded on the same form as her stomach ulcer. Although easy to initiate and maintain, this system presents some difficulty in tracking the progress of a specific ailment, such as the patient's ulcer. The doctor has to search the entire record to find information on that one problem.

Problem-Oriented Medical Records

One way to overcome the disadvantages of the conventional approach is to use the problem-oriented medical record (**POMR**) system of keeping charts. This approach, developed by Lawrence L. Weed, MD, makes it easier for the physician to keep track of a patient's progress. The information in a POMR includes the database; problem list; educational, diagnostic, and treatment plan; and progress notes.

Database. The database includes a record of the patient's history; information from the initial interview with the patient (such as "Patient unemployed—second time in past 12 months"); all findings and results from physical examinations (such as "Pulse 105 bpm, BP 210/80"), and any tests, x-rays, and other procedures.

Problem List. Each problem a patient has is listed separately, given its own number, and dated. You then identify a problem by its number throughout the record. You can also list work-related, social, or family problems that may be affecting the patient's health. For instance, the problem list for the patient described above might include, "Severe stomach pain, worse at night and after eating."

You can alert the doctor to the fact that the patient has lost two jobs within 1 year. Such radical life changes can often provoke strong physical reactions. In this patient's case the elevated blood pressure may be related to the job losses, and stress may be causing the stomach pain.

When you document problems, be careful to distinguish between patient signs and symptoms. **Signs** are objective, or external, factors—such as blood pressure, rashes, or swelling—that can be seen or felt by the doctor or measured by an instrument. **Symptoms** are subjective, or internal, conditions felt by the patient, such as pain, headache, or nausea. Together, signs and symptoms help clarify a patient's problem.

Educational, Diagnostic, and Treatment Plan. Each problem should have a detailed educational, diagnostic, and treatment summary in the record. The summary contains diagnostic workups, treatment plans, and instructions for the patient. Here is an example.

Problem 2, Stomach Pain, 2/2/XX [date]

- *Upper GI exam negative, CBC normal.*
- *Prescribed over-the-counter antacid, 2 tablets by mouth t.i.d. after each meal.*
- *Set up appointment for patient with Dr. R. Neil at stress-management clinic (Broughten Professional Center) for Monday, February 4, at 4:30 P.M.*
- *Patient's anxiety is high. Recheck in 1 week.*

Progress Notes. Progress notes are entered for each problem listed in the initial record. The documentation always includes—in chronological order—the patient's condition, complaints, problems, treatment, and responses to care. Here is an example.

Table 9-1

Common Medical Abbreviations

Abbreviation	Meaning	Abbreviation	Meaning
AIDS	acquired immunodeficiency syndrome	inj.	injection
a.m.a.	against medical advice	IV	intravenous
b.i.d./BID	twice a day	MI	myocardial infarction
BP	blood pressure	MM	mucous membrane
bpm	beats per minute	NPO	nothing by mouth
CBC	complete blood count	NYD	not yet diagnosed
C.C.	chief complaint	OOB	out of bed
CNS	central nervous system	OPD	outpatient department
CPE	complete physical examination	OR	operating room
CV	cardiovascular	PH	past history
D & C	dilation and curettage	PT	physical therapy
Dx	diagnosis	Pt	patient
ECG/EKG	electrocardiogram	q.i.d./QID	four times a day
ER	emergency room	ROS/SR	review of systems/systems review
FH	family history	s.c./subq.	subcutaneously
Fl/fl	fluid	SOB	shortness of breath
GBS	gallbladder series	S/R	suture removal
GI	gastrointestinal	stat	immediately
GU	genitourinary	t.i.d./TID	three times a day
GYN	gynecology	TPR	temperature, pulse, respirations
HEENT	head, ears, eyes, nose, throat	UCHD	usual childhood diseases
HIV	human immunodeficiency virus	VS	vital signs
I & D	incision and drainage	WNL	within normal limits
ICU	intensive care unit		

Problem 2, Stomach Pain, 2/9/XX. Patient enrolled in stress-reduction class. Reports stomach pain has diminished—"I can eat without pain; only a little discomfort at night." Vital signs improved: pulse 85 bpm, BP 115/70, respiration 20. Reduced antacid to one tablet by mouth two times daily after meals. Anxiety much reduced. Recheck anxiety level in 2 weeks.

SOAP Documentation

Many medical records, such as the POMR, emphasize the **SOAP** approach to documentation, which provides an orderly series of steps for dealing with any medical case. SOAP documentation lists the patient's symptoms, the diagnosis, and the suggested treatment. Information is documented in the record in the following order.

1. S = *S*ubjective data come from the patient; they describe his or her signs and symptoms and supply any other opinions or comments.
2. O = *O*bjective data come from the physician and from examinations and test results.
3. A = *A*ssessment is the diagnosis or impression of a patient's problem.
4. P = *P*lan of action includes treatment options, chosen treatment, medications, tests, consultations, patient education, and follow-up.

Whether you keep conventional or POMR charts, you can include all these steps for each problem. Figure 9-7 shows an example of SOAP notes. If you abbreviate any term when entering data into the records, use only approved medical abbreviations. For example, use "5 g" instead of "5 grams." Several resources, including those published by JCAHO and the American Medical Association, list approved medical abbreviations for measurements, instructions for taking medication, and other topics. Keep these references readily available in the office.

Appearance, Timeliness, and Accuracy of Records

You must ensure that the medical records are complete. They must also be written neatly and legibly, contain up-to-date information, and present an accurate, professional record of a patient's case.

Neatness and Legibility

A medical record is useless if the doctor or others have difficulty reading it. You should make sure that every word and number in the record is clear and legible. Follow these tips to keep charts neat and easy to read.

1. Use a good-quality pen that will not smudge or smear. Black ink is preferred, but blue is sometimes used to distinguish the original record from a photocopy. Use highlighting pens to call attention to specific items such as allergies. Be aware, however, that, unless the office has a color copier, most colored ink will photocopy black or gray. Highlighting-pen marks may not be visible on a photocopy.
2. If you type notes, be sure the typewriter ribbon is dark enough to make clear letters, as shown in Figure 9-8.
3. Make sure all handwriting is legible. Take time to write names, numbers, and abbreviations clearly.

Timeliness

Medical records should be kept up to date and should be readily available when a doctor or another health-care professional needs to see them. Follow these guidelines to ensure that a doctor can find the most recent information on a patient when it is needed.

1. Record all findings from examinations and tests as soon as they are available.
2. If you forget to enter a finding into the record when it is received, record both the original date of receipt and the date the finding was entered into the record.
3. To document telephone calls, record the date and time of the call, who initiated it, the information discussed, and any conclusions or results. You can either enter the telephone call directly into the record or make a note referring the doctor to a separate telephone log kept in the record.
4. Establish a procedure for retrieving a file quickly in case of emergency. Should the patient be in a serious accident, for example, the emergency doctor will need the patient's medical history immediately.

Accuracy

The physician must be able to trust the accuracy of the information in the medical records. You must make it a priority always to check the accuracy of all data you will enter in a chart. To ensure accurate data, follow these guidelines.

- Never guess at or assume knowledge of names, procedures, medications, findings, or any other information about which there is some question. Always check all the information carefully. Make the extra effort to ask questions of the physician or senior staff member and to verify information.
- Double-check the accuracy of findings and instructions recorded in the chart. Have all numbers been copied accurately? Are instructions for taking medication clear and complete?
- Make sure the latest information has been entered into the chart so that the physician has an accurate picture of the patient's current condition.

Professional Attitude and Tone

Part of creating timely, accurate records is maintaining a professional tone in your writing when recording information. As stated earlier in the chapter, record information from the patient in his own words. Also record the doctor's observations and comments, as well as any laboratory or test results. Do not record your personal, subjective comments, judgments, opinions, or speculations about a patient's words, problems, or test results. You may call attention to a particular problem or observation, for example, by attaching a note to the chart. Do not, however, make such comments part of the patient's record.

Computer Records

In some offices the computer is used for more than just storing financial, billing, and insurance information. Some hospitals, clinics, and even individual physicians use computer software to create and store patient records.

Advantages of Computerizing Records. In a setting in which several terminals in a network are connected to a

OUTLINE FORMAT PROGRESS NOTES

Patient Name *Hansen* (LAST) *Christopher* (FIRST) *M.* (MIDDLE) Date of Birth *3 / 1 / 65* Chart # *H234*

Prob. No. or Letter	DATE	S Subjective	O Objective	A Assess	P Plans
	6/16/99	Patient complaining of pain in lower right quadrant. Has been running fever of between 100.5°F and 101.3°F since Sunday morning. Has queasy feeling in stomach and has been unable to eat since yesterday morning.			
			BP 125/75. Temperature 101.2°F. Abdominal exam revealed rebound tenderness and distension in lower right quadrant.		
				Appendicitis	
					1. Admit to hospital 2. Surgically remove appendix.

Page *1*

Start each Progress Note (Subjective, Objective, Assessment, and Plans) at the appropriate shaded column to create an outline form. Write through the intervening columns to the right margin of the page.

PROGRESS NOTES

TO REORDER CALL TOLL FREE: (800)BIBBERO (800 242-2376) FORM # 26-7215-01

Figure 9-7. The SOAP approach to documentation is one way to organize information in a patient record.

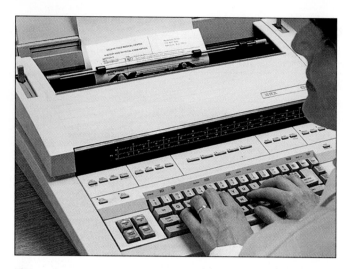

Figure 9-8. Typewritten notes and forms are clear and legible.

main computer, computerizing medical records presents several advantages. A physician can call up the record on her own or another computer monitor whenever the record is needed, review or update the file, and save it to the central computer again (see Figure 9-9).

Computerized records can also be used in teleconferences, where people in different locations can look at the same record on their individual computer screens at the same time. Records can also be sent by modem to the physician's home computer so that the physician will have a patient's records on hand for calls after hours. Computer access to patient records is also helpful for health-care providers with satellite offices in different cities or different parts of a city.

Computers are useful for tickler files (files that need periodic attention). For example, they can alert staff members about patients who are due for yearly checkups and patients who require follow-up care. Some hospitals have begun to use electronically scanned images of patients' thumbprints to keep track of records. This system saves time and helps maintain the security of patient records.

Security Concerns. Many health-care professionals have concerns about protecting the confidentiality of patient records in computer files. Each office must decide whether it will computerize the patient record system. Computer confidentiality was discussed in Chapter 6.

Medical Transcription

Your knowledge of abbreviations, medical terminology, and medical coding will be invaluable when transcribing a doctor's notes or dictation (either recorded or direct). **Transcription** means transforming spoken notes into accurate written form. These written notes are then entered into the patient record. As is the case with information in medical charts, all dictated materials are confidential and should be regarded as potential legal documents. They are part of the patient's continuing case history. They often include findings, treatment stages, prognoses, and final outcomes. Always date and initial all transcription pages.

Strive to make transcribed material accurate and complete. You must have a sound grasp of grammar, spelling, and medical abbreviations and terminology. If any medical word or term is unclear, look up its spelling, definition, and correct usage in a recognized reference source. Ask the physician only if you cannot find something in a reference source. Above-average typing or word processing accuracy and speed are also important.

Transcribing Recorded Dictation

Often the doctor or another health-care provider dictates into a recording device or voice mail type of dictation center. (This equipment is described in Chapter 5.) The following tips can help ensure fast, accurate transcription.

- Make sure that your workstation is free from clutter and that your desk and chair are at comfortable heights for proper support of your back, arms, and legs. Keep at hand all materials you may need for the transcription process—patient records, correspondence, and references for abbreviations and terminology.
- Adjust the transcribing equipment's speed, tone, and volume to obtain the best quality sound at a rate of speed that matches your abilities.
- Listen once all the way through the dictation tape, noting instructions, corrections, or special cues. This step helps you plan how to put the material in the correct order. It also ensures accuracy.
- Write down the exact elapsed time on the transcribing equipment's digital counter where difficult phrases, garbled statements, or other problems occur on the tape. Then you can quickly find the problems again and seek the correct information from the doctor.
- While transcribing, listen carefully to the rise and fall of the doctor's voice, which can provide clues about where to place punctuation and where to end sentences.

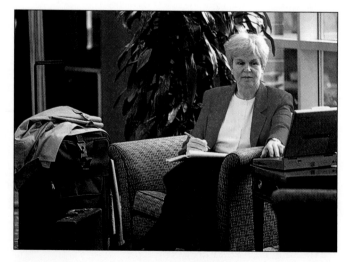

Figure 9-9. Computerized medical records provide physicians with easy access no matter where they are.

MULTISKILL FOCUS

Medical Transcriptionist

To gain medical assistant credentials, you must fulfill the requirements of either the American Association of Medical Assistants (for a Certified Medical Assistant) or the American Medical Technologists (for a Registered Medical Assistant). After obtaining your medical assistant certification or registration, you may wish to acquire additional skills in specialty areas through course work or on-the-job training. Although this course work or training may not lead to an additional certification or degree, it will enable you to expand your role in the medical office and advance your career as the demand for multiskilled health professionals increases.

Skills and Duties

A medical transcriptionist creates written health records for patients based on the physician's dictation or notes. The records may be typewritten or input on a computer. Some transcriptionists work for a single physician; others work for a small or large group.

To create a patient record, the transcriptionist listens to an audiocassette containing information dictated by the physician. Typical information on the tape includes the physician's diagnosis and treatment of the patient. Using dictation equipment, the transcriptionist can slow down or stop and start the cassette tape as she types.

The medical transcriptionist must have excellent typing skills and a good command of medical terminology to make sure that medical terms are used accurately and spelled correctly. She will often need to edit the physician's notes to make sure that the language follows Standard English grammar and usage. Sometimes she must also reorganize the physician's comments to create an understandable and easy-to-follow medical record. After she finishes transcribing the record, the medical transcriptionist checks it for correct spelling and punctuation. This last step is called proofreading.

Workplace Settings

Medical transcriptionists may work in the medical records department of a hospital or in a nursing home, clinic, laboratory, physician's practice, insurance company, or emergency or immediate health-care center. Some transcriptionists work for medical transcribing firms; others are self-employed and work out of their homes.

Education

Medical transcriptionists usually complete a training program at a 4-year college or university, junior or community college, vocational institute, or adult education center. They receive instruction in medical terminology, physiology, pharmaceuticals, laboratory procedures, and medical treatments. Some transcriptionists concentrate on a particular specialty area, such as pathology, and acquire specialized training in that area. Medical transcriptionists can become certified if they meet the qualifying standards of the American Association for Medical Transcription.

Where to Go for More Information

American Association for Medical Transcription
P.O. Box 576187
Modesto, CA 95355

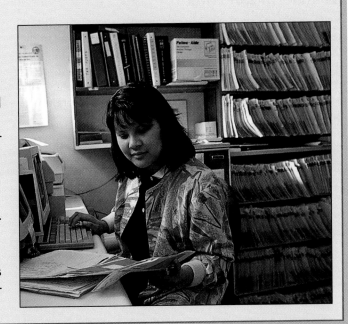

- If a statement is particularly long or highly technical, simply transcribe it word for word. It may make sense in written form. Never try to guess at the meaning of a word or phrase.
- Finally, reread the finished transcription to make sure that all punctuation, capitalization, spelling of names and terms, and paragraph indentions have been done correctly. You should be able to arrange ideas in their logical order and ensure proper sentence structure. Note any items that are still unclear, and ask the doctor to check them as soon as possible. Never enter questionable material into patient records. Any incorrectly transcribed information can become a legal liability for the doctor, should the records be used in a lawsuit.
- All transcribed doctor's notes for the patient's chart should be initialed by the doctor.

Transcribing Direct Dictation

At times the physician may wish to dictate material directly to you. He may want to get observations, comments, or treatment options into the record immediately rather than waiting until a more convenient time to dictate the material into a recorder. Follow these guidelines.

- Use a writing pad with a stiff backing or place the pad on a clipboard to make it easier to write quickly. Use a good ballpoint pen that will not smear or drag on the paper.
- Use incomplete sentences and phrases to keep up with the physician's pace. For example, say "Patient home Friday, recheck 2 wks" instead of "The patient is going home on Friday. We should see him again in 2 weeks."
- Use abbreviations for common phrases (*w/o* for "without," *s/b* for "should be," and so on); for medical terms (*q.d.* for "every day," *mg* for "milligrams," and so on); and for medications or chemicals.
- If a term, phrase, prescription, or name is unclear, ask for clarification right away (say "Excuse me, could you repeat that phrase, please?").
- If the physician speaks with a pronounced accent, ask her to speak more slowly than normal.
- Read the dictation back to the physician to verify all terms, names, figures, and other information for accuracy.
- Enter the notes into the patient record, and date and initial the notes.

Transcription Aids

Keep a library of medical, secretarial, and transcription reference books and medical terminology texts near the transcription workstation. Abbreviations can save time, but you should use only those that are accepted as standard. Reference books will help you find the correct word quickly and easily and help you apply proper grammar, style, and usage to the copy.

Correcting and Updating Patient Records

In legal terms, medical records are regarded as having been created in "due course." All information in the record should be entered at the time of a patient's visit and not days, weeks, or months later. Information corrected or added some time after a patient's visit can be regarded as "convenient" and may damage a doctor's position in a lawsuit.

Using Care With Corrections

If changes to the medical record are not done correctly, the record can become a legal problem for the physician. A physician may be able to more easily explain poor or incomplete documentation than to explain a chart that appears to have been altered after something was originally documented. You must be extremely careful to follow the appropriate procedures for correcting patient records.

Mistakes in medical records are not uncommon. The best defense is to correct the mistake immediately or as soon as possible after the original entry was made. Procedure 9-1 shows you how to correct the patient record.

Updating Patient Records

All additions to a patient's record—test results, observations, diagnoses, procedures—should be done in a way that no one could interpret as deception on the physician's part. In a note accompanying the material, the physician should explain why the information is being added to the record. In some cases the material may

PROCEDURE 9-1

Correcting Medical Records

Objective: To follow standard procedures for correcting a medical record

Materials: Patient file, other pertinent documents that contain the information to be used in making corrections (for example, transcribed notes, telephone notes, physician's comments, correspondence), good ballpoint pen

Method

1. Always make the correction in a way that does not suggest any intention to deceive, cover up, alter, or add information to conceal a lack of proper medical care.
2. When deleting information, never black it out, never use correction fluid to cover it up, and never in any other way erase or obliterate the original wording. Draw a line through the original information so that it is still legible.
3. Write or type in the correct information above or below the original line or in the margin. The location on the chart for the new information should be clear. You may need to attach another sheet of paper or another document with the correction on it. Note in the record "See attached document A" or similar wording to indicate where the corrected information can be found.
4. Place a note near the correction stating why it was made (for example, "error, wrong date; error, interrupted by phone call.") This indication can be a brief note in the margin or an attachment to the record. As a general rule of thumb, do not make any changes without noting the reason for them.
5. Enter the date and time, and initial the correction.
6. If possible, have another staff member or the physician witness and initial the correction to the record when you make it.

simply be a physician's recollections or observations on a patient visit that occurred in the past. Each item added to a record must be dated and initialed. Sometimes a third party may be asked to witness the addition.

Most hospitals and clinics have detailed guidelines for late entries to a patient's chart. You must follow these guidelines carefully to avoid potential legal problems. Procedure 9-2 shows you how to update a patient record.

Release of Records

All medical records, including x-rays and other test results, are created by the doctor and are considered the property of that doctor. The records and all they contain, however, are regarded as confidential. Even though the doctor owns the records, no one can see them without the patient's written consent. However, the law may require the doctor to release them, as in the case of contagious disease or when subpoenaed by a court.

Procedures for Releasing Records

Physicians often receive requests from lawyers, other physicians, insurance companies, government agencies, and the patient himself for copies of a patient's records. Use these guidelines for releasing medical information.

1. Obtain a signed and newly dated release from the patient authorizing the **transfer** of information—that is, giving information to another party outside the physician's office. Verbal consent in person or over the telephone is not considered a valid release. This release form should be filed in the patient's record.

PROCEDURE 9-2

Updating Medical Records

Objective: To document continuity of care by creating a complete, accurate, timely record of the medical care provided at your facility

Materials: Patient file, other pertinent documents (test results, x-rays, telephone notes, correspondence), good ballpoint pen, notebook, typewriter/transcribing equipment

Method

1. Verify that you have the right records for the right patient. You do not want to record information on the wrong patient chart.
2. Transcribe dictated doctor's notes as soon as possible, and enter them into the patient record. Delays increase the chance of making errors in transcribing and recording the information. Also, for legal reasons, medical information should be entered into the record in a timely fashion.
3. Spell out the names of disorders, diseases, medications, and other terms the first time you enter them into the patient record, followed by the appropriate abbreviation (for example: congestive heart failure [CHF]). Thereafter, you may use the abbreviations. Using only abbreviations could cause confusion.
4. Enter only what the doctor has dictated. Do *not* add your own comments, observations, or evaluations. Use self-adhesive flags or other means to call the doctor's attention to something you have noticed that may be helpful to the patient's case. Date and initial each entry. Should the file be examined later in a legal proceeding, your notes and comments will be taken as part of the official record.
5. Ask the doctor where in the file to record routine or special laboratory test results. He may ask you to post them in a particular section of the file or on a separate test summary form. If you use the summary form, make a note in the file that the results were received, and place the laboratory report in the patient's file with the record. Date and initial each entry. Whether or not test result printouts are posted in the record, always note in the chart the date of the test and the results.
6. Make a note in the record of all telephone calls to and from the patient. Date and initial the entries. These entries may also include the doctor's comments, observations, changes in the patient's medication, new instructions to the patient, and so on. If calls are recorded in a separate telephone log, you should note in the patient's record the time and date of the call and refer to the log.

   It is particularly important to record such calls when the patient is resisting treatment or has not made follow-up appointments. These entries can demonstrate that a doctor made every effort to provide quality care and to advise the patient of the risks of not following the treatment plan or not scheduling follow-up appointments.
7. Read over the entries for omissions or mistakes. Ask the doctor to answer any questions you have.
8. Make sure that you have dated and initialed each entry.
9. Be sure that all documents are included in the file.
10. Replace the patient's file in the filing system as soon as possible.

2. Make photocopies of the original material. Copy and send only those portions of the record covered by the release and only records originating from your facility (not records received from other sources). Do not send original documents. (If a record will be used in a court case, however, you must submit the original unless the judge specifies that a photocopy is acceptable.) If you cannot make copies, as in the case of x-rays, send the originals, and tell the recipient that they must be returned (see Figure 9-10). Follow up with the recipient until the originals have been returned and are placed in the patient's files.
3. Call the recipient to confirm that all materials were received. Avoid faxing confidential records. There is no way to tell who will see documents sent by fax.

Special Cases

It may not always be immediately clear who has the right to sign a release-of-records form. When a couple divorces, for example, both parents are still considered legal guardians of their children, and either one can sign a release form authorizing transfer of medical records. If a patient dies, the patient's next of kin or legally authorized representative, such as the executor of the estate, may see the records or authorize their release to a third party.

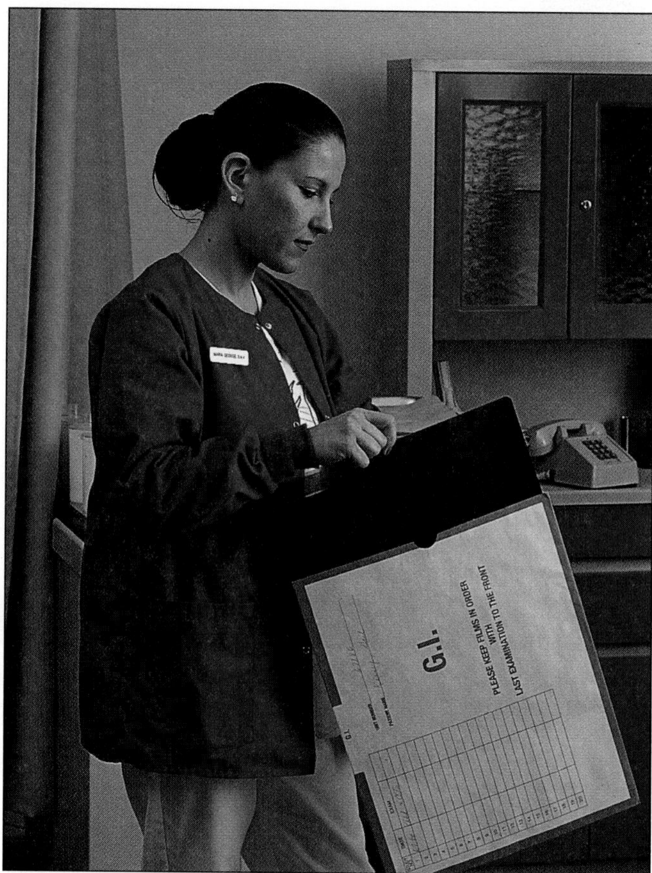

Figure 9-10. When you are preparing a patient record to be transferred, never send original material. One exception to this rule is x-rays, which should be sent with a request that the recipient return them as soon as possible.

Confidentiality

When children reach age 18, most states consider them adults with the right to privacy. No one, not even their parents, may see their medical records without the children's written consent. Some states extend this right to privacy to emancipated minors who are under the age of 18 and living on their own or are married, a parent, or in the armed services.

The main legal and ethical principle to keep in mind is that you must protect each patient's right to privacy at all times.

Summary

The medical assistant must properly prepare and maintain patient records. Patient records, also known as charts, contain important information about a patient's medical history and present condition. Patient records serve as communication tools as well as legal documents. They also play a role in patient and staff education and may be used for quality control and research. The six Cs of charting are the client's words, clarity, completeness, conciseness, chronological order, and confidentiality.

You should be familiar with the most common methods for documenting patient information, which include the conventional, or source-oriented, and problem-oriented medical records approaches. You must ensure not only that the medical records are complete but also that they are neat and written legibly, contain up-to-date information, and present an accurate, professional record of a patient's case. Part of maintaining patient records includes transcribing physician's notes—that is, transforming spoken notes into accurate written form. In addition, you must know the guidelines for how to correct and update a patient record and how to release it to a third party.

9 Chapter Review

Discussion Questions

1. What is your role in creating timely, accurate, and complete documentation for patient records?
2. Compare and contrast conventional, or source-oriented, medical records and problem-oriented medical records. What are the advantages and disadvantages of each type?
3. Why is confidentiality such a serious issue for patient medical records?

Critical Thinking Questions

1. Summarize the skills necessary for an employee who has been asked to assume responsibility for initiating and maintaining patient records.
2. Describe how a well-trained medical assistant could enhance the efficiency of a medical office's system of creating and maintaining patient records.
3. Evaluate how you would handle a situation in which a patient wants to take his medical test results and x-rays with him to a specialist's office.

Application Activities

1. After reading the following description of a patient's condition, list the patient's signs and symptoms.

   A 72-year-old man with no history of gastrointestinal problems was complaining of fatigue, back pain, appetite loss, and nausea. The patient had a hemoglobin of about 7g, indicating marked anemia. His blood pressure was low (95/70), his heartbeat erratic—from 55 to 85 bpm—and his white blood cell count elevated.

   While in the office he experienced a headache and ringing in his right ear. A CT scan taken the next day revealed an abdominal aortic aneurysm containing a large clot. The scan also revealed a small lesion in the lining of the stomach.
2. Copy the blank patient registration form shown in Figure 9-2. With a partner, take each other's medical history and make appropriate notes on the form.
3. Copy the blank combination medical history and physical examination form shown in Figure 9-3. Fill out the form by using the following patient information.

   For medical history section: Date: 2/14/96: The patient is Heather R. MacEntee, age 35, living at 344 Westwind Lane, Apartment 28, Round Tree, IL 60012; telephone (708) 333-5555. She is a real estate broker, married, with a 6-year-old child. Her father died at age 55; her mother is 62 and has congestive heart disease. She has no siblings. The family has a history of heart disease and diabetes. The patient had chickenpox and mumps at age 7 and surgery for an ovarian cyst at 22. She has an allergy to ragweed but is not taking any medications at present.

   For physical examination section: Ms. MacEntee weighs 142 lb, is 5 ft 10 in tall, and her temperature and respiration are normal. Her pulse is 74, her blood pressure is 110/75, and her chest sounds are normal. Her chief complaint is discomfort in the area of the gallbladder. She has intense pain after eating. Blood tests are normal. The doctor's initial impression is suspected gallstones, and an ultrasound scan of the gallbladder is ordered. Treatment plan depends on the scan results.

Further Readings

Eggland, Ellen Thomas. "Documenting the Details." *Nursing*, July 1995, 17.

Fisher, J. Patrick. *Basic Medical Terminology.* 4th ed. Columbus, OH: Glencoe/McGraw-Hill, 1993.

Fordney, Marilyn T., and Mary Otis Diehl. *Medical Transcription Guide: Do's and Don'ts.* Philadelphia: W. B. Saunders, 1990.

Hart, Linda J. "Alterations to Medical Records Can Be Detected." *The Professional Medical Assistant,* November/December 1994, 19–20.

Mandell, Marc. "Not Documented." *Nursing,* August 1994, 62–63.

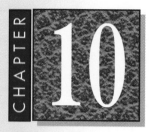

Managing the Office Medical Records

CHAPTER OUTLINE

- Importance of Records Management
- Filing Equipment
- Filing Supplies
- Filing Systems
- The Filing Process
- Storing Files

OBJECTIVES

After completing Chapter 10, you will be able to:

- Describe the equipment and supplies needed for filing medical records.
- List and describe the various types of filing systems.
- Discuss the benefits of each type of system.
- Discuss the advantages of color coding the files.
- Explain how to set up and use a tickler file.
- Describe each of the five steps in the filing process.
- Explain the steps to take in trying to locate a misplaced file.
- List and describe the basic file storage options and the advantages of each.
- Identify criteria for determining whether files should be retained, stored, or discarded.

AREAS OF COMPETENCE
1997 ROLE DELINEATION STUDY

ADMINISTRATIVE

Administrative Procedures

- Perform basic clerical functions

Key Terms

active file
alphabetic filing system
closed file
compactible file
cross-referenced
file guide
inactive file
lateral file
numeric filing system
out guide
records management system
retention schedule
sequential order
tab
tickler file
vertical file

Importance of Records Management

The information contained in the patient medical records is the most valuable information in a medical office. For a practice to operate smoothly and efficiently, it is critical that these records be organized in a way that makes them easily retrievable. Maintaining a well-organized, easy-to-use records management system is essential to providing good patient care. The **records management system** refers to the way patient records are created, filed, and maintained. When such a system is not in place, valuable time is wasted searching for important information. In addition, vital medical data can be lost.

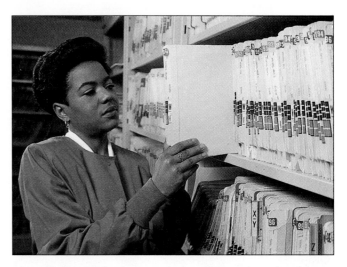

Figure 10-1. Files kept on shelves are easily accessible.

Filing Equipment

Filing equipment generally refers to the place where records, or files, are housed. Although there are various types of equipment, two of the most common options are shelves and cabinets. The choice of whether to use filing shelves or filing cabinets is often made according to space considerations and personal preference.

Filing Shelves

Files can be kept on shelves, which resemble traditional shelves, as shown in Figure 10-1. Files are stacked upright on the shelves in filing containers such as boxes or large heavy-duty envelopes. Some shelf systems have doors that slide from side to side or above or below the files. These doors can be locked for security. Other shelf systems have no front covers. Filing shelves are often long, sometimes extending the full length and height of an office wall or room. An advantage of keeping files on shelves is that it allows several people to retrieve and return files at one time.

Filing Cabinets

Filing cabinets are sturdy pieces of office furniture, usually made of metal or wood. They contain a series of pullout drawers in which files are hung. Filing cabinets, unlike shelves, are best used by one person at a time because the drawer setup provides limited maneuvering room. In addition, cabinets require more floor space than filing shelves. About twice the depth of the file drawer is needed to allow it to fully open.

Although shelves are horizontal by design, filing cabinets can stand vertically or horizontally. You are probably familiar with the more traditional filing cabinet, the vertical file. A **vertical file** features pullout drawers that usually contain a metal frame or bar equipped to handle letter- or legal-size documents. Hanging file folders are hung on this frame, with identifying names facing out. Vertical files usually have two, four, or six drawers.

Horizontal filing cabinets, called **lateral files,** often feature doors that flip up and pullout drawers. Files are arranged with sides facing out. Lateral files require more wall space but do not extend as far into the room as vertical file drawers.

Compactible Files

Some offices have limited space in which to house filing cabinets or shelves. These offices use a variation of shelf filing, called compactible files. **Compactible files** are kept on rolling shelves that slide along permanent tracks in the floor.

When not in use, these files can be stored close together—even one on top of another—to conserve space. When needed, they are rolled out into an open area so that the staff can easily use them. Compactible files can be moved manually or automatically with the touch of a button.

Rotary Circular Files

Rotary circular files are another option to consider when space is limited. These files are stored in a circular fashion, similar to a revolving door, and are accessed by rotating the files. They also can be operated either manually or electronically.

Tubs or Boxes

Some offices use tubs or boxes, in which files are suspended. These are organized like filing cabinet drawers but can be easily moved out of the way to accommodate office equipment or other needs. The one difficulty with housing files in boxes rather than in drawers is that they do not remain in one location. Therefore, they can easily be misplaced.

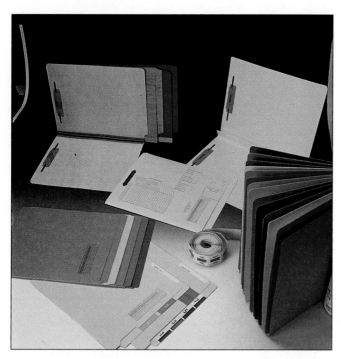

Figure 10-2. Medical offices use a wide variety of filing supplies.

Labeling Filing Equipment

Regardless of which type of filing equipment your office uses, files should be clearly labeled on the outside so that you do not have to open doors or drawers to know their contents. Labeling allows you to go directly to the appropriate place when retrieving a file. The label lists the range of files the drawer or shelf contains. For example, if the drawer includes all the files of patients whose last names begin with the letters A, B, C, and D, it should be labeled "A-D."

Security Measures

All filing equipment must be secure, to protect the confidentiality of medical records. *Never* place patient records in an unsecured filing system.

Most filing cabinets come with a lock and key. To protect filing shelves in a separate room, you can lock the file room. Security of the keys to that room then becomes an important issue. The number of staff members who have keys to that room should be limited—perhaps just to the head doctor and the office manager. Every staff member does not need a key to the filing equipment. When the office manager comes into the office each morning, she can unlock the files. Because the files remain open during the day, it is important to make sure they are not placed in areas where unauthorized people can obtain access to them. Posting a sign on the file room door stating "Authorized Personnel Only" helps ensure that files remain secure. To ensure office security after hours, some practices install alarm systems.

Equipment Safety

Safety is an important consideration for filing systems. For example, opening more than one drawer in a vertical file cabinet at the same time may cause it to fall forward. If the bottom drawer in a vertical file is left open, someone can easily trip over it. Shelves can be dangerous if staff members need to climb a ladder to retrieve files from the highest level.

Safety guidelines for each piece of equipment should be posted prominently in the office. Make sure that every staff member knows where the rules are posted. Then, make sure that everyone follows the rules to prevent possible injury.

Purchasing Filing Equipment

You may never have to buy filing equipment, because most medical offices already have filing systems in place. Occasionally, however, you may be responsible for setting up an office's filing system—for example, if your practice opens a new office. You may also need to buy equipment as the number of patients in the practice grows.

In either case you will need to determine where to position the files. When purchasing filing cabinets or shelves, you need to determine how much office space is available for files. This information, along with the number of file folders to be included, will help you figure out how many cabinets or shelves to purchase. An office-supply store or office-supply catalog can provide you with a list of available products.

Filing Supplies

Once you have chosen your filing equipment, you must select filing supplies. Figure 10-2 features an assortment of filing supplies commonly used by medical practices.

File Folders

The most basic filing supply is the file folder, often referred to as a manila folder. This folder is made of heavy paper folded in half to form a pocket that can hold papers. File folders come in two sizes: letter size, which is $8\frac{1}{2}$ by 11 inches, and legal size, which is $8\frac{1}{2}$ by 14 inches.

Tabs. An important feature of file folders is the **tab,** the tapered rectangular or rounded extension at the top of the folder. Tabs may extend the full length of the folder, as with straight-cut folders, but they are usually cut to extend partway across a folder.

Using folders with a variety of tab cuts makes it easier to read the names on the tabs. One common type of folder is the third-cut folder. Tabs are one-third the width of the folder and appear at the left, center, or right side.

Fourth-cut tabs are smaller. Tabs extend one-fourth the width of the folder and occupy one of four positions—left, left-center, right-center, or right.

Labeling File Folders. The tabs on file folders are used to identify the contents of the individual folder. You can write directly on the tab area in pen or pencil, or you can type a label and affix it to the tab area for a more professional appearance. Tabs can be covered with transparent tape to prevent smudging.

No matter what filing system your office uses, it is important to be consistent in preparing file labels. If all the files are labeled with the patient's last name, followed by the patient's first name and middle initial (for example, Brown, Emma L.), you should not prepare a label for a new folder giving the patient's name in a different order (for example, James P. Regan). Each member of a family should have a separate file.

File Jackets

By themselves, file folders cannot be suspended inside filing cabinet drawers. They must be placed inside file jackets, or hanging file folders. These jackets resemble file folders but feature metal or plastic hooks on both sides at the top, which hook onto the metal bars inside the drawers.

Plastic tabs, either colored or clear, and blank inserts are supplied to identify the contents of hanging file folders. The information is typed on the insert and placed in the plastic tab, which is inserted into the hanging file folder. Again, all inserts should be prepared in a consistent style.

File Guides

To identify a group of file folders in a file drawer, you may use **file guides,** which are heavy cardboard or plastic inserts. For example, if a drawer contains the files for patients whose last names begin with the letters A through C, the guides might separate A from B and B from C.

Out Guides

Another filing supply is an **out guide,** which is a marker made of stiff material and used as a placeholder when someone takes a file out of the filing system. Some out guides include pockets that can hold the name of the file that belongs in that place or the name of the individual who took the file and its due date for return. On another type of out guide, you write the information on the out guide and cross it out when the file is returned. Out guides can be used for both shelf and cabinet filing.

Although out guides are not essential, they are extremely helpful in ensuring that files are returned to their proper places. Out guides also save the time and effort necessary to go through files to determine where a particular file belongs.

File Sorters

File sorters are large envelope-style folders with tabs in which files can be stored temporarily. File sorters are used to hold patient records that will be returned to the files during the day or at the end of the day. The sorters help keep files in order and prevent them from being lost.

Binders

Some offices keep patient records in three-ring binders rather than in file folders. The binders are labeled on the outside spine. Documents are three-hole-punched and then placed inside the binder. Tab sheets are used to separate individual records. A binder can conveniently hold many records.

Purchasing Filing Supplies

Although you may never have to buy filing equipment, buying filing supplies may be one of your regular responsibilities as a medical assistant. (See Chapter 7 for a discussion of how to manage office supplies.)

Filing Systems

A filing system is a method by which files are organized. Any of a variety of filing systems may be used, but every system places patient records in some sort of **sequential order**—one after another in a pattern, or sequence, that can be predicted. It is important to find out which filing system your office is using and to follow it exactly. Any deviation can result in lost or misplaced records.

By far the most common filing system for maintaining patient files in sequential order is the alphabetic system. You would not, however, make any changes in your system without first consulting the doctors and other staff members in the practice.

Alphabetic

In the **alphabetic filing system,** files are arranged in alphabetic order, as shown in Figure 10-3. Files are labeled with the patient's last name first, followed by the first, or given, name and the middle initial.

There are specific rules to follow when filing personal names alphabetically (Table 10-1). If you have questions, consult a secretarial handbook or style manual. Although the alphabetic system is simple, you must know the exact spelling of a patient's name to retrieve a file.

Numeric

A **numeric filing system** organizes files by numbers instead of by names. In this system each patient name is assigned a number. New patients are assigned the next unused number in sequence. Then, instead of being filed by name, the files are arranged in numeric order—1, 2, 3,

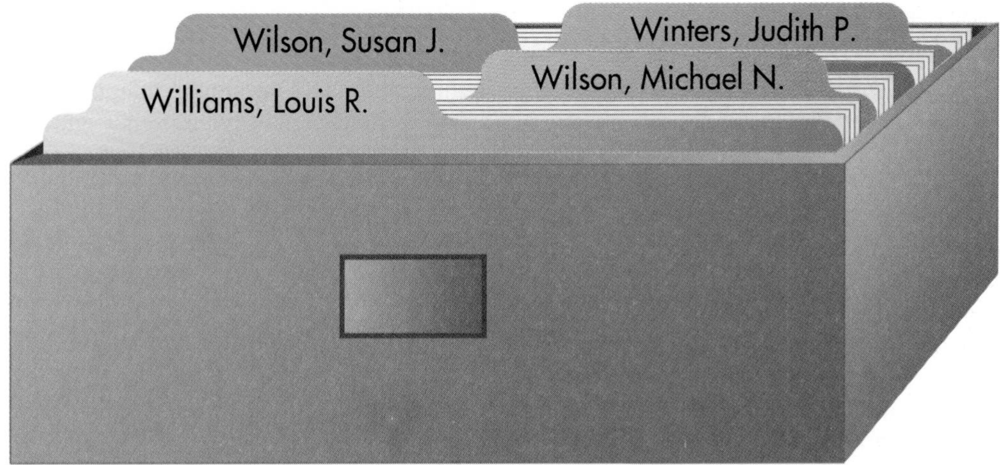

Figure 10-3. Most medical practices file patient records according to the alphabetic filing system.

4, and so on. The resulting files are sequential by the order in which patients have come to the practice.

Only the numbers are indicated on the files. Patient names are recorded elsewhere. Such a system is often used when patient information is highly confidential—as in the case of HIV-positive patients—and patients' identities need to be protected.

The numeric system can be expanded to indicate the location of files. For example, if the last three numbers represent the patient's number, the number 113306 may represent the file of the 306th patient, which can be found in the eleventh filing cabinet in the third drawer.

A numeric system must include a master list of patients' names and corresponding numbers. To ensure confidentiality, the office manager should keep the list in a secure place. The physician should hold a duplicate copy, which must also be kept under lock and key. Since folders are filed in numeric order, it should not be necessary for other staff members to have this list.

To find a patient's file number using a computer system, a staff member might input a password or access code, then type in the first three letters of the patient's last name. If the patient's last name were Mulligan, for example, the staff member would type in Mul. The computer would then show all patients whose last names begin with Mul. The staff member would scroll the names, find the patient, highlight the patient name, and hit the "Enter" key. The computer would then give the number of the patient's chart.

Color Coding

Color coding is used when there is a need to distinguish files within a filing system. For example, you may wish to find at a glance all the office's new patients, all patients on Medicare, or all patients whose last names begin with the letters WI. Coding by color can help you do so quickly and easily.

Patient records can be color-coded in a variety of ways. File folders are available in a range of colors, as are filing labels, plastic tabs, and stickers.

Using Classifications. To make the best use of color, you must first identify the classifications that are important to your office. For example, is it important to be able to identify all new patients easily? (A new patient is a patient who has never been seen in the practice or has not been seen at the practice in 3 years.) Once you select the classifications, choose a different color for each one.

Then file the information by color, within the filing system. For example, all new patients may be kept in red folders, or you can attach a red sticker or red filing label to the folders.

Some practices use the following color-coding system. Records of patients under the age of 18 are color-coded blue. Records of patients over the age of 65 are color-coded red. Records of patients who are insulin-dependent are color-coded green. Records of patients who are hemophiliacs are coded with a half-red/half-white sticker. In an emergency situation, as when a patient with diabetes passes out while in the office, the color coding gives staff members vital information at a glance.

After a color-coding system is finalized, the codes should be prominently posted on a chart in the file room so that all staff members are aware of them. This chart will help to ensure that records are filed correctly. Remember to update color-coded files consistently, coding new ones and revising older ones as a patient's status changes.

Using Color in an Alphabetic Filing System. One way to use color-coded filing is in conjunction with an alphabetic filing system. After files are organized alphabetically, each letter of the alphabet is assigned a color. Then the first two letters of each patient's last name are color-coded, usually with colored tabs.

The colored tabs are attached to the top of straight-edged or tabbed file folders. For example, if the letter S is coded as light blue and the letter M is coded as light green, all names starting with SM—like Smith—would have light-blue and light-green colored tabs at the top of the folders. The name Snyder would be filed under a different color combination, such as light blue (for S) and

Table 10-1

Rules for Alphabetic Filing of Personal Names

In alphabetizing, treat each part of a patient's name as a separate unit, and look at the units in this order: last name, first name, middle initial, and any subsequent names or initials. Disregard punctuation.

Name	Unit 1	Unit 2	Unit 3	Unit 4
Stephen Jacobson	JACOBSON	STEPHEN		
Stephen Brent Jacobson	JACOBSON	STEPHEN	BRENT	
B. T. Jacoby	JACOBY	B	T	
C. Bruce Hay Jacoby	JACOBY	C	BRUCE	HAY
Kwong Kow Ng	NG	KWONG	KOW	
Philip K. Ng	NG	PHILIP	K	

Treat a prefix, such as the O' in O'Hara, as part of the name, not as a separate unit. Ignore variations in spacing, punctuation, and capitalization. Treat prefixes—such as De La, Mac, Saint, and St.—exactly as they are spelled.

Name	Unit 1	Unit 2	Unit 3	Unit 4
A. Serafino Delacruz	DELACRUZ	A	SERAFINO	
Victor P. De La Cruz	DELACRUZ	VICTOR	P	
Irene J. MacKay	MACKAY	IRENE	J	
Walter G. Mac Kay	MACKAY	WALTER	G	
Kyle N. Saint Clair	SAINTCLAIR	KYLE	N	
Peter St. Clair	STCLAIR	PETER		

Treat hyphenated names as a single unit. Disregard the hyphen.

Name	Unit 1	Unit 2	Unit 3	Unit 4
Victor Puentes-Ruiz	PUENTESRUIZ	VICTOR		
Jean-Marie Vigneau	VIGNEAU	JEANMARIE		

A title, such as Dr. or Major, or a seniority term, such as Jr. or 3d, should be treated as the last filing unit, to distinguish names that are otherwise identical.

Name	Unit 1	Unit 2	Unit 3	Unit 4
Dr. George B. Diaz	DIAZ	GEORGE	B	DR
Major George B. Diaz	DIAZ	GEORGE	B	MAJOR
James R. Foster, Jr.	FOSTER	JAMES	R	JR
James R. Foster, Sr.	FOSTER	JAMES	R	SR

Adapted from William A. Sabin, *The Gregg Reference Manual,* 8th ed. (Columbus, OH: Glencoe/McGraw-Hill, 1996), 288–295.

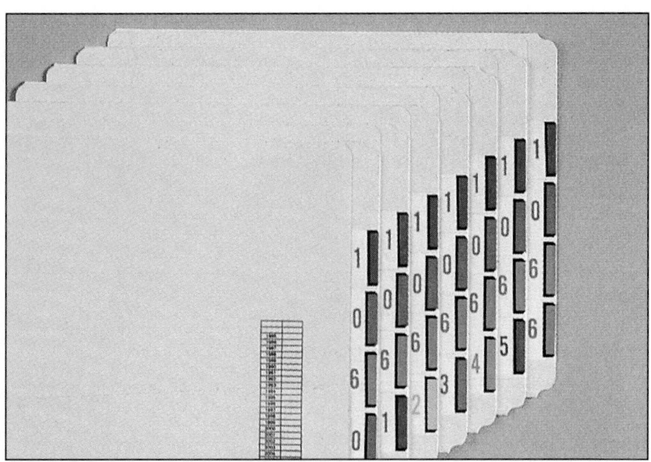

Figure 10-4. Using color coding can make it easy to find a misfiled record.

peach (for N). Because the colors will be the same in each segment of the file drawer, a color-coded system makes it easy to tell whether files are in their proper spots.

Using Color in a Numeric Filing System. Color can be used in a similar way with numeric systems. The numerals 1 to 9 may each be assigned a distinct color, as shown in Figure 10-4. Then, numerals 1, 21, 31, 41, and 51, for example, would share the same color in the ones place of their numeric designation.

As with the alphabetic system, color coding helps identify numeric files that are out of place. There are exceptions, however. For example, if a numeric system uses white stickers for the numeral 2 and red stickers for the numeral 3, the number 134 filed in place of 124 would be spotted immediately as a red sticker in a row of white, but the number 128 misfiled in the same spot could go unnoticed. Procedure 10-1 explains how to use your knowledge of alphabetic and numeric filing and color coding to set up a patient records system.

Tickler Files

To avoid losing track of important dates, many medical practices use tickler files. A **tickler file** is a reminder file. Any activity that needs to be scheduled ahead of time can be noted and a reminder placed in the file. For example, reminders to order supplies or send patient checkup cards can be entered. When the task has been completed, the note can be crossed off the list or removed from the file and thrown away. In some offices these notes are dated and placed in a separate "Completed" file for future reference.

Tickler files should be located by themselves in a prominent place in the office, such as in a plastic box mounted on the wall near the receptionist's desk. Someone in the office should be assigned the responsibility of regularly checking the tickler files. Tickler files can be checked daily or, at a minimum, once a week. It is important to check tickler files frequently because they work only if they are used regularly.

You can organize tickler files in a variety of ways. The most common method, discussed in Procedure 10-2, is to allot one file folder to each month of the year. Tickler files can also be organized by day of the week or week of the month. This method is most useful if there are responsibilities that occur regularly on a certain day of the week or in a certain week within the month. If there are so many notes in a monthly folder that it becomes cumbersome to deal with, it may be best to organize weekly files.

Tickler files are usually organized in file folders, but they can be set up in other ways. One way is to make notes on an office calendar or wall chart. Anyone walking by will be able to read the notes, however, and the number of activities you can include is limited by the space available.

Some offices keep their tickler files in three-ring binders, with tabs separating the months. Notes can be written on three-hole-punched sheets of paper, with pages added as needed. Binders offer essentially unlimited space.

Computers now offer tickler files. When the computer is turned on, it lists, for example, "Things to Do Today" with the tickler information posted for that date.

Supplemental Files

Occasionally you may need to set up additional files to supplement the medical records filing system. For example, you may wish to keep some information separate from the primary file, such as older patient records or insurance information. You may also be asked to create temporary files, such as copies of patient records in the primary files. In these cases you set up supplemental files. Supplemental files allow you to keep this additional information about each patient without cluttering up the primary filing cabinets and without making it difficult to find information.

Supplemental files are usually created using the same system as the primary files, but they are kept in a different location. Depending on frequency of use, they may be stored in a less accessible but equally secure area of the office.

If you are keeping supplemental files, it is important to distinguish their content from that of the primary files. For example, you may decide that all information pertaining to certain subjects—such as patient diagnosis and treatment—will be kept in the primary files and that all other information—such as insurance company payments for each patient—will be kept in the supplemental files. This designation will help you and other office staff members know exactly where to go to retrieve specific information.

PROCEDURE 10-1

Creating a Filing System for Patient Records

Objective: To create a filing system that keeps related materials together in a logical order and enables office staff to store and retrieve files efficiently

Materials: Vertical or horizontal filing cabinets with locks, file jackets, tabbed file folders, labels, file guides, out guides, filing sorters

Method

1. Evaluate which filing system is best for your office—alphabetic or numeric. Make sure the doctor approves the system you choose.
2. Establish a style for labeling files, and make sure that all file labels are prepared in this manner. Place records for different family members in separate files.
3. Set up a color-coding system to distinguish the files (for example, use blue for the letters A-C, red for D-F, and so on).
4. Use file guides to divide files into sections.
5. Use out guides as placeholders to indicate which files have been taken out of the system. Include a charge-out form to be signed and dated by the person who is taking the file.
6. To keep files in order and to prevent them from being misplaced, use a file sorter to hold those patient records that will be returned to the files during the day or at the end of the day.
7. Develop a manual explaining the filing system to new staff members. Include guidelines on how to keep the system in good order.

The Filing Process

Pulling and filing patient records and filing individual documents may be among your responsibilities as a medical assistant. Some practices require that records be returned to the files as soon as they are no longer needed. In other practices the timing is up to you. Still other offices schedule a specific time at the end of each day to file the current day's records and pull those for the next day.

Records waiting to be filed should be placed temporarily in a file return area, as shown in Figure 10-5. To protect patient privacy, this place should be in a secure area

PROCEDURE 10-2

Setting Up an Office Tickler File

Objective: To create a comprehensive office tickler file designed for year-round use

Materials: 12 manila file folders, 12 file labels, pen or typewriter, paper

Method

1. Write or type 12 file labels, 1 for each month of the year. Abbreviations are acceptable. Do *not* include the current calendar year, just the month.
2. Affix one label to the tab of each file folder.
3. Arrange the folders so that the current month is on the top of the pile. Months should follow in chronological order.
4. Write or type a list of upcoming responsibilities and activities. Indicate on the note the date by which the activity should be completed. Use a separate sheet of paper for each month.
5. File the notes by month in the appropriate folders.
6. Place the folders, with the current month on top, in a prominent place in the office, such as in a plastic box mounted on the wall near the receptionist's desk.
7. Check the tickler file at least once a week on a specific day, such as every Monday. Assign a backup person to check it in case you happen to be out of the office.
8. Complete the tickler activities on the designated days, if possible. Keep notes concerning activities in progress. Discard notes about completed activities.
9. At the end of the month, place that month's file folder at the bottom of the tickler file. If there are notes remaining in that month's folder, move them to the new month's folder.
10. Continue to add new notes to the appropriate tickler files.

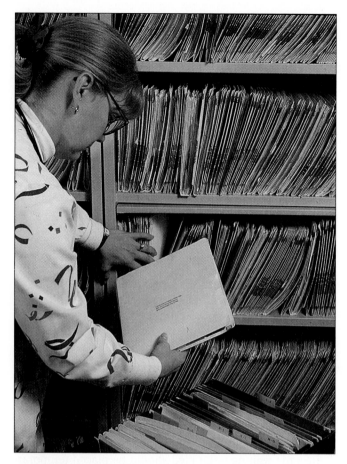

Figure 10-5. In some practices, patient records are filed once at the end of the day. Throughout the day, records are placed in a file sorter in a secure area of the office.

of the office. Clear rules should designate who may handle these files and in what situations.

How to File

Essentially, you will be filing three types of items: new patient record folders, individual documents that belong in existing patient record folders, and patient record folders that have previously been filed. There are five steps involved in filing: inspecting, indexing, coding, sorting, and storing.

Inspecting. The first step in the filing process is to make sure the item is ready to be filed. Inspect the document or patient record folder for a mark, notation, or stamp indicating that it is ready to be filed. For example, it may be initialed by the physician or stamped with the word *File* on a self-adhesive flag attached to the upper right corner. Some offices have staff members simply place folders ready for filing in a specially designated box or bin.

At this point, remove paper clips, rubber bands, and any extraneous material that does not need to be filed. Staple papers to keep them together. Documents are less bulky when stapled than when held together by clips or rubber bands.

If the document to be filed is much smaller than standard size, it may become lost in the file or even fall out. You may want to use tape or rubber cement to attach it to a standard-size piece of paper before filing it within the folder. When small documents have wording on both sides of the paper, they can be placed in standard-size clear plastic envelopes and then filed.

Indexing. *Indexing* is another term for naming a file. Names should be chosen carefully because that is how the file will be known, retrieved, and replaced. Patient names are traditionally used as the file names for patient records.

If you are using a numeric system, you can assign a number instead of a name. Most offices that use a numeric system use computer software to create new patient charts and assign numbers. As part of the indexing process, color-code the file (if you use color coding in your system).

Note that some files can logically be placed in more than one location. Such files should be **cross-referenced,** or filed in two or more places, with each place noted in each file. When cross-referencing a file, you may duplicate the exact contents of the file and place each file under a different heading, or you may create a cross-reference form that lists all the places to find the file. You would then place the form under any heading where it is appropriate to look for that file. You may wish to attach it to a blank file, cutting the file folder in half so that no other documents are mistakenly filed in it.

When filing folders that have previously been indexed, use this step as a way to check the indexing process. For example, take the opportunity to decide whether the name and color of the file folder are accurate or should be changed in any way.

Coding. This step can be skipped when filing patient record folders that have previously been filed. Coding means to put an identifying mark or phrase on a document to ensure that it is placed in the correct file. To code a record, simply mark the patient's name, the number, or the subject title of the file folder. If appropriate, you can underline or highlight key words on the document itself.

It is important to use a phrase or identifying code that anyone who will review the file can easily understand. Avoid medical jargon whenever possible because some terms may not be familiar to everybody. If you are unsure whether a code will be understood, attach a brief explanation to the front of the file folder for reference.

Sorting. If you have more than one folder to be filed, you must sort the files that have accumulated. Sort them in the order in which they are kept—such as alphabetically or numerically. Sorting saves you time later when you return the files to their proper places. If you will not be filing the folders immediately, store them in a temporary location, such as a file sorter.

Storing. The final step in the filing process is to store the files in the appropriate filing equipment. Documents should be stored neatly within their file folders in the proper sequence.

Careful attention to file storage will make your job easier in the long run. Make sure the folders are in good condition. Change them whenever they appear damaged or torn to prevent file contents from spilling out during the retrieval and filing process. If the file contains too many documents, divide it into two or more folders, and label each one (for example, Glass, Ann M.—Folder 1 of 2; Glass, Ann M.—Folder 2 of 2). Make sure to replace labels that are no longer legible.

Limiting Access to Files

Some offices restrict the number of people who can retrieve and return files. To obtain a file, staff members must fill out a requisition slip with their name and the name of the patient, as shown in Figure 10-6.

A record of who has the file is kept either in a notebook or on index cards in special boxes. The record includes the name of the file, the name of the borrower, the date the file was borrowed, and the date it is due back.

Under *no* circumstances should original patient medical records ever leave the practice. Photocopies can be made, if necessary. (Chapter 9 provides specific guidelines on releasing medical records to individuals and organizations outside your medical office.)

Springfield Medical Associates

Patient File Requisition Slip

Patient: ______________________

File Given to: ______________________

Date: ______________________

Time: ______________________

Due Back: ______________________

Figure 10-6. Some offices limit the personnel who have access to the file room. Staff members must fill out a requisition slip with their name and the name of the patient to obtain a patient record.

Filing Guidelines

There are specific rules for each filing system, as well as general guidelines, or helpful hints, applicable to any system. Following these guidelines will help you file more efficiently.

1. Each time you pull or file a patient record, glance at its contents. You should be familiar with the typical contents of a patient record folder to help avoid filing errors.
2. Keep files neat. Make sure that documents fit into the file folders and do not stick out or obscure file labels.
3. Do not overstuff file folders. Folders should be able to stay closed when laid on a flat surface.
4. When inserting documents into folders already in place in the drawer, lift the folders up and out of the drawer. Attempting to force documents into a folder inside the drawer can damage the documents or leave them sticking out of the folder.
5. Do not crowd the file drawer. Leave extra space to allow for leafing through the files and for retrieving and replacing files easily.
6. Where possible, use a combination of uppercase and lowercase letters to label folders. This format is easier to read than labels written completely in capital letters.
7. Choose file guides with a different tab position than your folders to help them stand out. Do not place guides so close together that they hide one another. A good rule of thumb is to position guides at least 5 inches apart.
8. If you are unsure whether to cross-reference a file, do it. It is better to err on the side of providing too many cross-references than too few.
9. File regularly so that you are not overwhelmed with too many folders to file.
10. Store only files in filing cabinets or on filing shelves. Do not store office equipment or supplies where files belong.
11. Train all staff members who will retrieve and replace files to make sure they have a thorough understanding of the system. Update them on any changes.
12. Periodically evaluate your office's filing system. "Tips for the Office" will help you with this task.

Locating Misplaced Files

Even in the best filing systems, there is a chance of temporarily misplacing or even losing patient medical records. No matter how good a system is, the people who do the filing are only human. If a file is misplaced, here are steps you can take to try to locate it.

1. Determine the last time you knew the file's location.
2. Go to that location, and retrace your steps. Look for the file along the way.
3. Look in the filing cabinet where the file belongs. Check neighboring files. Possibly the file was simply put in the wrong place.
4. Check underneath the files in the drawer or shelf to see if the file slipped out.

Tips FOR THE OFFICE

Evaluating Your Office Filing System

In a typical medical office, you retrieve and file documents daily using a filing system that may have been set up when the practice first opened. Now it is time to take a critical look at that system and determine how well it meets your needs.

The filing system you have probably does an adequate or better-than-average job of fulfilling the needs of the practice. Otherwise, retrieving and filing patient records would have become annoyingly inefficient. It is always beneficial to see where improvements can be made, however. Even a good filing system can be enhanced to increase office efficiency and save staff members valuable time.

Here are some simple guidelines for evaluating your filing system.

1. How well do you think your filing system meets your needs? Rate it on a scale of 1 to 10, with 10 representing the best. Survey staff members to determine their ratings, and calculate a composite number. *Based on this feedback, does your filing system seem to do a poor, adequate, or exceptional job?*
2. Note the type of system you use—for example, alphabetic or numeric. Then list the various reasons why files are retrieved from the system. *Would another system, a combination of systems (such as alphanumeric), or the addition of color coding save time or offer other benefits?*
3. Survey the office staff to determine whether there have been difficulties in retrieving or filing or problems with lost or misplaced files. Solicit suggestions for improvement. *If there have been problems, what steps can you take to avoid future difficulties?* (You might even ask your local office-supply representative for ideas.)
4. Consult personnel at other similar medical practices to determine which filing system works for them. Compare and contrast their systems with yours. How would their systems work in your office?

Before making any major changes to your filing system, evaluate each idea in terms of the time and effort it will require and the benefits it will deliver. For example, changing from an alphabetic to a numeric system may provide a relatively small benefit to your office but require a great deal of time to prepare new files and refile current documents. In that case implementing a numeric system is probably not worthwhile.

If you do make changes to your system, make sure that all staff members are retrained on how to file documents. It is well worth the extra time required at the start to prevent having to locate misplaced files in the future.

5. Check the pile of items to be filed or the file sorter envelope.
6. Consider possible cross-references or similar indexes (for example, similar patient names) for the file. Check those headings to see if the file was accidentally placed there.
7. Check with other staff members to determine if they have seen the file.
8. Even though files should always be kept in a secure area, occasionally individuals who are not part of the office staff, such as visiting physicians, may be in the area and may inadvertently pick up a file with their own materials. If you think someone could have taken the file, call the person immediately.
9. Ask another staff person to complete steps 1 through 7 to double-check your search.
10. Straighten the office, taking care to check through all piles of information where a file could be lodged.

If the misplaced file is not found within a reasonable time—24 to 48 hours—it may be considered lost. Losing a file has potentially devastating consequences. It may not be possible to duplicate the information within the file, but you can try to recreate it in a new file.

To do so, meet with the physician and office staff members to review the information needed. Record their recollections of information in the file. Note on the file document that it is a recollection and that the information is not official.

Then consult other office records that may include information related to the file. Contact insurance companies, laboratories, and other information providers for copies of original documents previously included in the lost file. Place copies of those records in the new file, or excerpt information. If the physician considers it appropriate, tell the patient whose file has been misplaced about its status and the steps you have taken to re-create it.

Active vs Inactive Files

At any given time, there are files that you use frequently and files that you use infrequently or not at all. Files that you use frequently are called **active files.** Files that you use infrequently are called **inactive files.** What constitutes an active, as opposed to an inactive, file? It depends on your individual practice. In a heart specialist's office, a patient who has not been seen for a year may be considered inactive, while in a dentist's office, a year may simply indicate one missed appointment.

There is a third category of files, called closed files. **Closed files** are files of patients who have died, have moved away, or for some other reason no longer consult the office. Although closed files could be moved immediately to storage, they are usually treated in the same manner as inactive files. That is, they are kept in the office for a certain length of time to make sure that there are no requests for the information in the file.

The physician must determine when a patient file is deemed inactive or closed. You and the physician can meet regularly, perhaps once a month or once a quarter, to review these files.

Storing Files

No office has unlimited space. Therefore, you will regularly need to transfer inactive and closed files from the office's filing area to a storage area.

Basic Storage Options

Before you can transfer files, you need to determine how and where they will be stored. The design and layout of file storage should make even older stored files easily accessible so that they can be periodically evaluated for retention or elimination.

There are many ways to store inactive files. For example, they can be stored in their original paper state or transferred into another format, such as onto a computer disk or tape or into microfilm or microfiche. Files can even be electronically coded with bar codes for immediate retrieval with a computer system. Regardless of the medium chosen for storing and preserving documents, keeping related material together and retrieving it should be made as easy as possible. Inactive files also must be kept secure, just as active ones are.

Paper Storage. If you choose to store files in their original form, you will be storing them as paper files. Paper files are often stored in boxes labeled with their contents. Choose boxes that are uniform in size so that they will stack well. Lift-off lids enable easy access to the contents of the box.

Paper files are bulky to store. They require roughly the same amount of space as they occupied in the office's primary files. Paper files preserve the original documents, however, and these documents can be important when providing evidence of medical treatment in legal proceedings. If paper files start to become brittle, they should be transferred to another storage medium.

Computer Storage. If storage space is limited, there are a number of paperless options for storing files. One such option is storing files on computer tapes or floppy disks, as shown in Figure 10-7. To do so, the office needs a computer system that can transfer documents to tapes or disks, then read them when they are retrieved from storage.

The easiest way to transfer documents directly into the computer is to use a scanner. This device copies a document onto the computer's hard drive. This process saves countless hours of rekeying (reentering) documents into the computer. Many scanners also have the capability of copying graphics and handwritten notes.

The document is then saved on a disk or on computer tape. Disks or tapes are labeled with the range of contents they contain. If documents were originally created on the computer, they can be similarly transferred to disk or tape, then deleted from the hard drive. Disks and tapes are dated and stored in file boxes or other containers.

Documents can be stored on the hard drive of the computer. The information should also be stored on disks, however, as a backup in case the hard drive crashes and information is lost.

If documents are stored directly on the hard drive, there are a variety of computer software programs that help in managing these records. This software checks files automatically using different criteria, such as the date the file was established or last updated. This software will help you make decisions about how long documents should be stored. When considering computer record management programs, look for user friendliness, speed and response time, and whether the features of the program meet your needs.

Microfilm, Microfiche, and Cartridges. Other paperless storage options include microfilm, microfiche, and film cartridges. (These storage options are discussed in Chapter 5.)

When considering transferring files to these formats, explore microfilm services, which index and transfer files for a fee. Using a service helps ensure that files are correctly indexed and thus easily found later on. Always have the microfilm service sign a confidentiality agreement.

Storage Facilities

Once you have determined the format for your stored files, you need to decide where to keep them. A number of options are available.

You may wish to store files in a remote area of your office building, such as an unused closet or office. Check to make sure that the area is secure, accessible, and safe for storing files (for example, do not store files where hazardous materials are stored). The practice may have to pay additional rent if the space is not within the confines of its office suite.

If there is no space in the building, consider a neighboring building, perhaps one in the same office complex. Many buildings rent space that can be used to store records. If you pursue this option, you will be responsible for managing the storage of records, including transporting them to the space, positioning them, and retrieving them as needed.

Certain storage facilities, called commercial records centers, will do some of the work for you (Figure 10-8). For a monthly fee, these centers typically house and manage stored documents. When evaluating commercial records centers, inquire about whether they will retrieve and/or deliver boxes or files and whether there is an onsite work area if someone needs to review the files at the storage location.

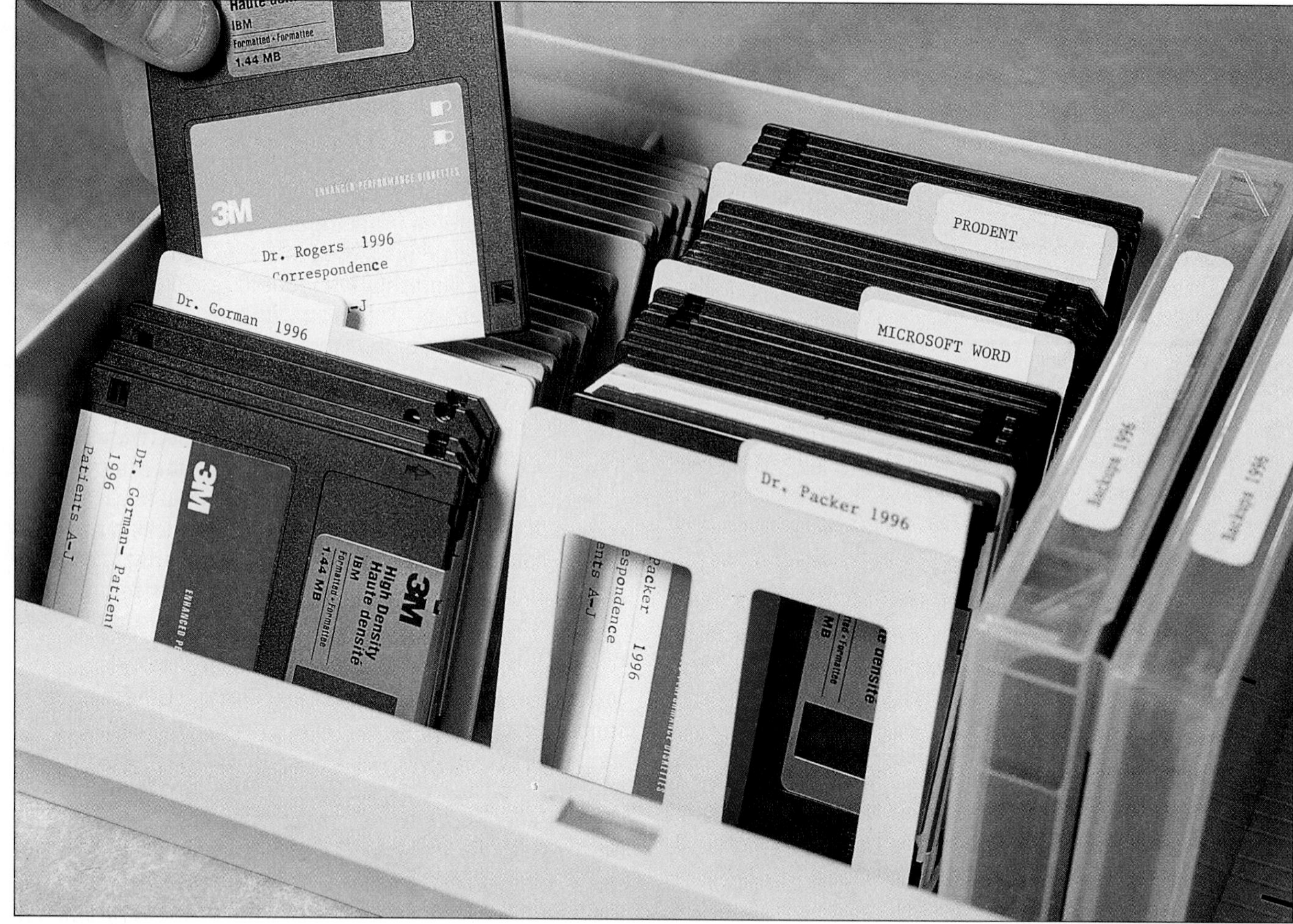

Figure 10-7. One paperless option for storing inactive files and closed files is on floppy disks.

Beware of general storage facilities that are not specially equipped for document management. These facilities may not address safety concerns, by taking precautions for fire or floods, for example.

Maintain a separate list of files stored off-site. This list can save a wasted trip to the storage site if a needed file is not housed there. The list also provides a valuable record if files are damaged or destroyed. Remember to update the list as new files are moved into storage and old files are taken out of storage and destroyed.

Storage Safety

No matter where you store files, you must consider the issue of safety, as well as security. Paper, computer, and film files are easily damaged and destroyed by fire, water, and extreme temperatures. Old, brittle paper files are particularly susceptible. Therefore, it is wise to evaluate the storage site and to take some basic precautions.

1. Choose a site with moderate temperatures year-round and adequate ventilation.
2. Select storage containers that can withstand intense heat and are waterproof. Look for metal or plastic boxes that are designated as fireproof and waterproof. Cardboard is not an option.
3. Choose a site equipped with a smoke alarm, sprinkler system, and fire extinguishers.
4. Select a site that is above ground and away from flood hazards. One way to find out if a site is susceptible to flooding is to inquire whether the facility has flood insurance, a requirement for sites at risk.
5. Choose a site that is kept locked, is regularly patrolled, or has an alarm system, to prevent theft or vandalism.
6. Remove old, brittle files as soon as possible, or transfer them into another format. They can then be placed in file storage again.
7. Ask for references from people at other offices who have stored files at the site. Talk to these people about what they like and dislike about the storage facility and any problems they have had in storing or retrieving documents.
8. If you are storing files in another form—on computer disk or microfiche—inquire about any special precautions the site owner takes to ensure safety.

Taking the time to thoroughly research storage options saves time and effort in the long run as you manage the stored files.

Retaining Files in the Office

You will not want to keep documents in storage forever, but how long should you keep them? To answer this question, most practices develop a records retention program.

Typically the doctor decides—based on the potential need for the information—how long to keep inactive or closed patient files in the office before sending them to storage. Working with the doctor, you should prepare a retention schedule. A **retention schedule** specifies how long to keep different types of patient records in the office after files have become inactive or closed. The schedule also details when files should be moved to a storage area (if outside the office) and how long they should be kept in storage before being destroyed. The retention schedule should be posted in the file room to make certain that all staff members are aware of it.

Although the doctor decides how long to keep inactive or closed patient records in the office, there are legal requirements for retaining certain types of information, which determine how long these documents must be stored.

1. According to the National Childhood Vaccine Injury Act of 1986, doctors must keep all immunization records on file in the office permanently. These records should not be put in storage.
2. The Labor Standards Act states that doctors must keep employee health records for 3 years.
3. The statute of limitations—the law stating the time period during which lawsuits may be filed—varies by state for civil suits. The most common length of time is 2 years. If a case involves a child or someone mentally incompetent, the statute of limitations extends the deadline. Regardless of the statute of limitations, it is always advisable for doctors to seek legal advice before destroying any records.
4. Many legal consultants advise that doctors maintain patient records for at least 7 years to protect themselves against malpractice suits.
5. The Internal Revenue Service usually requires doctors to keep financial records for up to 10 years.
6. Doctors are required to keep medical records of minors previously under their care for 2 to 7 years after the child reaches legal age, depending on the state. Some doctors keep these records indefinitely.
7. The American Medical Association, the American Hospital Association, and other groups generally suggest that doctors keep patient records for up to 10 years after a patient's final visit or contact.

For a complete list of federal regulations, contact the U.S. Superintendent of Documents in Washington, D.C., and request a copy of the *Guide to Record Retention Requirements.* This guide is updated annually and can be purchased for a small fee.

State and local retention requirements can be obtained from offices with which you regularly conduct business, such as insurance companies, state and local agencies, and medical associations. If you do business in more than one state, follow the schedule that requires the longest retention time for materials.

When counting years in a retention schedule, remember not to count the year in which the document was produced but to begin counting with the following year. This way, documents produced near the end of a calendar year will be tracked more efficiently. Procedure 10-3 summarizes the steps for setting up a records retention program.

When records can finally be eliminated, they cannot simply be thrown away. Even old records hold confidential information about patients. Therefore, they must be completely destroyed by shredding. Be careful not to destroy records prematurely, because they often cannot be re-created. You should keep for your records a list of documents that have been destroyed.

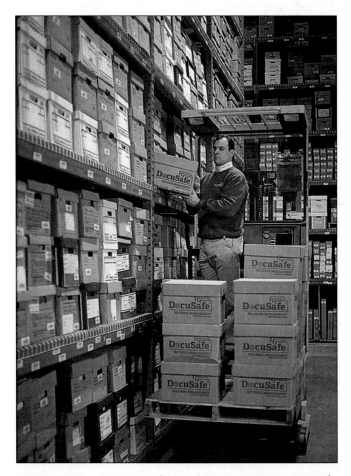

Figure 10-8. Commercial records centers manage stored documents for medical practices. Look for a center with personnel who retrieve and deliver boxes or files directly to your office.

PROCEDURE 10-3

Developing a Records Retention Program

Objective: To establish a records retention program for patient medical records that meets office needs as well as legal and government guidelines

Materials: *Guide to Record Retention Requirements* (published annually by the federal government), names and telephone numbers of local medical associations and state offices (including the state insurance commissioner and the medical practice's attorney), file folders, index cards, index box, paper, pen or typewriter

Method

1. On a piece of paper, list the types of information contained in a typical patient medical record in your office. For example, a file for an adult patient may include the patient's case history, records of hospital stays, and insurance information.
2. Research the state and federal requirements for keeping documents. Consult the *Guide to Record Retention Requirements* for federal guidelines. Contact the appropriate state office (such as the office of the insurance commissioner) for specific state requirements, such as rules for keeping records of insurance payments and the statute of limitations for initiating lawsuits. If your office does business in more than one state, be sure to research all applicable regulations. Consult with the attorney who represents your practice.
3. Compile the results of your research in a chart. At the top of the chart, list the different kinds of information your office keeps in patient records. Down the left side of the chart, list the headings "Federal," "State," and "Other." Then, in each box, record the corresponding information.
4. Compare all the legal and government requirements. Indicate which one is for the longest period of time.
5. Meet with the doctor to review the information. Work together to prepare a retention schedule. Determine how long different types of patient records should be kept in the office after a patient leaves the practice and how long records should be kept in storage. Although retention periods can vary based on the type of information kept in a file, it is often easiest to choose a retention period that covers all records. For example, all records could be kept in the office for 1 year after a patient leaves the practice and then kept in storage for another 9 years, for a total of 10 years. Determine how files will be destroyed when they have exceeded the retention requirements. Usually, records are destroyed by paper shredding. Purchase the appropriate equipment, as necessary.
6. Put the retention schedule in writing, and post it prominently near the files. In addition, keep a copy of the schedule in a safe place in the office. Review it with the office staff.
7. Develop a system for identifying files easily under the retention system. For example, for each file deemed inactive or closed, prepare an index card containing the following information:
   - Patient's name and Social Security number
   - Contents of the file
   - Date the file was deemed inactive and by whom
   - Date the file should be sent to storage (the actual date will be filled in later; if more than one storage location is used, indicate the exact location to which the file was sent)
   - Date the file should be destroyed (the actual date will be filled in later)

   Have the card signed by the doctor and by the person responsible for the files. Keep the card in an index box. This is your authorization to destroy the file at the appropriate time.
8. Use color coding to help identify inactive files. For example, all records that become inactive in 1997 could be placed in green file folders and moved to a supplemental file. Then, in January 1999 all the green files could be pulled and sent to storage.
9. One person should be responsible for checking the index cards once a month to determine which stored files should be destroyed. Before retrieving these files from storage, circulate a notice to the office staff stating which records will be destroyed. Indicate that the staff must let you know by a specific date if any of the files should be saved. You may want to keep a separate file with these notices.
10. After the deadline has passed, retrieve the files from storage. Review each file before it is destroyed. Make sure the staff members who will destroy the files are trained to use the equipment properly. Develop a sheet of instructions for destroying files. Post it prominently with the retention schedule, near the machinery used to destroy the files.
11. Update the index card, giving the date the file was destroyed and by whom.
12. Periodically review the retention schedule. Update it with the most current legal and governmental requirements. With the staff, evaluate whether the current schedule is meeting the needs of your office or whether files are being kept too long or destroyed prematurely. With the doctor's approval, change the schedule as necessary.

MULTISKILL FOCUS

Medical Record Technologist

To gain medical assistant credentials, you must fulfill the requirements of either the American Association of Medical Assistants (for a Certified Medical Assistant) or the American Medical Technologists (for a Registered Medical Assistant). After obtaining your medical assistant certification or registration, you may wish to acquire additional skills in specialty areas through course work or on-the-job training. Although this course work or training may not lead to an additional certification or degree, it will enable you to expand your role in the medical office and advance your career as the demand for multiskilled health professionals increases.

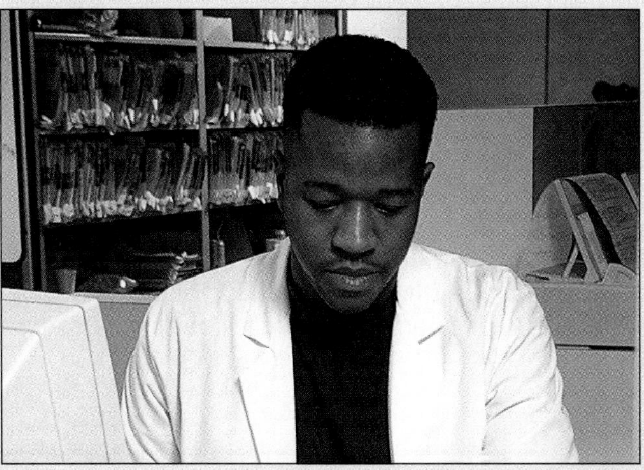

Skills and Duties

Also known as a medical record technician or a medical chart specialist, a medical record technologist maintains patient records for a physician or group of physicians. He is responsible for ensuring that all medical information is accurate and complete. In a hospital, a medical record technologist deals strictly with health information and has no patient contact. In a small office, however, he may have additional clerical duties such as answering the telephone.

A patient's medical record includes a medical history and statement of symptoms, as well as the results of examinations, laboratory tests, and x-rays. The physician's diagnoses and treatment plans are also included. The information in the patient's record may be needed for insurance purposes or to aid in further diagnosis and treatment. In addition, it may be used for research purposes.

The medical record technologist checks all patient charts for completeness and accuracy. He makes sure that all necessary forms related to the patient's care are included, properly filled out, and signed. He checks to see that all reports and test results are attached to the chart. If necessary, he speaks with the physician to clarify information about the patient's diagnosis or treatment.

The technologist must also code the medical record. He assigns a code to each clinical procedure and diagnosis if this coding has not already been done by another member of the health-care team. In the hospital setting, he assigns a diagnosis-related group (DRG) to the patient, using a special computer program. The DRG helps determine the reimbursement that the hospital will receive from Medicare or any other insurance provider that uses a DRG system. The medical record technologist may also use the coded records to set up a cross-reference index, a type of file that lists the same information under several different headings.

Some medical record technologists specialize in a particular area. Coding is one example. Another is registry, which involves keeping records of all occurrences of certain diseases like bone cancer. The information the registrar collects can be used by individual physicians or as part of a research study.

Workplace Settings

The majority of medical record technologists work in medical record departments of hospitals. Most of the rest work in nursing homes, group practices, and health maintenance organizations (HMOs). A few medical record technologists work in federal or state government offices, public health departments, health and property insurance companies, or accounting and law firms. Some record technologists are self-employed and work as consultants to nursing homes or physicians' offices.

Education

Most medical record technologists have completed a 2-year associate degree program at a junior or community college. Course work includes biology, anatomy and physiology, medical terminology, data processing, coding, and statistics. Record technologists can also be trained through the Independent Study Program in Medical Record Technology, a home-study program offered by the American Medical Record Association (AMRA).

To become certified as an Accredited Record Technician (ART), a technologist must take a written examination administered by the AMRA. In order to qualify for the examination, he must be a graduate of a 2-year associate degree program accredited by the Commission on Accreditation of Allied Health Education Programs (CAAHEP), or he must be a graduate of the Independent Study Program who has completed an additional 30 semester hours of academic credit.

Where to Go for More Information

American Medical Record Association
919 North Michigan Avenue, Suite 1400
Chicago, IL 60611

Summary

The organization of a practice's filing system depends on how files need to be retrieved. Alphabetic systems are the most common. Numeric systems are sometimes used in practices with patients who require a high level of confidentiality, such as those who are HIV-positive.

Color coding may be used to further identify files. In addition, special types of files, such as tickler files or supplemental files, are sometimes used.

The five steps in the filing process are inspecting, indexing, coding, sorting, and storing. Failure to follow each of the steps in order can result in misplaced or lost files.

Typically, only active files are kept in the practice's main file area. When patient records are determined to be inactive or closed, they are transferred to storage—either elsewhere in the office or outside the practice in a special storage facility. Files may be stored in a variety of formats: paper, microfilm or microfiche, or on the computer. Wherever files are stored and in whatever format, they must be kept safe and secure.

The amount of time that stored files are retained depends on legal, state, and federal guidelines. Offices manage the storage and destruction of files by developing a records retention program. Because even old files contain confidential information, they must be destroyed in an approved manner, not simply thrown away.

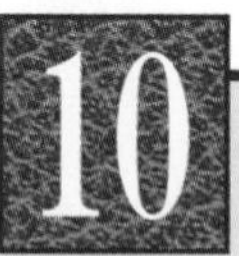

Chapter Review

Discussion Questions

1. Why is it important to use a filing system to keep medical records? What could happen if a filing system is not instituted or followed in a medical practice?
2. Compare and contrast the alphabetic filing system with the numeric filing system. What are the advantages and disadvantages of each method for filing medical records?
3. Why are safety and security critical issues for a patient record filing system?
4. Summarize the skills necessary for staff members whose primary responsibility is to file medical records.

Critical Thinking Questions

1. What special concerns might arise when storing records on the computer rather than in traditional paper files? What would you do to alleviate these concerns?
2. Why, do you think, should each member of a family have a separate medical file?
3. What filing system would you choose to file a series of numbered insurance claim forms for patients in your practice? Explain your reasoning.

Application Activities

1. Arrange these ten patient names in order as they would appear in an alphabetic filing system.

   Josephs, Leon S.
   Carl Jones
   Carly Jones
   Carl A. Jones
   Deirdre Anne Jones
   McCullough, Anthony L.
   E. Bruce Harrison
   Waters, Jamie H.
   Joan Carle
   James Waters
2. Using your class list, develop a numeric filing system and a master list that matches each number to a specific person. Then set up an alphabetic filing system based on students' last names. Discuss with your classmates which system is most useful in an educational setting and why.
3. Set up a personal tickler file for yourself, containing personal responsibilities—such as errands, appointments, and social engagements—for the coming week. Keep your notes in a file folder or on a calendar until all activities have been completed. At the end of the week, write a brief paragraph explaining whether or not you found the process helpful. Give several examples to support your answer.
4. Obtain an office-supply catalog that features filing supplies. Put together a product order to set up a patient records filing system for a midsized medical office serving approximately 100 patients. Assume that the practice has already purchased the appropriate equipment, such as filing cabinets or shelves.

continued

Chapter Review continued

Further Readings

"The Eyes Have It in Color Filing." *Managing Office Technology*, June 1994, 50.

Fernberg, Patricia. "Mobile Filing's on Track With Savings." *Modern Office Technology,* August 1991, 29.

"File Tracking." *Modern Office Technology,* April 1990, 38.

Frappaolo, Carl. "The Promise of Electronic Document Management." *Modern Office Technology,* October 1992, 38.

Gragg, Ellen. "Filing Systems Evolve as Office Technology Advances." *The Office,* July 1993, 12.

Haskins, David. "Indexicon Indexes Documents Quickly." *PC Magazine,* 13 September 1994, 48.

Lexington, Anne. "Organizing a System for Document Filing: The Key to Setting Up Proper Storage Is to Know the Legal Rules Regarding Document Archival and Retention." *The Office,* June 1992, 28.

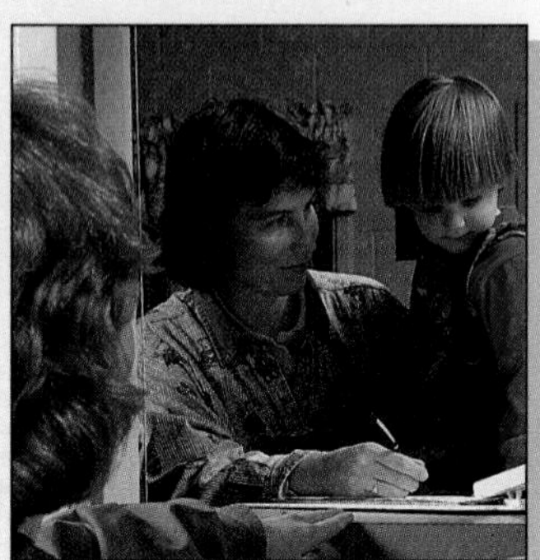

Section Two

Interacting With Patients

AREAS OF COMPETENCE

1997 ROLE DELINEATION STUDY

ADMINISTRATIVE

- Administrative Procedures

GENERAL (Transdisciplinary)

- Professionalism
- Communication Skills
- Legal Concepts
- Instructions
- Operational Functions

CHAPTER LIST

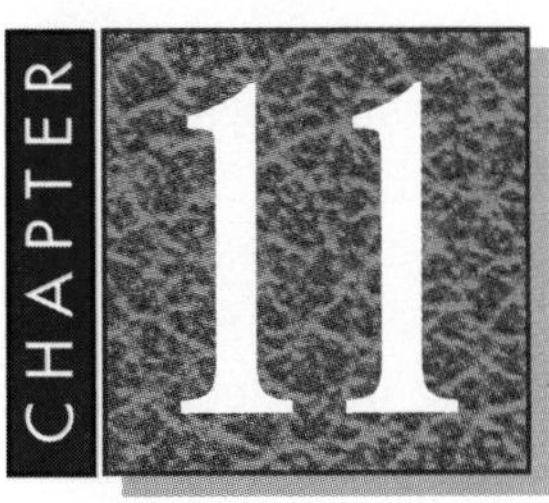

Telephone Techniques

CHAPTER OUTLINE

- Using the Telephone Effectively
- Managing Incoming Calls
- Types of Incoming Calls
- Using Proper Telephone Etiquette
- Taking Messages
- Telephone Answering Systems
- Placing Outgoing Calls
- Telephone Triage

OBJECTIVES

After completing Chapter 11, you will be able to:

- Explain how to manage incoming telephone calls.
- Compare the types of calls the medical assistant handles with those the physician or other staff members handle.
- Describe how to handle various types of incoming calls from patients and from others.
- Discuss the importance of proper telephone etiquette.
- Describe the procedures for taking telephone messages.
- Explain how to retrieve calls from an answering service.
- Describe the procedures for placing outgoing calls.
- Explain the function of telephone triage in the medical office.

AREAS OF COMPETENCE

1997 ROLE DELINEATION STUDY

GENERAL (Transdisciplinary)

Professionalism

- Prioritize and perform multiple tasks

Communication Skills

- Use professional telephone technique
- Receive, organize, prioritize, and transmit information

Key Terms

enunciation
etiquette
pitch
pronunciation
telephone triage

Using the Telephone Effectively

The telephone is an important tool for promoting the positive, professional image of a medical practice. When you answer the telephone, you may be the first contact a person has with the practice. The impression you leave can be either positive or negative. Your job is to ensure that it is positive.

Good telephone management leaves callers with a positive impression of you, the physician, and the practice. Poor telephone management can result in bad feelings, misunderstandings, and an unfavorable impression. The telephone image you present should convey the message that the staff is caring, attentive, and helpful. Showing concern for a patient's welfare is a quality that patients rate highly when evaluating health-care professionals. In addition, you must sound professional and knowledgeable when handling telephone calls. Learning and using proper telephone management skills will help keep patients informed and ensure their satisfaction with the medical practice.

Managing Incoming Calls

Telephone calls must always be answered promptly. The procedures for answering calls may vary. Guidelines are usually presented in the office policy and procedures manual. In general, you should greet callers with your name and the office name. Some people may feel awkward using their own name when answering the telephone. Introducing yourself to callers, however, lets them know that they are speaking to a real person, not simply an anonymous voice.

No matter how hurried you are, you should be courteous, calm, and pleasant on the telephone, devoting your full attention to the caller. If the caller does not give a name, ask for it. Identifying the caller enables you to pull the patient's file, if necessary.

Screening Calls

Part of the responsibility of answering the telephone involves screening calls before you transfer them. Each office has its own policy about calls that should be put through right away, those that should be returned later, and those that should be handled by other staff members. "Tips for the Office" describes some guidelines for screening calls.

Routing Calls

In general, there are three types of incoming calls to a doctor's office: calls dealing mainly with administrative issues, emergency calls that require immediate action by the doctor, and calls relating to clinical issues that require the attention of the doctor, nurse, nurse practitioner, or physician's assistant.

Calls Handled by the Medical Assistant. The most common calls to a medical office involve administrative issues. As a medical assistant, you will be able to handle most of these calls yourself. They will concern the following matters:

- Appointments (scheduling, rescheduling, canceling)
- Questions concerning office policies, fees, and hours
- Billing inquiries
- Insurance questions
- Other administrative questions
- X-ray and laboratory reports
- Reports from hospitals regarding a patient's progress
- Reports from patients concerning their progress
- Requests for referrals to other doctors

Tips FOR THE OFFICE

Screening Incoming Calls

Each medical office has its own policy about how to screen incoming calls before transferring them to the appropriate person. Calls come not only from patients, but also from other physicians, hospital personnel, pharmacists, insurance company personnel, sales representatives, and family members and friends of patients. Here are some general tips for screening calls.

Find out who is calling. A polite way to do this is to say, "May I ask who is calling?" Another option is, "May I tell Dr. ____ who is calling?"

Ask what the call is in reference to. When a caller asks to speak with the physician, you should ask the purpose of the call. Depending on the answer, you may determine that you or someone else in the office can handle the situation without disturbing the physician. The response may be as simple as solving a billing problem or clarifying instructions. Remember, however, that emergency calls should be transferred to the physician right away.

Decide whether the call should be put through. Although most calls are routed to the appropriate person, any callers who refuse to identify themselves should not be put through. In such a case suggest that the caller write a letter to the physician and mark it "Personal."

Determine what to do if the matter is personal. The physician may ask you to take a message in these instances. Inform the caller that the physician will return the call as soon as possible.

- Requests for prescription renewals, which must be approved by the doctor unless approval is indicated on the patient's chart
- Complaints from patients about administrative matters

Depending on the practice, the office manager or someone in the billing department may handle some administrative calls. The calls you handle may include scheduling appointments, receiving or requesting reports or information, insurance and billing questions, and general inquiries, such as those concerning office hours.

Calls Requiring the Doctor's Attention. Certain calls will require the doctor's personal attention. These include the following:

- Emergency calls
- Calls from other doctors
- Patient requests to discuss test results, particularly abnormal results
- Reports from patients concerning unsatisfactory progress
- Requests for prescription renewals (unless previously authorized on the patient's chart)

Occasionally the patient may prefer to discuss symptoms only with the doctor. These requests should be honored. Depending on the doctor's preference and availability, you may call the doctor to the telephone to handle calls of this nature as they are received. Otherwise, the calls will be returned later that day when the doctor has time available. (Most doctors have a set time, such as a half hour in the late morning or at the end of the day, for returning nonemergency patient calls.)

In certain practices some of these calls may be handled by others on the staff, such as a nurse practitioner or physician's assistant. For example, a nurse practitioner may be able to order a renewal of a regular prescription, provide advice for the care of a sprain, or answer well-baby questions or questions about the side effects of a drug.

The Routing List. Each medical office has a standard policy that documents how incoming telephone calls are to be routed and handled. A routing list, such as the one shown in Figure 11-1, specifies who is responsible for the various types of calls in the office and how the calls are to be handled. For example, the routing list indicates which calls should be put through to the doctor immediately and which ones can be returned later.

The routing procedure may simply identify the general title of the person responsible for handling a call. When

Handling Incoming Telephone Calls

	Route to doctor immediately	*Take message for doctor*	*Route to nurse or assistant*
Emergencies: bleeding, drug/allergic reaction, difficulty breathing, injury, pain, poisoning, shock, unconsciousness, incoherence or hysteria	X		
Calls from other physicians	if possible		
Patient progress report		X	
Patient request for laboratory report		X (if abnormal)	Melissa (if normal)
Patient questions re medication		X	
Patient questions re billing or insurance			Jerry
Patient complaints			Melissa
Appointments			Melissa
Prescription renewals or refills		X	
Office business			Jerry
Personal business		X	
Salespeople			Jerry

Figure 11-1. A routing list identifies which office staff member is responsible for each type of incoming call.

more than one person in the office has the same title, however, the name of the individual who has that particular responsibility should be specified.

Types of Incoming Calls

In dealing with incoming telephone calls, you will encounter a variety of questions and requests from numerous people. Many incoming calls are from patients. You will also receive calls from other people, including attorneys, other physicians, pharmaceutical sales representatives, and other salespeople.

Calls From Patients

As stated earlier in the chapter, patients call the medical office for a variety of reasons, including rescheduling appointments and requesting prescription renewals. If you will be discussing clinical matters over the telephone, it is a good idea to pull the patient's chart. The information in the chart may enable you to address any problems quickly. Having the chart handy also allows you to document the conversation immediately.

Always keep in mind that the physician is legally responsible for your actions, including relaying information to patients over the telephone. The office policy manual typically specifies what you may and may not discuss with patients. If you are uncertain about giving particular information to a patient, it is best to have the physician return the patient's call.

Appointment Scheduling. Follow office procedures for making or changing appointment times over the telephone. (Scheduling appointments is discussed in Chapter 12.)

Billing Inquiries. If a patient calls about a billing problem, you will need to pull the patient's chart and billing information. With this information, you can compare the charges with the actual services performed.

If a patient claims to have been overcharged, check to see if the correct fee was charged. If you find that an error was made, apologize, and tell the patient the office will send a corrected statement. Ask the patient to wait for the new statement before sending payment. If in fact the proper fee was charged, it may be helpful to speak to the physician before responding to the patient. The physician may be able to tell you if there were special circumstances regarding the visit or charge in question. Allowing the patient to pay the bill in installments is usually an acceptable option.

If a patient is dissatisfied, document all comments, and relay the information to the physician. If a bill has not been paid, ask if there are special circumstances affecting the patient's ability to pay. Always give this information to the physician or office manager.

Requests for Laboratory Reports. If a patient calls the office requesting the results of laboratory tests, pull the patient's chart to see if the report has been received. If it has not, suggest that the patient call back in a day or two. Some offices will call the laboratory for the results.

In some offices you may be authorized to give laboratory results by telephone if they are normal, or negative, so the patient does not have to wait for results to be mailed. Make a note on the patient's chart if you provide any information about test results. If a test result is abnormal, the physician will need to speak with the patient. In such a case tell the patient that the office has received the results and that the physician will call as soon as possible. Then place the patient's chart and the telephone message on the physician's desk.

Questions About Medications. One of the most common types of calls from patients involves questions about medication. A patient may ask about using a current prescription or may want to renew an existing prescription.

Prescription Renewals. Calls for prescription renewals occur frequently and may come from the patient's pharmacy or from the patient. A pharmacist usually calls to check before dispensing refills if more than a year has passed since the original prescription was written. If the physician has indicated on the patient's chart that renewals are approved, you may authorize the pharmacy to renew a prescription. In any other case, only the physician may authorize renewals. If the physician authorizes a renewal, you may be asked to telephone it in to the patient's pharmacy.

Old Prescriptions. Patients may call to ask if they can use a medication that was prescribed for a previous condition. In these instances, recommend that the patient come in for an appointment. Explain why the medication should not be used: it may be old and no longer effective, the current problem may not be the same as the previous one, the medication may not be helpful, and using the medication may mask the current condition's symptoms and make a diagnosis difficult.

If the patient does not want to make an appointment, relay the information to the physician. The physician will probably want to speak with the patient.

Reports on Symptoms. Sometimes patients call the office about symptoms they wish to discuss with the physician. Here are tips for handling such calls.

- Listen attentively to the patient.
- If the patient is in real distress, try to schedule an appointment that day or as soon as possible.
- Write down all the patient's symptoms completely, accurately, and immediately. In many instances the physician may be able to suggest simple emergency relief measures that you can relay to the patient. These measures may make the patient comfortable until the time of the appointment.

Progress Reports. Physicians often ask patients to call the office to let them know how a prescribed treatment is working. In these instances route the call to the physician, and log the call in the patient's medical record immediately. You may also be responsible for making routine follow-up calls to patients to verify that they are following treatment instructions.

Requests for Advice. Although a patient may ask you for your medical opinion, do not give medical advice of any kind. Explain that you are not trained to make a diagnosis or licensed to prescribe medication. Stress that the patient must see the physician. If the patient cannot come into the office, assure her that the physician will return the call or that you will call back after discussing the problem with the physician. Occasionally a patient wants to speak only with the physician, not other staff members. You must honor this request.

In some cases the physician may feel that a patient's symptoms warrant immediate attention and will insist on seeing the patient before prescribing any treatment. If the patient refuses to come to the office, note the reason on the chart, and suggest a visit to the emergency room or to a nearby physician. For legal reasons, it is important to document such conversations completely in the patient's chart, including the refusal of treatment.

Complaints. Even when an office provides the highest-quality care, complaints still occur. When a patient calls with a complaint, such as a billing error, it is important to listen carefully, without interrupting. Take careful notes of all the details, and read them back to the caller to ensure that you have written them down correctly. Let the caller know the person to whose attention you will bring the complaint and, if possible, when to expect a response.

Always apologize to the caller for any inconvenience the problem may have caused, even if the problem occurred through no fault of the office. Make sure the proper person receives the information about the complaint.

Sometimes a patient who calls with a complaint is angry. Responding to this type of call can be difficult and uncomfortable. Your first priority is to stay calm and try to pacify the caller. Follow these guidelines when dealing with an angry caller.

- Listen carefully, and acknowledge the patient's anger. By understanding the problem, you will be better able to work toward a solution.
- Remain calm, and speak gently and kindly. Do not act superior or talk down to the patient. Do not interrupt the patient. Do not return the anger or blame.
- Let the patient know that you will do your best to correct the problem. This message will convey that you care.
- Take careful notes, and be sure to document the call.
- Do not become defensive.
- Never make promises you cannot keep.
- Follow up promptly on the problem.
- Inform the physician immediately if an angry patient threatens legal action against the office.

Emergencies. Emergency calls must be immediately routed to the physician. Emergency situations include serious or life-threatening medical conditions, such as severe bleeding, a reaction to a drug, injuries, poisoning, suicide attempts, loss of consciousness, or severe burns. Figure 11-2 lists symptoms and conditions that require immediate help.

Symptoms and Conditions That Require Immediate Medical Help

- Unconsciousness
- Lack of breathing or trouble breathing
- Severe bleeding
- Pressure or pain in the abdomen that will not go away
- Severe vomiting or bloody stools
- Poisoning
- Injuries to the head, neck, or back
- Choking
- Drowning
- Electrical shock
- Snakebites
- Vehicle collisions
- Allergic reactions to foods or insect stings
- Chemicals or foreign objects in the eye
- Fires, severe burns, or injuries from explosions
- Human bites or any deep animal bites
- Heart attack. Symptoms include chest pain or pressure; pain radiating from the chest to the arm, shoulder, neck, jaw, back, or stomach; nausea or vomiting; weakness; shortness of breath; pale or gray skin color.
- Stroke. Symptoms include seizures, severe headache, slurred speech.
- Broken bones. Symptoms include being unable to move or put weight on the injured body part. The injured part is very painful or looks misshapen.
- Shock. Symptoms include paleness; feeling faint and sweaty; weak, rapid pulse; cold, moist skin; confusion or drowsiness.
- Heatstroke (sunstroke). Symptoms include confusion or loss of consciousness; flushed skin that is hot and dry; strong, rapid pulse.
- Hypothermia (a drop in body temperature during prolonged exposure to cold). Symptoms include becoming increasingly clumsy, unreasonable, irritable, confused, and sleepy; slurred speech; slipping into a coma with slow, weak breathing and heartbeat.

Figure 11-2. Emergency calls require swift but careful handling.

If someone calls the office on behalf of a patient who is experiencing any of these symptoms or conditions, you may instruct the caller to dial 911 to request an ambulance. Procedure 11-1 describes the steps for handling emergency calls. The physician should be called to the telephone immediately to offer assistance.

Other Calls

Besides calls from patients, a medical office receives many other types of calls. For example, family members and friends of patients may call the physician at the office. The physician will let you know how to handle these calls. The following are guidelines for managing calls from attorneys, other physicians, and salespeople.

Attorneys. Refer to the procedures listed in your practice's office policy manual regarding how to handle calls from attorneys. Follow the office guidelines closely, and ask the physician how to proceed if you receive a call that does not fall within the guidelines. Remember, never release any patient information to an outside caller unless the physician has asked you to do so.

Other Physicians. Patients at your practice may be referred to surgeons, specialists, and other physicians for

PROCEDURE 11-1

Handling Emergency Calls

Objective: To determine whether a telephone call involves a medical emergency and to learn the steps to take if it is an emergency call

Materials: Office guidelines for handling emergency calls; list of symptoms and conditions requiring immediate medical attention; telephone numbers of area emergency rooms, poison control centers, and ambulance transport services; telephone message forms or telephone message log

Method

1. When someone calls the office regarding a potential emergency, remain calm. This attitude will help calm the caller and enable you to gather necessary information in the most efficient manner.
2. Obtain the following information, taking accurate notes:
   a. The caller's name
   b. The caller's relation to the patient (if it is not the patient who is calling)
   c. The patient's name
   d. The patient's age
   e. A complete description of the patient's symptoms
   f. If the call is about an accident, a description of how the accident or injury occurred and any other pertinent information
   g. A description of how the patient is reacting to the situation
   h. Treatment that has been administered
   i. The caller's telephone number and the address from which the call is being made

It may be necessary for you to put the call on hold or to hang up so that you can call for medical assistance. Before you do so, however, be sure to read the information back to the caller to ensure that you have written it down correctly.

3. Read back the details of the medical problem to verify them.
4. If necessary, refer to the list of symptoms and conditions that require immediate medical attention to determine if the situation is indeed a medical emergency.

If the Situation Is a Medical Emergency

1. Put the call through to the doctor immediately, or handle the situation according to the established office procedures.
2. If the doctor is not in the office, follow established office procedures. They may involve one or more of the following:
   a. Transferring the call to the nurse practitioner or other medical personnel, as appropriate
   b. Instructing the caller to dial 911 to request an ambulance for the patient
   c. Instructing the patient to go to the nearest emergency room
   d. Instructing the caller to telephone the nearest poison control center for advice and supplying the caller with its telephone number
   e. Paging the doctor

If the Situation Is Not a Medical Emergency

1. Handle the call according to established office procedures.
2. If you are in doubt about whether the situation is a medical emergency, treat it like an emergency. It is better to be overly cautious than to let an emergency go untreated. The doctor should be the one to decide how to handle these situations. You must always alert the doctor immediately about an emergency call, even if the patient declines to speak with the doctor.

consultations. Consequently, you may receive calls from those physicians' offices. Route those calls to the physician if the caller requests that you do so. Always remember to ask if the call is about a medical emergency. Also keep in mind that you may not give out any patient information—even to another physician—unless you have a written, signed release from the patient.

Salespeople. As a medical assistant, you will probably be the contact for salespeople, unless the office policy manual states that another staff member should handle this duty. On the telephone, ask the salesperson to send you information about any new products or equipment. Pharmaceutical sales representatives may want to meet with the physician. Forward such messages to the physician with a request to let you know when to schedule the appointment. Many physicians see pharmaceutical sales representatives on certain days at certain times. Sometimes they limit the number of representatives they will see in one day. Make sure you know your office policy.

Using Proper Telephone Etiquette

Handle all telephone calls politely and professionally. Use proper telephone **etiquette,** or good manners, so you feel confident in your role of providing quality care and assistance. Adhering to the guidelines that follow will help ensure that your telephone conversations are pleasant and constructive.

Your Telephone Voice

When you speak on the telephone, your voice represents the medical office. It must effectively present your message. Because you cannot rely on body language or facial expressions to help you communicate over the telephone, it is important to make the most of your telephone voice. Use the following tips to make your voice pleasant and effective.

- Speak directly into the receiver. Otherwise, your voice will be difficult to understand.
- Visualize the caller, and speak directly to that person.
- Convey a friendly and respectful interest in the caller. You should sound helpful and alert.
- Use language that is nontechnical and easy to understand. Never use slang.
- Speak at a natural pace, not too quickly or too slowly.
- Use a normal conversational tone.
- Try to vary your pitch while you are talking. **Pitch** is the high or low level of your speech. Varying the pitch of your voice allows you to emphasize words and makes your voice more pleasant to listen to.
- Make the caller feel important.

Pronunciation. Proper **pronunciation** (saying words correctly) is one of the most important telephone skills. Sometimes last names are difficult to pronounce. Ask patients, "How do you pronounce your name?" to make them feel welcome and important.

Enunciation. **Enunciation** (clear and distinct speaking) is the opposite of mumbling. Good enunciation helps the person you are speaking to understand you, which is especially important when you are trying to convey medical information.

Making a Good Impression

In a sense your telephone duties include public relations skills. How you handle telephone calls will have an impact on the public image of the medical practice.

Giving Undivided Attention. Do not try to answer the telephone while continuing to carry out another task. This practice may lead to errors in message taking and may give the caller the impression that you are uncaring or uninterested. Give the caller the same undivided attention you would if the person were in the office. Listen carefully to get the correct information.

Putting a Call on Hold. Although you should try not to put a caller on hold, there will be times when it is unavoidable. You may receive a call on another line, or a situation in the office may prevent you from devoting your full attention to the caller. Sometimes you may have to check a file or ask someone else in the office a question on behalf of the caller. Before putting a call on hold, however, always let the caller state the reason for the call. This step is essential so that you do not inadvertently put an emergency call on hold.

The medical office may have a standard procedure for placing a call on hold. Typically you will ask the caller the purpose of the call, state why you need to place the call on hold, explain how long you expect the wait to be, and ask the caller if this wait is acceptable. If you think the wait will be long, offer to call back rather than asking the caller to hold. Being kept on hold too long or too often makes people think the staff is inattentive to their needs.

If you know you can return to the line shortly, you can put the caller on hold, then attend to the problem. If you need to answer a second call, get the second caller's name and telephone number, and put that call on hold until you have completed the first call. You can then return to the second call.

Handling Difficult Situations. At times it will be impossible to give your undivided attention to a caller because of a pressing issue or emergency in the office. If the call itself is not an emergency one, it is best to ask if you can call back. Explain that you are currently handling an urgent matter, and offer to return the call in a few minutes. Most people will appreciate your honesty. Return the call in a reasonable amount of time, and be sure to apologize for the inconvenience.

Remembering Patients' Names. When patients are recognized by name, they are more likely to have positive feelings about the practice. Using a caller's name during

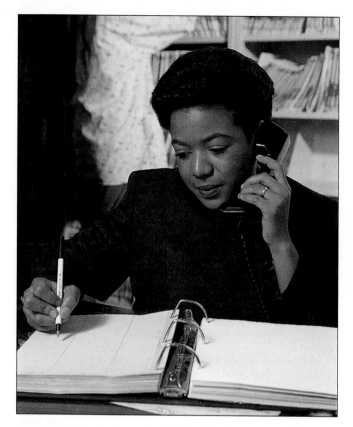

Figure 11-3. Use one hand or a telephone rest to hold the telephone so that the hand you write with is free to take messages.

a conversation makes the caller feel important. If you do not recognize a patient's name, it is better to ask "Has it been some time since you've seen the doctor?" rather than to ask if the patient has been to the practice before.

Checking for Understanding. When communicating by telephone, you do not have visual signals to convey the caller's feelings and level of understanding of the information you are discussing. Consequently, you must ask certain questions in the right way. If a call is long or complicated, summarize what was said to be sure that both you and the caller understand the information. Ask if the caller has any questions about what you have discussed.

Communicating Feelings. Whenever information is conveyed over the telephone, feelings are also communicated. When dealing with a caller who is nervous, upset, or angry, try to show empathy (an understanding of the other person's feelings). Communicating with empathy helps the caller feel more positive about the conversation and the medical office.

Ending the Conversation. It is not useful to let a conversation run on if you can effectively complete the call sooner. Before hanging up, however, take a few seconds to complete the call so that the caller feels properly cared for and satisfied. You can complete the call by summarizing the important points of the conversation and thanking the caller. Then let the caller hang up first. When you put the receiver down, never slam it—even if the caller has already hung up. Remember that all your actions reflect the professional image of the medical practice. Patients in the waiting room may see you when you are talking on the telephone.

Taking Messages

Always have paper and a pen or pencil near the telephone so that you are prepared to write down messages (Figure 11-3). Proper documentation protects the doctor if the caller takes legal action. A record of telephone calls should also be included in a patient's file as part of a complete medical history.

Documenting Calls

Documenting telephone calls is essential in a medical office. You can use telephone message pads or a telephone log book (Figure 11-4). Again, remember that many calls (for example, those concerning clinical problems or referrals) and the actions or decisions they lead to need to be documented in patients' charts. This documentation produces an accurate record and helps guard against lawsuits.

Telephone Message Pads. You can use telephone message pads, which often come in brightly colored paper, to record the following information:

- Date and time of the call
- Name of the person for whom you took the message
- Caller's name
- Caller's telephone number (including area code and extension, if any)
- A description or an action to be taken, including comments such as "Urgent," "Please call back," "Wants to see you," "Will call back," or "Returned your call"

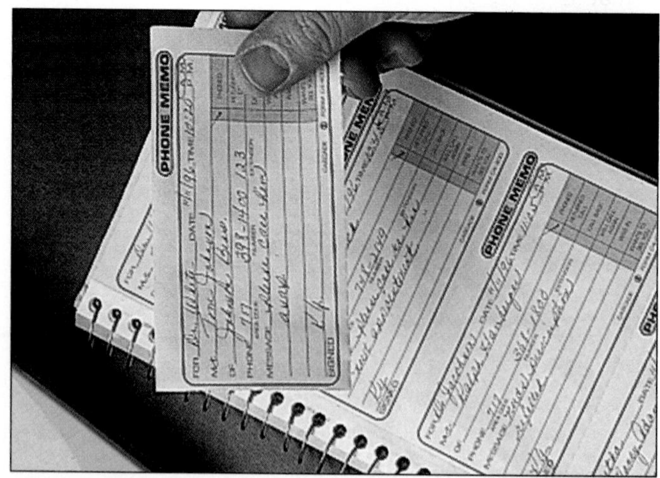

Figure 11-4. When using a telephone message pad or telephone log, be sure to fill out the form completely and accurately.

PROCEDURE 11-2

Retrieving Messages From an Answering Service

Objective: To follow standard procedures for retrieving messages from an answering service

Materials: Telephone message pad or telephone log

Method

1. Set a regular schedule for calling the answering service to retrieve messages. Having a regular schedule ensures that you do not miss any messages.
2. Call at the regularly scheduled time(s) to see if there are any messages.
3. Identify yourself, and state that you are calling to obtain messages for the practice.
4. Write down all pertinent information for each message on the telephone message pad or telephone log. Be sure to include the patient's name and telephone number, time of call, message or description of the problem, and action taken, if any.
5. Repeat the information, confirming that you have the correct spelling of all names.
6. When you have retrieved all messages, route them according to the office policy.

- The complete message, such as "Dr. Stephenson wants to reschedule the committee meeting."
- Name or initials of the person taking the call

The Telephone Log. Some medical offices use spiral-bound, perforated message books with carbonless forms to record messages. The top copy, or original, of each message is given to the appropriate person, and a copy is kept in the book for future reference.

Ensuring Correct Information

When you are taking a message, be sure to get the proper spelling of the caller's name. Repeat the spelling to the caller to make sure it is correct. When you have taken down all the necessary information, repeat the key points to the caller for verification.

Maintaining Patient Confidentiality

Do not repeat information over the telephone when the information is confidential. This point is especially important if patients or others in the office may overhear the conversation. You must also maintain patient confidentiality when handling written telephone messages. If a confidential message must be brought to the doctor's attention, do not leave it on the doctor's desk where it can be seen by someone else. Instead, put the message in a file folder marked "Confidential," and place the folder on the desk. Follow the same procedure when handling confidential faxes.

Telephone Answering Systems

An office telephone system can range from a single telephone line to a complex multiline system. Most medical offices use one or more of the following pieces of equipment and services to provide efficient management of telephone calls: an automated voice mail system, an answering machine, and an answering service. These systems are described in Chapter 5. One of your telephone responsibilities may be to retrieve messages from the practice's answering service. Procedure 11-2 describes how to do so.

Placing Outgoing Calls

You will often be required to place outgoing calls on behalf of the medical office. You may need to return calls, obtain information, or arrange patient consultations with other physicians.

Locating Telephone Numbers

Before you can place an outgoing call, of course, you must have the correct telephone number. If you are calling a patient, the telephone number should be in the patient's chart. To find other telephone numbers, you may need to consult a telephone directory or call for directory assistance.

The medical office should have at least one telephone directory, or telephone book, for the local calling area and perhaps additional directories for surrounding areas. Use these books to locate telephone numbers for outside calls. The office may also have a card file with commonly used telephone numbers, as shown in Figure 11-5, or these numbers may be listed in the office policy manual.

If you need to find a long-distance telephone number, many offices use the directory assistance service. You can reach this service by dialing 1-[area code]-555-1212. Use directory assistance only when you have exhausted other options, however, because most long-distance carriers charge a fee each time you use the service.

Applying Your Telephone Skills

You can apply the telephone skills you use for answering incoming calls when placing outgoing calls. Here are additional tips for handling outgoing calls.

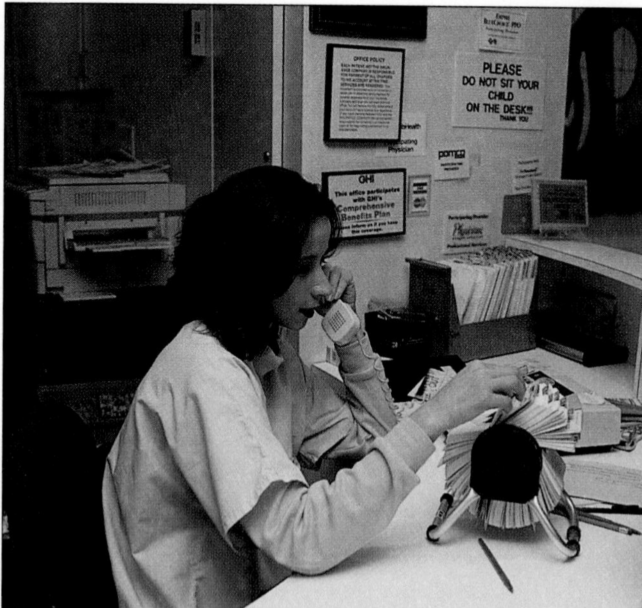

Figure 11-5. Keeping a card file on the desk allows you to easily find frequently used telephone numbers.

1. Plan before you call. Have all the information you need in front of you before you dial the telephone number. Plan what you will say, and decide what questions to ask so that you will not have to call back for additional information.
2. Double-check the telephone number. Before placing a call, always confirm the number. If in doubt, look it up in the telephone directory. If you do dial a wrong number, be sure to apologize for the mistake.
3. Allow enough time, at least a minute or about eight rings, for someone to answer the telephone. When calling patients who are elderly or physically disabled, allow additional time.
4. Identify yourself. After reaching the person to whom you placed the call, give your name, and state that you are calling on behalf of the doctor.
5. Ask if you have called at a convenient time and whether the person has time to talk with you. If it is not a good time, ask when you should call back.
6. Be ready to speak as soon as the person you called answers the telephone. Do not waste the person's time while you collect your thoughts.
7. If you are calling to give information, ask if the person has a pencil and piece of paper available. Do not begin with dates, times, or instructions until the person is ready to write down the information.

Arranging Conference Calls

It may be necessary for you to schedule conference calls with patients, hospitals, or other doctors to discuss tests or surgical results. When dealing with several people, suggest several time slots in case someone is not available at a particular time. Also keep in mind the various time zones in the country. Make sure that all the conference-call participants are given the proper time in their time zone to expect the call.

Telephone Triage

Some physicians delegate to other staff members some of the clinical decision making that is done over the telephone. In these instances, **telephone triage** is used as a process of deciding what necessary action to take. The word *triage* refers to the screening and sorting of emergency incidents. Performing triage correctly is an important skill. You should learn as much as possible about triage techniques.

Learning the Triage Process

Proper training of office staff is vital in providing safe, sound, and cost-effective medical care over the telephone. An increasing number of medical practices are preparing guidelines for the telephone staff to follow when patients call the office with specific medical problems or questions.

Guidelines are often written for common questions, such as how to deal with sniffles and fevers during cold and flu season or how to make a child with chickenpox more comfortable. Members of the telephone staff must realize, however, that their responsibility is to determine whether a caller needs additional medical care. They cannot diagnose or treat the patient's problem.

Office guidelines outline the specific information the telephone staff must obtain from the patient. In general, this information is the same type as that obtained during an office visit. It should include the patient's age, symptoms, when the problem began, and the patient's level of anxiety about the problem.

Categorizing Patient Problems

After the patient information is obtained, the guidelines help the staff categorize the problem according to severity. The telephone staff then decides if the problem can be handled safely with advice over the telephone, whether the patient needs to come into the office, or whether the problem requires immediate attention at an emergency room.

If a problem is deemed appropriate for telephone management, the guidelines may include recommendations for nonprescription treatment that may relieve symptoms and anxiety. Advise the caller that recommendations are based on the symptoms and are not a diagnosis. Remember that only the doctor is authorized to make a diagnosis and prescribe medication. Ask the caller to repeat any instructions you give, and tell the patient to call back within a specified time if symptoms worsen. Be sure to document the conversation in the patient's chart.

Taking Action

Clinical triage involves determining the extent of medical emergencies and deciding on the appropriate action. If a person calls who is having chest pains, you would be performing a type of triage by instructing him to go to the emergency room as soon as possible. Telephone triage is also used in handling common minor medical problems and questions. Whatever the nature of the problem, the situation must be dealt with appropriately to protect the health and safety of the patient.

Summary

The telephone is an important communication tool in the medical office. Your telephone manner will reflect the professionalism of the office. Medical offices commonly receive several types of calls, and there are varying ways to handle these calls.

Special attention should be given to documenting incoming telephone calls, ensuring accuracy, and maintaining patient confidentiality. Telephone etiquette involves practicing proper pronunciation and enunciation, giving undivided attention to callers, and accommodating patients' requests and needs. Placing outgoing calls requires the same careful attention as taking incoming calls. Telephone triage is the art of determining the level of urgency of each call and how it should be handled or routed.

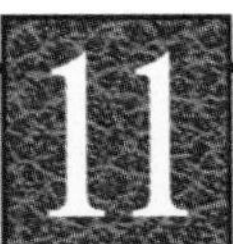

11 Chapter Review

Discussion Questions

1. What is the purpose of screening calls that come into the medical office?
2. Why is proper telephone etiquette so important in the medical office?
3. Name two of the nine most common types of calls received in the medical office, and give a specific example of each type.

Critical Thinking Questions

1. Outline the skills needed by a medical assistant who is responsible for answering incoming calls to a medical office.
2. Describe how you would handle a situation in which an angry patient calls to complain that he was overcharged for a recent office visit.
3. Imagine that you need to call a patient to tell her that she has to return to the office to have some blood redrawn because an insufficient amount of blood was drawn the first time. What would you say to the patient? What would you do if she refused to have the blood redrawn?

Application Activities

1. With a partner, role-play a scenario in which a patient calls the medical office to report symptoms. The patient then claims not to have time to come to the office for an appointment but instead asks for medical advice from the medical assistant. How should the medical assistant respond? When you have finished role-playing, discuss other ways the medical assistant could have dealt with the problem.
2. When speaking with patients on the telephone, how might you demonstrate the following qualities? Give several examples for each quality.
   a. concern
   b. attentiveness
   c. friendliness
   d. respect
   e. empathy
3. Create a one-page training sheet or chart for new personnel illustrating how to handle emergency calls coming into the medical office.

Further Readings

Barton, Ellen L., et al. "Making Phone Care Good Care." *Patient Care,* 15 December 1992, 103–106, 108, 110–117.

Bureau of Business Practice Editorial Staff. *The Secretary's Complete Self-Training Manual.* Englewood Cliffs, NJ: Prentice Hall, 1992.

Farrell, G. "Handling Patient Inquiries Over the Telephone." *Nursing Times,* 14–20 June 1995, 12.

"Handling Phone Calls Effectively." *Nursing 91,* September 1991, 98–100.

Johnson, Bruce E., Barton D. Schmitt, and John H. Wasson. "Taming the Telephone." *Patient Care,* 15 June 1995, 136–142, 149, 154–156.

Leebov, Wendy. *Telephone Tactics for Health-Care Professionals.* Chicago: American Hospital Publishing, 1990.

Wheeler, Sheila Q., and Judith H. Windt. *Telephone Triage: Theory, Practice, and Protocol Development.* Albany, NY: Delmar, 1993.

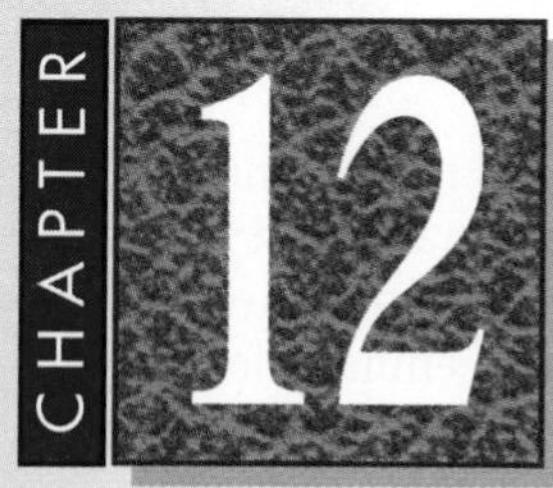

Scheduling Appointments and Maintaining the Physician's Schedule

CHAPTER OUTLINE

- The Appointment Book
- Appointment Scheduling Systems
- Arranging Appointments
- Special Scheduling Situations
- Scheduling Outside Appointments
- Maintaining the Physician's Schedule

OBJECTIVES

After completing Chapter 12, you will be able to:

- Explain the importance of the appointment book in maintaining the schedule in the medical office.
- Identify and describe different types of appointment scheduling systems.
- Discuss ways to arrange appointments for patients.
- Explain how to handle special scheduling situations.
- Describe how to schedule appointments that are outside the medical office.
- Discuss ways to keep an accurate and efficient physician schedule.

AREAS OF COMPETENCE

1997 ROLE DELINEATION STUDY

ADMINISTRATIVE

Administrative Procedures

- Schedule, coordinate, and monitor appointments
- Schedule inpatient/outpatient admissions and procedures

GENERAL (Transdisciplinary)

Professionalism

- Prioritize and perform multiple tasks

Key Terms

advance scheduling
agenda
cluster scheduling
double-booking system
itinerary
locum tenens
minutes
modified-wave scheduling
no-show
open-hours scheduling
overbooking
time-specified scheduling
underbooking
walk-in
wave scheduling

The Appointment Book

Time is a treasured commodity for both patients and physicians. Scheduling appointments in an organized fashion shows respect for everyone's time and creates an efficient patient flow. A well-managed appointment book is the key to establishing this efficiency.

Although most patients understand that they will probably have to wait in the reception area before they are seen by the physician, few patients are willing to wait more than 20 minutes. Offices that routinely have long waiting times can end up with dissatisfied patients and other problems. Some patients, in an attempt to avoid a long wait, may deliberately arrive after their scheduled appointment times. Accommodating these latecomers can throw the office schedule off track. Other patients may become resentful and decide to seek medical care with a competing practice.

Even in a well-run office, however, unexpected events can disrupt the schedule. Some patients arrive early, some arrive late, and others do not arrive at all. Some appointments take longer than expected, for example, if the physician needs to spend extra time with a patient. In addition, emergency appointments sometimes need to be squeezed into the schedule. For these reasons, making an office schedule flow smoothly can be a challenge.

Preparing the Appointment Book

Before you can begin scheduling appointments, you need to prepare the appointment book. The first step is to establish the matrix, or basic format, of the appointment book. You need to block off times on the schedule during which the doctor is not available to see patients. For example, you should block off times during which the doctor is scheduled to make hospital rounds or perform surgery (Figure 12-1). The day's schedule is then built around this matrix.

Obtaining Patient Information

When the matrix has been established, you can begin scheduling appointments. You must obtain and enter certain patient information for each appointment. At some practices personnel enter the information into both traditional paper appointment books and computerized systems. Then, if the computer fails to work for some reason, the office has the book for reference. Some doctors who have been in practice for many years are used to the appointment book method and do not want to give it up for a computer system. Other offices are completely computerized. Using either the book or computer method, obtain the necessary patient information:

- Patient's full name
- Home and work telephone numbers
- Purpose of the visit
- Estimated length of the visit

Commonly Used Abbreviations

If you are the person who maintains the appointment book, you will find that certain procedures and conditions occur frequently. To save space and time when entering information, use these abbreviations:

BP	blood pressure check
can	cancellation
cons	consultation
CPE	complete physical examination
ECG	electrocardiogram
FU	follow-up appointment
I & D	incision and drainage
inj	injection
N & V	nausea and vomiting
NP	new patient
NS	no-show patient
P & P	Pap smear (Papanicolaou smear) and pelvic examination
Pap	Pap smear
PT	physical therapy
re✓	recheck
ref	referral
RS	reschedule
sig	sigmoidoscopy
S/R	suture removal
surg	surgery
US	ultrasound

Determining Standard Procedure Times

If you are to schedule appointments efficiently, you must have an estimate of how long visits will take. Working with the physician or physicians in your practice, create a list of standard procedure times. Also indicate on the list how much time to allow for tests that are commonly performed in the practice. This list, kept beside the appointment book, helps you identify which openings are appropriate for the procedure or test involved. The lengths and types of tests and procedures will depend on the practice. Following are typical lengths of common procedures:

Complete physical examination	30–60 minutes
New patient visit	30 minutes or more
Follow-up office visit	5–10 minutes
Emergency office visit	15–20 minutes
Prenatal examination	15 minutes
Pap smear and pelvic examination	15–30 minutes
Minor in-office surgery, such as a mole removal	30 minutes

A Legal Record

The appointment book is considered a legal record. Some experts advise holding on to old appointment books for at least 3 years. Because the appointment book could be

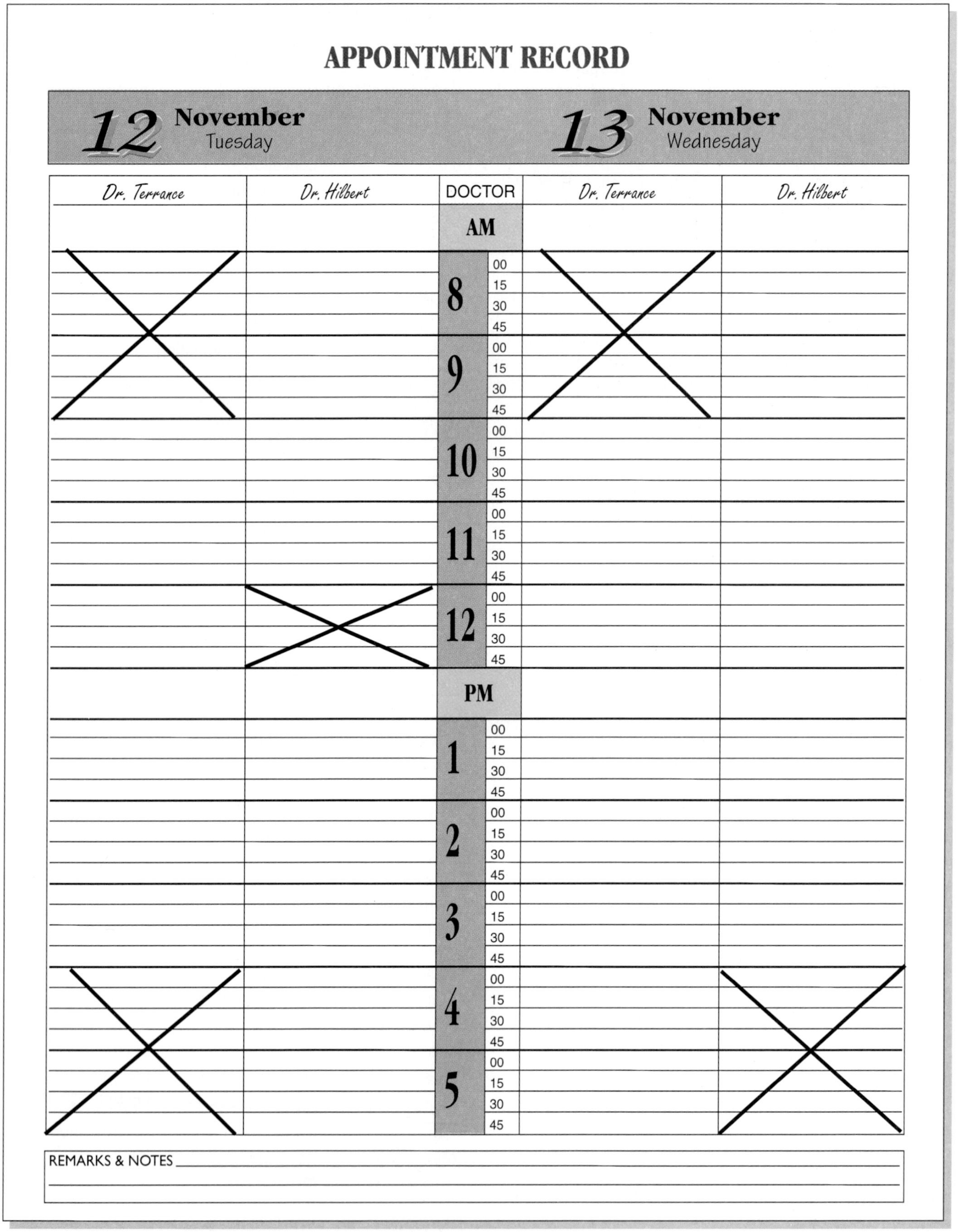

APPOINTMENT RECORD

12 November Tuesday			13 November Wednesday	
Dr. Terrance	Dr. Hilbert	DOCTOR	Dr. Terrance	Dr. Hilbert
		AM		
X		8 00 15 30 45	X	
X		9 00 15 30 45	X	
		10 00 15 30 45		
		11 00 15 30 45		
	X	12 00 15 30 45		
		PM		
		1 00 15 30 45		
		2 00 15 30 45		
		3 00 15 30 45		
X		4 00 15 30 45		X
X		5 00 15 30 45		X

REMARKS & NOTES

Figure 12-1. It is important to establish a matrix in the appointment book so that appointments are not scheduled for times when the doctor will be out of the office.

used as evidence in legal proceedings, entries must be clear and easy to read.

In some offices appointment entries are made only in ink so that information cannot be erased. Other offices permit the use of pencil to allow for changes or corrections if necessary. If pencil is used, at the end of each day you or another designated staff member should write directly over the penciled entries in ink to create a permanent document.

Appointment Scheduling Systems

There are several possible appointment scheduling systems. The method chosen usually depends on the type of practice and the physician's preferences. No matter which method your office uses, it should be regularly reviewed to see whether it is meeting its goals: a smooth flow of patients and minimal waiting time.

Open-Hours Scheduling

In the **open-hours scheduling** system, patients arrive at their own convenience with the understanding that they will be seen on a first-come, first-served basis. Depending on how many other patients are ahead of them, they may have a considerable wait. The open-hours system eliminates the problems caused by broken appointments (because there are no appointments), but it increases the possibility of inefficient downtime for the doctor. In addition, with this system the medical assistant cannot pull patients' charts before they arrive.

Most private practices have replaced the open-hours system with scheduled appointments. Open-hours systems are sometimes still used by rural practices and by practices specializing in urgent care, such as emergency centers. An open-hours system still requires the use of an appointment book, to record patients as they come into the office. You must also still establish a matrix so that you will know when a doctor is out of the office.

Time-Specified Scheduling

Time-specified scheduling (also called stream scheduling) assumes a steady stream of patients all day long at regular, specified intervals. A typical appointment slot might be 15 minutes (Figure 12-2). When a visit requires more time, you simply assign the patient additional back-to-back slots.

Wave Scheduling

Wave scheduling is based on the reality that some patients will arrive late and that others will require more or less time than expected with the physician. The goal of wave scheduling is to begin and end each hour with the overall office schedule on track. You determine the number of patients to be seen each hour by dividing the hour by the length of the average visit. If the average is 15 minutes, for example, you schedule four patients for each hour. You ask all four to arrive at the beginning of the hour and have the physician see them in the order of their actual arrival. The main problem with wave scheduling is that patients may realize they have appointments at the same time as other patients. The result may be confusion and possibly annoyance or anger.

Modified-Wave Scheduling

The wave system can be modified in several ways. With **modified-wave scheduling,** as shown in Figure 12-3, patients might be scheduled in 15-minute increments. Another option is to schedule four patients to arrive at planned intervals during the first half hour, leaving the second half hour unscheduled. This method allows time for catching up before the next hour begins.

Double Booking

With a **double-booking system,** two or more patients are scheduled for the same appointment slot. Unlike the wave or modified-wave system, however, the double-booking system assumes that both patients will actually be seen by the doctor within the scheduled period. If the types of visits are usually short (5 minutes, for example), it is reasonable to book two patients for one 15-minute opening. If both patients require the entire 15 minutes, however, the office falls behind schedule.

Double booking can be helpful if a patient calls with a problem and needs to be seen that day but no appointments are available. You could double-book this patient with an already scheduled patient. In such cases you should explain that the caller might have to wait a bit before being seen by the doctor.

Cluster Scheduling

As the name suggests, **cluster scheduling** groups similar appointments together during the day or week. (This system is also called categorization scheduling.) For example, you might cluster all physical examinations between 9:00 A.M. and 11:00 A.M. on Tuesdays and Thursdays. Cluster scheduling is also helpful in offices where specialized equipment or services (such as physical therapy or ultrasound) are available only at certain times. Procedure 12-1 explains how to create a cluster schedule.

Advance Scheduling

In some specialties patients might be booked weeks or months in advance, as for annual gynecologic examinations. In such practices **advance scheduling** is used. It is still advisable to leave a few slots open each day, however, for patients who call with unexpected or unusual problems.

Combination Scheduling

Some practices combine two or more scheduling methods. For example, they might use cluster scheduling for new patients and double booking for quick follow-ups.

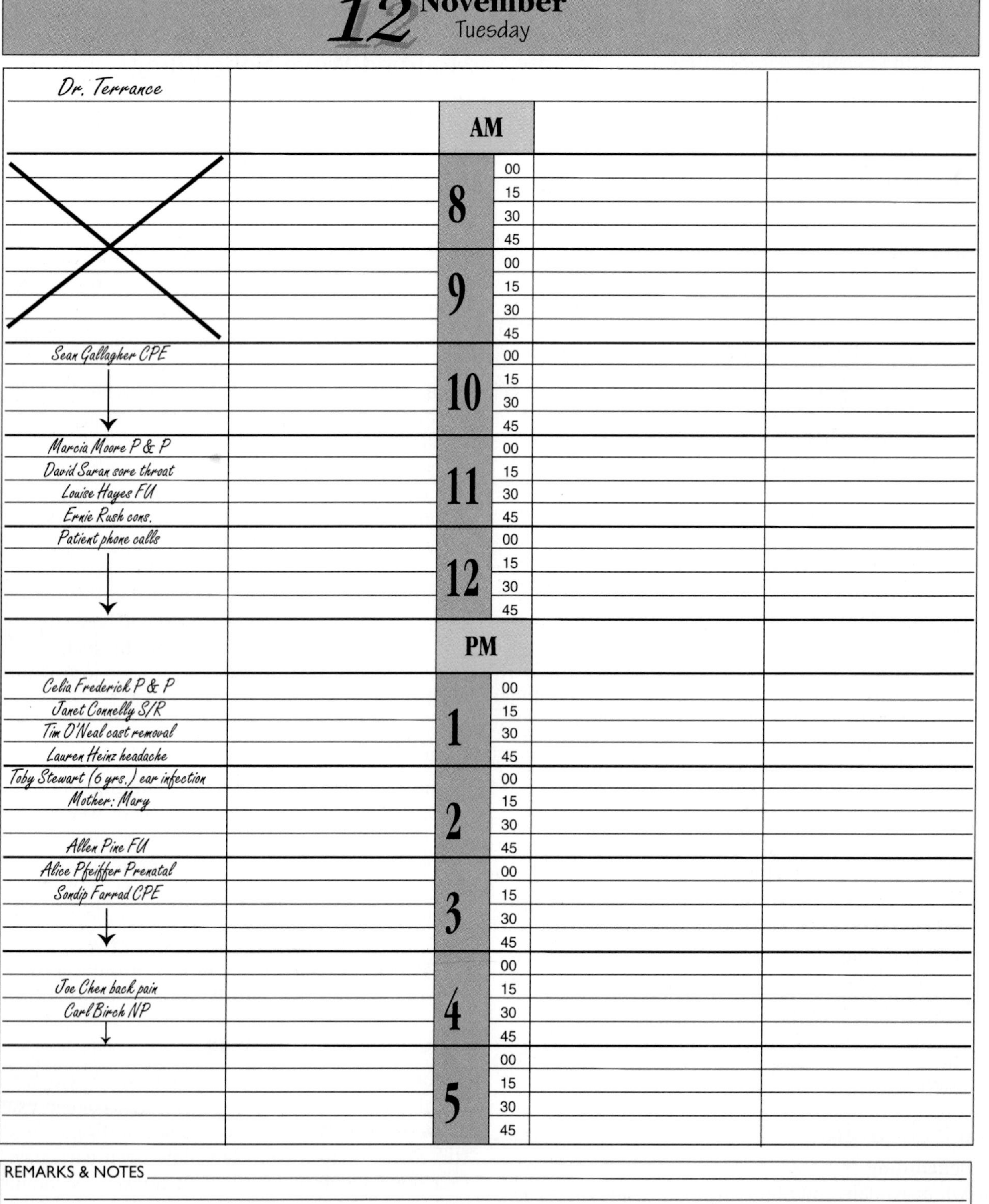

APPOINTMENT RECORD

12 November
Tuesday

	Dr. Terrance
AM	
8 00	
15	
30	
45	
9 00	
15	
30	
45	
10 00	Sean Gallagher CPE
15	
30	
45	
11 00	Marcia Moore P & P
15	David Suran sore throat
30	Louise Hayes FU
45	Ernie Rush cons.
12 00	Patient phone calls
15	
30	
45	
PM	
1 00	Celia Frederick P & P
15	Janet Connelly S/R
30	Tim O'Neal cast removal
45	Lauren Heinz headache
2 00	Toby Stewart (6 yrs.) ear infection
15	Mother: Mary
30	
45	Allen Pine FU
3 00	Alice Pfeiffer Prenatal
15	Sondip Farrad CPE
30	
45	
4 00	
15	Joe Chen back pain
30	Carl Birch NP
45	
5 00	
15	
30	
45	

REMARKS & NOTES

Figure 12-2. Time-specified appointment scheduling is commonly used in the medical office.

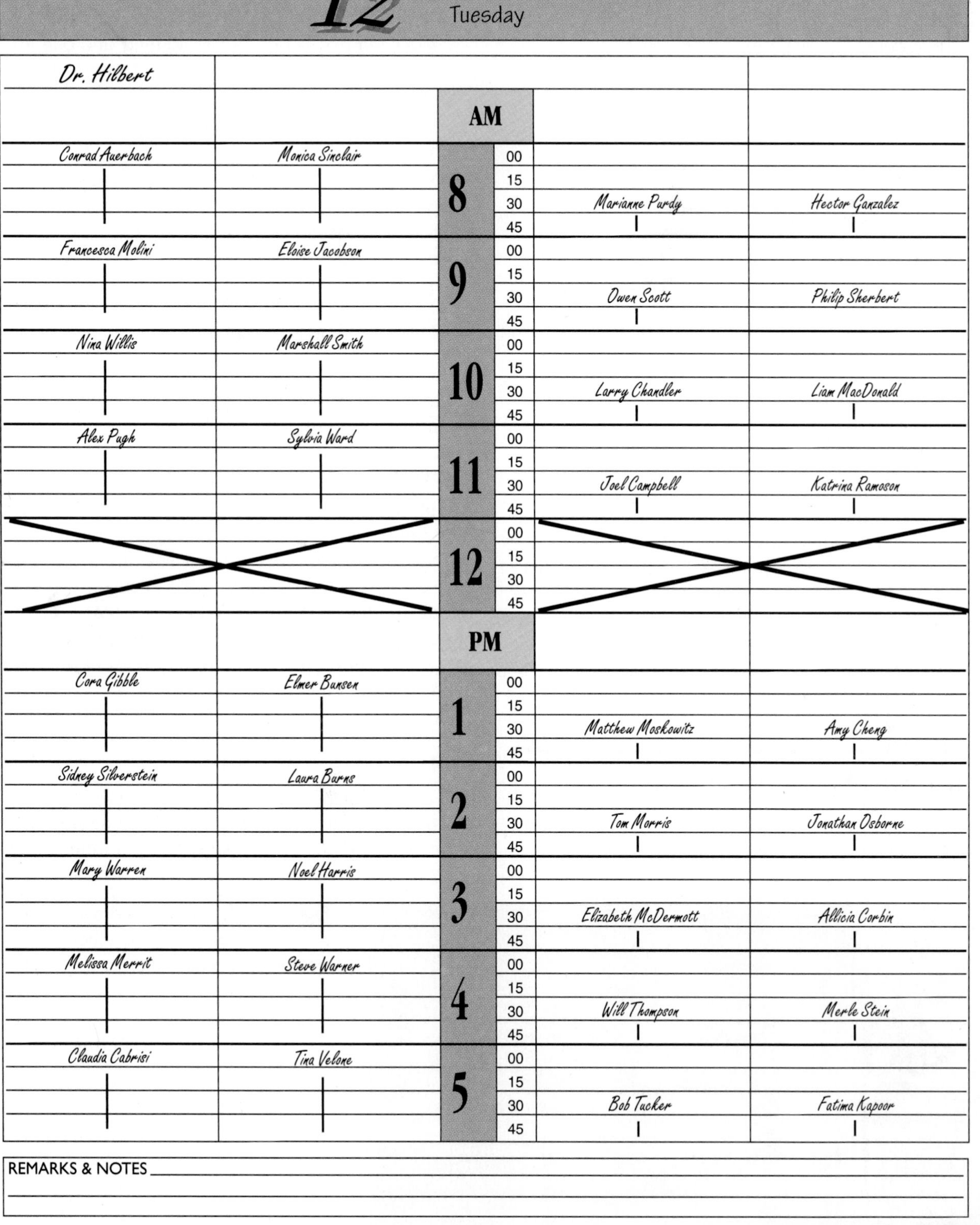

APPOINTMENT RECORD

12 November Tuesday

Dr. Hilbert				
		AM		
Conrad Auerbach	Monica Sinclair	8 00		
		15		
		30	Marianne Purdy	Hector Ganzalez
		45		
Francesca Molini	Eloise Jacobson	9 00		
		15		
		30	Owen Scott	Philip Sherbert
		45		
Nina Willis	Marshall Smith	10 00		
		15		
		30	Larry Chandler	Liam MacDonald
		45		
Alex Pugh	Sylvia Ward	11 00		
		15		
		30	Joel Campbell	Katrina Ramoson
		45		
X	X	12 00	X	X
		15		
		30		
		45		
		PM		
Cora Gibble	Elmer Bunsen	1 00		
		15		
		30	Matthew Moskowitz	Amy Cheng
		45		
Sidney Silverstein	Laura Burns	2 00		
		15		
		30	Tom Morris	Jonathan Osborne
		45		
Mary Warren	Noel Harris	3 00		
		15		
		30	Elizabeth McDermott	Allicia Corbin
		45		
Melissa Merrit	Steve Warner	4 00		
		15		
		30	Will Thompson	Merle Stein
		45		
Claudia Cabrisi	Tina Velone	5 00		
		15		
		30	Bob Tucker	Fatima Kapoor
		45		

REMARKS & NOTES

Figure 12-3. Modified-wave scheduling allows more flexibility than wave scheduling.

PROCEDURE 12-1

Creating a Cluster Schedule

Objective: To set up a cluster schedule

Materials: Calendar, tickler file, appointment book, colored pencils or markers (optional)

Method

1. Learn which categories of cases the physician would like to cluster and on what days and/or times of day.
2. Determine the length of the average visit in each category.
3. In the appointment book, cross out the hours in the week that the physician is typically not available (because of meetings, hospital rounds, lunch, teaching, days off, and so on).
4. Block out one period in midmorning and one in midafternoon for use as buffer, or reserve, times for unexpected needs.
5. Reserve additional slots for acutely ill patients. (The number of slots depends on the type of practice.)
6. Mark the appointment times for clustered procedures. If desired, color-code the blocks of time. For example, make immunization clusters pink, blood pressure checks green, and so forth.

Computerized Scheduling

Computerized scheduling systems are becoming more common in medical offices because they have several advantages over handwritten systems (Figure 12-4). For example, they can be programmed to "lock out" selected appointment slots so that those slots will always be available for emergencies. Computerized systems can also help staff members identify patients who often are late, forget their appointments altogether, or cancel. In addition, the computer can identify patients who may require additional time with the physician because of special needs.

Arranging Appointments

Whether you are arranging appointments in person or by telephone, be polite and courteous. Whenever possible, try to accommodate the patient's needs while still maintaining a smoothly flowing schedule.

New Patients

Appointments for new patients are most often arranged over the telephone. Be sure to obtain all the necessary information, including the correct spelling and pronunciation of the person's name, home address, daytime telephone number, and date of birth. When arranging the appointment, keep in mind that some physicians prefer to schedule new patients at certain times of the day, such as first thing in the morning.

Return Appointments

It is always good practice to ask patients returning to the reception area if they need to schedule another appointment. Getting them to make the appointment then will

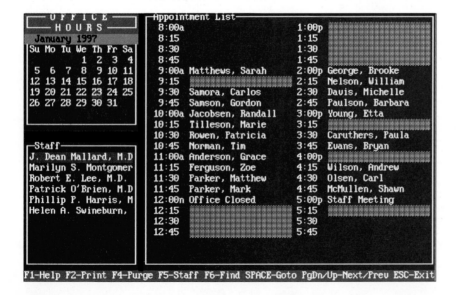

Figure 12-4. Many medical offices are now using computerized scheduling instead of or in addition to a traditional appointment book.

save you from having to do so by telephone later on. When patients call to arrange appointments, use the telephone techniques outlined in Chapter 11.

Appointment Reminders

Some patients may have trouble remembering their next appointment, especially if they arrange it far in advance. To help patients keep track of their appointments, you can use several types of appointment reminders.

Appointment Cards. In many offices the medical assistant fills out and hands the patient an appointment reminder card, like the one shown in Figure 12-5. To reduce the chance of error, enter the appointment in the appointment book first, then fill out the card. Otherwise, when the patient takes the appointment card, you have to rely on your memory when entering the appointment in the book.

Reminder Mailings. When making a follow-up appointment in person, you can ask the patient to address to himself a postcard on which you have written the next appointment's date and time. This postcard serves as a backup in case the patient loses the original appointment reminder card. Place the postcard in the tickler file under the day when it should be sent (usually a week before the appointment). Reminder mailings can also be sent to patients who make appointments over the telephone. In this case, of course, you must address the postcard for the tickler file yourself.

Reminder Calls. Depending on office policy and available time, you might also call patients 1 or 2 days before their appointments to confirm the scheduled time. This technique can be especially helpful for patients with a history of late arrivals or for **no-shows** (patients who do not call to cancel and do not come to the appointment).

Recall Notices. Many offices book appointments no more than a few weeks in advance. If your office has such a policy, you need a way to make sure patients do not forget to call for appointments that are 6 months—or even a year—away from their last appointments.

Suppose, for example, that the physician tells a patient she should have an annual breast examination. How can you help her remember to call to schedule one at the appropriate time? One way is to use a system of recall notices. In a tickler file enter the patient's name under the month when she should call the office. When the time arrives, send a form letter reminding her that she will soon be due for a breast examination and asking her to call for an appointment.

Special Scheduling Situations

Although a great deal of scheduling is routine, creativity and flexibility are necessary for scheduling some special cases. These special situations often involve patients, but they may also involve physicians.

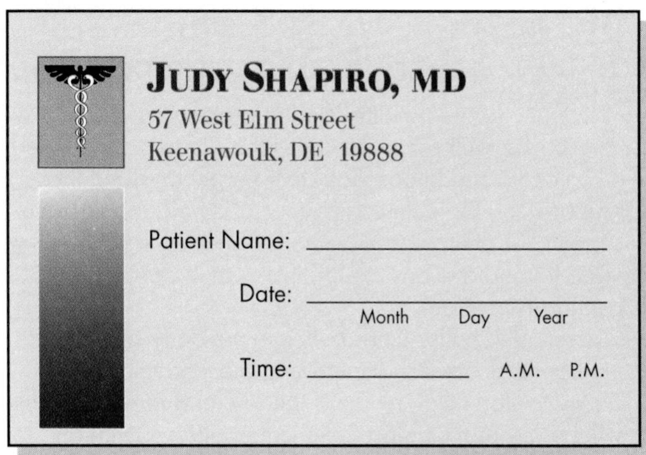

Figure 12-5. Before patients leave the office, be sure to give them an appointment card if they are scheduled to return to the office.

Patient Scheduling Situations

On some days all patients will keep their appointments and arrive on time. On many other days, however, patients may walk in without appointments, arrive late for scheduled appointments, or miss appointments entirely. Being prepared for these possibilities allows you to handle them better and to keep the office schedule running as smoothly as possible.

Emergencies. Your training as a medical assistant will help you recognize the signs of an emergency. In some instances you will refer the caller to the nearest hospital emergency room. In other instances you will ask the caller to come to the office right away. It is vital that doctors see emergency patients before patients who are already in the waiting area or on the schedule. It is best to explain to waiting patients that there has been an emergency (without giving details). This announcement helps them understand and accept the delay and also gives them an opportunity to reschedule their appointments. "Tips for the Office" provides guidelines for scheduling emergency appointments.

Referrals. Sometimes other doctors refer patients to the practice for second opinions or special consultations. Patients seeking second opinions before deciding on surgery should be fit into the schedule as soon as possible. Other referred patients should also be seen quickly, as a matter of professional courtesy to the referring doctor as well as good business practice.

Fasting Patients. Some procedures and tests require patients to fast (refrain from eating or drinking anything beginning the night before). Scheduling these patients as early in the day as possible shows consideration for their needs.

Patients With Diabetes. Like fasting patients, patients with diabetes can use extra consideration when you schedule their appointments. In general, patients who take

Tips FOR THE OFFICE

Scheduling Emergency Appointments

As a multiskilled medical assistant, you will be well prepared to tell the difference between acute conditions that are emergencies and those that are not. Guidelines on types of emergencies to be seen in the office and types to be referred elsewhere will vary. If you have any doubt, interrupt the physician to ask for instructions.

Even with buffer times built into the daily schedule, emergencies are still disruptive to most practices. Your ability to stay calm, respond quickly, and remain flexible will be of great comfort to the emergency patient and to others in the waiting area. Read the following story to see how an emergency situation can be handled skillfully.

The Situation

It is 4:15 P.M. in a busy family practice. The telephone rings. The caller is the father of a 10-year-old boy. Maria, the medical assistant, can hear the panic in his voice. His son Kyle has injured his knee while playing football with friends. Kyle cannot straighten the knee, and it is quite swollen.

Maria consults the physician, who suspects torn cartilage. The physician tells Maria to have the father wrap ice in a towel, apply it to Kyle's knee, and bring him in immediately. Maria relays this advice to the father and asks him how soon he can get to the office.

"It will take about 25 minutes," he replies.

The office schedule includes a buffer time opening at 4:30, but based on the father's estimate, Kyle cannot possibly arrive until 4:40. Maria notes that Mrs. Griffin, a good-natured retiree, is scheduled to come in for her weekly blood pressure check at 4:45 P.M. Hers is the last scheduled appointment of the day.

The Solution

Mrs. Griffin lives about 5 minutes from the office. Maria calls her home and explains that there has been an emergency. She offers Mrs. Griffin three choices: She can come in at 4:30 and be seen then; she can arrive at the usual time and expect to wait; or she can be rescheduled for tomorrow.

"No problem," Mrs. Griffin says cheerfully. "I'll come right over."

Mrs. Griffin arrives at 4:35. At 4:40, Kyle hobbles in, supported by his father. Maria greets them and offers Kyle a chair on which to prop his foot.

Mrs. Griffin's blood pressure check is complete at 4:45. Kyle waits only 5 minutes before he is seen.

Thanks to Maria's quick thinking, the office stays on schedule—essentially by switching one appointment for another.

insulin must eat meals and snacks at regular times. This routine keeps their blood sugar from dropping too low—a condition that can result in confused thinking or even loss of consciousness. Therefore, you might want to avoid scheduling patients with diabetes for slots in late morning, close to lunchtime. If the schedule is running late by the time these patients arrive, they will be waiting in your reception area at a time when they really need to eat.

If the physician sees several patients with diabetes, you might also ask him about keeping appropriate snacks on hand to offer these patients in emergencies. Most patients with diabetes, however, carry their own emergency snacks with them to treat low blood sugar.

Repeat Visits. Some patients need regular appointments, such as for prenatal checkups or physical therapy. If possible, schedule these appointments for the same day and time each week. Establishing a routine helps patients remember their appointments and simplifies the office schedule.

Late Arrivals. If the practice has patients who are routinely late, and gentle reminders to be on time have not helped, you might try booking them toward the end of the day. Even if a patient arrives late for a late-afternoon appointment, the doctor has already seen most of the day's patients, and the late patient will not disrupt the schedule.

Walk-Ins. From time to time, a patient (or a person who has not visited the practice before) may arrive without an appointment and still expect to see the doctor. These people are called **walk-ins.** Office policies on how to handle walk-ins vary. If the person is experiencing an emergency, handle the situation as you would handle any emergency. Otherwise, you might politely explain that the doctor is fully booked for the day and offer to schedule an appointment in the usual manner. If, by chance, the doctor is available and willing to see the walk-in, you should still ask the person to call to schedule appointments in the future.

Cancellations. When patients call to cancel appointments, thank them for calling, and try to reschedule the appointment while they are on the telephone. If patients say they will call later to reschedule, note this information in the appointment book.

You should also write "canceled" in the appointment book and cross out the patient's name. To avoid confusion, cancel the first appointment *before* entering the patient's rescheduled appointment. Remember that the appointment book is a legal record. If you forget to cross out the name at the time of the first appointment, it may later seem that the doctor saw the patient twice. It is also important to note the cancellation in the patient's medical record. This notation can protect the practice from possible legal action. For example, a patient whose incision became infected could not blame the doctor if the patient canceled an appointment for a dressing change.

You may be able to fill slots created by cancellations by calling patients who have appointments scheduled for later in the day or week. Some patients may be willing to come in earlier than planned. When you make appointments, you can ask patients if they would be interested in coming in earlier if openings occur. Placing the names of interested patients in a tickler file can save time later.

Missed Appointments. It is important for legal reasons to document a no-show in the appointment book and patient record. The physician may also want you to call the patient with a polite reminder that he has missed an appointment and needs to reschedule. There may have been a misunderstanding about the time, or the patient may simply have forgotten the appointment. If failure to keep the appointment could endanger the patient's health, mention this possibility to the patient, or ask the physician to tell the patient over the telephone.

Physician Scheduling Situations

Not all scheduling problems result from patients. Sometimes physicians disrupt the office schedule. They may be called away on an emergency, may be delayed at the hospital, or may simply arrive late. In any event, the appointment schedule may get off track.

Physicians are only human and may occasionally be late for appointments. Some physicians are frequently late, however, either when arriving in the morning or when returning from lunch or from regular meetings. If this situation occurs in your office, you might approach it in several ways.

At a staff meeting you could mention that the morning or afternoon schedule often seems to get off to a late start. Then you might ask if anyone has suggestions for improving this situation. The physician may recognize that she is the cause of the problem and decide to resolve it.

If the physician does not take responsibility for the problem, however, you may need to adjust the office schedule to handle the situation. Suppose, for example, that the first patient appointment slot is at 8:30 A.M., but the physician usually does not arrive until 8:35 A.M. You could simply avoid scheduling patients between 8:30 and 8:45 A.M. If a physician is often 15 minutes late returning from lunch or from meetings, you might leave open the first appointment slot after the normal arrival time. In effect, you build buffer time into the schedule.

Scheduling Outside Appointments

You may be responsible for arranging patient appointments outside the medical office. These appointments may include:

- Consultations with other physicians.
- Laboratory work.
- X-rays.
- Other diagnostic tests.
- Hospital stays.
- Surgeries.

Before scheduling these appointments, ask the doctor for an order that identifies the exact procedures to be performed and specifies when the results will be needed. Then talk with the patient to find convenient appointment times. This habit is not only courteous but also gives patients a sense of control over situations they may find a bit frightening. Some doctors' offices may have you call the outside laboratory or hospital with all information concerning the patient and then give the patient the number to call to set up the appointment. This approach is often easier for patients. They then have the telephone number in case they need to reschedule.

If you are calling to make the appointment for the patient, tell the medical assistant, scheduling secretary, or admissions clerk what consultation, test, or procedure is required. Then find out what your office or the patient must do to prepare for the appointment. For example, the admitting doctor may need to complete a preadmission evaluation for a patient who is to be hospitalized.

When arrangements have been made, inform the patient, and note on the chart that you have done so. You may also provide the patient with a completed referral slip or, in the case of laboratory work, a laboratory request slip. Procedure 12-2 explains how to schedule and confirm appointments for surgery. (You will find additional information on preparing patients for surgery in Chapter 14.)

Maintaining the Physician's Schedule

The schedules of busy physicians are not limited to office visits with patients and hospital rounds. Physicians also need to attend professional meetings, travel to conferences, present speeches to colleagues, complete paperwork, and perform other duties. Your job is to help physicians make the most efficient use of their time.

One way is to avoid overbooking appointments with patients. **Overbooking** (scheduling more patients than can reasonably be seen in the time allowed) creates stress for the physician and eventually causes the office schedule to fall behind.

The opposite problem, **underbooking**—leaving large, unused gaps in the schedule—does not make the best use of the physician's time. Of course, you have no control over patients who cancel appointments. If you cannot reschedule another patient for the empty slot, the physician can use the time to catch up on telephone calls to patients or to attend to other matters.

At times you will have to cancel appointments because the physician has been delayed or called away by an emergency. Apologize to waiting patients on behalf of the

PROCEDURE 12-2

Scheduling and Confirming Surgery at a Hospital

Objective: To follow the proper procedure for scheduling and confirming surgery

Materials: Calendar, telephone, notepad, pen

Method

1. Elective surgery is usually performed on certain days when the doctor is scheduled to be in the operating room and a room and an anesthetist are available. The patient may be given only one or two choices of days and times. (For emergency surgery the first step is to reserve the operating room.)
2. Call the operating room secretary. Give the procedure required, the name of the surgeon, the time involved, and the preferred date and hour.
3. Provide the patient's name (including maiden name, if appropriate), address, telephone number, age, gender, Social Security number, and insurance information.
4. Call the admissions office. Arrange for the patient to be admitted on the day of surgery or the day before (depending on the surgery to be performed). Ask for a copy of the admissions form for the patient record.
5. Some hospitals want patients to complete preadmission forms. In such cases request a blank form for the patient.
6. Confirm the surgery and the patient's arrival time 1 business day before surgery.

physician, and offer them a choice. Explain that they can wait in the office (give an estimated waiting time), leave to run errands and return later, or reschedule their appointments for another day. Always make sure patients who need immediate attention are seen by another physician.

Reserving Operating Rooms

If the doctor in your office plans to perform surgery at a hospital, you will need to call the operating room secretary to reserve the facility. Give the preferred days and times, the type of surgery, and the length of time the doctor will need the operating room. After the day and time are set, provide the secretary with all relevant patient information. Relay any requests from the doctor, such as the blood type and units of blood that may be needed. It may also be your responsibility to make arrangements for surgical assistants, an anesthetist, and a hospital bed for the patient following surgery.

Stocking the Medical Bag

Some physicians see patients at skilled nursing facilities and elsewhere outside the office. You must enter these visits on the appointment schedule, taking into account the necessary travel time. For these visits, you may be responsible for stocking the physician's medical bag, as shown in Figure 12-6. The supplies vary depending on the practice, but the following items are commonly included:

- Adhesive tape, bandages, dressings
- Biohazard container
- Sphygmomanometer and blood pressure cuff
- Containers for specimens
- Medications—antibiotics, epinephrine, digitalis
- Microscope slides and fixative
- Ophthalmoscope
- Otoscope
- Penlight
- Prescription pads and pens
- Scissors
- Sterile dressing forceps
- Sterile latex gloves
- Sterile swabs
- Sterile syringes and needles
- Stethoscope
- Thermometers

Post a list of all the necessary items in the area where you check, clean, and restock the medical bag.

Scheduling Pharmaceutical Sales Representatives

Drug manufacturers often send pharmaceutical sales representatives into medical offices with printed information about new drugs, as well as free samples that can be given to patients. These representatives are sometimes called detail persons. Some doctors do not want to meet with pharmaceutical representatives. Other doctors are willing to spend a few minutes if time permits and if the products are likely to be useful to the practice. Some doctors set aside a certain time 1 or 2 days a week to see detail persons. When a pharmaceutical representative who is unknown to you comes into the office, ask for a business card, and check with the doctor before scheduling an appointment (Figure 12-7). (Storing drug samples is discussed in Chapter 8.)

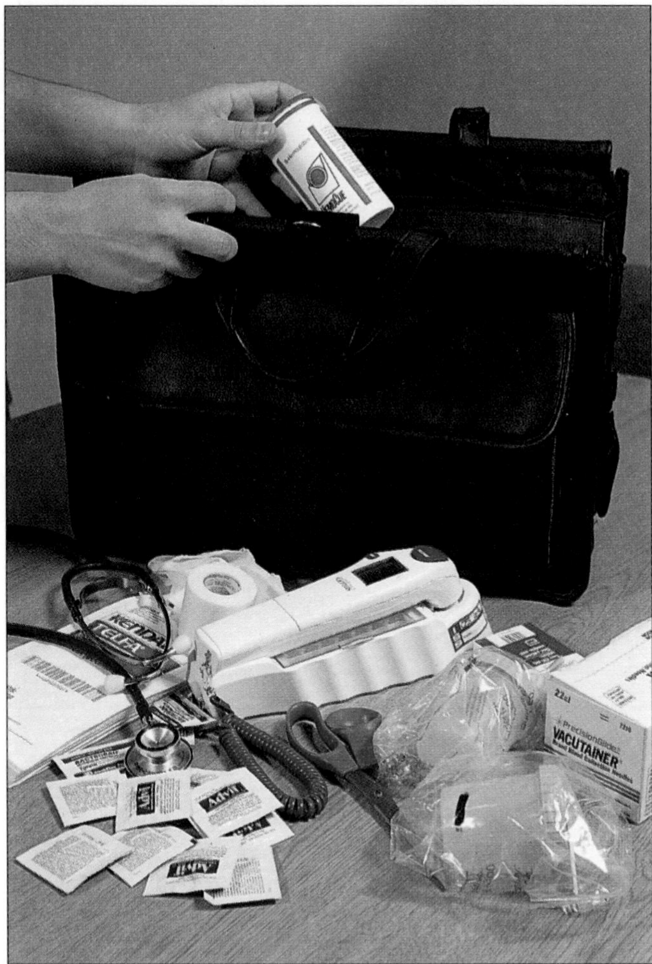

Figure 12-6. You may be responsible for keeping the physician's medical bag stocked with supplies.

Making Travel Arrangements

You may be responsible for arranging transportation and lodging when physicians attend meetings, speaking engagements, and other events out of town. You may contact the airline, car rental agency, hotel, or other services yourself, or you may work through a travel agent. In either case request confirmation of travel and room reservations. You may also be responsible for picking up tickets or seeing that they are mailed to the office if time permits before the trip.

Before the day of departure, obtain an itinerary from the travel agent, or create one yourself. An **itinerary** is a detailed travel plan, listing dates and times of flights and events, locations of meetings and lodgings, and telephone numbers. Give several copies to the physician, and keep one for the office.

You must schedule and confirm professional coverage of the practice during the physician's absence. This coverage may be important for legal reasons. A **locum tenens,** or substitute physician, may be hired to see patients while the regular physician is away. (*Locum tenens* is Latin for "one occupying the place of another.") You may have more than one locum tenens on call, depending on the practice. In some areas special firms provide a locum tenens and other temporary medical and nursing help.

Planning Meetings

You may help the doctor set up meetings of professional societies or committees. To do so, you will need to know how many people are expected to attend, how long the meeting will last, and the purpose of the meeting. In addition, ask the doctor if a meal is to be served.

Some groups always meet at the same location. If there is no established meeting place, you must choose and reserve one. Select a location with an adequately sized meeting room, sufficient parking, and, if needed, food services. Be sure also to arrange for necessary equipment, such as a microphone, podium, or overhead projector. Many conference centers and hotels have an on-site catering manager or conference manager to assist you with these arrangements. When the facility has been booked, mail a notice to all those expected to attend the meeting. On the notice provide the topic, names of the speakers, date, time, place, and admission costs or fees associated with attending.

With direction from the physician, you may also be responsible for creating the meeting's agenda. An **agenda** is a list of topics to be discussed or presented at a meeting in order of presentation. You may be asked to prepare the **minutes,** or the report of what was discussed and decided at the meeting.

Scheduling Time With the Physician

You and the physician should meet regularly to go through the tickler file and make sure necessary paperwork is prepared on time. Examples of recurring deadlines include those for state medical license renewal, Drug Enforcement Agency registrations, and documentation of the physician's continuing medical education (CME) requirements. Figure 12-8 lists items that are often part of a physician's schedule.

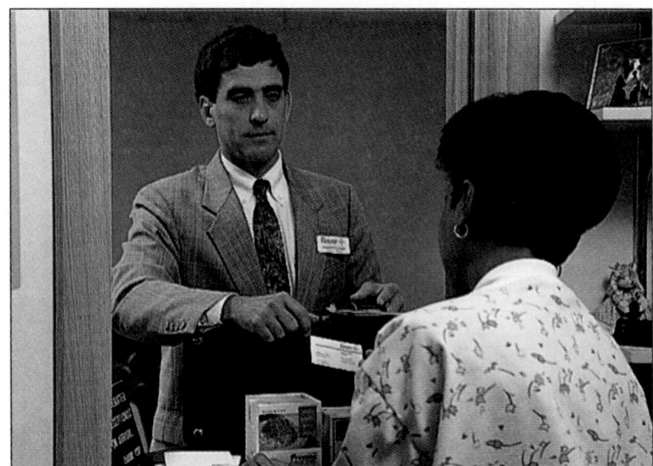

Figure 12-7. If pharmaceutical representatives come into the office without an appointment, you can ask them to leave a business card.

Common Items on a Physician's Schedule

Payments, Dues, and Fees

- Association dues
- Health insurance premium
- Payment for laundry service
- Liability insurance premium
- Life insurance premium
- Office rent
- Property insurance premium
- Paychecks for staff
- Payment for janitorial services
- Payment for leased equipment
- Taxes
  - *–Quarterly federal tax payments*
  - *–Quarterly state tax payments*
  - *–Annual federal and state tax filing deadline*

Time Commitments

- Committee meetings
- Conventions

Renewals and Accreditations

- Facility accreditation
  - *–State requirements*
  - *–Certificate of necessity*
  - *–Laboratory registration*
  - *–Federal requirements*
  - *–Ambulatory surgical centers*
  - *–Physician office laboratory*
- Medical license renewal
- Narcotics licenses renewal
- Drug Enforcement Agency registrations
- CME accreditations

Figure 12-8. Make time to meet with the physician regularly to review scheduling commitments.

Summary

Properly scheduling appointments in the medical office ensures a steady, efficient flow of patients. Setting up a matrix in the appointment book is the first step in scheduling appointments.

There are various appointment scheduling systems, including open-hours scheduling, wave scheduling, and cluster scheduling. Arranging appointments involves scheduling new and return patients and includes appointment reminder techniques. Special scheduling situations may occur, such as emergencies, referrals, and missed appointments. These situations may involve either patients or physicians. You may also be responsible for scheduling outside appointments for patients, as for testing or surgery.

Maintaining the physician's schedule includes such responsibilities as making travel arrangements and planning meetings. Meeting regularly with the physician helps ensure the smooth running of the office.

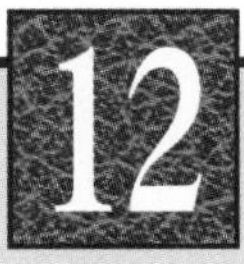

Chapter Review

Discussion Questions

1. Think about a time when you had a long wait after arriving for a medical appointment. How did you feel? What might the medical assistant have done to help you feel better about the wait?
2. Compare and contrast the four types of appointment reminders. What are the advantages and disadvantages of each?
3. Why is it important to note missed appointments and cancellations in the patient record and in the appointment book?

Critical Thinking Questions

1. Give an example of a medical office for which one type of appointment scheduling system is more efficient than another.
2. Summarize the skills needed by a medical assistant who is responsible for scheduling appointments.
3. Describe how you would handle a situation in which a patient calls for an appointment but is reluctant to disclose the purpose of the visit. What can you say to help the patient realize that it is advantageous to describe the nature of the visit?

Application Activities

1. An elderly patient uses public transportation to reach the medical office. At his last visit he seemed very tired. He commented that the bus was so full of commuters that he had to stand much of the way. How could you schedule future appointments to make them easier for this patient?
2. A patient calls to make an appointment for an annual Pap smear and pelvic examination. Although the office is open from 8:00 A.M. to 4:00 P.M., this procedure is usually performed in the afternoon at your practice. The patient says that she works from 9:00 A.M. to 5:00 P.M. and cannot take much time off from work. How can you help this patient arrange a convenient appointment time?
3. Dr. Thompson, the only physician in your office, is out of town at a medical meeting. She is due back tomorrow morning. At 4:00 P.M., Dr. Thompson calls to say that a blizzard has closed the airport, and she will be forced to stay away for another day. You look at tomorrow's schedule. She has a full patient load. What should you do?

Further Readings

Bean, Andrew G., and James Talega. "Predicting Appointment Breaking." *Journal of Health Care Marketing,* 22 March 1995, 29.

Buchholz, C. "My New Appointment Policy Gave Me Back My Practice." *The Wall Street Journal,* 23 June 1994, A1.

Eschenburg, Linda J. "How to Prioritize When Everything Is a Priority." *The Professional Medical Assistant,* May/June 1996, 8–10.

Johnson, Jan Leigh. "The Scheduled Appointment: Fact or Fiction?" *The Professional Medical Assistant,* November/December 1995, 8–10.

Lee, Nicholas, and Andrew Millman. "Hospital Based Computer Systems; ABC of Medical Computing." *British Medical Journal,* 14 October 1995, 1013.

Long, Mary Ann. "Scheduling Appointments for Ease and Accuracy." *The Professional Medical Assistant,* January/February 1995, 4–6.

Poorman-Douglas Corporation. "How to Reduce (Perceived) Waiting Time." *The Doctor's Office,* October 1993, 5.

Stein, Anne. "Getting Your Practice House in Order: Physician's Practice." *American Medical News,* 6 June 1994, 29.

Zeff, Patricia. "Delayed Reaction: Reducing Waiting Times for Patients." *American Medical News,* 27 February 1995, 14.

Patient Reception Area

CHAPTER OUTLINE

- First Impressions
- The Importance of Cleanliness
- The Physical Components
- Keeping Patients Occupied and Informed
- Patients With Special Needs

OBJECTIVES

After completing Chapter 13, you will be able to:

- Identify the elements that are important in a patient reception area.
- Discuss ways to determine what furniture is necessary for a patient reception area and how it should be arranged.
- List the housekeeping tasks and equipment needed for this area of the office.
- Summarize the OSHA regulations that pertain to a patient reception area.
- List the types of reading material appropriate to a patient reception area.
- Describe how modifications to a reception area can accommodate patients with special needs.
- Identify special situations that can affect the arrangement of a reception area.

Key Terms

access
Americans With Disabilities Act
color family
contagious
differently abled
infectious waste
interim room
Older Americans Act of 1965

AREAS OF COMPETENCE

1997 ROLE DELINEATION STUDY

GENERAL (Transdisciplinary)

Legal Concepts

- Follow federal, state, and local legal guidelines
- Comply with established risk management and safety procedures

Operational Functions

- Evaluate and recommend equipment and supplies

First Impressions

The reception area plays a significant role in a patient's experience at the doctor's office. It is the first area patients see when entering the office. It is also a place where they have to spend time waiting for their appointments.

The appearance of the reception area creates an impression of the practice. Is the office bright and cheerful, cool and modern, or warm and cozy? The impression created by the reception area reflects on the quality of care patients can expect to receive. For example, old, tattered, or dirty furniture in the reception area will give patients the impression that the medical practice is unsuccessful and outdated. A carefully designed and well-maintained patient reception area, on the other hand, can attract and keep patients in the practice. It also assures a pleasant and comfortable experience while they wait to receive medical care.

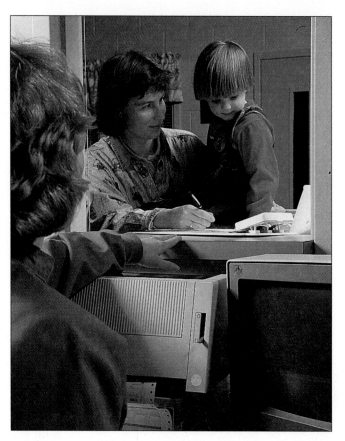

Figure 13-1. A receptionist's desk or window, where patients can check in, is part of every patient reception area.

Reception Area

The reception area includes a reception window or desk, as shown in Figure 13-1, where patients check in for their appointments. It also includes chairs and couches for patients to sit on while waiting. Most patient reception areas are arranged using the same basic organizational concepts. The impressions they create can vary widely, however, depending on the elements chosen to enhance this part of the office.

Lighting. Most medical offices use fairly bright lighting in the reception area, allowing patients to see their surroundings easily. Subdued lighting, like that sometimes used in restaurants, could be hazardous because it could cause patients to trip over or bump into hard-to-see objects. In addition, bright lighting is essential for reading, which is a common activity in the patient reception area. Bright lighting also conveys an impression of cleanliness.

Lighting should not be so bright that it becomes bothersome, however. Extremely bright light can be harsh on the eyes and create an annoying glare. A specialist, such as an electrician or lighting showroom salesperson, can help determine the appropriate level of lighting for the patient reception area.

Room Temperature. Patients will be uncomfortable if the reception area is too hot or too cold. In an uncomfortable setting, waiting time can seem much longer than it really is. Therefore, maintaining an average, comfortable temperature is important.

The thermostat should be kept at a temperature that feels comfortable to you and to the office staff. You might periodically survey patients to see if they are comfortable and adjust the setting accordingly. Many elderly people feel cold because of lowered metabolisms. You may want to increase the temperature setting for a geriatric practice or if the office sees a large number of elderly patients.

Music. Many medical offices pipe music through speakers to the reception area, as well as elsewhere in the office. The music provides a soothing background sound. Because the music is meant to calm patients, it should be chosen accordingly. Classical music, light jazz, and soft rock are appropriate choices, whereas heavy metal and rap music are not. Some offices use prepared tapes or compact discs. Others tune in to a local radio station.

The music should reflect the interests of the patients. If the office serves an older population, you might choose oldies or classical music. Try soft rock for an obstetrics/gynecology practice or children's folk music for a pediatric practice.

Decor

The patient reception area gets its distinctive look from the way it is decorated. With the appropriate elements, the decor can create whatever impression is desired—warm and friendly, modern and elegant, and so on. Some suggestions follow. It is wise to consult a professional decorator, if possible.

Colors and Fabrics. These are the primary elements that make up a room's decor. Colors can be used throughout the room—on walls, furniture, carpeting, and other items. Fabrics are used primarily on furniture and draperies.

When using several colors, it is important to decorate in color families to avoid a jarring, unprofessional look.

A **color family** is a group of colors that work well together. Colors fall within two basic areas, cool and warm. Using all cool colors—like white, blue, and mauve—creates a more harmonious impression in the reception area than mixing cool colors with warm ones like red, orange, and hot pink. When choosing the color family, consider the mood you want to create. Bright colors produce a lively atmosphere, whereas softer, muted colors create a relaxing one.

Fabrics, too, add to the atmosphere in the room. Heavy fabrics like velvet or brocade are more formal, whereas lightweight or sheer fabrics create a soft, delicate appearance. Patterns on fabrics or wallpaper can immediately change the mood of the room. No matter what the design, fabrics should be easy to clean and maintain.

Many medical offices are carpeted, and carpets come in a variety of colors and patterns. Carpeting is attractive, and it helps reduce noise. Carpet also provides a comfortable cushion when people walk through the office.

Carpeting should be easy to clean and durable enough to handle a large volume of patient traffic. Wall-to-wall carpeting is preferable to scatter rugs, which can cause injuries if someone slips on or trips over them and falls.

Specialty Items. Some offices include specialty items, or accessories, as part of the decor (Figure 13-2). Examples of such items include coatracks, aquariums, plants, paintings, sculptures, mobiles, and children's toys. Some items are meant to add a finishing touch, completing the desired atmosphere. Others may help to interest waiting patients by providing an activity, such as watching the fish in an aquarium.

Choosing Accessories. Although specialty items enhance the office decor, keep the number of accessories to a minimum. Too many pieces can give the room a cluttered look. Try to select specialty items that will be pleasing or helpful to patients. A clock is one example. Another useful item is a coatrack, which helps prevent clutter by providing a place for coats, umbrellas, and briefcases. Avoid accessories such as scented candles or potpourri that may be offensive to some people.

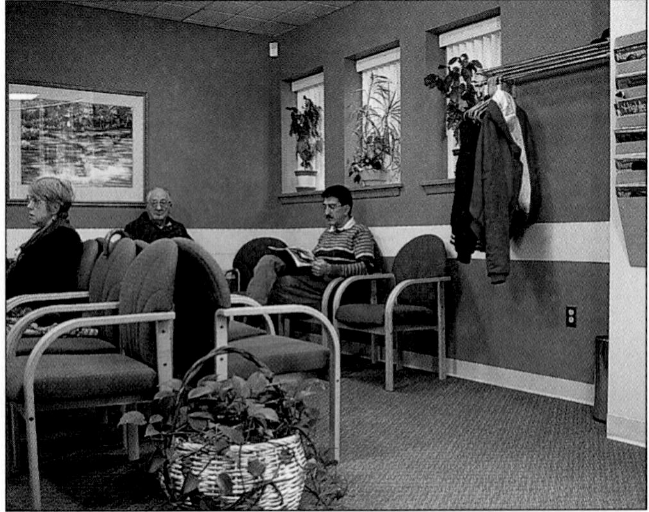

Figure 13-2. Specialty items—such as plants, paintings, and coatracks—enhance the patient reception area.

Keeping Safety in Mind. When selecting specialty items for the medical office, be sure to consider the issue of safety. Follow these guidelines to avoid potential hazards in the patient reception area.

1. Do not include any item smaller than a golf ball. Small items present a choking hazard for young children.
2. Avoid objects that can be easily pulled apart and then swallowed.
3. Avoid easily breakable items, such as glass vases, that might cause cuts or other injuries to patients.
4. Choose furniture with rounded, not sharp, corners. Coffee tables or other low tables with sharp corners can be a hazard especially to the elderly and to small children.
5. Secure heavy wall hangings, shelves, and coatracks to the wall so that there is no risk of their falling.
6. It is preferable to display artificial plants rather than living ones. Living plants may irritate patients who have allergies or present a poisoning hazard if parts of the plants are eaten by toddlers.

Furniture

Buying furniture for a patient reception room requires thoughtful planning. Although the office in which you work will no doubt be furnished already, it is a good idea to learn the steps and decisions involved in choosing furniture. You may be included in future purchasing decisions if the office expands or moves to a new location or if the doctor wants to redecorate.

Furniture styles vary to suit the office decor. Most important, seating furniture should be firm, comfortable, and easy to get in and out of. In addition, washable and fireproof fabric on the furniture minimizes care and maximizes safety.

The reception area should have enough furniture so that all patients and family members or friends who accompany them can sit, no matter how busy the office schedule. Forcing people to stand while they wait for an appointment makes the wait seem much longer. The American Medical Association (AMA) suggests that seating be sufficient to accommodate the number of patients, family members, and friends who may be in the office during a 2-hour time period. When calculating this number, be generous in allowing for family members. In some types of practices, such as pediatrics, all patients are accompanied by at least one parent or guardian and sometimes siblings as well.

Arranging Furniture. The furniture arrangement can make the office seem comfortable or uncomfortable. If furniture is too close together, patients do not have sufficient space to move around easily or to stretch their legs.

They may feel cramped. To ensure that patients have adequate room, a good rule of thumb is to allow 12 sq ft of space per person. By this measurement, a 120-sq-ft room (10 by 12 ft) can accommodate ten people comfortably.

The furniture arrangement should allow maximum floor space. Patients should be able to stretch out their legs when seated and to walk around the waiting room if they wish (Figure 13-3). Placing chairs against the wall usually produces the greatest amount of floor area. Additional seating in the middle of the room can be placed back-to-back to conserve space. Seats should be grouped so that families or friends can sit together.

Ensuring Privacy. Some patients come to the office alone and value their privacy. Placing single chairs or small groups of chairs in corners of the room offers patients some measure of privacy.

Some medical offices offer more complete privacy in the form of an **interim room,** a room in which people can talk or meet without being seen or heard from the patient reception area. This interim room provides an ideal location for medical staff to confer privately with patients about appointments or bills. It also allows patients to make private telephone calls and allows people to feed or diaper babies in privacy. Not every office has the luxury of space for such a room, but it provides a valuable service to patients when it is possible.

Accommodating Children. A pediatric waiting room caters to a unique age group of patients. Reception areas for children usually have the same basic setup as those for adults, but special accommodations for children are also made.

In addition to regular chairs, for example, child-size chairs may be available. Some waiting rooms include playhouses or play furniture, such as small tables. The decor may also be made appealing to young children by the use of bright colors and storybook characters. It is important to make the setting feel familiar and comfortable. The reception desk may stock rolls of stickers or other inexpensive prizes to give to young patients after they have seen the doctor. Later in the chapter, you will learn how to set up a pediatric reception area.

Some pediatricians' offices have a well waiting room and a sick waiting room to separate children who are contagious from well children. **Contagious** means having a disease or condition that can easily be transmitted to others.

The Importance of Cleanliness

No matter how tastefully it is decorated, the reception area will be unappealing if it is not clean. Patients expect a physician's office to maintain a high standard of cleanliness. The perception is that a messy or dirty reception area reflects a practice that does not meet minimum standards for cleanliness. A practice with a spotless, attractive reception area reassures patients they have chosen a practice with high standards of cleanliness.

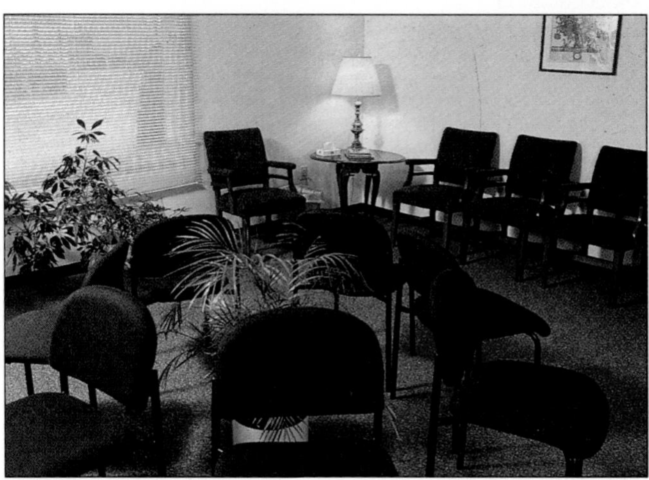

Figure 13-3. The furniture in a patient reception area can be arranged in a variety of ways.

Housekeeping

Keeping the patient reception area clean usually falls within the duties of the medical assistant. In most cases you will be responsible for supervising the work of a professional cleaning service. In a small medical office you may be required to clean the area yourself.

Because professional services generally clean in the evening after business hours, you will probably not be present while the housekeeping staff is working. You may be asked to provide feedback to the cleaning company, however. It may also be your responsibility to outline the tasks you expect workers to complete, including any special requests.

Tasks. Although housekeeping tasks vary from office to office, basic routines are applicable to areas such as the patient reception room. "Caution: Handle With Care" gives more information about maintaining a clean reception area.

Whether or not the office employs a professional cleaning service, you or another staff member will need to check for cleanliness throughout the day. As patients spend time in the office, items may become dirty or be moved out of place. Taking time between patient appointments or at midday to spot-clean small areas that have become dirty and straighten items will help keep the patient reception area in good condition.

Equipment. If you, and not a professional service, are responsible for cleaning, the person in charge of the office budget will approve the purchase of cleaning equipment and supplies. Examples of cleaning equipment include handheld and upright vacuums, mops, and brooms. Supplies include trash bags, cleaning solutions, rags, and buckets. It is a good idea to have some basic cleaning materials on hand in case an emergency cleanup job is needed during office hours.

CAUTION HANDLE WITH CARE

Maintaining Cleanliness Standards in the Reception Area

Cleanliness is one of the hallmarks of a medical office. Cleanliness is not only required in the examination and testing rooms. It is also expected in the patient reception area. A messy patient reception area reflects poorly on the physician and on the practice. Maintaining standards of cleanliness helps ensure that the reception area is presentable at all times.

As a medical assistant, you may be involved—along with the physician, office manager, and other staff members—in setting cleanliness standards for the office. Standards are general guidelines. In addition to setting standards, you will need to specify the tasks required to meet each standard. A checklist of the tasks required to meet all standards is a helpful document to create as well.

The following list outlines standards you may want to consider. Specific housekeeping tasks for meeting those standards are included in parentheses.

1. Keep everything in its place. (Complete a daily visual check for items that are out of place. Return all magazines to racks. Push chairs back into place.)
2. Dispose of all trash. (Empty trash cans. Pick up trash on the floor or on furniture.)
3. Prevent dust and dirt from accumulating on surfaces. (Wipe or dust furniture, lamps, and artificial plants. Polish doorknobs. Clean mirrors, wall hangings, and pictures.)
4. Spot-clean areas that become dirty. (Remove scuff marks. Clean upholstery stains.)
5. Disinfect areas of the waiting room if they have been exposed to body fluids. (Immediately clean and disinfect all soiled areas.)
6. Handle items with care. (Take precautions when carrying potentially messy or breakable items. Do not carry too much at once.)

After the standards have been established, type and post them in a prominent place for the office staff to see. The checklist of cleaning activities may be posted, but the person responsible for cleaning the office should also keep a copy.

You should also produce a schedule of specific daily and weekly cleaning activities. Less frequent housekeeping duties, such as laundering drapes, shampooing the carpet, and cleaning windows and blinds, can be noted in a tickler file so that they will be performed on a regular basis.

It is always a good idea to have a second staff member responsible for periodically working with the medical assistant on housekeeping responsibilities. That person may also be responsible for handling cleaning duties when the medical assistant is away from the office.

Cleaning Stains

If furniture, carpet, or other items in the reception area become stained, it is important to remove the stains quickly. Follow these tips for stain removal.

1. Try to remove the stain right away. The longer a stain remains, the more difficult it is to remove.
2. Blot as much of the stain as possible before rubbing it with a cleaning solution.
3. Take special precautions in handling stains involving blood, feces, and urine. Put on latex gloves before blotting or scraping up the stain.
4. Wipe the area with a cleaning solution and water. Blood, urine, and feces may require special cleaners with an enzyme that breaks down organic waste.
5. Use cold water instead of hot water because hot water often sets stains into the fabric.

Keep all cleaning materials within easy reach for quick action when a stain occurs.

Removing Odors

Odors are particularly offensive in a doctor's office because people expect a high level of cleanliness and cannot readily leave to escape the odor. Some odors that may occasionally be present in a medical practice include those of urine, feces, vomit, body odors, and laboratory chemicals. A good ventilating system with charcoal filters can help minimize odors. If the system has temporary high-speed blowers, they can be activated as well. Disinfectant sprays and deodorant scents may also help.

One odor that can be prevented is smoke. Display "Thank You for Not Smoking" signs prominently in the patient reception area. Do not provide ashtrays, and ask smokers to leave the office if they insist on smoking. Smoking not only produces an offensive odor: it also may affect the health of other patients in the waiting room. People who have asthma or other breathing disorders, or who are feeling unwell for any reason, are particularly sensitive to smoke.

Infectious Waste

There may be times when you will need to clean up infectious waste. **Infectious waste** is waste that can be dangerous to those who handle it or to the environment. Infectious waste includes human waste, human tissue, and body fluids, such as blood and urine. It also includes any potentially hazardous waste generated in the treatment of patients, such as needles, scalpels, cultures of human cells, and dressings.

Although infectious waste is not commonly generated in the patient reception area, it can be—as when a patient vomits or bleeds on the rug or on furniture. If that situation should occur, you must clean up the waste promptly.

Infectious waste must be handled in accordance with federal law. After cleaning infectious waste from the patient reception area, deposit it in a biohazard container. Disinfect the site to eliminate possible contamination of other patients.

OSHA Regulations

Federal safety precautions for the workplace are mandated by the Occupational Safety and Health Administration (OSHA), a government agency. OSHA has developed general guidelines for most businesses, as well as special rules for health-care practices. To determine whether the requirements are being met, OSHA periodically inspects medical offices. If the rules are not followed, medical offices may be required to pay penalties in addition to correcting the problem. All employees in a medical office must be thoroughly trained in following OSHA guidelines.

Among the OSHA requirements is regular cleaning of walls, floors, and other surfaces. OSHA requires the use of disinfectants to combat bacteria as part of a routine cleaning schedule. In addition, OSHA mandates that broken glass, which may be contaminated, be picked up using a dustpan and brush or tongs. It should not be picked up by hand, even if one wears gloves.

The Physical Components

No one arrangement of a reception area is necessarily better than another. As long as the arrangement provides clear pathways and comfortable places to wait, the reception area will be functional.

Office Access

The path patients must take to get from the parking area or street to the office and then back out again is called the office **access.** Some offices have easy access and some do not (Figure 13-4).

Parking Arrangements. Although some patients walk to the medical office or take public transportation, the majority of patients probably travel by car. Patients who drive to the office need a place to park.

The office can offer either on-street parking or a parking lot. On-street parking requires patients to fend for themselves. They may have to put money into parking meters, and parking spaces may be difficult to find. Both the money required and the potential problems in finding parking spots limit the ease with which patients can gain access to the office.

A free parking lot improves office access. Parking lots should be well lit for safety. To determine the number of parking spaces the office needs, calculate the average length of time a patient spends in the office from arrival to departure and the number of appointments scheduled during that time period. Allow one parking spot per appointment if most patients drive to the office and fewer if many use public transportation. In your count be sure to include parking spaces for office staff. Periodically reevaluate the office's parking needs because they may change over time.

Entrances. The entrance to the office should be clearly marked so that patients can find the office easily. The name of the practice and of the doctor or doctors should be on the door or beside the door. Just outside the doorway should be a doormat to help control the amount of dirt tracked into the office. If the office door opens directly to the outside, people inside will feel a sudden change in temperature each time the door is opened in hot or cold weather. A foyer or double door arrangement helps minimize the effects of the weather and helps keep the office at a consistent, comfortable temperature.

Doorways should be wide enough to accommodate patients using wheelchairs and walkers. Hallways should be extra wide to allow patients in wheelchairs to turn around or to allow two wheelchairs to pass one another. The Americans With Disabilities Act, discussed later in this chapter, requires that doorways have a minimum width of 32 inches and that hallways have a minimum width of 5 ft. Well-lit hallways, without obstructions, are a must.

Safety and Security

Safety and security are important concerns in any public building, and they are especially important in a doctor's office. To ensure safety of the patients and staff, such as protection from hazardous wiring or poorly lit hallways, there are guidelines for businesses, some of which pertain to the patient reception area. In addition, the medical office must be secure from burglary.

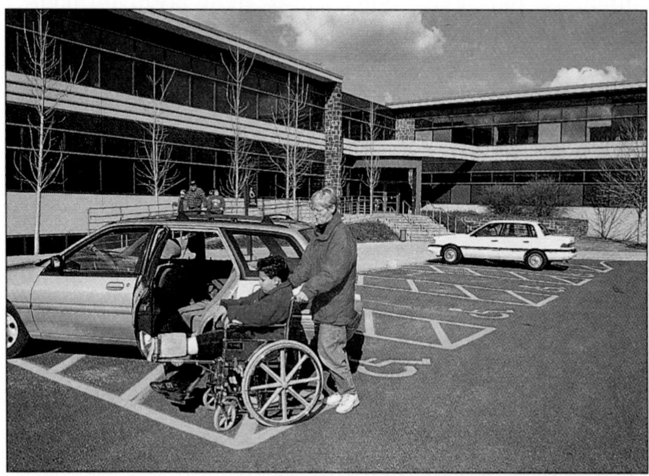

Figure 13-4. Patients should have easy, clear access from the parking lot to the medical office door.

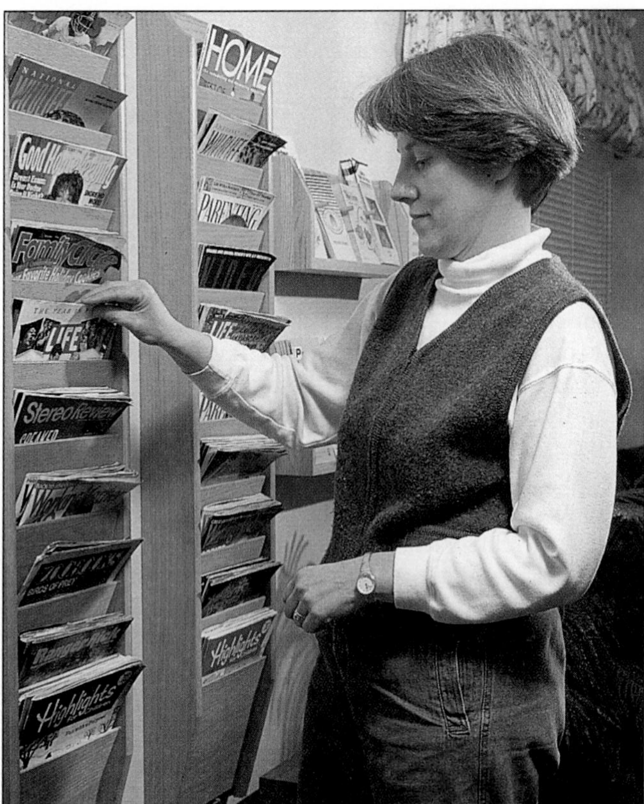

Figure 13-5. Reading materials can be organized on tables or in a wall rack.

Building Exits. Make sure you and the office staff are familiar with all building exits. It may be necessary to leave the office quickly, as during a fire, flood, or other emergency. You and other staff members must be prepared to assist and direct patients toward the exits in such a situation.

Ideally, the office should have at least two doorways that lead directly to the outside or to a hallway that leads to stairs. This arrangement affords patients and staff members the speediest, most direct route outside in case of an emergency. All exits must be clearly labeled with illuminated red "Exit" signs. These signs normally have a backup power system, such as a battery, so that they will remain lit even during a power outage.

Having two or more exits also allows staff members to enter and leave the office during nonemergency situations without disrupting people in the patient reception area. Deliveries can be made at the second entrance, further minimizing interruptions.

Smoke Detectors. By law, a medical office is required to install smoke detectors that sound an alarm when triggered by heat or smoke. The office staff should be trained in the proper procedure if the smoke alarm sounds—including how to evacuate patients from the building efficiently. Smoke detectors must be checked regularly to ensure that they are operating properly.

Security Systems. No matter where the medical office is located, a security alarm system is a wise investment, even if the office building is patrolled by security personnel. A security alarm system offers valuable protection for the confidential patient information housed in a medical office. After the alarm system is installed, all office staff members should thoroughly familiarize themselves with it. They should be able to arm and disarm it easily and know what to do if it is accidentally activated.

Keeping Patients Occupied and Informed

Many patients who come into a medical office are ill, anxious, and concerned about their health. While they wait in the reception area, they need a way to stay occupied so that the time seems to pass quickly. In addition, patients may want to be informed about a particular medical condition or about general health issues. To meet these patient needs, most medical offices provide reading materials in the patient reception area. They may also offer television or educational videotapes.

Reading Materials

The most common activity in a patient reception area is probably reading. Although some patients bring their own books or magazines, most patients expect to find reading materials at the medical office (Figure 13-5). Magazines and books are probably the most popular types of reading materials, but a variety of others may also be available.

Magazines and Books. Choosing the right mix of reading material to interest all patients is a challenge. You may know doctors' offices that have a wonderful selection of magazines and books and others that have a poor selection. Your judgment of the selection, however, is based on how those publications match your interests. "Tips for the Office" gives guidelines on selecting magazines for the medical office. In addition to reading materials for adults, most offices also have children's books and magazines for younger patients and family members.

You or someone on the office staff should be sure to screen publications for medical content. You can then alert the doctors to articles that might stimulate patients' questions.

Patient Information Packet. One type of reading material other than magazines is a patient information packet. This document is an easy way to inform patients about the practice. The packet can be designed in many ways, from a simple flyer to a formal folder with pockets to hold individual sheets of information. Topics covered in the packet can range from billing and insurance processing policies to biographical information on each physician in a group practice. Read Chapter 14 to learn more about how to develop the contents of a patient information packet.

Tips FOR THE OFFICE

Tailoring Office Magazines to Patient Interests

It is a common sight: patients waiting their turn for an appointment pick up one of the many magazines in the reception area. Sometimes it is hard to choose—because every magazine is interesting or because none of them are.

As a medical assistant, you may be responsible for selecting magazines for the office's reception area. The right selection can make the difference between a pleasant wait and a tedious one. Follow these guidelines to compile a suitable mix of magazines that will be of interest to a majority of patients.

1. Patients in some practices immediately share a common ground. They fall within the category of the practice's specialty—for example, geriatrics or pediatrics. Some magazines may be a natural "fit" for this category. A geriatric practice, for example, may provide publications geared toward senior citizens. A pediatric practice may offer parenting and children's magazines.
2. People waiting in a doctor's office usually have an interest in their health. Therefore, health magazines geared toward the general public are good choices. Of course, the waiting room is not the place for the highly technical medical journals the doctor may receive.
3. Make sure the magazines cover a variety of interests. The more topics available, the greater the chance that someone will be interested in one of them. Instead of subscribing to several magazines on one topic, try to limit subscriptions to one magazine per topic, unless the topic is of special interest to most patients.
4. Choose magazines that cover topics in a general way—travel, news, sports, fashion, or entertainment. Delving into these areas too specifically—as in a tennis magazine rather than one on a variety of sports—may not interest many patients.
5. Remove torn or out-of-date magazines from the patient reception area. Replenish them with a fresh supply as soon as possible.
6. The best way to determine patients' interests is to ask for feedback. Develop a form on which patients can indicate their hobbies, interests, and favorite types of magazines. Periodically display the form in the reception area, and encourage patients to make suggestions.

Medical Information. Another type of reading material commonly found in reception areas is medical brochures. Patients may be interested in information that pertains to their general health or to a specific condition. Brochures on a variety of topics are available to medical offices either free of charge or for a nominal fee. These brochures are usually produced by nonprofit associations that specialize in a disease or condition, such as the American Cancer Society, and by pharmaceutical companies.

Before displaying pamphlets and brochures in the reception area, be sure to read them thoroughly. They should provide accurate information. The physician may also want to review them for medical accuracy.

Bulletin Board. Most patient reception areas feature a bulletin board. Bulletin boards often highlight area meetings, such as those of support groups, and offer other current information. To encourage patients to look at the bulletin board, change the format and content frequently. An interesting design with bright colors and bold headlines attracts readers. Depending on your time and inclination, you might change the bulletin board every week, month, or season.

Items on a reception area bulletin board should be tailored to patient interests. For example, an obstetrics/gynecology practice specializing in infertility might display recent birth announcements from its patients. The bulletin board might also feature support groups for parents trying to conceive, information on the latest medical studies of fertility drugs, and magazine clippings on parenting issues.

Other more general items for display on any physician's bulletin board might include the following:

- Government reports on food and drugs
- Nutrition information
- Requests from the American Red Cross or the local blood bank for blood donors
- Pamphlets or flyers distributed by nonprofit health-care organizations, such as the American Heart Association
- Flyers on upcoming health fairs
- Blood pressure or other health screening notices
- Newspaper or magazine articles on interesting medical issues
- Community notices for food drives or similar charity events

The bulletin board might also feature information about staff members in the practice.

Finally, the bulletin board is an ideal place to display the office brochure. Put some extra copies of the brochure in an open envelope tacked to the bulletin board to encourage patients to take one home. To keep the bulletin board up to date, all time-sensitive materials, such as notices about a class or seminar, should be removed as soon as the date of the scheduled event has passed (Figure 13-6).

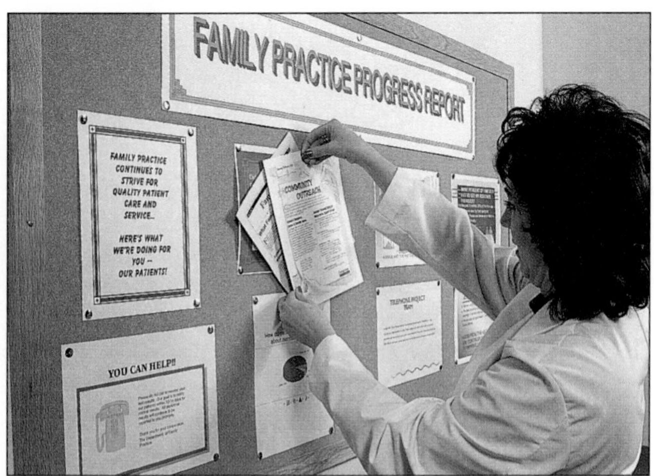
FAMILY PRACTICE PROGRESS REPORT
FAMILY PRACTICE CONTINUES TO STRIVE FOR QUALITY PATIENT CARE AND SERVICE.
HERE'S WHAT WE'RE DOING FOR YOU — OUR PATIENTS!
YOU CAN HELP!!

Figure 13-6. Check the office bulletin board frequently for outdated information.

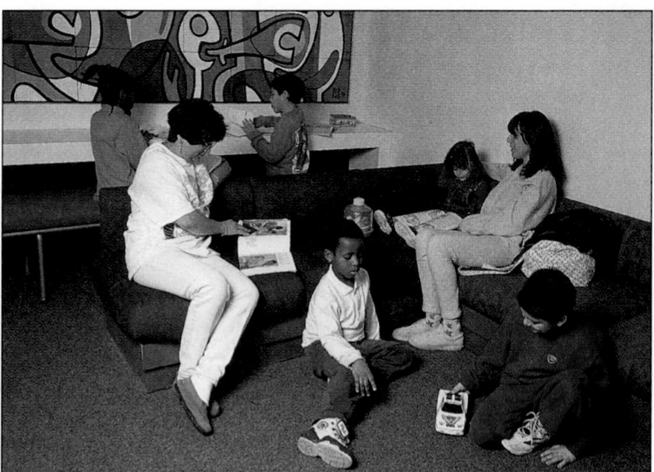

Figure 13-7. Toys and games that encourage quiet play are well suited to a reception area in a pediatric practice.

Television and Videotapes

Although reading remains the primary pastime in patient reception areas, watching television and videotapes is becoming a more common activity in physicians' offices across the country. Many patient reception areas now include a television, which can be tuned to regular stations or can play preselected videos. Physicians may provide informative health-care videos of general interest to their patients or videos that meet the more specific interests of the practice.

Items for Children

Many patient reception areas include items to occupy children while they wait. Because children—even sick ones—do not usually like to sit still for long periods, these items may include toys, games, videos, and books (Figure 13-7). If the pediatric reception area separates sick children from well children, the "well" side may include more active entertainment, such as an indoor slide or playhouse. The "sick" side may provide quieter games and activities, such as books and puzzles.

Choose toys carefully. You do not want children—even well ones—to be too active in the waiting room, because they might disrupt other patients and their families. Avoid balls, jump ropes, and other toys meant for outside use. Puzzles and blocks are good choices because they encourage quieter play. You might informally ask parents and children if they like the play items or if they would prefer other types of toys. Procedure 13-1 explains how to set up a pediatric playroom.

Patients With Special Needs

Some patients who come into the medical office will be **differently abled**—that is, they were born with or have acquired a condition that limits or changes their abilities. For example, people who are paralyzed from the waist down are differently abled; so are people who are visually impaired. This does not mean that these people cannot perform the same tasks that other people can. They may simply need special accommodations to do so.

Americans With Disabilities Act

Differently abled individuals are often singled out for their differences and are sometimes discriminated against. For example, if a company building does not have access ramps for wheelchairs, workers in wheelchairs cannot qualify for jobs there.

Preventing Discrimination. In 1990 a law was enacted to prevent certain types of discrimination. The **Americans With Disabilities Act** is a federal civil rights act forbidding discrimination on the basis of physical or mental handicap. This act maintains the rights of differently abled people in many areas, including jobs, transportation, and access to public buildings. The act relates to medical practices (and reception areas) in that an office must be able to accommodate any patient who wants to see the physician.

Differently Abled Patients. Differently abled patients may have special needs. With some forethought and planning, the office can accommodate these needs. Ensuring wheelchair access through doors and hallways, as mentioned earlier, is just one way. Using ramps instead of steps, as shown in Figure 13-8, allows easier access not only for wheelchair users but also for others who have limited mobility. Allowing additional space in the waiting room for wheelchairs, walkers, crutches, and guide dogs accommodates several types of differently abled patients. Procedure 13-2 explains how to organize the patient reception area to meet the special needs of patients who are physically challenged.

Although many offices do not make special accommodations for patients with vision or hearing impairments, you might consider doing so if there are several such patients in the practice where you work. Post prominent

PROCEDURE 13-1

Creating a Pediatric Playroom

Objective: To create a play environment for children in the patient reception area of a pediatric practice

Materials: Children's books and magazines, games, toys, nontoxic crayons and coloring books, television and videocassette recorder (VCR), children's videotapes, child- and adult-size chairs, child-size table, bookshelf, boxes or shelves, decorative wall hangings or educational posters (optional)

Method

1. Place all adult-size chairs against the wall. Position some of the child-size chairs along the wall with the adult chairs.
2. Place the remainder of the child-size chairs in small groupings throughout the room. In addition, put several chairs with the child-size table.
3. Put the books, magazines, crayons, and coloring books on the bookshelf in one corner of the room near a grouping of chairs.
4. Choose toys and games carefully. Avoid toys that encourage active play, such as balls, or toys that require a large area. Make sure that all toys meet safety guidelines. Watch for loose parts or parts that are smaller than a golf ball. Toys should also be easy to clean.
5. Place the activities for older children near one grouping of chairs and the games and toys for younger children near another grouping. Keep the toys and games in a toy box or on shelves designated for them. Consider labeling or color-coding boxes and shelves and the games and toys that belong there to encourage children to return the games and toys to the appropriate storage area.
6. Place the television and VCR on a high shelf, if possible, or attach it to the wall near the ceiling. Keep children's videos behind the reception desk, and periodically change the video in the VCR.
7. To make the room more cheerful, decorate it with wall hangings or posters.

signs in the reception area with information patients need to know. A staff member should offer to escort patients with hearing or vision impairments from the reception area to the examination room when it is their turn to see the doctor.

Older Americans Act of 1965

A growing proportion of the American population is elderly. Like those who are differently abled, many elderly people face discrimination. One reason for the discrimination may be that with age come medical conditions and disorders that create physical limitations.

The **Older Americans Act of 1965** was passed by Congress to eliminate discrimination against the elderly. Among other benefits, the act guarantees elderly citizens the best possible health care regardless of ability to pay, an adequate retirement income, and protection against abuse, neglect, and exploitation.

What does the Older Americans Act mean for the medical office reception area? If the practice serves elderly patients, the office staff must be sensitive to their special needs. The patient reception area should be as comfortable as possible for patients with arthritis, failing eyesight, and other common ailments of the elderly. Make sure there are a few straight-backed chairs, which are easier to get into and out of than soft sofas. Arms on chairs provide support when sitting and standing for patients who are unsteady. In addition, straight-backed chairs offer greater back support than low chairs or couches with sinking cushions. These chairs should be located near the front door and near the examination rooms.

Place reading materials within easy reach of the chairs so that elderly patients do not have to get up from their chairs for them. Have large-print books and magazines available, if possible, for patients with poor eyesight. You might also offer magnifying glasses for patients who like to use them. In addition, make sure that the print on all office signs is large and easy to read. The patient reception area should be well lit to help everyone, including elderly patients, see more clearly.

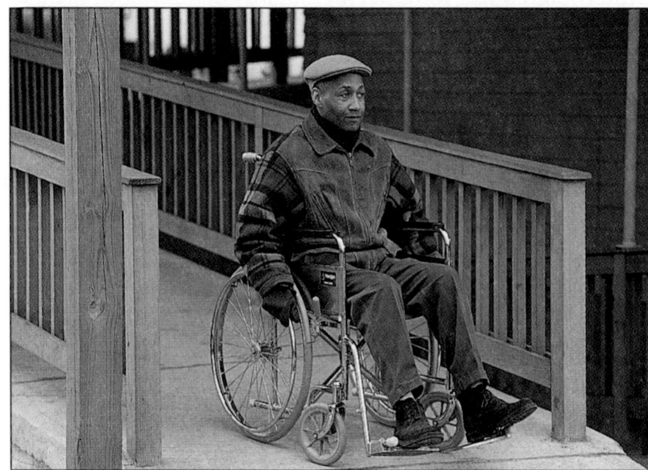

Figure 13-8. Ramps allow patients who use wheelchairs access to the medical office.

PROCEDURE 13-2

Creating a Waiting Room Accessible to Differently Abled Patients

Objective: To arrange elements in the reception area to accommodate patients who are differently abled

Materials: Chairs, bars or rails, adjustable-height tables, doorway floor coverings, magazine rack, television/VCR, ramps (if needed), large-type and braille magazines

Method

1. Arrange chairs, leaving gaps so that substantial space is available for wheelchairs along walls and near other groups of chairs. Keep the arrangement flexible so that chairs can be removed to allow room for additional wheelchairs if needed.
2. Remove any obstacles that may interfere with the space needed for a wheelchair to swivel around completely. Also remove scatter rugs or any carpeting that is not attached to the floor. Such carpeting can cause patients to trip and create difficulties for wheelchair traffic.
3. Position coffee tables at a height that is accessible to people in wheelchairs.
4. Place office reading materials, such as magazines, at a height that is accessible to people in wheelchairs (for example, on tables or in racks attached midway up the wall).
5. Locate the television and VCR within full view of patients sitting on chairs and in wheelchairs so that they do not have to strain their necks to watch.
6. For patients who have a vision impairment, include reading materials with large type and in braille.
7. For patients who have difficulty walking, make sure bars or rails are attached securely to walls 34 to 38 inches above the floor, to accommodate requirements set forth in the Americans With Disabilities Act. Make sure the bars are sturdy enough to provide balance for patients who may need it. Bars are most important in entrances and hallways. Consider placing a bar near the receptionist's window for added support as patients check in.
8. Eliminate the sill of metal or wood along the floor in doorways. Otherwise, create a smoother travel surface for wheelchairs and pedestrians with a thin rubber covering to provide a graduated slope. Be sure that the covering is attached properly and meets safety standards.
9. Make sure the office has ramp access.
10. Solicit feedback from patients with physical disabilities about the accessibility of the patient reception area. Encourage ideas for improvements. Address any additional needs.

Special Situations

Patients in a medical practice are usually a diverse group of people. Their interests, needs, and medical conditions can have an impact on the design of the reception area.

Patients From Diverse Cultural Backgrounds. The United States has long been called a melting pot because of its mixture of people and cultures. Each culture lends its own special qualities, and together the cultures combine to create a unique blend of people called Americans.

You may work in a neighborhood that has a distinct culture or one in which many cultures are represented. To help patients feel comfortable, make the reception area reflect aspects of their cultural backgrounds, whenever possible. This effort will help patients feel more welcome.

Suppose, for example, that the medical office where you work serves many Hispanic patients. Posting signs in Spanish and English acknowledges the fact that both languages are spoken in that neighborhood. Providing reading materials, such as newspapers and magazines, in a second language—for both adults and children—is another way to show respect and interest. Decorating the office for Spanish holidays, in addition to American ones, demonstrates that you care about what is important to patients. Displaying artwork created by local artists and artisans is another idea.

Patients Who Are Highly Contagious. Patients may have to come into the physician's office when they are highly contagious. This fact is a concern for all patients, but it is especially critical for patients who are immunocompromised. Immunocompromised patients have an immune system—which protects against disease—that is not functioning at a normal level. Because these patients do not have the normal ability to fight off disease, they are at greater risk than the average person for becoming sick. Patients undergoing chemotherapy and patients with AIDS, for example, have compromised immune systems.

To protect patients who are immunocompromised, as well as other patients and staff members, you may need to separate a highly contagious patient from them. Instead of having contagious patients wait in the reception area, for example, you might bring them directly into an examination room to wait. By screening patients for highly contagious conditions and taking precautions, you can minimize the chances of exposing other people unnecessarily.

Summary

The patient reception area is where patients wait before they are seen by the physician. The area's appearance creates an immediate and lasting impression on patients. Patients may notice elements such as temperature, lighting, decor, and cleanliness, all of which influence their perception of the practice.

Offices with well-planned, pleasant reception areas provide a comfortable experience for waiting patients. Important elements include easy access from the outside, safety measures that meet federal requirements, and appropriate furnishings, reading material, and other entertainment to make the wait as enjoyable as possible. Special accommodations for patients who are young, elderly, differently abled, and from diverse cultural backgrounds help create a welcoming environment.

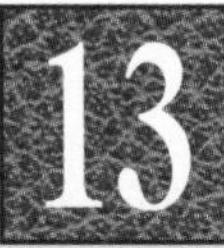

13 Chapter Review

Discussion Questions

1. Why is it important to make a patient reception area appear welcoming?
2. What elements of the patient reception area help make the wait to see the doctor as pleasant as possible?
3. What impact do the Americans With Disabilities Act and the Older Americans Act of 1965 have on the patient reception area?

Critical Thinking Questions

1. How many chairs would be needed for a waiting room in a pediatric practice that schedules three patients an hour? Explain your answer.
2. What difficulties might patients who use wheelchairs encounter if a medical office is not designed to accommodate them?
3. In what ways could you design the reception area of a medical office to reflect an African-American community? What specialty items might you include?

Application Activities

1. Design a reception area bulletin board for a family practitioner's office. List at least six items to include, and draw a rough sketch for placing these items on a rectangular bulletin board.
2. Develop a daily checklist for closing down a patient reception area at the end of the day. Be sure to include any housekeeping chores.
3. Visit a patient reception area at a clinic or a doctor's or dentist's office. Notice the decor, furniture arrangement, specialty items, and reading materials. Note what you like and dislike about the area. Then write down suggestions for improvement. Compare your results with those of your classmates.

Further Readings

Fader, Ellen G. "The Doctor's Office Collection." *School Library Journal,* June 1991, 48.

Favero, Martin S., and Richard Sadovsky. "Office Infection Control, OSHA, and You." *Patient Care,* 30 March 1993, 117.

Fenley, Gareth. "Cool Welcome." *Architectural Record,* February 1993, S34.

Gutfeld, Greg. "MTV Beats Anxiety." *Prevention,* October 1992, 22.

Maynard, Robert. "Could Your Shop Use a Face-Lift?" *Nation's Business,* August 1994, 47.

Oliver, Joan Duncan. "Rooms to Please Any I.D." *The New York Times,* 29 February 1996, C1.

Umlauf, Elyse. "The Bottom Line on Office Design." *Real Estate Today,* September 1995, 12.

Patient Education

Key Terms

consumer education
modeling
philosophy
screening

CHAPTER OUTLINE

- The Educated Patient
- Types of Patient Education
- Promoting Good Health Through Education
- The Patient Information Packet
- Educating Patients With Special Needs
- Patient Education Prior to Surgery
- Additional Educational Resources

OBJECTIVES

After completing Chapter 14, you will be able to:

- Identify the benefits of patient education.
- Explain the role of the medical assistant in patient education.
- Discuss factors that affect teaching and learning.
- Describe patient education materials used in the medical office.
- Explain how patient education can be used to promote good health habits.
- Identify the types of information that should be included in the patient information packet.
- Discuss techniques for educating patients with special needs.
- Explain the benefits of patient education prior to surgery, and identify types of preoperative teaching.
- List educational resources that are available outside the medical office.

AREAS OF COMPETENCE

1997 ROLE DELINEATION STUDY

GENERAL (Transdisciplinary)

Communication Skills

- Adapt communications to individual's ability to understand

Instruction

- Instruct individuals according to their needs
- Explain office policies and procedures
- Teach methods of health promotion and disease prevention
- Locate community resources and disseminate information

The Educated Patient

Patient education is an essential process in the medical office. It encourages patients to take an active role in their medical care. It results in better compliance with treatment programs. When patients are suffering from illness, disease, or injury, education can often help them regain their health and independence more quickly. Simply put, patient education helps patients stay healthy. Educated patients are more likely to comply with instructions if they understand the why behind the instructions. Also, educated patients are more likely to be satisfied clients of the practice.

Patients benefit from education, and the medical office benefits as well. Preoperative instruction of surgical patients, for example, lessens the chance that procedures will have to be rescheduled because surgical guidelines were not followed. Educated patients will also be less likely to call the office with questions. Thus, the office staff will have to spend less time on the telephone.

Patient education takes many forms and includes a variety of techniques. It can be as simple as answering a question that comes up during a routine visit. Patient education can involve printed materials. It can also be participatory, as with a demonstration of the procedure for changing a bandage or for giving oneself an insulin injection (Figure 14-1). No matter what type of patient education is used, the goal is the same—to help patients help themselves attain better health. Procedure 14-1 will help you make an educational plan.

As a medical assistant, you play a vital role in the process of patient education, primarily because of your constant interaction with patients in the office. Although the initial visit is a good time to assess the need for patient education, the educational process can and should be ongoing. Continue to assess patients' needs at every visit, and be aware of situations in which you can share meaningful and helpful information.

Types of Patient Education

Patient education can take many forms. Any instructions—verbal, written, or demonstrative—that you give to patients are a type of patient education. Most formal types of patient education involve some printed information. They may also include visual materials, such as videotapes. Patient educational materials inform patients and enable them to become involved in their own medical care.

Printed Materials

Printed educational materials come in a variety of formats. They can be as simple as a single sheet of paper, or they can be several sheets that are folded or stapled together to form a booklet.

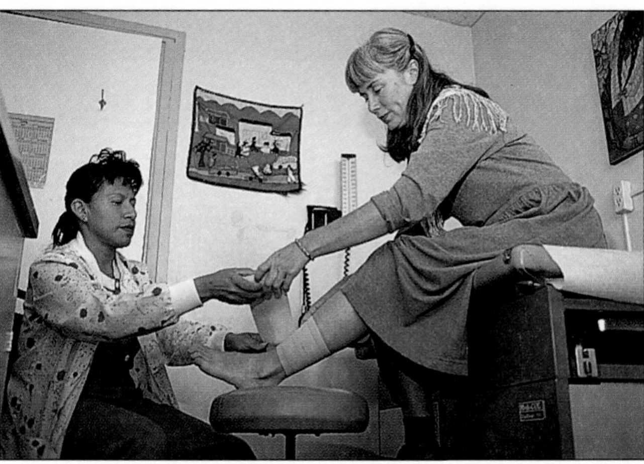

Figure 14-1. When helping patients learn through participation, you may demonstrate a technique, then ask the patient to demonstrate it for you.

Brochures, Booklets, and Fact Sheets. These materials often explain procedures that are performed in the medical office or give information about specific diseases and medical conditions. For example, women who have had a cesarean section delivery may be given a fact sheet describing simple exercises they can do in bed to help regain strength in the abdominal muscles. Some printed materials provide information to help patients stay healthy, such as tips for eating low-fat foods. Many educational aids are prepared by pharmaceutical companies and are provided free of charge to medical offices. Others may be written by the physician or members of the office staff. You may be asked to help prepare some of these materials.

Educational Newsletters. A popular patient education tool is the medical office newsletter. Newsletters contain timely, practical health-care tips. Regular newsletters can also offer updates on office policies, information about new diagnostic tests or equipment, and news about the office staff. Newsletters are often written by the doctor or office staff. Some publishing companies and medical groups also offer newsletters that can be customized to a particular practice.

Community-Assistance Directory. Patients often require the assistance of health-related organizations within the community. For example, an elderly patient may need the services of a visiting nurse or a meals-on-wheels food program. Other patients may need the services of a day-care center, speech therapist, or weight clinic. A written community resource directory prepared by the office is a valuable aid for referring patients to appropriate agencies.

Visual Materials

Many patients are better able to comprehend complicated medical information when it is presented in a visual format. When using visual educational materials, it is

PROCEDURE 14-1

Developing an Educational Plan

Objective: To create and implement a patient teaching plan

Materials: Pen, paper, various educational aids

Method

1. Identify the patient's needs for education. Consider the following:
   a. The patient's current knowledge
   b. Any misconceptions the patient may have
   c. Any obstacles to learning (loss of hearing or vision, limitations of mobility, language barriers, and so on)
   d. The patient's willingness and readiness to learn (motivation)
   e. How the patient will use the information
2. Develop and outline a plan using the various educational aids available. Include the following areas in the outline:
   a. What you want to accomplish (your goal)
   b. How you plan to accomplish it
   c. How you will determine if the teaching was successful
3. Write the plan. Try to make the information interesting for the patient.
4. Before carrying out the plan, share it with the physician to get approval and suggestions for improvement.
5. Perform the instruction.
6. Document the teaching in the patient's chart.
7. Evaluate the effectiveness of your teaching session. Ask yourself:
   a. Did you cover all the topics in your plan?
   b. Was the information well received by the patient?
   c. Did the patient appear to learn?
   d. How would you rate your performance?
8. Revise your plan as necessary to make it even more effective.

usually best to provide corresponding written materials that patients can keep for reference.

Videotapes. Videotapes are often used to educate patients about a variety of topics and to instruct them in self-care techniques (Figure 14-2). The use of videotapes is especially effective when teaching about complex subjects and procedures.

Seminars and Classes. Many physicians conduct or arrange educational seminars or classes for their patients. For example, an obstetrician might offer classes in childbirth preparation for patients and their partners.

Promoting Good Health Through Education

One of the most important goals of patient education is to promote good health. Health is not just the absence of illness. It is a complex concept that involves the body, mind, emotions, and environment. Health involves physical, mental, emotional, and social influences working together as a whole.

Maintaining or improving your health is the best way to protect yourself against disease and illness. **Consumer education**—education that is geared, both in content and language, toward the average person—has helped Americans become more aware of the importance of good health. As a result, many people are beginning to take greater responsibility for their own health and well-being.

There are many ways to achieve good health. You can develop healthful habits, take steps to protect yourself from injury, and take preventive measures to decrease the risk of disease or illness. Patient education in the medical office should help patients achieve these goals.

Healthful Habits

When educating patients about good health, you can recommend several specific guidelines. Encourage patients to incorporate the following healthful habits into their daily lives:

- Good nutrition, including limited fat intake and an adequate amount of fruits, vegetables, and fiber
- Regular exercise
- Adequate rest (7 to 8 hours of sleep a night)
- Not smoking and limiting alcohol consumption
- A balance of work and leisure activities

Whenever possible, these guidelines should be recommended to patients of all ages. Good health should be a top priority in life. Although it is best to incorporate healthful behavior before illness develops, remind patients that it is never too late to work toward improving their health.

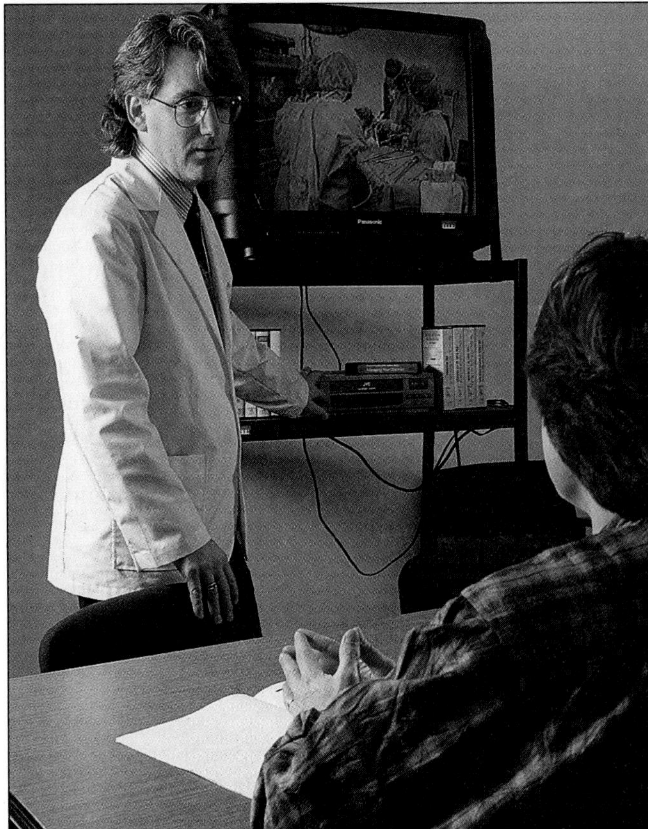

Figure 14-2. Videotapes are an excellent educational aid for the medical office because of their visual format.

Protection From Injury

Many accidents happen because people fail to see potential risks and do not develop plans of action. Following safety measures at home, at work, at play, and while traveling can help prevent injury. A discussion of ways to avoid accidents and injury should be part of the educational process. Tips for preventing injury at home and at work are listed in Figure 14-3.

Another essential aspect of educating patients about injury prevention is teaching them about the proper use of medications. A prescription includes specific instructions for taking the medication. Emphasize to the patient that these instructions must be followed exactly. In addition, the patient must not change the dosage or mix medications of any kind without first checking with the physician. Patients who do not adhere to these rules run the risk of potentially dangerous side effects. Tell patients to report to the physician any unusual reactions experienced when taking medications.

Preventive Measures

Preventive health care is an area in which patient education plays a vital role. Patients need to know that they can decrease their chances of getting certain illnesses and diseases by taking preventive measures. Preventive techniques can be described on three levels: health-promoting behaviors, screening, and rehabilitation.

Health-Promoting Behaviors. The first level of disease and illness prevention involves adopting the health-promoting behaviors mentioned earlier. This primary level of prevention also includes educating patients about the symptoms and warning signs of disease. One example is informing patients about the warning signs of cancer. The first letters of these warning signs spell the word *caution*. They are as follows:

- **C**hange in bowel or bladder habits
- **A** sore that does not heal
- **U**nusual bleeding or discharge
- **T**hickening or lump in a breast or elsewhere
- **I**ndigestion or difficulty in swallowing
- **O**bvious change in a wart or mole
- **N**agging cough or hoarseness

Screening. The second level of disease prevention is screening. **Screening** involves the diagnostic testing of a patient who is typically free of symptoms. Screening allows early diagnosis and treatment of certain diseases. Examples of screening tests include mammography and Pap for women and prostate examinations for men.

Rehabilitation. The third level of disease prevention involves the rehabilitation and management of an existing illness. At this level the disease process remains stable, but the body will probably not heal any further. The objective is to maintain functionality and avoid further disability. Examples of this level of prevention include stroke rehabilitation programs and pain management for a condition such as arthritis.

The Patient Information Packet

When patients come to the medical practice, they need to learn not only about health and medical issues but also about the medical office itself. The patient information packet explains the medical practice and its policies. Unlike most other patient education materials, the patient information packet deals mainly with administrative matters rather than with medical issues.

The patient information packet may be as simple as a one-page brochure or pamphlet. It may be a multipage brochure, however, or a folder with multiple-page inserts.

Benefits of the Information Packet

The patient information packet is a simple, effective, and inexpensive way to improve the relationship between the office and the patients. It provides important information about the practice and the office staff. This information

Tips for Preventing Injury

At Home

- Install smoke detectors, carbon monoxide detectors, and fire extinguishers.
- Keep all medicines, chemicals, and household cleaning solutions out of reach of children. Purchase products in childproof containers. Lock or attach childproof latches to all cabinets, medicine chests, and drawers that contain poisonous items.
- Keep chemicals in their original containers, and store them out of children's reach.
- Install adequate lighting in rooms and hallways. Install railings on stairs.
- Use nonskid backing on rugs to help prevent falls, or remove rugs altogether.
- In the bathroom use nonskid mats or strips that stick to the tub floor.
- Practice good kitchen safety: Store knives and kitchen tools properly. Unplug small appliances when not in use. Wipe up spills immediately.
- Shorten long electrical cords and speaker wires, or secure them with electrical tape. Avoid plugging too many electrical appliances into the same outlet.
- Never use appliances in the bathtub or near a sink filled with water.
- Exercise caution when using electrical appliances. Use outlet covers when outlets are not in use.
- To reach high places, use proper equipment, such as stepladders, not chairs.

At Work

- Use appropriate safety equipment and protective gear, as required.
- Lift heavy objects properly: Bend at the knees, not at the waist. As you straighten your legs, bring the object close to your body quickly. That way, strong leg muscles do the lifting, not weaker back muscles. Never attempt to move furniture on your own. Request that a member of the office building maintenance staff be engaged to do so.
- Use surge protectors on computer equipment to prevent overloading outlets.
- Make sure hallways, entrance areas, work areas, offices, and parking lots are well lit.
- If your job involves desk work, practice proper posture when sitting. Do not sit for long periods of time. Get up and stretch, or walk down the hall and back.

Figure 14-3. You can help patients stay healthy by instructing them about ways to avoid injury.

helps patients feel more comfortable with the qualifications of the health-care professionals involved in their care. The packet may help clarify the roles that each office staff member has in patient care.

The information packet also informs patients of office policies and procedures. Patients will learn the doctor's office hours, how to schedule appointments, the office's payment policies, and other administrative details. This information helps limit misunderstandings about these procedures.

The patient information packet also benefits the office staff. It is both an excellent marketing tool and an aid to running the office more smoothly. Providing patients with a prepared information packet saves staff time by answering a number of potential patient inquiries. The information packet is also a good way to acquaint new office staff members with office policies.

Contents of the Information Packet

Regardless of what material the information packet contains, it must be written in clear language so that patients are able to read and understand it. Information should not be presented in a technical medical style. Because you may be responsible for preparing portions of the policy packet, you should be familiar with the contents of a typical packet.

Introduction to the Office. A brief introduction serves to welcome the patient to the office. It may be helpful to summarize the office's philosophy of patient care. The office's **philosophy** means the system of values and principles the office has adopted in its everyday practices.

Physician's Qualifications. The packet commonly contains information about the physician's professional qualifications and training. It includes details about education, internship, and residency. It may list credentials such as board certification or board eligibility in a certain medical specialty. It may also list the physician's membership in professional societies. The information packet for a group practice may contain a paragraph or a page for each physician.

Description of the Practice. It is helpful to include a brief description of the practice, particularly if it is a specialty practice. Explaining the types of examinations or procedures that are commonly performed in the office may be useful. It may also be helpful to list any special services the office provides, such as physical examinations for employment, workers' compensation cases, or other occupational services.

Introduction to the Office Staff. Many patients are not familiar with the qualifications and duties of the various members of the office staff. It is a good idea, therefore, to identify the staff members according to their responsibilities and duties. Patients need to understand that some duties commonly thought to be a nurse's responsibilities may also be performed by a medical assistant. It may be helpful to include the professional credentials and licenses of key staff members.

Office Hours. This section should list the exact days and hours the office is open, including holidays. In addition, patients need to know what to do if an emergency occurs outside regular office hours. Tell the patient what number to call first (for example, the answering service, 911, or the hospital emergency room) and what to do next. Include the telephone number and address of the emergency room at the hospital with which the doctor is affiliated. Assure patients that the doctor can be reached at all times through the answering service.

Appointment Scheduling. This section of the packet should explain the procedure for scheduling and canceling appointments. You might suggest that patients can benefit by scheduling routine checkups and visits as far in advance as possible. Also note if certain times of the day are reserved for sudden or unexpected office visits.

In this section encourage patients to be on time for appointments. Explain the problems that result from late or broken appointments. If the office charges a fee for breaking an appointment without advance notice, mention it here.

Telephone Policy. Providing the office's telephone policies in the information packet can help reduce the number of unnecessary calls to the office and thus save time for the office staff. Explain which procedures can be handled over the telephone and which cannot. Explain procedures such as calling in for prescription renewals or laboratory test results. If the physician returns patients' calls at a certain time of day, mention that policy in this section. Some practices bill patients for telephone calls in which medical advice is given but not for follow-up calls. For example, if a parent of a child who was vomiting uncontrollably called the physician to get immediate medical advice, the call might be billed. If the physician called to inform a patient of test results, however, the call would not be billed.

Some offices (particularly pediatric offices) schedule a certain time of the day for patients (or parents and guardians) to call the physician for answers to their questions. This type of policy benefits both the office and the patients. The patients (or parents) have the assurance that they can speak with the physician about their concerns, and the office is spared interruptions during other times of the day.

Payment Policies. Inform patients of the office's policies regarding payment and billing. State whether payment is expected at the time of a visit or whether the patient can be billed. List accepted forms of payment (for example, cash, personal checks, and credit cards). It is not common practice to mention specific fees in an information packet.

Insurance Policies. Advise patients to bring proof of insurance coverage and the proper claim forms when they visit the office. State whether the office submits claim forms directly to the insurance company or whether the patient has this responsibility. Outline the practice's policy for handling Medicare coverage, including whether the office accepts patients who do not have supplemental insurance. Explain that the staff will help patients fill out insurance forms when necessary.

Patient Confidentiality Statement. The information packet may also include a statement to assure patients that their confidentiality will be maintained. It should state that no information from patient files will be released without signed authorization from the patient.

Other Information. The patient information packet may include the practice's policy on referrals. It may provide information about access to available community health resources or agencies. It may also include special instructions for common office procedures (for example, whether the patient needs to fast before a procedure or to avoid certain foods).

Distributing the Information Packet

For the information packet to be effective, you must make sure that new patients receive and read it. One way is to hand the packet to new patients at the time of their first office visit and briefly review the contents with them (Figure 14-4). Explain that they can find answers to many questions in the packet. Encourage patients to take the packet home, read the information, and keep it handy for future reference.

When new patients make an appointment, many offices send them a copy of the information packet if there is enough time before the appointment to get it to them

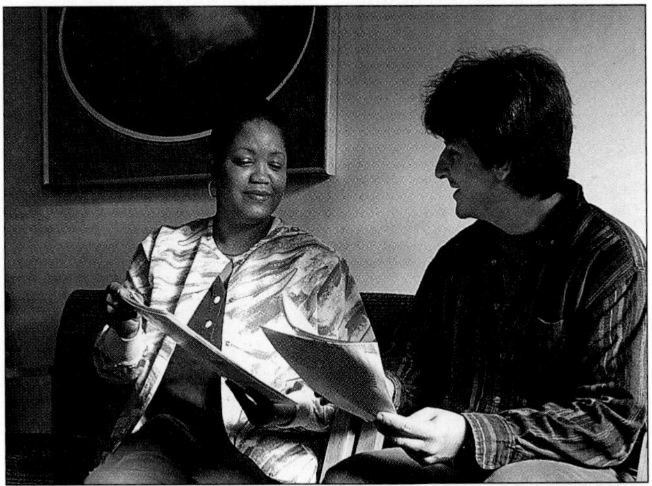

Figure 14-4. Give patients the patient information packet on their first visit to the office, or mail it prior to their first appointment.

by regular mail. (It is a nice gesture to include a detailed map or written directions to the office for new patients who are not familiar with the area.) Patients can review the packet before coming to the office and can ask questions during the visit. Additional copies of the packet should be placed in an accessible area in the office so that patients can take them home.

Special Concerns

Some practices serve patients who cannot read well or who do not speak or understand English. It may be necessary to create a second information packet written in very simple terms, which presents information through pictures and charts. The information packet can also be translated into one or more languages.

In any of these cases, make sure patients understand the office's policies and procedures. Additional one-on-one explanations may be required. Patients should still receive the printed materials to take home, however. Family members or friends may be able to read the materials for them, reinforcing what they learned in the office.

Educating Patients With Special Needs

During your career as a medical assistant, you will probably encounter many patients with special needs. Each patient's individual circumstances will affect your approach to patient education. In all cases try to see situations from the point of view of the patient. In many instances you can enlist the support of family or friends to aid in the educational process.

Elderly Patients

You will probably be called on to provide care for more and more elderly patients as the number of older people continues to grow (Figure 14-5). Patient education for elderly patients is especially valuable because it can help them prevent or manage health problems and thus feel capable and independent. You may need to educate some older people about the importance of taking measures to protect their health.

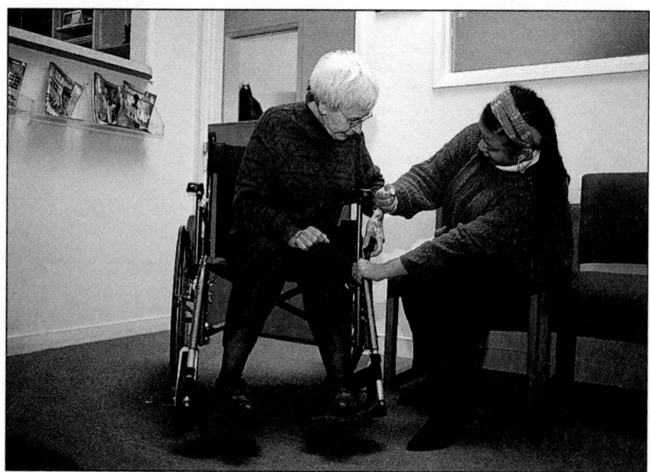

Figure 14-5. When instructing elderly patients, remember that each patient is an individual with unique needs.

You may work with elderly patients who have hearing or vision problems or physical limitations that restrict their ability to perform certain tasks. Keep the following suggestions in mind when working with elderly patients.

1. Treat each patient as an individual. This point is perhaps the most important to remember when dealing with elderly patients. Some older people have trouble understanding directions. Try to communicate with them at the highest level they can understand. Never talk down to patients.
2. Put instructions in writing. Because some elderly patients have problems with memory, detailed written instructions are an essential aspect of patient care. Patients can refer to the instructions as necessary or can ask a relative to do so.
3. Adjust procedures as needed. When demonstrating a procedure to elderly patients, keep in mind any physical limitations they may have, and adjust the procedure accordingly. Make sure patients understand the instructions by asking them to perform the procedure for you.

Patients With Mental Impairments

Patients with impaired mental functions include those with Alzheimer's disease, mental retardation, drug addictions, and emotional problems. These patients can be challenging to deal with because communication may be difficult. Tact and empathy are important. A key to dealing with these patients is to speak at their level of understanding. Again, you must try to meet patients' needs without talking down to them.

Patients With Hearing Impairments

Patients with hearing impairments may have conditions ranging from mild impairment to total hearing loss. It is a common mistake to treat these patients as though they have mental impairments. Although you may have difficulty communicating with these patients, remember that their inability to hear has nothing to do with their level of intelligence. "Educating the Patient" provides techniques for educating patients who have hearing impairments.

Patients With Visual Impairments

As with hearing impairment, the level of visual impairment can vary significantly from patient to patient. Determining the severity of a patient's condition allows you to tailor your instruction to the patient's needs.

EDUCATING THE PATIENT

Instructing Patients With Hearing Impairments

Educating patients who have hearing impairments need not be difficult if you pay a little extra attention in the following areas.

- Try to eliminate all background noise. Talk in a quiet room, if possible.
- Make sure the room is well lit.
- Face the patient, and make sure the patient can see your mouth. Having the patient watch your mouth movements can help him understand what you are saying.
- Speak loudly and clearly, but do not shout.
- Use visual aids as necessary.
- Tell patients to let you know right away if they cannot hear you or do not catch something you have said. Even patients who do not have hearing impairments often appear to understand what a medical professional is saying rather than admit they are confused. It is a good idea to ask patients to repeat information to you to check their understanding. Also, periodically ask if they would like you to go over any particular part of the explanation or instructions again.

An additional point to keep in mind when dealing with patients who have hearing impairments is that loss of hearing can cause them to withdraw and feel isolated. Being empathic and patient greatly enhances the educational process.

Elderly Patients With Hearing Loss

Most people experience a gradual loss of hearing as they get older. In addition to the preceding suggestions, try to talk in a lower pitch whenever possible. As people get older, they often have more trouble understanding higher tones.

Patients Who Wear Hearing Aids

When talking to a patient who wears a hearing aid, it is best to speak at a normal level. Many hearing aids make a normal voice louder but filter out loud noises. If you raise your voice, the hearing aid may filter it out. Consequently, the patient may hear only broken speech.

For those with mildly impaired vision, the approach may be as simple as providing instructional materials printed in large type. In addition, you can demonstrate procedures in a well-lit area and close to the patients. For more severe visual impairment, adjust the level of instruction appropriately. For example, to demonstrate how to use a particular knob on a wheelchair, you might actually place the patient's hand on the knob and discuss its function.

When speaking to someone who has a visual impairment, remember to use a normal tone of voice. A patient with a visual impairment does not necessarily also have a hearing impairment. Although you should never talk down to patients, you need to verify that they understand all verbal instructions. Have the patient repeat all instructions to you.

Giving procedural instructions may be a challenge, depending on the patient's ability to perform certain tasks. Suggest that patients ask a family member or friend to help them with procedures they have trouble doing on their own.

Multicultural Issues

Patients who come from diverse cultures often have different beliefs about the causes and treatment of illness. These differences may affect their treatment expectations and their willingness to follow instructions or agree to have certain procedures performed on them. There may also be communication problems if the patient does not understand English well. Communicating with patients in these situations is discussed in Chapter 4.

Patient Education Prior to Surgery

One instance in which patient education is vital to a successful outcome is the instruction given before a patient undergoes a surgical procedure. Although exact instructions vary according to the procedure, their purpose is to prepare the patient for the procedure and to aid the patient during the recovery period. Instructions may include verbal, written, and demonstrative techniques.

The Role of the Medical Assistant

Patients generally receive information about the need for surgery and its nature from the physician. Educating and preparing patients for surgery will probably be your responsibility, however. You may provide support and explanations to patients. You must verify that they understand any information they may have been given by other members of the health-care team. Preoperative instruction may include discussion of postoperative care issues, such as temporary dietary restrictions.

You may also be responsible for determining whether patients have all the information they need before surgery, from both an educational and a legal standpoint. All patients who are undergoing a surgical procedure must first sign an informed consent form. As stated in Chapter 9, this legal document provides specific information about the surgical procedure, including its purpose, the possible risks, and the expected outcome. The in-

PROCEDURE 14-2

Informing the Patient of Guidelines for Surgery

Objective: To inform a preoperative patient of the necessary guidelines to follow prior to surgery

Materials: Patient chart, surgical guidelines

Method

1. Review the patient's chart to determine the type of surgery to be performed.
2. Tell the patient that you will be providing both verbal and written instructions that should be followed prior to surgery.
3. Inform the patient about policies regarding makeup, jewelry, contact lenses, wigs, dentures, and so on.
4. Tell the patient to leave money and valuables at home.
5. If applicable, suggest appropriate clothing for the patient to wear for postoperative ease and comfort.
6. Explain the need for someone to drive the patient home following an outpatient surgical procedure.
7. Tell the patient the correct time to arrive in the office or at the hospital for the procedure.
8. Inform the patient of dietary restrictions. Be sure to use specific, clear instructions about what may or may not be ingested and at what time the patient must abstain from eating or drinking. Also explain these points:
   a. The reasons for the dietary restrictions
   b. The possible consequences of not following the dietary restrictions
9. Ask patients who smoke to refrain from or reduce cigarette smoking during at least the 8 hours prior to the procedure. Explain to the patient that reducing smoking improves the level of oxygen in the blood during surgery.
10. Suggest that the patient shower or bathe the morning of the procedure or the evening before.
11. Instruct the patient about medications to take or avoid before surgery.
12. If necessary, clarify any information about which the patient is unclear.
13. Provide written surgical guidelines, and suggest that the patient call the office if additional questions arise.
14. Document the instruction in the patient's chart.

formed consent form, along with documentation of all preoperative instruction, must be put in the patient's chart.

Benefits of Preoperative Education

Preoperative education has many benefits. It increases patients' overall satisfaction with their care. It helps reduce patient anxiety and fear, use of pain medication, complications following surgery, and recovery time. Letting the patient know what to expect during the surgery and afterward allows the patient to participate in all aspects of the surgical procedure.

Types of Preoperative Teaching

Three types of teaching should occur during the preoperative period: factual, sensory, and participatory. The combination of these teaching methods gives the patient an overall understanding of the surgical procedure.

Factual. Factual teaching informs the patient of details about the procedure. You should tell the patient what will happen during the surgery, when it will happen, and why the procedure is necessary. Factual information also includes restrictions on diet or activity that may be necessary both before and after surgery. Procedure 14-2 describes how to inform patients of guidelines for surgery.

Sensory. Give patients a description of the physical sensations they may have during the procedure. All five senses may be involved: feeling, seeing, hearing, tasting, and smelling.

Participatory. Participatory teaching includes demonstrations of techniques that may be necessary or helpful during the postoperative period. Aspects of postoperative care include cleaning the wound, changing the dressing, and applying ice packs.

During this phase of teaching, you need to first describe the technique to the patient and then demonstrate it. The patient should repeat the demonstration for you. If any aspects of the technique are unclear to the patient, you should demonstrate the technique again. The patient should be capable of performing the procedure properly. This process of teaching a new skill by having the patient observe and imitate is called **modeling.**

Using Anatomical Models

An anatomical model is a useful tool in preoperative education. As shown in Figure 14-6, looking at a lifelike model—and being able to see the actual body structures—helps patients better understand their condition. A model also allows patients to see how the surgical procedure will help correct their problem.

It may be difficult for a patient to visualize exactly what will take place in some surgical procedures. For example, think of arthroscopy of the knee. When told that the doctor will insert a viewing instrument into the knee, patients probably have no idea of the size of this scope. As a result, they may be particularly fearful of the procedure. Using a model to show exactly what will happen can ease patients' fears.

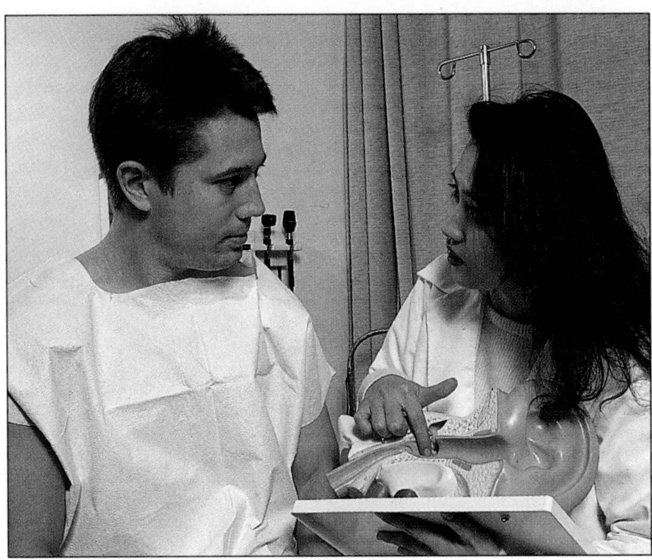

Figure 14-6. An anatomical model can help patients visualize what will happen during surgery.

Helping Patients Relieve Anxiety

When you provide preoperative education, be aware that the fear and anxiety of patients who are about to undergo a surgical procedure can adversely affect the learning process. Consequently, allow extra time for repetition and reinforcement of material.

Always consider your choice of words carefully, stressing the positive rather than the negative whenever possible. Involving family members in the educational process is often beneficial, particularly if the patient is especially apprehensive about the surgery. Remember to present your instructions and explanations in straightforward language that they can understand. Family members can often help relieve the patient's anxiety.

Verifying Patient Understanding

The key to the success of any educational process is verifying that patients have actually understood the information. A good way to check for understanding is to have patients explain in their own words what they have learned. In addition, have them repeat any demonstrations that you have given.

Additional Educational Resources

Besides the resources available in the medical office, a vast number of outside resources are available for patient education. You can use these resources to obtain information for your own use in patient education, or you can mention them to patients who are looking for additional information. Following are several sources of patient education materials:

1. Libraries and patient resource rooms. Most public libraries have an assortment of books, magazines, and electronic databases pertaining to health and medical topics. Many hospitals provide patient resource rooms, which include a variety of educational materials—such as books, brochures, and videotapes—for public use.
2. Computer resources. A great deal of up-to-date medical information can be accessed through on-line services and CD-ROM discs. The Internet is another widely used source of medical information.
3. Community resources. Many local social service agencies provide specialized health information related to such topics as nursing home care, visiting nurses' care, counseling, and rehabilitation. Most of these agencies are listed in the telephone book. Area hospitals, the library, and the local chamber of commerce are other good sources for these services.
4. Associations. Thousands of health organizations and associations can be contacted for information about preventive health care and virtually every known disease or disorder. The names, addresses, and telephone numbers of these organizations are provided in several directories, which are available at most libraries. Figure 14-7 provides a sample list of patient resource organizations.

Summary

Patient education plays a key role in many aspects of patient care. Knowledgeable patients are able to take an active approach to their own medical care. They are also likely to be aware of the benefits of activities that promote and protect their health.

There are many reasons for patient education in the medical office. Patients need to understand their medical conditions and to be prepared for necessary procedures. Many opportunities exist to educate patients about the benefits of good health. In addition, patients need to be informed of the policies of the medical office.

Many educational resources are available to both medical assistants and patients. The key for medical assistants is to take advantage of all opportunities to educate patients and to match this teaching to the needs of individual patients.

Outside Resources

Alzheimer's Association
70 East Lake Street
Chicago, IL 60601-5997
(800) 621-0379
(800) 572-6037 (in Illinois)
(312) 335-8882 (hearing-impaired)

American Academy of Pediatrics
Publications Department
P.O. Box 927
Elk Grove, IL 60009-0927
(708) 228-5005

American Cancer Society
777 Third Avenue
New York, NY 10017
(212) 586-8700

American Diabetes Association
Two Park Avenue
New York, NY 10016
(800) ADA-DISC
(212) 683-7444

American Dietetic Association
216 West Jackson Boulevard, Suite 800
Chicago, IL 60606-6995
(800) 366-1655

American Heart Association
7272 Greenville Avenue
Dallas, TX 75231-4596
(800) 242-8721
(214) 750-5300

American Red Cross
17th and D Street, NW
Washington, DC 20006
(301) 737-8300

The Arthritis Foundation
1314 Spring Street, NW
Atlanta, GA 30309
(800) 283-7800
(404) 872-7100

Asthma and Allergy Foundation of America
1717 Massachusetts Avenue, Suite 305
Washington, DC 20036
(800) 7-ASTHMA
(202) 265-0265

National AIDS Hotline
215 Park Avenue South, Suite 714
New York, NY 10003
(800) 342-AIDS
(800) 344-SIDA (Spanish)
(800) AIDS-TTY (hearing-impaired)

National Cancer Institute
Cancer Information Clearinghouse
Office of Cancer Communications
Building 31, Room 10A18
9000 Rockville Pike
Bethesda, MD 20205
(800) 4-CANCER

National Clearinghouse for
Alcohol and Drug Information
P.O. Box 2345
Rockville, MD 20852
(301) 468-2600

National Health Information Center
P.O. Box 1133
Washington, DC 20013-1133
(800) 336-4797
(301) 565-4167 (in Maryland)
(The information specialists at this agency can provide telephone numbers for associations that deal with specific diseases or problems.)

National Kidney Foundation
30 East 33d Street
New York, NY 10016
(212) 889-2210

National Organization for Rare Disorders (NORD)
100 Route 37, P.O. Box 8923
New Fairfield, CT 06812
(800) 999-NORD

President's Council on Physical Fitness and Sports
Department of Health and Human Services
Washington, DC 20001
(202) 272-3421

Figure 14-7. The addresses and telephone numbers listed are for national headquarters. Check your telephone book for local listings.

MULTISKILL FOCUS

Occupational Therapy Assistant

To gain medical assistant credentials, you must fulfill the requirements of either the American Association of Medical Assistants (for a Certified Medical Assistant) or the American Medical Technologists (for a Registered Medical Assistant). After obtaining your medical assistant certification or registration, you may wish to acquire additional skills in specialty areas through course work or on-the-job training. Although this course work or training may not lead to an additional certification or degree, it will enable you to expand your role in the medical office and advance your career as the demand for multiskilled health professionals increases.

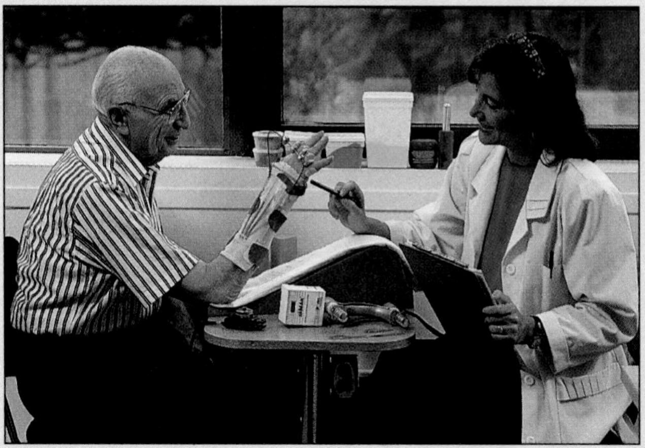

Skills and Duties

An occupational therapy assistant helps patients learn, or relearn, basic and special skills they need to function in their daily lives. Patient interaction is the focus of the occupational therapy assistant's job. An occupational therapy assistant works under the supervision of an occupational therapist.

Occupational therapists teach many different types of skills to many different types of patients. These skills include the following:

- Basic life skills, such as dressing and feeding oneself or moving about at home. For example, patients with partial paralysis or nerve damage resulting from a stroke may need this type of help.
- Vocational skills, such as typing. These skills will help patients with disabilities get jobs to support themselves.
- Designing and supervising arts and crafts activities. These activities serve as recreation and help patients develop fine motor skills in a nonthreatening, pleasant atmosphere.
- Helping accident victims who have an injured limb or a prosthetic device learn new ways to perform simple tasks. A patient with a prosthetic hand, for example, may need help learning to open jar lids.
- Working with patients who have behavioral or emotional disturbances. Occupational therapy may help these patients express their feelings in constructive ways, by building an interest in music, drama, or art.

The occupational therapy assistant also performs a number of clerical and administrative tasks. He checks inventories, orders supplies, and helps maintain the equipment in his workplace. He may also be responsible for paperwork, including writing reports on therapy sessions with patients.

Workplace Settings

Occupational therapy assistants often work in hospitals. They may also find work in clinics or long-term care facilities, such as retirement communities with assisted-care services, nursing homes, or rehabilitation centers. Some occupational therapists are employed in educational settings, including occupational workshops and schools for children with special needs.

Education

Community colleges and vocational schools offer 2-year programs for an associate degree in occupational therapy assisting. By completing a program approved by the American Occupational Therapy Association and passing a qualifying test, you can become a Certified Occupational Therapy Assistant (COTA).

Where to Go for More Information

The American Occupational Therapy Association
4720 Montgomery Lane
P.O. Box 31220
Bethesda, MD 20824-1220
(301) 948-9626

American Society of Hand Therapists
401 North Michigan Avenue
Chicago, IL 60611
(312) 321-6866

14 Chapter Review

Discussion Questions

1. Compare and contrast printed patient educational materials with visual materials. What are the advantages and disadvantages of each?
2. Why should the medical office take on the responsibility of helping to educate patients about health-promoting behavior?
3. In what ways can patient education prior to surgery benefit not only the patient but also the medical practice?

Critical Thinking Questions

1. Imagine that you are measuring the vital signs of an overweight 37-year-old woman. She becomes visibly upset when you ask her to step on the scale. The office has many brochures with tips on promoting good health. How might you bring up the subject of proper diet and exercise?
2. Describe some of the factual, sensory, and participatory information you would convey when educating a patient about postoperative care following surgical removal of a skin growth.
3. Describe the educational resources you might use to find information about a rare blood disorder that was recently discovered.

Application Activities

1. Develop an educational plan for the overweight patient mentioned in the first question of the previous section. Have another student assume the role of the patient, and practice implementing your plan. Ask the other student to evaluate your teaching method.
2. Write the section of a patient information brochure that describes the general roles of the medical office staff. Exchange your writing sample with that of another student, and critique each other's work.
3. With a partner, role-play a medical assistant giving procedural instructions to a patient with a hearing impairment. Then switch roles, and offer suggestions for improving each other's teaching techniques.

Further Readings

Anderson, Carolyn. *Patient Teaching and Communicating in an Information Age.* Albany, NY: Delmar, 1990.

Babcock, Dorothy E., and Mary A. Miller. *Client Education: Theory and Practice.* St. Louis, MO: Mosby–Year Book, 1994.

Frank, Robyn C., and Holly Berry Irving. *The Directory of Food and Nutrition Information for Professionals and Consumers.* 2d ed. Phoenix, AZ: Oryx Press, 1992.

Hancock, Lee, ed. *Key Guide to Electronic Resources: Health Sciences.* Medford, NJ: Learned Information, 1995.

Linton, Adrianne Dill, Mary Ann Matteson, and Nancy K. Maebius. *Introductory Nursing Care of Adults.* Philadelphia: W. B. Saunders, 1995.

Zipperer, Lorri A., and Brian P. Pace, eds. *Healthcare Resource and Reference Guide.* Chicago: American Medical Association, 1993.

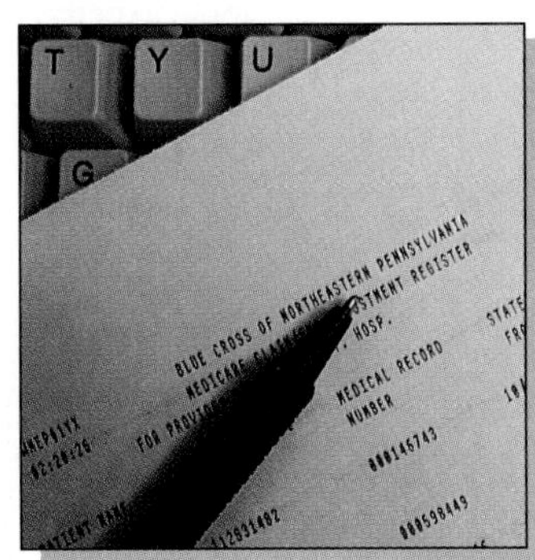

Section Three

Financial Responsibilities

AREAS OF COMPETENCE

1997 ROLE DELINEATION STUDY

ADMINISTRATIVE

- **Administrative Procedures**
- **Practice Finances**

CLINICAL

- **Patient Care**

GENERAL (Transdisciplinary)

- **Legal Concepts**
- **Operational Functions**

CHAPTER LIST

Processing Insurance Claims

CHAPTER OUTLINE

- Health Insurance: A Brief History
- Basic Insurance Terminology
- The Claims Process: An Overview
- Usual, Customary, and Reasonable Fees
- Universal Health Insurance Claim Form
- Cost-Saving Laws and Policies
- Types of Insurance
- Submitting Claims Electronically

OBJECTIVES

After completing Chapter 15, you will be able to:

- List the basic steps of the health insurance claim process.
- Describe your role in insurance claims processing.
- Explain the concept of usual, customary, and reasonable fees.
- Complete a universal health insurance claim form.
- Define Medicare and Medicaid.
- Discuss CHAMPUS/TRICARE and CHAMPVA health-care benefits programs.
- Define HMO, PPO, and IPA.
- Explain how to manage a workers' compensation case.
- Compare Blue Cross and Blue Shield coverage.
- Apply rules related to coordination of benefits.
- Explain how health maintenance organizations work.
- Define electronic claims processing.

AREAS OF COMPETENCE

1997 ROLE DELINEATION STUDY

ADMINISTRATIVE

Administrative Procedures

- Understand and apply third-party guidelines
- Obtain reimbursement through accurate claims submission
- Monitor third-party reimbursement
- Understand and adhere to managed care policies and procedures

Practice Finances

- Perform procedural and diagnostic coding

CLINICAL

Patient Care

- Coordinate patient care information with other health care providers

Key Terms

assignment of benefits
birthday rule
capitation
carrier
CHAMPUS/TRICARE
CHAMPVA
coinsurance
comorbidity
coordination of benefits
co-payment
deductible
diagnosis-related group (DRG)
disability insurance
eligibility
exclusion
explanation of benefits (EOB)
fee schedule
health insurance provider
health maintenance organization (HMO)
inpatient
managed care
Medicaid
Medicare
Medigap
outpatient
peer review organization (PRO)
premium
prognosis
provider of medical services
referral
subscriber
subscriber liability

continued

AREAS OF COMPETENCE continued

GENERAL (Transdisciplinary)

Legal Concepts

- Maintain confidentiality
- Use appropriate guidelines when releasing information
- Follow federal, state, and local legal guidelines
- Maintain awareness of federal and state health care legislation and regulations

Health Insurance: A Brief History

Health insurance was first offered in the United States in 1847. Accident insurance was created 3 years later, in response to overwhelming demand, to cover the frequent railroad and steamboat disasters of the era. By the turn of the century, almost 50 companies were selling accident insurance. At first health insurance replaced only income lost because of a disability, such as smallpox, typhus, scarlet fever, or other disease. It did not cover basic medical expenses. The emphasis remained on income replacement until 1929, when the first group coverage emerged.

First Group Coverage

In 1929 a group of schoolteachers in Dallas, Texas, joined forces to receive hospital care from Baylor Hospital on a prepaid basis. The concept of prepaid health care proved popular with hospitals and patients and later became the foundation of Blue Cross, a health insurance program that covers hospital-related costs. Later, Blue Shield was added as a nonprofit health insurance program covering the cost of doctors' care and other nonhospital-related expenses. The goal was to make health insurance accessible to as many people as possible. Today the Blue Cross and Blue Shield (BCBS) program is one of the largest insurers in the United States. The names of the Blue Cross and Blue Shield program vary by state, and in some states it is administered by a larger health-care organization. For example, Blue Cross/Blue Shield of Indiana is administered by the Associated National Group.

Health Insurance Becomes an Employment Benefit

The next major change took place during World War II. In 1943 President Franklin Roosevelt declared a "hold-the-line" wage freeze. Since all wages were frozen, workers looked for other ways to protect and increase their incomes. They began to negotiate for fringe benefits of employment, including group health insurance. After the war, group health insurance became a commonly accepted employment benefit. Today most employed people have health insurance through group plans.

Establishment of Medicare

In 1965 the federal government established **Medicare,** the first national health insurance for Americans aged 65 and older. Medicare, however, does not cover all health-care expenses (as discussed later in the chapter).

Development of Insurance Claim Filing

When health insurance was first introduced, many patients paid for their medical expenses and submitted a claim along with proof of payment. The insurer then processed the claim and reimbursed the patient according to the terms of the insurance policy. Today the medical assistant is most frequently the person who files insurance claims and handles insurers' payments to the medical practice. Some physicians still require patients to pay in full at the time of the visit and to file their own claims directly with their insurance company. Other physicians may charge a fee if the office files the claim for the patient.

Electronic Claims Processing: The New Standard

Today many practices process as many as 90% of their insurance claims electronically via computer. Medicare claims account for most electronic claims processed today. As the cost of new claims-processing software decreases, many more medical practices will file claims electronically. It is likely that all claims in the United States will eventually be filed electronically. Medicare strongly recommends that practices file Medicare claims electronically, if possible, primarily because filing electronically is a faster process than filing on paper.

Basic Insurance Terminology

The first step in understanding health and accident insurance is to learn some basic terminology. The **subscriber,** also known as the insured, is the person in whose name the insurance is carried. Sometimes the subscriber's policy also covers dependents of the subscriber, such as a spouse or children. If you are unsure whether a patient is a covered dependent, you must check with the subscriber before entering any claim.

An **assignment of benefits** is an authorization for the insurance carrier to pay the physician or practice directly. The **carrier** refers to the insurance company. In most cases, the subscriber pays the basic annual cost, or **premium,** of the health-care insurance. Some companies pay all or part of the premium for their employees. Depending on the type of insurance, the subscriber may pay a **deductible**—a fixed dollar amount that must be paid or "met" once a year before the insurer begins to cover expenses. The patient may also be required to make a **copayment,** a small fee paid at the time of service. The insurance company then pays the covered amount of the remainder of the fee. Finally, the patient may have to pay **coinsurance,** a fixed percentage of covered charges after her deductible is met.

Some expenses, such as routine eye examinations or dental care, may not be covered by an insurance company. Uncovered expenses are **exclusions.**

There are two kinds of providers. There is a **health insurance provider,** which is the insurance company. An insured person may have both a primary provider and a secondary provider. For example, some working patients older than 65 may choose to use their employers' health insurance. Medicare then becomes their secondary health insurance provider.

Another kind of provider is the **provider of medical services,** the doctor. Within certain insurance organizations, the primary care provider (PCP) is considered to be the first person patients go to for services, even if they are later referred to other providers, such as specialists.

The Claims Process: An Overview

From the time the patient enters a doctor's office until the time the insurer pays the practice for that office visit and associated services, several steps are carried out. In brief, the doctor's office performs the following services:

- Obtains patient information
- Delivers services to the patient and determines the diagnosis and fee
- Records payment from the patient and prepares insurance claim forms
- Reviews the insurer's processing of the claim, explanation of benefits, and payment

Obtaining Patient Information

You will need certain information to be able to file insurance claims for the patients of the medical practice where you work. This information is usually completed on a patient registration form, as shown in Chapter 9. When the patient first arrives, obtain or verify the following personal information:

- Name of patient
- Current home address
- Current home telephone number
- Date of birth
- Social Security number
- Next of kin or person to contact in case of an emergency

Obtain the following insurance information:

- Current employer (may be more than one)
- Employer address and telephone number
- Insurance carrier and effective date of coverage
- Insurance group plan number
- Insurance identification number (frequently the patient's Social Security number)
- Name of subscriber or insured

Obtain the following release signatures:

- Patient's signature on a form authorizing release of information to the insurance carrier (not required by Blue Shield; original contract is authorization)
- Patient's signature on a form for assignment of benefits

After you obtain personal and insurance information and release signatures from the patient, make a copy of the patient's insurance card, front and back, to include in the patient's record. Also record the effective date of insurance coverage because services performed before this date may be excluded from claims. To reduce possible payment problems, remind the patient before a service is performed if it might not be covered.

When obtaining insurance information, you must also determine whether the patient has more than one insurance policy. This information must be included on the claim form to avoid duplicate payment, which is a type of fraud. Avoiding duplicate payment is called coordination of benefits, discussed later in this chapter.

Delivering Services to the Patient

To ensure accuracy in claims processing, any services delivered to the patient in the office by the physician or other members of the health-care team must be entered into the patient record. Referrals to outside physicians or specialists must be entered into the record.

Physician's Services. The physician who examines the patient notes the patient's symptoms in the medical record. The physician also notes a diagnosis and treatment plan (including prescribed medications) and specifies if and when the patient should return for a follow-up visit. After completing the visit with the patient, the physician writes the diagnosis, treatment, and, sometimes, the fee on a charge slip and instructs the patient to give you the charge slip before leaving.

It will be your responsibility to translate the medical terminology on the charge slip into precise descriptions of medical services and procedural and diagnosis codes on the insurance claim form. The description (nomenclature) and codes are usually obtained from the *Physicians' Current Procedural Terminology* (CPT) manual, published annually by the American Medical Association (AMA). A sample page is shown in Figure 15-1.

Referrals to Other Services. You may be asked to secure authorization from the insurance company for additional procedures. If so, call the insurance company to explain the procedures and obtain approval and an authorization number. Write this number on a **referral** form, an authorization from your medical practice for the patient to receive the referred services. Send one copy of the referral form to the insurer and keep one copy for the practice records.

Frequently you will be asked to arrange an appointment for the referred services, particularly if the physician believes they are urgently needed. For example, a physician may send a patient for a specialist's evaluation or x-ray on the same day the patient visits your office.

Preparing the Insurance Claim Form

Everyone who receives services from a doctor in the practice where you work is responsible for paying the practice for those services. When the patient brings you the charge slip from the doctor, you may, depending on the policy of your practice:

- Accept payment from the patient for the full amount. The patient will submit a claim to the insurance carrier for reimbursement.
- Accept an insurance co-payment. A patient who participates in a health maintenance organization, discussed later in this chapter, will make a co-payment.
- File an insurance claim on behalf of the patient directly to the insurance company.

Filing the Insurance Claim. If you are going to submit the claim directly to the insurance company, you will fill out an insurance claim form, either manually or electronically. The physician will sign the form (except for Medicare claims filed by patients). You will then submit the form to the insurance carrier for payment and note in an insurance claim register, such as the one pictured in Figure 15-2, that you have filed a claim for this service. Sometimes the register is kept on the computer.

In spite of attempts to reduce paperwork in the health-care insurance field, insurers still require many forms. These are listed in Figure 15-3.

Time Limits. Claims must be filed in a timely manner. Time limits for filing claims vary from company to company. For example, some insurers will not pay a claim unless it is filed within 6 months of the date of service. The limits for Blue Cross and Blue Shield vary from state to state.

Medicare states that for services rendered from January 1 to September 30, claims must be filed by December 31 of the following year; for services rendered from October 1 through December 31, claims must be filed no later than December 31 of the second year following the service.

Medicaid states that claims must be filed no later than 1 year from the date of service. The time frame for refiling rejected claims varies by state. In Indiana, for example, if you filed a claim for a service performed on January 2, 1997, and the claim was rejected on May 31, 1997, you would have until May 31, 1998, to refile the claim.

Although Medicare and Medicaid allow quite a long time for claims to be filed, it is poor business practice to wait so long. In the typical medical practice, claims are filed 7 to 10 business days from the date of service. Some large practices file claims every day or twice a week.

Assisting the Patient With Forms. Many practices prefer to submit claims for the patient to ensure accurate submission. As a medical assistant with a strong working knowledge of claims submission, you can often help correct mistakes or misunderstandings and clarify matters for the patient. For example, suppose a patient receives a bill for $100 from your practice. She calls to say that she has paid her deductible for the year, so her insurance company should have paid 80% of the bill. You then call the patient's insurance company and learn that she still has to pay $100 to meet her deductible. If she pays the $100 bill in full, her deductible will then be met. You would then have to explain these facts to the patient.

Remember, no one can know everything about every insurance policy. You can always call the insurer to ask questions and obtain policy information. For example, suppose the doctor refers a patient to have a mammogram done at a particular hospital. You may need to call the patient's insurance company to see if it requires preauthorization for the procedure or if it requires the test to be done at a particular hospital or clinic. In either case, you may have to fill out a form from the insurance carrier and have the doctor sign it. The insurance company may instead assign the patient a preauthorization number, which must be included with the claim when it is submitted.

Do not try to interpret the patient's insurance policy or extent of coverage. Further, never assume that the patient knows how to fill out all the forms properly. It is extremely important to proofread and double-check a patient's insurance claim form. When claims are accurately

SURGERY

INTEGUMENTARY SYSTEM
Skin, Subcutaneous, and Accessory Structures

➤ INCISION AND DRAINAGE

(For excision, see 11400, et seq)

(10000–10020 have been deleted. To report, see 10060, 10061)

10040* Acne surgery (e.g., marsupialization, opening or removal of multiple milia, comedones, cysts, pustules)

10060* Incision and drainage of abscess (e.g., carbuncle, suppurative hidradenitis, cutaneous or subcutaneous abscess, cyst, furuncle, or paronychia); simple or single

10061 complicated or multiple

10080* Incision and drainage of pilonidal cyst; simple

10081 complicated

(For excision of pilonidal cyst, see 11770–11772)

(10100, 10101 have been deleted. To report, see 10060, 10061)

10120* Incision and removal of foreign body, subcutaneous tissues; simple

10121 complicated

(To report wound exploration due to penetrating trauma without laparotomy or thoracotomy, see 20100–20103, as appropriate)

10140* Incision and drainage of hematoma, seroma or fluid collection

(10141 has been deleted. To report, see 10140)

10160* Puncture aspiration of abscess, hematoma, bulla, or cyst

10180* Incision and drainage, complex, postoperative wound infection

(For secondary closure of surgical wound, see 12020, 12021, 13160)

➤ EXCISION—DEBRIDEMENT

(For dermabrasions, see 15780–15791)

(For nail debridement, see 11700–11711)

(For burn(s), see 16000–16042)

11000* Debridement of extensive eczematous or infected skin; up to 10% of body surface

11001 each additional 10% of body surface

11040 Debridement; skin, partial thickness

11041 skin, full thickness

11042 skin, and subcutaneous tissue

11043 skin, subcutaneous tissue, and muscle

11044 skin, subcutaneous tissue, muscle, and bone

➤ PARING OR CURETTEMENT

11050* Paring or curettement of benign hyperkeratotic skin lesion with or without chemical cauterization (such as verrucae or clavi) not extending through the stratum corneum (e.g., callus or wart) with or without local anesthesia; single lesion

11051 two to four lesions

11052 more than four lesions

(11060–11062 have been deleted. To report, see 11300–11313)

* = Service Includes Surgical Procedure Only • = New Code ▲ = Revised Code American Medical Association

Figure 15-1. To be sure of your coding on a claim form, you must check in the most recent edition of the *Physicians' Current Procedural Terminology* (CPT) manual.

Patient's Name	Insurance Company	Claim Filed		Payment Received		Difference (owed by patient)
		Date	Amount	Date	Amount	

Figure 15-2. After submitting a claim to an insurer, track each claim in an insurance claim register, such as the one pictured here.

filed, there is speedy reimbursement (for either the practice or the patient), which helps reduce frustration and friction in the professional environment.

Insurer's Processing and Payment

Your submitted claim for payment will undergo a number of reviews by the insurer. Currently, much of the review process occurs electronically.

Review for Medical Necessity. The insurance carrier reviews each claim to determine whether the diagnosis and accompanying treatment are compatible and whether the treatment is medically necessary. For example, if the diagnosis code indicated a sore throat and the treatment code indicated a cast for a broken leg, the claim would be denied because the treatment would not be medically necessary (or indeed appropriate) based on the diagnosis. (In this case, the error would probably have been an error in coding.)

If the diagnosis code indicated a sore throat caused by bacterial infection, however, and the treatment code indicated treatment with prescribed antibiotics, the claim would be approved because the treatment was medically necessary based on the diagnosis. You will need to know how to translate medical terminology into procedural and diagnosis codes to ensure payment for a claim.

Review for Allowable Benefits. The claims department also compares the fees the doctor charges with the benefits provided by the patient's health insurance policy. This review determines the amount of deductible or copayment the patient owes. This amount—that is, what the patient owes—is called **subscriber liability.**

Payment and Explanation of Benefits. After reviewing the claim, the insurer pays a benefit, either to the subscriber (patient) or to the practice, depending on what recipient the claim requested. With the payment, the insurer sends an **explanation of benefits (EOB)** form. If the patient receives the payment, he gets the original EOB form and the practice receives a copy (and vice versa). For each service submitted to an insurer, the EOB form gives the following information:

- Name of the subscriber and subscriber identification number

Types of Insurance Forms and Documents Used in a Medical Office

- Patient insurance identification card
- Universal health insurance claim form (HCFA-1500) (Form HCFA-1500 [12-90], Form OWCP-1500, Form RRB-1500; HCFA = Health Care Financing Administration)
- Lifetime Beneficiary Claim Authorization and Information Release
- Medicare Lifetime Assignment form
- Records Release Authorization form (for records only)
- Release and Assignment form (for records and payment)
- Assignment of Insurance Benefits form (payment and records necessary for payment)
- Release of Medical Information form (for electronic submission of claims)
- Insurance claim register (claims submitted)
- Insurance claim follow-up log (claims paid)
- Explanation of benefits form
- Explanation of Medicare benefits form (sent to patient)
- Medicare-approved Medical Necessity Statement

Figure 15-3. As a medical assistant, you will be expected to know how to use and process these types of forms.

- Name of the beneficiary
- Claim number
- Date, place, and type of service (coded)
- Amount billed by the practice
- Amount allowed (according to the subscriber's policy)
- Amount of subscriber liability (co-payment or deductible)
- Amount paid and included in the current payment
- A notation of any services not covered and an explanation of why they were not covered (for example, many insurance plans do not cover a woman's annual gynecologic examination and only a certain dollar amount of well-baby visits for infants)

Reviewing the Insurer's EOB and Payment

Verify all information on the EOB, line by line, using your records for each patient represented on the EOB. In a large practice, you will frequently receive payment and an EOB for several patients at one time. An example of a Medicare EOB is shown in Figure 15-4.

If all numbers on the EOB agree with your records, you can make the appropriate entries in the insurance follow-up log for claims paid. In a small practice, the insurance follow-up log is used to track filed claims, using such information as patient name, date the claim was filed, services the claim reflects, notations about the results of the claim, and any balance due from the patient. Larger practices tend to track claims on computer in a file called, for example, "Unpaid Claims." If all the numbers do not agree, you will need to trace the claim with the insurance company.

When a claim is rejected, the EOB states the reason. You will need to review the claim, examining all procedural and diagnosis codes for accuracy and comparing the claim with the patient's insurance information. You will probably need to speak with someone at the insurance company by telephone to resolve the claim problem.

Usual, Customary, and Reasonable Fees

The concept of usual, customary, and reasonable (UCR) fees was originally developed by Congress to pay medical insurance claims under Medicare. (Under Medicare Part B, the terms *customary* and *prevailing* correspond to *usual* and *customary*.)

- The *usual* fee is the average fee a physician charges for a service or procedure.
- The *customary* fee is the prevailing fee for that service or procedure in the geographic region.
- The *reasonable* fee is the generally accepted fee a physician charges for an exceptionally difficult or complicated service.

The UCR system meets the need for a flexible **fee schedule,** or price list, for medical services that can reflect regional cost differences and differences in medical education and specialty. A general practitioner (GP) in a rural practice, for instance, probably has fewer educational and overhead expenses than a neurosurgeon at a leading research-oriented hospital in a major city. Thus, the neurosurgeon's fee for examining a patient with a head injury will be higher than the GP's fee for a similar examination. Both fees may be considered appropriate if they meet the UCR standard. If the GP charges much more and the neurosurgeon charges much less for the examination than their regional peers do, the GP's fee may be the one that is considered unreasonable, even if it is still much lower than the neurosurgeon's fee.

The UCR rate is always the lowest of the following: the fee submitted, the provider's usual fee profile (total cost of all procedures performed by that provider, divided by total number of procedures performed), and the customary profile for the area. There is, however, a growing tendency to determine fees by national, rather than regional, trends.

Customary Fee

The customary fee is defined as either the average fee charged for the procedure by similar doctors in the same region or the ninetieth percentile of the fees charged for the procedure by similar doctors in the same area. The ninetieth percentile is usually calculated by the insurance company. The company determines the total number of doctors in a given geographic area, such as a county, who perform a particular procedure and the fee each doctor charges for that procedure. For example, suppose that a major city has 125 physicians who perform a particular in-office procedure. For this procedure, 30 doctors charge \$500, 30 charge \$600, 20 charge \$650, 20 charge \$700, 15 charge \$750, and 10 charge \$800. The customary fee listing, or profile, is as follows:

- Cases 1–30 billed at \$500
- Cases 31–60 billed at \$600
- Cases 61–80 billed at \$650
- Cases 81–100 billed at \$700
- Cases 101–115 billed at \$750
- Cases 116–125 billed at \$800

In this example, the ninetieth percentile of the 125 doctors is 112.5 ($125 \times 0.9 = 112.5$). The number 112.5 falls into the category of cases billed at \$750 (cases 101–115). All charges that are below that figure are said to be within the ninetieth percentile and are therefore covered by the UCR ninetieth percentile payment. All offices that charge above the ninetieth percentile are paid only the \$750 customary fee. Note, however, that the *average* fee for this procedure is much lower—\$634.

Calculating Customary Fees. In most cases, the insurance industry has already calculated average fees. Occasionally, however, you may need to calculate a customary fee. For example, you might calculate it at the doctor's re-

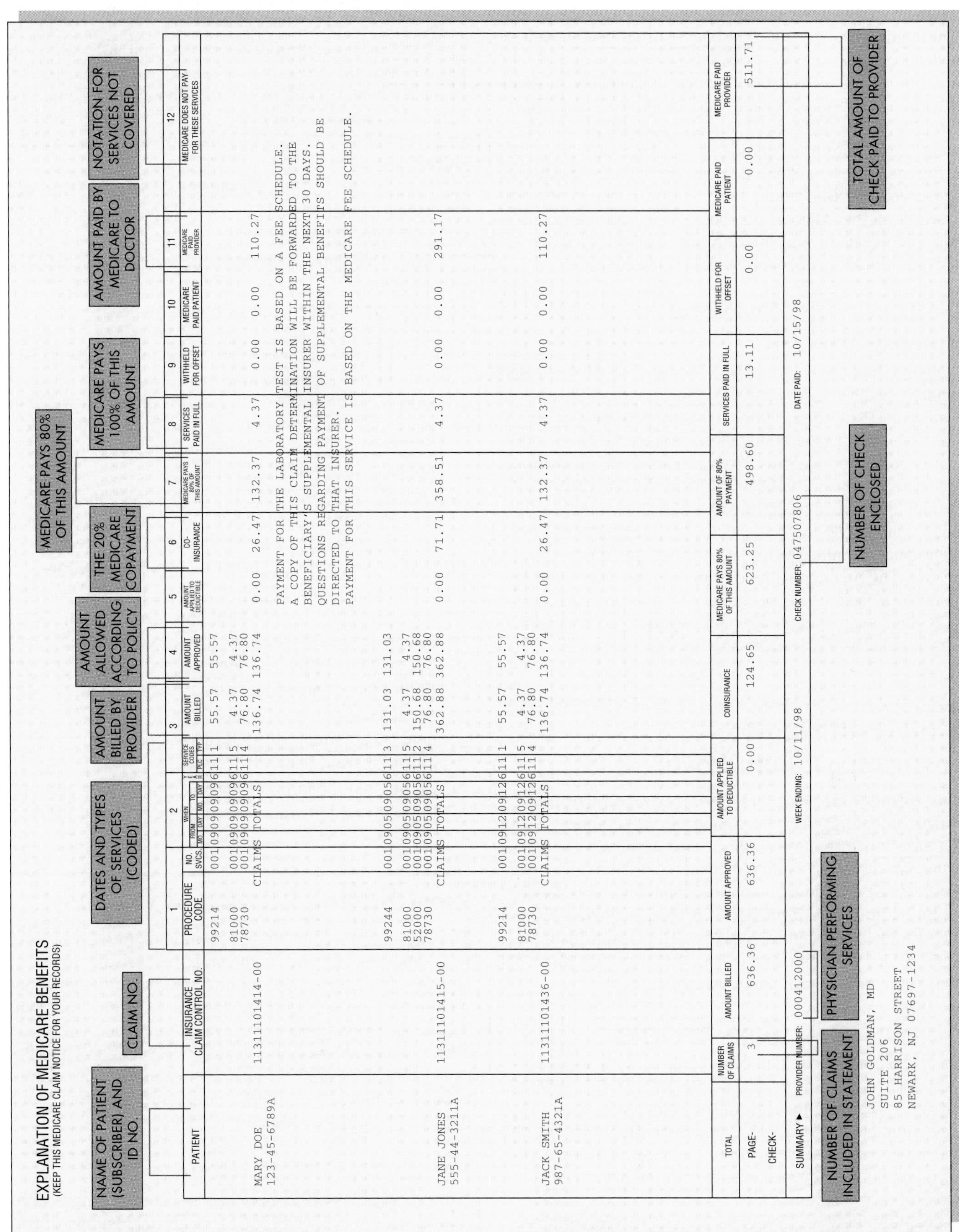

EXPLANATION OF MEDICARE BENEFITS
(KEEP THIS MEDICARE CLAIM NOTICE FOR YOUR RECORDS)

		1	2								3	4	5	6	7	8	9	10	11	12
PATIENT	INSURANCE CLAIM CONTROL NO.	PROCEDURE CODE	NO. SVCS.	WHEN FROM MO.	DAY	TO MO.	DAY	YEAR	SERVICE CODES PLC	TYP	AMOUNT BILLED	AMOUNT APPROVED	AMOUNT APPLIED TO DEDUCTIBLE	CO-INSURANCE	MEDICARE PAYS 80% OF THIS AMOUNT	SERVICES PAID IN FULL	WITHHELD FOR OFFSET	MEDICARE PAID PATIENT	MEDICARE PAID PROVIDER	MEDICARE DOES NOT PAY FOR THESE SERVICES
		99214	001	09	09	09	09	6	11	1	55.57	55.57								
		81000	001	09	09	09	09	6	11	5	4.37	4.37								
		78730	001	09	09	09	09	6	11	4	76.80	76.80								
MARY DOE 123-45-6789A	11311101414-00	CLAIMS TOTALS									136.74	136.74	0.00	26.47	132.37	4.37	0.00	0.00	110.27	
		99244	001	09	05	09	05	6	11	3	131.03	131.03								
		81000	001	09	05	09	05	6	11	5	4.37	4.37								
		52000	001	09	05	09	05	6	11	2	150.68	150.68								
		78730	001	09	05	09	05	6	11	4	76.80	76.80								
JANE JONES 555-44-3211A	11311101415-00	CLAIMS TOTALS									362.88	362.88	0.00	71.71	358.51	4.37	0.00	0.00	291.17	
		99214	001	09	12	09	12	6	11	1	55.57	55.57								
		81000	001	09	12	09	12	6	11	5	4.37	4.37								
		78730	001	09	12	09	12	6	11	4	76.80	76.80								
JACK SMITH 987-65-4321A	11311101436-00	CLAIMS TOTALS									136.74	136.74	0.00	26.47	132.37	4.37	0.00	0.00	110.27	

PAYMENT FOR THE LABORATORY TEST IS BASED ON A FEE SCHEDULE.
A COPY OF THIS CLAIM DETERMINATION WILL BE FORWARDED TO THE BENEFICIARY'S SUPPLEMENTAL INSURER WITHIN THE NEXT 30 DAYS.
QUESTIONS REGARDING PAYMENT OF SUPPLEMENTAL BENEFITS SHOULD BE DIRECTED TO THAT INSURER.
PAYMENT FOR THIS SERVICE IS BASED ON THE MEDICARE FEE SCHEDULE.

TOTAL	NUMBER OF CLAIMS	AMOUNT BILLED	AMOUNT APPROVED	AMOUNT APPLIED TO DEDUCTIBLE	COINSURANCE	MEDICARE PAYS 80% OF THIS AMOUNT	AMOUNT OF 80% PAYMENT	SERVICES PAID IN FULL	WITHHELD FOR OFFSET	MEDICARE PAID PATIENT	MEDICARE PAID PROVIDER
PAGE-	3	636.36	636.36	0.00	124.65	623.25	498.60	13.11	0.00	0.00	511.71
CHECK-											

SUMMARY ▶ PROVIDER NUMBER: 000412000 WEEK ENDING: 10/11/98 CHECK NUMBER: 047507806 DATE PAID: 10/15/98

JOHN GOLDMAN, MD
SUITE 206
85 HARRISON STREET
NEWARK, NJ 07697-1234

Figure 15-4. The insurer sends the explanation of benefits (EOB) form to both the subscriber and the medical practice.

quest to establish the fee for a new service or procedure. You might calculate it at the request of an insurer that is reviewing its fees.

Some practices use guidebooks published by medical consulting firms to set fees. One example is *The Physician Fee Guide,* published annually by Practice Management Information Corporation in Los Angeles. This guide lists fees for all current procedural terminology (CPT) codes. To use the guide, look up the location of your practice at the back of the book, find your geographic conversion factor, and multiply the fee by that factor to arrive at the recommended fee for your practice.

UCR Fees and Federally Funded Insurance

Congress has applied the UCR concept to all federally funded medical insurance programs, such as Medicare, Medicaid, CHAMPUS/TRICARE, and CHAMPVA. Physicians who participate in any of these federally funded programs opt to receive direct payment for services billed to Medicare, Medicaid, CHAMPUS/TRICARE, or CHAMPVA. By law, they must accept the UCR fee as payment in full. They cannot bill the patient for the difference between their usual fee and the UCR fee, as they can with a private insurer. The private insurance industry has recognized the value of a flexible fee schedule and has largely adopted UCR fees, even though federal law does not dictate the fees or policies of private insurance companies.

Universal Health Insurance Claim Form

The Health Care Financing Administration (HCFA), a congressional agency, designed form number 1500 (HCFA-1500) to handle Medicare and Medicaid claims. It is by far the most common insurance claim form (see Figure 15-5). It is so common that many practices stock it by the carton. The form has also been approved by the AMA Council on Medical Services. The Health Insurance Association of America (HIAA) recommends that its member insurance companies accept the form.

Acceptance by Many Insurers

Many insurance companies, although they may have their own claim forms, accept the HCFA-1500. When a patient gives you the insurance company's form, you may complete the HCFA-1500 and attach that form to the patient's form to be sent to the insurance carrier. If you have any doubt, however, check with the insurance company for its procedures.

Learning how to complete the HCFA-1500 properly represents a major step toward mastering insurance processing. As with all insurance claims, completing the HCFA-1500 is a simple process if you follow the directions shown in Procedure 15-1.

Optical Character Reader Scanning

The most recent edition of the HCFA-1500 form, which is the one you must use, has a special red ink for optical character reader (OCR) scanning. Photocopies cannot be scanned. Therefore, you must fill out an original form for each submission. Here are some tips for filling out the HCFA-1500 for an OCR.

1. Never enter data in a delete box, or field. This will cause the entire line to be deleted when scanned. The claim will be rejected.
2. Keep each entry inside its field, without touching the field lines.
3. Align the form in the printer or typewriter so that characters are entered in the proper field. Three boxes appear at the top left of the form marked PICA to help you align and size text. Clear, black, 10-point type (Courier or the equivalent) is preferred. Depending on the software program used in your office, electronic prompts may appear to remind you to align the form when entering data.
4. Do not enter any data by hand. OCRs may not be able to scan it. Clear, black, 10-point pica characters from a typewriter or laser printer are preferred.
5. Use all uppercase (CAPITAL) letters for all entries.
6. If you make an error, do not strike it out or delete it with correction tape or fluid and then retype it. OCRs cannot read items that are crossed out. Instead, reenter the data on the next line.
7. Do not use colored ink. OCRs cannot read it.
8. Do not use the abbreviation N/A to indicate that the field is "not applicable." If there is no information for a field, leave it blank.
9. Do not fold the form for mailing or any other purpose. If it is creased, it will not feed properly into an OCR.

Cost-Saving Laws and Policies

The rising cost of health care continues to be a leading economic, social, and political issue. Private insurers, federally funded program administrators, and health-care providers alike are working toward solutions that will control health-care costs for every American. There has been progress through the signing of several laws and the establishment of new national health-care policies. These policies include diagnosis-related groups, the prospective payment system, and utilization review.

Diagnosis-Related Groups

Congress has passed several laws to control rising health-care costs and has changed Medicare regulations drastically since the 1970s. At the same time, commercial insurers have also tried to cut costs where possible, and new insurers with innovative methods of reducing costs and paperwork have come into existence.

APPROVED OMB-0938-0008

PLEASE DO NOT STAPLE IN THIS AREA

CARRIER

PICA **HEALTH INSURANCE CLAIM FORM** PICA

1. MEDICARE (Medicare #) MEDICAID (Medicaid #) CHAMPUS (Sponsor's SSN) CHAMPVA (VA File #) GROUP HEALTH PLAN (SSN or ID) FECA BLK LUNG (SSN) OTHER (ID)

1a. INSURED'S I.D. NUMBER (FOR PROGRAM IN ITEM 1)

2. PATIENT'S NAME (Last Name, First Name, Middle Initial)

3. PATIENT'S BIRTH DATE MM DD YY SEX M F

4. INSURED'S NAME (Last Name, First Name, Middle Initial)

5. PATIENT'S ADDRESS (No., Street)

6. PATIENT RELATIONSHIP TO INSURED Self Spouse Child Other

7. INSURED'S ADDRESS (No., Street)

CITY STATE

8. PATIENT STATUS Single Married Other

CITY STATE

ZIP CODE TELEPHONE (Include Area Code) ( )

Employed Full-Time Student Part-Time Student

ZIP CODE TELEPHONE (INCLUDE AREA CODE) ( )

9. OTHER INSURED'S NAME (Last Name, First Name, Middle Initial)

10. IS PATIENT'S CONDITION RELATED TO:

11. INSURED'S POLICY GROUP OR FECA NUMBER

a. OTHER INSURED'S POLICY OR GROUP NUMBER

a. EMPLOYMENT? (CURRENT OR PREVIOUS) YES NO

a. INSURED'S DATE OF BIRTH MM DD YY SEX M F

b. OTHER INSURED'S DATE OF BIRTH MM DD YY SEX M F

b. AUTO ACCIDENT? YES NO PLACE (State)

b. EMPLOYER'S NAME OR SCHOOL NAME

c. EMPLOYER'S NAME OR SCHOOL NAME

c. OTHER ACCIDENT? YES NO

c. INSURANCE PLAN NAME OR PROGRAM NAME

d. INSURANCE PLAN NAME OR PROGRAM NAME

10d. RESERVED FOR LOCAL USE

d. IS THERE ANOTHER HEALTH BENEFIT PLAN? YES NO *If yes*, return to and complete item 9 a-d.

READ BACK OF FORM BEFORE COMPLETING & SIGNING THIS FORM.

12. PATIENT'S OR AUTHORIZED PERSON'S SIGNATURE I authorize the release of any medical or other information necessary to process this claim. I also request payment of government benefits either to myself or to the party who accepts assignment below.

SIGNED DATE

13. INSURED'S OR AUTHORIZED PERSON'S SIGNATURE I authorize payment of medical benefits to the undersigned physician or supplier for services described below.

SIGNED

PATIENT AND INSURED INFORMATION

14. DATE OF CURRENT: MM DD YY ILLNESS (First symptom) OR INJURY (Accident) OR PREGNANCY(LMP)

15. IF PATIENT HAS HAD SAME OR SIMILAR ILLNESS. GIVE FIRST DATE MM DD YY

16. DATES PATIENT UNABLE TO WORK IN CURRENT OCCUPATION FROM MM DD YY TO MM DD YY

17. NAME OF REFERRING PHYSICIAN OR OTHER SOURCE

17a. I.D. NUMBER OF REFERRING PHYSICIAN

18. HOSPITALIZATION DATES RELATED TO CURRENT SERVICES FROM MM DD YY TO MM DD YY

19. RESERVED FOR LOCAL USE

20. OUTSIDE LAB? YES NO $ CHARGES

21. DIAGNOSIS OR NATURE OF ILLNESS OR INJURY. (RELATE ITEMS 1,2,3 OR 4 TO ITEM 24E BY LINE)

1. ___ . __ 3. ___ . __

2. ___ . __ 4. ___ . __

22. MEDICAID RESUBMISSION CODE ORIGINAL REF. NO.

23. PRIOR AUTHORIZATION NUMBER

24. A DATE(S) OF SERVICE From MM DD YY To MM DD YY	B Place of Service	C Type of Service	D PROCEDURES, SERVICES, OR SUPPLIES (Explain Unusual Circumstances) CPT/HCPCS MODIFIER	E DIAGNOSIS CODE	F $ CHARGES	G DAYS OR UNITS	H EPSDT Family Plan	I EMG	J COB	K RESERVED FOR LOCAL USE
1										
2										
3										
4										
5										
6										

25. FEDERAL TAX I.D. NUMBER SSN EIN

26. PATIENT'S ACCOUNT NO.

27. ACCEPT ASSIGNMENT? (For govt. claims, see back) YES NO

28. TOTAL CHARGE $

29. AMOUNT PAID $

30. BALANCE DUE $

31. SIGNATURE OF PHYSICIAN OR SUPPLIER INCLUDING DEGREES OR CREDENTIALS (I certify that the statements on the reverse apply to this bill and are made a part thereof.)

SIGNED DATE

32. NAME AND ADDRESS OF FACILITY WHERE SERVICES WERE RENDERED (If other than home or office)

33. PHYSICIAN'S, SUPPLIER'S BILLING NAME, ADDRESS, ZIP CODE & PHONE #

PIN# GRP#

PHYSICIAN OR SUPPLIER INFORMATION

790-0115 (12/90) (OCR) 1 pt.

(APPROVED BY AMA COUNCIL ON MEDICAL SERVICE 8/88) *PLEASE PRINT OR TYPE* FORM HCFA-1500 (12-90) FORM OWCP-1500 FORM RRB-1500

Figure 15-5. The HCFA-1500 is the universal health insurance claim form accepted by most insurers, even if they have their own forms.

PROCEDURE 15-1

Completing the Universal Health Insurance Claim Form (HCFA-1500)

Objective: To complete the HCFA-1500 correctly

Materials: Patient record, HCFA-1500 form, typewriter or computer, patient ledger card

Method
The numbers below correspond to the numbered fields on the HCFA-1500.

Patient Information Section

1. Check the appropriate insurance box.

1a. Enter the patient's insurance number. Different insurers require you to fill out this field differently. CHAMPUS/TRICARE, for instance, requires the patient's Social Security number. For Medicaid or Medicare, use the patient's Medicaid or Medicare number. To be sure, ask to see the patient's insurance or Medicare card. For Medicaid, the recipient must always be the patient.

2. Enter the patient's name in this order: last name, first name, middle initial (if any).

3. Enter the patient's birth date using two digits each for the month, day, and year. For example, for a patient born on February 9, 1954, enter 02-09-54. Indicate the sex of the patient: male or female.

4. If the insured and the patient are the same person, enter SAME. If not, enter the policyholder's name. For CHAMPUS/TRICARE claims, enter the sponsor's (service person's) full name.

5. Enter the patient's mailing address, city, state, and zip code.

6. Enter the patient's relationship to the insured. If they are the same, mark SELF. For CHAMPUS/TRICARE, enter the patient's relationship to the sponsor.

7. Enter the insured's mailing address, city, state, zip code, and telephone number. If this address is the same as the patient's, enter SAME.

8. Indicate the patient's marital, employment, and student status by checking boxes.

9. Enter the last name, first name, and middle initial of any other insured person whose policy might cover the patient. If the claim is for Medicare and the patient has a Medigap policy, enter SAME.

9a. Enter the policy or group number for the other insured person. If this is a Medigap policy, enter MEDIGAP before the policy number.

9b. Enter the date of birth and sex of the other insured person (field 9).

9c. Enter the other insured's employer or school name. (Note: If this is a Medicare claim, enter the claims-processing address for the Medigap insurer from field 9. If this is a Medicaid claim and other insurance is available, note it in field 1a and in 2, and enter the requested policy information.

9d. Enter the other insured's insurance plan or program name. If the plan is Medigap and HCFA has assigned it a nine-digit number called PAYERID, enter that number here. On an attached sheet, give the complete mailing address for all other insurance information, and enter the word ATTACHMENT in 10d.

10. Check the appropriate YES or NO boxes in a, b, and c to indicate whether the patient's place of employment, an auto accident, or other type of accident precipitated the patient's condition. For PLACE, enter the two-letter state postal abbreviation.

For Medicaid claims, enter MCD and the Medicaid number at line 10d. For all other claims, enter ATTACHMENT here if there is other insurance information. Be sure the full names and addresses of the other insurer appear on the attached sheet. Also, code the insurer as follows:

MSP Medicare Secondary Payer
MG Medigap
SP Supplemental Employer
MCD Medicaid

11. Enter the insured's policy or group number. For Medicare claims, fill out this section only if there is other insurance primary to Medicare; otherwise, enter NONE.

11a. Enter the insured's date of birth and sex as in field 3, if the insured is not the patient.

11b. Enter the employer's name or school name here. This information will determine if Medicare is the primary payer.

11c. Enter the insurance plan or program name.

11d. Check YES or NO to indicate if there is another health benefit plan. If YES, you must complete 9a through 9d. Failure to do so will cause the claim to be denied.

12. Have the patient or an authorized representative sign and date the form here. If a representative signs, have the representative indicate the relationship to the patient.

13. Have the insured (the patient or another individual) sign here. This signature authorizes payment of Medigap benefits.

Physician Information Section

14. Enter the date of the current illness, injury, or pregnancy. Use two digits to indicate the month, day, and year, as you did in field 3.

15. *Do not complete this field.* Leave it blank for Medicare.
16. Enter the dates the patient is or was unable to work. This information could signal a workers' compensation claim.
17. Enter the name of the referring physician, clinical laboratory, or other referring source.
17a. Enter the physician's unique physician identifier number, or UPIN. (If there are several physicians involved in the claim, list their names in 17 and their UPINs in 17a. Then in field 24 list the procedure codes in the order corresponding to the order of the physicians listed in field 17.) Note that some medical professionals do not have UPINs. If so, enter one of the following, as appropriate:
    - BIA000, for a Bureau of Indian Affairs physician
    - INT000, for an intern
    - PHS000, for a Public Health Service physician
    - RES000, for a resident
    - RET00, for a retired physician
    - SLF000, for a self-referred patient
    - VAD000, for a Veterans Administration physician
    - OTH000, for anyone else
18. Enter the dates the patient was hospitalized, if at all, with the current condition.
19. Enter the date the patient was last seen by the referring physician or other medical professional.
20. Check YES if a laboratory test was performed outside the physician's office, and enter the test price. Ensure that field 32 carries the laboratory's exact name and address and the insurance carrier's nine-digit provider identification number (PIN). Check NO if the test was done in the office of the physician who is billing the insurance company.
21. Enter the multidigit *International Classification of Diseases, 9th edition, Clinical Modification* (ICD-9-CM) code number diagnosis or nature of injury. Enter up to four codes in order of importance.
22. Enter the Medicaid resubmission code and original reference number. (Note that this field is not required for Medicare.)
23. Enter the professional review organization prior authorization number for surgical procedures. (Different rules apply here for cataract surgery; check with the applicable carrier.)

24A. Enter the date of each service, procedure, or supply provided. Add the number of days for each, and enter them, in chronological order, in field 24G.

24B. Enter the two-digit place-of-service code. For example, 11 is for office, 12 is for home, and 25 is for birthing center. Your office should have a list for reference.

24C. Leave this field blank. It is reserved for insurance explanation of medicare benefits (EOMB) codes.

24D. Enter the CPT/HCPCS codes with modifiers for the procedures, services, or supplies provided.

24E. Enter the diagnosis code that applies to that procedure, as listed in field 21.

24F. Enter the dollar amount of fee charged.

24G. Enter the days or units on which the service was performed, using three digits. If a service took 3 days, as listed in 24A, enter 030. Note that 1 unit or service would be 010, 5.5 services 055, and 10 services 100.

24H. Leave this field blank.

24I. If the service was performed in an emergency room, check this field.

24J. Leave this field blank.

24K. Enter the insurance-company-assigned nine-digit physician PIN. For CHAMPUS/TRICARE, enter the physician's state license number.

25. Enter the physician's or care provider's federal tax identification number or, if he does not have one, Social Security number.
26. Enter the patient's account number assigned by your office.
27. Check YES to indicate that the physician will accept Medicare or CHAMPUS/TRICARE assignment of benefits.
28. Enter the total charge for the service.
29. Enter the amount already paid by the patient or insurance company.
30. Enter the balance due your office (subtract field 29 from field 28 to obtain this figure).
31. Have the physician or service supplier sign and date the form here.
32. Enter the name and address of the organization or individual who performed the services. If performed in the patient's home or the physician's office, leave this field blank.
33. List the billing physician's or supplier's name, address, zip code, and phone number.

Remember that the HCFA-1500 is not complicated, just detailed. If you keep that fact in mind, if you do not skip any boxes, and if you complete the fields properly, you should be able to submit claims with this form confidently and efficiently.

One law that is extremely important to you as a medical assistant is the Tax Equity and Fiscal Responsibility Act of 1982. This law uses **diagnosis-related groups (DRGs)** to set reimbursement. DRGs are groups of procedures or tests related directly to a given diagnosis that are likely to be covered by an insurer.

Relationship of Fees to DRGs. Congress passed a law in 1992 that strengthened and expanded the concept of paying a fixed amount according to DRGs. Originally intended for Medicare and now used by many insurers, these fees are based on the idea that similar medical diagnoses and similar hospital procedures should cost about the same. DRGs are assigned in the hospital *only* upon the patient's discharge from the hospital.

DRG Classification. There are almost 500 DRGs, based on the more than 10,000 codes in the *International Classification of Diseases, 9th edition, Clinical Modification* (ICD-9-CM). DRGs group ICD-9-CM codes into 25 major diagnostic categories based on organ systems.

DRGs are classified first by major diagnostic category. They are then classified by either a medical (M) or a surgical (S) code. The six variables for classifying a patient's DRG are:

- Principal diagnosis.
- Secondary diagnosis.
- Surgical procedures.
- **Comorbidity** (a preexisting condition, such as diabetes, that may cause the patient to need to stay in the hospital for at least 1 additional day) and any complications.
- Age and sex.
- Discharge status (a statement of patient condition that must be met before the patient can safely be discharged).

As stated earlier, DRGs are assigned in the hospital upon the patient's discharge. The DRGs are identified based upon primary and secondary diagnoses (and in some cases, third and fourth diagnoses), as well as any complications. For example, if the physician documents that a patient with a skull fracture was in a coma for less than 1 hour, DRG 28 is assigned. If the physician documents that the coma lasted for more than 1 hour, DRG 27 is assigned, with a resulting payment difference.

Prospective Payment System

In 1983 Congress passed the Social Security Amendment Act to reform Medicare. Title VI of this act was the prospective payment system, which greatly restructured the part of Medicare related to inpatient (hospital) services.

The objective of Title VI was to establish Medicare as a prudent buyer of health care while maintaining high-quality care. Thus, the prospective payment system pays hospitals a predetermined rate per discharge rather than a "reasonable-based" fee.

Peer Review Organizations. As a means of assuring high-quality care, the prospective payment system uses **peer review organizations (PROs).** These groups of health-care professionals check hospital diagnoses, quality of services, and patient admissions and discharges related to government-funded health care within each state. To receive payments from Medicare, a hospital must have a contract with a PRO and must undergo its periodic reviews. Medicare may make an exception if a state has a Medicare-approved hospital cost-control system.

The HCFA awards contracts to PROs to review hospitals within individual states. Although these physician-based organizations may operate slightly differently from state to state, they all perform the same basic function—checking the quality and accuracy of hospital services.

Advance Authorization. To control costs, many insurers require advance authorization from a PRO before a patient is hospitalized for some diagnoses. If the patient can be treated safely and effectively as an outpatient, the PRO will not approve payment for hospitalization. Thus, you must be aware of the diagnoses that require advance authorization for hospital admissions. To avoid nonpayment, you must check with the PRO for its current policy. For example, in the 1980s, cataract surgery often required hospitalization, but in the 1990s, the use of lasers has made cataract surgery a common outpatient procedure. Today insurers pay for hospitalization for cataract surgery only in rare instances.

Utilization Review

In addition to DRGs and PROs, there is another way medical services are reviewed to help control costs. An insurer may hire private companies to do a utilization review. In this review, company staff members examine the patient's course of treatment. For example, if a patient tore a ligament and was admitted to a hospital, the utilization review company would review the length of time the patient was in the hospital and the services that were provided there. If the length of hospitalization or list of services exceeded established standards, the review company would pass the physician's treatment plan on to an independent reviewing physician. This physician would then notify the treating physician that the treatment plan was excessive and must be reduced to acceptable cost levels.

Many insurers require that costly procedures be reviewed by a nurse or physician before authorizing payment for the procedure. As a medical assistant, you will be required to secure that authorization for any patient insured by those companies before sending the patient for the procedure.

There are exceptions in emergency cases, the procedures for which are specific to each insuring company or plan. Emergencies are usually handled in the hospital, and the hospital must request approval from the insurance company. Some insurance companies require patients to get their primary physician's approval before they can go to the emergency room. Those companies will not cover unauthorized emergency room visits. To prevent problems before they occur, document all patient information carefully, including the physician's care plan. In addition, keep this information available for utilization review.

Types of Insurance

All insurance groups or companies have their own rules and sometimes their own forms. Many companies have their own manuals, which you must keep handy in the office for reference. Representatives of the insurance companies are available to work with you, however, to answer questions and help ensure that claims are correctly filed. Their business depends on it. Never hesitate to contact an insurance company. Many have toll-free numbers for just this purpose.

Liability Insurance

Liability insurance covers injuries that are caused by the insured or that occurred on the insured's property. If an individual (or company) has home, business, automobile, or health liability insurance, the injured person can claim benefits under the insured's policy. To obtain details about coverage, contact the liability insurance company.

Disability Insurance

Disability insurance is a type of insurance that may be provided by an employer for its employees or purchased privately by self-employed individuals. Disability insurance is activated when the insured is injured or disabled. When the insured cannot work, the insurance company pays the insured a prearranged monthly amount that covers the insured's normal expenses. Generally, disability is far more expensive than life, home, or automobile insurance.

Federally Funded Programs

Several federally funded programs provide health-care insurance and assistance for specific categories of Americans. These programs include Medicare, Medicaid, CHAMPUS/TRICARE, and CHAMPVA.

Medicare. Medicare provides health insurance for citizens aged 65 and older. Certain patients under the age of 65 may also be entitled to Medicare. Such patients include those who are blind or widowed or who have serious long-term disabilities, such as chronic joint pain or kidney failure.

Medicare has two distinct parts. Part A is hospital insurance, which is billed by hospitals (or other health-care facilities). It pays most of the benefits for the following people:

- A patient who has been hospitalized (as an inpatient) up to 90 days for each benefit period. A benefit period begins the day a patient goes into the hospital and ends when that patient has not been hospitalized for 60 days.
- A patient who has been an inpatient in a skilled nursing facility (SNF) for no more than 100 days in each benefit period. A benefit period is usually 1 calendar year.
- A patient who is receiving medical care at home.
- A patient who has been diagnosed as terminally ill and needs hospice care. Medicare defines *terminally ill* as having a **prognosis** (prediction of the probable course of a disease in an individual and the chances of recovery) of 6 months or less to live. A hospice is a medical organization that provides pain relief to terminally ill patients and otherwise supports these patients and their families.
- A patient who requires psychiatric treatment. Currently Medicare covers only 190 days of psychiatric hospitalization in a patient's lifetime.
- A patient who requires respite care. Medicare provides for a respite, or short break, for the person who cares for a terminally ill patient at home. The terminally ill patient is moved to a care facility for the respite.

Medicare Part A has specific limitations and regulations governing payment. Here are just a few examples.

- Medicare Part A covers a hospital stay for most patients for 60 days. After 60 days, Medicare pays a flat rate per day for days 61–90 and a higher flat rate per day for days 91–150. After 150 days, Medicare pays nothing.
- Medicare Part A covers all SNF care for the first 20 days if the patient has been hospitalized for at least 3 days before entering the SNF. From days 21–100, Medicare requires the patient to pay a daily deductible amount. After 100 days of SNF care, Medicare pays nothing.
- Medicare has strict requirements for home health care, such as care provided by a home health aide. The patient must be unable to leave the home and must be in need of skilled nursing care, physical therapy, or speech therapy. Even then, Medicare pays for part-time care only. Any medical services or procedures for a patient receiving home health care must be ordered by a doctor and reviewed regularly by the same doctor.
- For a terminally ill patient, hospice care is covered for up to 210 days.

Medicare Part B pays most of a doctor's fee for performing a procedure or service. (It also covers care at home should a patient be confined to the home.) The remainder must be made up by the patient. The difference between the fee and the Medicare payment can amount to thousands of dollars. Instead of paying from their own pockets, recipients of Medicare Part A and Part B may purchase private insurance, called **Medigap,** to reduce the gap in coverage.

It is your responsibility to bill Medicare for Part B charges that patients incur. Legally, patients are not permitted to submit claims for reimbursement.

Part A Medicare expenses are paid for automatically by FICA (Federal Insurance Contributions Act), or Social Security, monies. These monies are provided by deductions from workers' paychecks and matching funds contributed by employers. Individuals who want Part B coverage voluntarily pay a monthly premium. A patient may qualify for Part A, Part B, or both. Whether enrolled in Part A or Part B, an individual must pay an annual or monthly deductible. The amount of this deductible is adjusted periodically by Congress.

Medicaid. **Medicaid** is a health-benefit program designed for low-income, blind, or disabled patients; families receiving aid to dependent children; foster children; and children born with birth defects. Medicaid is a health cost assistance program, not an insurance program. The federal government provides funds to all 50 states to administer Medicaid. Every state has a program to assist with medical expenses for citizens who meet its qualifications. Such programs may have different names and slightly different rules, but they provide basically the same assistance. This assistance includes:

- 12 days of **inpatient** hospital care per year (the patient is confined to the hospital and receives treatment there).
- 12 days of **outpatient** hospital care per year (the patient travels to the hospital for care).
- Laboratory services and x-rays.
- SNF care.
- Early diagnostic screening and treatment for minors (those aged 21 and younger).
- Contraception and other family planning services.

Accepting Assignment. A physician who agrees to treat Medicaid patients also agrees to accept the established Medicaid payment for covered services. This agreement is called accepting assignment. If the physician's fee is higher than the Medicaid payment, the patient cannot be billed for the difference. The physician can bill the patient for services that Medicaid does not cover, however.

Medi/Medi. Older or disabled patients who have Medicare and who cannot pay the difference between the bill and the Medicare payment may qualify for Medicare and Medicaid. This type of coverage is known as Medi/Medi. In such cases, Medicare is the primary payer, and Medicaid is the secondary payer.

False Billing or Fraud. In 1983 a law was passed that provided penalties for Medicare and Medicaid fraud. If you submit a false billing, the doctor may be fined or jailed. Doctors can also be fined for incorrectly coded procedures. To avoid these penalties, you must stay abreast of changing Medicare and Medicaid guidelines, and you must question any claim that looks suspicious.

Manuals are available from Medicare and Medicaid, and newsletters are sent to all medical practices that handle Medicare and Medicaid claims. You can contact the nearest regional Medicare, Medicaid, or Social Security office for information, booklets, or updated copies of the manuals. Updates of the Medicare and Medicaid manuals are sent in a timely manner to all medical practices that have Medicare and Medicaid patients. For example, if a Medicare policy change will go into effect in September, the agency tries to mail out updates regarding that policy in April or May.

Filing Medicare Claims

You can file Medicare claims using either the paper version or the electronic version of the HCFA-1500 form. All Medicare claims must be filed in the manner discussed earlier in this chapter in Procedure 15-1. Failure to do so may result in a reduced, suspended, or lost payment.

The patient's signature is required to process an HCFA-1500 for Medicare. In some cases, the physician's signature is also required. Often, both the patient's and the physician's signatures are on file. For example, a new patient may be asked to sign a paper copy of the HCFA-1500 in boxes 12 and 13. The copy, which is kept on file, is called a lifetime signature. If the patient is in a nursing home or hospital or is at home and cannot sign a claim form, her signature on a Lifetime Beneficiary Claim Authorization and Information Release will authorize release of information and payment. Figure 15-6 shows an example of a Lifetime Beneficiary Claim Authorization and Information Release. It is your responsibility to keep this release form in the patient's medical record. When you prepare the claim form, write or type SIGNATURE ON FILE in the patient signature field.

Because a physician cannot be assigned a Medicare number without having his signature on file, his signature is already technically on file. A physician's signature on file is essential for offices that submit claims electronically, because there is nowhere for him to sign. Many physicians appoint a representative in the office who can sign claim forms. Some have their signature made into a rubber stamp. If you use a rubber stamp for the physician's signature, you must guard the stamp with extreme care and keep it in a safe place.

Study the following tips for filing a Medicare claim electronically. (The section on electronic claims submission at the end of this chapter gives additional information.)

- Order the *Medicare Part B Reference Manual* if your office does not have it.
- Read Chapter 6 of this book, which covers electronic billing, in detail.
- Make sure that the physician or health-care provider has documented all medical services completely and correctly.
- Make sure that all diagnosis and procedural codes are correct.

Total Allowable Medicare Charge. The total allowable Medicare charge is always made up of the following two parts:

- The amount Medicare pays the physician or health-care provider (usually 80% of the bill) *after* the patient's $100 annual deductible is met
- The remaining 20% of the bill due from the patient (called a co-payment)

NEW CITY MEDICAL GROUP

787 Olden Street, Hastings, NY 10807   (914) 555-1599

LIFETIME BENEFICIARY CLAIM AUTHORIZATION AND INFORMATION RELEASE

Name of Patient: ______________________________

Medicare ID Number: ______________________________

I request that payment of authorized Medicare benefits be made either to me or on my behalf to (physician/supplier's name) or any services furnished me by that physician/supplier. I authorize any holder of medical information about me to release to the Health Care Financing Administration and its agents any information needed to determine these benefits or the benefits payable to related services.

I understand my signature requests that payment be made and authorizes release of medical information necessary to pay the claim. If other insurance is indicated in item 9 of the HCFA-1500 claim form or elsewhere on other approved claim forms or electronically submitted claims, my signature authorizes releasing of the information to the insurer or agency shown.

In Medicare assigned cases, the physician or supplier agrees to accept the charge determination of the Medicare carrier as the full charge, and the patient is responsible only for the deductible, coinsurance, and noncovered services. Coinsurance and the deductible are based upon the charge determination of the Medicare carrier.

Patient's Signature: ______________________   Date: ______________________

Figure 15-6. A Lifetime Beneficiary Claim Authorization and Information Release form is kept in a patient's medical record and is used when a doctor's office is unable to obtain signatures on insurance claim forms for a Medicare patient.

A patient may be billed for any services not covered by Medicare, provided that the patient has been informed in advance. It is your duty to inform the patient whenever Medicare will not cover a service.

Medicare Coding. Some claims are rejected because of incorrect coding. Medicare uses three systems of coding. They are:

- CPT codes, except for anesthesiology.
- HCFA's Common Procedure Coding System (HCPCS), known as "hic-pics," which are nationwide alphanumeric codes.
- State or regional contractors' alphanumeric codes.

HCFA's Common Procedure Coding System. HCFA's Common Procedure Coding System (HCPCS) was developed to code and describe the many services, materials, and drugs not covered by the CPT code book. HCPCS coding begins with A0000 and runs through V5999. Familiarize yourself with the basic groupings to avoid confusing national codes with regional codes. Regional codes begin with W, X, Y, and Z.

Special modifying codes for unusual services that are not adequately covered by HCPCS carry double letters, from AA through ZZ. To understand this coding in greater depth, you can obtain the HCPCS manual from the Superintendent of Documents, U.S. Government Printing Office, Washington, D.C. 20402. Most materials from the Government Printing Office are either free or inexpensive.

State or Regional Codes. State or regional codes for procedures and services are assigned and updated by each regional Medicare contractor. This coding system begins with W0000 and ends with Z9999. Special services or procedures are given a double alphabetic code, from WA through ZZ.

New Fee Schedule of the 1990s. To correct what Congress perceived as growing inequities in the Medicare system, a new fee schedule was established in phases from 1991 to 1996. Although many private insurers still use the former system, the new schedule replaces Medicare's former system of reasonable charges. Medicare's new fee schedule regulates payment for all services and procedures provided by doctors, based on the following factors:

- The doctor's work, office, and other overhead costs
- The geographic practice cost index (GPCI)—known as "gypsy"—which takes regional cost differences into account (A doctor in Billings, Montana, for instance, pays less to run a practice than a similar one in San Francisco, California.)
- Inflation

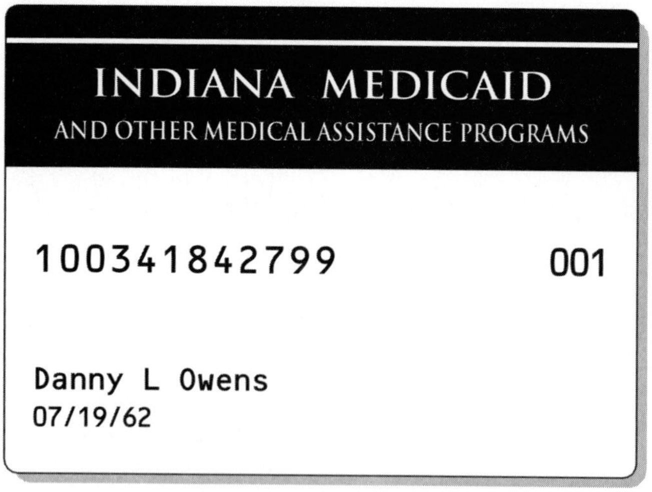

INDIANA MEDICAID
AND OTHER MEDICAL ASSISTANCE PROGRAMS

100341842799 001

Danny L Owens
07/19/62

Figure 15-7. A Medicaid card gives the patient's name and identification (or Social Security) number.

Participating Versus Nonparticipating. For participating doctors, Medicare sets what is called a "par fee" schedule. This schedule outlines the fees the participating doctors can charge. The practice submits these claims directly to Medicare, and Medicare sends the check to the practice. For nonparticipating doctors—doctors who do not accept Medicare assignment—Medicare sets a "non par fee" schedule. The patient pays the practice, and the patient receives reimbursement from Medicare. It is illegal for nonparticipating doctors to collect more than the non par fee schedule permits.

Filing Medicaid Claims

As with Medicare, you can file Medicaid claims using either the paper version or the electronic version of the HCFA-1500 form. Medicaid benefits can vary greatly from state to state. It is important to understand the Medicaid guidelines in your state so that your office's Medicaid reimbursement is prompt and trouble-free. Following are some suggestions.

1. Always ask for a Medicaid card from all patients who state that they are entitled to Medicaid. (Figure 15-7 shows an example of a Medicaid card. Medicaid cards vary from state to state.) Do not submit a claim to Medicaid if the patient cannot prove Medicaid membership. Doing so may constitute fraud. You may call Medicaid to verify eligibility.
2. Check the patient's Medicaid card, which is issued monthly and shows the patient's **eligibility**—whether the patient qualifies—for services or procedures. Eligibility is based on how much income the patient reported for the previous month.
3. Ensure that the physician signs all claims. Then send them to the state's Medicaid-approved contractor (which pays on behalf of the state) or to the state department that administers Medicaid (for example, the state department of social services or public health). Check the regulations with the state Medicaid office if you are unsure where to send the claim.
4. Unless the patient has a medical emergency, Medicaid often requires authorization before services are performed. Authorization must be obtained from the state Medicaid office in writing. You can obtain preliminary authorization by telephone, but you must follow up to get written approval.
5. Check the time limit on claim submissions. It can be as short as 2 months or as long as 1 year. Verify deadlines with your local Medicaid office.
6. Meet the deadlines. If a Medicaid claim is submitted after the time limit, the claim may be rejected.
7. Treat Medicaid patients with the same professionalism and courtesy that you extend to other patients. Simply because a patient qualifies for Medicaid assistance does not mean that the patient is in any way inferior to those with private insurance.

Programs Covering Members of the Military

The U.S. government provides health-care benefits to families of current military personnel, retired military personnel, and veterans through the CHAMPUS/TRICARE and CHAMPVA programs. CHAMPUS stands for Civilian Health and Medical Program of the Uniformed Services, and CHAMPVA stands for the Civilian Health and Medical Program of the Veterans Administration.

CHAMPUS/TRICARE. At the end of World War II, many medical facilities at government bases were closed. When the Korean War again created a need for medical services for families of military personnel, Congress filled that gap with CHAMPUS in 1956. In the 1980s, in an effort to control health-care costs within CHAMPUS, several states began to test out pilot programs offering families choices of ways in which they could use their military health-care benefits. The success of these programs led the Defense Department to establish a major reform in CHAMPUS, resulting in the **CHAMPUS/TRICARE** program. This program has been phased in gradually, beginning in the early 1990s, with completion by mid-1997.

CHAMPUS/TRICARE offers families three choices of health-care benefits:

- TRICARE Prime, based on the low-cost structure of a health maintenance organization, which you will read about later in this chapter
- TRICARE Extra, a network of health-care providers that families can use on a case-by-case basis, without a required enrollment
- TRICARE Standard, based on the same benefits and cost structure as the original CHAMPUS program

CHAMPUS/TRICARE is not a health insurance plan. Rather, it is a health-care benefit for families of uniformed personnel and retirees from the uniformed services (Figure 15-8). The uniformed services include the Army, Navy, Marines, Air Force, Coast Guard, Public Health Service, and National Oceanic and Atmospheric Administration.

The CHAMPUS/TRICARE sponsor, the person in uniform, is not eligible for CHAMPUS/TRICARE-paid medical care until he retires. Upon retirement, the sponsor receives prepaid medical care from a local physician's practice (under contract) or from a government health facility (usually, the nearest Army or Navy hospital).

CHAMPVA. Congress created **CHAMPVA** in 1973, using the original CHAMPUS program as a model. CHAMPVA covers the expenses of the families (dependent spouses and children) of veterans with total, permanent service-connected disabilities. It also covers surviving spouses and dependent children of veterans who died in the line of duty or as a result of service-connected disabilities.

Medical Services Covered by CHAMPUS/TRICARE and CHAMPVA. Unless you work in a military-related facility, you will probably see CHAMPUS/TRICARE and CHAMPVA patients only for emergency services or for nonemergency care that a military base cannot provide. Be aware, however, that CHAMPUS/TRICARE covers the following inpatient services:

- Anesthesia
- Blood treatments
- Chemotherapy and radiation therapy
- Computed tomography (CT) scans
- Hospice care
- Injections and intravenous infusions
- Intensive coronary unit treatment
- Laboratory tests
- Magnetic resonance imaging (MRI)
- Medical equipment, dressings, and supplies
- Medications
- Newborn care unit treatment
- Operating room and recovery room
- Oxygen therapy
- Physical therapy room expenses
- Semiprivate room
- Transplants (liver, heart, and lung)
- X-rays

CHAMPUS/TRICARE covers the following outpatient services: cardiac rehabilitation programs, consultations, infant care, mental health services, surgery (not all procedures), physicians' services, and other medical care. Within strict limits, CHAMPUS/TRICARE also covers family planning and biofeedback services. If in doubt about whether a procedure, service, or other item is covered, contact OCHAMPUS (the agency governing CHAMPUS/TRICARE) or OCHAMPVA (the agency governing CHAMPVA), both located in Aurora, Colorado.

CHAMPUS/TRICARE or CHAMPVA must authorize all nonemergency inpatient care in a civilian medical facility before admission. Otherwise CHAMPUS/TRICARE or CHAMPVA will not pay the claim. To document authorization, you must have a completed nonavailability

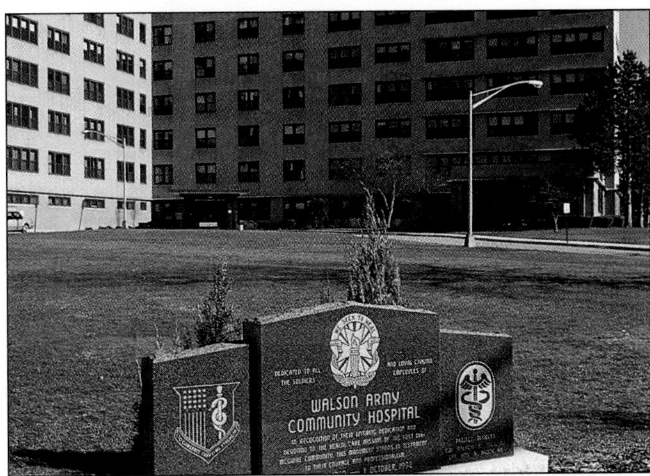

Figure 15-8. CHAMPUS/TRICARE covers health-care services for family members of military personnel and military retirees at facilities such as the military base hospital pictured here.

statement, Form DD1251, usually sent electronically from the nearest military base. This requirement is waived if the patient lives 40 miles or more from a base. No advance authorization is required in an emergency.

Following are examples of services that are *not* covered by CHAMPUS/TRICARE or CHAMPVA:

- Abortions
- Acupuncture
- Artificial insemination
- Chiropractic treatment
- Eyeglasses or contact lenses
- Food or vitamins outside the hospital setting
- Hearing examinations
- Orthopedic shoes
- Private hospital rooms
- Retirement homes

CHAMPUS/TRICARE and CHAMPVA Eligibility. You must verify CHAMPUS/TRICARE eligibility. All CHAMPUS/TRICARE patients should have a valid identification card. To receive CHAMPUS/TRICARE benefits, eligible individuals must be enrolled in the Defense Enrollment Eligibility Reporting System (DEERS), a computer database.

Eligibility for CHAMPVA is determined by the nearest Veterans Affairs medical center. Contact this center if any questions arise. Patients can choose the doctor they wish after CHAMPVA eligibility is confirmed.

CHAMPUS/TRICARE and CHAMPVA Participation Versus Nonparticipation. Under Medicare, participating doctors must see all Medicare patients who seek their care. Under CHAMPUS/TRICARE and CHAMPVA, participating doctors have the option of deciding whether to accept patients on a case-by-case basis. Make sure you know the policy of the doctor or doctors in your office on this issue.

Processing CHAMPUS/TRICARE and CHAMPVA Claims. Both CHAMPUS/TRICARE and CHAMPVA use the HCFA-1500 form. You must file a claim with this form no later than December 31 of the year after the year medical services were provided. When processing a claim, you must:

1. Determine eligibility. Ask to see the patient's identification card. Check the name on the card, card number, issue date, effective date, and expiration date.
2. Complete the HCFA-1500 correctly. Be sure to obtain the physician's and patient's (or authorized person's) signatures.
3. Note the patient's condition on entering the facility. In a nonemergency, verify that the patient has authorization for the service or procedure or that she lives more than 40 miles from the nearest base. Then determine whether the physician has accepted the case. In general, it is in a physician's best interest to accept assignment with CHAMPUS/TRICARE because he will be paid quickly.
4. Check about other insurance. If the patient has other insurance, it usually pays first. CHAMPUS/TRICARE pays first when the other insurance is Medicaid or supplemental CHAMPUS/TRICARE insurance.
5. Note whether the patient has been involved in an automobile or other accident in which another person may have been injured. If this has occurred, the patient must complete and present Form 2527 (Statement of Personal Injury—Possible Third-Party Liability). Send Form 2527 with the HCFA-1500. Form 2527 may indicate to CHAMPUS/TRICARE that the other party's insurance must cover some of the costs.

Blue Cross and Blue Shield

Many people think that Blue Cross and Blue Shield (BCBS) is one large corporation. Rather, it is a nationwide federation of local nonprofit service organizations that provide prepaid health-care services to BCBS subscribers. Each local organization operates under its own state laws, and specific plans for BCBS can vary greatly. For example, in one state a patient may have Blue Cross for hospital expenses and Blue Shield for physician's services. In another state both inpatient and outpatient costs may be covered by Blue Cross alone, by Blue Shield alone, or by a combined BCBS plan.

In some states BCBS helps the government administer Medicare, Medicaid, and CHAMPUS/TRICARE programs. For example, Blue Cross manages claims for Medicare Part A; Blue Shield manages claims for Medicare Part B.

Types of BCBS Policies. BCBS offers two basic types of policies: service benefit and indemnity benefit. A service benefit policy provides payment in full for all services it covers. With this type of policy, premiums may be relatively high, but the patient's out-of-pocket expenses are low. An indemnity benefit policy pays for a portion of covered services. With this type of policy, premiums may be relatively low, but the subscriber must pay a deductible plus a coinsurance amount (a fixed percentage of covered charges after meeting the deductible).

Several features make the BCBS plans unique. For example, BCBS cannot cancel a patient's policy because of poor health or greater-than-average benefit payments. BCBS must obtain the state insurance commissioner's approval for statewide rate or benefit changes. BCBS plans can be converted from group to individual coverage and can be transferred from state to state.

Blue Shield Reciprocity Plan. On a Blue Shield card, a double-headed arrow with a capital N and a three-digit number signifies membership in a permanent reciprocity plan. Under this plan the cardholder can be treated anywhere in the United States, and the plan will cover treatment expenses, whether for an emergency or not.

When a patient has membership in a permanent reciprocity plan, you must copy the N and the three-digit number onto the claim form. For referral information or authorizations, you can contact the local Blue Shield office. You then send the reciprocity plan claim form to the local Blue Shield office for processing.

BCBS Payments. BCBS plans typically pay participating physicians directly. The BCBS plans use various methods to determine payment. These include:

- Usual, customary, and reasonable (UCR) fees. This method is the primary method of payment.
- A fee schedule listing services and standard fees. BCBS pays a set amount for each service or procedure covered.
- A relative value scale (RVS). A five-digit number and a unit value are assigned to each procedure, based on the procedure's relative value compared with that of other common procedures. BCBS applies a conversion factor to the unit value to arrive at a payment.
- DRGs. BCBS pays a fixed fee based on the patient's diagnosis rather than on actual services rendered.

Reimbursement Procedures. You will need to explain BCBS reimbursement procedures to any BCBS patient because they vary with the specific plan. For example, the patient may pay the doctor directly and then apply to Blue Shield for reimbursement. The doctor may file a Blue Shield claim and then bill the patient for the difference between the Blue Shield payment and the actual fee.

If the Blue Shield plan requires it, you can file a claim using the HCFA-1500 or a Blue Shield service report form. Before filing any claim, however, determine the deductible, co-payment, and specific coverages of the patient's plan. Remember that BCBS plans can vary greatly in these aspects.

For services provided by nonparticipating physicians, the plans usually send payment to the subscriber. The subscriber must then endorse the payment to the nonparticipating physician. Like Medicare and Medicaid, BCBS sends an explanation of benefits (EOB) form after the claim is processed. Review this form to check for errors and to improve future claim submissions.

Workers' Compensation

Workers' compensation insurance covers accidents or diseases incurred in the workplace. In 1902 the state of Maryland enacted the first workers' compensation legislation because regular medical insurance did not cover job-related injuries or illnesses. Individual states adopted similar legislation through the 1940s. Federal law now requires employers to purchase and maintain a certain minimum amount of workers' compensation insurance for their employees.

Workers' compensation laws vary from state to state. In most states workers' compensation includes these benefits:

- Basic medical treatment for outpatient and inpatient care. This benefit can cover, for instance, stitching a shallow leg wound in the doctor's office or treating a severe head injury in the hospital.
- A weekly amount paid to the patient for a temporary disability. This amount compensates workers for loss of job income until they can return to work.
- A weekly or monthly sum paid to the patient. This payment is for a permanent disability.
- Death benefits. These benefits include a burial allowance and cash benefits paid to an employee's dependents when the employee dies because of a work-related illness or injury.
- Rehabilitation costs. These costs are incurred to restore an employee's ability to work again.

Managing Workers' Compensation Cases. Not all medical practices accept workers' compensation cases. Make sure you know your office's policy. Records management of workers' compensation varies by state. Typically, you will be responsible for the following administrative tasks when a workers' compensation patient contacts the practice for the first time.

- Call the patient's employer and verify that the accident occurred on the employer's premises.
- Obtain the employer's approval to provide treatment.
- Ask the employer for the name of his workers' compensation insurance company. (Employers are required by law to carry such insurance. It is a good policy to notify your state labor department about any employer you encounter that does not have workers' compensation insurance, although you are not required to do so.) You may wish to remind the employer that he must report any workplace accidents or injuries that result in a workers' compensation claim to the state labor department within 24 hours of the incident.
- Contact the insurance company and verify that the employer does indeed have a policy with the company and that the policy is in good standing.
- Obtain a claim number for the case from the insurance company. This claim number is used on all bills and paperwork.

Usually, these tasks can be completed quickly with a few telephone calls prior to the patient's first visit. If, however, the patient was first seen in a hospital emergency room, you have to find out the workers' compensation background information as quickly as possible after the patient is first treated (Figure 15-9).

At the time the patient starts treatment, create a patient record. If the patient is already one of the practice's regular patients, you may use the patient's existing chart. It is important to keep all patient information in one chart, primarily so the doctor has a historical context for treating a workers' compensation injury. You must, however, have a system in place for differentiating the workers' compensation visits from regular visits. If, for example, the office is computerized, it is common to have several codes to indicate regular visits, workers' compensation visits, car accident visits, and any other categories of visits the physician may wish to track.

Billing Workers' Compensation Claims. All bills for workers' compensation treatment must be filed with the patient's employer's workers' compensation insurance company every 30 days during treatment, using CPT standardized codes. It is also common practice to include the

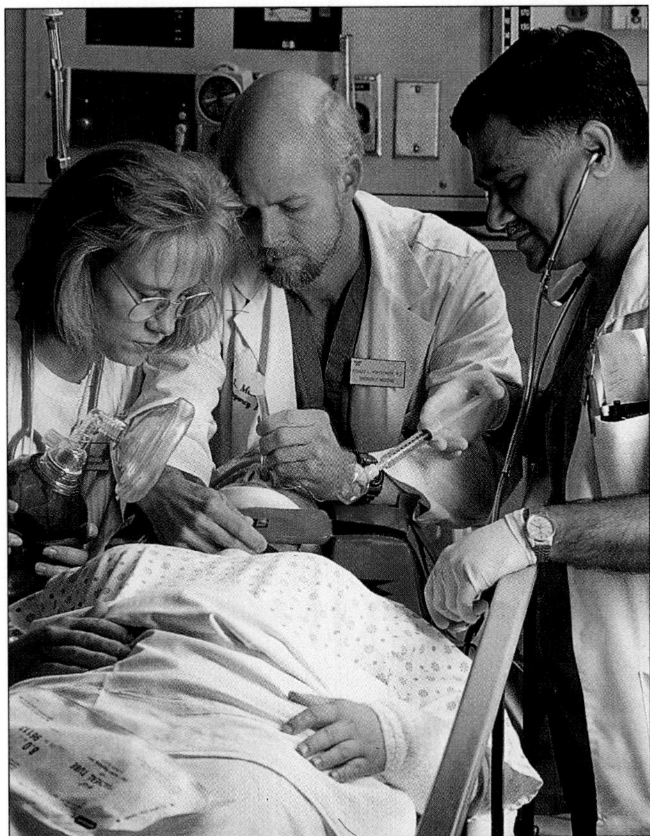

Figure 15-9. If a workers' compensation patient is first treated in a hospital emergency room, you must obtain insurance information from the patient's employer as quickly as possible.

doctor's notes about each patient visit. Doctors who agree to accept a patient covered under workers' compensation must accept the insurance company's payment in full. They cannot bill the insurance company for more and cannot bill the patient for any unpaid portion. Workers' compensation has no deductibles or co-payments for the patient. You must write off any unpaid portion on the ledger.

Health Maintenance Organizations

Health maintenance organizations (HMOs) are health-care organizations that provide specific services to individuals and their dependents who are enrolled in them. There are many types of HMOs, and new organizations are established every year. The payment relationship between HMOs and health-care providers varies, but most use a payment structure called **capitation.** For example, a physician who has ten HMO patients may be paid by the HMO a fee (called a capitation fee). A typical capitation fee is $100 per month per patient. This physician would receive $1000 per month from the HMO, whether she saw the HMO patients or not. If she provided services costing more than $100 to any of the HMO patients in any given month, she would not receive more money. Capitation fees may be paid quarterly or yearly, depending on the HMO.

Physicians enrolled in an HMO are called participating physicians, and their names are published in a directory of participating providers published by the HMO. The patient who is a member of the HMO chooses a provider from the published list. HMOs usually serve a limited geographic area (such as northern California or southeastern Pennsylvania), and the published lists are for the particular area in which the patient resides.

HMOs are often described as **managed care** organizations because they manage, negotiate, and contract for health care, with the goal of keeping health-care costs down. The philosophy of HMOs is different from that of other types of medical insurance programs. The focus of HMOs is not so much on medical procedures and services as on wellness, or preventive care. Thus, HMOs cover the cost of and encourage patients to have annual physical checkups by their primary care physicians to spot health problems before these problems become critical. This philosophy not only promotes wellness but also helps cut the rising cost of medical care.

Another goal of an HMO is to reduce the complexity of the health-care system for its subscribers. For example, most HMOs that use a capitation structure do not require subscribers to complete any paperwork or file claims for many routine procedures and services. As a medical assistant, you do file forms that reflect visits or procedures performed. The difference is that you do not need to track payments for claims.

Always try to keep your paperwork error-free. "Tips for the Office" provides some helpful suggestions.

HMO Co-Payment. Most HMOs charge their members a small co-payment, as little as $5 or $10, for each office visit. The patient is responsible for this fee and usually pays it at the time of the office visit. If it is not paid, you must bill the patient directly.

Special Billing Circumstances. Many Medicare and Medicaid recipients today receive their benefits through an HMO. If you work in a participating HMO practice, you must check the patient's Medicare or Medicaid status. In addition, hospitals may contract with HMOs for outpatient and inpatient care.

Some HMOs are self-contained, with all providers under one roof. Forms are needed then only if the patient is referred to outside HMO-approved specialists. If you work for such a specialist, you must bill the HMO. Check with the HMO to determine whether it accepts the HCFA-1500; most do.

In an emergency, or when patients are traveling outside their HMO area, you or the patient must contact the HMO for authorization of treatment. Many HMOs have toll-free numbers for this purpose.

Independent Practice Associations. Independent practice associations (IPAs) are HMOs that use only certain doctors at various different practices within a region. These doctors are under contract to provide procedures and services. IPAs are composed of doctors who practice independently. IPAs may pay each doctor a set amount per patient, or the doctors may bill the IPA for services or procedures.

Preferred Provider Organizations. Preferred provider organizations (PPOs) are another type of HMO. Physicians working under contract with PPOs agree to accept predetermined fees. Patients enrolled in PPOs, however, do not pay this predetermined amount. Rather, patients pay for services rendered. Some PPOs also require patients to pay large deductibles—up to 25%—of the predetermined charges. The PPOs pay the balance. If your employer is part of a PPO, you will bill patients for the deductible in the office's standard manner and bill the PPO for the balance.

HMO Treatment Sequence. Following is an example of how an HMO patient may receive treatment: A woman makes an appointment with her primary care physician because she has discovered a breast lump. For this visit, she makes a co-payment of $5. (The physician, remember, also receives that patient's capitation fee, as described earlier.) The physician directs her to have a mammogram and to see a specialist and gives her a written referral for each. The referrals state how many visits the primary care physician recommends, such as one visit to the radiology facility and perhaps two visits to the specialist, one for evaluation and one for follow-up. The patient makes co-payments of $5 to the radiology facility and $5 to the specialist's office. (The HMO pays the radiology facility and the specialist a capitation fee.)

If inpatient surgery becomes necessary, the patient may need to obtain authorization (preapproval) from her primary care physician and the HMO. If she suddenly

Tips FOR THE OFFICE

Following HMO Regulations for Paperwork

HMOs try to minimize paperwork, but there are still a certain number of necessary forms. Aetna US Healthcare, with 23 million members and many different HMOs, requires quite a large amount of paperwork. This company recommends that you follow these tips for more efficient claims processing.

- Make a copy of the patient's identification card, front and back. This is the single most important thing you can do to speed claims acceptance. The card will show the patient's exact subscriber number, the plan to which the patient subscribes, the patient's correct name, date of birth, and more.
- Review your copy of the card for the address to which to send claims.
- Determine whether any special form is required. This information may be on the insurance card. If not, call the insurer for clarification. Many insurers have toll-free telephone numbers for this purpose.
- Double-check the diagnosis code and CPT procedural code on the claim. Using the correct codes will speed acceptance.
- Ensure that you put the patient's correct membership identification number on the form. Most large insurers are fully automated, and their operators key in identification numbers—not names.
- Check to be certain that you correctly complete any referring physician information. One insurer requires that a primary physician make a referral for certain procedures, such as cardiac rehabilitation programs, and that the physician's name be used to process the claim.

Before the physician you work for sees a patient for a costly procedure, such as cardiac rehabilitation, some insurers strongly recommend that you:

- Check to make sure the patient's diagnosis is covered.
- Check the patient's policy for coverage.
- Open the case by calling the precertification nurse.
- Verify that precertification has been completed and that a certification number has been assigned.
- Write in *red ink* the number of visits allowed by the patient's policy.

Some insurers also recommend that you write the approved precertification number, number of allowed visits, and other information in an easily accessible place. You might use the registration sheet in the back of the patient's medical record.

Keep in mind that managed care organizations have different regulations. In addition to all of these, some insurers require formal written or verbal approval by a review nurse before certain procedures can be performed.

develops severe chest pain or another life-threatening emergency, however, she can receive care immediately. She must notify her primary care physician or the HMO as soon as possible (usually within 48 hours of the emergency).

Coordination of Benefits

Coordination of benefits clauses are legal clauses in insurance policies that prevent duplication of payment. These clauses restrict payment by insurance companies to no more than 100% of the cost of covered benefits. In many families, husband and wife are both wage earners. They and their children are frequently eligible for health insurance benefits through both employers' plans. In such cases the two insurance companies coordinate their payments to pay up to 100% of a procedure's cost. A payment of 100% includes the policyholder's deductible and co-payment. The primary, or main, carrier is the policy that pays benefits first. Then the secondary, or supplemental, carrier pays the deductible and co-payment.

Avoiding Fraud. Some patients with two insurance policies might be tempted to try to make money by telling both insurers that they have only one insurance policy. They might then receive double payments, which constitutes fraud and can lead to imprisonment. Try your best to determine whether a patient has more than one insurance policy.

Birthday Rule. Not all insurance policies have a coordination of benefits clause. Any policy without such a clause automatically becomes the primary payer. Laws to determine which policy is the primary insurer were passed in 1987. Chief among them is the **birthday rule,** which states that the insurance policy of the policyholder whose birthday comes first in the calendar year is the primary payer for all dependents.

For example, suppose a husband and wife are both employed and have work-sponsored insurance plans that cover their spouses and their three children. The husband's birthday is July 14 and the wife's birthday is June 11. Because of the birthday rule, the wife's insurance plan is the primary payer, and the husband's is the secondary payer. If a husband and wife were born on the same day, the policy that has been in effect the longest is the primary payer.

The birthday rule is applied in most states in which dependents are covered by two or more medical plans. Different states may have different rules, however. You should check with your state's insurance commission whenever you are in doubt.

Children of Separated or Divorced Parents. Rules for coordinating benefits are more complex for dependents of legally separated or divorced parents. For example, if a child's parents separate and move to different states, the original primary policy may no longer be primary, or the child may be covered by only one policy. The doctor or insurance company may ask you to determine which policy is the primary insurer, based on your updated records. You must determine:

1. Who has legal custody of the child. If the parent who has legal custody has not remarried, the policy of the parent whose birthday comes first is the primary payer. If the parent with legal custody has remarried, that parent's policy is primary.
2. Whether there is a legal document (court order or legal separation agreement) that dictates which parent is responsible for the children's medical expenses. Note that the responsible parent is not necessarily the custodial parent. The policy of the financially responsible parent is the primary insurer.
3. The states in which the policies originated. If one plan originated in a state without a coordination of benefits law and the other originated in a state with such a law, the plan from the state that has the law is the primary one.

Medicare Patients. An employee's company plan is primary for a patient aged 65 who is also eligible for Medicare benefits. In this case Medicare is the secondary payer. The patient can then submit expenses not paid by the company's plan to Medicare. For a retired individual who has private insurance and Medicare, Medicare is primary and private insurance is secondary.

Submitting Claims Electronically

Electronic claims transmission (ECT) is expected to increase because the process is easy, improves accuracy, and saves time. For example, using ECT, hundreds of claims can be submitted in one morning. Medicare claims can be reimbursed in 10 to 14 days rather than in the 3 to 4 weeks required with paper transactions. If errors or omissions occur in a paper claim, payment can be delayed for months. With ECT, errors can be detected as soon as they are entered, giving you the opportunity to correct them immediately.

Medicare encourages all practices to file electronically. As of July 1, 1996, all computer systems must use National Standard format or American National Standards Institute format to send claims electronically to Medicare.

Most health-care experts agree that all claims will eventually be handled electronically and that the same software and standards will be used nationally. However, ECT is just the beginning. In the near future, a device the size of a credit card will hold a patient's complete health record, including insurance data, medical history, and prescription history. Furthermore, all of that information will be easy to access, update, and transmit—possibly through machines similar to automated teller machines (Ouellette, 1995). These wallet-size medical records, which are currently being test-marketed, store up to 4 million characters of insurance data and medical information. Such a card will revolutionize insurance claims and the entire medical industry.

ECT provides three key benefits to the practice:

- Enhanced cash flow. Most major insurance companies can guarantee a 14-day turnaround time from submission to payment on error-free claims.
- Less paperwork, which saves time. Electronic processing takes hours instead of weeks.
- Accuracy and convenience. Errors and omissions that could cause a claim to be rejected are instantly identified on the screen. Problems identified on the insurer's screen are relayed to the practice within 1 or 2 days.

Necessary Equipment

To submit claims electronically, you need only three pieces of equipment: a personal computer, dependable electronic claims submission software, and a modem (as explained in Chapter 6). Practices that submit claims electronically usually submit more Medicare claims than any others. They may use software developed by Medicare or buy Medicare-approved software from a private vendor. Medicare's program automates only claims, whereas many commercial software programs will automate accounts payable, biographical patient data, and other data.

Other interactive computer software systems can link insurers, data clearinghouses, physicians, and hospitals within cities or states. These include the nationwide Health Care Information Network and BCBS's Internet site. Both provide instant on-line answers to your insurance questions. The Health Care Information Network gives authorized users data on patient eligibility, specialist referrals, and authorization for treatment and other information from a patient account. Check with your software provider, Medicare or other government agency, Internet provider, or other reputable data provider for information about local-access systems.

It is almost certain that insurance processing in the twenty-first century will be entirely on-line, with insurers, hospitals, and doctors all contributing electronically to a patient's record. In the next 10 years, you are likely to see rapid, extensive changes in insurance processing. You need to become familiar with today's new technologies because they are likely to become the standards of tomorrow. If you have difficulty using software or modems or transmitting insurance data to clearinghouses, ask another staff member for help, or consult the appropriate software and hardware manuals. You may wish to take a special computer course.

Types of Computer Systems

A medical practice may use one of several types of computer systems for electronic claims submission. The main types of systems are:

- In-house.
- Batch.
- Time-share.
- ECT.

An in-house system is an office computer system (it may be one personal computer or many) into which you enter insurance information to be stored, retrieved, edited, or printed out as needed. An in-house system cannot communicate with an insurer's system.

If your office uses the batch system, you will send insurance files by mail or messenger to a data processing center, which enters the data into its system. Then the center returns the information in the form of documents or disks, as needed.

A time-share system is an updated version of the batch system. In this system, the practice shares time with other users on a modem or computer system that transmits data to a data processing center. The center then sends documents or disks back to the practice.

Only ECT is completely electronic. An ECT system sends insurance information by modem directly to an insurance company's computers. The company's computers review the claim and either automatically approve it and provide reimbursement or electronically flag it for an employee's inspection. Increasing numbers of ECT systems reimburse by transferring funds electronically, without issuing paper checks. The ECT system is quick, uses no paper, and typically permits fewer mistakes and omissions than other methods of transmitting claims.

Signed Agreements and Compatibility

Insurance companies give special treatment to practices that file claims by modem because this system saves everyone so much time and money. However, you must be sure there is a signed agreement with the insurance company to submit claims electronically.

Also, determine if your practice's computer-generated claim form is compatible with the insurance company's system. To determine compatibility, do not rely on outside computer programmers or specialists. Rather, contact the insurance company directly. The insurance company may ask you to send samples of the form to see whether it is compatible with the company's computer system.

Procedures

In many ways, an electronic claim submission is like a handwritten or typed claim submission, but it is easier. No matter how a claim is filed, you must fill out every data field as precisely as possible, using the correct terminology and codes. Remember that you must have on hand and be familiar with CPT codes, Medicare's HCPCS national and regional codes, and ICD-9-CM diagnosis codes. For an example of how to submit an electronic Medicare claim, see Procedure 15-2.

If the practice where you work handles insurance claims electronically, you must obtain a signed Release of Medical Information form (Figure 15-13) from the patient. This form is signed by every new patient and is used by insurers, physicians, and any other qualified personnel who may need to examine the patient's records. For patients who began coming to the practice before electronic claims submission, obtain a blanket release statement at the earliest opportunity.

Maintaining Patient Confidentiality

Although computers have increased the speed and volume of data transmission, they have also increased the concern for security and patient confidentiality. Chapter 3 discusses patient confidentiality issues. To ensure that computerized insurance information is kept confidential, the AMA Council on Ethical and Judicial Affairs recommends that you:

- Verify the accuracy of all sources of information.
- Advise the patient and doctor that computer-based information exists and may be distributed to hospitals, employers, state agencies, and even private medical data gatherers who use the data for profit.
- Identify and verify all organizations that request information.
- Confine information releases to the specific information requested and the specific agency requesting it.
- Identify all individuals authorized to make changes to the insurance record.
- Keep on file original patient authorizations of release.
- Maintain stringent security measures at all times.

Security Measures. Keep magnetic computer disks or tapes in a secure place, such as a locked drawer or cabinet. Never leave them unattended when they are out of the locked cabinet. Computers in the medical practice should have passwords. Passwords are confidential and should not be released to unauthorized personnel for any reason. Passwords should be changed every few months (Medicare recommends every 90 days) to help maintain confidentiality. It is important to eliminate passwords of former employees. If a practice changes data processing services, the files held by the former processing service must be returned to the practice.

Releasing Information. Federal and state agencies, private companies, employers, attorneys, and other physicians may request insurance records. You must be familiar with state laws about the release of information, and you must ensure that the patient has signed a form authorizing release of information. If the authorization is a photocopy, you must obtain the patient's written approval or a new original authorization form. The only exception is in workers' compensation cases. In these

PROCEDURE 15-2

Submitting Medicare Claims Electronically

Objective: To submit an error-free insurance claim to Medicare via electronic transmission (Note: This exercise is a simulation. Submitting a claim for an imaginary person constitutes fraud.)

Materials: Patient medical record, personal computer, modem, claim submission software

Method

1. At the main menu prompt (usually this prompt is C:>), select the claim system.
2. Log on.
3. Enter the unique Medicare operator code given to you after passing the Medicare electronic claim test.
4. Enter your password. Medicare recommends that you change your password every 90 days or less for security reasons.
5. When the first screen comes up, enter the claim data (Figure 15-10). Be thorough; do not omit anything. The system will let you know what field you are in, show what data that field requires, pull up diagnosis codes, and even alert you if you make a mistake or leave something out. For example, it may beep and prompt you with INVALID ENTRY.
6. When you have finished filling out all the claims you wish to file electronically, back up the claims data on disk in case of error.
7. Print out the claims report (one is shown in Figure 15-11). This is for your own review, to check for any possible errors that might make Medicare reject the claim.
8. Print out any paper insurance claims required, using the standard HCFA-1500 form. These paper forms are for insurance organizations to which you are not connected electronically.

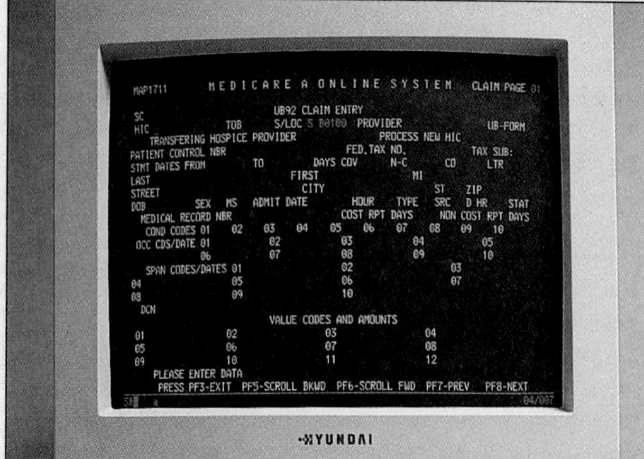

Figure 15-10. This is the first screen that shows Medicare claim data in an electronic claim transmission.

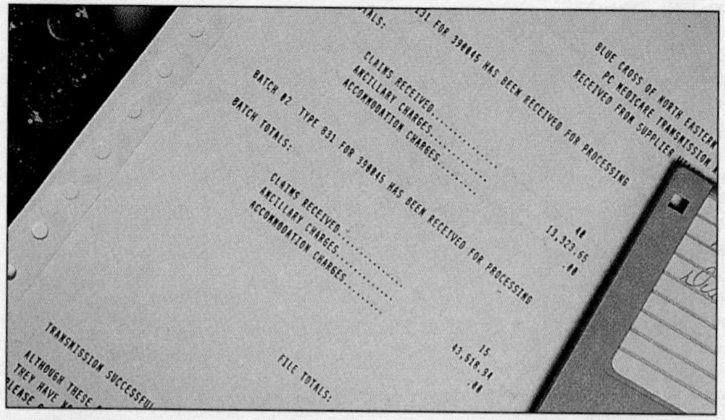

Figure 15-11. Print out the claims report to check for any errors that might make Medicare reject a claim.

(Note: You would take the remaining steps if you were actually going to submit the claim.)

9. Activate your modem. The modem will automatically open the port and dial Medicare's number. You may have to log on your operator code and password again, depending on the program.
10. When you are connected to Medicare's system, send the claims.
11. Obtain a confirmation report, such as the one shown in Figure 15-12.
12. Close out the system, and return to the main menu.

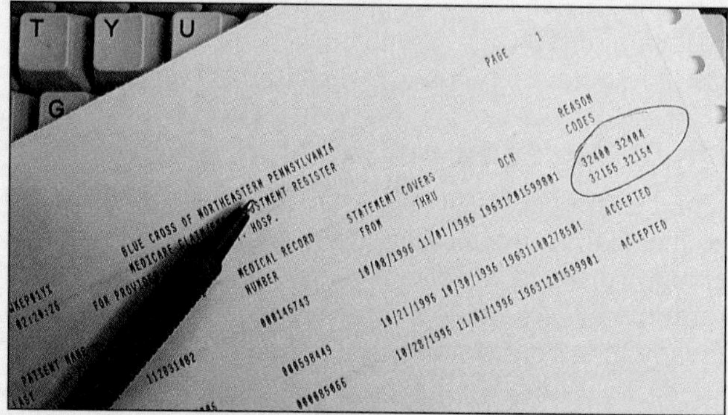

Figure 15-12. After you have sent the claims to Medicare's system, obtain a confirmation report for your records.

13. Carefully review Medicare's written confirmation of claims. This confirmation should be mailed to your practice within 2 to 4 days.
14. Review the explanation of benefits (EOB) that Medicare mails with the check in 10 to 14 days. If a claim is rejected, the EOB should review the claim—line by line—and explain why.
15. Contact Medicare immediately if either you or Medicare has made an error. Remember: Computers can make mistakes too.

RELEASE OF MEDICAL INFORMATION

Date ______________________

To (Insurance Company) ______________________

Group/Policy ID No. ______________________

I hereby authorize Dr. ______________________

to release to your company any information, including the diagnosis and the records of any examination or treatment given to me during the period of such medical or surgical care.

I also authorize and request your company to pay directly to the above-named doctor the amount due to me in my claim for treatment or services.

Signed (patient) ______________________

Signed (insured) ______________________

Witness ______________________

Figure 15-13. You must have a signed Release of Medical Information form before releasing any patient medical records.

cases, the contract is between the physician and the employer's insurance company, and insurance information can be released without patient authorization.

Releasing Information for HIV-Positive Patients. You must also exercise care when handling insurance information for HIV-positive patients. If a patient who is HIV-positive has applied for health or life insurance and requests that her records be sent to the insurance company, check your state law. Some states have ruled that HIV and AIDS information can be given only to a patient's spouse or to a partner, relative, or friend that the patient has specified in writing. This information includes coding, laboratory test results, and anything else indicating HIV status, such as ICD-9-CM code 795.8. All information released at the request of an HIV-positive patient should be accompanied by a statement requesting that the information be destroyed after viewing and a statement prohibiting disclosure to any other party without the patient's express written consent.

Documenting Claims Submission. You must document and secure every stage of electronic claims submission, just as you would do for written claims submission.

1. Log in each claim as it is submitted.
2. After entering a claim or batch of claims electronically, back it up on disk in case of system error.
3. Print out all claims for review, if applicable.
4. Make sure that Medicare and other insurers send a confirmation report of claims received. Receipt will be indicated by both an on-screen message and a written confirmation within 2 to 4 days.
5. Review the EOB line by line to detect errors or omissions.
6. Log in the check and detach it from the EOB, and send it to accounts receivable.
7. Compare the payment to the practice's fee, and enter any amount of payment not received.

Summary

As a medical assistant, you must learn the basic terminology of health insurance—such as usual, customary, and reasonable fees—and be able to use the universal health insurance claim form. You must also familiarize yourself with the various laws and policies related to insurance claims processing, the kinds of insurance with which you will be working, and the particular requirements that affect claims filing for each type of insurance. Learning about health insurance and claims processing is an ongoing experience. Take advantage of any workshops or classes that are held in your area.

Many of the procedures described in this chapter reflect the current emphasis on cost containment. The laws that govern the health insurance industry and your handling of health insurance claims are largely a response to rapidly rising health-care costs. Read professional publications to keep abreast of attempts to develop tools and policies that will streamline the insurance process. For example, much has been written about the universal health card, which would look much like a credit card, contain a person's whole medical history, and be read by a computer.

Lastly, as a medical assistant embarking on your career in an age of high technology, you must understand how to use medical office computer software for electronic claims processing. Again, take advantage of workshops and classes.

With all this knowledge of health insurance, claims processing, and medical terminology, you must not lose sight of the patient for whom you do this work. Your concern for the patient should be the primary motivating force for your continued learning and improvement as the medical office insurance expert.

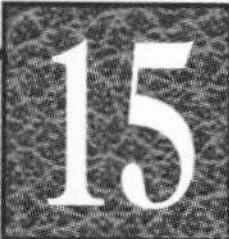

Chapter Review

Discussion Questions

1. How does CHAMPVA coverage compare with that of CHAMPUS/TRICARE?
2. What are the differences between Medicare Part A and Part B? How is each part funded?
3. Why do insurers coordinate benefits?
4. What are the advantages of electronic claims submission?

Critical Thinking Questions

1. How do you think the increasing cost of medical diagnoses and procedures is affecting the insurance industry?
2. How do you think utilization review helps control the cost of health insurance?
3. In what ways has new technology changed insurance claims submission?

Application Activities

1. Using a CPT manual, identify the codes for administering an allergy shot by a nurse, administering a complete examination of a new patient by a doctor, and performing a throat culture.
2. Using a modem and computer, log on to the BCBS Internet site. Use E-mail to post a question about insurance processing. Check back in a couple of days, and report to the class.
3. How would the birthday rule apply in a family with two working parents if the father's birthday is October 6 and the mother's is November 22?

Further Readings

Calabrese, Catherine M., and Cynthia A. Timko. "A User's Guide to the RBRVS Schedule." *The Professional Medical Assistant,* March/April 1996, 5–9.

Collins, R., et al. *From Patient to Payment: Insurance Procedures for the Medical Office.* Westerville, OH: Glencoe, 1993.

Covell, Alice. "Keeping Up With Coding Changes: Suggestions to Help You Cope." *The Professional Medical Assistant,* March/April 1995, 6–9.

"Electronic Billing of Medicare Claims." *Iowa Medicine,* March 1994, 105–106.

Enteen, R. *Health Insurance: How to Get It, Keep It, or Improve What You've Got.* New York: Paragon House, 1992.

Langreth, Robert. "Medical Records in Your Wallet." *Popular Science,* July 1993, 46.

Novack, Janet. "The Doctor's New Allies." *Forbes,* 18 February 1991, 85.

Ouellette, Tim. "Health Care at Your Fingertips: Blue Cross/Blue Shield of Massachusetts Unveils Health Care ATMs." *Computerworld,* 29 May 1995, 42.

Bookkeeping and Banking

CHAPTER OUTLINE

- The Business Side of a Medical Practice
- Bookkeeping Systems
- Banking for the Medical Office
- Planning for Retirement

OBJECTIVES

After completing Chapter 16, you will be able to:

- Describe traditional bookkeeping systems such as single entry and double entry.
- Define a pegboard system.
- Explain the benefits of performing bookkeeping tasks on the computer.
- List banking tasks in a medical office.
- Describe the logistics of accepting, endorsing, and depositing checks from patients and insurance companies.
- Reconcile the office's bank statements.
- Discuss different methods of financial planning for retirement.

AREAS OF COMPETENCE

1997 ROLE DELINEATION STUDY

ADMINISTRATIVE

Practice Finances

- Apply bookkeeping principles
- Document and maintain accounting and banking records

GENERAL (Transdisciplinary)

Operational Functions

- Apply computer techniques to support office operations

Key Terms

ABA number
accounts payable
accounts receivable
asset
benefit
bookkeeping
cashier's check
certified check
charge slip
check
endorse
401(k) plan
journalizing
money order
negotiable
patient ledger card
payee
payer
payroll deduction
pegboard system
pension plan
power of attorney
profit-sharing plan
reconciliation
third party check
vesting

The Business Side of a Medical Practice

A medical practice is a business. If it is to prosper, its income must exceed its expenses. In other words, it must produce a profit. To determine whether the business is making a profit, you may be asked to do **bookkeeping,** or systematic recording of business transactions. Your records will later be analyzed by an accountant or by a more experienced medical assistant.

Bookkeeping and banking are two key responsibilities of medical assistants. To fulfill these responsibilities, you need an understanding of basic accounting systems and certain financial management skills.

Importance of Accuracy

Whenever you do bookkeeping or banking, strive for 100% accuracy. Because bookkeeping records form a chain of information, an undetected error at the first link will be carried through all other links in the chain. Undetected errors can result in billing a patient twice for the same visit, omitting bank deposits, or making improper payments to suppliers. These actions can result in lost money—and patients—for the practice.

Establishing Procedures

A set procedure not only helps you remember important aspects of bookkeeping and banking but also helps ensure that your books are accurate. Here are some general suggestions for maintaining accuracy in bookkeeping and banking procedures for a medical practice.

1. Establish the practice's bookkeeping and banking procedures in a logical and organized way.
2. Be consistent. Always handle the same kinds of transactions in exactly the same way. For example, endorse all checks with the same information, regardless of who wrote them or when you will be depositing them.
3. Use check marks as you work to avoid losing your place if you are interrupted. For example, place a red check mark on each check stub as you reconcile the bank statement.
4. Write clearly, and always use the same type of pen. If more than one person performs bookkeeping and banking tasks, each person might use a different color ink to identify her work. It is recommended that as few people as possible perform these tasks, however. You may use pencil for trial balances and worksheets, but you should use pen for bookkeeping entries.
5. Double-check your work frequently to detect—and correct—any errors. To correct errors, draw a straight line through the incorrect figure, and write the correct figure above it. Do not erase errors or delete them with correction fluid or tape.
6. Keep all columns of figures straight, so that decimal points align correctly.

Using set procedures will help you organize your work, help ensure accuracy, and make you a more valuable member of the practice staff.

Bookkeeping Systems

Three types of manual accounting systems are commonly used in a medical practice: single entry, double entry, and pegboard. A computerized system may also be used. All bookkeeping systems record income, charges (money owed to the practice), disbursements (money paid out by the practice), and other financial information. The choice of system is based on the size and complexity of the practice.

Traditional Bookkeeping Methods

Even practices that use computers for many other administrative and clinical functions may still perform bookkeeping methods on paper. This choice is not old-fashioned but simply the preference of the physician/owner or the office manager. Some people believe that working with numbers on paper forces you to be especially careful and to pay close attention to detail—more so than working on a computer, which has built-in mechanisms for checking arithmetic, decimal alignment, and so on.

Single-Entry System. As the name implies, the single-entry system requires only one entry for each transaction. Therefore, it is the easiest system to learn and use. Unlike the double-entry system, however, the single-entry system is not self-balancing. In addition, it does not detect errors as readily and has fewer accuracy checkpoints. This system is also more likely to produce errors because information must be posted (copied) to the bookkeeping forms.

The single-entry system uses several basic records, as well as auxiliary records:

- A daily log (also called a general ledger, day sheet, or daily journal) to record charges and payments
- Patient ledger cards or an accounts receivable ledger, which shows how much each patient owes
- A checkbook register or cash payment journal, which shows the practice expenses
- Payroll records, which show salaries, wages, and payroll deductions
- Petty cash records, which show disbursements for minor office expenses

The double-entry and pegboard systems, discussed later in this chapter, also use these records.

Daily Log. The daily log is a chronological list of the charges to patients and the payments received from patients each day, as shown in Figure 16-1. In the daily log, you write the name of each patient seen that day. Across from the name, you record the service provided, the fee

Dr. ______________________ **Date** ______________________

Hour	*Patient*	*Service Provided*	*Charge*	*Paid*
	1			
	2			
	3			
	4			
	5			
	6			
	7			
	8			
	9			
	10			
	11			
	12			
	13			
	14			
	15			
	16			
		Totals		

Figure 16-1. A daily log is used to record charges and payments.

charged, and the payment received (if any). This process is called **journalizing.** You then post (copy) the charges and payments from the daily log to patient ledger cards (described below). Using a daily or monthly cash control sheet, you record checks and cash received, as well as deposits made each day.

Some physicians keep a daily log at their desks for entering information after they see each patient. In such cases, it may be helpful to write the name of each scheduled patient in the log to provide an appointment list. You may be responsible for this task.

In other offices, the medical assistants maintain the daily log. You can obtain the information for the log from charge slips and from checks received from patients or insurance companies. (Note: A **charge slip** is the original record of the doctor's services and the charge for those services. Some practices use a combination charge slip/receipt which automatically creates a receipt to tear off for the patient. Typically, a charge slip/receipt includes a duplicate copy underneath to use for bookkeeping purposes. Remember, you need to track charges *and* receipts for payment, regardless of whether the practice uses separate charge slips and receipts or a combination.) There may also be records of outside visits, such as to nursing homes or hospital emergency rooms.

Be sure to record any night calls or other unscheduled visits in the daily log. Simply check with the physician each morning. If the physician has not noted the charge amount on a charge slip/receipt or record of outside visits, remember to apply the correct fee.

Record in the daily log all payments that come in the mail. If a check from an insurance company includes payment for more than one patient (which frequently is the case), post the appropriate amount to each patient ledger card.

If extra columns are available, you can record additional financial information in the daily log. For example, in addition to showing the total amount charged to the patient, you can show a breakdown of that total into the amounts generated by different physicians in a group practice or by different functions of the office, such as laboratory or x-ray.

At the end of each day, total the charges and receipts in the daily log, and post these totals to the monthly summary of charges and receipts. To double-check your totals, perform the following procedures:

- Ensure that the day's total cash and check receipts are the same as the day's total bank deposit.
- Ensure that the sum of the day's charges for each type of service is the same as the total of the day's charges.

Patient Ledger Cards. Another bookkeeping task is preparing a patient ledger card for each patient. The **patient ledger card** includes the patient's name, address, home and work telephone numbers, and the name of the person who is responsible for the charges (if different from the patient). The ledger card also lists the patient's insurance information, Social Security number, employer's name, and any special billing instructions. Figure 16-2 shows an example of a patient ledger card.

You use the patient ledger card to record charges incurred by the patient, payments received, and the resulting balance owed to the doctor. Because these cards document the financial transactions of the patient account, they are sometimes called account cards. In some practices, they are photocopied for use as monthly statements.

The information for the patient ledger cards comes from the daily log or from charge slips. It is best to complete all the cards at the end of the day. If this is not possible, you may complete them as time permits during the day. To prevent double or omitted postings, put a small check mark next to each entry in the daily log after you post it to the proper ledger card.

Take great care when posting, because errors on ledger cards will be reflected on invoices. To ensure accuracy, add up the total charges and receipts from the ledger cards, and make sure the information matches the total charges and receipts in that day's daily log.

Accounts Receivable. Every day, you must also update the **accounts receivable** record, which shows the total owed to the practice. Total up the items on the accounts receivable record, and then total up the outstanding balances on the patient ledger cards. The two numbers should match. If they do not, recheck your work to find the cause of the discrepancy.

Accounts Payable. **Accounts payable** are the amounts the practice owes to vendors. If your responsibilities include accounts payable, keep careful records of equipment and supplies ordered, and compare orders received against the invoices. In the checkbook register, keep detailed and accurate records of accounts paid. (Accounts receivable and accounts payable are discussed in greater detail in Chapters 17 and 18.)

Record of Office Disbursements. The record of office disbursements is a list of the amounts paid for such items as medical supplies, office rent, office utilities, employee wages, postage, and equipment over a certain period of time. It shows the **payee** (the person who will receive the payment), the date, the check number, the amount paid, and the type of expense. Figure 16-3 is an example of a disbursement record.

A checkbook register may be used to record office disbursements. As an alternative, a disbursement journal or the bottom section of the daily log may be used to record office disbursements. For income tax purposes, this record should include only office expenses. The doctor's personal expenses should not be listed here.

Summary of Charges, Receipts, and Disbursements. Charges, receipts, and disbursements are usually summarized at the end of each month, quarter, or year, as shown in Figure 16-4. The summary is used to compare the income and expenses of the current period with the income and expenses from any previous period.

By analyzing summaries, a physician can see which functions of the practice are profitable, the total amount charged for services, the payments received for services, the total cost of running the office, and a breakdown of expenses into various categories. Based on this information, the physician can make vital business decisions. For example, after analyzing monthly summaries, the physician may decide to budget expenses differently, collect payments more promptly, cut unprofitable services, or expand profitable services.

Although an accountant may prepare these reports, an experienced medical assistant can prepare them. If you are asked to prepare them, follow these guidelines.

- Every business day, post the total charges and receipts from the daily log to the appropriate line and column of the monthly summary.
- Every business day, also post the disbursements from the record of office disbursements to the appropriate lines and columns of the monthly summary.
- At the end of the month, total the columns on the monthly summary.
- At the end of each quarter, post the charges, receipts, and disbursements for each of the previous 3 months to the quarterly summary. Then, total each column.
- At the end of the year, post the charges, receipts, and disbursements for each of the previous 12 months (or 4 quarters) to the annual summary. Then, total each column.

Remember that the total charges and total receipts in any summary should be almost the same. They may not be identical, because some bills may not have been fully collected. Procedure 16-1 offers a plan for setting up a medical practice bookkeeping system.

Double-Entry System. The double-entry accounting system is based on an accounting equation:

Assets = Liabilities + Owner Equity

Assets are goods or properties that have a dollar value, such as the medical practice building, bank accounts, office equipment, and accounts receivable. Owner equity (also called capital, net worth, or proprietorship) is the owner's right to the value of the assets. Liabilities are amounts owed by the practice to creditors, such as a mortgage on the building and accounts payable. Liabilities decrease the value of the assets. In other words, in a medical practice, the owner (the physician) has the rights to the value of the practice's assets, once the liabilities have been subtracted.

Because both sides of the accounting equation must always balance (agree), every transaction is recorded as an entry on each side of the equation. Thus, there are two entries, or a double entry. The double-entry system is accurate, detects errors easily, and provides the most complete information about the practice and its contribution to the physician's net worth. It is complex, however,

Patient's Name Jonathan Jackson

Home Phone (612) 555-9921 **Work Phone** (612) 555-1000

Social Security No. 111-21-4114

Employer Ashton School District

Insurance National Insurance Co.

Policy # 123-4-56-788

Person Responsible for Charges (if Different from Patient) ____________

JONATHAN JACKSON
123 Fourth Avenue
Ashton, MN 70809-1222

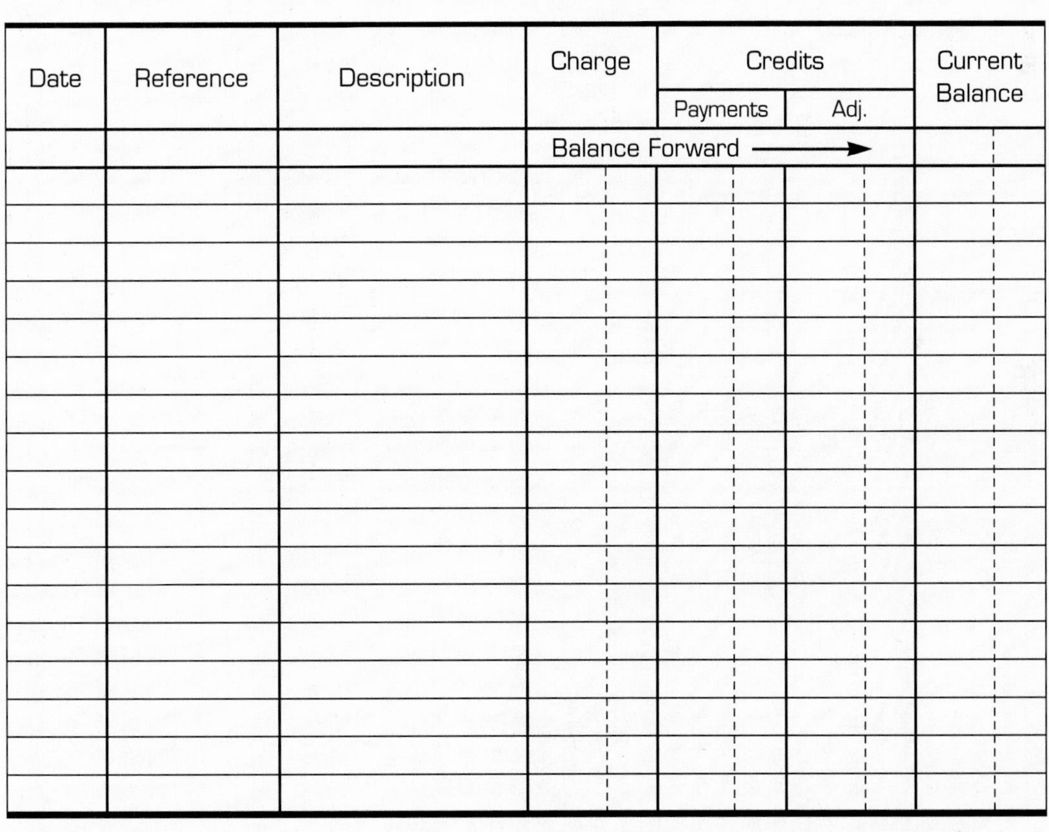

Date	Reference	Description	Charge	Credits		Current Balance
				Payments	Adj.	
			Balance Forward →			

Please Pay Last Amount in This Column ▲

OV—Office Visit
X—X-ray
ROA—Received on Account

C—Consultation
NC—No Charge
MA—Missed Appointment

EX—Examination
INS—Insurance

Figure 16-2. Patient ledger cards are used to show how much each patient owes.

Record of Office Disbursements

April 1998

DATE	PAYEE	CK. NO.	TOTAL AMOUNT	TYPES OF EXPENSES: RENT	UTILITIES	POSTAGE	LAB./ X-RAY	MEDICAL SUPPLIES	OFFICE SUPPLIES	WAGES	INSURANCE	TAXES	TRAVEL	MISC.
01	Philips' Med. Suppl.	1778	125.00					125.00						
01	Postage	1779	16.85			16.85								
02	Medi Path	1780	32.50				32.50							
02	Quik Service Co.	1781	82.40						82.40					
02	Philips' Med. Suppl.	1782	92.00					92.00						
02	Jean Medina	1783	77.06							77.06				
05	State Dept. of Rev.	1784	189.16									189.16		
06	General Insurance	1785	165.92								165.92			
07	Postage	(Cash)	5.19			5.19								
07	Micah Smith	(Cash)	15.00										15.00	
08	IRS	1786	419.41									419.41		
12	Quik Service Co.	1787	124.00						124.00					
13	City Laundry	1788	75.00											75.00
13	National Insurance	1789	189.00								189.00			
14	Broyer Assoc.	1790	1 500.00	1 500.00										
14	Postage	(Cash)	12.11			12.11								
15	City Gas Co.	1791	125.00		125.00									
19	Jean Medina	1792	85.92							85.92				
19	Postage	(Cash)	8.95			8.95								
21	Philips' Med. Suppl.	1793	85.00					85.00						
23	Medi Path	1794	67.90				67.90							
24	Micah Smith	(Cash)	10.00										10.00	
24	Elena Paxson	1795	126.00							126.00				
27	Postage	1796	17.32			17.32								
28	Johnson Assoc.	1797	123.45				123.45							
	Total		3770.14	1 500.00	125.00	60.42	223.85	302.00	206.40	288.98	354.92	608.57	25.00	75.00

Figure 16-3. A record of office disbursements lists the amounts paid over a certain period of time.

Quarterly Summary of Charges, Receipts, and Disbursements, 1999

	MONTH	1 CHARGES	2 RECEIPTS	3 DISBURSE-MENTS	4 WAGES	5 RENT & UTILITIES	6 OFFICE EXPENSES	7 GENERAL MEDICAL	8 X-RAY/ LAB.	9 TAXES	10 PERSONAL	11 MISC.
					Types of Disbursements							
1	Jan.	15400.00	14800.00	6218.14	3349.50	1625.00	129.86	93.45	241.86	589.02	100.00	89.45
2	Feb.	18255.00	18950.00	7050.40	3872.80	1683.08	235.00	118.72	266.00	611.20	186.60	77.00
3	Mar.	13850.00	13250.00	6530.14	3666.10	1702.85	43.85	243.11	187.02	577.00	88.11	22.10
4												
5	Subtotal	47505.00	47000.00	19798.68	10888.40	5010.93	408.71	455.28	694.88	1777.22	374.71	188.55
6												
7	Apr.											
8	May											
9	June											
10												
11	Subtotal											
12												
13	July											
14	Aug.											
15	Sept.											
16												
17	Subtotal											
18												
19	Oct.											
20	Nov.											
21	Dec.											
22												
23	Subtotal											
24												
25	Grand Total											
26												
27												
28												
29												
30												
31												
32												
33												
34												
35												
36												

Figure 16-4. Creating a summary of charges, receipts, and disbursements is a regular bookkeeping task, performed monthly, quarterly, or yearly.

PROCEDURE 16-1

Organizing the Practice's Bookkeeping System

Objective: To establish a bookkeeping system that promotes accurate record keeping for the practice

Materials: Daily log sheets; patient ledger cards; check register; summaries of charges, receipts, and disbursements

Method

1. Use a new daily log sheet each day. For each patient seen that day, record the patient name, the relevant charges, and any payments received.
2. Create a ledger card for each new patient, and maintain a ledger card for all existing patients. The ledger card should include the patient's name, address, home and work telephone numbers, and insurance company. It should also contain the name of the person responsible for the charges (if different from the patient) and the name of the person who referred the patient to the office. Update the ledger card every time the patient incurs a charge or makes a payment. Be sure to adjust the account balance after every transaction.
3. Record all deposits accurately in the check register. File the deposit receipt—with a detailed listing of checks and money orders deposited—for later use in reconciling the bank statement.
4. When paying bills for the practice, enter each check in the check register accurately, including the check number, date, payee, and amount.
5. Prepare a summary of charges, receipts, and disbursements every month, quarter, or year, as directed. Be sure to double-check the calculations from the monthly summary before posting them to the quarterly summary. Also, double-check the calculations from the quarterly summary before posting them to the yearly summary.

and requires a great deal of time and skill to master. If it is used in a medical practice, an accountant usually establishes and maintains the system, and the medical assistant simply keeps a daily log.

Pegboard System. The **pegboard system** lets you write each transaction once while recording it on four different bookkeeping forms. This technique reduces errors and saves time. The pegboard system, also called the one-write system, is the most widely used bookkeeping system in medical practices. It is accurate and easy to learn.

A pegboard system usually includes a lightweight board with pegs on the left or right edges (Figure 16-5). The pegs match holes that are punched in daily log sheets, patient ledger cards, charge slips/receipts, and deposit slips. The holes allow the forms to be aligned while stacked on top of each other. Information, entered on only one form, is simultaneously transferred to the form(s) below. Generally these forms are printed on NCR (no-carbon-required) paper. If not, you must place carbon paper between the forms.

Starting the Business Day. Place a daily log sheet on the pegboard at the beginning of each day. Then, place the stack of charge slips/receipts on the pegs, aligning the top line of the first charge slip/receipt with the daily log top line. Because the charge slips/receipts are shingled, or layered one over the other from top to bottom, alignment of the first aligns all the others. The charge slips/receipts are prenumbered. This numbering promotes good cash control and theoretically prevents embezzlement.

Upon Patient Arrival. As each patient comes into the office, place the patient's ledger card under the next available charge slip/receipt. Be sure to align the card's first blank line with the carbon strip on the charge slip/receipt. Write the date, the patient's name, and the patient's previous balance on the charge slip section. The information will automatically be recorded in the daily log and on the patient ledger card.

Attaching the Charge Slip/Receipt to the Patient Chart. Next, remove the charge slip/receipt and attach it to the patient chart so that the doctor will see it. After examining the patient, the doctor fills in the appropriate charges on the charge slip/receipt, indicates when the next appointment is needed, and gives the charge slip/receipt to the patient.

Before the Patient Leaves. The patient comes to you with the completed charge slip/receipt, and you again place the ledger card between the charge slip/receipt and the daily log. Check to be sure you align it properly. On the charge slip/receipt, write the charge slip/receipt number, date, procedure (or code), charges, payments, new balance, and the date and time of the next appointment (if any). As you write this information, it should be automatically transferred onto the ledger card and daily log. Finally, tear off the receipt, and give it to the patient. You can now return the patient ledger card to the file.

Payments After the Patient Visit. If you receive payments sometime after the patient visit, either by mail or in person, record them on the patient ledger card and daily log as you normally would. Record charges for doctor visits to hospitalized patients or other out-of-office visits in the same way. If required, you can use the pegboard system to record bank deposits and petty cash disbursements in the daily log, but you will need the appropriate overlapping forms.

End of the Day. At the end of each day, total and check the arithmetic (addition and subtraction) in all columns. If you find an error, correct it immediately by drawing a line through it and making a new entry on the next available writing line. Remember to make the correction on the patient ledger card also and to issue a new receipt to the patient.

Bookkeeping on the Computer

Physicians or office managers who choose to set up the practice's bookkeeping system on the computer enjoy several important benefits over traditional bookkeeping methods. Computerized bookkeeping saves time; many repetitive tasks are done by the computer. The computer also performs mathematic calculations. Most bookkeeping software programs include built-in tax tables, which can calculate tax liabilities and so on.

As discussed in Chapter 6, there are many bookkeeping software programs available on the market. Any bookkeeping software package performs the same tasks described earlier in this chapter under traditional bookkeeping systems. The practice in which you work may already have a computerized bookkeeping program in place. It is a good idea, however, to read current computer software magazines. You may learn about a new software program you might recommend to the physician or office manager, or you may read about a new or more efficient way to use the practice's current software program.

Banking for the Medical Office

Besides bookkeeping, you may be responsible for handling the banking for the practice. Because a practice may use traditional (manual) or electronic (computerized) banking methods, you should be familiar with both. Regardless of which method you use, remember to keep all banking materials secure because they represent the finances of the practice. For example, to prevent theft of checks, always put the checkbook in a securely locked place when it is not in use. Also, file deposit receipts promptly. If they are lost, you have no proof that a deposit was made. Lack of proof could cost the practice thousands of dollars.

Banking Tasks

Banking tasks for the medical practice include:

- Writing checks.
- Accepting checks.
- Endorsing checks.
- Making deposits.
- Reconciling bank statements.

To perform these tasks properly, you must be familiar with several terms and concepts related to banking.

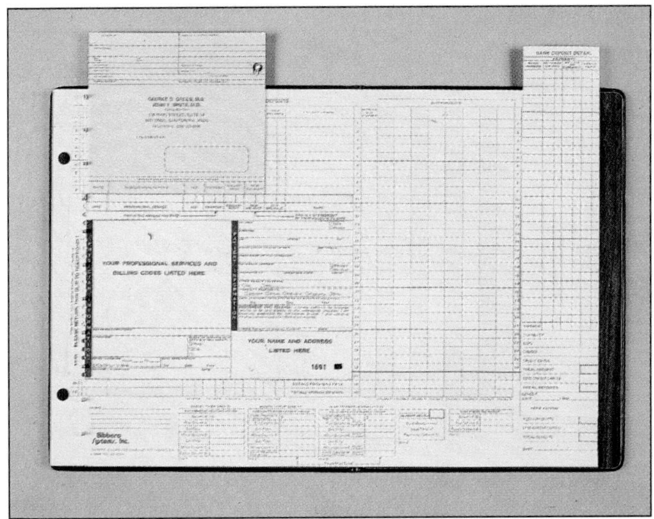

Figure 16-5. A pegboard system allows for simultaneous transfer of information while writing it only once.

Checks. A **check** is a bank draft or order for payment. The person who writes the check is called the **payer.** By writing a check, the payer directs the bank to pay a sum of money on demand to the payee. In order to be considered **negotiable** (legally transferable from one person to another), a check must:

- Be written and signed by the payer or maker.
- Include the amount of money to be paid, considered a promise to pay a specified sum.
- Be made payable to the payee or bearer.
- Be made payable on demand or on a specific date.
- Include the name of the bank that is directed to make payment.

Other Negotiable Papers. You may receive other negotiable paper in addition to standard personal and business checks.

1. A **cashier's check** is a check issued on bank paper signed by a bank representative. It is usually purchased by individuals who do not have checking accounts.
2. A **certified check** is a payer's check written and signed by the payer and stamped "Certified" by the bank. This certification means that the bank has already drawn money from the payer's account to guarantee that the check will be paid when submitted. (The money is set aside to cover this specific check.)
3. A **money order** is another kind of certificate of guaranteed payment. Money orders may be purchased from banks (bank money orders) or post offices (postal money orders) or from some convenience stores.

Check Codes. The face (front) of every check contains two important items: the American Banking Association (ABA) number and the magnetic ink character recogni-

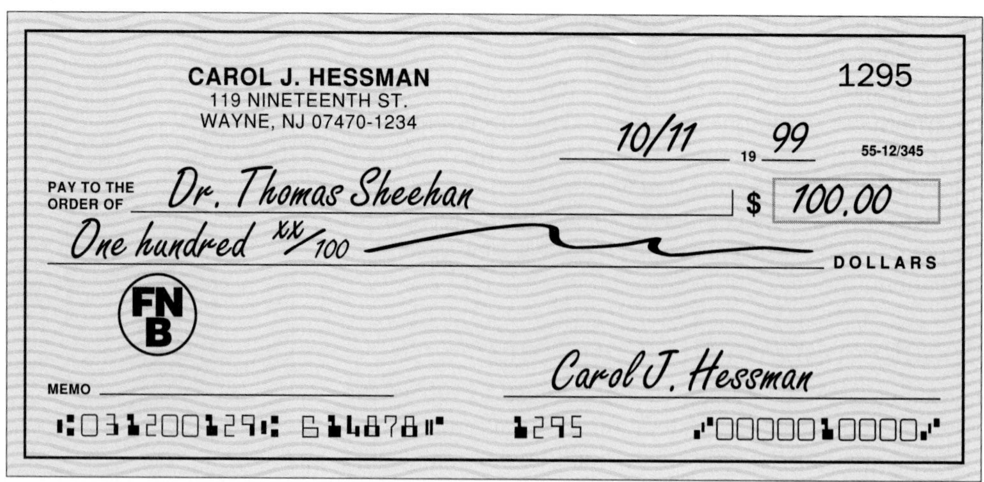

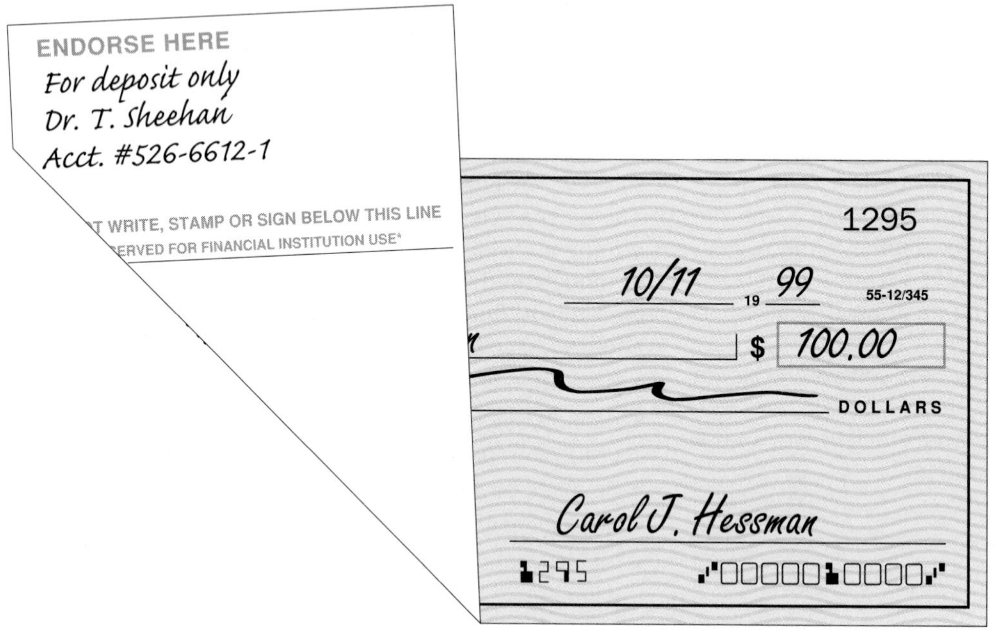

Figure 16-6. After verifying that a patient's check is correct, immediately endorse it with "For Deposit Only," the name of the practice, and the account number.

tion (MICR) code. The **ABA number** appears as a fraction, such as 60-117/310, on the upper edge of all printed checks. It identifies the geographic area and specific bank on which the check is drawn.

Found at the bottom of a check, the MICR code consists of numbers and characters printed in magnetic ink, which can be read by MICR equipment at the bank. This code enables checks to be read, sorted, and recorded by computer.

Types of Checking Accounts. A physician is likely to have three different types of checking accounts: a personal account, a business account for office expenses, and an interest-earning account. The interest-earning account will be used for paying special expenses, such as property taxes and insurance premiums. Most of your work will be with the business checking account. You may sometimes, however, make payments from, or transfer money to, the interest-earning account, as directed.

Accepting Checks. Before accepting any check, review it carefully. First be sure the check has the correct date, amount, and signature and that no corrections have been made. Figure 16-6 shows a correctly written and endorsed check. Do not accept a **third party check** (one made out to the patient rather than to the practice) unless it is from a health insurance company. Also, do not accept a check marked "Payment in Full" unless it actually does pay the complete outstanding balance. You may accept a check signed by someone other than the payer if the person who signed the check has power of attorney. **Power of attorney** gives a person the legal right to handle financial matters for another person who is unable to do so. Frequently power of attorney is granted to a patient's spouse, son, or daughter.

Be sure to follow the policy of your practice when accepting a check. For example, if a patient is new or unfamiliar, office policy may require you to request patient identification and to compare the signature on the identification with the signature on the check. Policy may also require that you not accept a check for more than the amount due.

Endorsing Checks. After accepting a check, immediately **endorse** it, that is to say, write the name of the doctor or the practice on the back. Include the words "For Deposit Only" and the account number. (For convenience, this statement may be made into a rubber stamp.) This type of endorsement prevents the check from being cashed if it is lost or stolen.

Be sure to endorse the check in ink, using a pen or rubber stamp. Place the endorsement in the 1.5-inch area indicated on the back of the check. Most personal and business checks have a number of lines or a shaded area preprinted on the checks for this purpose. Leave the rest of the back of the check blank for the use of the bank.

Completing the Deposit Slip. After endorsing the check, post the payment to the patient ledger card, and put the check with others to be deposited. Then, fill out a deposit slip, as shown in Figure 16-7. The account number is printed on deposit slips in MICR numbers that match those on the checks. As mentioned, these numbers enable checks and deposit slips to be read, sorted, and recorded by computer.

Banks will accept a list of deposited items on something other than the bank-provided deposit slip if the bank's deposit slip is attached. For example, if you are depositing 50 checks, you may create a computer printout listing the payers' names, check numbers, amount of each check, and total. You can then attach the printout to a deposit slip with the total written on the deposit slip. Another method is to attach a calculator or adding machine tape listing the individual check amounts and a total.

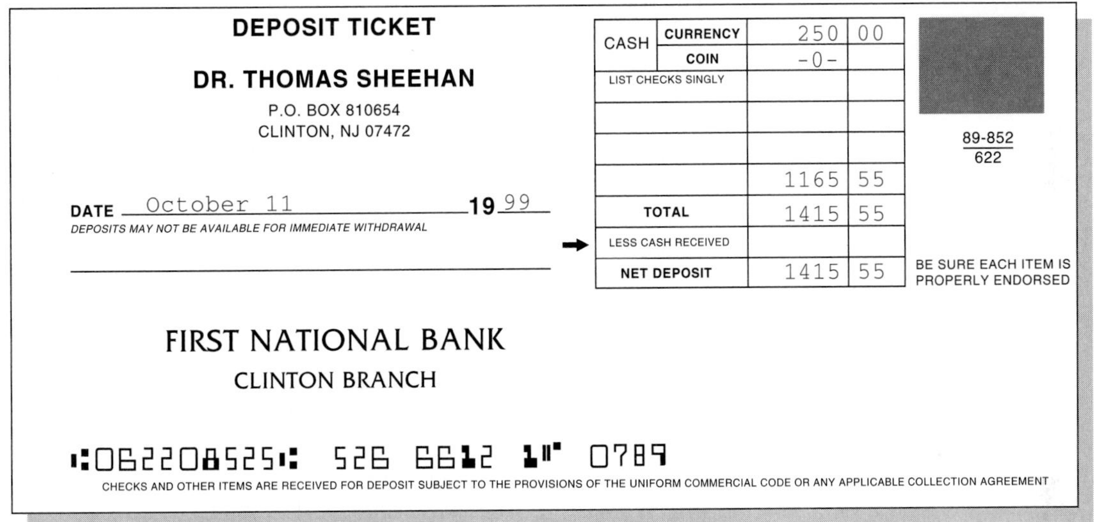

DEPOSIT TICKET

DR. THOMAS SHEEHAN
P.O. BOX 810654
CLINTON, NJ 07472

DATE October 11 19 99
DEPOSITS MAY NOT BE AVAILABLE FOR IMMEDIATE WITHDRAWAL

CASH	CURRENCY	250	00
	COIN	-0-	
LIST CHECKS SINGLY			
		1165	55
TOTAL		1415	55
LESS CASH RECEIVED			
NET DEPOSIT		1415	55

89-852
622

BE SURE EACH ITEM IS PROPERLY ENDORSED

FIRST NATIONAL BANK
CLINTON BRANCH

⑆062208525⑆ 526 6612 1⑈ 0789

CHECKS AND OTHER ITEMS ARE RECEIVED FOR DEPOSIT SUBJECT TO THE PROVISIONS OF THE UNIFORM COMMERCIAL CODE OR ANY APPLICABLE COLLECTION AGREEMENT

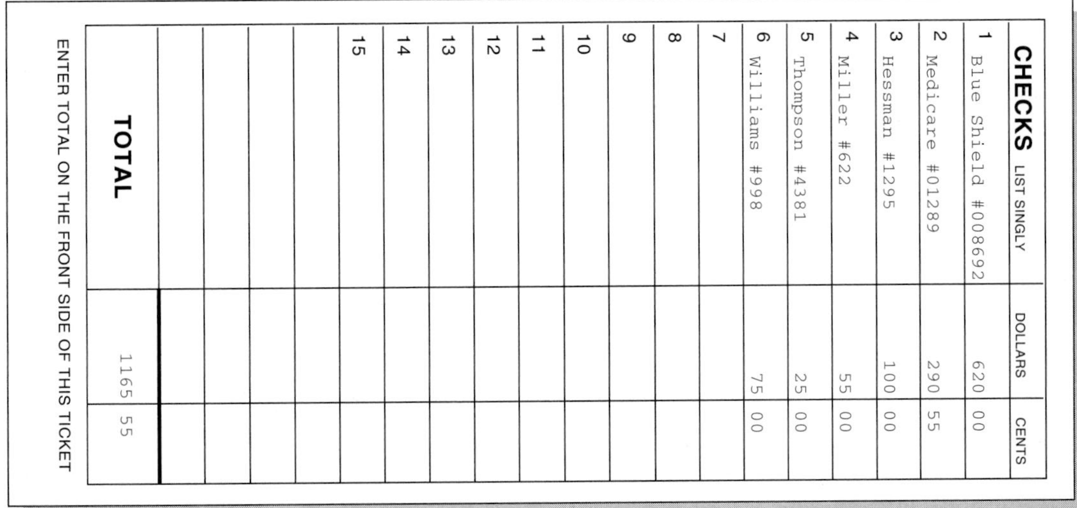

CHECKS LIST SINGLY	DOLLARS	CENTS
1 Blue Shield #008692	620	00
2 Medicare #01289	290	55
3 Hessman #1295	100	00
4 Miller #622	55	00
5 Thompson #4381	25	00
6 Williams #998	75	00
7		
8		
9		
10		
11		
12		
13		
14		
15		
TOTAL	1165	55

ENTER TOTAL ON THE FRONT SIDE OF THIS TICKET

Figure 16-7. List each check on the deposit slip, including the check number and amount.

PROCEDURE 16-2

Making a Bank Deposit

Objective: To prepare cash and checks for deposit and to deposit them properly into a bank account

Materials: Bank deposit slip and items to be deposited, such as checks, cash, and money orders

Method

1. Divide the bills, coins, checks, and money orders into separate piles.
2. Sort the bills by denomination, from largest to smallest. Then, stack them, portrait side up, in the same direction. Total the amount of the bills, and write this amount on the deposit slip on the line marked "Currency."
3. If you have enough coins to fill coin wrappers, put them in wrappers of the proper denomination. If not, count the coins, and put them in the deposit bag. Total the amount of coins, and write this amount on the deposit slip on the line marked "Coin."
4. Review all checks and money orders to be sure they are properly endorsed with a restrictive endorsement. List each check on the deposit slip, including the check number and amount. If you do not keep a list of the check writers' names in the office, record this information on the deposit slip also.
5. List each money order on the deposit slip. Include the notation "money order" or "MO" and the name of the writer.
6. Calculate the total deposit (total of amounts for currency, coin, checks, and money orders). Write this amount on the deposit slip on the line marked "Total." Photocopy the deposit slip for your office records.
7. Record the total amount of the deposit in the office checkbook register.
8. If you plan to make the deposit in person, place the currency, coins, checks, and money orders in a deposit bag. If you cannot make the deposit in person, put the checks and money orders in a special bank-by-mail envelope, or put all deposit items in an envelope and send it by registered mail.
9. Make the deposit in person or by mail.
10. Obtain a deposit receipt from the bank. File it in the office for later use when reconciling the bank statement.

Making the Deposit. Plan to deposit checks and cash into the practice's bank account in person at the bank, as described in Procedure 16-2. Avoid sending cash through the mail, but if it is absolutely necessary to do so, use registered mail. In any case, be sure to obtain a deposit receipt from the bank.

In a busy physician's office, you may need to make deposits every day. If the physician has a limited practice, you may make deposits less frequently. Keep in mind, however, that making deposits more frequently increases cash flow and reduces the risk of lost or bounced checks.

Reconciling Bank Statements. Another banking task is reconciling the bank statement. **Reconciliation** involves comparing the office's financial records with the bank records to ensure that they are consistent (all numbers agree) and accurate. In most practices this task is performed once a month when the practice receives the monthly checking account statement from the bank. An example of a bank statement is shown in Figure 16-8. The process of reconciliation is explained in Procedure 16-3.

Electronic Banking

Compared with traditional banking methods, electronic banking has several advantages. The previous chapter reviewed the use of the computer for submitting health insurance claims. Here we will discuss another use of the computer, showing how electronic banking can improve productivity, cash flow, and accuracy. The use of electronic banking can also speed up many banking tasks.

If your medical office uses electronic banking, your basic tasks will be the same as in an office that uses traditional banking methods. How these tasks are performed, however, may be quite different. When you use electronic banking, you are still responsible for recording and depositing checks, just as if you were using traditional methods, but you will see these differences.

- Rather than your recording each check in a paper checkbook and determining the new balance, the computer software calculates the new balance for you.
- Rather than your reconciling the office bank statement on paper, the computer software does it automatically.
- Rather than putting the checkbook and banking forms in a securely locked place at the end of the day, you use a computer password for security.

Many medical office software programs are available today. Each one has a different interface, uses different menus, and prompts you for information in different ways. Certain general concepts apply to all. For specific information, consult the user's manual that comes with your practice's computer software.

1st **First State Bank of Englewood**
CN 1
Englewood WI 54534-0001

PAGE 1

ACCOUNT NO. 518-833-3

STATEMENT PERIOD
07/19/98 TO 08/20/98

CAROL J CHARLESTON
APT 49
1013 HUGHES DR
LAWRENCE SQUARE WI 54690-1226

YOUR ACCOUNT SUMMARY

DEPOSIT ACCOUNTS	BALANCE
CHECKING ACCOUNT	2,088.08
SAVINGS ACCOUNT	6.54
TOTAL	2,094.62

CHECKING ACCOUNT

CAROL J CHARLESTON

SUMMARY OF ACCOUNT 518-833-3	
BEGINNING BALANCE ON 07/18/98	3,055.24
DEPOSITS AND CREDITS	+3,819.02
CHECKS & WITHDRAWALS	-4,786.18
ENDING BALANCE ON 08/20/98	2,088.08

CHECKS PAID: 38

CHECK	AMOUNT	DATE PAID	REFERENCE#
CHECK	450.00	07/19/98	81569110
2202	146.23	07/31/98	29521570
2203	122.03	07/29/98	29141271
2210*	43.00	07/29/98	07046380
2211	60.09	08/01/98	04597911
2214*	123.59	07/24/98	29470425
2215	47.70	07/19/98	12357289
2216	9.00	07/22/98	05479786
2217	30.00	07/26/98	29841864
2218	19.00	07/30/98	04330539
2219	12.00	07/24/98	04037820
2220	35.93	07/24/98	04068844
2221	10.00	08/12/98	05091269
2222	23.48	07/24/98	29465653
2223	242.43	07/26/98	29804419
2224	150.00	07/30/98	29405827
2225	830.00	08/07/98	02242873

CHECK	AMOUNT	DATE PAID	REFERENCE#
2226	181.00	08/12/98	05105878
2227	24.74	08/19/98	06120827
2228	140.00	08/12/98	05022086
2229	148.71	08/16/98	27248941
2230	53.16	08/13/98	27852752
2231	50.00	08/14/98	01018325
2232	50.00	08/13/98	05080148
2233	15.00	08/16/98	04709533
2234	13.95	08/19/98	06008593
2235	123.59	08/14/98	27050650
2236	50.00	08/13/98	05099115
2237	50.00	08/15/98	03014667
2238	20.00	08/16/98	04675854
2239	47.70	08/14/98	06172997
2240	24.74	08/19/98	06120925
2243*	400.00	08/14/98	29652307
2344	400.00	08/14/98	29652306

Figure 16-8. Each month you will receive a current bank statement, which you should reconcile with the previous statement and your checkbook register.

PROCEDURE 16-3

Reconciling a Bank Statement

Objective: To ensure that the bank record of deposits and withdrawals agrees with the practice's record of deposits and withdrawals

Materials: Previous bank statement, current bank statement, reconciliation worksheet (if not part of current bank statement), deposit receipts, red pencil, check stubs or checkbook register, returned checks

Method

1. Check the closing balance on the previous statement against the opening balance on the new statement. The balances should match. If they do not, call the bank.
2. Record the closing balance from the new statement on the reconciliation worksheet (Figure 16-9). This worksheet usually appears on the back of the bank statement.
3. Check each deposit receipt against the bank statement. Place a red check mark in the upper right corner of each receipt that is recorded on the statement. Total the amount of deposits that do *not* appear on the statement. Add this amount to the closing balance on the reconciliation worksheet.
4. Put the returned checks in numerical order.
5. Compare each returned check with the bank statement, making sure that the amount on the check agrees with the amount on the statement. Place a red check mark in the upper right corner of each returned check that is recorded on the statement. Also, place a check mark on the check stub or check register entry. Any checks that were written but that do not appear on the statement and were not returned are considered "outstanding" checks. You can find these easily on the check stubs or checkbook register because they have no red check mark.
6. List each outstanding check separately on the worksheet, including its check number and amount. Total the outstanding checks, and subtract this total from the bank statement balance.
7. If the statement shows that the checking account earned interest, add this amount to the checkbook balance.
8. If the statement lists such items as a service charge, check printing charge, or automatic payment, subtract them from the checkbook balance.
9. Compare the new checkbook balance with the new bank statement balance. They should match. If they do not, repeat the process, rechecking all calculations. Double-check the addition and subtraction in the checkbook register. Review the checkbook register to make sure you did not omit any items. Ensure that you carried the correct balance forward from one register page to the next. Double-check that you made the correct additions or subtractions for all interest earned and charges.

After the software has been installed and after you "boot up" (turn on the program), the computer screen displays the main menu. This menu offers several options. Among these options is "Banking" (or a similar term), which you should select.

The main menu then disappears, and another menu appears that offers several more options, including the following:

- Record Deposits
- Pay Bills
- Display Checkbook
- Balance Checkbook

Record Deposits. If you select "Record Deposits," a message on the computer screen prompts you to enter information about each check to be deposited that day. This information usually includes the check writer's name and the amount of the check. The check's ABA number may also be requested. After you enter this information, the computer gives you a chance to double-check it. If all the information is correct, you continue entering and checking the other deposits, one at a time. You can then select a command to print a deposit slip that contains the information you have just entered. To make the deposit, place the cash and checks in a deposit bag with the completed slip for deposit at the bank.

Pay Bills. The bill-paying function allows you to log checks that you write into a computerized checkbook register. For each check you want to write, a message on the computer screen should prompt you for information, such as the payee and the amount of the check. The computer should also give you a chance to verify and correct this information before moving on to the next check or printing the actual checks.

Some software programs automatically assign the next available check number to each new check you enter. To double-check that the computer-assigned check numbers match those on the actual checks, print a list of the checks you have entered, and compare it with the checks before mailing them.

10. If your work is correct, and the balances still do not agree, call the bank to determine if a bank error has been made. Contact the bank promptly because the bank may have a time limit for corrections. The bank may consider the bank statement correct if you do not point out an error within 2 weeks (or other period, according to bank policy).

HOW TO BALANCE YOUR CHECKING ACCOUNT

1. Subtract any service charges that appear on this statement from your checkbook balance.
2. Add any interest paid on your checking account to your checkbook balance.
3. Check off (✔) in your checkbook register all checks and pre-authorized transactions listed on your statement.
4. Use the worksheet to list checks you have written, ATM withdrawals, and Point of Sale transactions which are not listed on your statement.

5. Enter the closing balance on the statement.	$	.
6. Add any deposits not shown on the statement.	+	.
7. Subtotal	$	.
8. Subtract total transactions outstanding (from worksheet on right).	−	.
9. Account balance (should match balance in your checkbook register).	$	.

IF YOUR ACCOUNT DOES NOT BALANCE

a. Check your addition and subtraction first on this form and then in your checkbook.
b. Be sure the deposit amounts on your statement are the same as those in your checkbook.
c. Be sure all the check amounts on your statement agree with the amounts entered in your checkbook register.
d. Be sure all checks written prior to this reconcilement period but not listed on the statement are listed on the worksheet.
e. Verify that all MAC® ATM, Point of Sale, and other pre-authorized transactions have been recorded in your checkbook register.
f. Review last month's statement to be certain any corrections were entered into your checkbook.

WORKSHEET Transactions Outstanding	
Number or Date	Amount
TOTAL	

Figure 16-9. Use the reconciliation worksheet on the back of the bank statement to reconcile the statement with your checkbook register.

Display Checkbook. This function allows you to review the electronic checkbook register. Although you cannot change information that appears in the register, you can print it out. Thus, you can be sure the checks have been recorded properly, and you can check your latest balance.

If you select "Display Checkbook" from the "Banking" menu, the computer displays a list of all checks that have been entered into the register. Information includes check number, date, payee, and amount. Scrolling up and down reveals all the checks in the register. (Some banks also allow you to access this information by telephone. "Tips for the Office" gives more information about telephone banking.)

Balance Checkbook. The "Balance Checkbook" function electronically reconciles the monthly bank statement. After you enter the appropriate date or dates, the computer screen displays all the checks and deposits that were logged into the register in the order they were posted. Figure 16-10 shows an example of this function.

The next screen highlights each check or deposit that has not been seen on a previous bank statement. You are then prompted to indicate whether that item appears on the current statement, usually using Y for yes and N for no. After the computer queries these items, it may ask you to enter any items that appear on the current bank statement but are not in the checkbook, such as service charges.

Finally, a message on the screen prompts you to enter the current account balance from the bank statement. Then, the computer reconciles the bank statement. It will alert you if the system balance does not agree with the balance on the bank statement. If the balance does not agree, recheck the information you entered for possible error. If your work is correct, and the balances still do not agree, call the bank to determine if a bank error has been made.

Tips FOR THE OFFICE

Telephone Banking

Telephone banking is a form of electronic banking that enables you to access your bank's computer system by phone to obtain account information and perform simple banking tasks. To use telephone banking, you should have a push-button telephone, the telephone personal identification number (TPIN) assigned to your practice by the bank, and the telephone banking telephone number.

The telephone banking system prompts you for information. You use the push-button pad on the telephone to provide the information. For example, an automated voice may ask you to press 1 to inquire about deposits or 2 to inquire about withdrawals. Telephone banking is especially useful for the following banking tasks:

- Checking the current balance of an account
- Determining whether deposited funds are available
- Obtaining the date and amount of the last few deposits and the last few checks paid (usually the last three)
- Finding out if a specific check has been paid
- Transferring funds between accounts (if the practice has more than one account)
- Stopping payment on checks

Although this form of electronic banking is especially useful for some services, you cannot use it to manage all banking tasks. For example, you cannot use it to make deposits or reconcile a bank statement. However, it can be quite convenient for the day-to-day banking tasks listed above. If you have a hearing impairment and have a telecommunications device for the deaf (TDD) installed on the telephone, you can bank by phone.

Planning for Retirement

Many people—especially young people—do not make financial plans for their retirement. They may not be making much money at the start of their careers. "Just getting by" may take precedence over setting aside money for savings or retirement. They may assume that Social Security will cover their financial needs. They may not think about financial planning because retirement seems so far in the future. A knowledge of financial planning can be both personally and professionally useful, however. If you become an experienced medical assistant, you may manage the employee benefits records for your practice, including those for retirement plans.

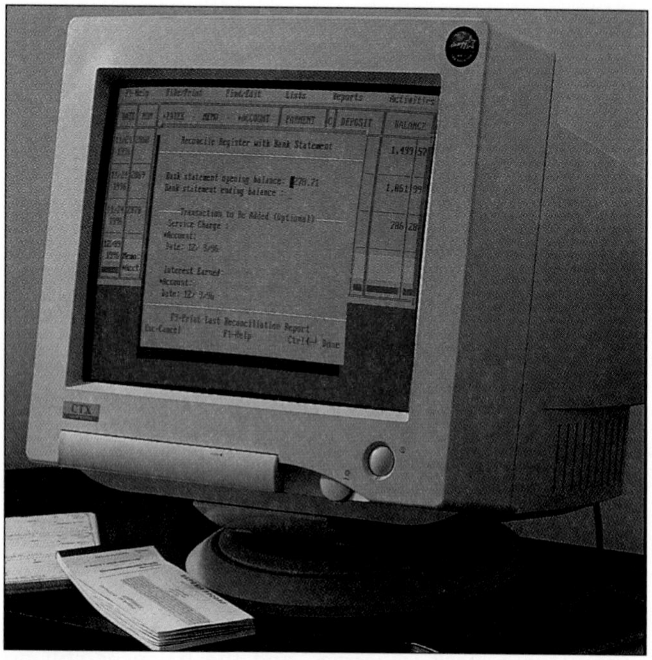

Figure 16-10. Electronic banking will allow you to see the "Balance Checkbook" function on the screen.

Starting Your Own Savings Program

Regardless of your age, you should think seriously about planning for your future financial security. In fact, the younger you are when you start planning, the more comfortable your retirement will be. Here is an example of the value of starting to save for retirement at an early age.

> *Judy and Joan are both medical assistants and have retirement plans that earn 6% interest. Judy started saving $100 a month at the age of 25, and Joan started saving $100 a month at the age of 35. By the time Judy is 65 years old, she will have $199,149. Joan will have $100,452 (approximately half of Judy's accumulated fund) by the time she is 65 years old.*

Because interest is compounded (that is, interest is paid on the initial investment *and* on the interest earned on the investment), Judy's fund is nearly twice Joan's because she started saving 10 years earlier.

Social Security

If you meet certain work requirements, Social Security will provide fixed monthly payments after you reach a certain age. It will not, however, pay enough to meet all your needs for housing, utilities, food, and clothing. Therefore, financial experts consider Social Security payments to be just one of three "pillars of economic security" (Allen, 1992).

Another pillar is personal savings, which may include insurance and investments. The third pillar is employer-sponsored retirement plans. A medical practice may offer various retirement plans to employees, along with other types of **benefits,** such as paid vacation, paid holidays, and disability and life insurance. Some practices provide an annual statement of compensation and benefits, which lists each benefit and its value along with the employee's salary.

Retirement Plans

Retirement benefits offer advantages for both employees and employers. For employees, retirement plans help build financial security for the future. Some plans also help reduce income taxes while the employee is working. For employers, retirement plans can reduce business taxes, reward long-term employees, and increase employee morale and productivity. Good retirement plans also enable employers to attract better employees and keep them longer.

Some retirement plans are paid for entirely by the employer. Others are paid for by the employee—usually through payroll deductions—or by both (Table 16-1).

Payroll Deductions. Amounts regularly withheld from your paycheck are called **payroll deductions.** Many deductions are required by law, such as federal, state, and local taxes. (Taxes will be discussed in Chapter 18.) However, FICA taxes deserve particular attention here. These taxes are required by the Federal Insurance Contributions Act and are used to fund Social Security, Medicare, and public disability insurance. Your employer must match the amount of FICA tax withheld from your paycheck and must send the combined amount to the federal government, usually every month.

Some payroll deductions are optional. These deductions may include the purchase of additional life insurance, savings bonds, or stocks; credit union deposits; payment for uniforms; or contributions to a retirement plan, such as a 401(k) plan or an individual retirement account (IRA). Eligibility for an optional payroll deduction plan depends on the policy of the practice for which you work.

If you have an IRA, payroll deductions are a convenient way to make regular contributions to it. Although the medical practice is not required to contribute to your IRA account, it may offer payroll deductions as a service. Depending on your income and marital status, you may deposit up to $2000 of your annual salary into an IRA, and your money will be 100% vested immediately. **Vesting** means that you have a legal right to all the money in your account.

Pension Plans. A **pension plan** is a retirement benefit that provides income (from an investment account) to an employee after retirement. (The age of retirement may vary from company to company, but is usually about 62 to 65.) The money to create pension plans usually comes from both employee and employer contributions. These funds are put into investment accounts that grow during the course of your career. Two common types of pension plans are 401(k) plans and profit-sharing plans.

401(k) Plans. Under a **401(k) plan,** your employer deposits part of your paycheck into a trust account. Your employer may also match a certain percentage of your contribution, say 10%, and add it to your trust account. Because your contributions to the 401(k) plan are taken out of your salary *before taxes are calculated,* you pay less in income tax while you save for retirement. Because the interest on your 401(k) contributions is tax-deferred, you pay no tax on that interest or on your contributions until you make a withdrawal.

Some restrictions apply to 401(k) plans. You may have to meet certain criteria to be eligible for a plan. For example, you may need to have worked for the practice for at least 1 year. You may contribute up to a maximum amount annually. In 1996 the amount was 15% of your salary or $9500, whichever was less. You are 100% vested for all of your payroll contributions. Also, you cannot withdraw money from your account without a tax penalty until you retire. You may, however, prior to retirement, withdraw money as a loan or if you need it because of heavy medical expenses or some other hardship. In these cases, your withdrawals are subject to income tax. If you terminate your employment, you must transfer, or "roll over," the funds in your 401(k) account to an individual retirement account (IRA). Otherwise, you will be taxed on the withdrawal.

Profit-Sharing Plans. In a typical **profit-sharing plan,** the practice every year adds an amount of money, usually based on profits, to your profit-sharing account. A medical practice can decide when you become eligible for its profit-sharing plan. For example, the practice may require you to be at least 21 years old, to work 1000 hours per year, and to have been an employee for at least 1 year.

The owners of many practices feel that profit-sharing plans motivate employees to increase productivity and decrease expenses. A few profit-sharing plans allow employees to add their own voluntary contributions to the profit-sharing account. As in a 401(k) plan, all deposited amounts accumulate interest tax-free until they are withdrawn.

Over time, as you participate in a profit-sharing plan, you become vested. The time required for vesting depends on your employer. For example, you may become fully vested (entitled to 100% of your account) after 5 years of employment, or you may be gradually vested over a period of 6 years (entitled to 20% after year 2, 40% after year 3, and so on). If you leave the practice before you are vested, you forfeit the employer-contributed amount in your account. Your employer may redistribute that amount among the remaining employees in the profit-sharing plan.

After you are vested, you can withdraw money from your profit-sharing account when you reach a certain age, retire, or experience certain events, such as a disability, illness, or job layoff.

Security for Your Pension Funds. The Employee Retirement Income Security Act of 1974 and various other laws regulate most pension plans and ensure that they are properly funded. The Department of Labor, the Internal Revenue Service, and the Pension Benefit Guaranty Corporation monitor pension plans. Because of these laws and agencies, you can be sure that your retirement benefits will be there when you need them.

If the practice where you work offers a pension plan, you may be able to add money to the account and even choose the investments in the plan. Therefore, you

Table 16-1

Financial Planning for Retirement

Type of Plan	Contributor to Plan	Plan Characteristics
Social Security	• Employee (50%) • Employer (50%)	• Required by federal law • Managed by the federal government • Provides payments upon retirement • Provides payments upon disability and to survivors upon death • Funds Medicare
Individual retirement account	• Employee • Employer (optional)	• Established through payroll deductions • Managed by the employee • Reduces the employee's taxable income by up to $2000 • Offers 100% vesting immediately • Accumulates interest and dividends tax-free • Transferable if the employee changes jobs
Profit-sharing plan	• Employer • Employee (optional)	• Provides monthly payment after retirement • Managed primarily by employer and usually based on profitability • Amount contributed by employer of up to 15% of employee's salary • Has eligibility and vesting requirements • Accumulates interest and earnings tax-free
401(k) plan	• Employee • Employer (optional)	• Provides monthly payment after retirement • Managed primarily by the employee through the employer • Has eligibility and vesting requirements • Reduces employee's taxable income • Accumulates interest and earnings tax-free

should become familiar with the pension plans available at your practice and consider them as part of your retirement planning.

Summary

The bookkeeping and banking responsibilities of a medical assistant involve managing the cash flow of the practice. To perform bookkeeping and banking tasks successfully, you must be familiar with basic financial concepts, such as income and expenses, and with bookkeeping and banking systems. You must also be able to use bookkeeping tools, such as the daily log of charges and receipts, patient's ledger card, and summary record of charges, receipts, and disbursements. In addition, you must be able to prepare and make bank deposits and to reconcile the monthly bank statement with the records of the practice.

In addition, it is important to know about the options for planning for financial security in your retirement. Because Social Security pays most retirees only a small amount, you will need other sources of income to meet your retirement needs. Retirement planning tools include payroll deductions for IRAs or other investments, as well as employer-sponsored pension plans, such as 401(k) plans.

16 Chapter Review

Discussion Questions

1. What types of business decisions might a doctor make based on a periodic summary of charges, receipts, and disbursements of the practice?
2. How does electronic banking compare with traditional banking methods?
3. Why do most practices offer retirement benefits, such as pension plans, to their employees?
4. Describe precautions you can take to keep the practice's financial records confidential. Discuss precautions for both paper records and computerized records.

Critical Thinking Questions

1. Why is accuracy so important to bookkeeping in a medical practice?
2. How can you stay up to date on electronic banking practices?
3. Why is it better to make retirement plans sooner rather than later?

Application Activities

1. Keep a daily log of your expenses and income for 1 month. Separate the expenses into categories, such as groceries, rent, utilities, and entertainment. At the end of the month, total your expenses and income. Calculate what percentage of your income you spent in each category. What changes, if any, might you make to your budget, based on this exercise?
2. Using a pegboard system, record the following transactions on a charge slip/receipt, a daily log sheet, and a patient ledger card.
   - Patient A has an outstanding balance of $65. She has blood work done in the practice laboratory, which costs $50. Before leaving, she writes a check for $20.
   - Patient B has no outstanding balance on his account. He sees the physician for an annual physical, which costs $80. As part of the physical, the following laboratory work is also ordered: Chem 21 for $65, CBC for $35, urinalysis for $20, and occult blood for $15. He gives the medical assistant $5 as his co-payment.
   - Patient C came in last week for an allergy shot from the nurse, which costs $20. Today the patient has an appointment for treatment of a urinary tract infection. She is charged for a brief examination, which costs $40, and urine tests, which cost $60. She plans to pay after she receives her next paycheck.
3. Reconcile your bank statement with your personal checking account, using the procedure described in this chapter.
4. Talk to a financial adviser, banker, or accountant about savings or investments that may be appropriate for you when planning your retirement. Report on the recommendations made.

Further Readings

Allen, Everett T., Jr., et al. *Pension Planning: Pensions, Profit-Sharing, and Other Deferred Compensation Plans.* Homewood, IL: Irwin Publishing, 1992.

Joel, Lewin G., III. *Every Employee's Guide to the Law.* New York: Pantheon Books, 1993.

Johnson, Joan M., and Marc W. Johnson. *Computerized Medical Office Management.* Albany, NY: Delmar, 1994.

Sack, Steven Mitchell. *The Employee Rights Handbook.* Rev. ed. New York: Facts On File, 1993.

White, Jane, and Bruce Pyenson. *J. K. Lasser's Employee Benefits for Small Business.* 2d ed. New York: Prentice Hall, 1993.

Yellin, Susan. "Preparing an Employment Contract." *The Vancouver Sun,* 13 October 1995.

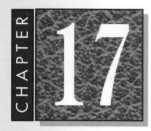

Billing and Collections

CHAPTER OUTLINE

- Basic Accounting
- Standard Payment Procedures
- Standard Billing Procedures
- Standard Collection Procedures
- Credit Arrangements
- Common Collection Problems

OBJECTIVES

After completing Chapter 17, you will be able to:

- Discuss the importance of accounts receivable to a medical practice.
- Explain how to accept and account for payment from patients.
- Prepare an invoice.
- Manage a billing cycle efficiently.
- Describe standard collection techniques.
- Explain how to perform a credit check.
- Identify credit arrangements.
- Recognize common collection problems.

AREAS OF COMPETENCE

1997 ROLE DELINEATION STUDY

ADMINISTRATIVE

Practice Finances

- Document and maintain accounting and banking records
- Manage accounts receivable

Key Terms

age analysis
class action lawsuit
collection percentage
credit
credit bureau
cycle billing
damages
disclosure statement
legal custody
open-book account
punitive damages
single-entry account
statement
statute of limitations
superbill
written-contract account

Basic Accounting

In any business, basic accounting involves managing accounts receivable and accounts payable. As stated in Chapter 16, accounts receivable is the term for income, or money, owed to the business. Accounts payable is the term for money owed by the business. In a medical practice, accounts receivable represents the money patients owe in return for medical services. Accounts payable describes the money the medical practice must pay out to run the practice.

Billing and collections are vitally important tasks because they convert the practice's accounts receivable into readily available income, or cash flow, from which the accounts payable can be paid. Unless billing and collections are carried out effectively, a practice might have plenty of money due in accounts receivable without having enough cash flow for accounts payable.

There are methods of improving billing and collection procedures to increase income for the practice. You will need to know about standard payment, billing, and collection procedures, as well as about credit arrangements and common problems in collecting payment.

Standard Payment Procedures

Most physicians prefer to collect payment from patients at each office visit. Immediate payment not only brings income into the practice faster, but it saves the cost of preparing and mailing bills and collecting on past-due accounts. For these reasons, many physicians' offices post a small sign at the reception desk that states, for example, "Payment is requested when services are rendered unless other arrangements are made in advance."

As a medical assistant, you are responsible for collecting these payments. If the patient cannot pay at the time of the visit, it is your responsibility to bill for the physician's services. A bill, the paperwork sent to patients to inform them of payment or balance due, is referred to as an invoice.

Determining Appropriate Fees

A fee schedule is a price list for the medical practice. Figure 17-1 shows an example. The fee schedule lists the services the doctor offers and the corresponding charges for those services. Fees are not randomly assigned. They

John Q. Davis, MD — *Adult and Pediatric Urology-Infertility*

SERVICE RENDERED	CPT	FEE
Initial OV	99204	$100.00
Follow-up Visit	99214	$65.00
Fertility Consultation	99243	$140.00
Office Consultation	99244	$140.00
Hospital Admission	99223	$150.00
Hospital Consultation	99254	$150.00
ER Visit	99284	$75.00–$150.00
Hospital Visit	99232	$55.00
Urinalysis w/ Micro	81000	$14.00
Culture	87086	$45.00
Stone Analysis	32360	$60.00
Venipuncture	36415	$10.00

SERVICE RENDERED	CPT	FEE
Condyloma Treatment	54050	$40.00
Cystoscopy	52000	$300.00
Catheterization	93975	$45.00
Vasectomy	55250	$775.00
Ultrasonic Guide Needle Biopsy	76942	$395.00
Prostate Biopsy	55700	$325.00
Biopsy Gun	A9270	$45.00
Uroflowmeter	51741	$80.00
Renal Ultrasound	76775	$295.00
Scrotal Ultrasound	76870	$295.00
Acidic Acid	99070	$20.00
Foley Catheter Starter Set	A4329	$35.00

Figure 17-1. The fee schedule shows the charges for services provided by the practice.

reflect the cost of services, the doctor's experience, charges of other doctors in the area, and other factors. Sometimes the fee allowed by insurance policies is a determining factor. The practice may use a particular system to determine how much to charge for each service. These systems are summarized below and are discussed in detail in Chapter 15.

Usual and Customary Fees. A usual fee is the fee a doctor charges for a service or procedure. A customary fee is either the average fee charged for a service or procedure by all comparable doctors in the same region or the ninetieth percentile of all fees charged by comparable doctors in the same region for the same procedure. There is a growing tendency, however, to determine fees by national rather than regional trends.

Resource-Based Relative Value System (RBRVS). RBRVS was created in response to the Omnibus Budget Reconciliation Act (OBRA), which was passed in 1989 to help reform Medicare payments to doctors. Before 1989, Medicare Part B paid doctors using customary, prevailing, and reasonable charges in a fee-for-service system.

Now, for each medical service, RBRVS assigns a code (relative value unit) that reflects the following factors:

- The doctor's skill and time required
- The professional liability expenses related to that service, such as malpractice insurance
- The overhead costs associated with that service

Based on the codes, the relative value units are converted to dollar amounts. These dollar amounts form the basis of the RBRVS fee schedule. This schedule creates uniform payments that are adjusted for geographic differences.

RBRVS began to be implemented in 1992. Since that time, it has reduced the growth rate of spending for doctors' professional services, related services and supplies, and other Medicare Part B services.

Processing Charge Slips

Fees must be determined in order to create a charge slip, the original record of the doctor's services and the charges for those services. Figure 17-2 shows an example of a charge slip. Charge slips are also called fee slips or transaction slips. They are usually numbered consecutively. They may be preprinted with common services and charges for the practice. Charge slips are used in several ways.

Some doctors keep a pad of charge slips on their desk. After seeing a patient, they fill in the services and charges on the charge slip. They give the charge slip to the patient and ask the patient to give it to you on the way out of the office.

In other offices, you may write the patient's name on the charge slip and give the slip to the doctor along with the patient's medical record. The doctor then fills

DATE	DESCRIPTION—CODE	CHARGE	PAYMENT	CURRENT BALANCE

(918) 555-9680

Tax ID No. 11-0004004

Patricia Belden, MD
111 Roosevelt Boulevard
Lawrence, OK 77527

99205	Office Visit, New Patient	36425	Venipuncture	59025	NST
99215	Office Visit, Established Patient	57454	Colposcopy with Biopsy	54150	Circumcision
99213	Office Visit, Established, Brief	57511	Cryosurgery	58300	IUD Insertion
88155	Pap	58100	Endometrial Biopsy	57170	Diaphragm Fitting
84703	Urine Pregnancy Test	56600	Vulva Biopsy		

NAME ____________________ DX ____________________ No. 0005807

Figure 17-2. A charge slip shows the services performed for a patient and the charges for those services.

in the services performed and asks you to fill in the charges according to the fee schedule. If questions arise about the fee for a particular service, you can refer to the fee schedule and tell the patient how much that service will cost.

Accepting Payment

When the patient comes to you with the charge slip, you complete the charge slip and ask for payment. There are several effective yet diplomatic ways to request payment. Two examples are, "For today's visit, the total charge is $50. How would you like to pay?" and "The charge for your laboratory work today is $80. Would you like to pay for that now?" Most practices accept several forms of payment, including cash, check, credit card, and insurance. Insurance payment is discussed in detail in Chapter 15.

Cash. If the patient chooses to pay in cash, count the money carefully to be sure you have received the proper amount. Next, record the payment on the patient's ledger card, and give the patient a receipt.

Some practices use a combination charge slip/receipt, as discussed in Chapter 16. If your practice does not, prepare a cash receipt manually, as shown in Figure 17-3. Then place the money in the cash drawer or cash box.

Check. If the patient pays by check, be sure the check is written properly, including the current date. The amount of the check should match the total amount listed on the charge slip, unless the patient has made prior arrangements to pay only part of the amount. The name of the doctor or practice should appear in the "Pay to the Order of" section and should be properly spelled. The check should be signed by the person whose name is printed on the check. After accepting the check, endorse it immediately, and deposit it in the practice bank account (using the procedure described in Chapter 16).

Credit Card. Many doctors' offices accept credit cards, such as Visa or MasterCard. This payment method offers advantages for both the practice and the patient. For the practice, it provides prompt payment from the credit card company, thus increasing cash flow. It also reduces the amount of time and money spent on preparing and mailing bills, thus decreasing expenses. For the patient, it is convenient and allows a large bill to be paid in several smaller amounts, usually once a month.

Credit cards have one major disadvantage for the practice—cost. The credit card company deducts a percentage of each charge for its collection service, usually between 1% and 5%. If a patient charges $100 in services on a credit card, for example, the practice receives only $95 to $99. The credit card company keeps the difference. A disadvantage for patients is the accrued interest charges on unpaid balances.

If the practice accepts credit card payments, the American Medical Association (AMA) suggests several guidelines.

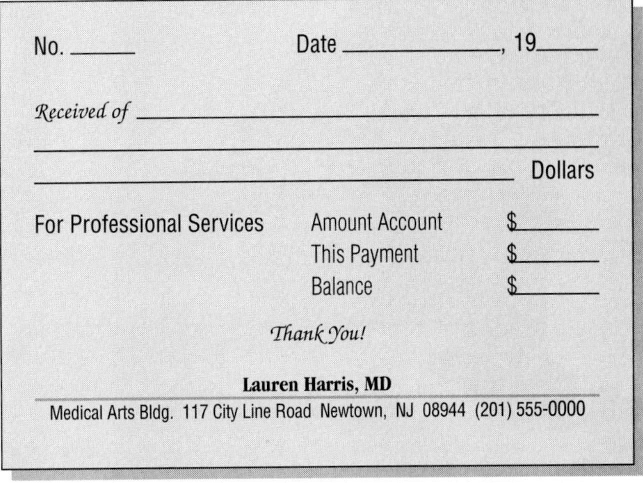
No. ______ Date ______________, 19______

Received of ______________________________

______________________________ Dollars

For Professional Services

Amount Account $______

This Payment $______

Balance $______

Thank You!

Lauren Harris, MD

Medical Arts Bldg. 117 City Line Road Newtown, NJ 08944 (201) 555-0000

Figure 17-3. After writing a receipt for cash, record the payment on the patient's ledger card.

- Do not set higher fees for patients who pay by credit card.
- Do not encourage patients to use credit cards for payment.
- Do not advertise outside the office that the practice accepts credit cards.

If a patient chooses to pay by credit card, process the transaction carefully to ensure that the credit card company charges the patient correctly. To begin, inform the patient of the amount due, and ask for the credit card.

Check the expiration date on the front of the credit card. If the card has not expired, put it in its spot on the credit card machine, and place a credit card voucher on top of it. Then, slide the imprint arm firmly to the right and back across the machine. Remove the voucher from the machine. Write in the date, and circle the type of credit card, such as Visa or MasterCard.

Next, obtain the authorization code from the credit card company. Some offices have devices that read the magnetic strip on the credit card and automatically transmit the information to the credit card company by telephone line (Figure 17-4). If your office has such a device, type in the amount to be charged on its keypad. Then, the credit card company issues an authorization code, which appears on the device's screen.

If your office does not have such a device, call the credit card company for the authorization code. Give the operator the patient's credit card number and the amount of the payment. The operator then gives you the authorization code.

Write the authorization code in the box marked "Authorization" on the credit card voucher. Initial the voucher in the appropriate box. Then, fill in the services provided and the amount of the charges. Enter the total charges in the box marked "Total."

Give the voucher to the patient to sign. Compare the patient's signature on the voucher with the signature on the back of the credit card (they should, of course, be

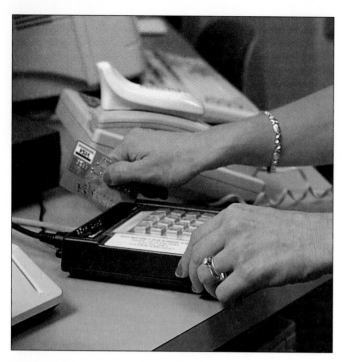

Figure 17-4. Using a device like this one, you can swipe the patient's card through the machine and obtain instant authorization from the credit card company.

identical). Keep one copy of the voucher for the office. Give the other copy, any carbon paper, and the credit card to the patient.

Using the Pegboard System for Posting Payments

Some physicians' offices use the pegboard system to post payments and generate receipts for patients, as described earlier, in Chapter 16. If your office uses the pegboard system, you may use the pegboard to record the payment on the ledger card and receipt simultaneously. You handle this task in basically the same way, whether the patient pays immediately or later, in response to a bill.

Determining Payment Responsibility

Generally the patient is responsible for payments for medical services. To help promote timely payments, however, you need to know exactly who is responsible for them.

Third Party Liability. Third party liability refers to the responsibility of the patient's insurance company to pay for certain medical expenses, which may include doctors' services. Each practice decides how to handle its patients' health insurance claims.

Some practices do not accept any insurance, although these practices are rare. The patient must pay the doctor directly and file an insurance claim for reimbursement. If you work in such a practice, you must give the patient the necessary medical information to fill out the insurance claim. A completed superbill (discussed later in this chapter) provides the information.

Practices increasingly handle all their patients' insurance paperwork to ensure accuracy, timely submission, and prompt payment. Some practices charge a fee for handling patients' insurance claims. Some practices handle paperwork only for patients who find it particularly difficult, such as those who are frail or disabled.

If you work in an office that handles insurance paperwork, you can submit insurance claims manually or electronically. Regardless of which method you use, be sure to use the proper forms, complete them correctly, and submit them within the time limits set by insurers. (Procedures for completing insurance forms and filing claims are discussed in Chapter 15.)

CHAMPUS/TRICARE, which provides health insurance for dependents of active-duty and retired military personnel, operates differently from other insurers. CHAMPUS/TRICARE pays the doctor through a local fiscal agent. Patients pay any co-payments and deductible amounts. You must adjust for the difference between the billed fees and the amounts received from CHAMPUS/TRICARE and the patient. If a CHAMPUS/TRICARE patient fails to pay the patient's portion, you may take steps to obtain payment just as you would with any other patient.

Responsibility for Minors. When a child's parents are married, either parent may consent (agree) to treatment for the minor child (child under age 18). Both parents are responsible for payment for the minor's treatment. If you must send them a bill, you should address it to both parents to ensure payment. There is one exception to this process. Anyone under the age of 18 who is no longer living at home and is self-supporting is considered an emancipated minor and is responsible for payment. For example, a 16-year-old girl who is pregnant and leaves her parents' home to set up a household with her boyfriend is considered an emancipated minor.

Divorce or separation can create confusion about which parent can consent to the child's treatment and which of the two is responsible for payment. The parent who has **legal custody,** or the court-decreed right to make decisions about a child's upbringing, is the parent who has consent ability and payment responsibility. A divorced couple's legal and financial arrangements are considered private information, however. Therefore, you should assume that the parent who brings the child for treatment has consent ability and payment responsibility. The physician should inform the responsible parent of this assumption before providing treatment.

Professional Courtesy. As a matter of professional courtesy, a doctor may treat some patients free of charge or for just the amount covered by the patient's insurance. These patients often include other doctors and their families, the practice's staff members (including medical assistants) and their families, other health-care professionals (including pharmacists and dentists), clergy members, and hospital employees.

Be sure you know the doctor's policy so that you do not bill these patients in error. If, for example, the doctor agrees to accept only the amount paid by the patient's insurance, note this professional courtesy on the patient's ledger card, and do not request co-payment.

Standard Billing Procedures

If the physician extends credit to patients, you need to know how to prepare invoices. You also have to manage related billing responsibilities, such as establishing and maintaining billing cycles.

Preparing Invoices

As a medical assistant, part of your job is to prepare an invoice to mail to the patient who does not pay when services are rendered or who makes only a partial payment. Figure 17-5 shows an invoice with an itemized list of services. You can obtain most of the information for the invoice from the patient ledger card. The invoice should include the following information:

- Physician's name, address, and telephone number
- Patient's name and address
- Balance (if any) from the previous month(s)
- Itemized list of services and charges, by date, for the current month
- Payments from the patient or insurer during the month
- Total balance due

Whatever invoicing procedure you use, enclose a self-addressed envelope with the invoice, to encourage prompt payment.

Using Codes on the Invoice. Write the name of each procedure on the itemized list, or use codes for common procedures, such as OV for office visit. If you use codes, be sure that an explanation of the codes appears with the invoice. (Many practices use invoices with a key to the codes printed at the bottom.) Using an itemized list on invoices is standard procedure in most physicians' offices and is required by all health insurance plans. After completing the invoice, fold it in thirds, and mail it in a typewritten business envelope.

Using the Patient's Ledger Card as an Invoice. As an alternative to writing or typing the invoice, you may photocopy the patient's ledger card and fold the photocopy so that the patient's address shows through the window in a window envelope. If you prepare invoices this way, be sure there are no stray marks or comments written on the card. Also, be sure the photocopy is clean and easy to read.

Generating the Invoice by Computer. In computerized offices, you may print out an invoice for each patient account that has a balance due. Follow the instructions in the software manufacturer's manual. You can then fold the printouts and mail them in window envelopes.

Using an Independent Billing Service. Large practices may have invoices handled by an independent billing service. The billing service may rapidly copy ledger cards for patients with balances due. Then it mails the copies to patients, usually with an envelope for sending payment directly to the physician's office.

Sending Invoices Electronically to Insurance Companies. Invoices to insurance companies may be prepared using one of the methods described above. Physicians' offices that have a computer and modem may bill insurance companies electronically, as discussed in Chapter 15.

Using the Superbill

Some doctors' offices use a **superbill,** which includes the charges for services rendered on that day, an invoice for payment or insurance co-payment, and all the information for submitting an insurance claim. Figure 17-6 shows an example of a superbill. Having all this information on one form saves time and paperwork. These forms are often printed on NCR (no-carbon-required) paper with copies for the practice, patient, and insurance company.

Complete as much of the superbill as possible at the beginning of the patient's visit. (See Procedure 17-1 for specific instructions.) Some practices use a computerized version of the superbill, printing it out instead of completing the initial information by hand. Attach the superbill to the patient's medical record, and give them both to the doctor before he sees the patient.

Managing Billing Cycles

Many practices send out their bills just after the end of each month. You can send out bills at any regular time, however, such as once a week or twice a month. You may also send bills at a particular time of the month at the patient's request.

Cycle billing is a common billing system that bills each patient only once a month but spreads the work of billing over the month. Using this system, you send invoices to groups of patients every few days.

For example, you may bill on the fifth of the month for patients whose last names begin with A through D. Then, on the tenth of the month, you may bill patients whose names begin with E through H, and so on. In a larger office with more patients, you may prefer to bill more frequently but to smaller groups of patients.

Standard Collection Procedures

Although most patients pay invoices within the standard 30-day period, some do not. When a patient does not pay an invoice during the standard period, you need to take steps to collect the payment. For example, you may need

INVOICE

PLEASE SEND ALL PAYMENTS TO:
FAMILY MEDICAL ASSOCIATES
1007 WASHINGTON BLVD.
ROBBINSVILLE, PA 19173-1299
(717) 555-4344
TAX ID#: 11-31700002

CLOSING DATE
08/12/98
ACCOUNT NUMBER
1364
DUE FROM PATIENT
10.00

CHARGES OR PAYMENTS MADE AFTER CLOSING DATE WILL APPEAR ON NEXT STATEMENT.

RESPONSIBLE PARTY NAME

MELISSA WINSTON
400 MOUNTAIN ROAD
HAMILTON, PA 19181

☐ PLEASE CHANGE ADDRESS IF INCORRECT

AMOUNT ENCLOSED

DETACH THIS STUB AND RETURN WITH PAYMENT

DATE OF SERVICE	PROCEDURE CODE	DIAGNOSTIC CODE	SERVICE DESCRIPTION	ORIGINAL CHARGE	INSURANCE PAID	ADJ.	PATIENT PAID	AMOUNT DUE	DUE FROM
5/13/98	99213	473.9	EXT PAT-INTER	50.00	40.00	.00	.00	10.00	PAT
5/13/98	92567	473.9	TYMPANOGRAM	35.00	35.00	.00	.00	.00	INS
5/02/98	99203	706.2	NEW PAT-INTER	80.00	70.00	.00	10.00	.00	INS

PLEASE NOTE: ANY BALANCE NOW DUE BY THE PATIENT HAS BEEN SUBMITTED TO THE PATIENT'S INSURANCE (IF ANY) AND PROCESSED AND IS NOW THE RESPONSIBILITY OF THE PATIENT.

ACCOUNT NO.	SOCIAL SECURITY #	CURRENT	OVER 30 DAYS	OVER 60 DAYS	OVER 90 DAYS	OVER 120 DAYS	INSURANCE PENDING	DUE FROM PATIENT
1364	140-62-0000	10.00	.00	.00	.00	.00	.00	10.00

Figure 17-5. The invoice shows an itemized list of services and charges, organized by date, for the current month.

Lakeridge Medical Group
262 East Pine Street, Suite 100
Lakeridge, NJ 07500

☐ **PRIVATE** ☐ **BLUECROSS** ☐ **IND.** ☐ **MEDICARE** ☐ **MEDI-CAL** ☐ **HMO** ☐ **PPO**

PATIENT'S LAST NAME	FIRST	ACCOUNT #	BIRTHDATE / /	SEX ☐ MALE ☐ FEMALE	TODAY'S DATE / /
INSURANCE COMPANY	SUBSCRIBER		PLAN #	SUB. #	GROUP

ASSIGNMENT: I hereby assign my insurance benefits to be paid directly to the undersigned physician. I am financially responsible for non-covered services. SIGNED: (Patient, or Parent, if Minor) DATE: / /	RELEASE: I hereby authorize the physician to release to my insurance carriers any information required to process this claim. SIGNED: (Patient, or Parent, if Minor) DATE: / /

✔	DESCRIPTION	M/Care	CPT/Mod	DxRe	FEE
	OFFICE CARE				
	NEW PATIENT				
	Brief		99201		
	Limited		99202		
	Intermediate		99203		
	Extended		99204		
	Comprehensive		99205		
	ESTABLISHED PATIENT				
	Minimal		99211		
	Brief		99212		
	Limited		99213		
	Intermediate		99214		
	Extended		99215		
	Comprehensive		99215		
	CONSULTATION-OFFICE				
	Focused		99241		
	Expanded		99242		
	Detailed		99243		
	Comprehensive 1		99244		
	Comprehensive 2		99245		
	Case Management		98900		
	Post-op Exam		99024		

✔	DESCRIPTION	M/Care	CPT/Mod	DxRe	FEE
	PROCEDURES				
	Tread Mill (In Office)		93015		
	24 Hour Holter		93224		
	If Medicare (Set up Fee)		93225		
	Physician Interpret		93227		
	EKG w/Interpretation		93000		
	EKG (Medicare)		93005		
	Sigmoidoscopy		45300		
	Sigmoidoscopy, Flexible		45330		
	Sigmoidos. , Flex. w/Bx.		45331		
	Spirometry, FEV/FVC		94010		
	Spirometry, Post-Dilator		94060		
	LABORATORY				
	Blood Draw Fee		36415		
	Urinalysis, Chemical		81005		
	Throat Culture		87081		
	Occult Blood		82270		
	Pap Handling Charge		99000		
	Pap Life Guard		88150-90		
	Gram Stain		87205		
	Hanging Drop		87210		
	Urine Drug Screen		99000		
	SUPPLIES				

✔	DESCRIPTION	M/Care	CPT/Mod	DxRe	FEE
	INJECTIONS/IMMUNIZATIONS				
	Tetanus		90718		
	Hypertet	J1670	90782		
	Pneumococcal		90732		
	Influenza		90724		
	TB Skin Test (PPD)		86585		
	Antigen Injection-Single		95115		
	Multiple		95117		
	B12 Injection	J3420	90782		
	Injection, IM		90782		
	Compazine	J0780	90782		
	Demerol	J2175	90782		
	Vistaril	J3410	90782		
	Susphrine	J0170	90782		
	Decadron	J0890	90782		
	Estradiol	J1000	90782		
	Testosterone	J1080	90782		
	Lidocaine	J2000	90782		
	Solumedrol	J2920	90782		
	Solucortef	J1720	90782		
	Hydeltra	J1690	90782		
	Pen Procaine	J2510	90788		
	INJECTIONS - JOINT/BURSA				
	Small Joints		20600		
	Intermediate		20605		
	Large Joints		20610		
	Trigger Point		20550		
	MISCELLANEOUS				

DIAGNOSIS:	ICD-9								
___ Abdominal Pain	789.0	___ Gout	274.0	___ C.V.A. - Acute	436.	___ Electrolyte Dis.	276.9	___ Herpes Simplex	054.9
___ Abscess (Site)	682.9	___ Asthma	493.90	___ Cere. Vas. Accid. (Old)	438	___ Fatigue	780.7	___ Herpes Zoster	053.9
___ Adverse Drug Rx	995.2	___ Asthmatic Bronchitis	493.90	___ Cerumen	380.4	___ Fibrocys. Br. Dis	610.1	___ Hydrocele	603.9
___ Alcohol Detox	291.8	___ Atrial Fib.	427.31	___ Chestwall Pain	786.59	___ Fracture (Site)	829.0	___ Hyperlipidemia	272.4
___ Alcoholism	303.90	___ Atrial Tachi.	427.0	___ Cholecystitis	575.0	___ Open/Close		___ Hypertension	401.9
___ Allergic Rhinitis	477	___ Bowel Obstruct.	560.9	___ Cholelithiasis	574.00	___ Fungal Infect. (Site)	110.8	___ Hyperthyroidism	242.9
___ Allergy	995.3	___ Breast Mass	611.72	___ COPD	492.8	___ Gastric Ulcer	531.90	___ Hypothyroidism	244.9
___ Alzheimer's Dis.	290.1	___ Bronchitis	490	___ Cirrhosis	571.5	___ Gastritis	535.0	___ Labyrinthitis	386.30
___ Anemia	285.9	___ Bursitis	727.3	___ Cong. Heart Fail.	428.9	___ Gastroenteritis	558.9	___ Lipoma (Site)	214.9
___ Anemia - Pernicious	281.0	___ Cancer, Breast (Site)	174.9	___ Conjunctivitis	372.30	___ G.I. Bleeding	578.9	___ Lymphoma	202.8
___ Angina	413.9	___ Metastatic (Site)	199.1	___ Contusion (Site)	924.9	___ Glomerulonephritis	583.9	___ Mit. Valve Prolapse	424.0
___ Anxiety Synd.	300.00	___ Colon	153.9	___ Costochondritis	733.99	___ Headache	784.0	___ Myocard. Infarction (Area)	410.9
___ Appendicitis	541	___ Cancer, Rectal	154.1	___ Depression	311.	___ Headache, Tension	307.81	___ M.I., Old	412
___ Arterioscl. H.D.	414.0	___ Lung (Site)	162.9	___ Dermatitis	692.9	___ Migraine (Type)	346.9	___ Myositis	729.1
___ Arthritis, Osteo.	715.90	___ Skin (Site)	173.9	___ Diabetes Mellitus	250.00	___ Hemorrhoids	455.6	___ Nausea/Vomiting	787.0
___ Rheumatoid	714.0	___ Card. Arrhythmia (Type)	427.9	___ Diabetic Ketosis	250.1	___ Hernia, Hiatal	553.3	___ Neuralgia	729.2
___ Lupus	710.0	___ Cardiomyopathy	425.4	___ Diverticulitis	562.11	___ Inguinal	550.9	___ Nevus (Site)	216.9
		___ Cellulitis (Site)	682.9	___ Diverticulosis	562.10	___ Hepatitis	573.3	___ Obesity	278.0

DIAGNOSIS: (IF NOT CHECKED ABOVE)

SERVICES PERFORMED AT: ☐ Office ☐ E.R. ☐ ☐   ☐ CLAIM CONTAINS NO ORDERED REFERRING SERVICE   REFERRING PHYSICIAN & I.D. NUMBER

RETURN APPOINTMENT INFORMATION: 5 - 10 - 15 - 20 - 30 - 40 - 60 [DAYS] [WKS.] [MOS.] [PRN]	NEXT APPOINTMENT M - T - W - TH - F - S DATE / / TIME: AM PM	ACCEPT ASSIGNMENT? ☐ YES ☐ NO	DOCTOR'S SIGNATURE

INSTRUCTIONS TO PATIENT FOR FILING INSURANCE CLAIMS:

1. Complete upper portion of this form, sign and date.
2. Attach this form to your own insurance company's form for direct reimbursement.

MEDICARE PATIENTS - DO NOT SEND THIS TO MEDICARE.
WE WILL SUBMIT THE CLAIM FOR YOU.

☐ CASH ☐ CHECK # ______ ☐ VISA ☐ MC ☐ CO-PAY	
TOTAL TODAY'S FEE	
OLD BALANCE	
TOTAL DUE	
AMOUNT REC'D. TODAY	

Figure 17-6. A superbill is a form that can also be used as a charge slip and invoice and can be submitted with insurance claims.

PROCEDURE 17-1

How to Bill With the Superbill

Objective: To complete a superbill accurately

Materials: Superbill, patient ledger card, patient information sheet, fee schedule, insurance code list, pen

Method

1. Make sure the doctor's name and address appear on the form.
2. From the patient ledger card and information sheet, fill in the patient data, such as name, sex, date of birth, and insurance information.
3. Fill in the place and date of service.
4. Attach the superbill to the patient's medical record, and give them both to the doctor.
5. Accept the completed superbill from the patient after the patient sees the doctor. Make sure that the doctor has indicated the diagnosis and the procedures performed.
6. If the doctor has not already recorded the charges, refer to the fee schedule for procedures that are marked. Then fill in the charges next to those procedures.
7. In the appropriate blanks, list the total charges for the visit, and the previous balance (if any). Deduct any payments or adjustments received before this visit.
8. Calculate the subtotal.
9. Fill in the amount and type of payment (cash, check, money order, or credit card) made by the patient during this visit.
10. Calculate and enter the new balance.
11. Have the patient sign the authorization-and-release section of the superbill.
12. Keep a copy of the superbill for the practice records. Give the original to the patient along with one copy to file with the insurer.

to call or write the patient to determine the reason for nonpayment or to set up a payment arrangement.

Whether you use telephone calls, notes, or letters, there are laws, such as statutes of limitations, and professional standards to guide your efforts to collect overdue payments from patients.

State Statute of Limitations

A **statute of limitations** is a state law that sets a time limit on when a collection suit on a past-due account can legally be filed. The time limit varies with the type of account.

Open-Book Account. An **open-book account** is one that is open to charges made occasionally as needed. Most of a physician's long-standing patients have this type of account. An open-book account uses the last date of payment or charge for each illness as the starting date for determining the time limit on that specific debt.

Written-Contract Account. A **written-contract account** is one in which the physician and patient sign an agreement stating that the patient will pay the bill in more than four installments. Some states allow longer time limits for these accounts than for open-book accounts. Written-contract accounts are regulated by the Truth in Lending Act, discussed later in this chapter.

Single-Entry Account. A **single-entry account** is an account with only one charge, usually for a small amount. For example, someone vacationing in your area might come in for treatment of a cold. This person's account would list only one office visit. If the vacationer did not become a regular patient, the account would be considered a single-entry account. Some states impose shorter time limits on single-entry accounts than on open-book accounts.

Using Collection Techniques

Individual practices have their own ways of approaching the task of collection. Most begin the process with telephone calls, letters, or statements.

Initial Telephone Calls or Letters. When calling a patient or sending a letter about collections, be friendly and sympathetic. (Do not call a patient at work and leave a message. That type of phone call is an invasion of privacy. Call the patient at home.) Assume that the patient forgot to pay or was temporarily unable to pay. If you do not receive a response to your telephone call or initial collection letter, your next letters may need to be more urgent in tone. Standard collection letters, such as the one shown in Figure 17-7, are available for you to fill in the details, or you can create a letter to reflect the style of the practice.

Preparing Statements. You might send the patient a statement for an account that is 30 days past due. A **statement** is similar to an invoice except that it contains a courteous reminder that payment is due. This reminder can be a typewritten note on the statement, a brightly colored sticker, or a separate handwritten note attached to the statement.

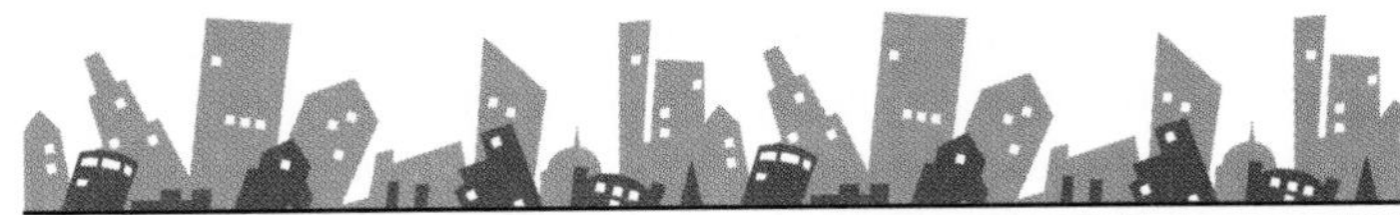

City Medical Group

1234 Wayne Street
Smithtown, OR 93689
(503) 555-1217

Internal Medicine
Marianne Harris, MD
Karen Payne-Johnson, MD

May 5, 1999

Mr. J. J. Andrews
1414 First Avenue
Smithtown, OR 93668

Dear Mr. Andrews:

It has been brought to my attention that your account in the amount of $240.00 is past due.

Normally at this time the account would be placed with a collection agency. However, we would prefer to hear from you regarding your preference in this matter.

( ) Payment in full is enclosed.

( ) Payment will be made in ______ days.

( ) I would like to make regular weekly/monthly payments of $ ______ until this account is paid in full. My first payment is enclosed.

( ) I would prefer that you assign this account to a collection agency for enforcement of collection. (Failure to return this letter within 30 days will result in this action.)

( ) I don't believe I owe this amount for the following reason(s):

Signed: ________________________________

Please indicate your preference and return this letter within 30 days. Please do not hesitate to call if you have any questions regarding this matter.

Sincerely,

Diana Sanchez
Office Manager

Figure 17-7. Standard collection letters are available for you to fill in the details.

If an account is 60 days past due, you could send a collection letter that says, for example, "If you are unable to pay your account in full this month, please telephone our office at [number] to make payment arrangements."

If an account is 90 days past due, your collection letter can contain stronger wording. For example, it might say, "Please let us know when you plan to pay the $250 past-due balance. We have sent you three monthly reminders. If you cannot pay in full now, please contact us at [number] to make payment arrangements. We want to be understanding but need your cooperation."

If an account is 120 days or more past due, you can send a final letter. It might state, "Every courtesy has been extended to you in arranging for payment of your long overdue account. Unless we hear from you by [date], the account will be given to [name of collection agency] for collection." Be sure to note the cutoff date on the patient's ledger card. By law, you cannot threaten to send an account to a collection agency unless it will actually be sent on that cutoff date. Therefore, you must be sure you are ready to do so before you send such a letter.

If you still cannot collect payment, the physician may indeed choose to hire an outside collection agency. Once an agency has taken over the account, there should not be any more correspondence on this matter between the physician's office and the patient.

Preparing an Age Analysis

Age analysis is the process of classifying and reviewing past-due accounts by age from the first date of billing. A quarterly or more frequent age analysis, such as that shown in Figure 17-8, helps you keep on top of past-due accounts and determine which ones need follow-up.

You can do an age analysis by computer or by hand. An age analysis should list all patient account balances, when the charges originated, the most recent payment date, and any special notes concerning the account.

ACCOUNTS RECEIVABLE–AGE ANALYSIS

Date: October 1, 1999

Patient	Balance	Date of Charges	Most Recent Payment	30 days	60 days	90 days	120 days	Remarks
Black, K.	120.00	5/24	5/24			75.00	45.00	3rd Notice
Brown, R.	65.00	8/30	8/30	65.00				
Green, C.	340.00	8/25						Medicare filed
Jones, T.	500.00	6/1	6/30		125.00	125.00	250.00	3rd Notice
Perry, S.	150.00	7/28	7/28	75.00	75.00			1st Notice
Smith, J.	375.00	6/15	7/1			375.00		2nd Notice
White, L.	200.00	6/24	7/5	20.00	30.00	150.00		2nd Notice

Figure 17-8. An age analysis organizes past-due accounts by age.

In a single doctor's office or a small group practice, information for the age analysis may come from the patient ledger cards. You may place color-coded tags on the patient ledger cards to indicate the number of days past due. For example, a yellow tag might be placed on the ledger card of an account that is 60 days past due. An orange tag might be used for an account that is 90 days past due. A red tag might be used for an account that is 120 days or more past due. In a large practice, however, age analysis is typically done on the computer. Use of patient ledger cards will be phased out as more practices become computerized.

Following Laws That Govern Debt Collection

Federal and state laws govern debt collection. Table 17-1 outlines the penalties for violating laws that regulate credit and debt.

Fair Debt Collection Practices Act of 1977. This act (also called Public Law 95–109) governs the methods that can be used to collect unpaid debts. It prevents you from threatening to take an action that is either illegal or that you do not actually intend to take. The aim of this law is to eliminate abusive, deceptive, or unfair debt collection practices. For example, the law requires that after you have said you are going to give an account to a collection agency if it is not paid within 1 month, you must actually do so. Not doing what you threaten to do can be construed as harassment, and your practice can be liable for a harassment charge. Following are guidelines for sending letters and making calls requesting payment from patients.

1. Do not call the patient before 8 A.M. or after 9 P.M. Calling outside those hours can be considered harassment.
2. Do not make threats or use profane language. For example, do not state that an account will be given to a collection agency in 7 days if it will not be.
3. Do not discuss the patient's debt with anyone except the person responsible for payment. If the patient is represented by a lawyer, discuss the problem only with the lawyer, unless the lawyer gives you permission to talk to the patient.
4. Do not use any form of deception or violence to collect a debt. For example, do not pose as a government employee or other authority figure to try to force a debtor to pay.

Telephone Consumer Protection Act (TCPA) of 1991. This act protects telephone subscribers from unwanted telephone solicitations, commonly known as telemarketing. The act prohibits autodialed calls to emergency service providers, cellular and paging numbers, and patients' hospital rooms. It prohibits prerecorded calls to homes without prior permission of the resident, and it prohibits unsolicited advertising via fax machine.

These regulations do not apply to people who have an established business relationship with the telemarketing firm or people who have previously given the telemarketing firm permission to call. The law also does not apply to telemarketing calls placed by tax-exempt nonprofit organizations, such as charities.

Although most provisions of this federal law do not apply to medical practices, you should be aware of the law. One way to avoid an unknowing violation of this law is to limit your calls to patients to the hours between 8 A.M. and 9 P.M. (some states, however, have exceptions for the TCPA provisions). Also, place your calls yourself. Do not use an automated dialing device for calls to patients.

Observing Professional Guidelines for Finance Charges and Late Charges

According to the AMA, it is appropriate to assess finance charges or late charges on past-due accounts if the patient is notified in advance (Council on Ethical and Judicial Affairs, 1994). Advance notice may be given by posting a sign at the reception desk, giving the patient a pamphlet describing the practice's billing practices, or including a note on the invoice.

The physician must adhere to federal and state guidelines that govern these charges. The physician should also use compassion and discretion when assigning charges, especially in hardship cases (Council on Ethical and Judicial Affairs, 1994).

Using Outside Collection Agencies

If your collection efforts do not result in payment, the doctor may wish to select a collection agency to manage the account. Because doctors adhere to the humanitarian and ethical standards of the medical profession, they must be careful to avoid collection agencies that use harsh or harassing collection practices. "Tips for the Office" gives information about selecting an outside collection agency.

When giving a patient's account to an agency, supply the following information about the patient:

- Full name and last known address
- Occupation and business address
- Name of spouse, if any
- Total debt
- Date of last payment or charge on the account
- Description of actions you took to collect the debt
- Responses to collection attempts

Color-coded tabs on the patient ledger cards make this information easy to gather. Note on the patient ledger card that the account has been given to a collection agency. When the agency reports progress toward a settlement, record that information on the card too.

After the account is given to the agency, do not send bills to or contact the patient in any way. If the patient

Table 17-1

Laws That Govern Credit and Collections

Law	Requirements	Penalties for Breaking Law
Equal Credit Opportunity Act (ECOA)	• Creditors may not discriminate against applicants on the basis of sex, marital status, race, national origin, religion, or age. • Creditors may not discriminate because an applicant receives public assistance income or has exercised rights under the Consumer Credit Protection Act.	• If an applicant sues the practice for violating the ECOA, the practice may have to pay **damages** (money paid as compensation), penalties, lawyers' fees, and court costs. • If an applicant joins a class action lawsuit against the practice, the practice may have to pay damages of up to $500,000 or 1% of the practice's net worth, whichever is less. (A **class action lawsuit** is a lawsuit in which one or more people sue a company that wronged all of them the same way.) • If the Federal Trade Commission (FTC) receives many complaints from applicants stating that the practice violated the ECOA, the FTC may investigate and take action against the practice.
Fair Credit Reporting Act (FCRA)	• This act requires credit bureaus to supply correct and complete information to businesses to use in evaluating a person's application for credit, insurance, or a job.	• If one applicant sues the practice in federal court for violating the FCRA, the practice may have to pay damages, **punitive damages** (money paid as punishment for intentionally breaking the law), court costs, and lawyers' fees. • If the FTC receives many complaints from applicants stating that the practice violated the FCRA, the FTC may investigate and take action against the practice.
Fair Debt Collection Practices Act (FDCPA)	• This act requires debt collectors to treat debtors fairly. It also prohibits certain collection tactics, such as harassment, false statements, threats, and unfair practices.	• If one debtor sues the practice in a state or federal court for violation of the FDCPA, the practice may have to pay damages, court costs, and lawyers' fees. • If the debtor joins a class action suit against the practice, the practice may have to pay damages of up to $500,000 or 1% of the practice's net worth, whichever is less. • If the FTC receives many complaints from debtors stating that the practice violated the FDCPA, the FTC may investigate and take action against the practice.
Truth in Lending Act (TLA)	• This act requires creditors to provide applicants with accurate and complete credit costs and terms, clearly and obviously.	• If one applicant sues the practice in a federal court for violation of the TLA, the practice may have to pay damages, court costs, and lawyers' fees. • If the FTC receives many complaints from applicants stating that the practice violated the TLA, the FTC may investigate and take action against the practice.

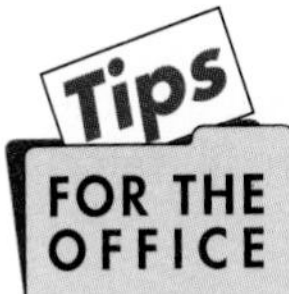

FOR THE OFFICE

Choosing a Collection Agency

If a patient does not respond to your final collection letter or has twice broken a promise to pay, the doctor may choose to seek the help of a collection agency. This step should be taken carefully, however. Some collection agencies use illegal and unethical tactics to obtain payment. For example, some collectors have made repeated, profane phone calls to frighten debtors. Others have threatened debtors with prison for nonpayment. A good collection agency reflects the humanitarian and ethical standards of the medical profession.

To help select an effective—and ethical—collection agency, ask for a referral from the doctor's colleagues, fellow specialists, or hospital associates. You may also contact one of the following organizations:

American Collectors Association
4040 West 70th Street
Minneapolis, MN 55434

Associated Credit Bureaus of America
Collection Division
6767 Southwest Freeway
Houston, TX 77074

Medical-Dental-Hospital Bureaus of America
111 East Wacker Drive
Chicago, IL 60601

After obtaining a referral, contact the agency, and request samples of its letters, reminder notices, and other print material for debtors. Be sure this material is courteous and reflects the way you would handle the collection. Also, be sure the agency uses a persuasive approach rather than simply suing debtors. Ask if the agency reports cases that deserve special consideration to the doctor's office.

Determine what methods the agency uses for out-of-town accounts. For example, it may use out-of-town services to help with those collections. Ask the agency about its collection percentage and fees for large, small, and out-of-town accounts. Be sure the percentages and fees are appropriate for the collection amounts.

After selecting a collection agency, supply all pertinent data to the agency, such as the patient's name, address, and full amount of the debt. Mark the patient's ledger card so that you do not call or write to the patient about the debt. If the patient contacts the office about the account, refer the patient to the collection agency.

If you receive any payments from the debtor, alert the collection agency immediately. (The agency takes a portion of any payments it collects.) Also, contact the agency if you learn anything new about the patient's address or employer.

wants to discuss payment, refer the patient to the agency. If the patient sends a payment, forward it to the agency; or, if the agency and the practice agree, keep the payment for the practice, and forward the collection fee to the agency.

The arrangement with the agency should give the doctor the final word on the uncollected account. In other words, the doctor should decide whether to write off the debt or take the matter to court.

Computing a Collection Percentage

The **collection percentage** is the total amount of payments received by the practice compared with the total amount of charges assessed for the year. It also reflects your success in handling collections. There are two types of collection percentages: gross and adjusted (or net).

Gross Collection Percentage. The gross collection percentage is the total payments received divided by the total charges assessed. In multispecialty practices in 1995, the gross collection percentage was 73.1% (Medical Group Management Association, 1996). For every $10,000 the average practice billed, it received $7310 in payments.

Adjusted Collection Percentage. The adjusted collection percentage is the total payments divided by the total charges, minus the total adjustments made. An adjustment is the difference between the practice's charges and the insurer's payment for a given procedure.) In 1995 the adjusted collection percentage was 96% (Medical Group Management Association, 1996). Only 4% of the average practice's charges were not paid or accounted for through adjustments.

Insuring Accounts Receivable

To protect the practice from lost income because of nonpayment, the practice may buy accounts receivable insurance. One type of accounts receivable policy pays when a large number of patients do not pay and the physician must absorb the lost income. It protects the practice's cash flow and helps ensure that the practice will have sufficient income to cover expected expenses.

Credit Arrangements

Sometimes a doctor agrees to extend credit to a patient who is unable to pay immediately. This situation is not uncommon when a patient's medical bills are high. By extending **credit,** the doctor gives the patient time to pay for services, which are provided on trust. If the doctor knows the patient well, he may offer credit without checking the patient's credit history. Otherwise, the doctor may ask you to perform a credit check.

Performing a Credit Check

To perform a credit check, be sure you have the most current information. You will need the patient's address, telephone number, and Social Security number and the patient's employer's name, address, and telephone number. With this information you can verify employment and generate a credit bureau report.

Employment Verification. Explain to the patient that you will be calling his employer to verify employment. Many employers have someone designated to handle such calls. The patient may be able to give you that name before you call the place of employment.

After calling, record the updated information on the patient's registration card, along with any credit references you obtain from the patient.

Credit Bureau Report. A **credit bureau** is a company that provides information about the creditworthiness of a person seeking credit. If a patient's credit history is in question, you may request a report from a credit bureau. A sample credit report is shown in Figure 17-9. A credit bureau collects information about an individual's payment history on credit cards, student loans, and similar accounts. Three leading national credit bureaus are TRW Inc., Equifax Inc., and Trans Union Credit Information Company.

The physician may decide not to extend credit, based on the credit report. If so, the Fair Credit Reporting Act states that you must inform the patient in writing of the reason credit was denied. You must also provide the name and address of the credit bureau. This information

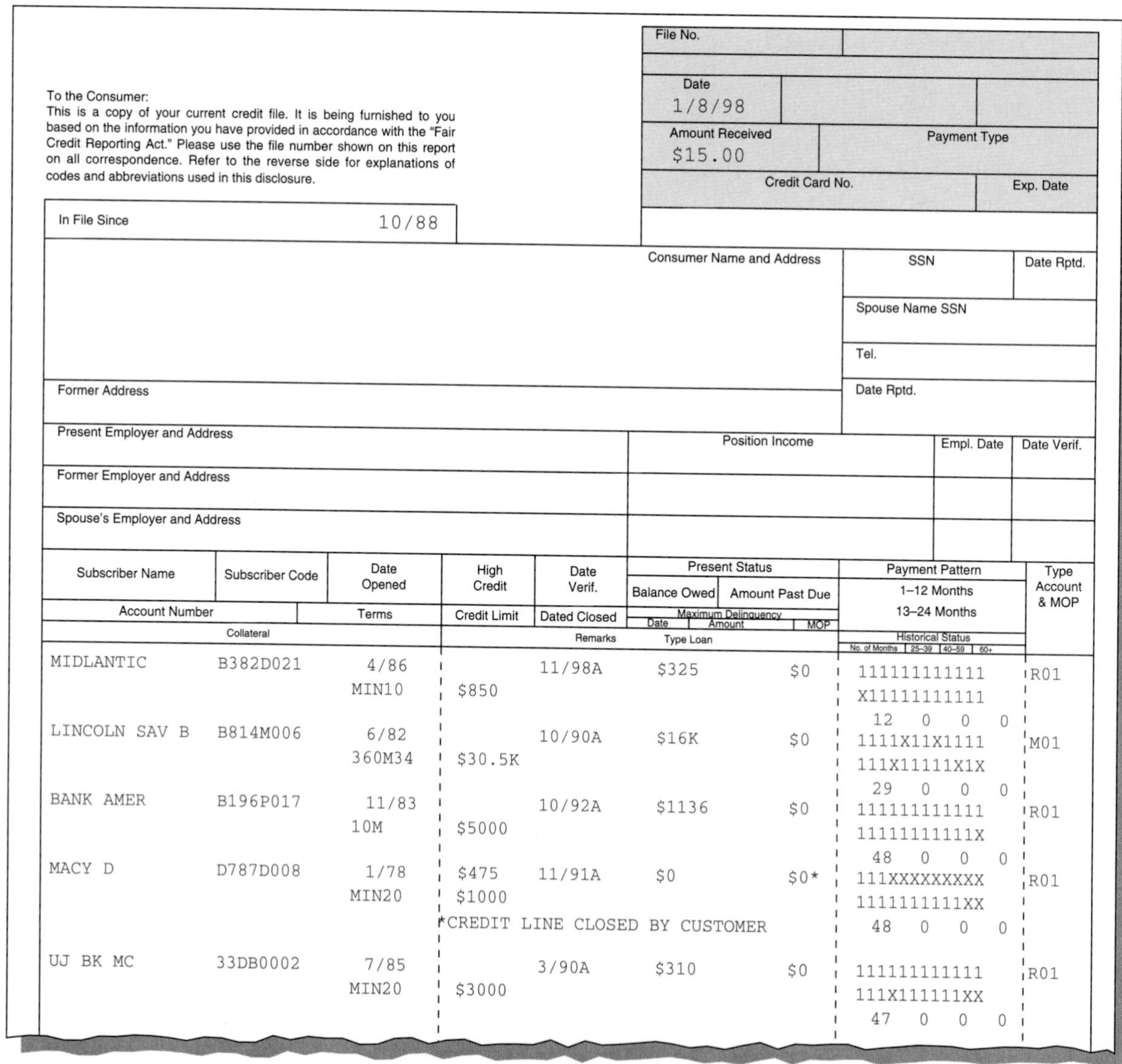

To the Consumer:
This is a copy of your current credit file. It is being furnished to you based on the information you have provided in accordance with the "Fair Credit Reporting Act." Please use the file number shown on this report on all correspondence. Refer to the reverse side for explanations of codes and abbreviations used in this disclosure.

File No.

Date: 1/8/98

Amount Received: $15.00 — Payment Type

Credit Card No. — Exp. Date

In File Since: 10/88

Consumer Name and Address — SSN — Date Rptd.

Spouse Name SSN

Tel.

Former Address — Date Rptd.

Present Employer and Address — Position Income — Empl. Date — Date Verif.

Former Employer and Address

Spouse's Employer and Address

Subscriber Name / Account Number	Subscriber Code / Collateral	Date Opened / Terms	High Credit / Credit Limit	Date Verif. / Dated Closed / Remarks	Present Status: Balance Owed / Type Loan	Amount Past Due / Maximum Delinquency (Date, Amount, MOP)	Payment Pattern: 1–12 Months / 13–24 Months / Historical Status (No. of Months, 25–39, 40–59, 60+)	Type Account & MOP
MIDLANTIC	B382D021	4/86 MIN10	$850	11/98A	$325	$0	111111111111 X11111111111 12 0 0 0	R01
LINCOLN SAV B	B814M006	6/82 360M34	$30.5K	10/90A	$16K	$0	1111X11X1111 111X11111X1X 29 0 0 0	M01
BANK AMER	B196P017	11/83 10M	$5000	10/92A	$1136	$0	111111111111 11111111111X 48 0 0 0	R01
MACY D	D787D008	1/78 MIN20	$475 $1000	11/91A	$0	$0*	111XXXXXXXXX 1111111111XX 48 0 0 0	R01
			*CREDIT LINE CLOSED BY CUSTOMER					
UJ BK MC	33DB0002	7/85 MIN20	$3000	3/90A	$310	$0	111111111111 111X111111XX 47 0 0 0	R01

Figure 17-9. Credit reports are generated by credit bureaus.

allows the patient to contest the credit report and to correct any incorrect information the credit bureau may have.

Following Laws Governing Extension of Credit

When you help the doctor decide whether to grant credit to a patient, you must comply with certain laws governing extension of credit.

Equal Credit Opportunity Act. This act states that credit arrangements may not be denied based on a patient's sex, race, religion, national origin, marital status, or age. Also, credit cannot be denied because the patient receives public assistance or has exercised rights under the Consumer Credit Protection Act, such as disputing a credit card bill or a credit bureau report.

Under the Equal Credit Opportunity Act, the patient has a right to know the specific reason that credit was denied. Some reasons might include having too little income or not being employed for a certain period of time. Vague reasons about not meeting minimum standards or not receiving enough points on a credit-scoring system are not acceptable.

Truth in Lending Act. This act is Regulation Z of the Consumer Credit Protection Act. The Truth in Lending Act covers credit agreements that involve more than four payments. It requires the physician and patient to discuss, sign, and retain copies of a **disclosure statement** (frequently called a federal Truth in Lending statement), which is a written description of the agreed terms of payment (Figure 17-10).

According to the Truth in Lending Act, a disclosure statement must meet the following requirements.

1. The agreement must be discussed with the patient when the terms are first determined. The physician and the patient must agree on the payment terms.
2. Both the physician and the patient must sign the document to indicate mutual agreement on the written terms.

Further, a disclosure statement must include:

1. The amount of total debt (the amount for which the patient is receiving credit).
2. The amount of the down payment (which is sometimes greater than the weekly or monthly payments that follow).
3. The amount of each payment (which may be weekly or monthly or for another period) and the date it is due. (Frequently the total number of payments to be made after the down payment is also included.)
4. The due date for the final payment.
5. The interest rate, if interest is to be paid, expressed as an annual percentage.
6. The total finance charges, if any. (If interest is charged, the total amount of interest accrued during the course of the debt will be entered here.)

The practice and the patient should each keep a copy of the signed disclosure agreement.

Under the Truth in Lending Act, you must send the patient a statement of account at the end of each billing cycle. This statement must include the previous balance, any payments or charges, the periodic and annual interest rates, finance charges (if any) for the billing cycle, the new balance, and a description of how the new balance was obtained.

Extending Credit

If the doctor decides to extend credit, several possible arrangements can be made. Two common arrangements are the unilateral decision and the mutual agreement.

Unilateral Decision. The doctor may decide that the patient will be billed every month for the full amount owed and should make whatever payment is possible each month. This type of arrangement is considered a unilateral decision of the doctor and is not regulated by the Truth in Lending Act.

Mutual Agreement. Another option is a mutual, or bilateral, agreement between physician and patient. They might agree that the patient will be billed for the full amount owed each month and will pay a minimum amount each month. If the physician does not assess finance charges, and if the total number of payments is four or fewer, this type of agreement is also not covered by the Truth in Lending Act. If the physician and patient make a bilateral agreement that includes more than four payments, or if the physician assesses finance charges, the agreement is subject to the requirements of the Truth in Lending Act.

Common Collection Problems

There are two common collection problems that medical practices encounter. The first is patients who cannot pay—also called hardship cases—and the second is patients who have moved and have not received an invoice.

Hardship Cases

A physician may decide to treat some patients without charge—or at a deep discount—simply because they cannot pay. These patients may be poor, uninsured or underinsured, or elderly and on a limited income. They may be patients who have suffered a severe financial loss or family tragedy. Medical ethics require physicians to provide care to individuals who need it, regardless of their ability to pay. Nevertheless, free treatment for hardship cases is at the physician's discretion.

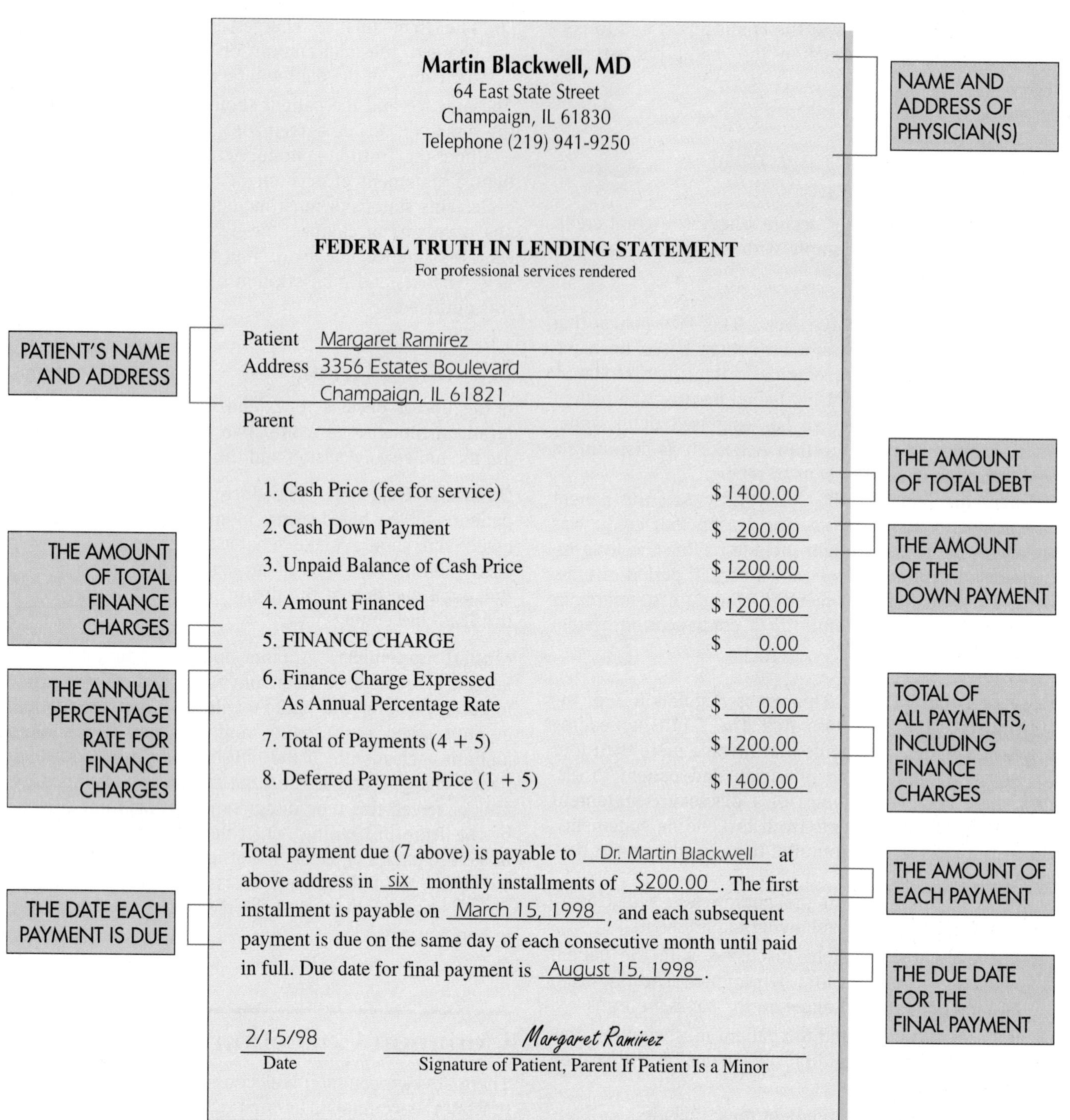
Martin Blackwell, MD
64 East State Street
Champaign, IL 61830
Telephone (219) 941-9250

FEDERAL TRUTH IN LENDING STATEMENT
For professional services rendered

Patient Margaret Ramirez
Address 3356 Estates Boulevard
Champaign, IL 61821
Parent ______

1. Cash Price (fee for service)	$ 1400.00
2. Cash Down Payment	$ 200.00
3. Unpaid Balance of Cash Price	$ 1200.00
4. Amount Financed	$ 1200.00
5. FINANCE CHARGE	$ 0.00
6. Finance Charge Expressed As Annual Percentage Rate	$ 0.00
7. Total of Payments (4 + 5)	$ 1200.00
8. Deferred Payment Price (1 + 5)	$ 1400.00

Total payment due (7 above) is payable to Dr. Martin Blackwell at above address in six monthly installments of $200.00. The first installment is payable on March 15, 1998, and each subsequent payment is due on the same day of each consecutive month until paid in full. Due date for final payment is August 15, 1998.

2/15/98 — Date
Margaret Ramirez — Signature of Patient, Parent If Patient Is a Minor

Figure 17-10. The federal Truth in Lending Act mandates that a written disclosure statement be completed and signed by the physician and patient.

Patient Relocation and Address Change

Sometimes an invoice remains unpaid because the patient has moved and has not received the invoice. Obviously, you will have a problem if you are trying to call such a patient about an invoice.

Remember not to discuss a debt with anyone except the person responsible for the charges. When you make a telephone call for collection, however, you may ask a third party for the patient's new address. If the third party claims not to know the new address, do not call again unless there is reason to believe that the third party has learned of the person's address since the first inquiry.

MULTISKILL FOCUS

Coding, Billing, and Insurance Specialist

To gain medical assistant credentials, you must fulfill the requirements of either the American Association of Medical Assistants (for a Certified Medical Assistant) or the American Medical Technologists (for a Registered Medical Assistant). After obtaining your medical assistant certification or registration, you may wish to acquire additional skills in specialty areas through course work or on-the-job training. Although this course work or training may not lead to an additional certification or degree, it will enable you to expand your role in the medical office and advance your career as the demand for multiskilled health professionals increases.

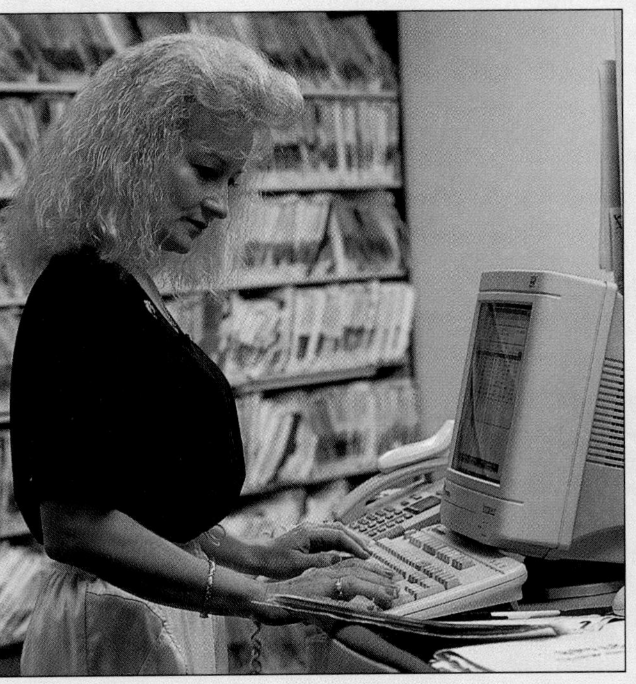

Skills and Duties

A coding, billing, and insurance specialist analyzes the data in patients' charts to provide accurate information for insurance claims. She is also responsible for processing insurance forms and obtaining fees for procedures performed, either from patients or from their insurance companies.

For the purpose of processing insurance claims, there is a code for every recognized disease, condition, problem, and diagnosis. The codes used in medical records come from the International Classification of Disease (ICD) system, issued by the World Health Organization (WHO). There is also a separate system of codes for medical procedures, known as the *Physicians' Current Procedural Terminology,* released annually by the AMA. Coders are encouraged to take a course each year to stay informed about coding changes and updates.

After coding the medical record, the specialist bills the responsible party for the charges incurred by the patient's diagnosis and treatment. She may bill the patient, Medicare or Medicaid, and/or an insurance company. If the insurance company has questions about a bill, it may request the patient's medical records to verify that a particular procedure was medically necessary.

The coding, billing, and insurance specialist may also assist patients with the claims process. She can explain what information the patient must provide to streamline the process. When patients are responsible for submitting claims to their insurance companies, the coding, billing, and insurance specialist may tell the patient what forms to use.

The coding, billing, and insurance specialist also processes responses from the insurance companies, including the explanation of benefits (EOB) form. She checks the EOB against the claim form to make sure that the insurance company addressed all procedures that were performed. Sometimes a balance remains because the insurance company did not pay the total amount due on all procedures. In those cases the coding, billing, and insurance specialist sends a bill to the patient or responsible party. She may discover an error in the EOB. In such instances she looks for the source of the error and then contacts the insurance company to correct it.

Workplace Settings

Coding, billing, and insurance specialists work in many health-care settings, including hospitals, nursing homes, and physicians' practices. Some are employed by insurance companies.

Education

Coding specialists receive part of their training on the job and the rest through workshops, seminars, and courses. A high school diploma or its equivalent is required to be eligible for this training. After completing the training, a coding specialist may take the American Health Information Management Association (AHIMA) certification examination to become a Certified Coding Specialist.

Where to Go for More Information

American Health Information Management Association
919 North Michigan Avenue, Suite 1440
Chicago, IL 60611-1683
(312) 787-2672

Summary

Most doctors prefer to obtain payment by cash, check, or credit card at the time medical services are provided. As a medical assistant, you may assign the fee for these services and collect payment. For various reasons, however, some patients cannot pay immediately. To accommodate these patients, the doctor may want to extend credit. If so, you may be asked to check credit references or to obtain a credit report.

When patients have made credit arrangements with the doctor, you must regularly prepare invoices from information on the patient ledger cards. To simplify this task, you may use a multipurpose superbill and send out invoices in billing cycles.

If patients do not pay their bills within 30 days, you may be asked to act as the doctor's collection agent. Through telephone calls and collection letters, you can try tactfully to collect payments. Federal and state laws govern collections and carry harsh penalties for infractions.

If your efforts to collect a payment are not effective, the doctor may ask you to help find an outside collection agency. A good collection agency should reflect the humanitarian standards of the medical profession. You will need to supply the agency with the pertinent account information.

Chapter Review

Discussion Questions

1. Why do physicians prefer to obtain payment from a patient at the time of the visit rather than sending an invoice?
2. Name an advantage and a disadvantage for a medical practice that accepts credit cards for payment.
3. How can you encourage patients to pay invoices in a timely manner?

Critical Thinking Questions

1. Why, do you think, are there laws that govern the tactics of collection agencies? Give an example to support your answer.
2. What might be some particular billing considerations in a pediatrician's practice?
3. What should you do if you receive a call from a patient claiming that another employee has made a rude or threatening collection phone call?

Application Activities

1. With a partner, role-play a scenario in which you, as a medical assistant, are making an initial request for payment over the phone to a patient who is late in paying a bill but has not yet been sent any collection letters. Your partner should act as the patient, offering any information or explanation she wants.
2. Give a fictional example of a "special consideration" collection case for which you might set up a payment schedule. How would you handle the case?
3. Using the guidelines described in this chapter, write a collection letter to a fictional patient. The patient owes the doctor $125, and the account is 60 days past due. Share your letter with a classmate to analyze how well you complied with federal collection guidelines.

Further Readings

Cain, Rita Marie. "Call Up Someone and Just Say 'Buy.'" *American Business Law Journal* 31 (1994): 641.

Cost Survey: 1996 Report Based on 1995 Data. Englewood, CO: Medical Group Management Association, 1996.

Council on Ethical and Judicial Affairs. *Code of Medical Ethics: Current Opinions With Annotations.* Chicago: American Medical Association, 1994.

Office of Consumer Affairs. *Credit and Financial Issues: Responsive Business Approaches to Consumer Needs.* Washington, DC: U.S. Department of Commerce, May 1995.

Terkel, Susan Neiburg. *Understanding Child Custody.* New York: Franklin Watts, 1991.

Accounts Payable, Payroll, and Contracts

CHAPTER OUTLINE

- Managing Accounts Payable
- Managing Disbursements
- Handling Payroll
- Calculating and Filing Taxes
- Managing Contracts

OBJECTIVES

After completing Chapter 18, you will be able to:

- Give several examples of disbursements.
- Record disbursements in a disbursement journal.
- Set up and maintain a petty cash fund.
- Create employee payroll information sheets.
- Compute an employee's gross earnings, total deductions, and net earnings.
- Prepare an employee earnings record and payroll register.
- Set up the practice's tax liability accounts.
- Complete federal, state, and local tax forms.
- Submit employment taxes to government agencies.
- Describe the basic parts of an employment contract.

Key Terms

cash flow statement
counter check
dependent
employment contract
gross earnings
limited check
net earnings
pay schedule
petty cash fund
quarterly return
tax liability
tracking
traveler's check
voucher check

AREAS OF COMPETENCE

1997 ROLE DELINEATION STUDY

ADMINISTRATIVE

Practice Finances

- Apply bookkeeping principles
- Manage accounts payable
- Process payroll

Managing Accounts Payable

As you know from Chapter 17, accounts payable are the practice's expenses (money leaving the business), and accounts receivable reflect a practice's income (money coming into the business). This chapter focuses on accounts payable, including payroll. A basic accounting principle to bear in mind is that when a practice's income exceeds its expenses, it has a profit. When a practice's expenses exceed its income, it has a loss.

Because of this relationship between income and expenses, most practices try to reduce expenses by controlling accounts payable. As a medical assistant, you play an important role in helping control accounts payable and maximize profits.

Accounts payable fall into three main groups:

- Payments for supplies, equipment, and practice-related products and services
- Payroll, which may be the largest of the accounts payable
- Taxes owed to federal, state, and local agencies

A practice's accounting system usually consists of several elements. These elements include the daily log, patient ledger cards, the checkbook, the disbursements journal, the petty cash record, and the payroll register.

Because the daily log and patient ledger cards are used primarily for accounts receivable, they are discussed in Chapter 16, along with the checkbook. The disbursements journal, petty cash record, and payroll register are used primarily in accounts payable. Procedure 18-1 tells you how to set up and use these accounting tools effectively.

Managing Disbursements

A disbursement is any payment the physician's office makes for goods or services. One of the most common disbursements is payment for office supplies. Other disbursements include payments for equipment, dues, rent, taxes, salary, and utilities. No matter what type of disbursement you make on behalf of the practice, you must keep accurate records of the purchase and the payment.

Managing Supplies

In most practices, the physician authorizes one person to handle the purchasing of supplies and other products. This person is usually the office manager or medical assistant.

Guidelines for purchasing supplies are discussed in detail in Chapter 8. When buying clinical or office supplies, keep these principles in mind to control expenses.

1. Order only the necessary supplies, and order them only in the proper amounts. Buying too much reduces cash flow. Buying too little may cause you to run out of needed items and you may have to reorder too often.

PROCEDURE 18-1

Setting Up the Accounts Payable System

Objective: To set up an accounts payable system

Materials: Disbursements journal, petty cash record, payroll register, pen

Method

Setting Up the Disbursements Journal

1. Write in column headings for the basic information about each check: date, payee's name, check number, and check amount.
2. Write in column headings for each type of business expense, such as rent and utilities.
3. Write in column headings (if space is available) for deposits and the account balance.
4. Record the data from completed checks under the appropriate column headings.

Setting Up the Petty Cash Record

1. Write in column headings for the date, transaction number, payee, brief description, amount of transaction, and type of expense.
2. Write in a column heading (if space is available) for the petty cash fund balance.
3. Record the data from petty cash vouchers under the appropriate column headings.

Setting Up the Payroll Register

1. Write in column headings for check number, employee name, earnings to date, hourly rate, hours worked, regular earnings, overtime hours worked, and overtime earnings.
2. Write in column headings for total gross earnings for the pay period and gross taxable earnings.
3. Write in column headings for each deduction. These may include federal income tax, Federal Insurance Contributions Act (FICA) tax, state income tax, local income tax, and various voluntary deductions.
4. Write in a column heading for net earnings.
5. Each time you write payroll checks, record earning and deduction data under the appropriate column headings on the payroll register.

2. Combine orders when possible. You may save money and time by placing a larger order for several items at once rather than placing a smaller order each time an item is needed.
3. Follow your practice's purchasing guidelines, if any. For example, you may have to get the physician's approval for purchases over a specific dollar amount. Employees may have to submit purchase orders (formal requests for goods or services).
4. Buy from reputable suppliers. They are more likely to provide on-time delivery and satisfactory handling of your order. If your office does not already have a list of reliable suppliers, ask for recommendations from other practices.
5. Get the best-quality supplies for the best price.
6. For clinical supplies, consider the amount for which insurance companies will reimburse the practice. For example, if your office does only a few throat cultures a year, it might make more sense to send those patients elsewhere for the test than to stock the supplies required. The small reimbursement amount for a few throat cultures may not justify purchasing the supplies. Also consider shelf life. Do not buy large amounts of clinical supplies that will expire before use.

Writing Checks

Virtually all disbursements are made by check. Paying by check gives the practice complete, accurate records of all financial transactions.

Before writing a check, make sure the checking account balance is up-to-date and large enough to cover the check you want to write. (Chapter 16 discusses writing checks and managing the checkbook register.) Subtract the amount of each check from the previous balance, enter the new balance, and carry that balance forward to the next stub.

If you use a pegboard system, you will automatically record the date, check number, payee, and check amount on the check register as you write out the check. You must note the reason for payment and the new balance manually, however. Record that information in the appropriate spaces on the register.

If you make an error when completing a check, write VOID in ink across the front of the check in large letters so that it cannot be used again. Then file the voided check in numerical order with the returned checks.

After filling out the check properly, detach it from the checkbook, and give it to the doctor to sign, along with the invoice to be paid. (With experience, you may be trusted to sign checks under a certain amount.) Mark the date, check number, and amount paid on the invoice. Make a copy of the invoice for your records. Keep these copies with supporting documents, such as order forms or packing slips, in a paid-invoice file. Then, mail the check and the original invoice to the payee in a neatly hand-addressed or typewritten envelope. If you use a window envelope, be sure the payee's address shows through the window.

Commonly Used Checks. Most practices use checks from a standard checkbook, or they use **voucher checks,** business checks with stubs attached. Voucher checks come in several styles. A common style is a large, ring-bound checkbook, with three checks to a page. A perforation divides each check from its matching stub, which the practice retains.

Limited checks are sometimes used for payroll. A **limited check** states that it is void after a certain time limit. Many practices use checks that are void after 90 days.

Other Types of Checks. You or the physician may sometimes need to use other types of checks. The physician may use a cashier's check to pay certain types of taxes. A cashier's check is purchased from a bank, written on the bank's own checking account, and signed by a bank official.

The physician may use a certified check to pay certain taxes or to buy property. A certified check is a standard check that the bank verifies and certifies before it is used. This certification means that funds have been set aside to guarantee payment of the check.

A **counter check** is a special bank check that allows the depositor to withdraw funds from her account only. It states, "Pay to the Order of Myself Only." The physician may use a counter check when she wants to withdraw money but has forgotten her checkbook.

A physician may use **traveler's checks** when attending an out-of-town conference or whenever using a personal check or carrying a lot of cash is not appropriate. Printed in $10, $20, $50, and $100 denominations, these checks must be signed at the location where they are purchased (usually a bank). To use traveler's checks, the physician fills in the payee's name and signs it in a second place. She must sign it in the payee's presence so the payee can ensure that the signatures match.

Recording Disbursements

As described in Chapter 16, you may record disbursements in a check register, in a disbursements journal, or on the bottom section of the daily log.

If you use a disbursements journal, follow these steps to record disbursements.

1. When beginning a new journal page, give each column a heading to reflect the type of expense, such as utilities or rent.
2. For each check, fill in the date, payee's name, check number, and check amount in the appropriate columns.
3. Determine the expense category of the check.
4. Record the check amount in the column for that type of business expense.
5. If you must divide a check between two or more expense columns, record the total in the check amount

column. Then record the amount that applies to each type of expense in the appropriate column.

Recording disbursements in columns for each type of expense allows you to total and track expenses by category. **Tracking** (watching for changes) is important because it helps control expenses. Before tracking, check your calculations by performing a trial balance.

1. Total the check amount column.
2. Find the total for each expense column.
3. Add together all the expense column totals. The combined expense column total should match the total in the check amount column.
4. If the amounts do not match, recheck every entry until you find the error. When you find it, draw a line through it, and record the correct information neatly above it or to the side.
5. When the two amounts match (or balance), carry forward all column totals to the disbursements journal for the next month. Remember to prepare summaries and perform balances at the end of every month, quarter, and year.

Managing Petty Cash

Occasionally, you may need to make small (petty) cash disbursements for minor expenses such as postage-due fees or holiday decorations (Figure 18-1). To avoid writing checks for such small amounts, you may pay for them from the **petty cash fund,** cash kept on hand in the office for small purchases. The doctor should determine the amount of the petty cash account (usually $50) and the minimum amount of cash to be kept on hand (such as $15).

Starting and Maintaining a Petty Cash Fund. To start the fund with $50, write a check to "Petty Cash" or "Cash" for that amount. Enter the check in the miscellaneous column of the monthly disbursement record. Then, cash the check. Because this money will be used for small disbursements, be sure to get some of it in pennies, nickels, dimes, quarters, and dollar bills. Put this money in a special petty cash box, along with a stack of petty cash vouchers.

For each payment from the petty cash fund, obtain a receipt, or create a petty cash voucher. The voucher should record the transaction number, date, amount paid, purpose of the expense, your signature (as the person issuing the money), and the signature of the person receiving it. Keep the receipt for any item purchased, along with the completed voucher, in the petty cash box to verify expenses later.

Also, document each petty cash withdrawal on a petty cash record form. Include the transaction number, date, payee, a brief description, amount, and type of expense (such as office expense, auto expense, or miscellaneous expense). If a space is provided, calculate and record the new balance in the petty cash fund.

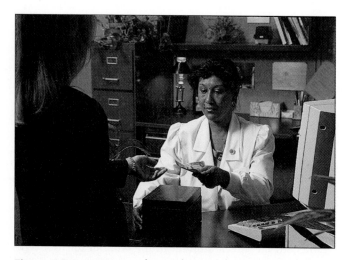

Figure 18-1. You may be in charge of maintaining the practice's petty cash fund. Count cash carefully, and keep accurate records about purchases made.

Replenishing the Petty Cash Fund. At the end of the month (or whenever the fund is low), compare the latest petty cash balance to the money in the petty cash box. If you have not kept a running balance, total the receipts and vouchers, then count the cash on hand. Subtract the total amount on the receipts and vouchers (for example, $35) from the original balance (for example, $50). The difference ($15) should equal the cash on hand in the petty cash box ($15).

To replenish the account, write a check to "Cash" or "Petty Cash" for the amount spent ($35). Cash the check and add the money to the box, bringing the total back up to the original amount of $50. Record the check for $35 on the disbursement record. Also, total the receipts and vouchers by expense category. Record those totals in the appropriate columns on the disbursement record.

Understanding Financial Summaries

The physician may periodically analyze the income and expenses of the practice. Financial summaries provide an easy-to-read report on the business transactions for a given period, such as a month or a year.

An accountant usually prepares financial summaries. Although you will probably not have to create these summaries, you should understand how they are prepared.

Statement of Income and Expense. Also called a profit-and-loss statement, a statement of income and expense highlights the practice's profitability. It shows the physician the practice's total income and then lists and subtracts all expenses.

Cash Flow Statement. A **cash flow statement** shows how much cash is available to cover expenses, to invest, or to take as profits. The cash flow statement begins with the cash on hand at the beginning of the period and shows the income and disbursements made during that period. It concludes with the new amount of cash on hand at the end of the period.

Trial Balance. The doctor may review trial balances periodically to ensure that the books balance. The combined expense column total should match the total in the check amount column. If the amounts do not match, recheck every entry until you find the error.

Handling Payroll

You may be responsible for handling the office payroll (Table 18-1). If so, your duties may include:

- Obtaining tax identification numbers.
- Creating employee payroll information sheets.
- Calculating employees' earnings.
- Subtracting taxes and other deductions.
- Writing paychecks.
- Creating employee earnings records.
- Preparing a payroll register.
- Submitting payroll taxes.

Applying for Tax Identification Numbers

Every employer—whether a single physician or a corporate practice—must have an employer identification number (EIN). An EIN is required by law for federal tax accounting purposes. An EIN is obtained by completing Form SS-4 (Application for Employer Identification Number)

Table 18-1

Payroll Duties

Frequency	Duties
Upon assuming payroll responsibilities	• Apply for an employer identification number (EIN) with Form SS-4 if the physician does not already have an EIN.
Whenever a new employee is hired	• Have the employee complete an Employee's Withholding Allowance Certificate (Form W-4) and Employment Eligibility Verification (Form I-9). • Record the employee's name and Social Security number from the Social Security Card.
Every payday	• Withhold federal income tax as well as state and local income taxes (if any). • Withhold the employee's share of FICA taxes (for Social Security and Medicare). Record a matching amount for the employer's share. • Calculate how much the practice must pay for each employee's federal and state unemployment tax.
Monthly or biweekly (depending on your deposit schedule)	• Deposit withheld income taxes, withheld and employer Social Security taxes, and withheld and employer Medicare taxes.
Quarterly (by April 30, July 31, October 31, and January 31)	• File Employer's Quarterly Federal Tax Return (Form 941). With the return, pay any taxes that were not deposited earlier. • Deposit federal unemployment tax, if over $100.
At least once a year	• Have all employees update their W-4 forms.
On or before January 31	• Give employees their Wage and Tax Statements (Form W-2), which show total wages and various withheld taxes. • File Employers Annual Federal Unemployment (FUTA) Tax Return (Form 940) with tax amount due.
On or before February 28	• File Transmittal of Wage and Tax Statements (Form W-3) along with the government's copies of the W-2 forms.

and submitting it to the Internal Revenue Service (IRS). Some states also require employer tax reports, for which the practice must have a state identification number, obtained from the proper state agency.

Creating Employee Payroll Information Sheets

The practice must maintain up-to-date, accurate payroll information about each employee. You should prepare a payroll information sheet for each employee. Each sheet should have the following information:

1. The employee's name, address, Social Security number, and marital status
2. An indication that the employee has completed an Employment Eligibility Verification (Form I-9), verifying that the employee is a U.S. citizen, a legally admitted alien, or an alien authorized to work in the United States
3. The employee's pay schedule, number of dependents, payroll type, and voluntary deductions

Pay Schedule. On the payroll information sheet, list the employee's **pay schedule,** showing how often he is paid. Common pay schedules are weekly, biweekly, and monthly.

Number of Dependents. Also, record the number of **dependents** (people who depend on the employee for financial support). Dependents may include a spouse, children, and other family members.

You can find the number of dependents on the Employee's Withholding Allowance Certificate (Form W-4), which should have been completed when the employee was hired (Figure 18-2). Remember to keep the completed W-4 forms in the physician's personnel file, and update them at least annually.

Payroll Type. List the employee's payroll type—hourly wage, salary, or commission—on the payroll information sheet. An hourly wage is a set amount of money per hour of work. A salary is a set amount of money per pay period, regardless of the number of hours worked. A commission is a percentage of the amount an employee earns for the employer. Salespeople, for example, are often paid by commission.

Voluntary Deductions. Finally, document the voluntary deductions to be taken from the employee's check. These may include additional federal withholding taxes, contributions to a 401(k) plan, or payments to a company health insurance plan. If the employee wants additional federal taxes taken out of her paycheck, she will indicate this deduction on the W-4 form.

Gross Earnings

Gross earnings refers to the total amount of income earned before deductions. Gross earnings must be calculated for each employee as a first step in the payroll process.

Calculating Gross Earnings. For every payroll period, use data from the payroll information sheet to compute each employee's gross earnings. For an hourly employee, use this equation:

$$\text{Hourly Wage} \times \text{Hours Worked} = \text{Gross Earnings}$$

If an employee earns \$8 per hour and works 35 hours, for example, her gross earnings are \$280 (\$8 × 35 hours) per week.

For a salaried employee, use the salary amount as the gross earnings for the pay period, no matter how many hours she worked. If an employee earns a weekly salary of \$400, for example, she receives that amount whether she worked 30, 40, or 50 hours during that week.

Fair Labor Standards Act. The Fair Labor Standards Act primarily affects employees who earn hourly wages. It limits the number of hours they may work, sets their minimum wage, and regulates their overtime pay. It also requires the employer to record the number of hours they work, usually on a time card or in a time book.

For hourly employees, this act mandates payment of:

- Time and a half (1½ times the normal hourly wage) for all hours worked beyond the normal 8 in a regular workday.
- Time and a half for all hours worked on the sixth consecutive day of the work week.
- Twice the normal wage (double time) for all hours worked on the seventh consecutive workday.
- Double time, plus normal holiday pay, for all hours worked on a company-approved holiday.

The Fair Labor Standards Act also requires overtime payments for part-time hourly employees for every hour worked beyond the normal 8 in a day or 40 in a week.

Making Deductions

The law requires all employers to withhold money from employees' gross earnings to pay federal and state and local (if any) income taxes and certain other taxes. In addition, employees may wish you to make certain voluntary deductions. For example, you might be asked to deduct an amount for child care, if the practice or hospital provides on-site child care. You might also deduct employee contributions to health insurance premiums.

You must deposit all employee deductions and employer payments into separate accounts. Monies from these **tax liability** accounts are used to pay taxes to appropriate government agencies.

Income Taxes. You must withhold enough money to cover the employee's federal income tax for the pay period. You can determine this amount by finding the employee's number of exemptions (from Form W-4) and referring to the tax tables in *Circular E, Employer's Tax Guide,* published by the IRS.

Consult the state and local tax tables for other income taxes. These taxes may be simpler to calculate. For exam-

Form W-4 (1996)

Want More Money In Your Paycheck? If you expect to be able to take the earned income credit for 1996 and a child lives with you, you may be able to have part of the credit added to your take-home pay. For details, get Form W-5 from your employer.

Purpose. Complete Form W-4 so that your employer can withhold the correct amount of Federal income tax from your pay. Because your tax situation may change, you may want to refigure your withholding each year.

Exemption From Withholding. Read line 7 of the certificate below to see if you can claim exempt status. *If exempt, only complete lines 1, 2, 3, 4, 7, and sign the form to validate it.* No Federal income tax will be withheld from your pay. Your exemption expires February 18, 1997.

Note: *You cannot claim exemption from withholding if (1) your income exceeds $650 and includes unearned income (e.g., interest and dividends) and (2) another person can claim you as a dependent on their tax return.*

Basic Instructions. If you are not exempt, complete the Personal Allowances Worksheet. Additional worksheets are on page 2 so you can adjust your withholding allowances based on itemized deductions, adjustments to income, or two-earner/two-job situations. Complete all worksheets that apply to your situation. The worksheets will help you figure the number of withholding allowances you are entitled to claim. However, you may claim fewer allowances than this.

Head of Household. Generally, you may claim head of household filing status on your tax return only if you are unmarried and pay more than 50% of the costs of keeping up a home for yourself and your dependent(s) or other qualifying individuals.

Nonwage Income. If you have a large amount of nonwage income, such as interest or dividends, you should consider making estimated tax payments using Form 1040-ES. Otherwise, you may find that you owe additional tax at the end of the year.

Two Earners/Two Jobs. If you have a working spouse or more than one job, figure the total number of allowances you are entitled to claim on all jobs using worksheets from only one W-4. This total should be divided among all jobs. Your withholding will usually be most accurate when all allowances are claimed on the W-4 filed for the highest paying job and zero allowances are claimed for the others.

Check Your Withholding. After your W-4 takes effect, use **Pub. 919,** Is My Withholding Correct for 1996?, to see how the dollar amount you are having withheld compares to your estimated total annual tax. Get Pub. 919 especially if you used the Two Earner/Two Job Worksheet and your earnings exceed $150,000 (Single) or $200,000 (Married). To order Pub. 919, call 1-800-829-3676. Check your telephone directory for the IRS assistance number for further help.

Sign This Form. Form W-4 is not considered valid unless you sign it.

Personal Allowances Worksheet

A Enter "1" for **yourself** if no one else can claim you as a dependent . . . . **A** ____

B Enter "1" if:
- You are single and have only one job; or
- You are married, have only one job, and your spouse does not work; or
- Your wages from a second job or your spouse's wages (or the total of both) are $1,000 or less.

. . **B** ____

C Enter "1" for your **spouse.** But, you may choose to enter -0- if you are married and have either a working spouse or more than one job (this may help you avoid having too little tax withheld) . . . . **C** ____

D Enter number of **dependents** (other than your spouse or yourself) you will claim on your tax return . . . . **D** ____

E Enter "1" if you will file as **head of household** on your tax return (see conditions under **Head of Household** above) . **E** ____

F Enter "1" if you have at least $1,500 of **child or dependent care expenses** for which you plan to claim a credit . . **F** ____

G Add lines A through F and enter total here. **Note:** This amount may be different from the number of exemptions you claim on your return ▶ **G** ____

For accuracy, do all worksheets that apply.
- If you plan to **itemize or claim adjustments to income** and want to reduce your withholding, see the Deductions and Adjustments Worksheet on page 2.
- If you are **single** and have **more than one job** and your combined earnings from all jobs exceed $30,000 OR if you are **married** and have a **working spouse or more than one job,** and the combined earnings from all jobs exceed $50,000, see the Two-Earner/Two-Job Worksheet on page 2 if you want to avoid having too little tax withheld.
- If **neither** of the above situations applies, **stop here** and enter the number from line G on line 5 of Form W-4 below.

---------- **Cut here and give the certificate to your employer. Keep the top portion for your records.** ----------

Form **W-4**
Department of the Treasury
Internal Revenue Service

Employee's Withholding Allowance Certificate

▶ **For Privacy Act and Paperwork Reduction Act Notice, see reverse.**

OMB No. 1545-0010
1996

1 Type or print your first name and middle initial	Last name	2 Your social security number
Home address (number and street or rural route)		3 ☐ Single ☐ Married ☐ Married, but withhold at higher Single rate. **Note:** *If married, but legally separated, or spouse is a nonresident alien, check the Single box.*
City or town, state, and ZIP code		4 If your last name differs from that on your social security card, check here and call 1-800-772-1213 for a new card . . . . . ▶ ☐

5 Total number of allowances you are claiming (from line G above or from the worksheets on page 2 if they apply) . **5** ____

6 Additional amount, if any, you want withheld from each paycheck . . . . **6** $ ____

7 I claim exemption from withholding for 1996 and I certify that I meet **BOTH** of the following conditions for exemption:
- Last year I had a right to a refund of **ALL** Federal income tax withheld because I had **NO** tax liability; **AND**
- This year I expect a refund of **ALL** Federal income tax withheld because I expect to have **NO** tax liability.

If you meet both conditions, enter "EXEMPT" here . . . . ▶ **7** ____

Under penalties of perjury, I certify that I am entitled to the number of withholding allowances claimed on this certificate or entitled to claim exempt status.

Employee's signature ▶ **Date ▶** , 19

8 Employer's name and address (Employer: Complete 8 and 10 only if sending to the IRS)	9 Office code (optional)	10 Employer identification number

Cat. No. 10220Q

Figure 18-2. Update all Employee's Withholding Allowance Certificates (W-4 forms) at least once a year.

ple, they may be 4% and 1% of the employee's gross earnings, respectively.

FICA Taxes. For FICA tax, withhold from the employee's check half of the tax owed for the pay period. Pay the other half from the practice's accounts. The amount of FICA tax that funds Social Security differs from the amount that funds Medicare. Report these two amounts separately. Check IRS *Circular E* for the latest FICA tax percentages and level of taxable earnings.

Unemployment Taxes. Federal unemployment tax is not a deduction from employees' paychecks, but it is based on their earnings. It is paid by the practice. The Federal Unemployment Tax Act (FUTA) requires employers to pay a percentage of each employee's income, up to a certain dollar amount. The percentage may be reduced if the employer also pays state unemployment taxes.

States calculate unemployment taxes differently. Some states tax employers and employees; others tax only employers. State unemployment tax usually varies with the employer's past employment record. Employers with few layoffs, such as physicians, have lower tax rates than those with many layoffs. To compute state unemployment tax, apply the assigned tax rate to each employee's earnings, up to a maximum for the calendar year. For details, consult your state unemployment insurance department.

Workers' Compensation. Some states require employers to insure their employees against possible loss of income resulting from work-related injury, disability, or disease. Although state laws vary, they typically require doctors to carry this insurance with a state insurance fund or state-authorized private insurer. Usually, a medical practice's insurance agent will audit the payroll books annually and then issue a bill for the workers' compensation premium due.

Calculating Net Earnings

Add each employee's required and voluntary deductions together to determine the total deductions. Then, subtract the total deductions from the gross earnings to get the employee's **net earnings,** or take-home pay. Use the following equation:

Gross Earnings – Total Deductions = Net Earnings

Preparing Paychecks

The way you prepare the practice's payroll will depend on the system the practice uses. In a small practice, you may write paychecks manually, following the standard check-writing procedure discussed in Chapter 16. In this case, write the check amount for the employee's net earnings, and deduct the check amount from the office checkbook.

If the practice uses a payroll service, you may supply time cards or payroll data to the service by mail or electronically. The service calculates all the deductions, prepares paychecks, and mails them to the practice for distribution.

No matter how paychecks are prepared, they should include information about how the check amount was determined. This information usually appears on the check stub. It should match the information on the employee earnings records and payroll register. Procedure 18-2 explains the process for generating payroll.

Maintaining Employee Earnings Records

You need to keep an employee earnings record for each employee (Figure 18-3). When you create the record, list the employee's name, address, phone number, Social Security number, birth date, spouse's name, number of dependents, job title, employment starting date, pay rate, and voluntary deductions.

Then, for each pay period, record the employee's gross earnings, individual deductions, net earnings, and related information. Properly completed earnings records show each employee's earning history.

Maintaining a Payroll Register

A payroll register summarizes vital information about all employees and their earnings (Figure 18-4). At the end of each pay period, record each employee's earnings to date, hourly rate, hours worked, overtime hours, overtime earnings, and total gross earnings. Also, list the gross earnings subject to unemployment taxes and FICA, all required and voluntary deductions, net earnings, and the paycheck number.

Handling Payroll Electronically

Manual payroll preparation and related tasks may take an hour per week for each employee (Payroll Store, 1995). To save time and to provide the convenience for employees of having their paychecks automatically deposited, some practices handle payroll tasks electronically. "Tips for the Office" discusses this topic.

If you work in a relatively small practice, you may handle all payroll tasks in the office, using accounting or payroll software. If you work in a large practice, you may prepare payroll information on the computer and transmit it by modem to an outside payroll service for processing. Depending on which system and software the practice has, you may use the computer to:

- Create, update, and delete employee payroll information files.
- Prepare employee paychecks, stubs, and W-2 forms.
- Update and print employee earnings records.
- Update all appropriate bookkeeping records, such as the payroll ledger and general ledger, with payroll data.

To perform these payroll functions electronically, follow the specific instructions in the software manual or get instructions from the payroll service. Generally, you would follow these steps.

PROCEDURE 18-2

Generating Payroll

Objective: To handle the practice's payroll as efficiently and accurately as possible for each pay period

Materials: Employees' time cards, employees' earnings records, payroll register, IRS tax tables, check register

Method

1. Calculate the total regular and overtime hours worked, based on the employee's time card. Enter those totals under the appropriate headings on the payroll register.
2. Check the pay rate on the employee earnings record. Then multiply the hours worked (including any paid vacation or paid holidays, if applicable) by the rates for regular time and overtime (time and a half or double time). This yields gross earnings.
3. Enter the gross earnings under the appropriate heading on the payroll register. Subtract any nontaxable benefits, such as health-care programs.
4. Using IRS tax tables and data on the employee earnings record, determine the amount of federal income tax to withhold based on the employee's marital status and number of exemptions. Also compute the amount of FICA tax to withhold for Social Security (6.2%) and Medicare (1.45%).
5. Following state and local procedures, determine the amount of state and local income taxes (if any) to withhold based on the employee's marital status and number of exemptions.
6. Calculate the employer's contributions to FUTA and to the state unemployment fund, if any. Post these amounts to the employer's account.
7. Enter any other required or voluntary deductions, such as health insurance or contributions to a 401(k) fund.
8. Subtract all deductions from the gross earnings to get the employee's net earnings.
9. Enter the total amount withheld from all employees for FICA under the headings for Social Security and Medicare. Remember that the employer must match these amounts. Enter other employer contributions, such as for federal and state unemployment taxes, under the appropriate headings.
10. Fill out the check stub, including the employee's name, date, pay period, gross earnings, all deductions, and net earnings. Make out the paycheck for the net earnings.
11. Deposit each deduction in a tax liability account.

First, select an option from the "Payroll" menu. Wait for the prompt, then select the appropriate employee from a list of employees.

To create an employee payroll information file for a new employee, input the same information that you would record manually on an employee payroll information sheet: name, address, Social Security number, marital status, pay schedule, number of dependents, payroll type, and voluntary deductions. Print two copies of the employee payroll information file—one for the employee and one for the physician's personnel file.

To update an employee payroll information file when an employee moves, marries, has a child, or wants to change deductions, select "Update Employee File." After making the changes, print out two copies of the file. Show one to the employee to confirm that the information is correct. Then have the employee sign and date it. Keep the signed copy for the physician's personnel file, and give the other to the employee. To ensure that payroll information is always correct and current, you should update it once a year for every employee.

To delete an employee payroll information file when an employee leaves the practice, select "Terminate Employee." Remember to print out and file a copy of this information before deleting it, because the physician is required to keep employees' payroll records for 4 years.

To generate paychecks and stubs, select the employee from the list of employees and choose the "Print Paycheck" option. Then, answer each prompt displayed by the computer (for example, hours worked). The computer has the employee's pay rate, payroll type, and deductions on file and automatically calculates the employee's net earnings, generates a paycheck, and prints a pay stub with the appropriate information.

To create an employee earnings record, select this option and follow the prompts for the needed information. Depending on the software used, each employee's earnings record may be updated automatically every time you generate a paycheck or make changes to other payroll files.

Calculating and Filing Taxes

In many practices, medical assistants set up tax liability accounts for money withheld from paychecks. These accounts are used to submit this money to appropriate agencies.

Name ______________________ Soc. Sec. No. ______________ Dependents __________ Year ________

Address ______________________ Birth Date ______________ Deductions __________

______________________ Job Title ______________

Employed on ______________ Pay Rate

Spouse ______________________ Terminated on ______________

Phone Reason

Record of Changes	Date	Rate

Check Number	Period Number	Earnings			Deductions					Net Pay	Cumulative FICA
		Regular	OT	Total	FICA	Fed. Tax	State	SUI	SDI		
1st Quarter Total											
2d Quarter Total											
3d Quarter Total											
4th Quarter Total											

Figure 18-3. Earnings records show the earning history of each employee at your practice.

Pay Period 6/1–6/14

Emp. No.	Name	Earnings to date	Hrly. Rate	Reg. Hrs.	OT Hrs.	OT Earnings	TOTAL GROSS	Earnings Subject to Unemp.	Earnings Subject to FICA	Social Security (FICA)	Medicare	Federal W/H	State W/H	Health Ins.	Net Pay	Check No.
0010	Scott, B.	9,823.14	14.00	70.00			980.00	980.00	980.00	60.50	14.10	147.92	15.10	25.00	717.38	11747
0020	Wilson, J.	14,290.38	17.00	70.00	6.50	153.00	1343.00	1343.00	1343.00	83.26	19.47	160.45	15.85	67.50	996.47	11748
0030	Diaz, J.	2,750.26	5.50	46.25			254.37	254.37	254.37	15.77	3.68	38.20	3.75		192.97	11749
0040	Ling, W.	2,240.57	6.80	30.00			204.00	204.00	204.00	12.66	2.96	26.02	3.12		159.54	11750
0050	Harris, E.	2,600.98	10.00	23.50			235.00	235.00	235.00	14.57	3.41	33.52	3.36		180.14	11751

Figure 18-4. A payroll register is designed to summarize information about all employees and their earnings.

Setting Up Tax Liability Accounts

You must set up at least two bank accounts to hold the money deducted from paychecks until it can be sent to the appropriate government agencies. One account will hold deductions from employees' paychecks for federal, state, and local income taxes and FICA taxes. Another account will hold employer payments based on payroll, such as federal and state unemployment taxes. For these accounts, choose a bank that is authorized by the IRS to accept federal tax deposits. If the practice makes other paycheck deductions, as for workers' compensation or a 401(k) plan, set up an account for each of these also.

Each time you prepare paychecks, deposit the withheld money into the proper account. Then, record the deposited amounts as debits in the practice's checking account.

Understanding Federal Tax Deposit Schedules

You will probably deposit federal income taxes and FICA taxes (which together are known as employment taxes) on a quarterly, monthly, or biweekly (every-other-week) schedule. Every November IRS personnel decide which deposit schedule your office should use for the next year.

If the IRS does not notify you about this matter, determine your deposit schedule based on the total employment taxes your office reported on the previous year's Employer's Quarterly Federal Tax Returns (Form 941). For example, if your office reported $50,000 or less in employment taxes during the past year, you would make monthly employment tax deposits the present year. If your office reported more than $50,000 during the past year, you would make semimonthly tax deposits.

There are exceptions to the monthly or semimonthly tax deposit schedules: the $500 rule and the $100,000 rule. The $500 rule applies to employers who owe less than $500 in employment taxes during a tax period (such as a quarter). These employers do not have to make a deposit for that period. The $100,000 rule applies to employers who owe $100,000 or more in employment taxes on any one day during a tax period. These employers must deposit the tax by the next banking day after the day that ceiling is reached.

Submitting Federal Income and FICA Taxes

Some businesses must submit federal income taxes and FICA taxes to the IRS by electronic funds transfer (EFT). The EFT program, known as TAXLINK, began in 1995. Since then, more taxpayers have been required to use it each year. If your practice is not required to use EFT but wishes to do so voluntarily, contact the IRS, Cash Management Site Office, to enroll.

If your practice does not use EFT, you must submit these employment taxes with a Federal Tax Deposit (FTD) Coupon (Form 8109) (see Figure 18-5). FTD Coupons are supplied by the IRS. They are printed with the physician's name, address, and EIN. They have boxes for filling in the type of tax and the tax period for which the deposit is being made.

To make the deposit, write a single check or money order for the total amount of federal income taxes and FICA taxes withheld during the tax period. Make the check payable to the bank where you make the deposit. This must be a Federal Reserve Bank or another bank authorized to make payments to the IRS. Also, complete the FTD Coupon. Then, mail or deliver the check and FTD Coupon to the bank. The bank will give you a deposit receipt.

If you work in a practice with a large payroll, you may need to make deposits every few days. In most practices, however, you will probably make deposits once a month. Then, every 3 months, a more complete accounting is required on a **quarterly return,** called the Employer's Quarterly Federal Tax Return (Form 941).

Tips FOR THE OFFICE: Handling Payroll Through Electronic Banking

An electronic funds transfer system (EFTS) enables you to handle the practice's payroll without writing payroll checks manually. The physician must sign up for EFTS with the bank, and employees must supply their bank account numbers to the employer. Then, the bank electronically deposits employees' paychecks into their bank accounts, as directed.

Most employees like to have their paychecks deposited automatically. The money is available on the day of deposit, and no one has to worry about losing a paycheck, getting to the bank before it closes, or carrying a paycheck around. Also, employees still receive a check stub along with a notification of deposit, so they can track their earnings and deductions.

Contact your bank for more information and specific procedures for setting up EFTS and electronic payroll.

Submitting FUTA Taxes

FUTA taxes provide money to workers who are unemployed. If the practice owes more than $100 in federal unemployment tax at the end of the quarter, deposit the tax amount with an FTD Coupon (Form 8109). At the end of the year, file an Employer's Annual Federal Unemployment (FUTA) Tax Return (Form 940) with any final taxes owed (Figure 18-6).

Generally, an employer must pay FUTA taxes if employees' wages total more than $1500 in any quarter (3-month period) and if those employees are not seasonal or household workers. The FUTA tax, which is 6.2%, is applied to the first $7000 of income for a year.

Filing an Employer's Quarterly Federal Tax Return

Each quarter, file an Employer's Quarterly Federal Tax Return (Form 941) with the IRS (Figure 18-7). This tax return summarizes the federal income and FICA taxes (employment taxes) withheld from employees' paychecks.

As a general rule, you should file Form 941 at the nearest IRS office by the last day of the first month after the quarter ends. If the practice has deposited all taxes on time, you have an additional 10 days after the due date to file.

Handling State and Local Income Taxes

Send withheld state and local income taxes to the proper agencies, using their forms, procedures, and schedules. If required, prepare quarterly or other tax forms for the state and local governments.

Filing Wage and Tax Statements

After the end of each year, file a Wage and Tax Statement (Form W-2) with the appropriate federal, state, and local government agencies for each employee who had federal income and FICA taxes withheld during the previous year (Figure 18-8). Also, supply copies of Form W-2 to each employee.

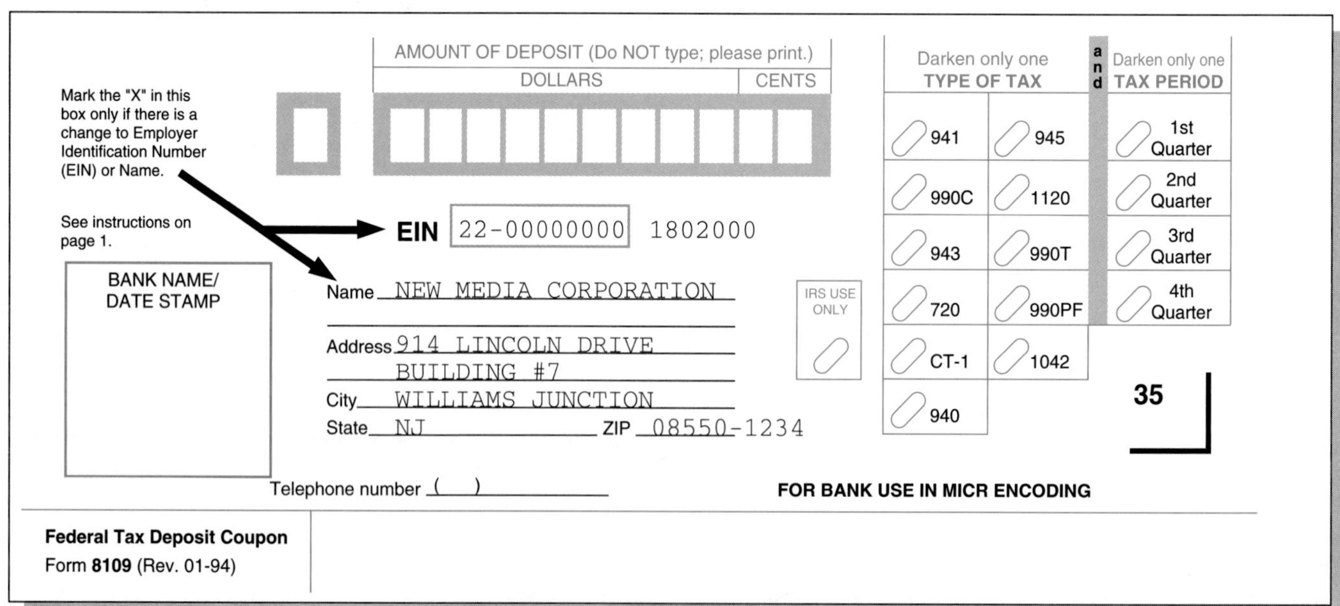

AMOUNT OF DEPOSIT (Do NOT type; please print.)
DOLLARS | CENTS

Mark the "X" in this box only if there is a change to Employer Identification Number (EIN) or Name.

See instructions on page 1.

EIN 22-00000000 1802000

BANK NAME/ DATE STAMP

Name NEW MEDIA CORPORATION

Address 914 LINCOLN DRIVE
BUILDING #7

City WILLIAMS JUNCTION

State NJ ZIP 08550-1234

Telephone number ( )

IRS USE ONLY

Darken only one TYPE OF TAX: 941, 945, 990C, 1120, 943, 990T, 720, 990PF, CT-1, 1042, 940

and

Darken only one TAX PERIOD: 1st Quarter, 2nd Quarter, 3rd Quarter, 4th Quarter

35

FOR BANK USE IN MICR ENCODING

Federal Tax Deposit Coupon
Form 8109 (Rev. 01-94)

Figure 18-5. Practices that do not use TAXLINK to submit taxes electronically must submit federal income and FICA taxes with a Federal Tax Deposit (FTD) Coupon (Form 8109).

Form **940**

Department of the Treasury
Internal Revenue Service (O)

Employer's Annual Federal Unemployment (FUTA) Tax Return

▶ For Paperwork Reduction Act Notice, see separate instructions.

OMB No. 1545-0028

1995

T	
FF	
FD	
FP	
I	
T	

Name (as distinguished from trade name) Calendar year

Trade name, if any

Address and ZIP code Employer identification number

A Are you required to pay unemployment contributions to only one state? (If no, skip questions B and C.)	☐ **Yes**	☐ **No**
B Did you pay all state unemployment contributions by January 31, 1996? (If a 0% experience rate is granted, check "Yes.") (If no, skip question C.)	☐ **Yes**	☐ **No**
C Were all wages that were taxable for FUTA tax also taxable for your state's unemployment tax?	☐ **Yes**	☐ **No**

If you answered "No" to any of these questions, you must file Form 940. If you answered "Yes" to all the questions, you may file Form 940-EZ, which is a simplified version of Form 940. You can get Form 940-EZ by calling 1-800-TAX-FORM (1-800-829-3676).

If you will not have to file returns in the future, check here, complete, and sign the return . . . ▶ ☐
If this is an Amended Return, check here . . . ▶ ☐

Part I Computation of Taxable Wages

		Amount paid		
1	Total payments (including exempt payments) during the calendar year for services of employees		**1**	
2	Exempt payments. (Explain each exemption shown, attach additional sheets if necessary.) ▶	**2**		
3	Payments of more than $7,000 for services. Enter only amounts over the first $7,000 paid to each employee. Do not include payments from line 2. The $7,000 amount is the Federal wage base. Your state wage base may be different. **Do not use the state wage limitation**	**3**		
4	Total exempt payments (add lines 2 and 3)		**4**	
5	**Total taxable wages** (subtract line 4 from line 1) ▶		**5**	

Be sure to complete both sides of this return and sign in the space provided on the back. Cat. No. 11234O Form **940** (1995)

DETACH HERE

Form **940-V**

Department of the Treasury
Internal Revenue Service

Form 940 Payment Voucher

For Paperwork Reduction Act Notice, see Form 940 instructions.

OMB No. 1545-0028

1995

Complete boxes 1,2,3, and 4. Make your check or money order payable to the **Internal Revenue Service.** Include your employer identification number on your check or money order. Do not send cash.

1 Enter the amount of the payment you are making ▶ $	**2** Enter the first four characters of your business name	**3** Enter your employer identification number
Do not staple your check or money order to the voucher or the return.	**4** Enter your name Enter your address Enter your city, state, and ZIP code	

Figure 18-6. Tax dollars filed with FUTA tax returns (Form 940) provide money to workers who are unemployed.

Form **941** (Rev. January 1996) Department of the Treasury Internal Revenue Service (O)

4141

Employer's Quarterly Federal Tax Return

▶ See separate instructions for information on completing this return.

Please type or print.

Enter state code for state in which deposits made . ▶ ☐ (see page 3 of instructions).

Name (as distinguished from trade name) | Date quarter ended

Trade name, if any | Employer identification number

Address (number and street) | City, state, and ZIP code

OMB No. 1545-0029

T
FF
FD
FP
I
T

If address is different from prior return, check here ▶ ☐

IRS Use

1	1	1	1	1	1	1	1	1	1	2	3	3	3	3	3	3	4	4	4

5	5	5	6	7	8	8	8	8	8	8	9	9	9	10	10	10	10	10	10	10	10	10	10

If you do not have to file returns in the future, check here ▶ ☐ and enter date final wages paid ▶

If you are a seasonal employer, see **Seasonal employers** on page 1 of the instructions and check here ▶ ☐

1 Number of employees (except household) employed in the pay period that includes March 12th ▶

2	Total wages and tips, plus other compensation	2	
3	Total income tax withheld from wages, tips, and sick pay	3	
4	Adjustment of withheld income tax for preceding quarters of calendar year	4	
5	Adjusted total of income tax withheld (line 3 as adjusted by line 4—see instructions)	5	
6a	Taxable social security wages . . . $ × 12.4% (.124) =	6a	
b	Taxable social security tips . . . $ × 12.4% (.124) =	6b	
7	Taxable Medicare wages and tips . . . $ × 2.9% (.029) =	7	
8	Total social security and Medicare taxes (add lines 6a, 6b, and 7). Check here if wages are not subject to social security and/or Medicare tax ▶ ☐	8	
9	Adjustment of social security and Medicare taxes (see instructions for required explanation) Sick Pay $ ______ ± Fractions of Cents $ ______ ± Other $ ______ =	9	
10	Adjusted total of social security and Medicare taxes (line 8 as adjusted by line 9—see instructions)	10	
11	**Total taxes** (add lines 5 and 10)	11	
12	Advance earned income credit (EIC) payments made to employees, if any	12	
13	Net taxes (subtract line 12 from line 11). **This should equal line 17, column (d) below** (or line D of Schedule B (Form 941))	13	
14	Total deposits for quarter, including overpayment applied from a prior quarter	14	
15	**Balance due** (subtract line 14 from line 13). See instructions	15	

16 **Overpayment,** if line 14 is more than line 13, enter excess here ▶ $ ______
and check if to be: ☐ Applied to next return **OR** ☐ Refunded.

- **All filers:** If line 13 is less than $500, you need not complete line 17 or Schedule B.
- **Semiweekly schedule depositors:** Complete Schedule B and check here ▶ ☐
- **Monthly schedule depositors:** Complete line 17, columns (a) through (d), and check here. ▶ ☐

17 **Monthly Summary of Federal Tax Liability.**

(a) First month liability	(b) Second month liability	(c) Third month liability	(d) Total liability for quarter

Sign Here Under penalties of perjury, I declare that I have examined this return, including accompanying schedules and statements, and to the best of my knowledge and belief, it is true, correct, and complete.

Signature ▶ Print Your Name and Title ▶ Date ▶

For Paperwork Reduction Act Notice, see page 1 of separate instructions. Cat. No. 17001Z Form **941** (Rev. 1-96)

Figure 18-7. Most practices make tax deposits monthly and then make a more complete accounting once every 3 months on the Employer's Quarterly Federal Tax Return (Form 941), the first page of which is shown here.

a Control number		OMB No. 1545-0008	
b Employer's identification number		1 Wages, tips, other compensation	2 Federal income tax withheld
c Employer's name, address, and ZIP code		3 Social security wages	4 Social security tax withheld
		5 Medicare wages and tips	6 Medicare tax withheld
		7 Social security tips	8 Allocated tips
d Employee's social security number		9 Advance EIC payment	10 Dependent care benefits
e Employee's name, address, and ZIP code		11 Nonqualified plans	12 Benefits included in box 1
		13	14 Other
		15 Statutory employee ☐ Deceased ☐ Pension plan ☐ Legal rep. ☐	Hshld. emp. ☐ Subtotal ☐ Deferred compensation ☐

16 State	Employer's state I.D. No.	17 State wages, tips, etc.	18 State income tax	19 Locality name	20 Local wages, tips, etc.	21 Local income tax

Department of the Treasury—Internal Revenue Service

Form **W-2** **Wage and Tax Statement** **1995**

Copy 1 For State, City, or Local Tax Department

Figure 18-8. A Wage and Tax Statement (Form W-2) records the total amount of taxes withheld during the previous year for each employee.

Form W-2 shows the employee's total taxable income for the previous year. It also shows the exact amount of federal income taxes and FICA taxes (for Social Security and Medicare) withheld, along with the amounts of state and local taxes withheld (if any).

Along with the W-2 forms, submit Form W-3, a Transmittal of Wage and Tax Statements (Figure 18-9). This form lists the employer's name, address, and EIN and summarizes the amount of all employees' earnings and the federal income taxes and FICA taxes withheld.

Managing Contracts

An **employment contract**—a written agreement of employment terms between employer and employee—may be considered a benefit because it increases employee job security. It also allows the employer to attract and keep the best employees. Although contracts are rarely offered to medical assistants, you should be aware of them because they may be used for doctors and executive management of a practice and because they may be used for medical assistants in the future.

Legal Elements of a Contract

An employment contract is a legal agreement between two or more people to perform an act in exchange for payment. To be binding, the contract must include these main elements:

- An agreement between two or more competent people to do something legal
- Names and addresses of the people involved
- Consideration (whatever is given in exchange, such as money, work, or property)
- Starting and ending dates, as well as date(s) the contract was signed
- Signatures of the employer and employee

A Medical Assistant Contract

Some medical practices use employment contracts for medical assistants. This type of contract would include these elements:

- A description of your duties and your employer's duties
- Plans for handling major changes in job responsibilities
- Salary, bonuses, and other forms of compensation

DO NOT STAPLE

a Control number	33333	For Official Use Only ▶ OMB No. 1545-0008	
b Kind of Payer: 941 ☐ Military ☐ 943 ☐ CT-1 ☐ Hshld. ☐ Medicare govt. emp. ☐		1 Wages, tips, other compensation	2 Federal income tax withheld
		3 Social security wages	4 Social security tax withheld
c Total number of statements	d Establishment number	5 Medicare wages and tips	6 Medicare tax withheld
e Employer's identification number		7 Social security tips	8 Allocated tips
f Employer's name		9 Advance EIC payments	10 Dependent care benefits
		11 Nonqualified plans	12 Deferred compensation
		13 Adjusted total social security wages and tips	
g Employer's address and ZIP code		14 Adjusted total Medicare wages and tips	
h Other EIN used this year		15 Income tax withheld by third-party payer	
i Employer's state I.D. No.			

Under penalties of perjury, I declare that I have examined this return and accompanying documents, and, to the best of my knowledge and belief, they are true, correct, and complete.

Signature ▶ Title ▶ Date ▶

Telephone number ( )

Form **W-3 Transmittal of Wage and Tax Statements 1995**

Department of the Treasury Internal Revenue Service

Paperwork Reduction Act Notice

We ask for the information on this form to carry out the Internal Revenue laws of the United States. You are required to give us the information. We need it to ensure that you are complying with these laws and to allow us to figure and collect the right amount of tax.

The time needed to complete and file this form will vary depending on individual circumstances. The estimated average time is 27 minutes. If you have comments concerning the accuracy of this time estimate or suggestions for making this form simpler, we would be happy to hear from you. You can write to the **Internal Revenue Service,** Attention: Tax Forms Committee, PC:FP, Washington, DC 20224. **Do NOT** send the form to this address. Instead, see **Where To File.**

Item To Note

Change to Kind of Payer Box.—The 942 box was retitled "Hshld." for household because **Form 942,**Employer's Quarterly Tax Return for Household Employees, is obsolete for wages paid after 1994. For more details, get **Pub. 926,** Employment Taxes for Household Employers.

Need Help?

Information Reporting Call Site.—The IRS operates a centralized call site to answer questions about reporting on Forms W-3, W-2, 1099, and other information returns. If you have questions related to reporting on information returns, you may call (304) 263-8700 (not a toll-free number).

Bulletin Board Services.—Using a personal computer and a modem, you can get information from either of two electronic Bulletin Board Systems (BBS)—the SSA-BBS or the IRP-BBS (IRS). You can access the SSA-BBS by dialing (410) 965-1133 or the IRP-BBS (IRS) by dialing (304) 263-2749.

Information available includes magnetic media and paper filing information, some IRS and SSA forms and publications, correct social security number information, information on electronic filing, and general topics of interest about information reporting. You can also use the bulletin board systems to ask questions about magnetic media or electronic filing programs, and reporting on information returns.

Substitute Forms.—Employers filing privately printed Forms W-2 must file Forms W-3 that are the same width as Form W-2. The forms must meet the requirements in **Pub. 1141,** General Rules and Specifications for Private Printing of Substitute Forms W-2 and W-3.

Forms and Publications.—You can get any of the forms and publications mentioned in these instructions by calling 1-800-TAX-FORM (1-800-829-3676).

Cat. No. 10159Y

Figure 18-9. Submit a Transmittal of Wage and Tax Statements (Form W-3) with the W-2 forms.

- Benefits, such as vacation time, sick days, life insurance, and participation in pension plans
- Grievance procedures
- Exceptional situations under which the contract may be terminated by either you or your employer
- Termination procedures and compensation

- Special provisions, such as job sharing, medical examinations, or liability coverage

If you are offered an employment contract, study it closely. Consider any local laws that may apply, and have a lawyer or business adviser review the contract.

Summary

Accounts payable are the practice's expenses—money leaving the business, including payroll. You may deal with accounts payable when ordering supplies, writing checks for disbursements, and recording them in a disbursements journal. To pay for and track small expenses, you may set up and maintain a petty cash fund.

A large part of accounts payable is payroll management. Your payroll duties may include applying for tax identification numbers, creating employee payroll information sheets, calculating employees' gross earnings, making deductions, calculating net earnings, and writing paychecks. To track payroll data, you may create employee earnings records and a payroll register.

Because taxes are so closely related to payroll, you may set up the practice's tax liability accounts. You may also complete federal, state, and local tax forms and send the taxes to the appropriate government agencies.

An employment contract is a written agreement of employment terms between employer and employee. Contracts may be used for physicians and executive management of a practice and are sometimes used for medical assistants as well.

18 Chapter Review

Discussion Questions

1. List several examples of common disbursements in a medical practice, and number them in order of importance. Be prepared to defend your ranking to the rest of the class or to your group.
2. Describe situations in which medical assistants might need to use voucher checks, certified checks, and traveler's checks.
3. Give the name and number of the tax form that should be used in each of the following situations. Discuss the components of each form. Explain why one form cannot be used for another tax task.
   - Inform employees of the amount of tax withheld from their earnings during the past year.
   - Verify that an employee is legally eligible to work in the United States.
   - Inform the IRS of the total taxes withheld from all employees' earnings during the quarter.

Critical Thinking Questions

1. When ordering office supplies and equipment, why should you buy high-quality products that are not necessarily the least expensive ones available?
2. Why should you calculate a trial balance of the disbursements journal monthly?
3. Why, do you think, does the IRS require both employers and employees to file Wage and Tax Statements (Form W-2)?

Application Activities

1. Record the following disbursements made on September 9, 1998, in a disbursements journal:
   - Check no. 1234, payee—Tom Jones (electrician), check amount—$125
   - Check no. 1235, payee—Postmaster (postage), check amount—$32
   - Check no. 1236, payee—Gateway Property Management (rent), check amount—$900
2. Simulate an office petty cash account, using your own personal expenses. Determine a starting amount, and use it for 2 weeks to buy small items. For each purchase, obtain a receipt, or write a petty cash voucher. Record each withdrawal you make from the petty cash account, using a petty cash record. At least once during the 2-week period, write a check to replenish the account.
3. Prepare your personal federal income tax return, using information from the Wage and Tax Statement (Form W-2) and the Employee's Withholding Allowance Certificate (Form W-4) provided by your employer.

Further Readings

Ernst & Young. *The Ernst & Young Tax Guide 1997.* New York: John Wiley, 1997.

Internal Revenue Service. *Circular E, Employer's Tax Guide.* Rancho Cordova, CA: Government Printing Office, 1996.

Internal Revenue Service. *Federal Employment Tax Forms.* Rancho Cordova, CA: Government Printing Office, 1995.

Payroll Store. "Electronic Payroll Services." Rochester, NY: Cyberplex, 1995.

Roberson, Cliff. *The McGraw-Hill Small Business Tax Advisor.* 2d ed. New York: McGraw-Hill, 1992.

Part Three

Clinical Medical Assisting

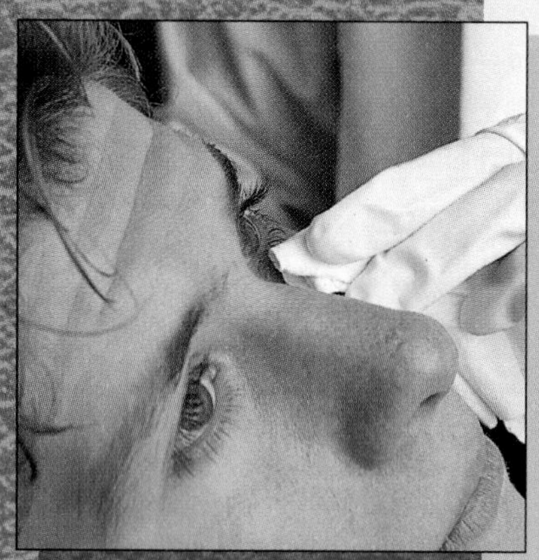

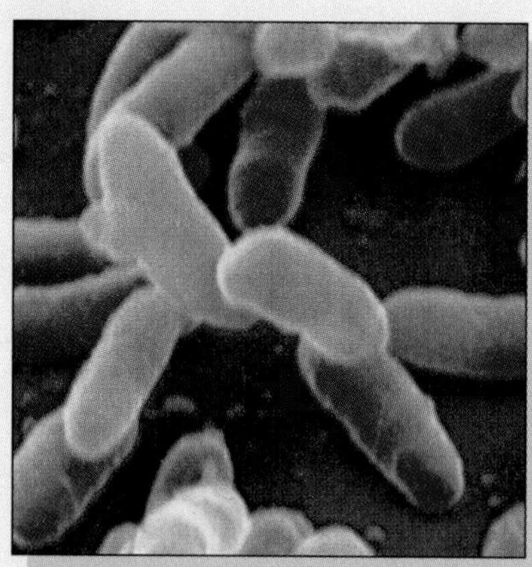

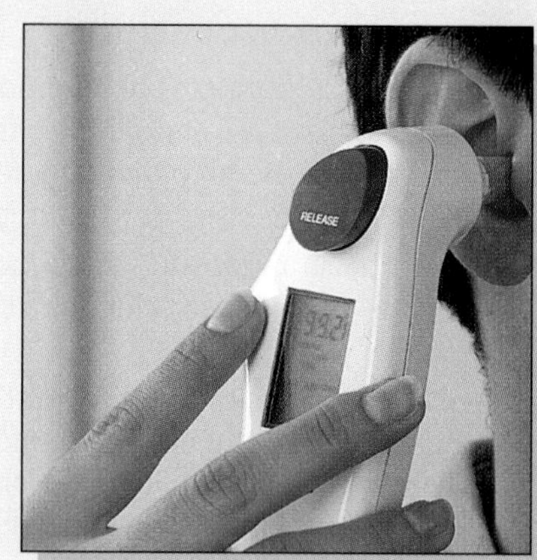

"One of the most important things you must remember when assisting with patients is to put yourself in the patient's place. How would you feel if you were told to do something you didn't know how to do? Wouldn't you want to know ahead of time what will be expected of you?

"As a medical assistant, it is your job to anticipate the physician's every need during a physical exam. Compare the process with that of surgery, where the doctor is handed an instrument even before he asks for it. You should try to make as smooth a transition as possible from one step to the next; everyone benefits."

Diane Morlock,
Medical Assisting Instructor
Stautzenberger College
Toledo, Ohio

Section One

The Medical Office Environment

Section Two

Understanding the Body and Assisting With Patients

Section Three

Specialty Practices and Medical Emergencies

Section Four

Physician's Office Laboratory Procedures

Section Five

Nutrition, Pharmacology, and Diagnostic Equipment

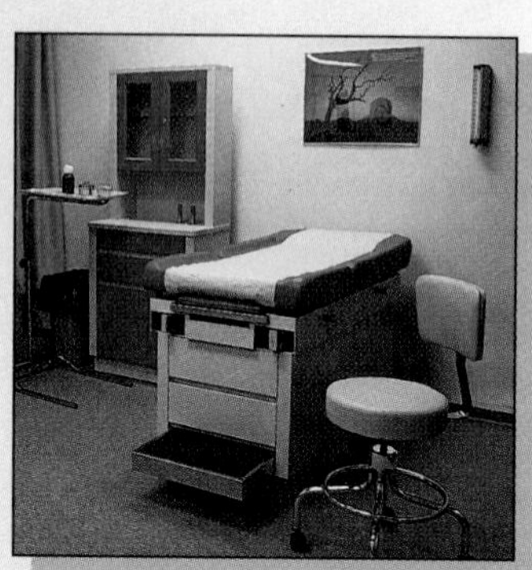

Section One

The Medical Office Environment

AREAS OF COMPETENCE

1997 ROLE DELINEATION STUDY

CLINICAL

- **Fundamental Principles**
- **Patient Care**

GENERAL (Transdisciplinary)

- **Professionalism**
- **Communication Skills**
- **Legal Concepts**
- **Instruction**

CHAPTER LIST

Principles of Asepsis

CHAPTER OUTLINE

- History of Infectious Disease Prevention
- Microorganisms and Disease
- The Disease Process
- The Body's Defenses
- The Cycle of Infection
- Breaking the Cycle
- Medical and Surgical Asepsis
- OSHA Bloodborne Pathogens Standard and Universal Precautions
- Educating Patients About Preventing Disease Transmission

OBJECTIVES

After completing Chapter 19, you will be able to:

- Explain the historical background of infectious disease prevention.
- Identify the types of microorganisms that cause disease.
- Explain the disease process.
- Explain how the body's defenses protect against infection.
- Describe the cycle of infection.
- Identify and describe the various methods of disease transmission.
- Explain how you can help break the cycle of infection.
- Compare and contrast medical and surgical asepsis.
- Describe how to perform aseptic hand washing.
- Define Bloodborne Pathogens Standard and Universal Precautions as described in the rules and regulations of the Occupational Safety and Health Administration (OSHA).
- Explain the role of Universal Precautions in the duties of a medical assistant.
- List the procedures and legal requirements for disposing of hazardous waste.
- Explain how to educate patients in preventing disease transmission.

Key Terms

antibody
antigen
asepsis
bacterial spore
biohazardous material
biohazardous waste container
carrier
disinfection
endogenous infection
exogenous infection
fomite
immunity
macrophage
microorganism
normal flora
opportunistic infection
pathogen
phagocyte
reservoir host
sanitization
Standard Precautions
sterilization
subclinical case
susceptible host
Universal Precautions
vector
virulence

AREAS OF COMPETENCE

1997 ROLE DELINEATION STUDY

CLINICAL

Fundamental Principles

- Apply principles of aseptic technique and infection control

Patient Care

- Prepare and maintain examination and treatment areas

continued

AREAS OF COMPETENCE continued

GENERAL (Transdisciplinary)

Instruction

- Teach methods of health promotion and disease prevention

History of Infectious Disease Prevention

Throughout history, doctors have tried to solve the problem of infection: what causes it, how it spreads, how to prevent it, and how to treat it. Some infections, such as the plague in the Middle Ages, have changed the course of history.

During the past century, remarkable advances have taken place in knowledge regarding the causes, prevention, and treatment of infectious disease. The threat of infection, however, is as great as it has ever been. Medical science still wrestles with relatively new infectious diseases, such as acquired immunodeficiency syndrome (AIDS) and Ebola virus disease. In addition, some older diseases (such as methicillin-resistant *Staphylococcus aureus,* or MRSA, and tuberculosis) continue to challenge researchers because they have become resistant to established medications.

As a medical assistant, you need to understand how to perform specific tasks to control infection and prevent disease transmission. First, however, you need to understand the disease process and how infection spreads.

Hippocrates

The Greek physician Hippocrates (circa 460 to 377 B.C.) made the first recorded attempt to control infection. Although Hippocrates is usually associated with the Hippocratic oath, a code of ethics for physicians, his scientific beliefs were as influential as his ethical beliefs. Instead of basing his practice of medicine on religion, he used logic. He believed that environmental and natural forces, such as diet, exercise, climate, and occupation, play the greatest role in disease and health. He taught his students to study disease by observing with the senses and by keeping careful records of patients' symptoms.

Hippocrates believed in simple and natural treatments, using strong drugs and surgery only as a last resort. He often prescribed a diet of basic foods, such as barley gruel. Some of his treatments—for example, honey in vinegar or boiled water—alleviated the symptoms of infection by causing the body to expel phlegm and urine. One of his innovations, the treatment of wounds with coal tar, was effective in controlling infection. Centuries after Hippocrates' time, scientists discovered that coal tar contains carbolic acid, a natural germ-killing chemical. Carbolic acid, also known as phenol, is a common chemical ingredient in today's antiseptics and disinfectants. It is now used in low concentrations (1.0% to 1.5%) because it is readily absorbed by the body and is carcinogenic at higher levels.

Joseph Lister

Joseph Lister was a British surgeon, scientist, and researcher who lived from 1827 to 1912 (Figure 19-1). He discovered how to use chemical antiseptics to control surgery-related infections caused by invisible organisms known as microorganisms. **Microorganisms** are simple forms of life commonly made up of a single cell. These organisms are so small that they can be seen only through a microscope.

Lister practiced in the Glasgow Royal Infirmary in Scotland, where 45% to 50% of people who had amputations died as a result of infection. The saw used for amputations was simply wiped with a towel or on someone's sleeve and put back in its case. At the time, even simple operations had similar rates of infection and death, and surgery was often fatal. Because people did not yet understand that microorganisms cause infection, almost no one made an effort to destroy the organisms, let alone to keep a sterile environment and sterile surgical instruments.

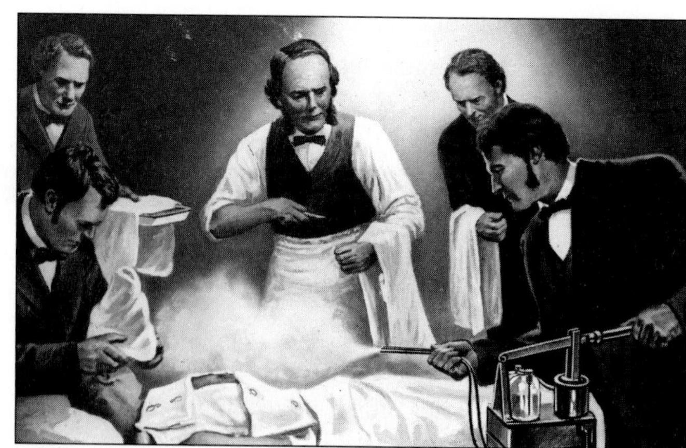

Figure 19-1. Joseph Lister pioneered the study and practice of eliminating as many microorganisms as possible during medical procedures.

Lister worked to lower the rate of infection and death. He had heard of the work of Louis Pasteur (1822–1895), the French chemist and microbiologist who had developed the germ theory. Pasteur, shown in Figure 19-2, had discovered that microorganisms, which he called germs, cause particular types of fermentation in certain liquids, such as milk and wine. He suggested that specific germs might also grow in humans and cause specific diseases. He believed that all microorganisms multiply from previously existing ones (biogenesis) rather than spontaneously growing or coming to life from nowhere (abiogenesis). Pasteur worked to increase the practices of hygiene, sanitation, and direct means of destroying microorganisms as ways to fight the spread of disease.

Joseph Lister used Pasteur's germ theory to conclude that microorganisms cause the infection of surgical wounds. He thought that the key is to keep germs from getting into a wound.

In 1865 Lister tried treating wounds with a type of carbolic acid that had been shown to cure infections in cattle. Unsatisfied with the results, he tried a purer form of carbolic acid. Like Pasteur, Lister believed that germs travel mainly through the air, so he tried spraying the acid into the air above the wounds. Later he realized that the germs that come into direct contact with a wound through hands and instruments do more damage than germs in the air. He then applied the acid directly on wounds, cleansing and dressing them with it. As a result, the death rate among the amputees dropped to 15%. Eventually, the death rate from operations went down to 2% to 3%, and surgeons were able to perform a wider variety of operations more safely.

Lister also used antiseptics to disinfect surgical equipment and supplies. His work led to the practice of sterile technique: making an operating room germ-free. This technique includes such measures as having workers wear protective, sterile clothing and draping patients to expose only the area being operated on.

Oliver Wendell Holmes and Ignaz Semmelweis

The American physician and essayist Oliver Wendell Holmes (1809–1894) was another key figure in solving the puzzle of infection. In 1843 he published *The Contagiousness of Puerperal Fever.* This paper demonstrated that puerperal fever, a disease that was responsible for the deaths of many women in childbirth, was carried from patient to patient by doctors. This concept was harshly criticized, but Holmes did not back down. He reprinted the paper, with additions, in 1855, after serving as the dean of Harvard Medical School.

About the same time, in Vienna a Hungarian physician, Ignaz Semmelweis (1818–1865), also concluded that puerperal fever was a communicable disease. He ordered students in his hospital ward to scrub their hands with a chlorinated lime solution before moving from one patient to another. Although the hospital's mortality rate from puerperal fever fell dramatically, Semmelweis's views were not widely accepted during his lifetime.

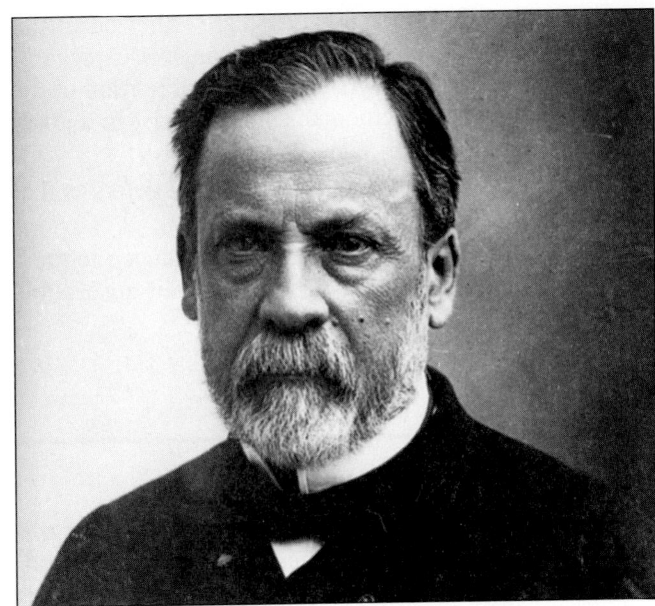

Figure 19-2. Louis Pasteur developed the germ theory and suggested that germs (microorganisms) might cause disease in humans.

These and other contributions to knowledge about infection have evolved into the current techniques for keeping infectious microorganisms out of the medical office and operating room. These techniques are now widely accepted and are legally required in the practice of medicine. You will apply these techniques in your daily work as a medical assistant.

Microorganisms and Disease

Microorganisms live all around us. They are found in and on our bodies, in the air we breathe, in the water we drink, and on almost every surface we touch. Types of microorganisms include:

- Viruses, the smallest infectious agents, many of which cause disease.
- Bacteria, single-celled organisms that reproduce quickly and are a major cause of disease.
- Protozoans, single-celled organisms found in soil and water, most of which do not cause disease.
- Fungi, organisms with a complex cell structure, most of which do not cause disease.
- Very small multicellular organisms, a few of which are parasitic (living on or in another organism) and cause disease.

Although everyone is surrounded by microorganisms, people are able to escape infection most of the time for the following reasons.

1. The majority of microorganisms are either beneficial or harmless. **Pathogens,** microorganisms capable of causing disease, comprise only a small portion of the total number of microorganisms that exist in a given environment.
2. The human body has a wide variety of defenses that allow people to resist infection.
3. Conditions must be favorable for a pathogen to grow and to be transmitted to a person who is susceptible (sensitive) to infection.

The Disease Process

Many types of diseases affect humans. An infectious disease is one that is caused by the action of a microorganism. The infection begins when the microorganism finds a human host, that is, a body in which it can survive, multiply, and thrive. To grow, a microorganism requires specific conditions. These conditions include the proper temperature, pH (a measure of the body's acid-base balance), and moisture level. The temperature within the human body (98.6°F, or 37°C), the body's neutral pH, and the body's dark, moist environment are prime conditions for the growth of microorganisms.

Some pathogens nearly always cause disease, whereas others cause disease less often or only under certain circumstances. A microorganism's disease-producing power is called **virulence.** When microorganisms damage the body, they do so in many ways:

- By depleting nutrients or other materials needed by the cells and tissues they invade
- By reproducing themselves within body cells
- By making body cells the targets of the body's own defenses
- By producing toxins, or poisons, that damage cells and tissues

The Body's Defenses

Daily life constantly exposes people to multitudes of pathogens, but the bodies of healthy individuals have built-in defenses against them. The condition of being resistant to pathogens and the diseases they cause is called **immunity.** When these defenses are not functioning properly (as when people have poor health, inadequate nutrition, or poor hygiene habits), people become particularly susceptible to invasion, setting the stage for infection to occur.

There are other reasons that a person's defenses may be weak. A break in the skin caused by injury can leave a person especially vulnerable to microorganisms. This type of opening in the body provides the organisms with an unprotected point of entry. Drugs can also weaken the body's ability to fight infection. For example, cancer drugs may kill healthy cells along with the cancer cells. Disorders of the immune system, such as AIDS, interfere with the body's natural ability to fight infection.

Because people are constantly, and quite literally, surrounded by pathogens, the body's natural defenses against pathogens are crucial to survival. If people do not have these defenses, they are potentially vulnerable to infection by every microorganism they encounter, including those naturally found in the body. Infections by microorganisms that can cause disease only when a host's resistance is low are called **opportunistic infections.** Examples of opportunistic infections are pneumonia caused by *Pneumocystis carinii* (a protozoan) and oral candidiasis, caused by *Candida* (a yeastlike fungus found commonly in the mouth as well as the intestinal tract and vagina). Both of these infections are common in AIDS patients.

The human body has many types of defense mechanisms that work to fight off pathogens. **Normal flora** are beneficial bacteria found in the body that create a barrier against pathogens. These bacteria produce substances that can harm invaders and starve them by using up the resources pathogens need to live. Normal flora colonize the skin, nose, mouth, vagina, rectum, and intestines. For example, some staphylococci bacteria are normally present on the skin and in the upper respiratory tract. The normal flora in any given area are specific (indigenous) to those areas, different from flora in or on other parts of the body.

Intact skin is the best first-line defense people have against disease. Skin secretions also serve as a barrier to invaders. Other body fluids and functions protect people from disease as well. Tears, saliva, and internal secretions such as prostatic fluid and cervical mucus have a mild germ-killing acidity. The respiratory tract is lined with cilia, tiny projections that continuously beat upward to expel foreign substances trapped in mucus (Figure 19-3). Coughing and sneezing rid the respiratory tract of excess mucus. Urine washes out pathogens from the bladder and urinary tract, and urine's high acidity also helps prevent bacterial growth. Contractions of smooth muscle along the intestinal tract help rid the body of infectious microorganisms as well.

When microorganisms succeed in invading body tissues, the immune system immediately begins to neutralize and destroy them. The immune system includes nonspecific defenses, which are often used in conjunction with the two main types of specific defenses: humoral defenses (fluid mechanisms) and cell-mediated defenses. The immune system also involves the spleen, lymph nodes, tonsils, thymus, lungs, liver, and kidneys, all of which contain lymphatic tissue. Lymphatic tissue is a filtering network of connective tissue containing large numbers of lymphocytes. Lymphocytes are specialized white blood cells that combat infectious agents.

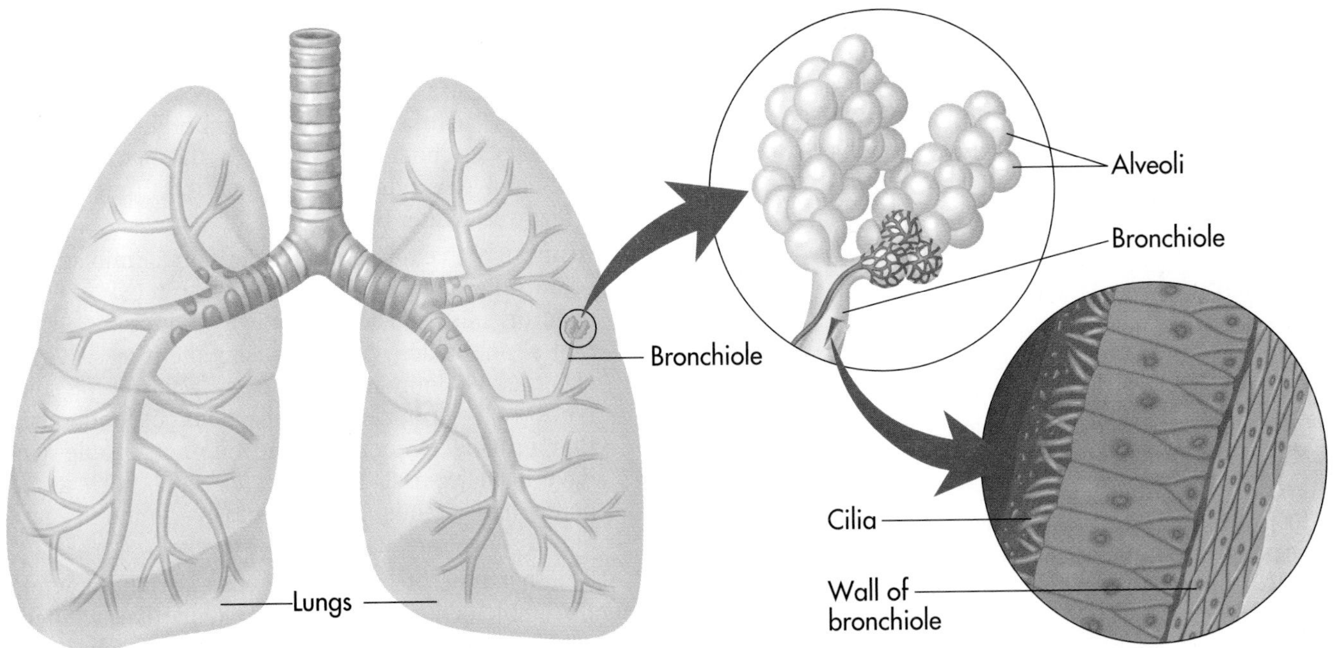

Figure 19-3. The sweeping motion of cilia that line the respiratory tract helps rid the body of foreign particles and some microorganisms.

Nonspecific Defense

One type of nonspecific defense is the process known as phagocytosis, which occurs when special white blood cells called **phagocytes** engulf and digest pathogens. (Figure 19-4 shows how a phagocyte "swallows" a pathogen.) A pouch forms around the pathogen as it is engulfed. The phagocyte secretes enzymes and metabolites into the pouch, destroying the trapped material. Phagocytes are the cells that form pus as they go to the site of infection to help destroy microorganisms.

There are several varieties of phagocytes, two of which are of particular importance. Neutrophils are phagocytes that move on their own and can act quickly to destroy an invading microorganism. **Macrophages,** which are known

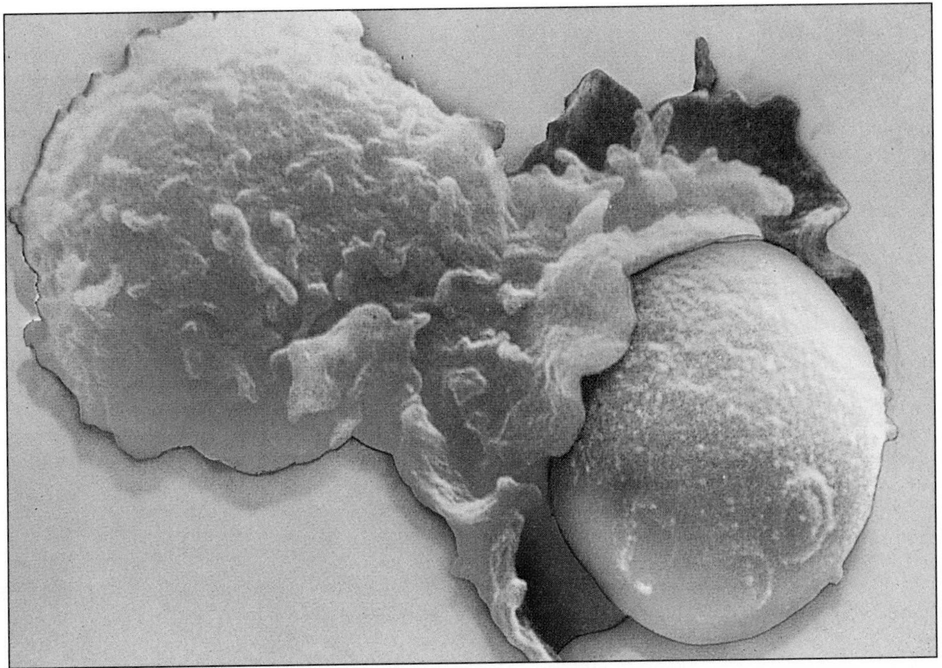

Figure 19-4. Phagocytes protect the body from infection by finding, surrounding, and digesting intruding microorganisms.

as monocytes while in the bloodstream, are phagocytes found in the lymph nodes, liver, spleen, lungs, bone marrow, and connective tissue. They are larger and generally slower-moving than neutrophils, but they live longer. Macrophages also play several roles in humoral and cell-mediated immunity, including presenting the antigens to the lymphocytes involved in these defenses.

Humoral Immunity

One type of humoral protection is provided by **antibodies,** highly specific proteins that attach themselves to foreign substances. This type of defense involves two types of lymphocytes: B cells (also called B lymphocytes) and T cells (also known as T lymphocytes). When the body is invaded by an **antigen** (a foreign substance), helper T cells activate B cells to produce antibodies, which combine with the antigens to neutralize them. Although the initial response to a major invasion by an antigen may not be a highly effective defense, memory B cells are produced for the appropriate antibody. A later invasion by the same antigen will be quickly and effectively countered. Specific antibodies are produced in response to specific antigens. These antibodies act as a homing device to attract phagocytes, which then engulf and destroy the antigen.

The formation of antibodies gives the body immunity from a particular disease. Immunity can be natural or artificial, active or passive (Figure 19-5).

1. Active immunity is a long-term immunity in which the body produces its own antibodies. Active immunity can be natural or artificial.
2. Passive immunity results when antibodies produced outside the body enter the body. Passive immunity can be natural or artificial.
3. Natural active immunity results from exposure to organisms that cause a disease, such as mumps. Although the person becomes sick with the disease, her body produces antibodies that prevent her from having the disease again if she is reexposed to it. A fetus acquires natural passive immunity when the mother's antibodies move across the placenta. Natural passive immunity lasts only a short time, usually a few weeks after birth.
4. Artificial active immunity results from administration of an immunization or vaccine with killed or weakened organisms. These organisms induce the formation of antibodies without causing the disease. Artificial passive immunity occurs as a result of some types of immunizations (injections of antibodies) that provide temporary protection for people who have been exposed to serious diseases, such as hepatitis and tetanus. Artificial passive immunity lasts only a short time, usually a few weeks.

The other type of humoral defense is called complement. Complement is a group of proteins that circulates in the blood and body fluids and is always present in low amounts. When it is activated by antibodies, however, complement can multiply rapidly and destroy pathogens. It helps the white blood cells ingest microorganisms, sometimes making a hole in the microorganisms' cells to spill out the contents and kill the cells. The main reason that most bacteria do not cause disease is that these proteins can destroy many species of bacteria.

Cell-Mediated Immunity

In addition to their role in humoral immunity, T cells are instrumental in cell-mediated immunity. Cell-mediated immunity differs from humoral immunity in that T cells do not form antibodies to combat antigens. Instead, they directly attack the invader. Several different types of T cells are involved in the attack process. Helper T cells activate the killer T cells, which bind with the antigen and kill it.

Immunity

Active Immunity	**Passive Immunity**
Body produces its own antibodies; provides long-term immunity	Antibodies produced outside of the body are introduced into the body; provides only temporary immunity
Natural Active Immunity	**Natural Passive Immunity**
Results from exposure to disease-causing organism	Results when antibodies from the mother cross the placenta to the fetus
Artificial Active Immunity	**Artificial Passive Immunity**
Results from administration of a vaccine with killed or weakened organisms	Results from immunization with antibodies to a disease-causing organism

Figure 19-5. Immunity to a disease can be acquired in a variety of ways: naturally, artificially, actively, and passively.

Suppressor T cells slow down or stop the attack after the antigen is destroyed. Memory T cells are formed and will respond quickly to another attack by the same antigen.

Cell-mediated defenses against infection often result in inflammation of the affected area. Inflammation occurs when phagocytes enter the area, stick to the lining of the blood vessels, and come out of the vessels to attack the infecting agent. Small blood vessels then dilate and leak fluid, resulting in swelling, redness, and warmth. This process often causes fever, which is a common response to many infections and may play a part in fighting infection. The fever results when endogenous pyrogen, a product of phagocytic cells, acts on the area of the brain that controls the body's temperature.

The Cycle of Infection

Five elements must be present for infection to occur: a reservoir host, a means of exit, a means of transmission, a means of entrance, and a susceptible host. These elements make up the cycle of infection (Figure 19-6).

Reservoir Host

The cycle of infection begins with establishment of the pathogen in the reservoir host. The **reservoir host** is an animal, insect, or human whose body is susceptible to growth of the pathogen. Most pathogens require a reservoir host to provide nutrition and a place to multiply.

The presence of the pathogen in the reservoir host may cause an infection in the host. At times, however, the host escapes full infection. A human **carrier** is a reservoir host who is unaware of the presence of the pathogen and so spreads the disease. The carrier exhibits no symptoms of infection. A human host also may have a **subclinical case,** which is a manifestation of the infection that is so slight as to be unnoticeable. The host experiences only some of the symptoms of the infection or milder symptoms than in a full case. A wide range of diseases can be manifested subclinically.

An infection in the reservoir host may be one of two types. The first is an **endogenous infection,** one in which an abnormality or malfunction in routine body processes has caused normally beneficial or harmless microorganisms to become pathogenic. The second type is an **exogenous infection,** one that is caused by the introduction of a pathogen from outside the body.

Means of Exit

To continue the cycle of infection, the pathogen must exit from the reservoir host. Common routes of exit from this host include the following:

- Through the nose, mouth, eyes, or ears
- In feces or urine
- In semen, vaginal fluid, or other discharge through the reproductive tract
- In blood or blood products from open wounds

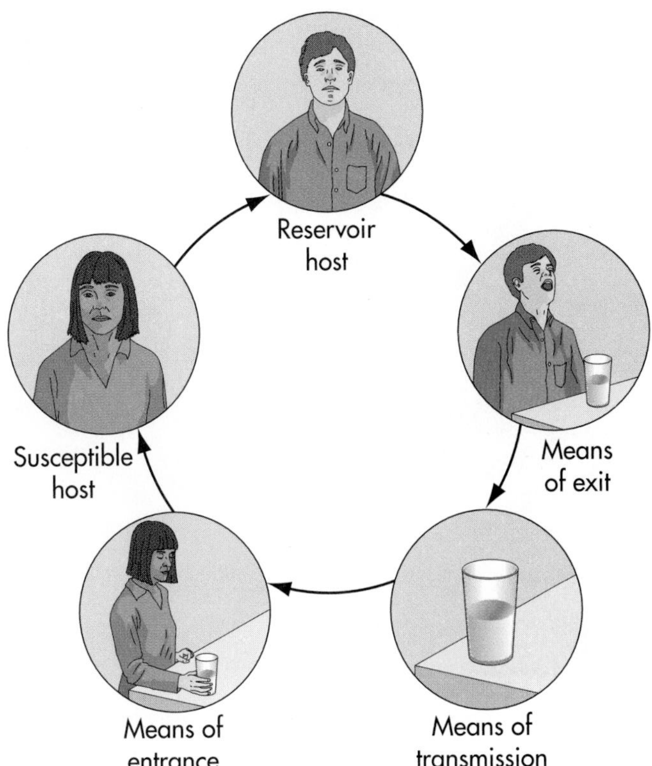

Figure 19-6. The cycle of infection must be broken at some point to prevent the spread of disease.

Means of Transmission

To reproduce after it has exited from the reservoir host, the pathogen must spread to another host by some means of transmission. The means may be direct or indirect. Direct transmission occurs when the pathogen moves immediately from one host to another. This type of transmission may happen through contact with the infected person or with the discharges of the infected person, such as saliva or blood.

Indirect transmission is possible only if the pathogen is capable of existing independently of the reservoir host. In this case, the pathogen survives until a new host encounters it and the pathogen takes up residence in that new host. Indirect transmission can occur by the following means:

- **Vectors,** which are living organisms, such as insects, that carry microorganisms from an infected person to another person
- **Fomites,** or inanimate objects, such as clothing, body fluids, water, food, or even a stethoscope, which may be contaminated with infectious organisms and thus serve to transmit disease
- Droplets expelled into the air by sneezing, coughing, speaking, or breathing
- Contaminated food or drink

Airborne Transmission. Pathogens can be transmitted to a new host through the air. For example, microorganisms may enter the respiratory tract of a new host by in-

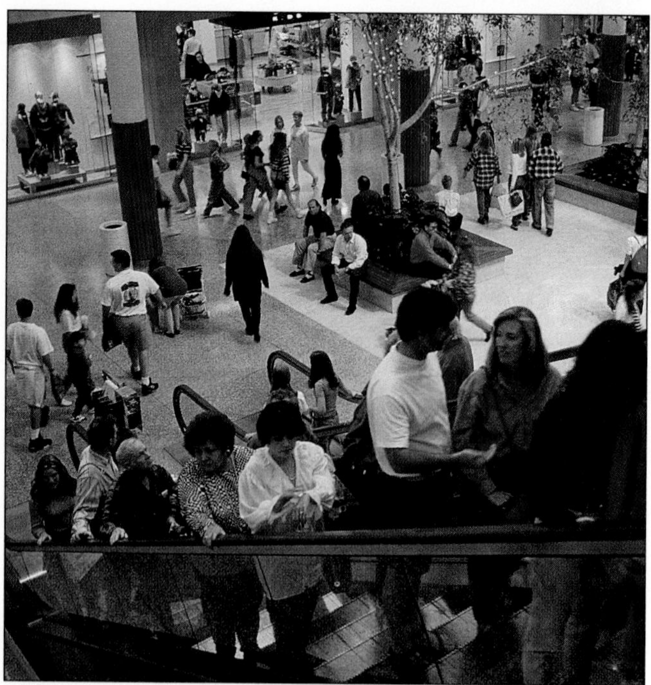

Figure 19-7. Because many people touch escalator railings, they are common fomites for disease transmission.

halation. Respiratory diseases such as influenza, or flu, are often transmitted this way.

Pathogens may be inhaled from a variety of sources, such as soil particles or secretion droplets. If people inhale contaminated soil particles, they may contract fungal diseases. If people inhale contaminated droplets, they may contract a wide variety of diseases, including influenza and chickenpox. Because pathogens can spread relatively rapidly through airborne transmission, they may cause large epidemics among susceptible people.

Blood-Borne Transmission. Pathogens can also enter a new host through contact with blood or blood products. Blood-borne pathogens (discussed in greater detail in Chapter 21) may be transmitted in a variety of ways:

- Directly, as when the contaminated blood of one person comes into contact with another person's broken skin or a pregnant woman transmits a disease to her fetus across the placenta
- Indirectly, as when pathogens are transferred through blood transfusions, needle sticks, or improperly sterilized dental equipment

Ingested Transmission. A new host may be exposed to pathogens by ingesting contaminated food or liquids. Food can become contaminated when it is handled by an infected person who has poor hygiene habits, such as a customer at a self-service salad bar who did not wash his hands. The amount of contamination needed in a food to make someone ill varies. People who produce less stomach acid may become infected with a smaller dose of pathogens than those with higher acid production because stomach acid kills many microorganisms. An example of a pathogen transmitted by ingestion is a strain of *Escherichia coli* bacteria, which can cause severe food poisoning. Another pathogen, *Giardia lamblia,* is an intestinal parasite that causes symptoms such as diarrhea, gas, weight loss, and fatigue. This parasite is generally found in contaminated water sources, but it can also be transmitted through food.

Transmission by Touching. Direct or indirect contact through touch is another method of transmitting infection. This type of transmission can occur by touching the hands of someone who has sneezed or coughed on them. It can occur by kissing, by sharing a drinking glass or lipstick with someone who is infected, or by touching something that an infected person has touched (Figure 19-7).

Contact with an infected person's mucous membranes is especially dangerous. Some organisms can be transmitted by this route even though they are unable to penetrate intact skin. Sexually transmitted diseases are spread through the direct contact of one mucous membrane with another (in the penis, vagina, urethra, mouth, anus) during sexual activity.

Infection can also occur on intact skin. For instance, skin that is normal or slightly irritated may break out in boils if infected with pathogenic staphylococci bacteria. Some species of another type of bacteria—streptococci—can produce inflammation or lesions on intact skin.

Transmission During Pregnancy or Birth. If a mother becomes infected during her pregnancy, she can pass on pathogens to her unborn child (fetus). An infection may be transmitted while the fetus is in the mother's uterus, and this infection may result in damage to the fetus. This transmission is a form of blood-borne transmission.

Some blood-borne infections that produce only mild symptoms in the mother may be devastating to the fetus (for example, rubella). Other infections, such as herpes, gonorrhea, syphilis, or streptococcal infections, may infect the baby during passage through the birth canal. An infection that is present in a child at the time of birth is said to be congenital.

Means of Entrance

Just as the pathogen requires a means of exit from the reservoir host, it also needs a means of entrance into the new host. Pathogens can enter a new host through any cavity lined with mucous membrane, such as the mouth, nose, throat, vagina, or rectum. They can also enter through the ears, eyes, intestinal tract, urinary tract, reproductive tract, or breaks in the skin. Most pathogens can take advantage of any means of exit and entry. For example, the droplets from an infected person's sneeze can land on a small abrasion on the skin of another person, spreading the infection.

Susceptible Host

A final requirement must be met for the infection cycle to remain intact. The person into whom the pathogen has been transmitted must be an individual who has little or no immunity to infection by that organism. This individual is called a **susceptible host.**

Susceptibility is determined by a variety of factors, some related to the host, some to the pathogen, and some to the environment. Factors related to the host include the following:

- Age
- Genetic predisposition to certain illnesses
- Nutritional status
- Other disease processes
- Stress levels
- Hygiene habits
- General health

Factors related to the pathogen include the number and concentration of pathogens, the strength (virulence) of the pathogen, and the point of entry. Environmental factors, such as the living conditions of the host and the host's exposure to hazardous substances, also affect susceptibility.

Once a new host has been infected, the cycle can continue. This host becomes the reservoir host and eventually transmits the pathogen to yet another host.

Environmental Factors in Disease Transmission

The climate, food, water, animals, insects, and people in a community may greatly influence the types and courses of infection there. In a highly dense population, the infection rate may be higher than in a low-density population because pathogens spread more quickly from person to person when people are in closer proximity. The proximity factor is one reason for the increase in respiratory disease during seasons when people are indoors for long periods.

Animals play a role in infection. Unpasteurized milk from an infected cow may cause disease. Infections related to pathogens are found in domestic and wild animals. Some pathogens can infect animals and people. Butchers, hunters, and people in occupations dealing with animals may be at greater risk than other individuals for infection by those pathogens.

The environment affects the incidence of diseases carried by insects. Whether a potentially disease-carrying insect is in a certain area depends on whether that area has the appropriate climate and environment the insect needs to live. For instance, in tropical regions, malaria is spread by the female *Anopheles* mosquito (Figure 19-8). In other areas, ticks may carry Rocky Mountain spotted fever or Lyme disease.

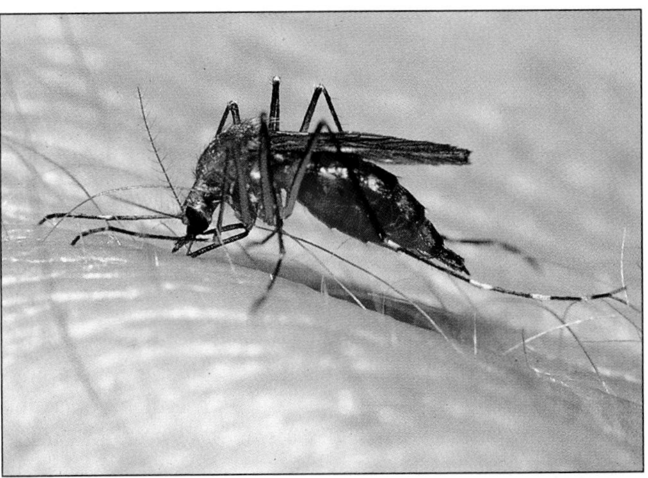

Figure 19-8. The female *Anopheles* mosquito carries malaria-causing parasites, transmitting them to humans when it bites.

Economic and political factors influence the pattern of infection transmission. They help determine the cleanliness of an area, the availability of medical care, and people's knowledge about preventing infection. Other factors that influence infection transmission include the availability of transportation, urbanization, population growth rates, and sexual behavior.

Breaking the Cycle

As a medical assistant, you will apply the principles of asepsis to break the cycle of infection and prevent infections from spreading. **Asepsis** is the condition in which pathogens are absent or controlled. In medical settings, where many people are hosts to pathogens and many others are susceptible, asepsis can break the cycle by preventing the transmission of pathogens.

You can help break the cycle of infection in your office by taking specific measures that include the following:

- Maintaining strict housekeeping standards to reduce the number of pathogens present
- Adhering to government guidelines to protect against diseases caused by pathogens
- Educating patients in hygiene, health promotion, and disease prevention

Medical and Surgical Asepsis

You will take measures to eliminate the elements that must be present for disease to occur. To do so, you must have a thorough knowledge of the two types of asepsis:

- Medical asepsis, or clean technique, which is based on maintaining cleanliness to prevent the spread of microorganisms and to ensure that there are as few microorganisms in the medical environment as possible

- Surgical asepsis, or sterile technique, which depends on a completely sterile environment that eliminates all microorganisms

Medical Asepsis

The medical office can be the host to many pathogens. Therefore, strict, controlled asepsis is crucial. All employees in the medical office must observe and practice the principles of asepsis to ensure a safe environment for patients and staff.

You can promote asepsis through vigilant cleanliness. In fact, part of your job is to perform daily cleaning tasks in addition to those performed by an outside cleaning service. The office should be well stocked with housekeeping equipment, including a vacuum cleaner, brooms, dustpans, mops, buckets, sponges, bleach, dust cloths, trash bags, glass cleaner, paper towels, disinfectant spray, disposable emesis basins, and cleaning solutions.

Every day before patients arrive, you must inspect the office, dust, and clean any surfaces or objects that may be dirty or contaminated. Keeping the office clean reduces the number of microorganisms on surfaces.

Office Procedures. Other physical aspects of the medical office also contribute to asepsis (Figure 19-9). They include:

1. A reception room that has designated waiting areas for well and sick people. If there is not enough space, sick patients should be led immediately to an examination room. You may need to explain this policy to well people who have been waiting so that no one thinks other patients are getting preferential treatment.
2. An office that is well lit and ventilated, has no drafts, and has a temperature of approximately 72°F.
3. Furniture that is kept in good repair and is replaced when necessary.
4. A strict "no eating or drinking" policy.
5. Trash that is emptied as necessary.
6. An insect-free environment.
7. A posted sign asking that any safety or health hazard be reported to the receptionist.
8. A posted sign asking that patients use tissues for coughs or sneezes, put all waste in the trash can, and tell the receptionist if they are nauseated or have to use the rest room. (Ideally, the waiting room should be equipped with a rest room for emergencies.)

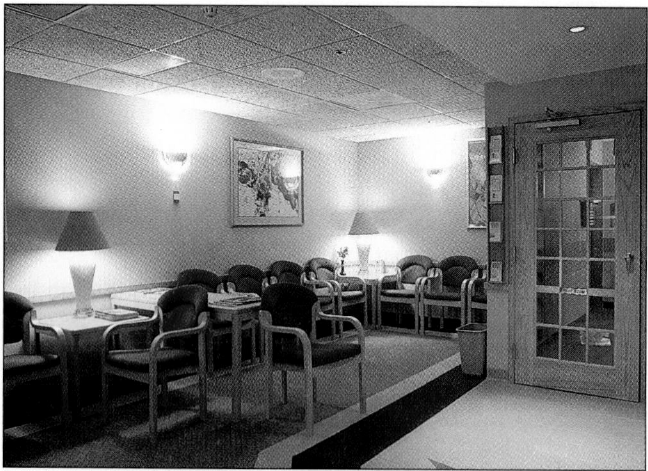

Figure 19-9. Asepsis begins in the reception area and waiting room of a medical office. These areas should be kept well lit, well ventilated, and free from dust and dirt. A rest room should be accessible to patients from the waiting area.

Asepsis During Medical Assistant Procedures. Many of the procedures you perform require aseptic techniques to prevent cross contamination from one place to another. For instance, when opening a sterile container, you should rest its lid faceup instead of facedown. Placing it facedown would contaminate the inside of the lid and make it unsuitable to be put back on the sterile container. When administering tablet or capsule medications, you should pour them into the bottle cap or a cup rather than into your hand. This technique prevents the transfer of microorganisms from your hand onto the medication. To prevent cross contamination, you must also follow guidelines about the types of protective gear to wear during a procedure. (Personal protective equipment is discussed later in this chapter.)

Hand Washing. The most important aseptic procedure for a medical assistant is hand washing. You must wash your hands at the following times:

- At the beginning of the day, after breaks, before and after using the rest room, before and after lunch, and before leaving for the day
- Before and after using gloves, handling specimens or waste, seeing each patient, handling clean or sterile supplies, and performing any procedure
- After blowing your nose or coughing

Aseptic hand washing removes accumulated dirt and microorganisms that could cause infection under the right conditions. Procedure 19-1 describes how to perform aseptic hand washing.

Other Aseptic Precautions. You need to make certain precautions part of your daily routine. For example, take these safeguards.

PROCEDURE 19-1

Aseptic Hand Washing

Objective: To remove dirt and microorganisms from under the fingernails and from the surface of the skin, hair follicles, and oil glands of the hands

OSHA Guidelines: This procedure does not involve exposure to blood, body fluids, or tissues.

Materials: Liquid soap, nailbrush or orange stick, paper towels

Method

1. Remove all jewelry (plain wedding bands may be left on and scrubbed).
2. Turn on the faucets using a paper towel, and adjust the water temperature to moderately warm.
3. Wet your hands and apply liquid soap. (Liquid soap, especially when dispensed with a foot pump, is preferable to bar soap. There is less available area for dirt to accumulate on a liquid soap dispenser than on bar soap, and there is a smaller chance of dropping the soap dispenser into the sink or onto the floor.)
4. Work the soap into a lather, making sure that all of both hands are lathered. Rub vigorously in a circular motion for 2 minutes. Keep your hands lower than your forearms so that dirty water flows into the sink instead of back onto your arms. The fingertips should be pointing down. Interlace your fingers to clean between them, and use the palm of one hand to clean the back of the other (Figure 19-10).
5. Use a nailbrush or orange stick to dislodge dirt around your nails and cuticles (Figure 19-11).
6. Rinse your hands well, keeping the hands lower than your forearms and not touching the sink or faucets.
7. With the water still running, dry your hands thoroughly with clean, dry paper towels, and then turn off the faucets using a clean, dry paper towel. Discard the towels.

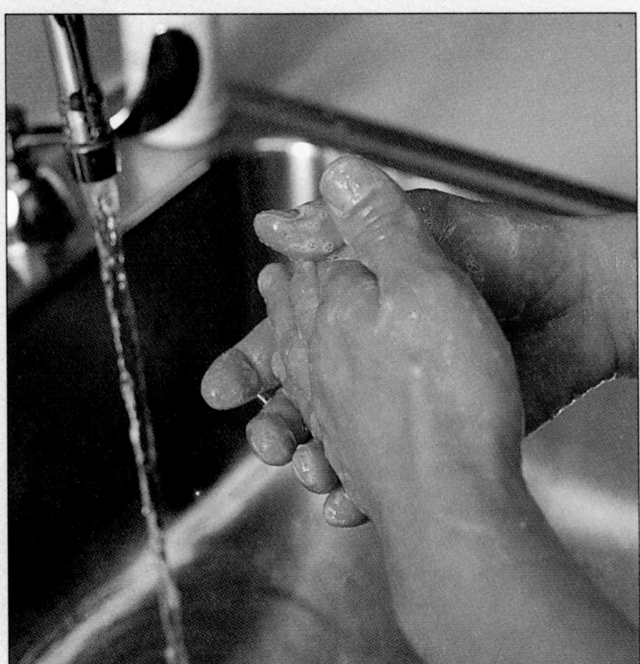

Figure 19-10. When you wash your hands, be sure to clean all surfaces, including the palms and between the fingers.

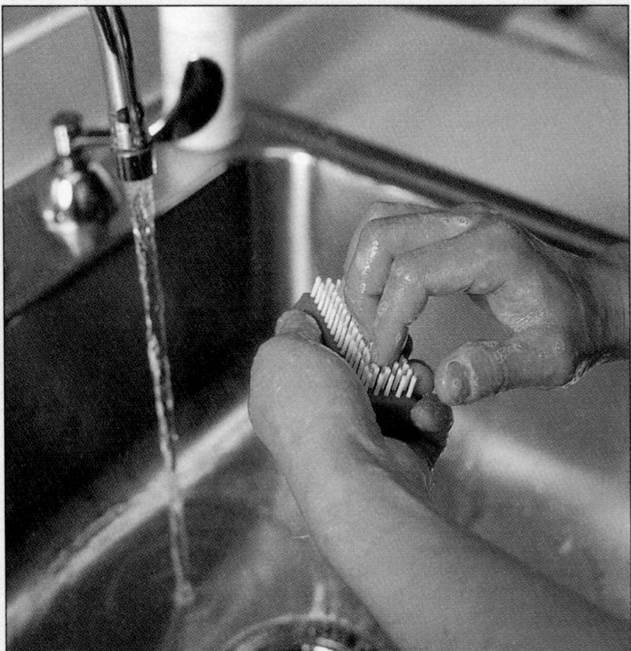

Figure 19-11. The nails and cuticles require additional attention to ensure that all dirt is removed.

- Avoid leaning against sinks, supplies, or equipment.
- Avoid touching your face or mouth.
- Use tissues when you cough or sneeze, and always wash your hands afterward.
- Whenever possible, avoid working directly with patients when you have a cold.
- Wear gloves and a mask if you have a cold and must work with patients.
- Stay home if you have a fever, and remain there until you have maintained a normal temperature for 24 hours.

Surgical Asepsis

Surgical asepsis takes medical asepsis to a higher level. The aim of surgical asepsis is to keep the surgical environment completely free of all microorganisms. In a typical medical office, you may be asked to assist with various surgical procedures, such as closing a wound or removing a cyst. The sterile technique of surgical asepsis must be maintained for even simple, minor operations and injections. Keep in mind, however, that the more extensive the procedure, the greater the risk of infection.

Sterile Technique. Sterile technique requires strict adherence to a set order of procedures. If there is any interruption in this order, you must start the procedures again from the beginning. An object or area is considered either sterile or not sterile, and if there is any question, you must consider the object or area contaminated. To prevent interruptions in the technique, you must also ensure that when objects touch one another, clean goes against clean, unclean goes against unclean, and sterile goes against sterile.

The surgical scrub is of primary importance in surgical asepsis. Surgical scrub procedures are similar to those for aseptic hand washing, but there are several distinctions. Differences include the following.

1. A sterile scrub brush is used instead of a nailbrush.
2. Both hands and forearms are washed.
3. The hands are kept above the elbows to prevent water from running from the arms onto washed areas.
4. Sterile towels are used instead of paper towels.
5. Sterile gloves are put on immediately after the hands are dried.

Surgical Asepsis During a Surgical Procedure. Chapter 29 describes assisting with minor surgery. Several points concerning surgical asepsis, however, are introduced here. Before performing a surgical procedure, the doctor may ask you to help prepare the skin. Your goal is to remove as many microorganisms as possible from around the area that is to undergo surgery so that you reduce the chances of these organisms entering the surgical opening. The skin and body openings, particularly the nose, mouth, and perineum, cannot be considered sterile. Nevertheless, the principles of aseptic technique require that you try to keep the area as contamination-free as possible.

Asepsis also involves keeping instruments and supplies sterile for use during the surgical procedure. After the sterile field has been created, handle items as little as possible to minimize the chance of contamination. Cover items that are not being used immediately with a sterile towel. If you are not wearing sterile gloves during a procedure (as when you are the only medical assistant and you must hand the doctor items from outside the sterile field), you must use transfer forceps to handle a sterile instrument. Transfer forceps look like big scissors or tweezers. Although the handles are not sterile, the tips that touch the instruments are. Procedure 19-2 explains how to move items using transfer forceps.

If you are wearing sterile gloves, you handle sterile items directly and carefully avoid touching anything that is not sterile. Throughout the procedure, you are responsible for maintaining the sterile field (in this case, the area of surgery).

After the procedure, you continue using aseptic technique in caring for the patient's surgical wound. Typically, you need to apply dressings and keep the wound clean in an aseptic manner to prevent infection. You will also instruct the patient in how to care for the wound.

After you instruct the patient and guide her out of the room, immediately place any supplies and disposable instruments that were used during the surgery into the appropriate **biohazardous waste containers.** These are leakproof, puncture-resistant containers that are color-coded red or labeled with a special biohazard symbol to show that they contain **biohazardous materials** (biological agents that can spread disease to living things). These containers are used to store and dispose of contaminated supplies and equipment in a way that preserves aseptic techniques and complies with the law.

Sanitizing, Disinfecting, and Sterilizing Instruments

After disposing of biohazardous waste, you must sanitize, disinfect, and sterilize reusable surgical instruments. **Sanitization** involves reducing the number of microorganisms on an object or a surface to a fairly safe level. To sanitize instruments after surgery, rinse them under warm, running water. If you cannot rinse them with water immediately, soak them in a disinfectant solution that has anticoagulant properties.

After rinsing the instruments, scrub them using hot, soapy water. Use a neutral-pH detergent that does not cause stains, corrosion, scratching, or a high level of suds and that is an effective blood solvent. Always wear utility gloves, use plastic brushes (never steel wool or wire), and keep different types of instruments (sharp, hinged, or of different metals) apart from each other when sanitizing them. After removing all visible stains and

PROCEDURE 19-2

Moving Sterile Items Using Transfer Forceps

Objective: To move sterile items onto a sterile field using transfer forceps

OSHA Guidelines: This procedure does not involve exposure to blood, body fluids, or tissues.

Materials: Sterile transfer forceps, forceps container with sterile solution, sterile 4- x 4-inch gauze packet (opened to expose the gauze), sterile supplies or equipment, Mayo stand with sterile field of instruments

Method

1. Grasp the forceps by the handles. Do not open the forceps.
2. Lift the forceps slowly in a vertical position, letting the sterile solution run toward the tips.
3. Lift the forceps out of the solution, taking care not to touch the sides of the container.
4. Carefully open and close the forceps to remove excess solution from them; then dry the tips by touching them to the sterile gauze in the opened packet.
5. Grasp the sterile supplies or instrument, pointing the forceps downward and avoiding touching the sterile container or field (Figure 19-12).
6. Place the sterile supplies or instrument on the sterile field, well inside the imaginary 1-inch border that is considered not sterile.
7. Place the forceps back into the forceps container, being careful to avoid touching the sides.

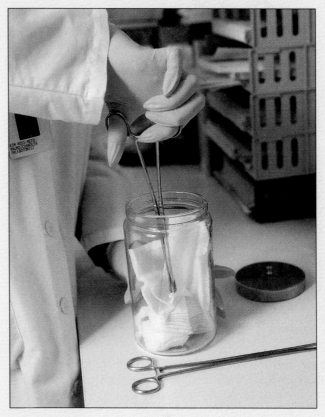

Figure 19-12. When using transfer forceps, touch only the handles.

residue, rinse the instruments under running water, and roll them in a clean towel to dry them. Examine all instruments closely to make sure that they are in working order.

Disinfection is the destruction of infectious agents on an object or surface by direct application of chemical or physical means. Common disinfectants include chemical germicides, boiling water, and steam. You use disinfectants only on objects and surfaces because they are too strong to use on human tissue. Although disinfection kills a great many pathogens, **bacterial spores** (primitive, thick-walled reproductive bodies capable of developing into new individuals) and some viruses are not eliminated through disinfection.

To kill spores and viruses resistant to disinfection on instruments, you must sterilize them. **Sterilization** is the destruction of all microorganisms, including bacterial spores, by specific means. (For detailed information and procedures on instrument sanitization, disinfection, and sterilization, see Chapter 20.)

Disinfecting Work Surfaces

Another postsurgical aseptic procedure you will perform is disinfecting all work surfaces that were exposed to contamination (Figure 19-13). For this process, you must use bleach or a germ-killing solution approved by the U.S. government's Environmental Protection Agency (EPA). If protective coverings on surfaces or equipment were exposed to contamination during a procedure, you must replace them.

Medical asepsis and surgical asepsis are required by law. Each individual who works in a medical setting must recognize the importance of asepsis and strictly adhere to aseptic procedures in daily routines.

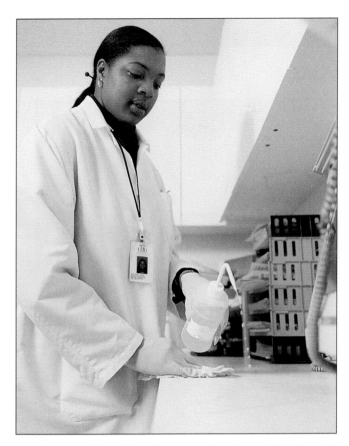

Figure 19-13. Work surfaces must be thoroughly cleaned with an EPA-approved chemical disinfectant.

OSHA Bloodborne Pathogens Standard and Universal Precautions

You must know the laws that require basic practices of infection control in a medical office. You must also know how to apply these laws in your office. Federal regulations related to infection control and asepsis were developed by the Department of Labor's Occupational Safety and Health Administration (OSHA) and described in the OSHA Bloodborne Pathogens Standard of 1991. These laws aim to protect health-care workers from health hazards on the job, particularly from accidentally acquiring infections. They also help protect from health hazards patients and any other people who may come into the medical office.

OSHA Bloodborne Pathogens Standard

To ensure that biohazardous materials do not endanger people or the environment, laws set forth in the OSHA Bloodborne Pathogens Standard of 1991 dictate how you must handle infectious or potentially infectious waste generated during medical or surgical procedures. According to these rules, any potentially infectious waste materials must be discarded or held for processing in biohazardous waste containers. These wastes include the following:

- Blood products
- Body fluids
- Human tissues
- Vaccines
- Table paper, linen, towels, and gauze with body fluids on them
- Used scalpels, needles, sutures with needles attached, and other sharp instruments (known as sharps)
- Used gloves, disposable instruments, cotton swabs, and disposable applicators

Many medical offices today use only disposable paper gowns, drapes, coverings, and towels. Some offices, however, use cloth linens, which must be laundered. Certain rules apply to the laundering of cloth linens that are soiled with potentially infectious materials.

Most medical offices use outside, licensed waste management services approved by the EPA to dispose of medical waste. A waste management service can provide your office with instructions for preparing items before they are taken away.

The disposition and handling of contaminated sharps are of special concern because these instruments can easily puncture the skin and expose you to extremely dangerous viruses. Used sharps must never be bent, broken, re-capped, or otherwise tampered with. After use, place them in a rigid, leakproof, puncture-resistant biohazardous waste container for sharps. Disposable and reusable sharps are kept in separate containers. Metal basins containing disinfectant are often used to store reusable sharps until they can be processed. The outside waste management company may supply containers for the disposable items, sterilize them on its premises, and discard them in the city trash dump or incinerate them. You may sanitize, disinfect, and sterilize reusable sharps in your office, particularly if the practice is in a rural area without an outside waste management company nearby. See "Caution: Handle With Care" for a discussion of the guidelines you must follow when disposing of biohazardous waste and potentially infectious laundry waste.

OSHA's laws for hazardous waste disposal, as well as other OSHA regulations about measures to prevent the spread of infection, provide a margin of safety, ensuring that medical facilities meet at least the minimal criteria for asepsis. These laws include requirements for training personnel, keeping records, housekeeping, wearing protective gear, and other measures.

Although federal laws exist, individual states have some discretion in applying them. You should become familiar with the laws in your state to ensure that you are helping your medical office comply. Penalties for failing to comply with regulations can be severe (see Table 19-1).

Universal Precautions

OSHA requires medical professionals to follow specific "universal blood and body fluid precautions" as set forth by the Department of Health and Human Services' Centers for Disease Control and Prevention (CDC). These **Universal Precautions** prevent health-care workers from exposing themselves and others to infections. Following Universal Precautions means assuming that all blood and body fluids are infected with blood-borne pathogens. Universal Precautions apply to:

- Blood and blood products.
- Human tissue.
- Semen and vaginal secretions.
- Saliva from dental procedures.
- Cerebrospinal, synovial, pleural, peritoneal, pericardial, and amniotic fluids, which bathe various internal structures in the body.
- Other body fluids, if visibly contaminated with blood or of questionable origin in the body.

Breast milk, while not on the list of fluids covered by Universal Precautions, is generally treated as such because it has been shown that mothers can pass along the human immunodeficiency virus (HIV) to their infants through breast milk (*Surgeon General's Report,* June 1994).

Hospitals now use **Standard Precautions,** which are a combination of Universal Precautions and rules to reduce the risk of disease transmission by means of moist body substances (known as Body Substance Isolation guidelines). Standard Precautions apply to:

- Blood.
- All body fluids, secretions, and excretions except sweat.
- Nonintact skin.
- Mucous membranes.

Standard Precautions are used in hospitals for the care of all patients. They are an important measure for preventing the transmission of disease in the hospital setting. In medical offices you use Universal Precautions

CAUTION

HANDLE WITH CARE

Proper Use of Biohazardous Waste Containers and Handling of Infectious Laundry Waste

Biohazardous waste containers are available in a variety of designs. Frequently, more than one design is used in the clinical setting. These containers are often provided by outside sterilization and waste management companies. Examples of biohazardous waste containers include:

- Bags or containers that are red or have a biohazardous waste label (for any material contaminated with blood or body fluids, such as used dressings or gloves).
- Boxes with biohazardous waste labels (sometimes lined with red bags and used for disposable gowns, examination table covers, and similar items that may be contaminated with blood or body fluids).
- Rigid, leakproof sharps containers that are red or have a biohazardous waste label (for lancets, needles, and other sharp objects).

Every biohazardous waste container has a lid that you must replace immediately after use. In addition, you may not overfill the container, and you must replace it when it is full. All biohazardous waste containers must have a fluorescent orange or orange-red label with the biohazard symbol and the word *BIOHAZARD* in a contrasting color (Figure 19-14). Red bags or red containers may be substituted for containers with biohazardous waste labels.

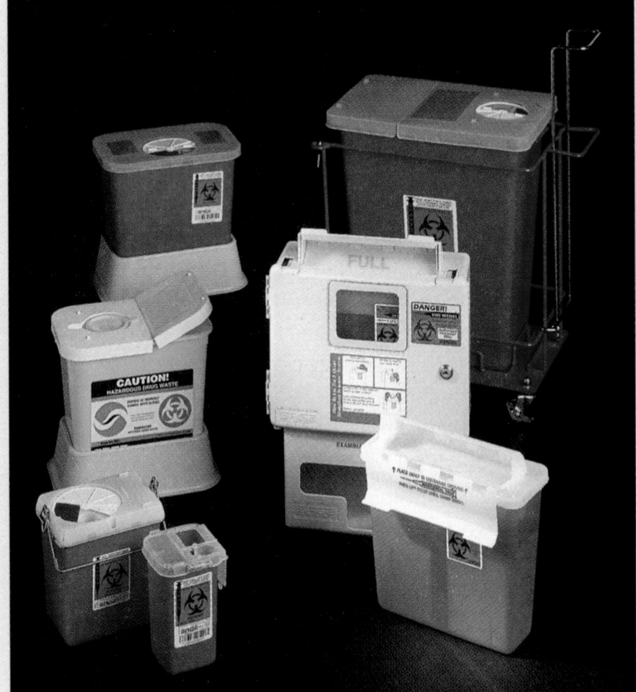

Figure 19-14. All biohazardous sharps containers should be rigid, leakproof, and labeled with the biohazard symbol.

continued

CAUTION HANDLE WITH CARE

Proper Use of Biohazardous Waste Containers and Handling of Infectious Laundry Waste continued

You must follow these guidelines when handling hazardous waste.

1. Always wear gloves.
2. Place hazardous waste in the appropriate biohazardous waste container immediately or as soon as possible.
3. Keep biohazardous waste containers close to the place where the waste material is generated.
4. Keep the containers closed when not in use, close them before removing them from the area of use, and keep them upright to avoid any spills.
5. If outside contamination of the primary container occurs, place that container in a secondary container to prevent leakage during handling, processing, storage, and transport.
6. Drop—do not push—intact contaminated needles into the biohazardous waste container for sharps.
7. To avoid accidental puncture wounds, never break off, re-cap, reuse, or handle needles after use.
8. If there is a danger of hazardous waste puncturing the primary container, place that container in a secondary container.
9. Do not open, empty, or clean reusable sharps containers by hand.
10. When they are two-thirds full, discard disposable sharps containers in large biohazardous waste containers.

When cleaning up spills, place the resulting contaminated material in a biohazardous waste bag. The bag must be leakproof on the sides and bottom and be closed tightly. Then place the plastic bag in a cardboard box also marked with the biohazard symbol. The outside waste management agency will pick up the box for incineration before disposing of it in a public landfill.

Potentially infectious laundry waste must also be handled in a specific manner. OSHA has issued regulations for handling this type of waste. You must be sure to:

1. Place contaminated laundry in a laundry bag that is red, marked with the biohazard symbol, or recognizable to facility employees as contaminated material to be handled using Universal Precautions (Figure 19-15).
2. Pack any laundry to be transported so that it does not leak in transit.
3. Have the laundry washed in a designated area on-site or at a professional laundry facility.

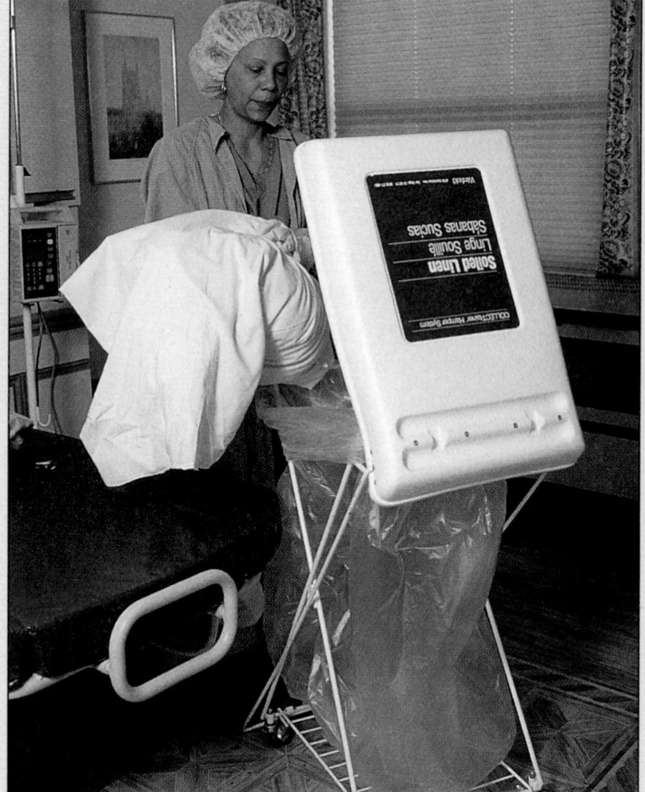

Figure 19-15. Place soiled linens and other laundry in an appropriate bag as soon as possible.

Any laundry service the medical office uses should abide by all OSHA regulations. For example, anyone handling laundry must wear gloves and handle contaminated materials as little as possible.

when dealing with patients. The application of Universal Precautions is expanding, in practice, to include all body fluids, secretions, and excretions and moist body surfaces.

As mentioned earlier, some types of pathogens can be transmitted when the host's infected blood comes in contact with another person's skin. Skin that has been broken from a needle puncture or other wound and mucous membranes, such as those lining the nose and throat, are the areas that need the most protection. If a patient's (or coworker's) blood or body fluids come in contact with such areas, pathogens can be transferred from the patient's body to that of the medical worker.

OSHA outlines the routine safeguards to take when performing each medical procedure or task, depending on that task's level of risk. The degree of risk is determined by how much exposure to potentially infectious

Table 19-1

Infectious Waste Disposal: Penalties for Not Following Regulations, as Set Forth by OSHA

Type of Violation	Characteristics of Violation	Penalties for Violation
Other than serious violation	Direct relationship to job safety and health but would probably not result in death or serious physical	Fine of up to $7,000 (discretionary)
Serious violation	Substantial probability that death or serious physical harm could result; employer knew, or should have known, of the hazard	Fine of up to $7,000 (mandatory)
Willful violation	Violation committed intentionally and knowingly	Fine of up to $70,000, with a $5,000 minimum; if violation resulted in death of employee, additional fine and/or up to 6 months' imprisonment
Repeated violation	Substantially similar (but not the same) violation found upon reinspection; not applicable if initial citation is under contest	Fine of up to $70,000
Failure to correct prior violation	Initial violation was not corrected	Fine of up to $7,000 for each day the violation continues past the date when it was supposed to stop

substances you are likely to encounter. When a procedure is explained, particular icons will be used to represent each of the OSHA guidelines. These icons are shown in Figure 19-16.

OSHA divides tasks into the following three categories.

1. Category I tasks are those that expose a worker to blood, body fluids, or tissues or those that have a chance of spills or splashes. These tasks always require specific protective measures.
2. Category II tasks do not usually involve risk of exposure. Because they may involve exposure in certain situations, however, OSHA requires that precautions be taken.
3. Category III tasks do not require any special protection. These tasks, such as taking a patient's blood pressure, involve no exposure to blood, body fluids, or tissues. (Observe patients for open wounds before you touch them to perform such tasks.)

Category I Tasks

A Category I task you might perform would be assisting with a minor surgical procedure in the office, such as the removal of a cyst. This procedure requires that you wash your hands before and after the procedure and that you wear protective gloves, a mask and protective eyewear or a face shield, and protective clothing. After the

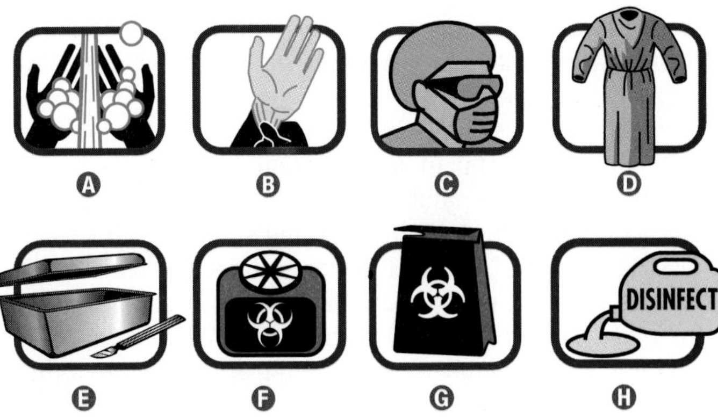

Figure 19-16. These icons will appear at the beginning of each Procedure to let you know which OSHA guidelines you should follow. They represent (a) hand washing, (b) gloves, (c) mask and protective eyewear or face shield, (d) laboratory coat or gown, (e) reusable sharps container, (f) sharps disposal, (g) biohazardous waste container, and (h) disinfection.

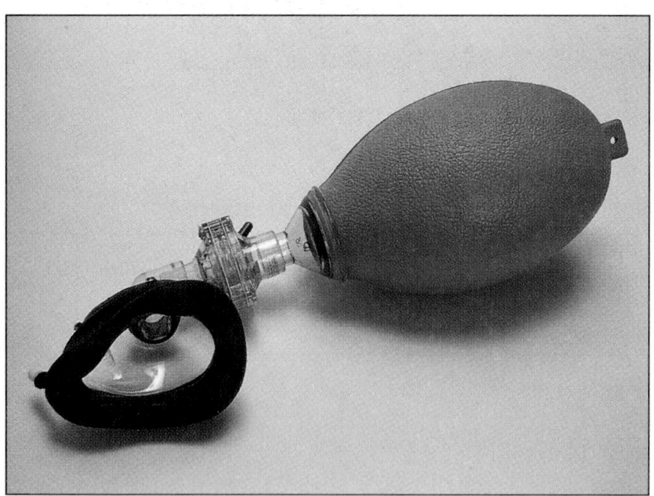

Figure 19-17. Resuscitation bags are sometimes used when a person requires mouth-to-mouth resuscitation. You must use one of these bags if blood is visible in the person's mouth or airway.

procedure, you must follow the guidelines for dealing with disposable and nondisposable sharp equipment and decontaminating work surfaces.

Category II Tasks

A Category II task you might perform would be giving mouth-to-mouth resuscitation to a patient. Because blood is usually not visible in such situations, the task is not classified as Category I. Gloves are still recommended, however, although you may not have time to get them in an emergency. Because you will be exposed to saliva in such a procedure, OSHA recommends using disposable airway equipment and resuscitation bags (shown in Figure 19-17), which medical offices are required to supply.

OSHA recommends taking these precautions to decrease the risk of transmitting infectious diseases through mouth-to-mouth resuscitation. Of particular concern to health-care workers is HIV, which causes AIDS, and the hepatitis B virus (HBV).

AIDS damages the body's ability to fight disease, and it is ultimately fatal in most instances. Hepatitis B is a highly contagious and potentially fatal disease that causes inflammation of the liver and sometimes liver failure. Health-care workers become infected with these viruses at work every year. Hepatitis B infection occurs far more frequently on the job than HIV infection. (See Chapter 21 for detailed information on these and other blood-borne pathogens.)

Category III Tasks

A Category III procedure you may perform is giving a patient medicated nose drops. This task involves tilting the patient's head and holding the dropper above the patient's nostril. Although you must perform aseptic hand washing before and after the procedure, there are no other protective requirements. Some Category III tasks require no precautions. Examples of these tasks are instructing a patient in how to use a heating pad or how to take care of a cast for a broken leg.

Personal Protective Equipment

Employers are required by law to supply personal protective equipment (PPE) at no charge to their employees. Health-care workers require many kinds of personal protective equipment to do their jobs, including gloves, masks and protective eyewear or face shields, and protective clothing (Figure 19-18). During each procedure, keep in mind that the greater your chances of exposure to blood, the more protective equipment you need to wear.

Gloves. You must wear gloves for all procedures that involve exposure to blood, other body fluids, or broken skin. There are several kinds of gloves for different situations.

1. Disposable gloves are worn once and then discarded. They cannot be used if they are torn, punctured, or otherwise damaged. Both examination and sterile gloves are disposable.
2. Examination gloves are worn during procedures that do not require a sterile environment.
3. Sterile gloves are used for sterile procedures such as minor surgery or urinary catheterization.
4. Utility gloves (used when cleaning up) are stronger than disposable gloves and may be decontaminated and reused if they show no signs of deterioration (including discoloration) after use.

Masks and Protective Eyewear or Face Shields. You must wear appropriate masks and protective eyewear or face shields for procedures in which your eyes, nose, or mouth may be exposed. These procedures are ones that have a potential for spraying or splashing blood, such as surgery or the collection or examination of blood.

Protective Clothing. If you are likely to have blood or body fluids sprayed or splashed on your clothing during a procedure, you must wear a protective laboratory coat, gown, or apron. You may also wear a hair covering and/or shoe coverings for such procedures. You should always have a change of work clothing available in the event that blood or body fluids reach your regular clothes around or through the protective clothing.

OSHA Procedures for Postprocedure Cleanup

After a procedure, personnel in every medical office must follow specific steps to clean and decontaminate the environment. The cleanup steps OSHA requires are as follows.

1. Decontaminate all exposed work surfaces with bleach or with a germ-killing solution approved by the EPA.
2. Replace protective coverings on surfaces or equipment if they have been exposed.

3. Decontaminate receptacles, such as bins, pails, and cans, on a regular basis as part of routine housekeeping procedures.
4. Pick up any broken glass with tongs—never by hand—even when wearing gloves, because the sharp edges may cut the gloves and expose the skin to infecting organisms.
5. Discard all potentially infectious waste materials in appropriate biohazardous waste containers.

Applying the Law to Daily Work

In the course of daily work, you and other medical personnel may come in contact with patients who carry dangerous or fatal infectious disease. You are at risk for accidental exposure to these types of disease with every patient. Pathogens may be present in a patient's blood or other body fluids.

A patient or anyone who comes in contact with infectious waste generated by another patient or a health-care worker is at risk for infection. To minimize the risk of cross contamination, you need to become familiar with the OSHA regulations that describe the precautions medical office personnel must take in matters such as clothing, housekeeping, record keeping, and training.

Exposure Incidents

The OSHA Bloodborne Pathogens Standard also specifies what to do in case of an exposure incident. An exposure incident is one in which a worker, despite all precautions, has reason to believe that he has come in contact with a substance that may transmit infection. Contact may occur when a medical worker accidentally sticks himself with a used needle. This "puncture exposure incident" is the most common kind of exposure.

The basic rules covering exposure incidents apply to all serious infections, such as HBV and HIV. The rules covering HBV also include vaccination.

When an exposure incident occurs, the physician or employer must be notified immediately. This prompt action is extremely important because quick and proper treatment can help prevent the development of many diseases, such as hepatitis B. Timely action can also prevent the worker from exposing other people to a potentially acquired infection. Reporting the incident increases the chance of preventing the same type of accident from happening again.

After such an exposure, the employer must offer the exposed employee a free medical evaluation. The employer must refer the employee to a licensed health-care provider who can counsel the employee about what happened as well as about how to prevent the spread of any potential infection. The health-care provider also takes a blood sample and prescribes appropriate treatment. If the employee does not want to participate in the medical evaluation and treatment, he has the right to refuse it. (The employee's refusal should be documented.)

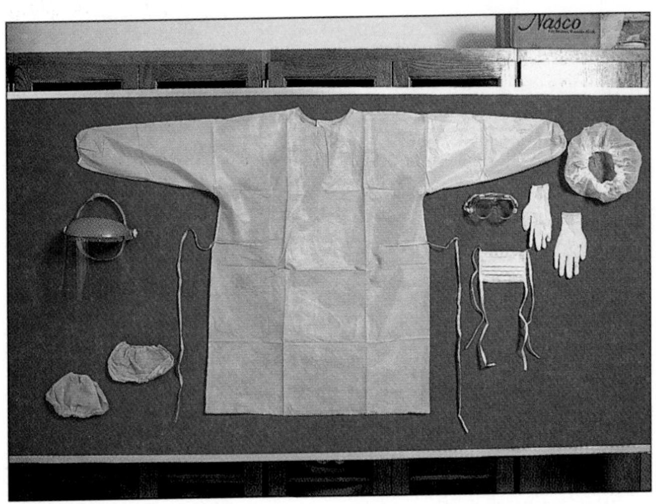

Figure 19-18. Health-care workers may need to use various types of personal protective equipment including gloves, masks and protective eyewear or face shields, gowns, and other protective clothing.

If an employee who has not received the HBV vaccination and is not known to be immune is exposed to any infected person—especially someone who is HBV-positive or at high risk—it is recommended that the employee be tested for HBV and receive the vaccination if necessary. This vaccination may prevent infection. When the source person's HBV status is unknown and she does not wish to be tested, the employee should be tested. If the source person agrees to be tested, the law requires that the employee be informed of the test results. The employee may agree to give blood but not to be tested. In such a case, the blood sample must be kept for 90 days in case the employee later develops symptoms of HBV or HIV infection and decides to be tested then.

The health-care provider who performs the postexposure evaluation must give the employer a written report stating whether HBV vaccination was recommended and received and that the employee was informed of the results of any blood tests. Any additional information must be kept confidential.

Other OSHA Requirements

OSHA also requires that all health-care workers who have occupational exposure to blood or other potentially infectious materials have the opportunity to receive the HBV vaccine, free of charge, as needed throughout employment. Within 10 days of a medical worker's starting a job, the doctor or employer is required to offer the worker the opportunity to receive this vaccination. The vaccine is recommended for all health-care workers unless:

- They have received it in the past.
- A blood test shows them to be immune to the virus.
- There are medical reasons for which the vaccine is contraindicated.

In most cases, the employee is permitted to decline the vaccination if he signs a form accepting all the conditions. (A few employers require HBV vaccination as a condition for employment.) Even if the health-care worker declines the vaccination when beginning employment, he still has the opportunity to receive the free vaccine and any necessary booster shots throughout his employment.

Transmission From Health-Care Workers to Patients

There may be times when a health-care worker has a serious infection that she could transmit to a patient. For this reason, OSHA has special recommendations for workers who perform procedures that could result in a patient's exposure to disease. Although the risk of a health-care worker's transmitting an infection to a patient is small if OSHA standards are followed, these additional precautions are advised for high-risk procedures. High-risk procedures include the following:

- Those that are thought to have caused the transmission of infection from a medical worker to a patient in the past
- Those that may carry that risk, such as oral or obstetric or gynecologic procedures
- Those that involve needles, especially if a needle is in a body cavity or a body space that is difficult to see and the health-care worker's fingers are nearby (if the worker's skin was cut, the patient could be exposed to the worker's blood)

Workers who perform high-risk procedures should know their HIV and HBV status. HBV vaccination is strongly recommended. Also, workers who have skin conditions characterized by sores that secrete fluid should forgo direct patient care and the handling of equipment used for exposure-prone procedures until their condition has healed.

If a member of the medical staff is infected with HIV or HBV, he should not perform procedures that might result in exposure for the patient without the advice of an expert review panel. This panel could include the health-care worker's own physician, someone with expert knowledge about the transmission of infectious disease, a medical professional with expert knowledge about the procedures in question, public health officials, and a member of the infection-control committee of the institution, if applicable.

The panel advises the worker on when he is allowed to perform these procedures. The advice includes requiring the worker to inform potential patients of the infection before the procedure. The panel must otherwise protect the health-care worker's confidentiality.

Although great controversy has surrounded the subject of required testing of all health-care workers for HIV or HBV, no recommendations are in place for such testing. The risk of infection transmission from worker to patient is not considered great enough to justify the extensive resources that mandatory testing would require.

Educating Patients About Preventing Disease Transmission

As a medical assistant, you can be influential in educating patients about ways to protect themselves from disease. Whenever you have the opportunity for patient education, you should stress the basic principles of hygiene and disease prevention.

1. Wash your hands frequently, especially before eating and after using the toilet, touching dirty objects, coming into contact with bodily fluids (including one's own), and touching doorknobs, railings, and handles.
2. Take a daily shower or bath, maintain daily dental care, and use clean clothes and bedding.
3. Thoroughly wash dirty drinking glasses, dishes, and utensils, especially when someone in the household is ill.
4. Use tissues when coughing or sneezing, and discard them properly after one use.
5. Maintain adequate light and ventilation in the home.
6. Routinely use a commercial disinfectant to clean rooms in the home, especially the bathroom and kitchen.
7. Use condoms if you have sexual intercourse with more than one partner or with people whose HIV or HBV status is unknown.
8. Adhere to immunization schedules.
9. Eat nutritious foods and keep physically fit.
10. Avoid stress.
11. Protect against exposure to ticks or any other potentially harmful insects or animals.

Educating patients about health promotion and disease prevention is an important part of your job. Patients with adequate knowledge can work to keep their defenses functioning properly. They can also avoid exposing themselves to infections and transmitting infections when they are ill. In addition, they are more likely to have a successful recovery from illness. To provide patients with the knowledge they need, you should educate them in the following subjects:

- Nutrition and diet
- Exercise and weight control
- Prevention of sexually transmitted diseases
- Smoking cessation
- Alcohol and drug abuse prevention and treatment
- Proper use of medications and prescribed treatments for an infection already acquired
- Stress-reduction techniques

The goal of patient education is to help patients take care of themselves. In fact, many patients expect this kind of education along with their treatment. Thus, you should encourage patients to play an active part in their own health care. A variety of patient education tools are available to help you with this task. Charts, diagrams, brochures, videotapes, audiotapes, and anatomical models can be excellent teaching resources. You may find it helpful to develop or design some resources that deal with issues of particular importance to the patients with whom you work routinely. Figure 19-19 shows examples of brochures you could use to educate patients about infection control.

In addition to educating patients about disease prevention, you will also need to educate them about disease treatment. Some patients do not follow their doctor's instructions, and they may prolong their illness or experience a relapse as a result. You will need to stress to patients the important role they play in their own treatment. See "Educating the Patient" for more information about patient compliance.

Your extensive interaction with patients and your key role in managing the office provide you with many opportunities for patient education. You will share the responsibility for educating patients with the doctor and other health-care personnel. On average, doctors spend 25% of their total office time providing information to, instructing, and counseling patients. Your role is to

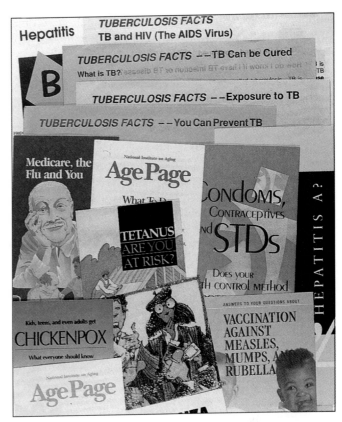

Figure 19-19. Brochures and other visual aids are effective means of educating patients about infection control.

EDUCATING THE PATIENT

Following the Doctor's Instructions

Patients' visits do not always end with the doctor's diagnosis. Occasionally, you will need to clarify the doctor's instructions or explain procedures that patients will need to perform at home. As you take part in patient education, follow these steps when you begin and end procedures.

1. Begin by identifying yourself as a medical assistant, and identify patients by name.
2. Ask patients to repeat the highlights of their sessions to determine their level of understanding.
3. As patients are leaving, encourage them to call the office with any problems or questions. Briefly document educational sessions and their topics in patients' records, dating and initialing each entry.

Patient compliance with treatment is often a problem, particularly for treatment of infection. One study found that more than half of all patients stop taking antibiotic medications too early ("Patients Misuse Antibiotics," 1996). After the physician informs a patient that medication is being prescribed, you should emphasize the importance of completing the course of treatment in the exact way it was prescribed. Explain that even if symptoms of the illness disappear before the treatment is finished, the patient must complete the full course of medication. Also instruct patients to do the following.

- Call the office immediately if you experience any unexpected reaction.
- Eat a balanced diet and drink plenty of fluids.
- Avoid sharing medication.
- Keep medication out of the reach of children.
- Refrain from activities that will interfere with healing.
- Stay away from substances that would interact poorly with the prescribed medication.

Teach patients any relevant procedures, such as how to take a temperature. After teaching sessions, have patients demonstrate the procedures to ensure that they are performing them correctly. For patients who have had minor surgery, teach simple concepts of asepsis to use in caring for the surgical wound at home.

reinforce and explain the doctor's instructions. If you encounter patient concerns, questions, or problems that you are not equipped to deal with, refer them to the doctor.

Summary

As doctors and scientists have learned more about the causes of infection, they have developed principles and practices of asepsis. You will be responsible for using these techniques to keep patients, yourself, and your workplace free from contamination. The two levels of asepsis used today are medical asepsis and surgical asepsis. You must also follow federal regulations related to infection control and asepsis, including the OSHA Bloodborne Pathogens Standard, Universal Precautions, and Standard Precautions (if you work in a hospital).

To protect patients and yourself, you need to know how pathogens cause disease, how disease is transmitted, and how to prevent the spread of infection. You will also use this knowledge to help your employer educate patients about ways they can remain healthy and reduce their risk of contracting diseases.

19 Chapter Review

Discussion Questions

1. A patient expresses concern about the possibility of acquiring HIV from other patients who may be HIV-positive. What could you say about the office to reassure this patient?
2. What should you do if you accidentally stick yourself with a used needle?
3. What techniques and materials can you use to educate an illiterate patient?

Critical Thinking Questions

1. Which part of the cycle of infection is the easiest to break? Explain your answer.
2. What special areas or situations at home or in public need extra aseptic precautions?
3. How has modern technology contributed to knowledge and technique concerning asepsis?

Application Activities

1. Rub your fingers across a culture plate. Then perform aseptic hand washing. Rub your fingers across another culture plate. Place the two plates in a warm area. After 24 hours, compare the microorganisms that have grown on each plate. Record your results.
2. Make a chart showing specific types of procedures you might perform and what safeguards you should take to protect yourself from exposure to potentially infectious substances during those procedures. Below the chart, list general precautions you should take during or after procedures.
3. With another student, role-play a scenario involving a medical assistant and a patient. The medical assistant should use various media to explain and teach the patient about a specific infectious disease.

Further Readings

Dedhar, J., and G. Enquist. "Practical Guidelines for Body Substance Precautions in Long Term Care." *Canadian Journal of Infection Control,* Autumn 1992, 77–80.

Gruninger, U. J. "Patient Education: An Example of One-to-One Communication." *Journal of Human Hypertension,* January 1995, 15–25.

Knabe, S. L., and J. West. "Asepsis—Transplant Infection Control in the OR." *Today's OR Nurse,* February 1992, 19–25.

Luthi, Theres. "The Global Village of Germs: Once Conquered Diseases Are Reappearing." *World Press Review,* May 1995, 39.

Nichols, Ronald Lee, and Jeffrey W. Smith. "Bacterial Contamination of an Anesthetic Agent (Propofol)." *New England Journal of Medicine,* July 1995, 184.

"Patients Misuse Antibiotics." *The Professional Medical Assistant* 29, no. 1 (January/February 1996): 4.

Pfeiffer, Naomi. "Stubborn Pathogens Require New Weapons." *Medical World News,* 15 December 1993, 33.

Surgeon General's Report to the American Public on HIV Infection and AIDS. Washington, DC: U.S. Public Health Service, June 1994.

U.S. Department of Labor, Occupational Safety and Health Administration. "Occupational Exposure to Bloodborne Pathogens: Final Rule." *Federal Register,* December 1991, 64,003–64,182.

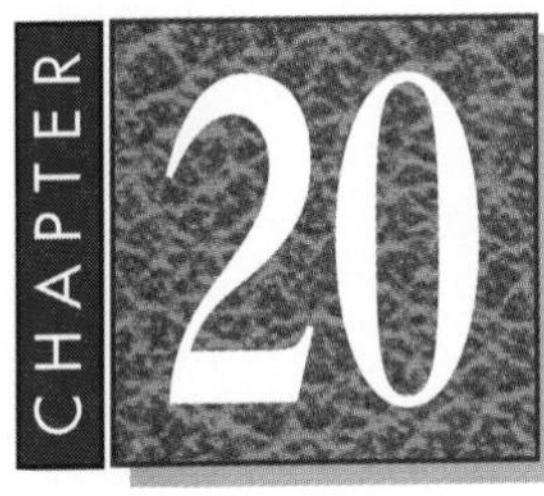

Infection-Control Techniques

CHAPTER OUTLINE

- The Medical Assistant's Role in Infection Control
- The Three Levels of Infection Control
- Sanitization: The First Level of Infection Control
- Disinfection: The Second Level of Infection Control
- Sterilization: The Third Level of Infection Control
- Some Infectious Diseases
- Reporting Guidelines
- Guideline for Isolation Precautions in Hospitals
- Immunizations: Another Way to Control Infection

Key Terms

antiseptic
autoclave
contraindication
disinfectant
immunization
nosocomial infection
sterilization indicator
ultrasonic cleaning

OBJECTIVES

After completing Chapter 20, you will be able to:

- Describe the three levels of infection control.
- Compare and contrast the procedures for sanitization, disinfection, and sterilization.
- Describe measures used in sanitization.
- List various methods used in disinfection and the advantages and disadvantages of each.
- Explain what an autoclave is and how it operates.
- List the steps in the general autoclave procedures.
- Explain how to wrap and label items for sterilization in an autoclave.
- Describe how to complete the sterilization procedure using an autoclave.
- Describe four other methods for sterilizing instruments.
- List some infectious diseases, and identify their signs and symptoms.
- Describe Centers for Disease Control and Prevention (CDC) requirements for reporting cases of infectious disease.
- Describe CDC guidelines for patient isolation.
- Explain the purpose of immunization.
- Describe your role in educating patients about immunizations.

AREAS OF COMPETENCE
1997 ROLE DELINEATION STUDY

CLINICAL

Fundamental Principles

- Apply principles of aseptic technique and infection control

continued

AREAS OF COMPETENCE continued

GENERAL (Transdisciplinary)

Legal Concepts

- Document accurately
- Follow federal, state, and local legal guidelines
- Maintain awareness of federal and state health care legislation and regulations

Instruction

- Teach methods of health promotion and disease prevention

The Medical Assistant's Role in Infection Control

As you learned in Chapter 19, the cycle of infection is one in which pathogens grow and are transmitted from one host to another. To control infectious diseases, this cycle must be broken. You can help break the cycle by applying information you have learned to specific tasks in the office setting. These tasks include:

- Following correct sanitization, disinfection, and sterilization procedures.
- Helping patients understand basic disease prevention techniques and recognize infectious diseases.
- Administering immunizations and educating patients about the importance of immunizations and schedules for obtaining them.

The Three Levels of Infection Control

Three levels of infection control are used in a medical office setting. The following are the three levels and guidelines for determining which level to use.

1. Sanitization is the process of cleaning and scrubbing instruments and equipment, generally by washing with detergents and scrubbing as needed. Sanitization removes contaminated materials and some microorganisms from surfaces. It is the means of cleaning equipment that touches only intact skin, such as reflex hammers and blood pressure cuffs.
2. Disinfection is the second level of infection control. It is used on instruments and equipment that come in contact with intact mucous membranes or other surfaces not considered sterile. Instruments that normally require only sanitization but that are visibly contaminated with blood, body fluid, or tissue must be disinfected. Disinfection kills many, but not all, microorganisms on surfaces. (It does not destroy spore-forming organisms.) To disinfect instruments such as nasal specula and endotracheal tubes, you would use a chemical approved by the Environmental Protection Agency (EPA).
3. Sterilization is the complete destruction of all microorganisms—pathogenic, beneficial, and harmless—from the surface of instruments and equipment. It is required for all instruments that penetrate the skin (needles) or that come in contact with normally sterile areas of the body, such as muscle tissue and internal organs. You would use a special device, such as an autoclave, to sterilize equipment.

Sanitization: The First Level of Infection Control

Sanitization is the scrubbing of instruments and equipment with special brushes and detergent to remove blood, mucus, and other contaminants or media where pathogens can grow. Sanitization is used to clean items

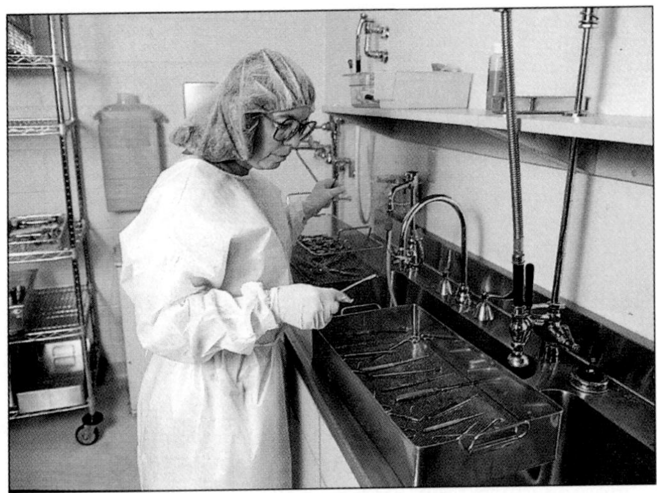

Figure 20-1. When working with instruments and equipment, separate pointed or sharp-edged instruments from all others.

that touch only healthy, intact skin. For other equipment, sanitization is the first step before disinfection and sterilization. Instruments and equipment that you can sanitize and reuse without further disinfection or sterilization include the following:

- Blood pressure cuff
- Ophthalmoscope (an instrument containing a mirror and lenses used to examine the interior of the eye)
- Otoscope (an instrument used for inspecting the ear)
- Penlight
- Reflex hammer
- Stethoscope
- Tape measure
- Tuning fork

Collecting Instruments for Sanitization

Sanitize instruments as soon as possible after use. If you cannot sanitize them immediately, place them in a sink or container filled with water and a neutral-pH detergent solution that has anticoagulant properties. In a surgical setting, use a special receptacle of disinfectant solution for collecting contaminated instruments. In an examination setting, place instruments in a sink or a container that can be transported to a sink. Take care when placing instruments in sinks or basins. You can damage pieces of equipment if you drop them carelessly into a receptacle. Nicks or scratches can affect their function and can provide opportunities for bacterial contamination.

When you are ready to begin the sanitization procedure, put on properly fitting, intact utility gloves. They are the barrier between your skin and any infectious material on the instruments and equipment to be cleaned. When you work with instruments that may be contaminated with blood, body fluids, or tissue, you may want the additional protection of a mask, eye protection, or protective clothing.

Separate the sharp instruments from all other equipment (Figure 20-1). Separating them reduces the risk of blunting sharp edges or points, damaging other equipment, and injuring yourself.

Scrubbing Instruments and Equipment

Begin by draining the disinfectant or detergent solution in which the equipment was soaking. Rinse each piece of equipment in hot running water, and handle only one item at a time (by its handles where applicable). Scrub each item using hot, soapy water and a small plastic scrub brush. Never use metal brushes or steel wool, which can scratch and damage instruments. Pay careful attention to hinges, ratchets, and other nooks and crannies where it is possible for contaminated material to collect (Figure 20-2). Use brushes of different sizes to clean all areas of each item.

Use a detergent specially formulated for medical instruments and equipment. This type of detergent is low-sudsing, has a neutral pH, and is formulated to dissolve blood and blood products. Equipment and instrument manufacturers provide guidelines for sanitizing various types of products. For example, stainless steel items must be sanitized differently from chrome-plated instruments. Follow manufacturers' guidelines when you are working with their products.

After scrubbing all surfaces and removing all visible stains and residue, rinse instruments individually, and place each one on a clean towel. Roll the instrument in the towel to remove most of the moisture. Then dry the instrument thoroughly, and examine it closely to be sure that it is operating correctly. Be sure that all moving parts operate smoothly and that surfaces are free from nicks, scratches, and other imperfections. Instruments that need only to be sanitized can be returned to trays or bins for storage. Wrap items that require disinfection and sterilization in a clean covering, and set them aside for those processes.

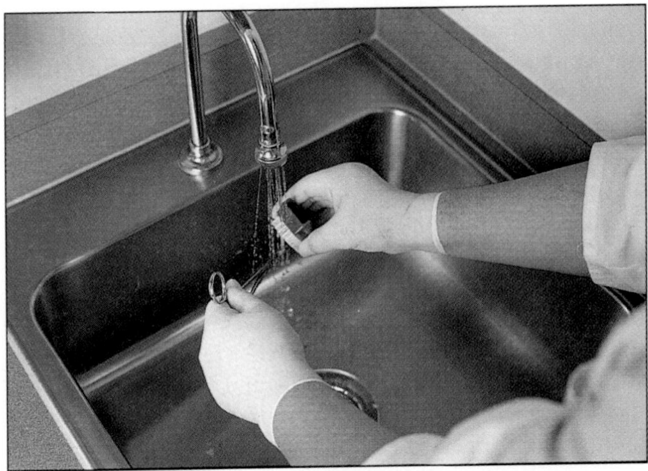

Figure 20-2. Clean all areas of an instrument, using a brush for hard-to-reach surfaces.

Rubber and Plastic Products

To sanitize rubber and plastic products, you may need to soak them only for a short period or not at all. Some rubber and plastic products fade or discolor if left in a detergent solution. When you sanitize these products, be sure to follow manufacturers' guidelines.

Syringes and Needles

Disposable syringes and needles have replaced reusable ones in most medical offices. Current medical practice encourages the use of disposable products during procedures that involve blood. Using disposable instruments helps reduce the risk of infection to both patients and health-care personnel.

If your office reuses syringes, be sure to sanitize them as soon as possible after use. Fill the syringe with cool water, and flush the water through the needle. Flushing helps prevent blood or medication from coagulating inside the syringe.

Take the syringe apart, and place the needle in a high-temperature water bath (at least 250°F, or 121°C) for further cleaning. Soak the needle in the bath for at least 20 minutes, then remove it. Handle each needle individually, using forceps. Never handle needles by hand, even though you will be wearing gloves, because of the infection danger posed by needle sticks. Clean each needle's point, lumen, shaft, and hilt and the inside of the hub (Figure 20-3). Rinse the needle, then use a clean syringe to flush first tap water and then distilled water through the needle. Inspect all needles for damage, such as blunted points or bent shafts. Discard needles with imperfections. After inspection, wrap the sanitized needles for sterilization as described later in this chapter.

Wash each syringe with detergent and warm water, using small brushes to reach all the way inside. Rinse the syringe thoroughly. Flush clear water through it at least twice. Use distilled water for the final flush. Wrap the syringe for sterilization.

Ultrasonic Cleaning

Delicate instruments or those with moving parts should be sanitized by using ultrasonic cleaners. **Ultrasonic cleaning** involves placing instruments in a special bath. The cleaner generates sound waves through a cleaning solution, loosening contaminants. Ultrasonic cleaning is safe for even very fragile instruments. If your medical office sanitizes instruments with an ultrasonic cleaner, follow the manufacturer's guidelines for operating the device.

Separate instruments with points or sharp edges from other equipment. Also separate instruments made of different types of metal. The ultrasonic cleaning process can cause one metal to disintegrate and fuse with another metal, rendering all instruments useless. Place all instruments with hinges or ratchets in the ultrasonic cleaner in the open position. If you place such an instrument in the cleaner in the closed position, contaminated material can become trapped between the two surfaces.

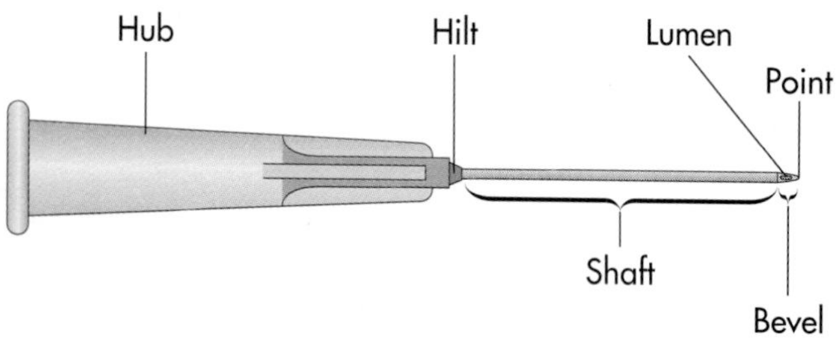

Figure 20-3. Be sure to clean all parts of reusable needles adequately.

After the instruments have been in the ultrasonic cleaner for the recommended cleaning time, remove them and rinse them under cool running water. Be sure to remove all the ultrasonic cleaning fluid. Then dry the instruments, and wrap them for storage or for disinfection and sterilization.

You can reuse ultrasonic cleaning solution for several cleaning baths. Replace it according to the care and maintenance procedures outlined by the manufacturer of the cleaning device.

Disinfection: The Second Level of Infection Control

Sanitization is often only the beginning of the process of eliminating microorganisms. After sanitization, some instruments and equipment require only disinfection before being used again. Disinfection of other items, however, is merely the second step in infection control, performed before the process of sterilization. You must wear gloves when handling instruments during disinfection procedures because instruments requiring disinfection are considered to be contaminated.

To destroy microorganisms, a disinfectant solution must reach every surface of an instrument. Even when it does reach every surface, however, disinfection cannot kill all microorganisms. Bacterial spores and certain viruses have been known to survive disinfection with strong chemicals and boiling water. It is essential to understand this limitation of disinfection when you work with instruments and equipment.

Disinfection is usually sufficient for instruments that do not penetrate a patient's skin or that come in contact only with a patient's mucous membranes or other surfaces not considered sterile. Instruments and equipment that you can disinfect and reuse without sterilization include the following:

- Enamelware
- Endotracheal tubes (tubes used to establish an artificial airway through the nose, mouth, or direct tracheal route)
- Glassware

- Laryngoscopes (tubes equipped with lighting and used to examine the interior of the larynx through the mouth)
- Nasal specula (instruments used to enlarge the opening of the nose to permit viewing)

Note that you must sterilize any instrument or piece of equipment—including those listed above—if there is visible contamination with blood or blood products before another use, even if disinfection is commonly considered sufficient. Sterilization is the only reliable measure you can take to eliminate blood-borne pathogens.

Using Disinfectants

Disinfectants are cleaning products applied particularly to instruments and equipment to reduce or eliminate infectious organisms. They are used primarily on inanimate materials. In contrast, cleaning products that are used on human tissues as anti-infection agents are called **antiseptics.**

There are no clear indications that an item has been properly and completely disinfected. To ensure optimum effectiveness of disinfectants, follow the manufacturers' guidelines carefully when using them.

Other factors may also have an impact on the effectiveness of a disinfectant. For example, if the disinfectant solution has been used many times, it may not be as powerful as a fresh solution. When wet items are put in the disinfectant bath, the surface moisture may dilute the solution. Traces of the soap used in the sanitization process can alter the chemical makeup of the disinfectant, making it nonlethal to pathogens. Evaporation can also alter the chemical makeup of the solution.

Choosing the Correct Disinfectant

Manufacturers' guidelines are the most accurate and up-to-date sources of information about the type of disinfectant to use on a given product. Generally, disinfect instruments and equipment by using one or more of the following agents:

- Boiling water
- Germicidal soap products
- Alcohol
- Acid products
- Formaldehyde
- Glutaraldehyde
- Household bleach
- Iodine and iodine compounds

Each of these disinfectants has advantages and disadvantages. Before using any disinfectant product or procedure, it is important to understand some general guidelines about disinfectant use as well as specific concerns with each approach.

Boiling Water. It was long considered sufficient to boil instruments and equipment to achieve sterilization. Research has proved that boiling water is not sufficient to sterilize a surface. Boiling water is, however, an effective means of disinfection. A special unit is used for boiling instruments and equipment for disinfection purposes.

When boiling items, place them in the unit in the open position. Do not preheat the instruments. Place them in the unit at room temperature. Use distilled water in the unit to reduce the formation of mineral deposits on the instruments as well as on the unit itself. Empty the unit, and clean it according to the manufacturer's instructions.

After boiling, allow the instruments to cool. Then remove them, using sterile transfer forceps. Store the instruments carefully according to recommended procedures to prevent contamination.

Germicidal Soap Products. Research has shown that the use of soap in the process of disinfection is less important than the scrubbing and rinsing steps. Germ-killing additives may increase the effectiveness of soap products, however, and a soap-and-water disinfection may be sufficient for items that do not come in contact with a patient's skin or mucous membranes.

Alcohol. Alcohol (70% isopropyl) is commonly used to clean instruments and equipment that would be damaged by immersion in soap and water or other disinfectant solutions. It is a corrosive product, however, and can cause damage to the skin if it is used excessively.

Acid Products. The killing power of concentrated acid products such as phenol (carbolic acid) is quite high. In a concentrated form, acid products are also extremely corrosive and toxic to tissue and should be used with care.

Formaldehyde. Formaldehyde is a corrosive and an irritant to body tissue. It is commonly used as a preservative in a 10% solution, whereas in a 5% solution it can be used as a germicidal agent and a sporicidal agent. Formaldehyde must be used at room temperature because its effectiveness is reduced in cooler environments. After disinfecting items with formaldehyde, rinse them thoroughly with distilled or sterile water before using them on patients.

Glutaraldehyde. Glutaraldehyde (known more commonly by the trade names Cidex, Cidexplus, and Glutarex) is used in chemical sterilization processes, but you can also use it as a disinfectant. Immersing instruments or equipment in a bath of glutaraldehyde for 10 to 30 minutes is sufficient for disinfection. Any chemical used in this "cold disinfection" method must be rated as a sterilant and registered with the EPA.

Household Bleach. Bleach (sodium hypochlorite) is commonly used in laboratory settings to provide a measure of protection against transmission of the human immunodeficiency virus (HIV). It is an effective disinfectant when used in a 10% solution. Bleach is used to disinfect surfaces and to soak rubber equipment before sanitization. Ventilation may be necessary when you use bleach because the fumes should not be inhaled for a prolonged period.

Iodine and Iodine Compounds. Iodine products are used as both disinfectants (solutions stronger than 2%) and antiseptics (solutions weaker than 2%). They are somewhat corrosive, however, and their effectiveness is limited by the presence of blood products, mucus, or soap.

Handling Disinfected Supplies

After disinfecting equipment, handle it with care to prevent contamination of any surface that may later come in contact with a patient. Use sterile transfer forceps, or sterilizing forceps, to remove items from whatever disinfection unit is used. Always wear gloves to handle disinfected items, and make sure you store disinfected equipment in a clean, moisture-free environment.

Sterilization: The Third Level of Infection Control

Sterilization is required for all instruments or supplies that will penetrate a patient's skin or come in contact with any other normally sterile areas of the body. Sterilization is also required for all instruments that will be used in a sterile field, even if they will not actually be used on a patient. An item is considered either sterile or unsterile. If you doubt the status of an item, consider it unsterile.

Before sterilizing an item, you must first sanitize it and, sometimes, disinfect it. Instruments and equipment that need to be sterilized include the following:

- Curettes (spoon-shaped instruments for removing material from the wall of a cavity or other surface)
- Needles
- Syringes
- Vaginal specula (instruments used to enlarge the opening of the vagina and allow examination of the vagina and cervix)

Sterilize instruments and equipment by one of the following methods:

- Autoclaving
- Chemical (cold) processes
- Dry heat processes
- Gas processes
- Microwave processes

The Autoclave

The primary method for sterilizing instruments and equipment is the use of pressurized steam in an **autoclave** (Figure 20-4). This device forces the temperature of steam above the boiling point of water (212°F, or 100°C). There are two reasons why sterilization by autoclave is such a widely accepted method of sterilization.

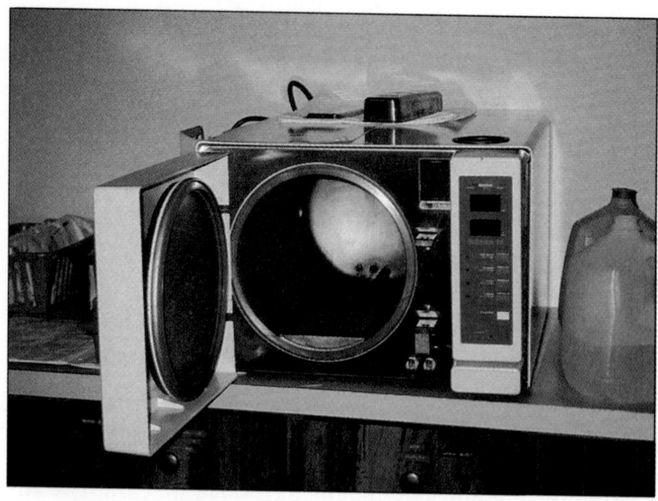

Figure 20-4. Steam autoclaving is the most common method of sterilizing instruments and equipment.

First, steam autoclaves can operate at a lower temperature than is required for dry heat sterilization. The moist heat from steam more quickly permeates the clean, porous wrappings in which all instruments are placed prior to loading them into the unit. Second, the moisture causes coagulation of proteins within microorganisms at a much lower temperature than is possible with dry heat. When cells containing coagulated protein cool, their cell walls burst, resulting in the death of the microorganisms.

General Autoclave Procedures. In general, the autoclave process involves your taking the following steps.

1. Prepare sanitized and disinfected instruments and equipment for loading into the autoclave by wrapping them in muslin or special porous paper or plastic bags or envelopes and labeling each pack. (Include sterilization indicators according to office policy.)
2. Clean the autoclave, and preheat it according to the manufacturer's guidelines. (Some models require putting instruments in before preheating.)
3. Perform any quality control procedures (besides including sterilization indicators in instrument packs) required by office policy.
4. Load the instruments and equipment into the autoclave. Allow adequate space around the items to ensure that steam reaches all areas.
5. Set the autoclave for the correct time after the correct temperature and pressure have been reached.
6. Run the autoclave through the sterilization cycle, including drying time.
7. Remove the instruments and equipment from the autoclave.
8. Store the instruments and equipment properly for the next use. Rotate stored items so that packages with the oldest date are used first.
9. Clean the autoclave and the surrounding work area.

During each step of the process, assume that the instruments and equipment are contaminated, and follow Universal Precautions.

- Wear gloves to avoid contamination by blood, body fluids, or tissues.
- Take measures to protect against needle sticks or cuts—for example, by using forceps to handle sharps.
- Wash your hands thoroughly after all cleaning procedures.

Wrapping and Labeling All Items. Wrap items in porous fabric, paper, or plastic when placing them in the autoclave. This material helps surround the items with the correct levels of moisture and heat. Instruments and equipment that are to be used immediately after autoclaving or that do not have to be sterile when used can be placed on trays with material above and below the items. Items that are to be stored or that must be sterile when used must be wrapped and sealed before autoclaving. Refer to Procedure 20-1 for wrapping and labeling instructions.

A number of products are available for wrapping items for sterilization. Muslin (140 count) is the most commonly used wrapping fabric. Other products include permeable paper or plastic bags or envelopes, disposable nonwoven fabric, and clear plastic envelopes with one side made of fabric or other permeable material. Figure 20-6 shows several common wrapping products.

Instruments that will be used together must be wrapped together to form a sterile pack. Take care to wrap the pack loosely so that the steam can reach the instruments inside. Position the instruments so they do not touch each other inside the pack. When using a pack later, consider all items (even those not used) unsterile, and return them for sanitization, disinfection, and sterilization.

Clearly label each pack to identify the item or items inside the wrapping and the person who completed the procedure. The label must also include the date so that packs are not used after their expiration dates. A 30-day period is generally considered the maximum shelf life for a sterile pack.

Cleaning and Preheating the Autoclave. Clean the autoclave before every load. Be careful to check for solution that may have boiled over and for the formation of deposits on any of the inner surfaces. Make sure the water reservoir is filled to the proper level with distilled water. Also check the discharge lines and valves to make sure there are no obstructions. If lines or valves are blocked, air may remain trapped inside the chamber, rendering the load unsterile.

Once the unit is clean, preheat it according to the manufacturer's guidelines. Loading cold instruments into an overheated chamber can cause excess condensation, so be sure to understand and follow the preheating instructions.

Understanding Autoclave Settings. Modern autoclaves are designed to operate as automatically as possible. Because you are responsible for the sterility of the items processed by the autoclave, however, you must be able to identify the various gauges and interpret their readings correctly.

Most autoclaves have three gauges and a timer (Figure 20-7). The jacket pressure gauge shows the outer chamber's steam pressure. The chamber pressure gauge shows the inner chamber's steam pressure. The temperature gauge shows the temperature inside the inner, or sterilization, chamber. The timer allows you to control the number of minutes that the load is exposed to the high-temperature, pressurized steam.

Exact temperature and pressure requirements vary with the model and type of autoclave, as well as with the instruments and packaging in the load. In general, the temperature must reach 250° to 270°F (121° to 132°C), and the chamber pressure gauge must show 15 to 30 lb of pressure. Follow the manufacturer's instructions precisely for each autoclave load. Procedure 20-2 describes the general steps to follow for running a load through the preheated autoclave.

Storing Sterilized Supplies. After packs and instruments are sterilized in the autoclave, you must store them in a clean, dry location. The method you use to wrap an item for sterilization determines the item's sterile shelf life. As a general rule, double-layer, fabric- or paper-wrapped packages are considered sterile for 30 days. The manufacturers of other wrapping products provide their own guidelines for sterile shelf life.

Return items for sanitization, disinfection, and sterilization after the sterile shelf life period has elapsed. Do not reuse any wrapping or labeling products. Instead, process each item as if it had never been cleaned.

Cleaning the Autoclave and Work Area. Clean the autoclave after each use to prevent accumulation of deposits that might affect the unit's operation. You may use an all-purpose cleaner, although specific cleaning products are available for use with autoclaves.

You are responsible for ensuring that routine cleaning is done correctly and thoroughly. When you clean the unit, also check for signs of cracking or wear in gaskets, drain valves, and tubing. Check the level of distilled water in the reservoir. Service representatives who specialize in the maintenance of your unit should periodically clean and check all seals and gauges.

The work area around the autoclave unit should be divided into two areas: one for unsterile, not-yet-autoclaved items and one for sterile equipment as it is removed from the unit. Each area should be clearly marked. Do not use supplies from one area in the other. Be sure to move any sterile packs or equipment to the correct storage areas when cleaning the counters and other work surfaces. If anything is spilled on a sterile pack or instrument, return the item for sanitization, disinfection, and sterilization.

Performing Quality Control. From time to time, personnel at an independent testing facility should check the

PROCEDURE 20-1

Wrapping and Labeling Instruments for Sterilization in the Autoclave

Objective: To enclose instruments and equipment to be sterilized in appropriate wrapping materials to ensure sterilization and to protect supplies from contamination after sterilization

OSHA Guidelines

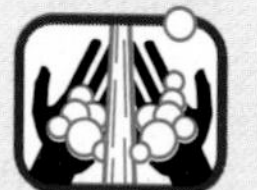 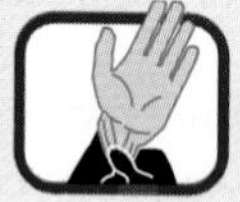 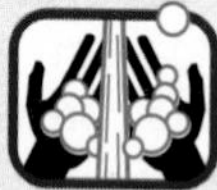

Materials: Dry, sanitized, and disinfected instruments and equipment; wrapping material (paper, muslin, gauze, bags, envelopes); sterilization indicators; autoclave tape; labels (if wrapping does not include space for labeling); pen

Method

For wrapping instruments or equipment in pieces of paper or fabric:

1. Wash your hands and put on gloves before beginning to wrap the items to be sterilized.
2. Place a square of paper or muslin on the table with one point toward you. With muslin, use a double thickness. The paper or fabric must be large enough to allow all four points to cover the instruments or equipment you will be wrapping and to provide an overlap, which will be used as a handling flap.
3. Place each item to be included in the pack in the center area of the paper or fabric "diamond" (Figure 20-5a). Items that will be used together should be wrapped together. Take care, however, that surfaces of the items do not touch each other inside the pack. Inspect each item to make sure it is operating correctly. Place hinged instruments in the pack in the open position. Wrap a small piece of paper, muslin, or gauze around delicate edges or points to protect against damage to other instruments or to the pack wrapping.
4. Place a sterilization indicator inside the pack with the instruments. Position the indicator correctly, following the manufacturer's guidelines.
5. Fold the bottom point of the diamond up and over the instruments in to the center (Figure 20-5b). Fold back a small portion of the point (Figure 20-5c). This "handle" will be used later, when the sterile pack is opened.
6. Fold the right point of the diamond in to the center. Again, fold back a small portion of the point to be used as a handle (Figure 20-5d).

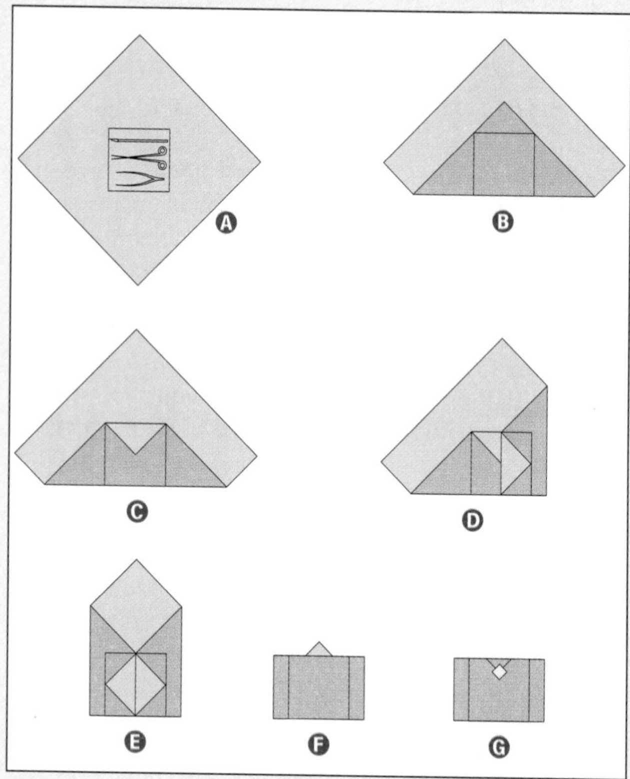

Figure 20-5. Follow this sequence when you wrap instruments in a paper or fabric pack for sterilization in an autoclave.

7. Fold the left point of the diamond in to the center, folding back a small portion to form a handle. The pack should now resemble an open envelope (Figure 20-5e).
8. Grasp the covered instruments (the bottom of the envelope) and fold this portion up, toward the top point (Figure 20-5f). Fold the top point down over the pack, making sure the pack is snug but not too tight.
9. Secure the pack with autoclave tape (Figure 20-5g). A "quick-opening tab" can be created by folding a small portion of the tape back onto itself. The pack must be snug enough to prevent instruments from slipping out of the wrapping or damaging each other inside the pack but loose enough to allow adequate circulation of steam through the pack.
10. Label the pack with your initials and the date. List the contents of the pack as well. If the pack contains syringes, be sure to identify the syringe size(s).

continued

PROCEDURE 20-1 continued

Wrapping and Labeling Instruments for Sterilization in the Autoclave

11. Place the pack aside for loading into the autoclave.
12. Remove gloves, dispose of them in the appropriate waste container, and wash your hands.

For wrapping instruments and equipment in bags or envelopes:

1. Wash your hands and put on gloves before beginning to wrap the items to be sterilized.
2. Insert the items into the bag or envelope, as indicated by the manufacturer's directions. Hinged instruments should be opened before insertion into the package. Needles may need to be inserted into special holders before being placed inside the bag or envelope.
3. Close and seal the pack. Make sure the sterilization indicator is not damaged or already exposed.
4. Label the pack with your initials and the date. List the contents of the pack as well. If the pack contains syringes, be sure to identify the syringe size(s).
5. Place the pack aside for loading into the autoclave.
6. Remove gloves, dispose of them in the appropriate waste container, and wash your hands.

operation of the autoclave. Commonly, this check is done by running a regular load through the complete cycle and sending one or more samples from the load to a testing laboratory. The laboratory examines the articles and tests them for sterility. You may be required to process the test load and prepare it for submission to the test facility.

Preventing Incomplete Sterilization. Although the autoclave is generally considered the simplest and most effective method for sterilizing instruments and equipment, certain pitfalls can cause incomplete sterilization. The three leading factors that cause incomplete sterilization are incorrect timing, insufficient temperature, and inadequate steam levels. Once again, the manufacturer's

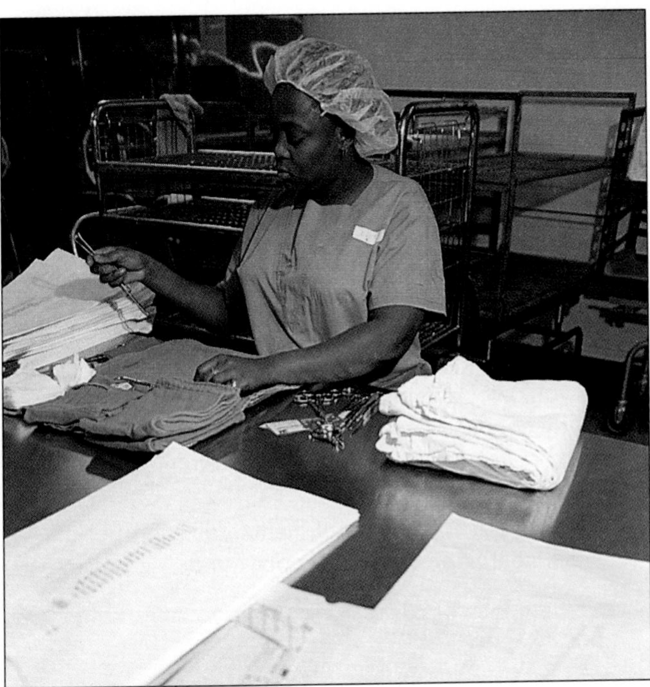

Figure 20-6. Many wrapping products are available for use when instruments or equipment are autoclaved.

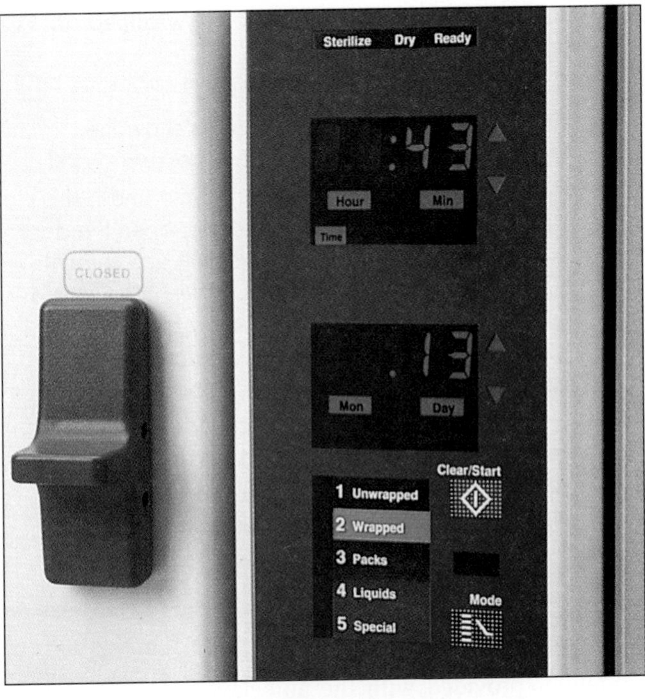

Figure 20-7. Understanding the gauges and timer is essential to proper operation of an autoclave.

PROCEDURE 20-2

Running a Load Through the Autoclave

Objective: To run a load of instruments and equipment through an autoclave, ensuring sterilization of items by properly loading, drying, and unloading them

OSHA Guidelines

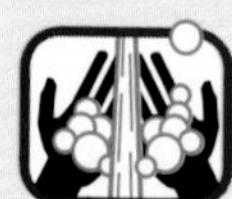
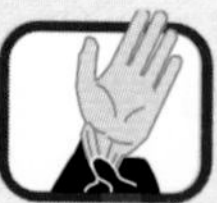
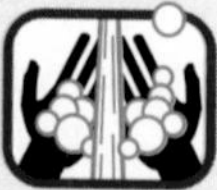

Materials: Dry, sanitized, and disinfected instruments and equipment, both individual pieces and packs; oven mitts; sterile transfer forceps; storage containers for individual items

Method

1. Wash your hands and put on gloves before beginning to load items into the autoclave.
2. Rest packs on their edges, and place jars and containers on their sides.
3. Place lids for jars and containers with their sterile sides down.
4. If the load includes plastic items, make sure no other item leans against them. (Pressure that results from the high temperatures can cause plastic items to bend or warp.)
5. If your load is mixed—containing both wrapped packs and individual instruments—place the tray containing the instruments below the tray containing the wrapped packs (Figure 20-8). (This arrangement prevents any condensation that forms on the instruments from dripping onto the wrapped packs, saturating the wrapping.)
6. Close the door and start the unit.
7. Start the timer when the indicators show the recommended temperature and pressure.
8. Right after the end of the steam cycle and just before the start of the drying cycle, open the door to the autoclave slightly (between $\frac{1}{4}$ and $\frac{1}{2}$ inch). (Opening the door more than $\frac{1}{2}$ inch causes cold air to enter the autoclave, possibly resulting in excessive condensation in the chamber. This condensation would cause incomplete drying.)
9. Dry according to the manufacturer's recommendations. (Packs and large items may require up to 45 minutes to dry completely.)
10. Unload the autoclave after the drying cycle is finished. (Do not unload any packs or instruments with wet wrappings, or the object inside will be considered unsterile and must be processed again.)
11. Unload each package carefully. Wear oven mitts to protect yourself from burns when removing wrapped packs. Use sterile transfer forceps to unload unwrapped individual objects.
12. Inspect each package or item, looking for moisture on the wrapping, underexposed sterilization indicators, and tears or breaks in the wrapping. (Consider the pack unsterile if any of these conditions is present.)
13. Place sterile packs aside for transfer to storage.
14. Place individual items that are not required to be sterile in clean containers.
15. Place items that must remain sterile in sterile containers, being sure to close the container covers tightly.
16. As you unload items, avoid placing them in an overly cool location because the cool temperature could cause condensation on the instruments or packs.
17. Remove gloves, dispose of them in the appropriate waste container, and wash your hands.

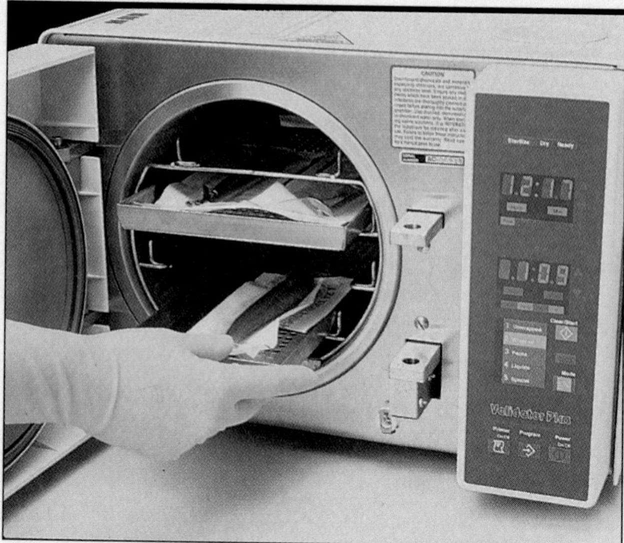

Figure 20-8. Properly loaded trays allow steam to reach all instruments and equipment.

guidelines provided with the autoclave unit are the best source for accurate information about how to operate it correctly.

Timing Guidelines. After loading the autoclave, make sure the heating cycle lasts long enough to allow the steam to permeate all wrappings to reach the instruments

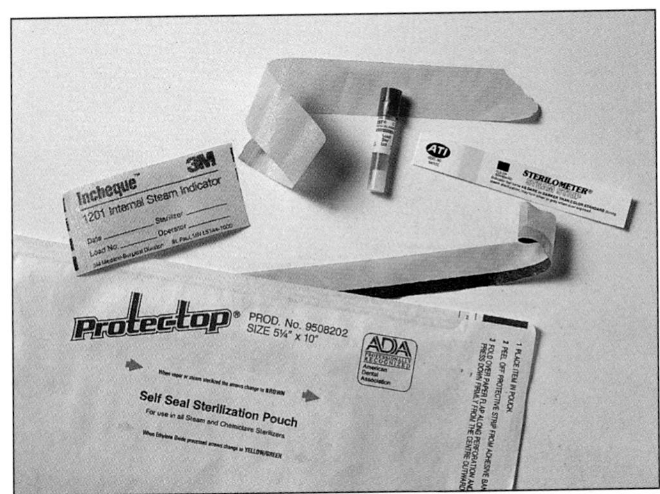

Figure 20-9. Sterilization indicators are manufactured in many sizes and shapes.

and equipment inside. Although following timing guidelines helps ensure sterilization, you should also use sterilization indicators. **Sterilization indicators** are tags, inserts, tapes, tubes, or strips that confirm that the items in the autoclave have been exposed to the correct volume of steam at the correct temperature for the correct length of time. Several types of indicators are available (Figure 20-9).

You place tags or inserts within the load, whereas you affix tapes to the outside of wrapped instrument packs. These types of indicators have designated areas or words that change color when the correct temperature has been reached. Some also show when the proper temperature, pressure, and duration have occurred. Although it is generally acceptable to rely on these indicators as a guarantee of sterility, they are, in reality, only indicators that the load has been exposed to conditions that usually result in sterile surfaces. They do not guarantee that the contents of the autoclave are actually sterile.

Other sterilization indicators are bioindicator tubes and strips. These tubes and strips contain live microorganisms or bacterial spores. After being run through a sterilization cycle, the microorganisms in the indicator should be dead. If they are still alive, you know that the sterilization cycle is not working. Some of these indicators must be sent to a laboratory for testing, whereas others can be cultured in the office. It is important to remember that, although these indicators show more conclusively than others that bacteria have been killed, items in a given load may still be unsterile.

In general, place indicators in a sufficient number of places in the load so that you can be reasonably confident of the sterility of all items in the chamber. The following locations are suitable for indicator positioning:

- Within instrument packs
- On the outside of wrapped instrument packs
- Inside containers, especially those that cannot be positioned so that steam surrounds the item
- Near the air exhaust valve
- In any other areas into which steam might not be able to flow freely

If you have any doubt about the sterility of an instrument or piece of equipment, do not use it. Instead, put it aside for another cycle of sanitization, disinfection, and sterilization. The risks to patients and to you are too great to take chances.

Temperature Guidelines. The length of the sterilization cycle is only one factor that has an impact on the final quality of autoclave operations. You must also be sure that the unit is operating at the correct temperature. Unit thermometers and sterilization indicators help confirm that correct temperatures have been reached.

Temperatures that are too high can cause problems as easily as those that are too low. If the temperature is too high inside the autoclave compartment, the steam does not have the correct level of moisture. The heat and moisture will not penetrate wrapped packs of instruments, and the result will be an unsterilized load.

If the temperature is too low, the steam contains too much moisture. Packs will be oversaturated, and the drying cycle will be insufficient. Wet packs can easily pick up contaminants from surfaces they touch after you unload them from the autoclave. Common causes of low temperature are failing to preheat the autoclave chamber, loading cold instruments into an overheated chamber, opening the unit door too wide during drying, and overfilling the water reservoir.

Steam Level Guidelines. Even with correct time and temperature levels, if the correct level of steam is not present during the autoclave cycle, items will not be sterile at the end of the cycle. It is vital that the unit force all air out of the chamber at the beginning of the sterilization cycle. It is also essential that you place items in the chamber in positions that will not cause formation of air pockets.

To help ensure proper operation of the unit, check all release valves and discharge lines to make sure they are free from obstruction. Clogged valves and lines may prevent elimination of all air from the chamber.

To prevent the formation of air pockets, load items in the autoclave so that the steam can circulate freely around all sides of the items. Place containers on their sides to avoid trapping air. Besides allowing the free flow of steam, careful positioning helps ensure that all items dry thoroughly before you remove them from the autoclave.

Other Methods of Sterilization

Although steam autoclaving is the most common method of instrument and equipment sterilization, other methods may be used. In fact, the autoclave is not recommended for some instruments because of the extreme temperatures used.

Chemical Processes. Sterilization using chemical solutions is sometimes called cold sterilization because this method does not use heat to kill microorganisms. The chemical sterilization process is generally used on instruments that can be damaged by prolonged exposure to the high temperatures of a steam autoclave. The time required for cold sterilization is generally about 10 hours, however, and you must be sure to follow the manufacturer's guidelines exactly to ensure sterilization.

One chemical process uses an unsaturated chemical vapor sterilizer, or, as it is known by its trade name, the Chemiclave (Figure 20-10). This unit combines chemical sterilization with steam autoclaving techniques. A measured amount of bactericidal solution is released into a cleaning chamber. The temperature inside the unit is raised to 270°F (132°C), and the pressure is raised to 20 to 40 lb. This unit has the advantage of fast operation (about 20 minutes) because there is no need to preheat the inner chamber.

Dry Heat Processes. Dry heat processes are used when the items to be sterilized would be damaged by immersion in chemical solutions or by exposure to steam. Operating essentially the same way as a household oven, the dry heat unit raises the temperature in the sterilizing chamber to 250° to 320°F (121° to 160°C). Sterilization is accomplished in about an hour at the upper end of the temperature range; however, time requirements increase dramatically for lower temperatures (about 9 hours at 250°F).

Gas Processes. Gas sterilization uses ethylene oxide, a gas that is hazardous to humans and to the environment. Because of this potential danger, gas sterilization is commonly used only in hospital and manufacturing environments. Instruments that can be damaged by exposure to heat and moisture can be effectively sterilized by this method. Gas sterilization usually takes longer than steam autoclaving (about 2 to 3 hours) because the gas process includes a mandatory aeration step to remove residual gas from the items being cleaned.

Microwave Processes. The newest method of instrument sterilization is microwaving. This method uses low-pressure steam with radiation to produce localized heat that kills microorganisms. The cycle, which may be as short as 30 seconds, is faster than other methods of sterilization. Current models, however, have a small chamber size: 1 to 3 cu ft. You can sterilize metal instruments in a microwave unit by placing them under a partial vacuum in a glass container.

Waste Disposal

The sanitization, disinfection, and sterilization processes generate some waste products. For example, when sterilizing needles and syringes, you will discard needles that are bent or blunted. If you are resterilizing equipment whose shelf life has expired, the old wrappings should be considered unsterile and should be handled appropriately. Follow correct disposal procedures for biohazardous waste when discarding any supplies or equipment during the sterilization process.

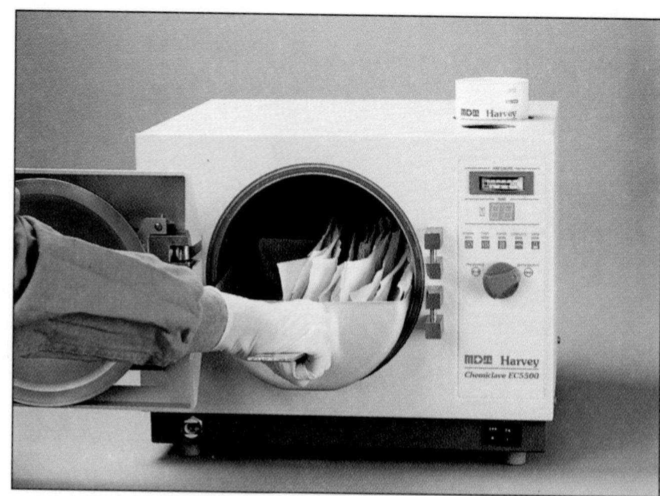

Figure 20-10. The Chemiclave is an unsaturated chemical vapor sterilizer.

Some Infectious Diseases

Sanitization, disinfection, and sterilization are crucial to infection control. Infection control is not limited to these procedures, however. Identifying signs and symptoms of some infectious diseases can also help protect health-care workers and patients from exposure to pathogens. Signs are objective findings as measured or perceived by an examiner. They may include a fever or a rash. Symptoms are subjective indications of a disease or a change in condition as perceived by the patient. Nausea and dizziness are examples of symptoms. Table 20-1 summarizes characteristics of some infectious diseases.

You can help break the cycle of infection by recommending guidelines for patients to follow to limit the spread of infectious disease in general. In Chapter 19, you learned about ways to educate patients in the prevention of disease transmission. It is also helpful to teach patients to recognize the symptoms of infectious diseases they may encounter. Early recognition may prompt early treatment and measures to protect others who are vulnerable to transmission of the disease from the infected patient. In a hospital setting, follow additional guidelines to prevent infection. Several guidelines to follow in hospitals are discussed in "Diseases and Disorders."

Chickenpox (Varicella)

Chickenpox, or varicella, is a contagious viral infection with an incubation period of 7 to 21 days. Patients with chickenpox experience an itchy rash that begins as tiny, red bumps and eventually becomes fluid-filled blisters. The blisters break and dry into scabs, usually within a few days. The rash may cover most of the body. Patients may also run a slight fever, have a headache, and experience general malaise. The infection is spread through direct or indirect transmission, as well as by droplets, or airborne secretions. Patients should be isolated for about

Table 20-1

Characteristics of Some Infectious Diseases

Disease	Infecting Agent	Transmission Method	Incubation Period	Isolation Period	Reporting Required
Chickenpox	Virus	D/I/DR	7–21 days	Until all blisters have scabbed over	By some states
Common cold	Various viruses	D/I	2–3 days	None	No
Croup	Various bacteria, viruses	D/I	2–3 days	None	No
Diphtheria	Bacteria	D/I/DR	2–5 days	Two negative tissue samples	Yes
Hib infections	Bacteria	D/I/DR	3 days	Varies	No
Influenza	Various viruses	D/I	1–3 days	As patient can be isolated	No
Measles	Virus	D/DR	8–14 days, until rash appears	7 days after rash onset	Yes
Mumps	Virus	D/DR	2–3 weeks	Until swelling stops	Yes
Pertussis	Bacteria	D/I/DR	1 week	3 weeks after cough onset	Yes
Poliomyelitis	Virus	D	Usually 7–14 days	1 week after onset	Yes
Roseola	Possibly virus	Unknown	5–15 days	Unknown	No
Rubella	Virus	D/DR	Usually 16–18 days	None except to protect pregnant women	Yes
Scarlet fever	Bacteria	D/DR	1–3 days	7 days	No
Tetanus	Bacteria	D (through contamination of puncture wound)	3–21 days	None	Yes
Tuberculosis	Bacteria	DR	4–12 weeks	Variable	Yes

Note: D = direct; I = indirect; DR = droplet

a week following the initial eruption of the rash, until all the blisters have scabbed over. In 1996 the Food and Drug Administration (FDA) approved a live vaccine for chickenpox, and it was recently added to the immunization schedule for children. Many states require reporting chickenpox cases to the state or county department of health, although there are no national requirements for reporting them.

Common Cold

Common colds are viral infections of the upper respiratory tract. They are transmitted from person to person through direct or indirect contact. The patient does not have to be isolated. It is important, however, that commonsense precautions be taken to avoid spreading the infection to others. For example, advise the patient to use tissues whenever he coughs or sneezes, and have the

DISEASES AND DISORDERS

Preventing Nosocomial Infections

Patients in hospital settings are at risk not only from the disease or injury that caused the hospitalization but also from **nosocomial**, or hospital-related, **infection**. The Centers for Disease Control and Prevention (CDC) publishes a seven-part series discussing techniques for control of nosocomial infections. The guidelines cover the following topics:

- Catheter-associated urinary tract infections
- Hand washing and environmental control
- Infection control in hospital personnel
- Intravascular device-related infections
- Isolation precautions in hospitals (discussed later in this chapter)
- Nosocomial pneumonia
- Surgical wound infections

Researchers at the CDC have found that if hospital personnel pay careful attention to the care of instruments and devices used to deliver care to patients, significant improvements can be made regarding patients' chances for avoiding infection. In addition, new, less-invasive techniques for delivering medications are promising an even greater reduction in patient risk.

To obtain a copy of these guidelines, contact:

National Technical Information Service (NTIS)
5285 Port Royal Road
Springfield, VA 22161
703-487-4650

The CDC can also be found on the World Wide Web at http://www.cdc.gov.

patient and his family wash their hands frequently and, if possible, use disposable dishware while the patient is ill. Incubation normally lasts for 2 to 3 days.

Croup

Croup is a condition that occurs when an allergy, a foreign body, an infection, or a new growth obstructs the upper airway. It is characterized by a harsh, barking cough, difficulty breathing, hoarseness, and low-grade fever. Croup is most common in infants and young children. Symptoms of croup may be lessened by humidifying the air in the child's room, encouraging rest, and giving clear, warm fluids. If croup accompanies a bacterial respiratory infection, the doctor may prescribe antibiotics. As with the common cold, have the patient and her family take commonsense precautions to prevent spreading the respiratory infection to others.

Diphtheria

Diphtheria is a bacterial infection, primarily of the nose, throat, and larynx. The patient may experience pain, fever, and respiratory obstruction. Untreated, diphtheria is generally fatal. The incubation period is between 2 and 5 days. The patient must be isolated from others and undergo antibiotic therapy until tissue cells taken from the nose and the throat show negative results. Once a leading cause of death among young children, diphtheria is now rare in the United States because of widespread immunization. Cases of diphtheria must be reported to the state or county health department.

Haemophilus Influenzae Type B

Haemophilus influenzae type B (Hib) is a frequent cause of bacterial infections, including blood infections, epiglottitis, and pneumonia, in infants and young children in the United States. It is spread through direct, indirect, and droplet transmission. The incubation period is approximately 3 days. The patient may experience upper respiratory symptoms, fever, drowsiness, body aches, and diminished appetite. The infection can also cause bacterial meningitis (a swelling or inflammation of the tissue covering the spinal cord and brain) and should be carefully monitored.

Influenza (Flu)

Nearly everyone has experienced symptoms of influenza, or the flu: fever, chills, headaches, body aches, and upper respiratory congestion. Isolation and other commonsense precautions can greatly reduce transmission of this viral infection.

Measles (Rubeola)

Measles, also called rubeola, is an infectious viral disease spread through droplets or direct transmission. Normally, the disease requires 8 to 13 days for the initial symptom of fever to appear. The characteristic itchy rash appears 14 days after exposure. Patients should follow isolation procedures for 7 days after the rash first appears. Children under the age of 3 are especially at risk for contagion and should be kept apart from family members who have contracted the disease. The CDC requires reporting measles to the state or county health department.

Mumps

Mumps is a viral infection that primarily affects the salivary glands. The incubation period lasts from 2 to 3 weeks. The patient may experience pain, especially related to parotitis (inflammation of the parotid gland near the ear), and fever. Isolation procedures should be followed until glandular swelling stops. You must report all cases of mumps to the state or county health department.

Pertussis (Whooping Cough)

Pertussis, or whooping cough, is an acute, highly contagious bacterial infection of the respiratory tract. Symptoms include slight fever, sneezing, runny nose, and quick, short coughs. The characteristic "whoop" occurs during the inhaled breath that follows a severe coughing fit. The patient should be isolated for 3 weeks after the onset of the spasmodic coughs. Whooping cough cases must be reported to the state or county health department.

Poliomyelitis (Polio)

Poliomyelitis, also called polio, is an acute viral disease involving the gray matter of the spinal cord. It is caused by any of three related viruses, and it occurs in three different forms:

1. Inapparent, in which a patient may experience fever, sore throat, headache, and vomiting
2. Nonparalytic, in which a patient experiences the same symptoms as with the inapparent type, but in a more severe form, and in which pain and stiffness occur in the neck, back, and legs
3. Paralytic, in which a patient has the same symptoms as with the nonparalytic form, followed by recovery and then signs of central nervous system paralysis

Although polio outbreaks occur worldwide, polio's current incidence in the United States is limited to fewer than ten cases each year. Since the 1950s, the incidence of polio has decreased as a result of the routine immunization of most children. Vaccinations may be administered orally or by injection to protect against all three types of polio viruses. There is no drug treatment once the disease begins. Report all cases of polio to the state or county health department.

Roseola

Roseola is a rose-colored rash thought to be caused by a human herpes virus. The disease affects infants and young children; its incubation period lasts between 5 and 15 days. Symptoms include sudden, high fever; sore throat; swollen lymph nodes; and, after several days, a rash. Although seizures may sometimes accompany cases involving a very high fever, the disease is usually not serious.

Rubella (German Measles)

Rubella, or German measles, is a highly contagious viral disease. It is transmitted through direct or droplet transmission, and incubation normally occurs in 16 to 18 days, although periods as long as 23 days have been recorded. Symptoms are mild and include fever and an itchy rash. Because of effective vaccination programs, the occurrence of rubella is diminishing. Fetuses of pregnant women who are not immune to rubella are at the greatest risk because the disease can cause birth defects in a fetus during the first trimester of pregnancy. Report rubella to the state or county department of health.

Scarlet Fever (Scarlatina)

Scarlet fever, also known as scarlatina, commonly accompanies strep throat (a bacterial infection). In addition to the symptoms of strep throat (fever, sore throat, and swollen glands), the patient experiences the characteristic "strawberry rash" (tiny, bright-red spots) that progresses from the trunk and neck to the face and extremities, along with nausea and vomiting. Incubation occurs in 1 to 3 days, and the patient may be kept isolated for 7 days, although a shorter period may be allowed if symptoms indicate the infection is not severe.

Tetanus

Tetanus is an acute, often fatal infectious bacterial disease. The infection follows the introduction of pathogenic spores, which enter the body through a contaminated puncture wound. If the disease process is not halted, the patient can experience lockjaw (a motor disturbance resulting in difficulty opening the mouth) and, eventually, paralysis. Incubation of the disease is normally 3 to 21 days. Patients with tetanus do not need to be isolated, but you must report cases to the state or county health department.

Tuberculosis

Tuberculosis, also called TB, is an infectious bacterial disease that mainly affects the lungs but can also involve other organs. A patient infected with tuberculosis may not have any symptoms. The body's immune system often destroys the bacteria, leaving only a scar or spot on the lungs. Sometimes, however, the infection spreads, and the patient exhibits these symptoms:

- Night sweats
- Productive and prolonged cough
- Fever
- Chills
- Fatigue
- Unexplained weight loss
- Diminished appetite
- Bloody sputum

Incidence of Tuberculosis. After a rise in the nationwide number of tuberculosis cases between 1985 and 1992, the incidence in the United States began to decline. Incidence remains high or on the increase in many states, however, particularly in some urban centers. You may encounter patients with tuberculosis, and you can never relax your vigilance when working in environments where there is any risk of infection.

Many factors contribute to the continued high incidence of tuberculosis. You may work with patients who are affected by some or all of these factors.

- Infection with HIV increases the risk for developing tuberculosis after exposure to the pathogen.
- The population of the United States is shifting to include a larger percentage of people from countries where there is a higher incidence of tuberculosis.
- The number of people living in environments known to pose increased risk, such as long-term institutional settings, homeless centers, and medically underserved neighborhoods, has increased.
- The public health-care system is unable to meet the needs of its constituents, resulting in patients who remain untreated.
- New drug-resistant strains of the tuberculosis pathogen are appearing, requiring longer and more potent therapy regimens, which are harder to enforce and with which many patients do not comply.

Understanding how tuberculosis is transmitted and managed will help you apply the principles of infection control.

Transmission of Tuberculosis. *Mycobacterium tuberculosis,* the microorganism responsible for tuberculosis infection, is spread through droplet transmission. The bacteria can spread through the air near an infected person when the person breathes, coughs, sneezes, or talks. When another person inhales the bacteria, they travel through that person's respiratory system to lodge in the alveoli. From there, the bacteria eventually spread throughout the body.

The most effective way to break the growth cycle of the tuberculosis pathogen is to contain the bacteria at the source. Containing the pathogen at this point prevents its entrance into another host. Containment measures include the following.

- Instruct patients in the correct procedure for covering the mouth when sneezing, coughing, laughing, or yawning. Explain that patients should properly dispose of tissues or other materials that have been used to block a sneeze or a cough and should thoroughly wash their hands afterward.
- When you must perform a procedure that induces coughing, conduct the procedure in an area with negative air pressure, such as inside a protective booth. Negative air pressure acts to draw contaminated air out of the immediate area and into a filtration system.
- When you work with a patient who is infectious, wear a personal respirator to prevent inhalation of the bacteria. Be sure also to apply standard sanitization, disinfection, and sterilization techniques to instruments and equipment.

Increasing Resistance to Tuberculosis. Another way to break the pathogenic growth cycle is to decrease the susceptibility of the host. Early diagnosis, prompt treatment, and compliance with the treatment regimen have a positive impact on the outcome of tuberculosis. Risk factors for infection include the following:

- HIV infection or another state that weakens the immune system
- Intravenous drug use
- Previous tuberculosis infection
- Diabetes mellitus, a disorder characterized by a deficiency of the hormone insulin
- End-stage renal disease, a type of kidney disease
- Low body weight

Treating Tuberculosis. Tuberculosis infection must be confirmed by a Mantoux tuberculin skin test, in which you administer tuberculin intradermally with a needle and syringe. If the test results are positive, the skin area turns red and becomes raised and hard. A positive test result reveals that a patient has had previous exposure to tuberculosis, either from immunization (common outside the United States) or from coming in contact with the tuberculosis bacteria. If a patient tests positive for tuberculin sensitivity, further tests, including chest x-rays and sputum examination, are performed.

The specific treatment of a patient with active tuberculosis depends on the part of the body affected and the type of tuberculosis involved. In all cases, however, drug therapy must be initiated immediately. Emphasize to patients the importance of completing the entire course of treatment (12 to 18 months on medication). Help patients comply with the treatment by providing education about the disease, the expected course of treatment, the anticipated outcome, and measures patients can take to prevent the spread of the disease.

Patients with active pulmonary tuberculosis should be hospitalized in a facility approved for treating the disease. They should also be placed in an isolation room with negative air pressure. Visitors should be kept to a minimum. Patients may be discharged to their homes after starting TB therapy, even though they may still be infectious. Transmission is less likely to occur after treatment has begun (*TB Care Guide,* 1994).

Reporting Guidelines

The CDC requires reporting of certain diseases to the state or county department of health. This information, which is forwarded to the CDC, helps research epidemiologists control the spread of infection. Figure 20-11 lists diseases that must be reported.

The Notifiable Disease Surveillance System

Acquired immunodeficiency syndrome (AIDS)	Lymphogranuloma venereum
Amebiasis	Malaria
Anthrax	Measles
Aseptic meningitis	Meningococcal infections
Botulism, foodborne	Mumps
Botulism, infant	Pertussis
Botulism, wound	Plague
Botulism, unspecified	Poliomyelitis, paralytic
Brucellosis	Psittacosis
Chancroid	Rabies, animal
Cholera	Rabies, human
Congenital rubella syndrome	Rheumatic fever
Diphtheria	Rocky Mountain spotted fever
Encephalitis, post-chickenpox	Rubella
Encephalitis, postmumps	Salmonellosis
Encephalitis, postother	Shigellosis
Encephalitis, primary	Syphilis, all stages
Gonorrhea	Syphilis, primary and secondary
Granuloma inguinale	Syphilis, congenital
Hansen disease	Tetanus
Hepatitis A	Toxic shock syndrome
Hepatitis B	Trichinosis
Hepatitis C	Tuberculosis
Hepatitis, unspecified	Tularemia
Legionellosis	Typhoid fever
Leptospirosis	Yellow fever
Lyme disease	

Note: The National Notifiable Disease Surveillance System does not require the reporting of varicella (chickenpox) cases. Many state agencies do, however, and the Council of State and Territorial Epidemiologists recommends the reporting of varicella cases to the CDC.

Figure 20-11. These diseases must be reported to the National Notifiable Disease Surveillance System of the CDC, through your state or county health department.

Guideline for Isolation Precautions in Hospitals

In early 1996 the CDC issued the current Guideline for Isolation Precautions in Hospitals. If you work in a hospital, it is essential to understand and apply these precautions. You must always ensure that you create an environment that protects people from disease-causing microorganisms. The guideline is made up of three major parts.

1. The first part combines the important features of Universal Precautions and Body Substance Isolation guidelines into one comprehensive set of precautions. This combined guideline is called Standard Precautions, and it is required in hospital settings.
2. The second part lists precautions designed to prevent the spread of infection through droplet, airborne, or contact transmission. These guidelines, called Transmission-Based Precautions, must be applied when you know the infectious status of patients. These Transmission-Based Precautions are applied in addition to Standard Precautions.
3. The third part describes specific syndromes you may encounter that are highly indicative of infection. When you do not know a patient's status but observe characteristics of infectious disease, follow the precautions described in this section of the guideline to prevent droplet, airborne, or contact transmission of pathogens until a diagnosis can be made.

Immunizations: Another Way to Control Infection

One of the necessary elements in the cycle of infection is the transmission of the pathogen to a susceptible host. You have already learned how to reduce the risk of infection by altering environmental conditions so that microorganisms find it difficult or impossible to survive. In addition, the risk of infection can be decreased by reducing the susceptibility of the host to infection. This reduction can be accomplished through **immunization** (administration of a vaccine or toxoid to protect susceptible individuals from infectious diseases).

When a healthy patient is vaccinated with a weakened strain of a virus, the lymphocytes manufacture antibodies against that virus. These antibodies remain in the body, making it immune to that virus in the future. Live-virus vaccines are used to immunize against measles and poliomyelitis. Immunization with a related virus can also be effective against some diseases. For example, immunization with cowpox virus has completely eradicated the incidence of smallpox, a contagious disease that leaves permanent scars on the skin.

Killed-virus vaccines, which are used to immunize against influenza and typhoid fever, do not provide protection for as long a period as that provided by live-virus vaccines. Weakened toxins, called toxoids, are used to produce active immunity against diseases such as tetanus and diphtheria.

Immunization Recommendations

The Advisory Committee on Immunization Practices, the American Academy of Pediatrics, and the American Academy of Family Physicians jointly publish immunization schedules for children. The National Coalition for

Adult Immunization (NCAI) publishes similar schedules for adults. You should be familiar with the current guidelines regarding these vaccination schedules. The pediatric schedule is shown in Figure 20-12. The adult schedule is shown in Figure 20-13.

Many patients think of immunization requirements as existing only for children; however, there are also immunizations every adult should have. According to the NCAI, more than half of Americans over the age of 50 are not properly immunized against two potent diseases: tetanus and diphtheria.

Administering Immunizations

In many states, medical assistants may administer immunizations. Most immunizations are given as injections. (Chapter 38 describes administration of various types of injections.) Some vaccines, such as live polio, are given orally.

Whether or not you administer vaccines, you must explain the need for immunization to patients, as well as describe what side effects, if any, they may experience. Common side effects of immunizations include soreness near the injection site, low-grade fever, and general malaise.

Special Immunization Concerns

Patients who are young, pregnant, or elderly, as well as those who have a weakened immune system, may require special handling related to immunizations. Health-care workers have special immunization needs too.

Pediatric Patients. Encourage parents to bring their children to the office at the recommended times for all immunizations. If a child has a fever, however, postpone the immunization until the fever has subsided. Do not postpone the visit if the child has an upper respiratory infection *without* a fever. Remember that the child does not need to restart a series of immunizations. He can simply receive the next scheduled immunization as soon as possible.

Informed Consent. As with any drug, the physician may ask you to explain the benefits and risks of immunization. For a pediatric patient, provide this information to the parents. Explain that the side effects of immunizations are usually mild, such as a slight fever or soreness, and of short duration. Advise parents that the benefits of immunity greatly outweigh the risks. Then obtain informed consent for the child's immunization. Remember that religious beliefs may prohibit parents from consenting to immunizations for their child. Record this information in the patient's chart.

Contraindications. Before administering a childhood immunization, check for any contraindications to its use. A **contraindication** is a symptom that renders use of a remedy or procedure inadvisable, usually because of risk. For example, pertussis vaccine must not be given to a child with a progressive neurological disorder. It also must not be administered to a child who developed seizures, persistent crying, or a fever of 104°F or higher after receiving a previous pertussis vaccine. In such a situation, the doctor would direct you to administer diphtheria and tetanus toxoids instead of diphtheria and tetanus toxoid and pertussis vaccine (DTP).

Immunization Records. Under the National Childhood Vaccine Injury Act of 1988, you must record certain information about immunizations in a child's permanent medical record. Required information includes:

- The vaccine's type, manufacturer, and lot number.
- The date of administration.
- The name, address, and title of the health-care professional who administered the vaccine.

You must also document:

- The administration site and route.
- The vaccine's expiration date.

Parents should maintain an accurate, up-to-date immunization record for each child. Each state issues an immunization record form, which may be available in languages other than English, depending on the state. You can obtain copies from your state's department of health. Complete a form after each child's first immunization. Instruct the parents to keep the form and bring it with the child for each subsequent immunization so that you can update the record.

Advise parents that this record is important to keep because it acts as proof of immunization, required by day-care centers, schools, the military, and other organizations. This record may also be helpful when parents consult another doctor, in case of emergency, or when moving to a new location.

Pregnant Patients. Because pregnancy may increase a woman's susceptibility to diseases and because some maternal diseases can endanger the fetus, certain immunizations may be recommended during pregnancy. Other immunizations, such as that for rubella, however, should not be administered to pregnant women because they can cause fetal defects. In general, vaccines that are based on a live virus should not be given to pregnant patients.

Before administering any immunization or other drug to a pregnant patient, determine the fetal risks associated with it. One method is to find out the drug's pregnancy risk category. The FDA has established five categories to indicate the results of clinical tests performed on animals and humans:

- Category A, which indicates that there is no known risk to the fetus
- Categories B, C, and D, which indicate some potential risk, which may be outweighed by the benefits of the drug
- Category X, which indicates an unacceptable degree of risk to the fetus

For a more detailed discussion of pregnancy risk categories, see Table 38-7 in Chapter 38. Each drug's package insert should indicate its pregnancy risk category and

Recommended Childhood Immunization Schedule
United States, January - December 1997

Vaccines[1] are listed under the routinely recommended ages. Bars indicate range of acceptable ages for vaccination. Shaded bars indicate *catch-up vaccination:* at 11-12 years of age, hepatitis B vaccine should be administered to children not previously vaccinated, and Varicella vaccine should be administered to children not previously vaccinated who lack a reliable history of chickenpox.

Age ▶ / Vaccine ▼	Birth	1 mo	2 mos	4 mos	6 mos	12 mos	15 mos	18 mos	4-6 yrs	11-12 yrs	14-16 yrs
Hepatitis B[2,3]	Hep B-1									Hep B[3]	
		Hep B-2			Hep B-3						
Diphtheria, Tetanus, Pertussis[4]			DTaP or DTP	DTaP or DTP	DTaP or DTP		DTaP or DTP[4]		DTaP or DTP	Td	
H. influenzae type b[5]			Hib	Hib	Hib[5]	Hib[5]					
Polio[6]			Polio[6]	Polio		Polio[6]			Polio		
Measles, Mumps, Rubella[7]						MMR			MMR[7] or	MMR[7]	
Varicella[8]						Var				Var[8]	

Approved by the Advisory Committee on Immunization Practices (ACIP), the American Academy of Pediatrics (AAP), and the American Academy of Family Physicians (AAFP).

(For **necessary footnotes** and important information, see reverse side.)

IS 5081

[1] This schedule indicates the recommended age for routine administration of currently licensed childhood vaccines. Some combination vaccines are available and may be used whenever administration of all components of the vaccine is indicated. Providers should consult the manufacturers' package inserts for detailed recommendations.

[2] **Infants born to HBsAg-negative mothers** should receive 2.5 μg of Merck vaccine (Recombivax HB) or 10 μg of SmithKline Beecham (SB) vaccine (Engerix-B). The 2nd dose should be administered $\geq$ 1 mo after the 1st dose.
Infants born to HBsAg-positive mothers should receive 0.5 mL hepatitis B immune globulin (HBIG) within 12 hrs of birth, and either 5 μg of Merck vaccine (Recombivax HB) or 10 μg of SB vaccine (Engerix-B) at a separate site. The 2nd dose is recommended at 1-2 mos of age and the 3rd dose at 6 mos of age.
Infants born to mothers whose HBsAg status is unknown should receive either 5 μg of Merck vaccine (Recombivax HB) or 10 μg of SB vaccine (Engerix-B) within 12 hrs of birth. The 2nd dose of vaccine is recommended at 1 mo of age and the 3rd dose at 6 mos of age. Blood should be drawn at the time of delivery to determine the mother's HBsAg status; if it is positive, the infant should receive HBIG as soon as possible (no later than 1 wk of age). The dosage and timing of subsequent vaccine doses should be based upon the mother's HBsAg status.

[3] Children and adolescents who have not been vaccinated against hepatitis B in infancy may begin the series during any childhood visit. Those who have not previously received 3 doses of hepatitis B vaccine should initiate or complete the series during the 11-12 year-old visit. The 2nd dose should be administered at least 1 mo after the 1st dose, and the 3rd dose should be administered at least 4 mos after the 1st dose and at least 2 mos after the 2nd dose.

[4] DTaP (diphtheria and tetanus toxoids and acellular pertussis vaccine) is the preferred vaccine for all doses in the vaccination series, including completion of the series in children who have received $\geq$1 dose of whole-cell DTP vaccine. Whole-cell DTP is an acceptable alternative to DTaP. The 4th dose of DTaP) may be administered as early as 12 months of age, provided 6 months have elapsed since the 3rd dose, and if the child is considered unlikely to return at 15-18 mos of age. Td (tetanus and diphtheria toxoids, absorbed, for adult use) is recommended at 11-12 years of age if at least 5 years have elapsed since the last dose of DTP, DTaP, or DT. Subsequent routine Td boosters are recommended every 10 years.

[5] Three *H. influenzae* type b (Hib) conjugate vaccines are licensed for infant use. If PRP-OMP (PedvaxHIB [Merck]) is administered at 2 and 4 mos of age, a dose at 6 mos is not required. After completing the primary series, any Hib conjugate vaccine may be used as a booster.

[6] Two poliovirus vaccines are currently licensed in the US: inactivated poliovirus vaccine (IPV) and oral poliovirus vaccine (OPV). The following schedules are all acceptable by the ACIP, the AAP, and the AAFP, and parents and providers may choose among them:

1. IPV at 2 and 4 mos; OPV at 12-18 mos and 4-6 yr
2. IPV at 2, 4, 12-18 mos, and 4-6 yr
3. OPV at 2, 4, 6-18 mos, and 4-6 yr

The ACIP routinely recommends schedule 1. IPV is the only poliovirus vaccine recommended for immunocompromised persons and their household contacts.

[7] The 2nd dose of MMR is routinely recommended at 4-6 yrs of age or at 11-12 yrs of age, but may be administered during any visit, provided at least 1 month has elapsed since receipt of the 1st dose and that both doses are administered at or after 12 months of age.

[8] Susceptible children may receive Varicella vaccine (Var) at any visit after the first birthday, and those who lack a reliable history of chickenpox should be immunized during the 11-12 year-old visit. Children $\geq$ 13 years of age should receive 2 doses, at least 1 mos apart.

Immunization Protects Children

Regular checkups at your pediatrician's office or local health clinic are an important way to keep children healthy.

By making sure that your child gets immunized on time, you can provide the best available defense against many dangerous childhood diseases. Immunizations protect children against: hepatitis B, polio, measles, mumps, rubella (German measles), pertussis (whooping cough), diphtheria, tetanus (lockjaw), *Haemophilus influenzae* type b, and chickenpox. All of these immunizations need to be given before children are 2 years old in order for them to be protected during their most vulnerable period. Are your child's immunizations up-to-date?

The chart on the other side of this fact sheet includes immunization recommendations from the American Academy of Pediatrics. Remember to keep track of your child's immunizations—it's the only way you can be sure your child is up-to-date. Also, check with your pediatrician or health clinic at each visit to find out if your child needs any booster shots or if any new vaccines have been recommended since this schedule was prepared.

If you don't have a pediatrician, call your local health department. Public health clinics usually have supplies of vaccine and may give shots free.

American Academy of Pediatrics

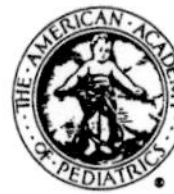

The information contained in this publication should not be used as a substitute for the medical care and advice of your pediatrician. There may be variations in treatment that your pediatrician may recommend based on individual facts and circumstances.

Figure 20-12. This schedule shows recommended ages for various childhood immunizations.

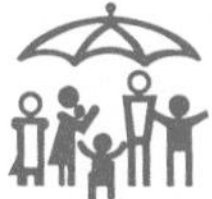

National Coalition for Adult Immunization

4733 Bethesda Avenue • Suite 750 • Bethesda, MD 20814-5228
(301) 656-0003 • Fax: (301) 907-0878 • E-mail: adultimm@aol.com

ADULT IMMUNIZATION SCHEDULE

Timing of Immunizations				
Hepatitis A (Hep A) for those at risk*	Two doses are recommended for persons requiring long-term protection.			
	first dose		second dose 6 to 12 months later	
Hepatitis B (Hep B) for those at risk*	first dose	second dose 1 month later	third dose 5 months after second dose	
Measles, Mumps, Rubella (MMR)	One dose is recommended for adults born in 1957 or later if that person is not previously immunized. (Second dose may be required in some work or school settings.)			
Tetanus, Diphtheria (Td) if initial series not given during childhood	first dose	second dose 1 month later	third dose 6 months after second dose	booster shot every 10 years
Varicella (Chickenpox)	Two doses are recommended for persons 13 and older who have not had chickenpox.			
	first dose		second dose 1 to 2 months later	

IMMUNIZATIONS FOR OLDER ADULTS AND FOR THOSE WITH CHRONIC ILLNESSES

Timing of Immunizations	
Influenza (Flu)	Given yearly in the fall to people age 65 or older. Also recommended for people younger than 65 who have medical problems such as heart disease, lung disease, diabetes, and other conditions, and for others who work or live with high-risk individuals.*
Pneumonia	Usually given once at age 65 or older. A repeat dose 5 years later may be given to those at highest risk.* Also recommended for people younger than 65 who have chronic illnesses such as those listed for influenza, and also those with kidney disorders and sickle cell anemia.* Can be given at any time during the year.

***Consult your doctor to determine your level of risk.**

8/96

Adapted from the Immunization Action Coalition, 1573 Selby Avenue, St. Paul, MN 55104

Figure 20-13. Adult immunizations are recommended for adults who did not receive vaccines as children and for older adults with chronic illnesses. (National Coalition for Adult Immunization. Reprinted with permission.)

specific contraindications or precautions for taking the drug during pregnancy.

Elderly Patients. Influenza and influenza-related pneumonia represent a serious health risk for patients over the age of 65. Although elderly patients can be immunized against influenza each year and influenza-related pneumonia one time, they may have common misconceptions about vaccinations. They may worry about the expense, about getting the disease from the vaccine, or about the need for vaccination when they do not feel ill.

Explain to patients who are concerned about the cost of vaccinations that if they are not enrolled in one of the many insurance plans that covers immunization, Medicare Part B covers the cost. For those worried about the potential side effects of immunization, describe the mild symptoms they may encounter, and emphasize that the symptoms are short-lived. You might also mention that, compared to the potential dangers of contracting a serious infection, the symptoms are quite mild.

Because older patients are much more likely than younger patients to develop side effects as a result of immunizations, instruct older patients so that they recognize and immediately report any adverse effects. That way, the physician can treat elderly patients before their illness becomes severe.

Immunocompromised Patients. Patients who have an impaired or weakened immune system (are immunocompromised) include those with acquired immunodeficiency syndrome (AIDS) or other immune disorders and those undergoing chemotherapy. Infants may also be considered immunocompromised if they have mothers who are infected with HIV or have AIDS or an unknown immune status.

All immunizations affect the immune system. A patient with a compromised immune system can experience minimal to dangerous effects, depending on the vaccine. Before administration of any immunization, the physician should check the patient's medical history. If the patient is immunocompromised, the dosage may need to be adjusted or administration postponed.

Immunization for immunocompromised patients depends on exactly what disease is present. For example, inactive poliomyelitis vaccinations should be given to patients with altered immune systems, whereas the oral form that is based on the live virus can be given to patients with healthy immune systems. Also consider the immunization status of the patients' families and caregivers. All family members and caregivers of patients with AIDS should receive only inactive poliomyelitis vaccinations and should receive annual flu vaccinations.

Health-Care Workers. Health-care workers are at risk of contracting infectious diseases and should pay careful attention to their own immunization status. Regulations of the Occupational Safety and Health Administration (OSHA) require employers to offer medical workers vaccination against hepatitis B at no cost to employees. Health-care workers may choose to decline this service, but if they do, they must sign a waiver.

Summary

You have many opportunities to break the cycle of infectious disease transmission while carrying out your duties as a medical assistant. Your own safety and the safety of both patients and colleagues depend on your knowledge and skills as you handle instruments and equipment, recognize symptoms of infectious diseases, and teach patients about the importance of immunization.

Sanitization, disinfection, and sterilization break the pathogen growth cycle by eliminating microorganisms on the surface of instruments and equipment. The steam autoclave is the most effective method for controlling infections transmitted by unsterile instruments. Familiarity with all aspects of the autoclave operation is essential, including preparing instruments for sterilization, running the load through the autoclave, removing and inspecting sterilized items, and storing supplies to ensure sterility.

In addition to recognizing the symptoms of infectious diseases, you can teach patients about symptoms of infectious diseases that are likely to affect them. Informed patients are more likely than the uninformed to seek medical aid quickly and less likely to spread illness to others. You can play a vital role in reducing patient vulnerability by encouraging patients to maintain a correct immunization status and by remaining aware of special immunization concerns for certain patients.

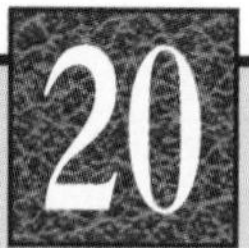

Chapter Review

Discussion Questions

1. As you are unloading the autoclave, you notice that a small container is sitting upright in the load. The sterility indicators on items surrounding the container are correctly exposed. What should you do with the container?
2. You are preparing to disinfect a tray of assorted equipment. At the bottom of the tray, you discover several pieces of gauze stained with what appears to be dried blood. What should you do with the instruments? What should you do with the gauze?
3. Identify several common childhood illnesses that must be reported to the state or county department of health. What might occur if you were to neglect reporting such illnesses?

Critical Thinking Questions

1. You are taking the general history of a 13-year-old female patient. You discover that she never had a second measles-mumps-rubella (MMR) vaccination. What special considerations, if any, should be taken into account before administering the vaccination?
2. A 26-year-old woman has recently tested positive for HIV. She is discussing her desire to return to her job as a housing advocate at a local women and children's shelter. Besides reviewing general hygiene practices, what other topics should you discuss with her?
3. In what way are you attempting to break the pathogen growth cycle when you recommend flu vaccines to patients?

Application Activities

1. Prepare a receptacle of sanitized and disinfected instruments and equipment for steam autoclaving. Demonstrate the correct method for handling sharps and instruments with hinges or ratchets.
2. Load an autoclave with wrapped instrument packs and other equipment. Demonstrate the correct placement of open glass containers, plastic items, instrument packs, and a tray of loose instruments.
3. Work with another student to role-play a situation in which you explain the recommended immunizations for the following people: a 4-month-old baby, a 5-year-old boy who has never received any immunizations, a 15-year-old boy who has never had chickenpox, and an adult female who was born in 1958 and was never immunized for measles, mumps, and rubella.

Further Readings

All About OSHA. Washington, DC: U.S. Department of Labor, 1995.

Fackelman, Kathleen. "100-Day Cough." *Science News* 150, no. 3 (20 July 1996): 46–47.

"Germs and Chronic Illness." *U.S. News and World Report* 118 (27 March 1995): 58.

Guideline for Prevention of Nosocomial Pneumonia. Atlanta, GA: Centers for Disease Control and Prevention, December 1994.

Immunization of Adults: A Call to Action. Atlanta, GA: Centers for Disease Control and Prevention, May 1994.

Luthi, Theres. "The Global Village of Germs." *World Press Review* 42 (May 1995): 39.

Nichols, Ronald Lee, and Jeffrey W. Smith. "Bacterial Contamination of an Anesthetic Agent." *New England Journal of Medicine,* 20 July 1995, 184.

Pfeiffer, Naomi. "Stubborn Pathogens Require New Weapons." *Medical World News* 34 (15 December 1993): 33.

TB Care Guide: Highlights From Core Curriculum on Tuberculosis. Atlanta, GA: Centers for Disease Control and Prevention, 1994.

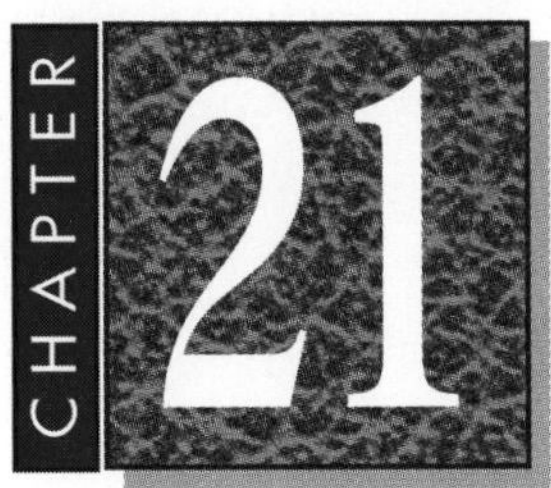

HIV, Hepatitis, and Other Blood-Borne Pathogens

CHAPTER OUTLINE

- Transmission of Blood-Borne Pathogens
- Universal Precautions
- Disease Profiles
- AIDS Patients
- Other Blood-Borne Infections
- Reporting Guidelines
- Patient Education
- Special Issues With Terminal Illness

OBJECTIVES

After completing Chapter 21, you will be able to:

- Describe ways in which blood-borne pathogens can be transmitted.
- Explain why strict adherence to Universal Precautions is essential in preventing the spread of infection.
- Describe the symptoms of hepatitis and AIDS.
- List and describe the blood tests used to diagnose HIV infection.
- Identify chronic disorders often found in patients who have AIDS.
- Compare and contrast drugs used to treat AIDS/HIV infection.
- Describe the symptoms of infection by other common blood-borne pathogens.
- Explain how to educate patients about minimizing the risks of transmitting blood-borne infections to others.
- Describe special issues you may encounter when dealing with patients who have terminal illnesses.

Key Terms

anergic reaction
blood-borne pathogen
chancre
clinical drug trial
enzyme-linked immunosorbent assay (ELISA) test
hairy leukoplakia
helper T cell
immunocompromised
immunofluorescent assay (IFA) test
jaundice
Kaposi's sarcoma
mucocutaneous exposure
percutaneous exposure
protease inhibitor
terminal
Western blot test

AREAS OF COMPETENCE

1997 ROLE DELINEATION STUDY

CLINICAL

Fundamental Principles

- Apply principles of aseptic technique and infection control
- Screen and follow up patient test results

GENERAL (Transdisciplinary)

Professionalism

- Adhere to ethical principles

Communication Skills

- Treat all patients with compassion and empathy

continued

AREAS OF COMPETENCE continued

Legal Concepts

- Follow federal, state, and local legal guidelines
- Use appropriate guidelines when releasing information

Instruction

- Instruct individuals according to their needs
- Teach methods of health promotion and disease prevention
- Locate community resources and disseminate information

Transmission of Blood-Borne Pathogens

As discussed in Chapter 19, infectious diseases are spread through a cycle that involves transmission of pathogens from host to host. When you use medical and surgical asepsis and various techniques and procedures to sanitize, disinfect, and sterilize instruments, equipment, and surfaces, you help prevent the transmission of all types of pathogens. You also need to know about specific types of pathogens—how they are transmitted and what measures you can take to prevent their transmission. **Blood-borne pathogens** are disease-causing microorganisms carried in the host's blood. They are transmitted from one host to another through contact with infected blood, tissue, or body fluids.

The Centers for Disease Control and Prevention (CDC) has identified specific substances that can serve as transmission agents for blood-borne diseases. (Although breast milk is not included, it has been implicated in the transmission of the human immunodeficiency virus [HIV]. Breast-feeding is contraindicated for women who have HIV infection.) The following substances can serve as transmission agents:

- Blood
- Blood products (such as plasma)
- Human tissue
- Semen
- Vaginal secretions
- Saliva from dental procedures
- Cerebrospinal fluid (from around the brain and spinal cord)
- Synovial fluid (from joints and around tendons)
- Pleural fluid (from around the lungs)
- Peritoneal fluid (from the abdominal cavity)
- Pericardial fluid (from around the heart)
- Amniotic fluid (from the sac containing a fetus)

Some substances are not considered a viable means for transmitting blood-borne disease, even though they may transmit other types of disease. If any of these substances contain visible traces of blood, however, their status shifts because they may then serve as transmission agents for blood-borne diseases. The substances are as follows:

- Feces
- Nasal secretions
- Perspiration
- Sputum
- Tears
- Urine
- Vomitus
- Saliva

The growth cycle of pathogenic microorganisms requires a means of exit from the host. In the case of a blood-borne disease, the means of exit can be any of the substances identified as transmission agents or potential transmission agents. The cycle also requires a means of entrance into a new host. Blood-borne pathogens can be introduced into a new host through several routes, including:

- Needle sticks from needles used on an infected patient.
- Cuts or abrasions on the skin of the uninfected person.
- Any body opening of an uninfected person.
- A transfusion with infected blood.

People at Increased Risk

People who are at increased risk for developing an infectious disease caused by blood-borne pathogens are those who come in contact with substances that may harbor the pathogens. Besides health-care professionals, people in certain other careers are at increased risk for exposure to blood-borne pathogens, including members of these groups:

Table 21-1

Cases of Health-Care Workers With AIDS/HIV Infection

Health-care workers with documented and possible occupationally acquired AIDS/HIV infection, by occupation, reported through June 1996, United States[1]

Occupation	Documented Occupational Transmission[2] Number	Possible Occupational Transmission[3] Number
Dental worker, including dentist	—	7
Embalmer/morgue technician	—	3
Emergency medical technician/paramedic	—	10
Health aide/attendant	1	12
Housekeeper/maintenance worker	1	7
Laboratory technician, clinical	16	16
Laboratory technician, nonclinical	3	—
Nurse	20	27
Physician, nonsurgical	6	11
Physician, surgical	—	4
Respiratory therapist	1	2
Technician, dialysis	1	2
Technician, surgical	2	1
Technician/therapist, other than those listed above	—	5
Other health-care occupations	—	1
Total	**51**	**108**

Source: Centers for Disease Control and Prevention.

[1]Health-care workers are defined as those persons, including students and trainees, who have worked in a health-care, clinical, or HIV laboratory setting at any time since 1978. See *MMWR* 1992; 41:823–25.

[2]Health-care workers who had documented HIV seroconversion after occupational exposure or had other laboratory evidence of occupational infection: 44 had percutaneous exposure, 5 had mucocutaneous exposure, 1 had both percutaneous and mucocutaneous exposures, and 1 had an unknown route of exposure. Forty-six exposures were to blood from an HIV-infected person, 1 to visibly bloody fluid, 1 to an unspecified fluid, and 3 to concentrated virus in a laboratory. Twenty-four of these health-care workers developed AIDS.

[3]These health-care workers have been investigated and are without identifiable behavioral or transfusion risks; each reported percutaneous or mucocutaneous occupational exposures to blood or body fluids, or laboratory solutions containing HIV, but HIV seroconversion specifically resulting from an occupational exposure was not documented.

- Law enforcement officers
- Mortuary or morgue attendants
- Firefighters
- Medical equipment service technicians
- Barbers
- Cosmetologists

Of all the blood-borne microorganisms, the pathogens posing the greatest risk are HIV, which causes acquired immunodeficiency syndrome (AIDS), and two variants of the hepatitis virus (hepatitis B virus [HBV] and hepatitis C virus [HCV]). The CDC records information about the occurrence of many blood-borne diseases, including AIDS/HIV infection and hepatitis. Table 21-1 shows

MULTISKILL FOCUS

HIV/AIDS Instructor

To gain medical assistant credentials, you must fulfill the requirements of either the American Association of Medical Assistants (for a Certified Medical Assistant) or the American Medical Technologists (for a Registered Medical Assistant). After obtaining your medical assistant certification or registration, you may wish to acquire additional skills in specialty areas through course work or on-the-job training. Although this course work or training may not lead to an additional certification or degree, it will enable you to expand your role in the medical office and advance your career as the demand for multiskilled health professionals increases.

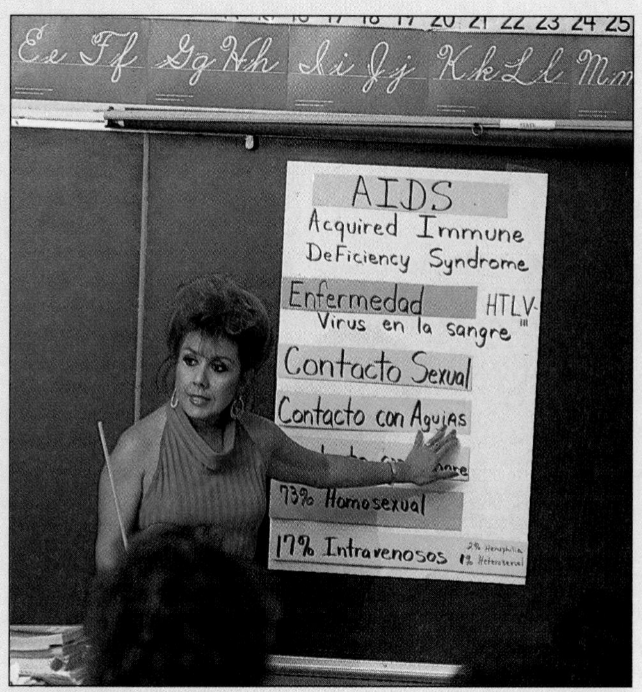

Skills and Duties

An HIV/AIDS instructor educates people about HIV infection and AIDS. Trained and certified by the American Red Cross, the HIV/AIDS instructor presents factual information in an age-appropriate, nonjudgmental, and culturally sensitive manner. She educates the community about HIV transmission and prevention and personalizes the facts about HIV and AIDS. She also emphasizes the importance of showing compassion toward people who are living with HIV or whose family members, friends, or partners may be HIV-positive.

The HIV/AIDS instructor may be certified in a number of Red Cross programs, including:

- The Basic HIV/AIDS Program, which presents a variety of interactive educational activities to educate the community.
- The African American HIV/AIDS Program, which was developed by African American staff of the Red Cross in partnership with the National Urban League to present culturally affirming information.
- The Hispanic HIV/AIDS Program, which was developed by the Red Cross with national Hispanic organizations and is available in both Spanish and English.
- The Workplace HIV/AIDS Program, which is tailored for each specific work site and covers topics such as rights and responsibilities, disability laws, local resources, and other issues of interest to employers and employees.
- Act SMART, developed by the Red Cross and the Boys & Girls Clubs of America to provide prevention knowledge and skills through age-appropriate activities for people ages 6 through 17.

Workplace Settings

HIV/AIDS instructors work in a variety of settings. They may run programs in schools, universities, offices, places of worship, community meeting rooms, clinics, hospitals, and people's homes.

Education

To become an HIV/AIDS instructor, you must be trained and certified by your local American Red Cross chapter. There are no specific educational requirements to be eligible for the training. This is often an unpaid volunteer position.

More than 26,000 instructors were teaching one or more of the Red Cross HIV/AIDS programs in 1995. To date, instructors trained by the Red Cross have reached more than 12 million people through HIV/AIDS education sessions. With the increasing awareness of AIDS and other sexually transmitted diseases, this field is expected to grow.

Where to Go for More Information

The American Red Cross
HIV/AIDS Education, Health and Safety Services
8111 Gatehouse Road, 6th Floor
Falls Church, VA 22042
703-206-7180

reported cases of AIDS/HIV infection in health-care workers to whom the virus was or may have been transmitted during the performance of their jobs.

Researching the Spread of Infectious Diseases

Health-care workers across the country file reports on the incidence of infectious diseases, such as AIDS and hepatitis, to state health departments. These state health departments pass the information on to the CDC. Epidemiologists at the CDC use this information to research trends in the spread of infectious diseases. Their research into the trends and patterns of disease outbreaks helps identify effective disease control tactics and allocate resources to especially hard-hit areas.

Universal Precautions

The most effective means of preventing the spread of HIV, hepatitis, and other blood-borne pathogens is to avoid contamination in the first place. As a medical assistant, you have a responsibility to help prevent infection in your patients, yourself, and your coworkers.

Following Universal Precautions, as required by the Department of Labor's Occupational Safety and Health Administration (OSHA), is critical to fulfillment of that responsibility. In recent years the application of Universal Precautions has been broadened in medical offices to include all body fluids, secretions, excretions, and moist body surfaces. This broadening is more like the application of Standard Precautions, which must be used in hospitals. (See Chapter 19 for more information on Universal Precautions and Standard Precautions.) Your best course of action is to assume that every patient is contaminated with blood-borne pathogens. Procedure 21-1 explains how to apply Universal Precautions to prevent transmission of blood-borne pathogens during any procedure or treatment in your medical facility.

Disease Profiles

You must understand infectious diseases, especially hepatitis and AIDS, to help prevent their spread. Because researchers continue to identify new diseases, you need to keep up-to-date on developments in the area of infectious diseases to perform your job effectively. This knowledge about diseases is useful to you for several reasons.

- You can identify symptoms that may indicate patients are infected with a blood-borne disease.
- You can provide patients with education they can use to limit their risk of contracting such a disease.
- You can identify habits your patients have that may increase their risk of spreading disease and educate them in different techniques to limit their risk.

Hepatitis

Hepatitis is a viral infection of the liver that can lead to cirrhosis and death. There are several hepatitis virus variants that differ in their means of transmission as well as in the presenting symptoms of infection. These variations include the following:

- Hepatitis A, caused by hepatitis A virus (HAV). Hepatitis A is spread mainly through the fecal-oral route. People can be infected with HAV by drinking contaminated water, eating contaminated food, or having intimate contact with an infected person. HAV can spread in day-care settings when an attendant changes the diaper of an infected child, then helps another child with feeding before performing adequate hand washing. The disease is rarely fatal (the recovery rate is 99%), and there is a vaccine that prevents infection.
- Hepatitis B, which is the most common blood-borne hazard health-care workers face. It is spread through contact with contaminated blood or body fluids and through sexual contact. Most patients recover fully from HBV infection, but some patients develop chronic infection or remain carriers of the pathogen for the rest of their lives. Adults and children with hepatitis B who develop lifelong infections may experience serious health problems, including cirrhosis (scarring of the liver), liver cancer, liver failure, and death. Preventing the spread of the infection is the most effective means of combating the disease. Following Universal Precautions and receiving HBV vaccination are the most effective ways to control the spread of the infection.
- Hepatitis C (also referred to as non-A/non-B), which is also spread through contact with contaminated blood or body fluids and through sexual contact. There is no cure for this variant, which has resulted in more deaths than hepatitis A and hepatitis B combined. Many people become carriers of hepatitis C without knowing it, because they do not experience any symptoms of the virus. If the infection causes immediate symptoms, they often resemble the flu. Although treatment exists to suppress the virus, nothing can prevent or stop the virus from replicating. Over time, it is likely to damage the liver, causing cirrhosis, liver failure, and cancer. As with hepatitis B, preventing the spread of the infection is the best way to combat the disease.
- Hepatitis D (delta agent hepatitis), which occurs only in people infected with HBV. Delta agent infection may make the symptoms of hepatitis B more severe, and it is associated with liver cancer. The HBV vaccine also prevents delta agent infection.
- Hepatitis E, caused by hepatitis E virus (HEV). Hepatitis E is transmitted by the fecal-oral route, usually through contaminated water. Chronic infection does not occur, but acute hepatitis E may be fatal in pregnant women.

Risk Factors. Risk factors for HBV and HCV infection are the same. Although both infections can be spread

PROCEDURE 21-1

Applying Universal Precautions

Objective: To take specific protective measures when performing tasks in which a worker may be exposed to blood, body fluids, or tissues

OSHA Guidelines

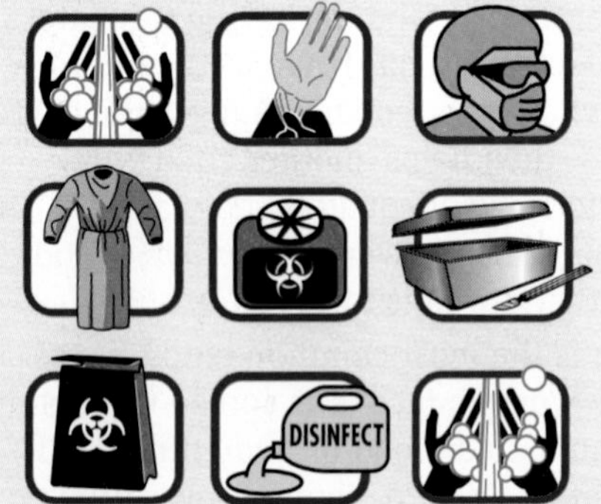

Materials: Items needed for the specific treatment or procedure being performed

Method

1. Perform aseptic hand washing. (See Procedure 19-1 in Chapter 19.)
2. Put on gloves and a gown or a laboratory coat and, if required, eye protection and a mask or a face shield.
3. Assist with the treatment or procedure as your office policy dictates.
4. Follow OSHA procedures (outlined in Chapter 19) to clean and decontaminate the treatment area (Figure 21-1).
5. Place reusable instruments in appropriate containers for sanitizing, disinfecting, and sterilizing, as appropriate (see Chapter 20).
6. Remove your gloves and all personal protective equipment. Place them in waste containers or laundry receptacles, according to OSHA guidelines (see Chapter 19).
7. Wash your hands.

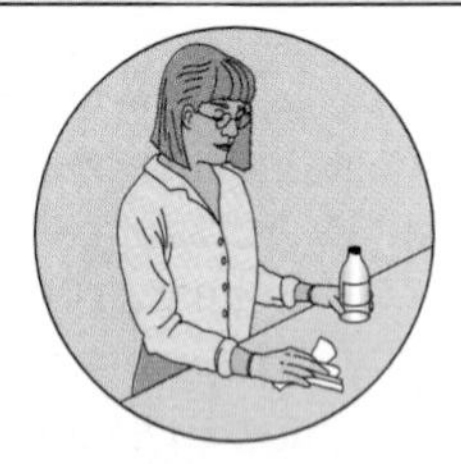

❶ Decontaminate exposed work areas.

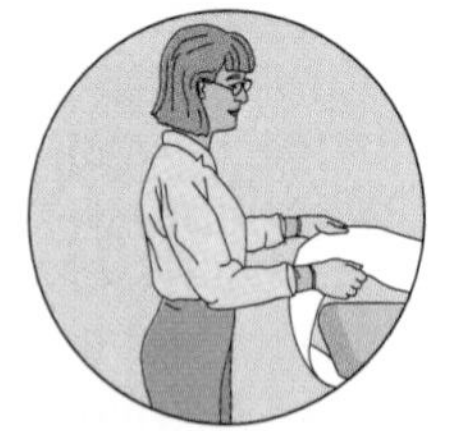

❷ Replace exposed protective coverings.

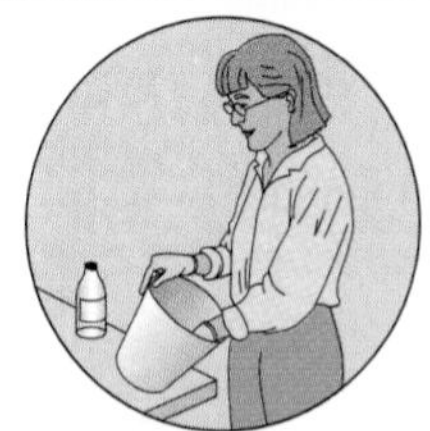

❸ Decontaminate receptacles.

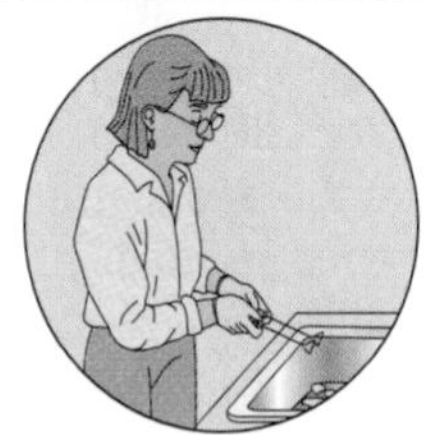

❹ Pick up broken glass.

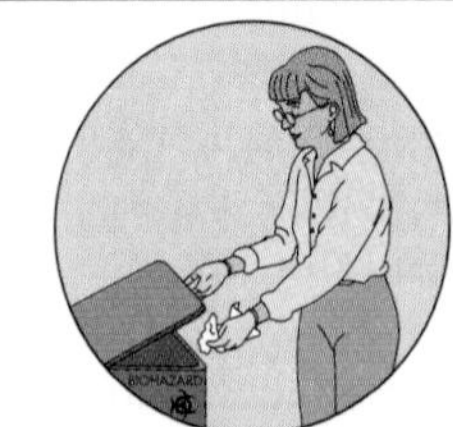

❺ Discard infectious waste.

Figure 21-1. Follow these OSHA guidelines to clean and decontaminate the medical environment after each procedure or treatment.

through sexual contact—and high-risk sexual activity is a risk factor for hepatitis—the main risk factor is working in an occupation that requires exposure to human blood and body fluids. Other risk factors include:

- Using intravenous drugs.
- Having hemophilia, a disorder characterized by a permanent tendency to bleed and requiring blood transfusions.
- Traveling internationally to areas with a high prevalence of hepatitis B.
- Having received blood transfusions before screening for HBV/HCV was in place.
- Receiving hemodialysis, a procedure in which toxic wastes are removed from a patient's blood.
- Living with a partner who has hepatitis B or hepatitis C.
- Having multiple sexual partners.

Risk in the Medical Community. As described, the primary risk factor for HBV and HCV infection is occupational exposure to the virus. In fact, although exposure to HIV has received more publicity and causes the greatest fear, your risk of contracting hepatitis, particularly hepatitis B, is actually considerably greater. Studies show that the risk of contracting HIV from a single needle-stick exposure is approximately 0.5%, whereas the risk of contracting hepatitis B from a single needle-stick exposure varies from 6% to as much as 33%. Several variables are responsible for the broad range of measured risk in HBV infection, including the immune status of the recipient and the efficiency of the virus transmission.

Progress of the Infection. Infection with hepatitis is a multistage process. The stages are as follows:

1. The prodromal stage, in which patients may experience general malaise, specific symptoms such as nausea and vomiting, or no symptoms at all
2. The icteric, or **jaundice,** stage, characterized by yellowness of the skin, eyes, mucous membranes, and excretions (Figure 21-2), which usually appears 5 to 10 days after initial infection
3. The convalescent stage, which occurs after the two acute infection stages and can last from 2 to 3 weeks as symptoms gradually abate

The acute illness lasts approximately 16 weeks for hepatitis B and hepatitis C. Although patients recover, they may remain infected with the virus for life.

Symptoms. People infected with hepatitis may show no symptoms, may experience such mild or subtle symptoms that they do not realize they are seriously ill, or may experience severe symptoms. When you treat patients with hepatitis infection, any of these signs and symptoms may be present:

- Jaundice
- Diminished appetite
- Fatigue
- Nausea
- Vomiting
- Joint pain or tenderness
- Stomach pain
- General malaise

Diagnosis. Diagnosis of hepatitis is made through an investigation of risk factors and exposure incidents as well as through several blood tests. Most of the blood tests indicate the presence of antigen-antibody systems that relate to infection by hepatitis. They can also be used to determine the stage of the disease.

Preventive Measures. The best prevention against hepatitis is avoiding contact with contaminated substances. Follow Universal Precautions when working with all patients, and be especially careful with patients who have unknown or hepatitis-positive status.

A vaccine is available to prevent HBV infection. In fact, OSHA has established guidelines that require your employer to offer you this vaccine at no charge. If you decline the offer, you must sign a waiver. Current standard medical practice recommends against declining the vaccine. (For more information on this vaccination, see Chapter 19.)

Vaccination against HBV does not protect you from other strains of hepatitis. There are currently no vaccines for HCV, for example.

In the past, HBV vaccination was recommended only for high-risk individuals, such as medical personnel, dialysis patients, homosexual men, and intravenous drug users. This program of vaccinating only selected individuals did not greatly reduce the incidence of infection. Today the CDC recommends routine vaccination for everyone.

If you are exposed to hepatitis B and have not been vaccinated, you can receive a postexposure inoculation of hepatitis B immune globulin (HBIG). HBIG is given in large doses during the 7-day period after exposure. Shortly after beginning the treatment, you would also receive HBV vaccination. The HBIG inoculation is also used for infants born to HBV-infected mothers.

AIDS/HIV Infection

HIV is a virus that infects and gradually destroys components of the immune system. AIDS is the condition that results from the advanced stages of this viral infection.

Over a period of time and in most cases, HIV infection develops into AIDS, which results in death. The pathogen gradually destroys helper T cells. **Helper T cells** are white blood cells that are a key component of the body's immune system and that work in coordination with other white blood cells (B cells, macrophages, and so on) to combat infection.

The virus also attacks neurons, causing demyelination (destruction of the myelin sheath of a nerve), which results in neurological problems, including dementia. Most patients with AIDS acquire various opportunistic infections. Opportunistic microorganisms do not ordinarily cause disease in a person with a properly functioning immune system. Examples of opportunistic infections are *Pneumocystis carinii* pneumonia and oral candidiasis.

Virtually everyone is at risk for contracting AIDS. Although the initial outbreak of the disease in the United States appeared in the male homosexual population and currently homosexual and bisexual men comprise a large percentage of AIDS cases, the disease knows no limits. The incidence of HIV infection in homosexual men, how-

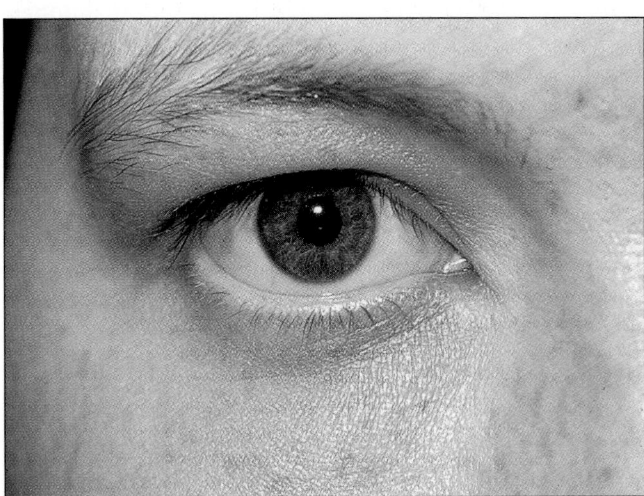

Figure 21-2. Jaundice is caused by excess bilirubin, which is produced in the liver and deposited throughout the body and which results in the yellow appearance of the patient's eyes and skin.

ever, has leveled off and even declined slightly in some areas of the United States. At the same time, the incidence of infection in heterosexual men and women and teenagers is increasing rapidly. The incubation period in adults is between 8 and 15 years, and the majority of adults with the disease are between the ages of 25 and 45.

Risk Factors. The greatest risk factor for contracting HIV infection is unprotected sexual activity. The virus can be found in blood, semen, and vaginal secretions and can be transmitted to an uninfected person through mucous membranes in the vagina, rectum, or mouth, especially if there are cuts or open sores in those areas. Some strains of the virus are more likely to infect the cells in the female reproductive tract (Langerhans cells). The HIV strain most common in the United States, however, targets the monocyte or lymphocyte white blood cells and is more prone to being passed along through anal sex and blood-to-blood contact.

The virus can also be spread by the sharing of needles used by intravenous drug users. The minute amount of blood left on a needle after injection provides an ample supply of the virus to transmit the infection to another host. Needles used in tattooing and ear piercing can also pose a risk. In all cases needles should be new or sterile.

The virus can pass from mother to fetus during pregnancy, as well as to an infant during delivery or through breast-feeding. Not every infant born to an infected mother contracts the disease, and some infected infants have cleared the virus from their systems within a year after birth. Scientists are studying these children in an effort to determine how their immune systems allow them to escape infection altogether or to eradicate the virus after infection (Toufexis, 1996). Scientists suspect that either the immune systems of the infants in the study fought off an HIV invasion or the infants developed a permanent tolerance for it.

At one time the virus was also being spread through the nation's blood supply. Transmission was occurring through transfusion of HIV-contaminated blood products. This form of transmission has virtually stopped as a result of an aggressive screening program that began in 1985. All blood donations are tested for the virus, and contaminated donations are destroyed. People who received blood prior to 1986 (especially between 1978 and 1985) are at risk for coming down with AIDS. Because of the long incubation period of the virus (8 to 15 years), infected people may not yet exhibit any symptoms of infection.

Risk in the Medical Community. Health-care workers have contracted HIV infection as a direct result of occupational activities (see Table 21-1). Investigations showed that infection in most of the cases occurred as a result of **percutaneous exposure,** that is, exposure through a puncture wound or needle stick. **Mucocutaneous exposure,** or exposure through a mucous membrane, resulted in infection in a few cases.

Further analysis identified that in most cases the infecting substance was HIV-infected blood. Concentrated virus cultures in the laboratory and visibly bloody body fluid caused a few of the cases.

Progress of the Infection. Current research has shown that development of AIDS occurs in three main stages:

- Initial infection
- Incubation period
- Full-blown AIDS

Initial infection by the virus can occur years before any symptoms appear to arouse suspicions about HIV infection. In some cases the initial infection is marked by severe flulike symptoms. Identification of the initial infection, however, is almost always through hindsight. The virus attacks helper T cells during this initial phase.

During the initial phase of infection by HIV, the virus enters the cell, and the host cell produces multiple copies of the virus. As a result helper T cells die or are disabled. The body's immune system responds to the attack at this point, cleansing the blood supply of the virus, and the virus enters an inactive phase.

The incubation period begins when the virus incorporates its genetic material into the genetic material of the helper T cells. The virus is trapped within the lymph system, and the host experiences few, if any, symptoms of the disease. Many doctors discover the infection in patients during this period when treating them for other illnesses. This incubation period, in which people are HIV-positive but do not have AIDS, generally lasts 8 to 15 years.

Sometime during the incubation period, HIV becomes active again and continues to attack and destroy helper T cells. As the number of helper T cells dwindles, the patient becomes more prone to opportunistic infections.

The threshold at which a patient is officially diagnosed with AIDS is the point at which there are 200 or fewer helper T cells per milliliter of blood. Once a person has full-blown AIDS—the third phase of infection—opportunistic infections take hold as the overall immune system undergoes deterioration. Neurons are destroyed, resulting in neurological problems, including dementia.

Diagnosis. To know for certain whether a person is infected with HIV, that person must have blood tested specifically for HIV infection. (All HIV testing is anonymous.) The **enzyme-linked immunosorbent assay (ELISA) test** confirms the presence of antibodies developed by the body's immune system in response to an initial HIV infection. ELISA is only about 85% accurate because of cross-reactivity from other viruses. Therefore, positive specimens are confirmed by a different method—the **Western blot test** or the **immunofluorescent antibody (IFA) test.** These tests are more accurate because they are specific to individual viruses.

These HIV tests were first developed for use on blood samples, but the ELISA and Western blot tests can also be run on oral fluid samples obtained in the medical office. Positive results from two of the three HIV tests (ELISA plus one other) yield an accurate diagnosis in almost 100% of patients tested.

Home tests are available that involve an ELISA test followed by either a Western blot test or an IFA test if the ELISA results are positive. These tests are performed on a drop of the patient's blood, which is collected on a specially treated card. Patients are identified only by a number, which they use to obtain their test results. (Keep in mind that people who perform home tests may not report positive results to the proper authorities.)

In all cases involving testing for HIV, you must follow measures to ensure protection of the patient's confidentiality. Knowledge about a patient's test results should be limited to those who will be treating the patient and appropriate authorities as required by law. The patient's decision on whether or not to reveal test results to family and friends should be respected at all times.

Symptoms. HIV infection can cause a variety of problems as it progresses to AIDS. Patients with AIDS may complain of any of the following symptoms:

- Systemic complaints, such as weight loss, fatigue, fever, chills, and night sweats
- Respiratory complaints, such as sinus fullness, dry cough, shortness of breath, difficulty swallowing, and sinus drainage
- Oral complaints, such as gingivitis, oral lesions, and **hairy leukoplakia,** which is a white lesion on the tongue
- Gastrointestinal complaints, such as diarrhea and bloody stool
- Central nervous system complaints, such as depression, personality changes, concentration difficulties, and confusion or dementia
- Peripheral nervous system complaints, such as tingling, numbness, pain, and weakness in the extremities
- Skin-related complaints, such as rashes, dry skin, and changes in the nail bed
- **Kaposi's sarcoma,** abnormal tissue occurring in the skin and sometimes in the lymph nodes and organs manifested by reddish purple to dark blue patches or spots on the skin

Because many other diseases can cause these symptoms, the occurrence of any one symptom is not necessarily indicative of AIDS. Be aware, however, that patients exhibiting a combination of symptoms should be tested. The two symptoms most indicative of AIDS are hairy leukoplakia and Kaposi's sarcoma.

Preventive Measures. The only way to prevent the spread of HIV infection is to avoid specific activities or to take safety precautions when engaging in these activities. Activities requiring preventive measures can be divided into three groups, based on the means of transmission of the disease:

- Sexual contact
- Sharing of intravenous needles
- Medical procedures

Prevention and Sexual Contact. The most effective method for preventing the spread of AIDS/HIV infection through sexual contact is to avoid high-risk sexual activity. Such high-risk activities or situations include:

1. Having unprotected vaginal, oral, or anal sex, either homosexual or heterosexual, *unless* the individuals are involved in a long-term, monogamous relationship, they both have been tested and received negative results, and they have not engaged in any unsafe sexual activity 6 months before the test or anytime after the test.
2. Having multiple sexual partners, even when using protection against infection.
3. Experiencing a concurrent infection with another sexually transmitted disease.

In addition, precautions must be taken when using a condom as a means of protection against infection. Proper use of a condom requires adherence to the following guidelines.

- A condom must be used every time the individual has sex and must never be reused.
- Only latex condoms provide protection against spread of the HIV pathogen. Lambskin condoms provide birth control only, not protection against disease.
- If lubrication is required, the lubricant must be water-based, not petroleum-based (such as petroleum jelly). Lubricants other than those specifically formulated for use with latex condoms can damage the condom, rendering it permeable and eliminating its usefulness as a barrier against disease.
- Condoms should be placed on the penis before any risk of leakage of seminal fluid occurs. Space should be left at the tip to act as a reservoir for ejaculated semen.
- Intercourse should not be attempted unless the penis is fully erect, and the penis should be withdrawn while it is still erect.
- The condom must remain in place from the beginning to the end of intercourse and should be held in place during withdrawal to prevent slippage. After withdrawal the condom should be disposed of properly.

Prevention and Intravenous Drug Use. Intravenous drug users are at risk for infection when they share needles. The most effective means of preventing the spread of the pathogen among drug users is to avoid sharing or reusing needles.

Prevention and Medical Procedures. Preventing the spread of AIDS/HIV infection in the medical environment involves taking many precautions. You must take precautions to prevent the spread of infection between patients, between yourself and the patient, and when you are working with equipment, supplies, or instruments that may be contaminated.

Strict adherence to Universal Precautions (Standard Precautions in a hospital) when working with patients is the best method for preventing the spread of disease among patients and between the patient and you. You must use gloves whenever there is a risk of contact with blood, tissue, or body fluids, and you must dispose of gloves properly after use. (See Chapter 19 for specific disposal guidelines.)

You must wash your hands carefully and thoroughly between patients. Wear additional personal protective equipment in situations where there is a risk of being splashed or sprayed by blood or body fluids.

Although gloves and other personal protective equipment provide adequate protection in many situations, they provide only limited protection against injury. Be especially careful when handling pointed or sharp-edged instruments or equipment. Do not attempt to break or recap needles, and make sure they are disposed of in a puncture-proof biohazardous waste container. Pick up broken glass with tongs, and dispose of it in a puncture-proof biohazardous waste container.

Education as Prevention. As a medical assistant, you will encounter many opportunities to inform and educate patients about the dangers of HIV infection and AIDS, the ways in which the disease is spread, the ways in which it is not spread, and methods for preventing its spread. Use these opportunities to educate patients, because one of the best preventive measures is providing accurate and thorough information to people.

AIDS Patients

Treating patients infected with HIV and those who have developed AIDS is one of today's most challenging areas of medicine. New research findings occur frequently and may change treatment and diagnostic procedures. Because HIV infection is nearly always fatal, patients—and their families and caregivers—usually experience extreme psychological stress.

The AIDS Patient Profile

Although there are certain high-risk populations, such as intravenous drug users and homosexual men, virtually no one is immune to AIDS. Research evidence shows that HIV has been in the United States since approximately 1970. This conclusion is based on knowledge about the incubation period of the disease and the initial reports of *Pneumocystis carinii* pneumonia and Kaposi's sarcoma in homosexual men beginning in 1978. These diseases, which had been quite rare, are now considered hallmarks of HIV infection.

Because the infection seemed to occur exclusively in homosexual men, it was originally called gay-related infectious disease, or GRID. Rapidly, however, it became apparent that the disease could be passed not only through male-to-male sexual contact but also through blood transfusion, through the sharing of intravenous drug paraphernalia, through occupational exposure, through male-to-female sexual contact, through female-to-female sexual contact, and from mother to fetus as well as from mother to infant during breast-feeding.

As of December 1996, 22.6 million men, women, and children were HIV-infected worldwide. That number is expected to increase to 200 million by the year 2000.

Homosexual men still constitute a large percentage of people with HIV infection and AIDS in the United States. Growth in infection of people in this group has slowed, however, as a result of educational campaigns and the population's adherence to "safer sex" practices. Data show that the disease occurs primarily among young people, especially those in large metropolitan areas. AIDS incidence rates for large metropolitan areas are approximately three times as high as rates for small metropolitan areas and nearly five times as high as rates in rural areas. Rural areas are, however, starting to show an increase in incidence.

Two groups of people who are contracting HIV infection in increasing numbers are intravenous drug users (especially African Americans and Hispanics in large metropolitan areas) and women. Because of the increase in infection among women, there has also been an increase in the number of infected children.

The CDC publishes a quarterly report, *The HIV/AIDS Surveillance Report,* which contains data about the incidence of HIV infection and AIDS nationwide. Information about age, gender, sexual orientation, race, occupation, residence, and source of infection are some of the facts collected in an effort to help epidemiologists generate an accurate picture of the patterns of the disease. Data also help identify the prevention programs most likely to succeed with a given population and help community leaders make decisions about the care of people with HIV infection and AIDS.

Chronic Disorders of the AIDS Patient

The impaired immune system of the AIDS patient permits opportunistic infections, which further reduce the body's ability to fight off infection. These infections attack many different parts of the body (Figure 21-3).

One of the cornerstones of the care of patients who have AIDS is to prevent opportunistic infections and identify such infections as quickly as possible when they occur. Identifying malignancies, if they occur, is also of utmost importance. If you are familiar with the common disorders an AIDS patient faces, you will be better able to identify early signs of infection or malignancy and point them out to the doctor. He may then initiate early treatment, which is usually most effective. You can help patients who have been diagnosed with HIV to understand the risks they face, as well as the measures best suited to preventing particular infections.

***Pneumocystis Carinii* Pneumonia.** The most common opportunistic infection in AIDS patients is *Pneumocystis carinii* pneumonia, or PCP. Nearly 75% of AIDS patients experience this protozoal infection, with symptoms of fever, cough, and breathing difficulties. These symptoms are often very general, may not be very severe, and can be overlooked or attributed to other problems. Diagnosis is made through chest radiographs (x-ray film records of the

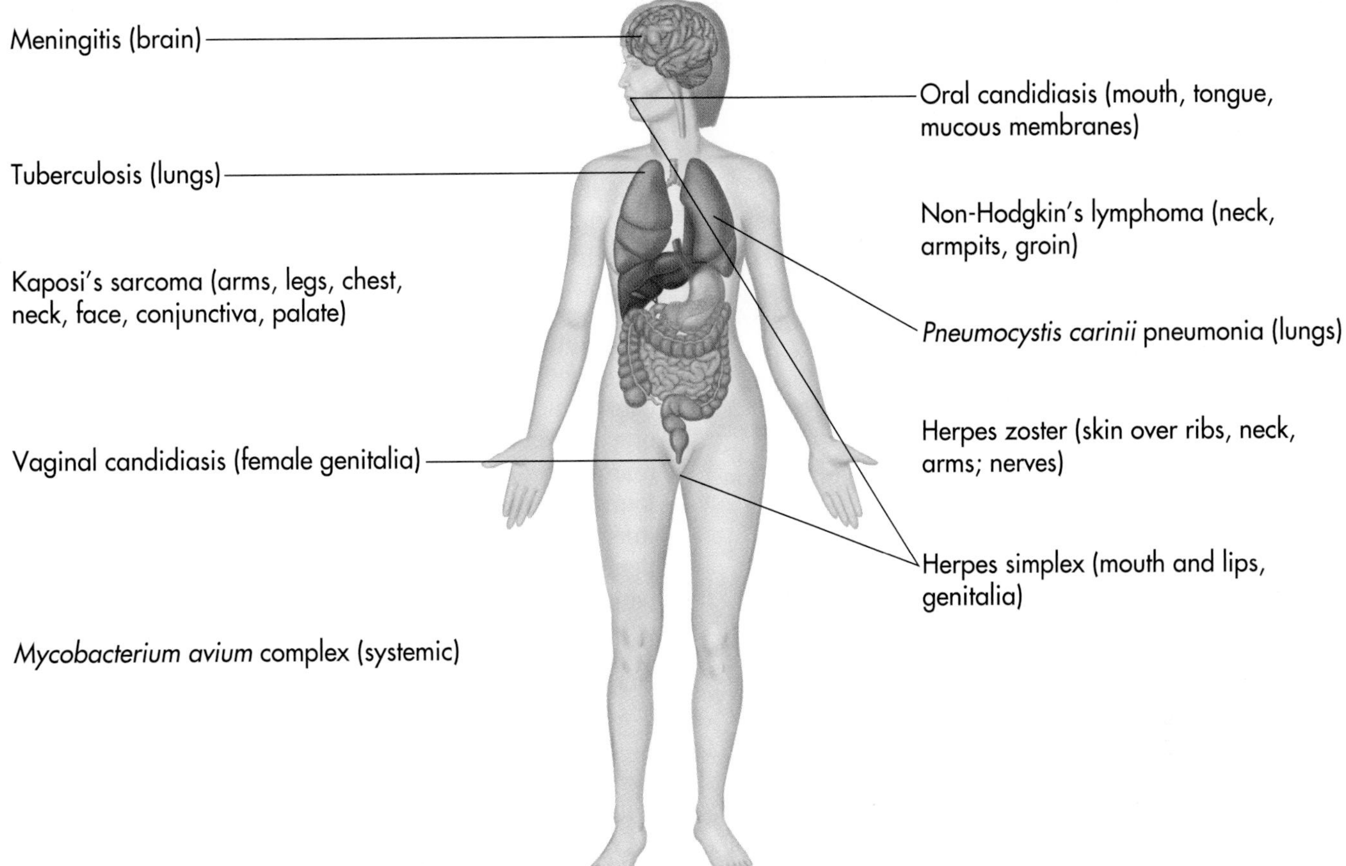

Figure 21-3. The AIDS patient may contract a variety of opportunistic infections, which affect many different parts of the body.

chest), the Wright-Giesma sputum stain (substances that impart color so sputum can be studied), and bronchoalveolar lavage (a technique by which cells and fluid from alveoli, tiny sacs in the lungs, are removed for diagnosis).

AIDS patients should avoid contact with people who have colds or the flu. If contact is unavoidable, ill people should wear surgical masks to reduce the risk of spreading infection to AIDS patients. Everyone who comes in regular contact with AIDS patients should have a current flu immunization. Flu immunizations must be renewed every year.

Treatments for *Pneumocystis carinii* pneumonia can cause side effects. Some of the side effects are measurable only through laboratory tests, whereas some may be reported by the patient. Side effects include the following:

- Nausea
- Rash
- Hypotension (abnormally low blood pressure)
- Anemia
- Neutropenia (diminished number of neutrophils in the blood)
- Hepatitis
- Colitis (inflammation of the colon)
- Leukopenia (reduction in the number of leukocytes in the blood)

Kaposi's Sarcoma. Kaposi's sarcoma is a particularly aggressive form of tumor. Although it is uncommon in the general population (it is found in males averaging age 89 in the Mediterranean Sea region), it is the most common HIV-related malignancy. Kaposi's sarcoma appears as reddish purple to dark blue skin lesions that are found anywhere on the body (Figure 21-4). They are usually first found on the arms and legs, then on the chest, neck, and face. The lesions may appear in areas such as the conjunctiva or the eyelids, between the toes, behind the ears, and on the palate.

Treatment for Kaposi's sarcoma includes chemotherapy. Chemotherapy may cause flulike symptoms accompanied by fever.

Non-Hodgkin's Lymphoma. The second most common malignancy associated with HIV infection is non-Hodgkin's lymphoma (NHL). Because NHL can appear in multiple sites, it is difficult to predict the problems HIV-infected patients will encounter with it. The symptoms vary, depending on which, if any, opportunistic infections are present. Other considerations are the rate of tumor growth and the location of the malignancy.

Tuberculosis. Tuberculosis is often a curable disease when treatment regimens are followed exactly and completely. (See Chapter 20 for more information on tubercu-

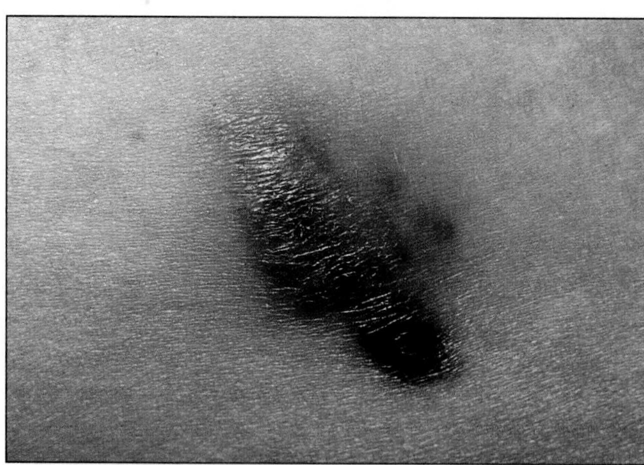

Figure 21-4. Kaposi's sarcoma is a rare form of skin cancer associated with AIDS.

losis.) There has, however, been a rise in the number of cases in recent years as a result of HIV infection and antibiotic resistance. HIV infection is by far the single largest risk factor for the development of tuberculosis infection into the active form of the disease. HIV infection reduces the effectiveness of the immune system and makes it possible for tuberculosis bacilli to multiply and spread infection more easily. AIDS patients who have symptoms of tuberculosis should receive the Mantoux skin test (TB scratch test), a chest x-ray, and possibly a sputum culture. These tests are the only means of definitive diagnosis. AIDS patients should be tested yearly for tuberculosis infection. If they suspect they have been exposed to the pathogen through contact with a known or suspected source, they should undergo testing at the earliest opportunity.

The Mantoux skin test yields false negative results in some people with AIDS. In fact, as the number of helper T cells decreases, the more likely it is for patients to exhibit negative results. When two or more other antigens are combined with the tuberculin units used in the Mantoux test, a more accurate picture of infection emerges.

If patients do not respond to any of the substances injected for the test, they are considered to have an **anergic reaction.** An anergic reaction occurs when the body is unable to mount a normal response to invasion by a pathogen. Patients who respond to the other substances but not to the tuberculin units are considered free of tuberculosis infection. People with AIDS who exhibit an anergic reaction to the test should be considered for preventive therapy designed to halt development of the tuberculosis infection into disease.

Mycobacterium Avium **Complex (MAC) Infection.** *Mycobacterium avium* complex (MAC) is responsible for 97% of the nontuberculous bacterial infections in AIDS patients, although it is difficult to detect in these patients. Postmortem studies of AIDS patients indicate that the disease is undetected in more than 50% of cases. The pathogen can be acquired orally or through inhalation. Symptoms include the following:

- Systemic illness
- Fever
- Night sweats
- Fatigue
- Weight loss
- Diarrhea
- Stomach pain

Meningitis. The pathogens that cause many of the common opportunistic infections in patients with AIDS can result in several forms of meningitis. Diagnosis is often difficult because the presenting symptoms and laboratory results are not always consistent with those found in patients without compromised immune systems. Infection of the central nervous system in an AIDS patient can lead to AIDS dementia complex, in which the patient's mental and motor functions gradually and irreversibly decline.

Oral Candidiasis. More than half the patients diagnosed with AIDS develop oral candidiasis (*Candida albicans*), or thrush. The infection in an AIDS patient takes one of three primary forms:

- Reddened, atrophic patches on the hard mucous membranes
- Coating of the tongue
- Patches on the tongue, soft palate, tonsils, and mucous membranes toward the cheek

Vaginal Candidiasis. Women who have AIDS are predisposed to vaginal candidiasis. Those who develop the infection often experience a severe case that is difficult to cure. Symptoms include these:

- Pruritus (extreme itching)
- Dysuria (painful or difficult urination)
- Labial excoriations (abrasions of the genital labia)
- Thick, adherent discharge

Herpes Simplex. One of the most common infections experienced by humans, herpes simplex virus (HSV), can manifest in a range of forms, from mild to life-threatening. People with compromised immune systems are especially at risk for infection by HSV. There are two forms of the virus: HSV-1 and HSV-2. HSV-2 is transmitted primarily through sexual exposure, whereas HSV-1 is transmitted primarily through exposure to oral secretions. It is possible, however, for HSV-2 to be transmitted through oral contact and for HSV-1 to be transmitted sexually.

Herpes Zoster. The herpes virus that causes chickenpox may become dormant in the body and may return as shingles, or herpes zoster. Generally the patient experiences pain followed by the appearance of reddened, raised lesions on one side of the body. In a patient who has a healthy immune system, the lesions last from 3 to 5 days and clear up within 15 days, although it can take an additional month for the patient's skin to return to its preinfection condition. In a patient who is **immunocompromised** (having an impaired or weakened immune system), however, the formation of lesions can last as long as 2 weeks, and clearing may not occur for 21 to 28 days. Herpes zoster rarely proves fatal, even in immunocompromised patients.

Treating Opportunistic Infections

The wide variety of opportunistic infections that may afflict AIDS patients makes treatment management a challenge. In some instances drug side effects that patients with intact immune systems would easily tolerate pose major problems for the immunocompromised patient. Repeated episodes of infection can leave a patient allergic to treatment medication or with a tolerance to the medication, requiring higher and higher doses for effectiveness. The pathogen itself may mutate into a strain that is resistant to treatment. Treatment for one set of symptoms may conflict with treatment for another set or may exacerbate other symptoms.

Testing Regulations

Currently the CDC does not recommend mandatory HIV testing for health-care workers. Health-care professionals emphasize that a health-care worker's chances of being infected by a patient are much higher than a patient's chances of being infected by a health-care worker. Although there have been well-publicized incidents of infection from health-care worker to patient, no required testing programs exist today. (Refer to Chapter 19 for additional precautions for avoiding transmission of disease from health-care workers to patients.)

Drug Treatments

Pharmaceutical companies are devoting resources to research and development of vaccines to prevent HIV infection and medications to cure the disease once patients are infected. For example, leading pharmaceutical companies have developed several drugs called **protease inhibitors,** which block the production of a key enzyme, protease, that is required for the host cell to replicate the virus. One of these drugs, ritonavir, reduced the death rate of a

Table 21-2

FDA-Approved Drugs for HIV/AIDS Patients

Classification	Purpose	Examples of Drugs
Antibacterial	Treatment and prevention of mycobacterial infections; also treatment of *Pneumocystis carinii* pneumonia (PCP)	Azithromycin (1996), clarithromycin (1993/1995), rifabutin (1992), sulfamethoxazole (1981/1994)
Antiemetic	Treatment of anorexia	Dronabinol (1992)
Antifolate	Treatment of PCP	Trimetrexate glucuronate (1993)
Antifungal	Treatment of oral candidiasis and meningitis	Fluconazole (1990), itraconazole (1992)
Antimalarial	Treatment of toxoplasmosis	Pyrimethamine (1988)
Antimycobacterial	Prevention of *Mycobacterium avium* complex (MAC)	Rifabutin (1992)
Antineoplastic	Treatment of Kaposi's sarcoma	Daunorubicin (liposomal) (1996), doxorubicin hydrochloride (1995), interferon alfa-2a (1988), interferon alfa-2b (1988), megestrol acetate (1993), trimetrexate glucuronate (1993)
Antineutropenic	Treatment of neutropenia	Filgrastim (1991), sargramostim (1991)
Antiprotozoal	Treatment of PCP	Atovaquone (1992), pentamidine (IM + IV) (1984), pentamidine (aerosolized) (1989), trimetrexate glucuronate (1993)

continued

Table 21–2 continued

FDA-Approved Drugs for HIV/AIDS Patients

Classification	Purpose	Examples of Drugs
Antiretroviral	Treatment of adult and pediatric patients who are intolerant to or deteriorating on approved therapies, or for use with AZT; prevention of perinatal transmission in HIV+ pregnant women and in newborns	Didanosine (1991/1992), indinavir sulfate (1996), lamivudine (1995), nevirapine (1996), ritonavir (1996), saquinavir mesylate (1995), stavudine (1994), zalcitabine (1992/1994), zidovudine (1987/1990/1994)
Antiviral	Treatment of cytomegalovirus (CMV) retinitis	Cidofovir (1996), foscarnet (1991), ganciclovir (IV) (1989), ganciclovir (oral) (1994/1995), ganciclovir (implant) (1996), interferon alfa-2a (1988), interferon alfa-2b (1988/1991)
Appetite stimulant	Treatment of patients with significant weight loss	Dronabinol (1992), megestrol acetate (1993)
Folic acid antagonist	Treatment of toxoplasmosis	Pyrimethamine (1988)
Hematinic	Treatment of anemia related to AZT therapy	Erythropoietin (1990)
Hematopoietic stimulant	Treatment of cancer patients	Filgrastim (1991), sargramostim (1991)
Immunomodulator	Prevention of infections	Filgrastim (1991), immune globulin (IV) (1993), interferon alfa-2a (1988/1991), interferon alfa-2b (1992)
Protease inhibitor	Blocking of production of enzyme needed for HIV replication	Indinavir sulfate (1996), ritonavir (1996), saquinavir mesylate (1995)
Red blood cell growth	Treatment of anemia	Erythropoietin (1990)

Source: Centers for Disease Control and Prevention.

Note: Numbers in parentheses represent the date or dates the drugs were approved for the specified purpose.

group of patients with advanced AIDS by 50% during a 7-month study period. Another drug, indinavir, when used in combination with two other AIDS drug treatments, reduced the level of the virus in blood samples by a factor of 1000. Table 21-2 identifies different classifications of drugs currently approved by the FDA for treatment of diseases associated with HIV infection and AIDS.

Researchers are looking for ways to determine which diseases a patient is likely to develop and how well a patient will respond to antiviral medications. Current research indicates that the amount of HIV present in the bloodstream may be a good indicator of the patient's condition. The host cell can mutate the virus into resistant strains if the infection is not treated early enough with medication of sufficient strength. Testing for the amount of HIV that has escaped from the lymph system into the bloodstream can help doctors determine the best time at which to begin antiviral therapy and the appropriate dosage.

Zidovudine. The first drug approved for use against AIDS was zidovudine (azidothymidine [AZT]). In general, doctors prescribe AZT therapy, in combination with other drugs, when the patient's T-cell count dips below 500 cells per milliliter of blood. They use several drugs to provide a multilayered defense against the virus. If the dosage is not strong enough, the host cell may mutate the virus into a superresistant strain. If only one drug is used, the virus may mutate into a strain resistant to that particular drug.

There are, however, many side effects common to the use of this drug, including the following:

- Anemia
- Nausea
- Malaise
- Headache
- Insomnia
- Neutropenia
- Dementia

Approximately 40% of patients using zidovudine experience some or all of these side effects. Side effects ease for most patients within 6 weeks of starting the therapy. For other patients, doctors need to adjust or interrupt the dosage, especially if patients experience anemia, neutropenia, or dementia.

Patients who are receiving zidovudine therapy must be closely monitored during the first 2 months of therapy. Monthly monitoring should include physical examinations, patient interviews, and complete blood counts, including platelet counts and differential counts. After the 2-month period, these tests, as well as liver function tests and phosphokinase levels, should be completed quarterly.

Didanosine and Zalcitabine. Zidovudine is effective in patients for only a limited time. Eventually the disease resumes its progression despite the use of zidovudine. When the disease progresses, most patients are switched to didanosine (dideoxyinosine or ddI) or zalcitabine (dideoxycytidine or ddC), which are chemically related to zidovudine. These medications are also used for patients who are intolerant of zidovudine.

Didanosine users commonly suffer from diarrhea caused not by the drug itself but by the buffering agent used to carry the drug. The drug is dispensed in pill or powder form and must be taken 2 to 3 hours before eating. The powder form contains more of the buffering agent; therefore, patients who use this form are more likely to encounter diarrhea as a side effect. The following are other side effects:

- Peripheral neuropathy (a disorder affecting the central nervous system)
- Pancreatitis (inflammation of the pancreas)
- Hepatitis
- Neutropenia
- Dry mouth

Tell patients not to use alcohol while taking didanosine and to be alert for symptoms of pancreatitis, such as abdominal pain, nausea, and vomiting. Tell patients that if these symptoms occur, they should stop taking the medication until tests can be completed to rule out or identify pancreatitis.

Zalcitabine is easier to administer than didanosine and is less expensive. Although zalcitabine may also cause peripheral neuropathy, the patient's risk of pancreatitis is lower. Side effects related to zalcitabine but not to didanosine include a skin rash and ulcers on mucous membranes.

Patients who receive either didanosine or zalcitabine should be monitored each month. At that time you may assist in conducting various tests, including a complete blood count and a neurological examination.

Stavudine. Some patients cannot tolerate zidovudine, didanosine, or zalcitabine. Stavudine (d4T) may be an alternative for them. Patients who receive this drug should receive a monthly neurological examination as well as various other tests.

Other Medications. New drugs are being approved for the treatment of AIDS on an ongoing basis. One of your responsibilities as a medical assistant is to stay informed about possible therapies for patients. Then if the physician begins using a new therapy, you can communicate information to patients at a level they can understand. The CDC is one good source of information about available medications.

Continuing Research. Research in several areas has demonstrated that some people appear to be immune to infection by HIV, are able to coexist with the virus, or have the ability to clear the virus from their systems. One study of 58 female prostitutes in Nairobi, Kenya, is seeking to determine why these women, after repeated exposure to the virus through unprotected sexual contact, show no evidence of infection (Toufexis, 1996). This elimination of the virus from the human system has led epidemiologists to study these cases to make new vaccines or treatments to boost the immune system's ability to defend against the virus.

Other Blood-Borne Infections

Hepatitis and HIV infections are the best known of the blood-borne pathogens you may encounter working in the medical field. There are also several other blood-borne diseases of which you should be aware. Some of these diseases pose particular risk to patients already infected with HIV. For this reason, you should advise HIV-positive patients about symptoms and preventive measures related to the diseases.

Cytomegalovirus

People with compromised, or impaired, immune systems and infants (whose immune systems undergo additional development after birth) are especially at risk for cytomegalovirus (CMV). CMV is an extremely common infection. Blood tests show that nearly 80% of adults tested have antibodies for the virus. The presence of these antibodies indicates an infection at some point in the person's life. The infection rarely causes noticeable symptoms in adults with normal immune systems.

The disease sometimes takes a form similar to infectious mononucleosis in otherwise healthy adults, however. It may develop into severe lung disease in immunocompromised adults. Symptoms of the infection may include swollen glands, fever, and fatigue.

Pregnant women can pass the disease on to their newborns. Infants with CMV present signs of jaundice, a rash, and low birth weight. In severe cases CMV can cause brain damage, mental retardation, deafness, blindness, and death.

Erythema Infectiosum (Parvovirus B19)

Erythema infectiosum, or fifth disease, is a moderately contagious disease seen mainly in children and caused by human parvovirus B19. The term *fifth disease* was assigned to this "fifth" eruptive disease found in children in the late 1800s. (Sources vary on which diseases were considered first through fourth, but all include measles and rubella. Popular knowledge adds mumps and chickenpox to the list, while some more formal sources include scarlet fever and Dukes' disease.) The disease is characterized by the abrupt onset of a rash. The virus may be transmitted from mother to fetus, and although it does not cause birth defects, there is some risk of fetal death from infection. More severe signs of infection may be seen in immunocompromised patients.

Human T-Cell Lymphotrophic Virus

Infection with the human T-cell lymphotrophic virus (HTLV-1) often appears in intravenous drug users, in people who have received multiple blood transfusions, and in the sexual partners, children, and household contacts of infected people. The virus attacks T cells, an important component of the body's immune system, by penetrating the cells and incorporating its genetic material into the cells' genetic material.

Some people who are infected with HTLV-1 show no symptoms, while others exhibit severe symptoms. Infection with HTLV-1 most commonly leads to adult T-cell leukemia/lymphoma (ATLL), although patients can also contract disturbances of the spinal cord or partial paralysis.

Physical findings in cases of ATLL include skin lesions, disease of the lymph nodes, fever, abdominal distress, arthritis, and sometimes hypercalcemia (an excess of calcium in the blood). Diagnosis is confirmed when the virus is found in blood or other body tissues.

Listeriosis

Listeriosis is an infectious disease caused by the bacterium *Listeria monocytogenes.* Once infected, an individual can pass the infection to others through contact with blood or blood products, and a pregnant woman can pass the infection to her fetus.

If the infection is passed to a fetus during the later stages of pregnancy, the infant may be stillborn. Infected infants who survive may develop meningitis (inflammation of the membranes covering the brain and spinal cord), pneumonia, or septicemia (blood poisoning).

Symptoms in infected adults may include fever, shock, rash, and generalized aches, but most people do not notice any symptoms. The disease can rapidly cause death in elderly or immunocompromised patients through circulatory collapse.

Listeriosis is diagnosed by blood tests. If symptoms are present and the patient is at high risk, however, antibiotic therapy is sometimes initiated before positive identification of the pathogen.

Malaria

Malarial infection is spread from person to person primarily through the bite of infected mosquitoes. There have also been cases of transmission from mother to fetus, as well as from an infected to an uninfected person through an accidental needle stick. Malaria is mainly a tropical infection present in parts of Africa, Asia, and Central and South America.

The parasite usually enters the bloodstream through the mosquito's bite. It invades the liver, moving from there into red blood cells. Within a red blood cell, the parasite multiplies and eventually causes rupture of the cell. When the cell ruptures, new parasites are released to continue the cycle of infection, growth, rupture, and release. An infected person does not exhibit symptoms until several of these cycles have occurred. Symptoms are caused by the pigments released from the red blood cells and metabolic toxins from the parasites.

A 4- to 8-hour, three-part cycle marks infection with malaria. In the first stage of the cycle, the patient experiences shaking chills. In the second stage, the patient experiences high fever that spikes as high as 104° or 105°F. The third stage is marked by excessive perspiration. The patient may also report nausea, vomiting, headache, and gastrointestinal symptoms and may exhibit an enlarged spleen and liver tenderness. Laboratory results will show normal or decreased white blood cell counts and decreased platelet count.

Avoidance of infection is the best means of preventing the spread of malaria. Once infected, most people recover from the disease if treated quickly. When malaria is suspected, blood tests are performed every few hours until the diagnosis is confirmed or another reason is discovered for the patient's symptoms.

Syphilis

Syphilis is a sexually transmitted disease caused by the spirochete *Treponema pallidum.* A pregnant woman can pass this disease to her fetus. An affected infant experiences the most severe form of syphilis. An infant born with congenital syphilis may exhibit nail exfoliation (the nails falling off), hair loss, rhinitis (inflammation of the nose), lesions, anemia, failure to thrive, and paralysis of one or more limbs.

Syphilis in adults and adolescents occurs in the following three stages.

1. In the first stage, infection is indicated by the initial appearance of a painless ulcer, called a **chancre.** This ulcer may appear on the tongue, lips, genitalia, rectum, or elsewhere.
2. Patients in the second stage may experience nontender swelling of the lymph nodes. This stage may also include a generalized skin rash, fever, and the presence of mucous-membrane lesions. Condylomas (wartlike lesions of the skin) may appear in areas of moist skin.
3. The third stage may occur between several years and 2 or 3 decades after initial infection. During this stage, the patient may exhibit tumors of the skin, bones, and liver, as well as central nervous system manifestations such as dementia, abnormal reflexes, and psychosis.

Table 21-3

States' Reporting Guidelines for HIV Infection

States Requiring Reports by Name	States Requiring Anonymous Reports	States Not Requiring Reports
Alabama	Georgia	Alaska
Arizona	Iowa	California
Arkansas	Kansas	Connecticut
Colorado	Kentucky	Delaware
Idaho	Maine	Florida
Illinois	Montana	Hawaii
Indiana	New Hampshire	Louisiana
Michigan	Oregon	Maryland
Minnesota	Rhode Island	Massachusetts
Mississippi	Texas	Nebraska
Missouri		New Mexico
Nevada		New York
New Jersey		Pennsylvania
North Carolina		Vermont
North Dakota		Washington
Ohio		District of Columbia
Oklahoma		
South Carolina		
South Dakota		
Tennessee		
Utah		
Virginia		
West Virginia		
Wisconsin		
Wyoming		

Source: Centers for Disease Control and Prevention, AIDS Clearinghouse, Rockville, MD.

Between the first two stages and the final stage is a period of latency during which the patient exhibits no symptoms and appears to be disease-free. Blood tests will still show indications of infection, and treatment is usually administered in an effort to prevent the disease from reaching the late stage.

Identifying and treating syphilis in an HIV-positive individual are difficult tasks. Because the presence of the HIV pathogen alters the function of the immune system, test results that normally indicate the presence of syphilis may yield false-negative findings. Additional tests are required to confirm diagnosis. With the presence of HIV, the course of the syphilis infection may be accelerated, and the benefits of drug therapy to combat the infection may be reduced.

Toxoplasmosis

The primary source of the pathogen *Toxoplasma gondii* is cat feces. Although undercooked meat products are another source, most cases appear in people who have handled cat litter boxes. For that reason pregnant women and those with compromised immune systems, such as patients with AIDS, should not handle cat litter boxes.

Most people infected with toxoplasmosis experience no symptoms. Symptoms may, however, include fever, malaise, sore throat, rash, stiff neck, disease of the lymph nodes, and fatigue. A pregnant woman may pass the infection to her fetus, and the infection may result in spontaneous abortion, malformation, or retardation (depending on the trimester in which the organism enters). Infants who survive may also suffer from deafness, blindness, brain damage, and seizures. Diagnosis is confirmed through blood tests.

Reporting Guidelines

Each state formulates requirements for reporting HIV infection and AIDS. That information is then sent to the Centers for Disease Control and Prevention. Table 21-3 lists states that require reporting of HIV infection by name of patient, states that accept anonymous reporting, and states that do not require reporting. Follow your employer's guidelines or procedures when you must report cases of HIV infection.

When you report a communicable disease, you must fill out a report form. Your state health department may have a different form for each reportable disease. You must obtain the correct form and a disease identification number from the health department every time you report a communicable disease. To fill out such a form, you need access to the following information:

- Disease identification (usually a code number, as well as the name of the disease)
- Patient identification (including name, address, date of birth, sex, ethnic origin, and occupational or educational status) if required (as already noted, some states require only anonymous reporting of some diseases)
- Infection history (date of onset, vaccination history, laboratory results)
- Reporting-institution information (name of person completing report, title, contact information)

Each state and each medical facility have specific guidelines that you must adhere to when filling out such a form. Procedure 21-2 describes, in general, how to notify state and county agencies about reportable diseases.

Reporting guidelines must also be followed if a worker comes in contact with a substance that may transmit infection. These guidelines, which are explained in OSHA's Bloodborne Pathogens Standard, include reporting exposure incidents to employers immediately. (See Chapter 19 for specific guidelines on handling exposure incidents.)

Patient Education

Patient education is one of the most effective means of preventing disease transmission. As a medical assistant, you are in a pivotal position in relation to your patients. You can assess patients' understanding of their risk for infection, measures they must take to eradicate an infection (if possible), potential dangers posed by treatments, and methods for controlling an infection's spread. Staying up-to-date on new information will help you provide patients with effective, relevant education.

Drug Trials

New drug treatments for HIV infection and AIDS are being tested every day. Some patients may be interested in information about clinical drug trials. **Clinical drug trials** are internationally recognized research protocols designed to evaluate the efficacy or safety of drugs and to produce scientifically valid results. According to your institution's protocol, you may be required to introduce certain patients to such programs or to monitor patients involved in drug trial programs. You can obtain information about drug trials from the AIDS Clinical Trials Information Service at 800-874-2572.

Patients With Special Concerns

You will be responsible for educating patients with a variety of needs and concerns. Some patients, particularly teenagers and patients about to be discharged from the hospital, may have specific concerns involving HIV and HBV infection.

Teenagers. You may work with teenagers who have come in to obtain a means of birth control or receive treatment for sexually transmitted diseases (STDs). During the patient interview, you are in a position to educate the teenagers about the dangers of HIV and HBV infection. Most teenagers think that they are invincible and that disease happens only to "other people." You can effectively educate teenagers about HIV and HBV infection by helping them realize that disease can happen to anyone. Begin by establishing a trusting relationship with them and by providing them with facts rather than lectures or moral appeals. Figure 21-7 shows how commonly various risk factors, or exposure categories, are implicated in the transmission of AIDS to male adolescents aged 13 to 19. Figure 21-8 provides similar information for females aged 13 to 19. Armed with data such as these, you can stress to teenage patients the importance of preventive behaviors in avoiding HIV infection.

The Patient About to Be Discharged. When a patient has been hospitalized with HBV or HIV infection, the disruption in his life often lingers long past the discharge date. He must make changes and continue some treatment when he goes home. Your job as a medical assistant is to make sure that the patient comes to the medical office for follow-up care, reports any adverse reactions to therapy or treatment, and knows which signs and symptoms to report to the doctor. You must also ensure that the patient knows what precautions to take to avoid transmitting the infection to others.

As part of the education process, the patient may request additional information from you, or you may need to provide information to the patient's family members or other caregivers. See "Educating the Patient" for suggestions on where to obtain information for patients and their families.

Multicultural Concerns

Although you must be sensitive to and respectful toward patients from all backgrounds, you may need to target your education efforts toward certain groups. For example, according to the CDC's quarterly report, the incidence of HIV infection is increasing more in some groups than in others. Data in the report on the pattern of the disease can help you ascertain which groups need improved education. If you work with patients who are in these high-risk groups or who know people in them, you are in a unique position to provide them with information on preventive measures they can follow to avoid exposure to blood-borne pathogens. Because some patients

PROCEDURE 21-2

Notifying State and County Agencies About Reportable Diseases

MICHIGAN DEPARTMENT OF PUBLIC HEALTH
Division of Disease Surveillance

ENTERIC ILLNESS CASE INVESTIGATION
(Please check appropriate illness)

_______Shigellosis
_______Non-typhoid Salmonellosis
_______Campylobacter enteritis
_______Giardiasis
_______Amebiasis

CASE INFORMATION

Name: ______________ Age or Birthdate: ______________ Sex: ________ Race: ________

Address: ______________ (Street) (City) (County) (Zip) Phone: ______________

Occupation: ______________ (What) (Where) *High Risk: Y N
(If infant or student list school, nursery or day care center)

Attending Physician: ______________ Address or Phone: ______________ Was the patient hospitalized: Y N

Hospital: ______________ Dates: ______________ (Admission) (Discharge)

Onset: ______________ Date recovered: ______________ Symptom Summary: ______________

Suspected Causative Agent: ______________
(include species or serotype if known)

HOUSEHOLD CONTACTS INFORMATION

Name	Age	Family Relationship	Occupation	*High Risk Y N	Provide date of onset for all household members with concurrent similar illness
1)					
2)					
3)					
4)					
5)					
6)					
7)					
8)					
9)					
10)					

*"High Risk" = occupation as food handler, direct patient care worker, day care center worker or person attending day care or who is institutionalized. Stool specimens should be obtained on "high risk" cases and "high risk" household contacts as appropriate for the illness. Results may be recorded in Laboratory Information Section of this form (see over).

Name of the person who completed this form: ______________ County: ______________

Information obtained from: ______________ Date: ______________

Telephone Interview: ______________ Home Visit: ______________ Outbreak Investigation: ______________

C-30 Rev. 10/83 AUTH: Act 368, P.A. 1978

Figure 21-5. Some states have specific forms for use with particular communicable diseases or diseases of a certain type.

continued

PROCEDURE 21-2 continued

Notifying State and County Agencies About Reportable Diseases

Objective: To report cases of infection with reportable disease to the proper state or county health department

OSHA Guidelines: This procedure does not involve exposure to blood, body fluids, or tissues.

Materials: Communicable disease report form, pen, envelope, stamp

Method

1. Check to be sure you have the correct form. Some states have specific forms for each reportable infectious disease or type of disease (Figure 21-5), as well as a general form (Figure 21-6). CDC forms may also be used for reporting specific diseases.
2. Fill in all blank areas unless they are shaded (generally for local health department use).
3. Follow office procedures for submitting the report to a supervisor or physician before sending it out.
4. Sign and date the form. Address the envelope, put a stamp on it, and place it in the mail.

NON-HOUSEHOLD CONTACTS WITH A CONCURRENT SIMILAR ILLNESS

Name	Approximate date of onset of symptoms	Address and/or Phone	Relationship to case (Nature of contact)
1)			
2)			
3)			
4)			
5)			

ADDITIONAL EXPOSURES OR COMMENTS

Home Sewage System: Municipal Septic Tank Other________

Home drinking Water Type: Municipal Private Well Other________

As appropriate for the illness, ask about meals eaten away from home, stores where groceries bought, brand of poultry, meat, dairy products consumed, overnight travel, recent foreign travel, group functions, exposure to raw milk, untreated water, animals, etc. within one incubation period before onset.

(shigellosis to 7 days, salmonellosis - up to 3 days, Campylobacter enteritis - up to 10 days)

Be specific, provide place name(s) and date(s).

FOLLOW-UP FECAL CULTURE RESULTS FOR "HIGH RISK" CASE AND/OR CONTACTS.

Name or Initials	Date(s) Obtained and Findings
1)	
2)	
3)	
4)	
5)	

Figure 21-5. Continuation of form.

ARIZONA DEPARTMENT OF HEALTH SERVICES
COMMUNICABLE DISEASE REPORT
Important Instructions on Reverse Side
PLEASE PRINT OR TYPE

County/IHS ID Number/Chapter	State ID Number

PATIENT'S NAME (Last) (First)	DATE OF BIRTH	SEX ☐ Male ☐ Female	ETHNICITY ☐ Hispanic ☐ Non-Hispanic
STREET ADDRESS	CENSUS TRACT	CITY	RACE ☐ White ☐ Am. Indian ☐ Asian ☐ Black ☐ Other ☐ Unknown
COUNTY / STATE	ZIP CODE	PHONE NO.	
DIAGNOSIS OR SUSPECT REPORTABLE CONDITION			COUNTY USE ONLY: LAB CONFIRMATION DATE:______ ☐ Negative ☐ Positive ☐ Not Done ☐ Unknown
DATE ONSET / DATE OF DIAGNOSIS	LAB RESULTS		
PATIENT OCCUPATION OR SCHOOL			
PHYSICIAN OR OTHER REPORTING SOURCE	PHONE NUMBER		COUNTY USE ONLY: ☐ Confirmed case ☐ Probable case ☐ Outbreak Associated ☐ Ruled Out
STREET ADDRESS	CITY	STATE / ZIP CODE	

Original and 1st copy to County Health Department ☐ CHECK IF ADDITIONAL FORMS ARE NEEDED (Quantity)________

REPORTABLE DISEASES

Arizona Revised Statutes and Arizona Administrative Code require the following diseases to be reported to the County Health Department or Indian Health Services within 5 business days of diagnosis or treatment.

AIDS[3]
Amebiasis[1]
Anthrax
Aseptic meningitis
Botulism*
Brucellosis
Campylobacteriosis[1]
Chancroid[3]
Chlamydial infections (genital)[3]
Cholera*
Coccidioidomycosis
Colorado tick fever
Conjunctivitis, acute[2]
Cryptosporidiosis
Dengue
Diphtheria*
Ehrlichiosis
Encephalitis, viral
Foodborne illness/ Waterborne illness*
Giardiasis[1]
Gonorrhea[3]
Haemophilus influenzae*
Hemolytic Uremic Syndrome[1]
Hepatitis A[1]
Hepatitis B, Delta Hepatitis
Hepatitis Non-A, Non-B
Herpes Genitalis[3]
HIV[3]
Lead Poisoning[3]
Legionellosis
Leprosy
Listeriosis
Lyme Disease
Malaria
Measles*
Meningococcal disease*
Mumps
Pediculosis[2]
Pertussis*
Pesticide poisoning[3]
Plague*
Poliomyelitis*
Psittacosis
Q Fever
Rabies in humans*
Relapsing fever
Reye's Syndrome
Rocky Mt. spotted fever
Rubella*
Congenital rubella syn.
Salmonellosis[1]
Scabies[2]
Shigellosis[1]
Staphylococcal disease[1,2]
Streptococcal diseases[1,2]
Syphilis[3]
Tetanus
Toxic Shock Syndrome
Trichinosis
Tuberculosis[3]
Tuberculosis infection in children <6 yrs of age
Tularemia
Typhoid Fever[1]
Typhus fever
Varicella
Yellow Fever*

*Telephone report required to the County Health Department or Indian Health Services within 24 hours.

[1] Report within 24 hours of diagnosis if in food handler.

[2] Outbreak reports only

[3] These conditions are reported on other forms, call 1-800-334-1540 for a supply

ADHS/DPS/OIDS/IDES-1 (Rev. 11-94)

Figure 21-6. Each state has its own communicable disease report.

Exposure Categories Reported for Adolescent Males With AIDS, by Percentage (through December, 1995)

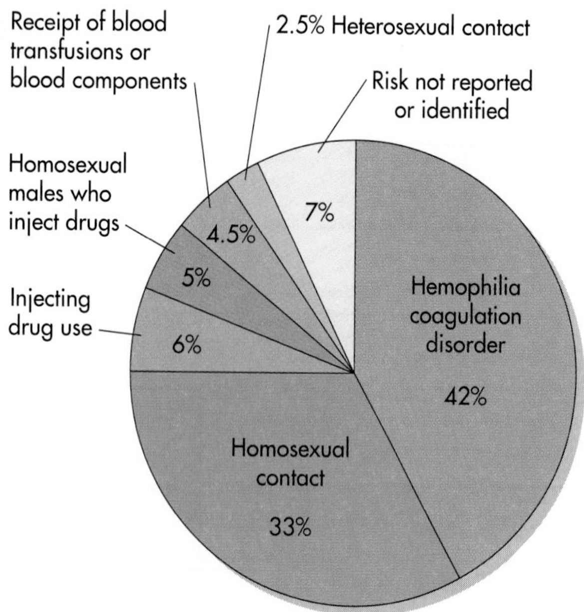

Figure 21-7. These percentages provide insight into the types of exposure male teenagers should guard against.
Source: *HIV/AIDS Surveillance Report.* Vol. 7, no. 2. Atlanta, GA: Centers for Disease Control and Prevention, December 1995.

may be reluctant to discuss sensitive subjects, be sure to have brochures available (in several languages) for them to take home and read.

Special Issues With Terminal Illness

In this chapter you have learned about a variety of blood-borne diseases. One of these diseases is almost always fatal, and others may be fatal in certain situations. Just as you need to educate patients about preventing such diseases and about methods of treatment, you need to provide support and counsel to patients, their families, and their loved ones when they are informed that their illnesses are **terminal,** or fatal. You must understand something of people's reactions to a terminal diagnosis to help them cope with the situation.

Patients react to the idea of dying in different ways. Some are angry that death is coming to them. Others are grateful that relief from pain and suffering is near. Many terminal patients respond by denying that they are dying. After patients fully realize that they are going to die, depression is a common reaction. The only thing you can be certain of is that no two patients respond to a terminal diagnosis in exactly the same way.

You can help patients come to terms with the fact that they are going to die by:

- Supporting and accepting them no matter how they react.
- Encouraging them to express their feelings and thoughts freely.
- Communicating respect through your use of nonverbal communication, including your posture and touch.
- Meeting reasonable needs and demands as quickly as possible.
- Providing referrals to hospices, which offer a variety of services, including personal care for patients who are dying and emotional support for them and their families.

Summary

Infectious diseases are transmitted in many different ways. Medical and surgical asepsis and various techniques and procedures for sanitizing, disinfecting, and sterilizing instruments, equipment, and surfaces all help prevent disease transmission. Specific transmission methods dictate which approaches work best for which diseases. The focus of this chapter has been blood-borne transmission.

The transmission of blood-borne pathogens is a particular concern for medical assistants as well as for people in many other professions. The pathogens that pose the greatest risk are HIV, HBV, and HCV. Infection with these pathogens can result in death or chronic disease.

Your role as a medical assistant is to help prevent the spread of such infectious diseases. The preventive measures you will take at work include following Universal

Exposure Categories Reported for Adolescent Females With AIDS, by Percentage (through December, 1995)

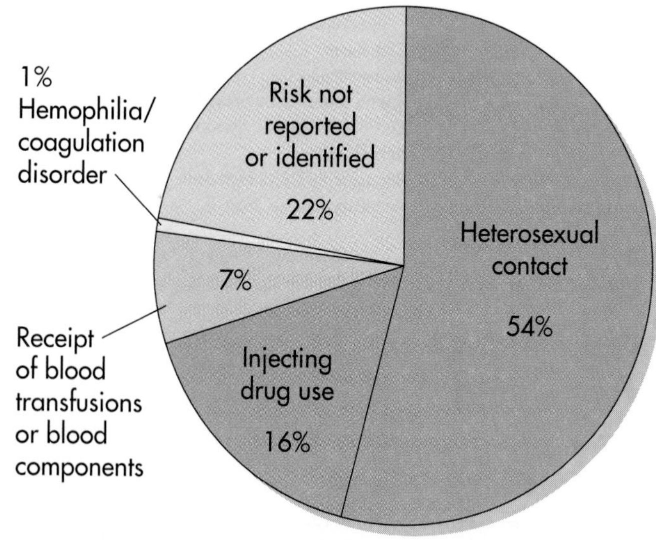

Figure 21-8. Female teenagers face greater risk of HIV infection from heterosexual contact than male teenagers do.

EDUCATING THE PATIENT

Obtaining Information About AIDS and Hepatitis

Some patients who have AIDS or hepatitis may want additional information about care options, drug treatments and clinical trials, prevention guidelines, risk factors, and therapy management. Many high-quality resources are available for these patients.

One of the best places to direct patients is to the Centers for Disease Control and Prevention, located in Atlanta, Georgia. The CDC offers a variety of services, such as the following:

- CDC National AIDS Clearinghouse, telephone number 800-458-5231
- CDC National AIDS Hotline, telephone number 800-342-2437
- AIDS Clinical Trials Information Service, telephone number 800-874-2572
- HIV/AIDS Treatment Information Service, telephone number 800-448-0440

The Consumer Information Center (CIC), in Pueblo, Colorado, offers a variety of free and low-cost booklets about many health matters, including topics such as HIV/AIDS, hepatitis, and other sexually transmitted diseases. The CIC can be reached at:

Consumer Information Center
Pueblo, CO 81009
303-544-5277, Ext. 370

Patients who are comfortable using computers and who have access to the World Wide Web can find a variety of resources there. The Web sites for both the CDC (www.cdc.gov) and the CIC (www.pueblo.gsa.gov) are very comprehensive.

Many local support and resource organizations may also be available to the patient. In your position you can serve both the patient, by helping him contact these organizations, and the organizations, by publicizing their efforts.

Precautions, watching patients for signs of infectious diseases, and educating patients about the risk factors associated with blood-borne diseases.

Information about infectious diseases changes constantly. You can best serve your patients and your employer if you keep up-to-date on research, advances in treatment, and general information. Your efforts with patient education may include information about preventive measures, drug trials, follow-up care, and hospices for terminally ill patients.

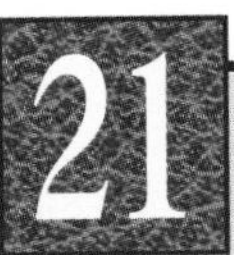

21 Chapter Review

Discussion Questions

1. Identify preventive measures you might recommend to a patient to limit her risk for acquiring HIV infection.
2. As a medical worker, what preventive measures can you take to avoid acquiring HBV infection? HCV infection?
3. Why do opportunistic infections pose such a risk to the HIV-infected patient?

Critical Thinking Questions

1. One of your patients brings his teenage son in for an examination. The son admits to engaging in sexual foreplay with a woman who has since been diagnosed with HIV infection. What questions would you ask the son to discover whether he is at risk? What tests might your office run to determine whether he has HIV infection? How long might he have to wait to find out whether he has contracted the infection?
2. Pair up with a classmate. Each of you should choose to debate one side of the following issue: All health-care personnel should be required to undergo testing for HIV infection.
3. While talking with one of your patients, an HIV-positive individual, you learn that friends have recently purchased a kitten for her. What will you do or say?

Application Activities

1. Working in a small group, have all members role-play a situation in which a patient and his family have just learned that he has HIV infection. Have one member of the group assume the role of the medical assistant and offer support and understanding to them. Then have other students in the class critique your approach.

continued →

21 Chapter Review

2. Contact your local legislature to determine what, if any, pertinent legislation is being considered that would have an impact on HIV-positive patients. Present your findings to the class in an oral report.
3. Identify resources in your area that a person might use if she is exposed to HIV. Explore what is available to patients at various points in the disease process. Prepare a brochure in which you identify the resources and what they provide.

Further Readings

Centers for Disease Control and Prevention. "U.S. Public Health Service Recommendations for Human Immunodeficiency Virus Counseling and Voluntary Testing for Pregnant Women." *Morbidity and Mortality Weekly Report (MMWR)* 44, no. RR-7 (2 July 1995): 1–15.

"Hepatitis." *Current Health 2*, December 1995, 20–21.

HIV/AIDS Surveillance Report. Vol. 7, no. 2. Atlanta, GA: Centers for Disease Control and Prevention, December 1995.

"H.I.V. and TB Join to Form Deadly Spiral." *New York Times*, 4 June 1995, sec. 1, p. 4.

Landau, Elaine. *Tuberculosis.* New York: Franklin Watts, 1995.

"Man of the Year: Dr. David Ho, AIDS Researcher." *Time*, 30 December 1996, 55–87.

Miller, Chris. "Information on Transmission of Hepatitis C Incomplete." *The Professional Medical Assistant* 27, no. 1 (January/February 1994): 4.

Ray, M. Catherine. "Seven Ways to Empower Dying Patients." *American Journal of Nursing* 96, no. 5 (May 1996): 56–57.

Schoub, Barry D. *AIDS and HIV in Perspective.* New York: Cambridge University Press, 1994.

Toufexis, Anastasia. "Are Some People Immune?" *Time*, 12 February 1996, 65.

Preparing the Examination and Treatment Area

CHAPTER OUTLINE

- The Medical Assistant's Role in Preparing the Examination Room
- The Examination Room
- Cleanliness in the Examination Room
- Room Temperature, Lighting, and Ventilation
- Medical Instruments and Supplies
- Physical Safety in the Examination Room

Key Terms

accessibility
consumable
fixative
general physical examination
occult blood
transcutaneous absorption

OBJECTIVES

After completing Chapter 22, you will be able to:

- Explain the medical assistant's role in preparing the examination room.
- Describe the layout and features of a typical examination room.
- Describe steps to prevent the spread of infection in the examination room.
- Explain how and when to disinfect examination room surfaces.
- Describe the importance of such factors as temperature, lighting, and ventilation in the examination room.
- Identify instruments and supplies used in a general physical examination, and tell how to arrange and prepare them.
- Explain how to eliminate hazards to physical safety in the examination room.

AREAS OF COMPETENCE

1997 ROLE DELINEATION STUDY

CLINICAL

Fundamental Principles

- Apply principles of aseptic technique and infection control

Patient Care

- Prepare and maintain examination and treatment areas
- Assist with examinations, procedures, and treatments

GENERAL (Transdisciplinary)

Legal Concepts

- Comply with established risk management and safety procedures

continued

The Medical Assistant's Role in Preparing the Examination Room

When a patient enters an examination room, the patient expects to find it clean and neat. The doctor assumes that all medical instruments and supplies necessary for an examination or treatment are ready to use. Preparing the examination room for patients and doctors is your responsibility. You must keep this room not only spotlessly clean and in good order but also free from obstacles that might cause an accidental injury. Safety, efficiency, and comfort are the main concerns in the examination room.

The Examination Room

The examination room is the area where the physician observes the patient, listens to the patient's description of symptoms, performs a general physical examination, and dispenses treatment. A physician performs a **general physical examination** to confirm a patient's health or diagnose a medical problem. Figure 22-1 shows a typical examination room.

Number and Size of Rooms

The number of examination rooms in a medical office depends on the number of doctors who work there and on each doctor's patient load. Ideally, each doctor in a medical office has at least two examination rooms for her exclusive use. A minimum of two rooms per doctor enables the medical assistant to prepare one room while the doctor examines a patient in the other room.

The customary size for an examination room is 8 by 12 ft. The room should be large enough to accommodate the doctor, the patient, and one assistant comfortably. At the same time, it should be small enough that instruments and supplies will be within easy reach. Doors and interior walls should be soundproofed to ensure privacy for patients.

Some examination rooms have dressing cubicles in one corner. Other rooms have screens in one corner, behind which the patient may disrobe. Regardless of a room's layout, you should provide privacy for patients whenever they need to disrobe and put on gowns.

A rack for the patient's medical records usually hangs on the wall directly outside the examination room or on the outside of the door. A light or other device on the wall or door may be used to signal that the room is occupied.

Furnishings

Furnishings should be arranged for efficiency, the convenience of the physician, and the comfort of the patient. The examining table is the key piece of equipment in the examination room. It should be positioned in the center of the room or coming out from the wall. This arrangement allows the physician and an assistant to attend to the patient on at least three sides. The examining table usually contains a pullout step for the patient to use when getting onto the table. It may also contain drawers for storing instruments and table coverings.

Examining tables are usually adjustable to enable the patient to assume the various positions that the physical examination may require. The physician will probably tell you beforehand if you need to adjust the table in a particular way.

Most examination rooms also have a writing surface large enough to spread out the patient's records, a sink, and a countertop. Shelves, cupboards, and drawers store routine supplies such as dressings, adhesive tape, and bandages.

The examination room may also include the following items:

- One or more chairs
- A rolling stool

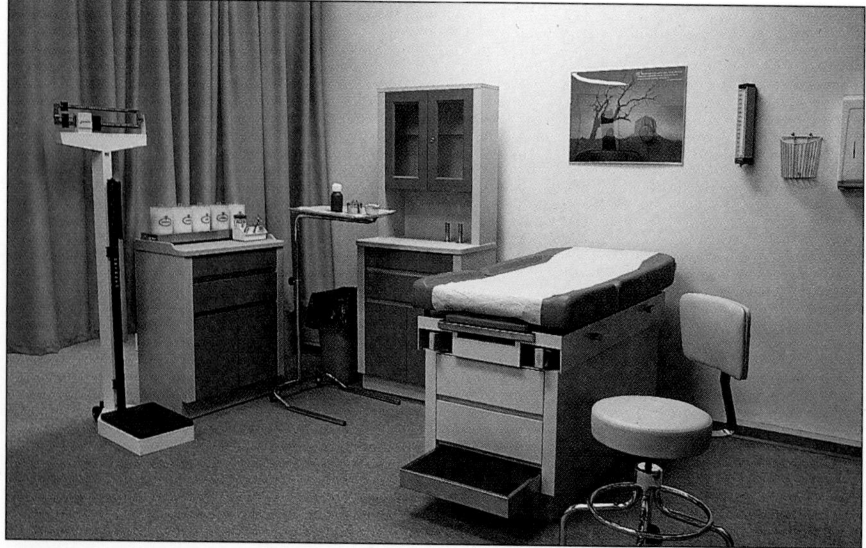

Figure 22-1. You are responsible for making sure the examination room is clean and orderly.

- A weight scale with height bar
- A metal wastebasket with a lid
- Biohazardous waste containers for disposal of biohazardous materials (biological agents that can spread disease to living things)
- Puncture-proof containers for disposal of biohazardous sharps
- A high-intensity lamp
- Wall brackets for hanging instruments

Special Features

The Americans With Disabilities Act of 1990 (ADA) requires that businesses, services, and public transportation provide "reasonable accommodations" for the disabled. To comply with this act, the examination room in a medical office must have features that make the area accessible to patients who use wheelchairs or who have visual or other types of physical impairments. **Accessibility** refers to the ease with which people can move in and out of a space. The ADA accessibility guidelines require the following:

- A doorway at least 36 in (915 mm) wide to allow a person in a wheelchair to pass through
- A clearance space in rooms and hallways that is 60 in (1525 mm) in diameter to allow a person in a wheelchair to make a 180° turn
- Stable, firm, slip-resistant flooring
- Door-opening hardware that can be grasped with one hand and does not require the twisting of the wrist to use
- Door closers adjusted to allow time for a person in a wheelchair to enter or exit through the door
- Grab bars in the lavatory

Cleanliness in the Examination Room

As you learned in Chapter 19, you can follow specific measures to achieve medical asepsis and prevent the spread of pathogenic microorganisms in the medical office. These measures involve strict housekeeping standards and adherence to government guidelines.

A clean examination room is extremely important in preventing the spread of infectious diseases to patients and health-care workers. Part of your job is to carefully follow infection-control procedures in the medical office and to keep the examination room clean and neat.

Infection Control

People with a variety of contagious diseases visit medical offices every day. The potential for the spread of infection is thus higher in medical offices than in most other places. For that reason, you must be especially careful to follow infection-control procedures at work. You can safeguard the health of staff members and patients by:

- Making hand washing a priority.
- Keeping the examining table clean.
- Disinfecting all work surfaces.

Hand Washing. Clean hands are the first step in preventing infection transmission in the examination room. Wash your hands with disinfectant soap and warm water at the following times:

- At the beginning of the day
- Before and after having contact with each patient
- Before and after using gloves or performing any procedure
- Before and after eating or taking a break
- Before and after using the bathroom
- After blowing your nose or coughing
- Before and after handling specimens, waste, or clean or sterile supplies
- Before leaving for the day

After washing your hands, use a clean paper towel to handle faucets or doorknobs. The paper towel helps you avoid contaminating your clean hands with microorganisms. (See Procedure 19-1 in Chapter 19 for the steps in performing aseptic hand washing.)

Examining Table. The disposable paper that covers the examining table provides a barrier to infection during an examination. Always change the covering after each use (Figure 22-2). Your office might use precut lengths, or you might need to tear off a piece from a roll of paper. Cover pillows with fresh paper. Also, provide paper towels for patients who need to wipe away excess lubricants after certain procedures.

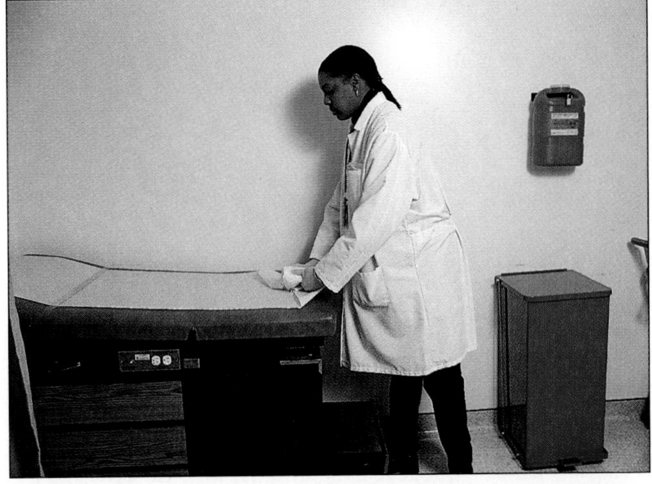

Figure 22-2. When you remove the cover from the examining table, roll it up tightly and quickly. Then carefully prepare it for disposal.

PROCEDURE 22-1

Guidelines for Disinfecting Examination Room Surfaces

Objective: To reduce the risk of exposure to potentially infectious microorganisms in the examination room

OSHA Guidelines

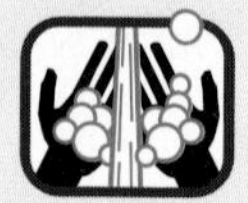
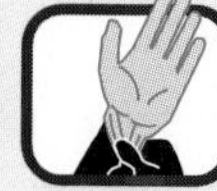
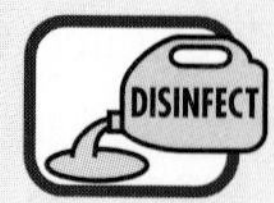

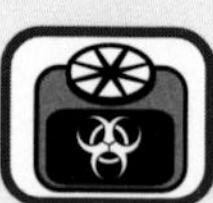

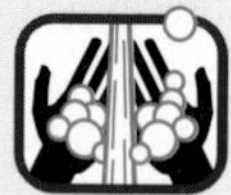

Materials: Utility gloves, disinfectant (10% bleach solution or EPA-approved disinfecting product), paper towels, dustpan and brush, tongs, forceps, clean sponge or heavy rag

Method

1. Wash your hands and put on utility gloves.
2. Remove any visible soil from examination room surfaces with disposable paper towels or a rag.
3. Thoroughly wipe all surfaces with the disinfectant.
4. In the event of an accident involving a broken glass container, use tongs, a dustpan and brush, or forceps to pick up shattered glass, which may be contaminated (Figure 22-3).
5. Remove and replace protective coverings, such as plastic wrap or aluminum foil, on equipment if the equipment or the coverings have become contaminated. After removing the coverings, disinfect the equipment and allow it to air-dry. (Follow office procedures for the routine changing of protective coverings.)
6. When you finish cleaning, dispose of the paper towels or rags in a biohazardous waste receptacle. (This step is especially important if you are cleaning surfaces contaminated with blood, body fluids, or tissues.)
7. Remove the gloves and wash your hands.
8. If you keep a container of 10% bleach solution on hand for disinfection purposes, replace the solution daily to ensure its disinfecting potency (Figure 22-4).

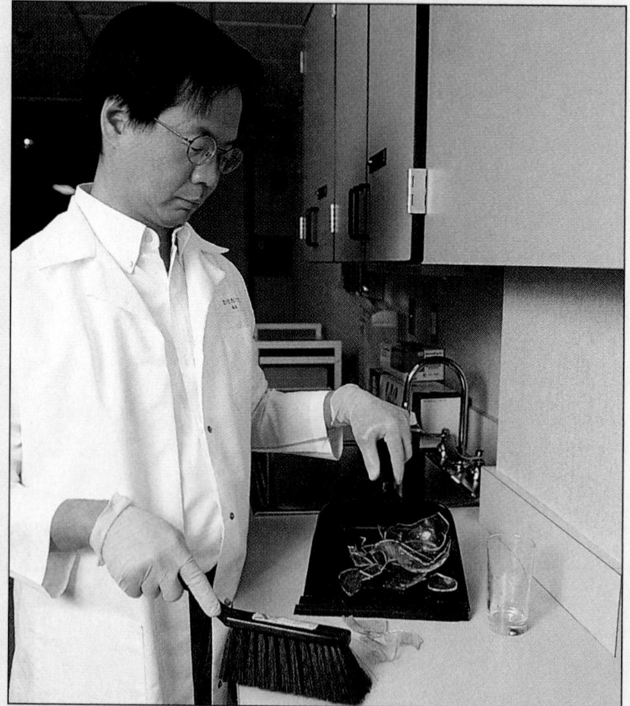

Figure 22-3. Because broken glass may be contaminated, never pick it up directly with your hands. Use a brush and dustpan, tongs, or forceps to clean it up.

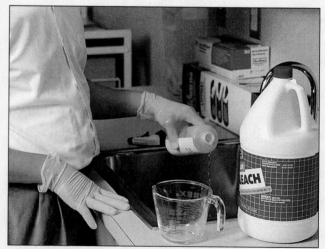

Figure 22-4. Replace the bleach solution each day to ensure its disinfecting potency.

When you remove the used covering from the examining table, roll it up quickly and carefully. You should have a small, tight bundle of paper when you finish. Crumpling the paper haphazardly or shaking it in the air stirs up dust and microorganisms and can spread infection.

Dispose of used paper coverings soiled by body fluids, especially blood, in a biohazardous waste container. (Refer to Chapter 19 for specific guidelines for disposing of hazardous items.) Used coverings with no visible fluids may be disposed of according to the procedures established by your office. Place soiled linen cloths and pillowcases in biohazard-labeled bags for sending to a laundry for cleaning.

Surfaces. You are responsible for disinfecting work surfaces in the examination room, including the examining table, sink, and countertop. As you learned in Chapter 20, disinfection involves exposing all parts of a surface to a disinfectant such as a 10% solution of household bleach in water or a product approved by the Environmental Protection Agency (EPA). Surfaces must be disinfected at the following times:

- After an examination or treatment during which surfaces have become visibly contaminated with tissues, blood, or other body fluids
- Immediately following accidental blood or body fluid spills or splatter
- At the end of your work shift

Clean and disinfect the toilet and sink in the patient lavatory, and inspect and disinfect reusable receptacles such as wastebaskets on a regular basis. In most offices these tasks are performed once a day. You must, however, follow the schedule established by your office. Procedure 22-1 describes how to disinfect work surfaces, floors, and equipment in the examination room. Replace protective coverings on equipment or surfaces that were exposed to blood, other body fluids, or tissues during the examination.

Storage. During the examination, you may need to collect biohazardous specimens, such as blood or urine, from the patient for testing. You are responsible for storing these specimens properly. See "Caution: Handle With Care" for guidelines to follow when storing biohazardous materials.

CAUTION

HANDLE WITH CARE

Storing Biohazardous Materials

During a general physical examination, the physician may ask you to collect various types of specimens from the patient for testing in the laboratory. These specimens must be handled and stored properly because they have the potential to be biohazards. Exposure that can spread disease may occur through the following routes:

- Inhalation (breathing)
- Ingestion (swallowing)
- **Transcutaneous absorption** (absorption through a cut or crack in the skin)

Occupational Safety and Health Administration (OSHA) regulations require storing biohazardous materials separately from food and beverages. You must not place food and beverages in refrigerators, freezers, or cabinets where blood or other potentially infectious materials are present or put specimens in a refrigerator that is otherwise used to store food and beverages.

There are several reasons why it is dangerous to put food or beverages in the laboratory refrigerator. If a biohazardous substance is not clearly labeled and you are in a hurry, you might accidentally grab it and ingest it. There is always the possibility that containers of biohazardous substances might leak or spill or that residue from the hazardous material might not have been thoroughly cleaned from the outside of containers. This residue could lead to contamination of food or beverages.

OSHA regulations require that a warning label containing the biohazard symbol be clearly and securely posted on the outside of refrigerators, freezers, and cabinets where biohazardous materials are stored. The government also recommends keeping the laboratory refrigerator and the refrigerator for the employees' personal use in separate rooms. These measures help prevent employees from accidentally putting food and beverages in the wrong place.

OSHA regulations also prohibit medical personnel from doing any of the following activities in a room where potentially infectious materials are present:

- Eating
- Drinking
- Smoking
- Chewing gum
- Applying cosmetics
- Handling contact lenses
- Chewing pencils or pens
- Rubbing eyes

These work practice controls, like all OSHA regulations, represent safeguards to protect workers against the health hazards of blood-borne pathogens.

CAUTION HANDLE WITH CARE

Refrigerator Temperature Control

Health inspectors visit medical facilities periodically to check that health and safety standards are being upheld. One of the first things they check is the temperature of refrigerators. To prevent spoilage or deterioration of testing kits, blood specimens, and other stored materials, the temperature of the laboratory refrigerator should be maintained between 36° and 46°F (2° and 8°C). Keep a thermometer in the laboratory refrigerator to monitor the temperature.

Similar guidelines apply to the refrigerator in the employee area. Food spoils quickly in a refrigerator if the temperature is not low enough. The temperature of the food refrigerator should be maintained between 32° and 40°F (0° and 4.4°C). In addition to monitoring the temperature, make sure that food is not stored in the refrigerator too long. All food containers—including brown bags containing lunches—should be dated and thrown out when their freshness has expired. You can prevent the growth of bacteria by wiping up food spills immediately and cleaning the interior and exterior of the refrigerator routinely.

Follow office procedures for the routine cleaning of both refrigerators and for the proper maintenance of the temperature of the refrigerators' contents while the refrigerators' interiors are cleaned. Specimens, for example, must be kept at a specific temperature at all times. For documentation purposes, keep a log of dates when the laboratory refrigerator is cleaned.

Storage of testing kits and specimens often involves refrigeration as a means of preservation. Adequate preservation requires maintaining careful control of the temperature in a refrigerator. Read "Caution: Handle With Care" for more information on preventing spoilage by controlling refrigerator temperature.

Putting the Room in Order

After ensuring that the examining table is clean, all surfaces are properly disinfected, and all necessary items are stored, take time to straighten the examination room and put things in order. A neatly arranged room boosts patient confidence and supports the impression of a well-run office. It also contributes to the physical safety of patients and staff. Tasks include the following:

- Putting the rolling stool back where it belongs
- Pushing in the examining-table step
- Returning supplies to containers
- Putting away prescription pads and sample medications that may have been left out

Housekeeping

Medical offices usually contract with a janitorial service for after-hours cleaning. Janitorial services perform general cleaning tasks such as emptying wastebaskets, vacuuming carpets, scrubbing floors, dusting furniture, washing windows, and cleaning blinds. To be sure that the service cleans and sanitizes all areas adequately, you need to work with your employer to develop and implement a cleaning schedule. Take into account the types of surfaces to be cleaned, the type of contamination present, and the tasks or procedures to be performed.

You may be responsible for assigning housekeeping chores to janitorial workers. If so, you will need to monitor their work and let the service know if there are any lapses in cleanliness. You may also do some housekeeping chores yourself, such as damp dusting an open shelf. Because dust harbors bacteria and allergens, it is important to keep the examination rooms as dust-free as possible.

Room Temperature, Lighting, and Ventilation

No patient wants to sit in an examination room that looks unkempt. Nor do patients feel comfortable in a room that is cold, dimly lit, or stuffy. Adjusting the temperature, lighting, and ventilation is part of keeping the examination room in good order and fit for use.

Room Temperature

Because patients may be wearing only a thin paper gown or drape while in the examination room, you must be sure the examination room is warm enough. Set the thermostat to maintain the temperature at approximately 72°F, and make sure there are no drafts from windows or doors. Patients often feel anxious while waiting for the doctor, and a warm room can help them relax.

Lighting

Good lighting is required to make accurate diagnoses, to correctly carry out medical procedures, and to read orders and instructions. A well-lit room also helps prevent accidents.

Adjust room lights and blinds or drapes as necessary in preparation for an examination. If there is an examination lamp with a movable arm, be sure the arm is positioned appropriately. Replace all burned-out lightbulbs as soon as possible.

Ventilation

The air in the examination area should smell fresh and clean. From time to time, you may have to deal with offensive odors from urine, vomitus, body odors, or laboratory chemicals. First you must eliminate the source of the odor, especially if the source is potentially infectious or toxic. Then you can take steps to remove the odor.

Some examination rooms have a ventilation system with a filter that absorbs odors. If the rooms in your office do not, you may be able to turn on a high-speed blower to vent room air to the outside. In some cases an open window and a fan may be sufficient to freshen the air. Remember to check the room temperature after using fresh-air approaches to odor control.

If necessary, you can temporarily mask unpleasant odors with a room deodorizer or spray. Some sprays also help kill germs.

Medical Instruments and Supplies

Doctors require various instruments and supplies to perform an examination or procedure. Instruments are tools or implements doctors use for particular purposes. Disposable instruments are often referred to as supplies.

You must maintain all instruments and supplies needed in the examination room. This responsibility involves the following three tasks:

1. Ordering and stocking all supplies needed for examinations and treatment procedures
2. Keeping the instruments sanitized, disinfected, or sterilized (as appropriate) and in working order
3. Ensuring that all instruments and supplies are placed where the doctor can easily reach them

Instruments Used in a General Physical Examination

Many of the instruments physicians use are made of fine-grade stainless steel and are reusable. Some of these instruments may have disposable parts.

Physicians also use a number of disposable instruments, such as curettes and needles, because these instruments are both convenient and sanitary. As discussed in Chapter 19, you must discard used disposable instruments and supplies according to OSHA guidelines. Place any such items contaminated with blood or other body fluids in biohazardous waste containers.

Commonly used instruments are shown in Figure 22-5 and are described on the following pages.

- An anoscope is an instrument used to open the anus for examination.
- An examination light provides an additional source of light during the examination. It is usually on a flexible arm to permit light to be directed to the area being examined.
- A laryngeal mirror reflects the inside of the mouth and throat for examination purposes.
- A nasal speculum is an instrument used to enlarge the opening of the nose to permit viewing. This type of speculum may consist of a reusable handle with a disposable speculum tip, or it may be a disposable one-piece unit.
- An ophthalmoscope is a lighted instrument that is used to examine the inner structures of the eye.
- An otoscope is an instrument used to examine the ear canal and the tympanic membrane. The otoscope consists of a light source, a magnifying lens, and an ear speculum.
- A penlight is a small flashlight used when additional light is necessary in a small area. It may also be used to check pupil response in the eye.
- A reflex hammer has a hard-rubber triangular head. It is used to check a patient's reflexes.
- A sphygmomanometer is a piece of equipment used to measure blood pressure.
- A stethoscope is used to listen to body sounds. It is described in more detail in Chapter 24.
- A tape measure is a long, narrow strip of fabric, marked off in inches and sometimes in centimeters, used to measure size or development of an area or part of the body.
- A thermometer is used to measure body temperature.
- A tuning fork tests patients' hearing.
- A vaginal speculum is used to enlarge the vagina to make the vagina and the cervix accessible for visual examination and specimen collection.

Inspecting and Maintaining Instruments. Prior to the examination, make sure that all instruments are sanitized, disinfected, or sterilized (as appropriate) and that they are in good working order. (See Chapter 20 for a description of the types of instruments requiring sanitization, disinfection, or sterilization and of the methods used for each.) For example, test the lights on the otoscope and ophthalmoscope to make sure that the lights work. Place all rechargeable batteries in a battery charger when the instruments are not in use.

Medical instruments are expensive and are designed to work in precise ways. Read the manufacturers' directions so that you are familiar with the care and maintenance of various instruments. Routinely check instruments for

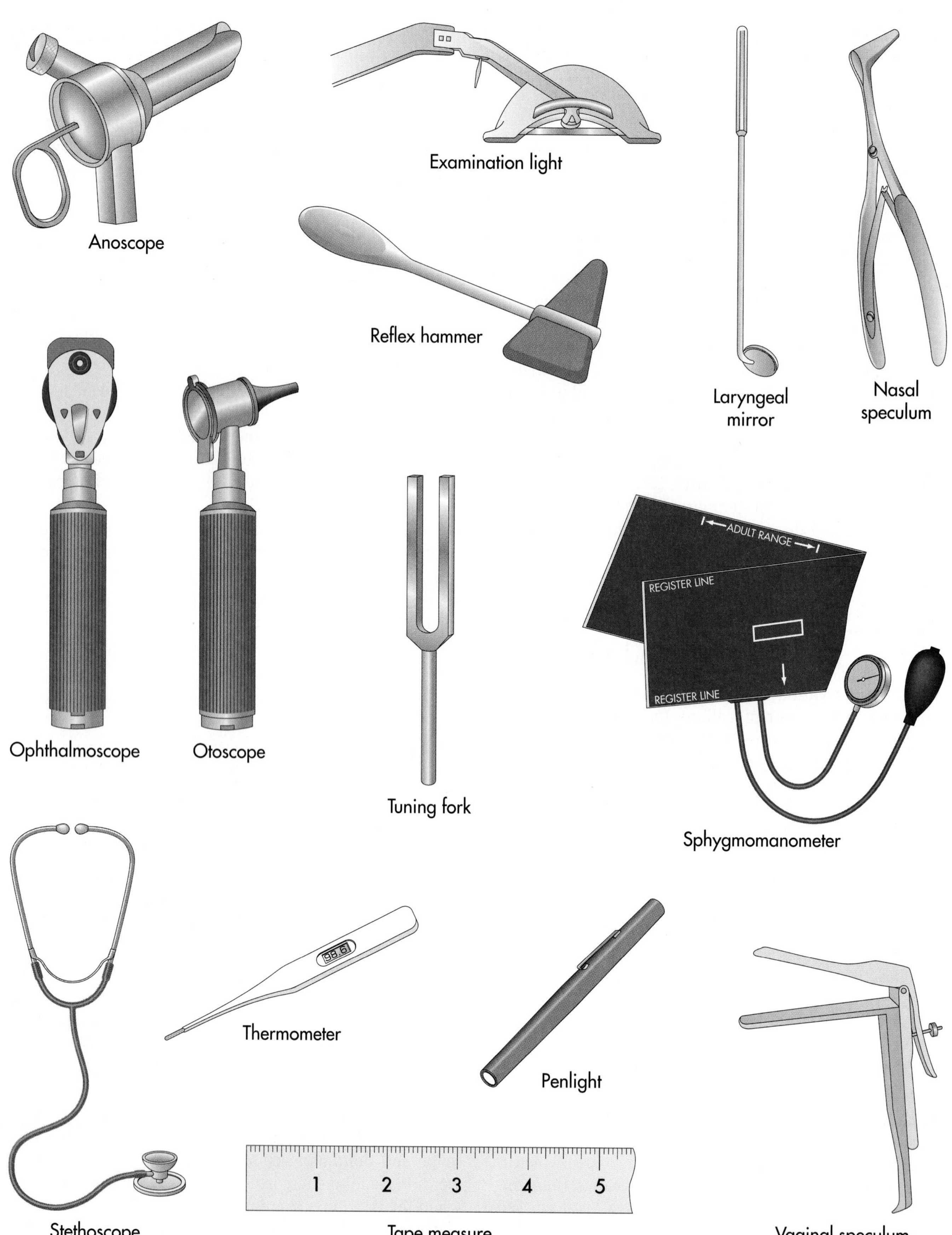

Figure 22-5. These instruments may be used in a general physical examination.

Table 22-1

General Guidelines for Cleaning Instruments

Process	Guidelines*	Instruments
Sanitization	• Use detergent, or as indicated by the manufacturer • Applies to instruments that do not touch the patient or that touch only intact skin • Disinfect these instruments if contaminated with blood or body fluids	Ophthalmoscope Otoscope Penlight Reflex hammer Sphygmomanometer Stethoscope Tape measure Tuning fork
Disinfection	• Use an EPA-approved chemical or a 10% bleach solution to kill infectious agents outside the body • Applies to instruments that touch intact mucous membranes but do not penetrate the patient's body surfaces	Laryngeal mirror Nasal speculum
Sterilization	• Use an autoclave or other approved method to kill all microorganisms • Applies to instruments that penetrate the skin or contact normally sterile areas of the body	Anoscope Curette Needle Syringe Vaginal speculum

*Keep in mind that these guidelines are general. Each office may have its own methods and schedule for cleaning instruments, depending on the office's specialty.

chipping and rusting, and report to the doctor any instruments that need repair or replacement.

Arranging Instruments. The doctor must be able to find and reach instruments easily during an examination. You can assist by placing instruments in the same place for every examination or by arranging them in the order the doctor will use them.

Doctors usually begin a general physical examination by examining the patient's head and face and working down the body. They may want instruments placed in that order. Other doctors may have individual preferences about how they want instruments arranged. In any case, make certain you know each doctor's preferences.

With the exception of the stethoscope, which most doctors carry with them, instruments are kept in one of three places during an examination:

- Mounted on the wall (sphygmomanometer, some otoscopes and ophthalmoscopes)
- Set out on the countertop (penlight, reflex hammer, tape measure, tuning fork, thermometer, some otoscopes and ophthalmoscopes)
- Set on a clean (or sterile, if appropriate) towel or tray (anoscope, laryngeal mirror, nasal speculum, vaginal speculum)

Preparing Instruments. You must prepare some instruments before they can be used. For example, you may need to warm a vaginal speculum by holding it under warm water just prior to the examination. You might warm the mirrored end of the laryngeal mirror with water or over an alcohol lamp. You can also spray it with a special spray that prevents fogging. Any time you will be handling instruments, you must first wash your hands. If the instruments are sterile, you must also wear sterile gloves.

Cleaning Instruments. After the examination, put used instruments in a container, and take them to the cleaning area. Always handle instruments carefully, because mishandling can alter their precision. Dispose of supplies in the appropriate containers, and use approved procedures for sanitizing, disinfecting, and sterilizing reusable instruments and equipment. Refer to Table 22-1 for general guidelines on cleaning instruments. (See Chapter 20 for detailed information on this topic.)

Supplies for a General Physical Examination

Supplies for a general physical examination may be either disposable or consumable. Figure 22-6 shows various types of supplies.

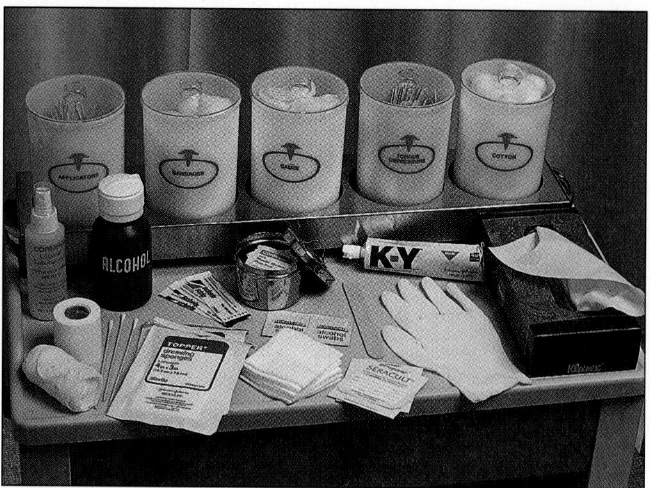

Figure 22-6. These supplies may be used in a general physical examination.

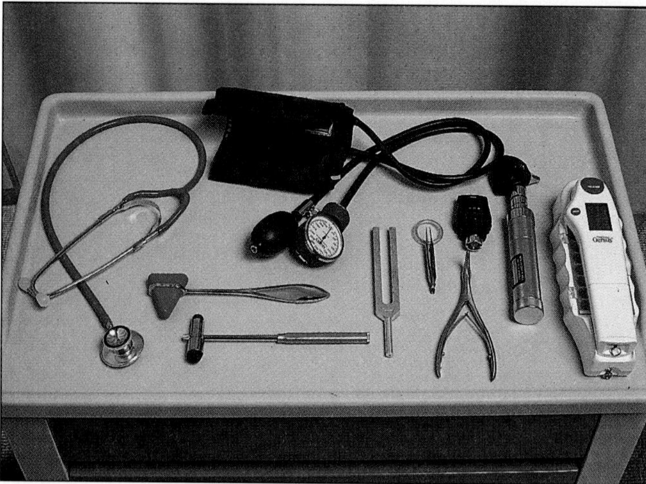

Figure 22-7. Arrange the instruments for a general physical examination so that they are convenient for the doctor.

Disposable supplies are items that are used once and discarded. They include the following:

- Cervical scraper (a wooden scraper used to obtain samples of cervical secretions)
- Cotton balls
- Cotton-tipped applicators
- Curettes
- Disposable needles
- Disposable syringes
- Gauze, dressings, and bandages
- Glass slides
- Gloves, both sterile and examination (unsterile) types
- Paper tissues
- Prepared paper slides used to test the stool for the presence of **occult blood** (blood not visible to the naked eye)
- Specimen containers
- Tongue depressors

Consumable supplies are items that can be emptied or used up in an examination. These items include the following:

- **Fixative** (a chemical spray used for preserving a specimen obtained from the body for pathologic examination)
- Isopropyl alcohol (for cleansing skin)
- Lubricant (a water-soluble gel used during examination of the rectum or vaginal cavity)

As they do with instruments, doctors may have a preferred arrangement of supplies for the general physical examination. Figure 22-7 shows a typical arrangement of instruments.

Keep supplies such as prescription blanks, drugs (especially narcotics), and needles in a locked cabinet away from the patient examination areas. Make sure that patients do not have access to these items.

Storing Supplies. You can use the cabinets and drawers in the examination room to store nonperishable supplies. You should store every item in its own place so that you can find it quickly. You might even color-code or label drawers so that you can easily locate items. You should store supplies that come in various sizes, such as bandages, according to size. You need to routinely straighten and clean the insides of all cabinets and drawers in the examination room.

Restocking Supplies. To be sure you have a sufficient quantity of items on hand, order new supplies well in advance of needing them. A good guideline to follow is to order a new supply when the first half of a box, tube, or bottle has been used up. You may want to use a record-keeping system to help you determine which supplies you need to restock most frequently and how long it takes for new supplies to arrive. The information you should keep track of to develop such a system includes the following:

- The types of supplies your office uses
- The quantities of each type of supply you use in a given amount of time, such as a month
- The frequency with which you must reorder particular supplies
- The names of various suppliers, along with the amount of time it takes to receive your orders

Physical Safety in the Examination Room

Accidents can happen in the examination room. For example, patients and staff members can fall or cut themselves. You have an important responsibility to remove or correct hazards that might cause injury to patients, physicians, or staff members.

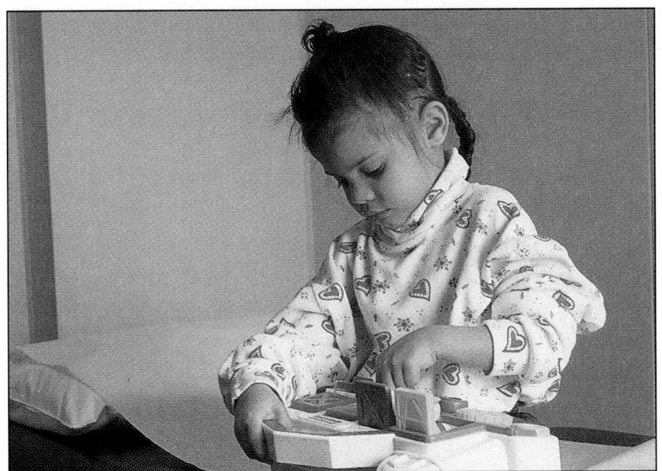

Figure 22-8. Toys provided must be safe for children of all ages.

Maintaining a Safe Environment

It is easier to maintain a safe environment if you pay special attention to the following areas in the examination room:

- Floor
- Cabinets and drawers
- Furniture
- Cords and cables

Floor. You can take several measures to prevent falls. Wipe or mop up spills immediately. Clear the floor of dropped objects. If the floor is carpeted, make sure there are no snags or tears that could cause someone to trip and fall. Spilled medications, chemicals, and other substances pose a threat to young children, who may ingest anything they find on the floor. Destroy and dispose of medications that are accidentally dropped on the floor.

Cabinets and Drawers. Close overhead cabinet doors promptly after removing supplies. Leaving cabinet doors open can result in injury. In addition, an open cabinet door leaves supplies exposed to patients. Make sure drawers are kept closed so that no one bumps into them.

Furniture. Routinely inspect the furniture in the examination room and reception area. Make sure there are no rough edges or sharp corners on the examining table, countertop, chairs, or other furniture. If you are not authorized to repair or replace unsafe pieces of furniture, bring them to the attention of your supervisor.

Cords and Cables. Electrical cords and medical and office equipment cables should run along the walls and should be taped or fastened down securely. Replace tape on cords and cables when it becomes worn.

Special Safety Precautions

Some patients, such as children and people with disabilities, may be particularly susceptible to accidents in your office. You need to take special precautions to ensure their safety.

Children. Keep sharp instruments out of the reach of children, and store toxic items in high cabinets. Also, keep all medications and objects out of the reach of young children, because children are likely to pick up items and put them in their mouths and could choke or be poisoned.

If children's toys and books are kept in the reception area or examination room, make sure they are picked up when not in use and stored safely. Toys should be washable and made of safe materials. (Sanitize daily those toys that children put in their mouths; sanitize other toys weekly. If well children and sick children use the same reception area or examination room, sanitize and disinfect toys after sick children play with them.) Periodically check toys for sharp edges that might cause cuts. Make sure toys do not have small parts or pieces that could cause choking if swallowed. Figure 22-8 shows appropriate toys for the medical office reception area or examination room.

Patients With Physical Disabilities. Patients with disabilities are more likely than other patients to fall. Some patients may use walkers or canes for support, whereas others may simply be unsteady on their feet. Patients with vision impairments may have difficulty seeing obstacles, stairs, and other potential hazards. Safe flooring and handrails in the reception area, bathroom, hallways, and examination room help ensure the safety of patients with impaired mobility or vision. Procedure 22-2 explains how to make the examination room safe for visually impaired patients.

Fire Safety

Fire is a safety hazard anywhere, but it is especially likely where there is sophisticated, high-voltage medical equipment—such as an x-ray machine. Any electrical instrument in the examination room, however, is a potential fire hazard. Other potentially hazardous items are gas tanks and flammable chemicals.

Fire Prevention. Be aware of anything that might cause a fire in the examination room. If you cannot correct the situation yourself, report the hazard to your supervisor.

Be alert to the following potential hazards:

- Frayed electrical wires, overloaded outlets, and improperly grounded plugs. These present a danger of electric shock and fire. Contact a licensed electrician to remedy these problems.

PROCEDURE 22-2

Making the Examination Room Safe for Patients With Visual Impairments

Objective: To ensure that patients with visual impairments are safe in the examination room

OSHA Guidelines: This procedure does not involve exposure to blood, body fluids, or tissues.

Materials: Reflective tape, if needed

Method

1. Make sure the hallway leading to the examination room is clear of obstacles.
2. Increase the amount of lighting in the room. Adjust the shades on windows in the room—if there are any windows—to allow for maximum natural light. Turn on all lights, especially those under cabinets, to dispel shadows.
3. Clear a path along which the patient can walk through the room. Make sure the chairs are out of the way. If there is a scale in the room, position it out of the path. If there is a step stool for the examining table, place it right up against the table.
4. Make sure the floor is not slippery.
5. Remove furniture that might be easily tipped over, such as a visitors' chair that is lightweight. If the physician will use an examination chair, push it out of the way.
6. Provide a sturdy chair with arms and a straight back to make it easier for the patient to sit down and stand up.
7. A wide strip of reflective tape will make the examining-table step visible for all patients. Apply it to the step's edge if tape is not there already. If your office uses a step stool instead of a step, make sure the tape on the stool is facing out.
8. Alert the patient to protruding equipment or furnishings.
9. Arrange the supplies for the patient, such as gowns or drapes, with the following guideline in mind: It is easier to see light objects against dark objects or dark objects against light objects than light objects against light objects or dark objects against dark objects. If, for example, there is a dressing cubicle, lay the light-colored gown or drape against a dark bench instead of hanging the gown or drape against a light wall.

- Materials that are extremely flammable, including alcohol and some disinfectants. Supplies such as paper table coverings can also ignite and spread flames quickly in the event of a fire. Check to make sure that all such items are stored and disposed of properly to minimize the fire danger. Flammable liquids should never be kept near a heat source. If you are not sure whether a chemical is flammable, read the manufacturer's label or Material Safety Data Sheet. (Material Safety Data Sheets are discussed in Chapter 32.)
- Smoking. Smoking should not be permitted anywhere in a medical facility. In addition to causing health problems, smoking is a fire hazard. "No Smoking" signs should be posted prominently throughout the office.
- Inoperative smoke detectors. Make sure that smoke detectors throughout the office are working properly. Replace batteries promptly. If smoke detectors are wired into the building's electrical system, report any malfunction to the building manager.

In Case of Fire. Despite the precautions that you and your coworkers take, a fire may break out. Be prepared to use fire safety equipment and to evacuate the building safely.

Using Safety Equipment. The number of fire extinguishers in the office depends on the size and number of rooms in the office. Regardless of the total number of extinguishers, you should locate an all-purpose fire extinguisher in or close to each examination room. Figure 22-9 shows how to operate a typical fire extinguisher. Have the fire extinguisher professionally serviced once a year to ensure its effectiveness.

If there is a fire blanket in the examination room, be sure that you know how to use it and that it is stored so as to be easily accessible in an emergency. To use a fire blanket to smother burning clothing, wrap the victim in the blanket and roll him on the floor.

Planning an Evacuation Route. An evacuation route provides a safe way out of a building during an emergency. Learn the location of fire alarms, fire doors, and fire escapes in relation to the examination room. Use exit signs as a guide in unfamiliar areas of the building. Stage fire drills with your coworkers so that you can evacuate the facility and lead patients to safety. Plan what you will do if your route becomes blocked.

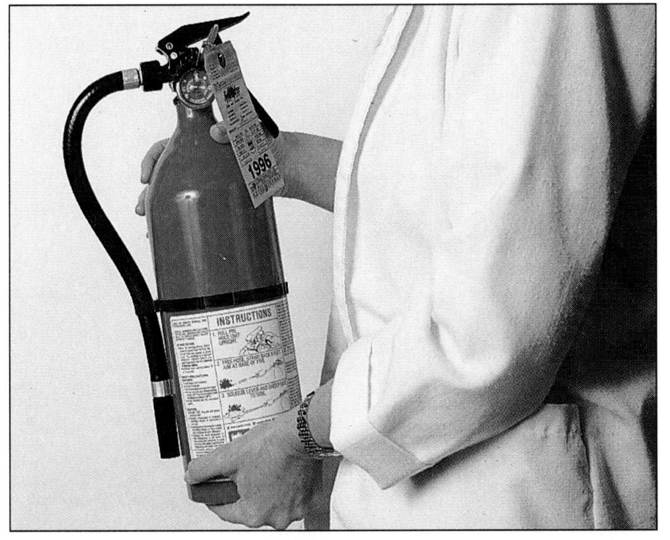

1

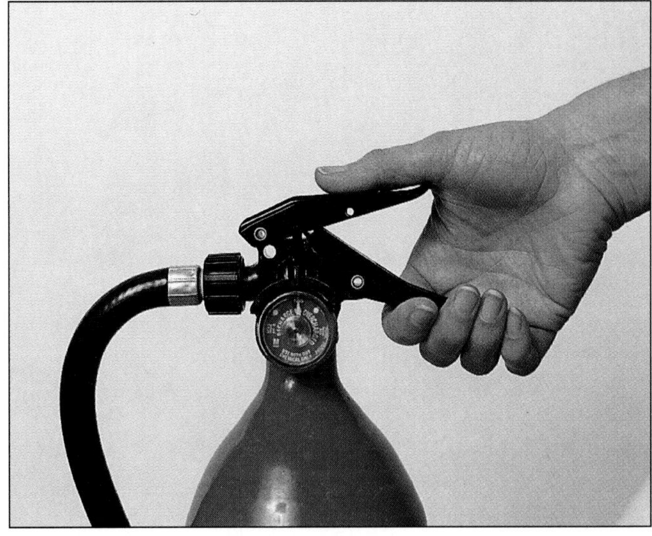

3

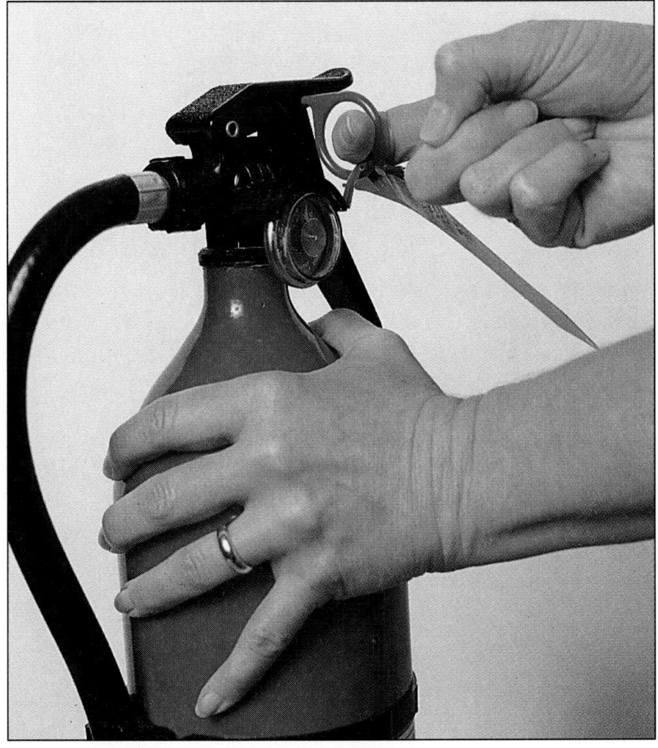

2

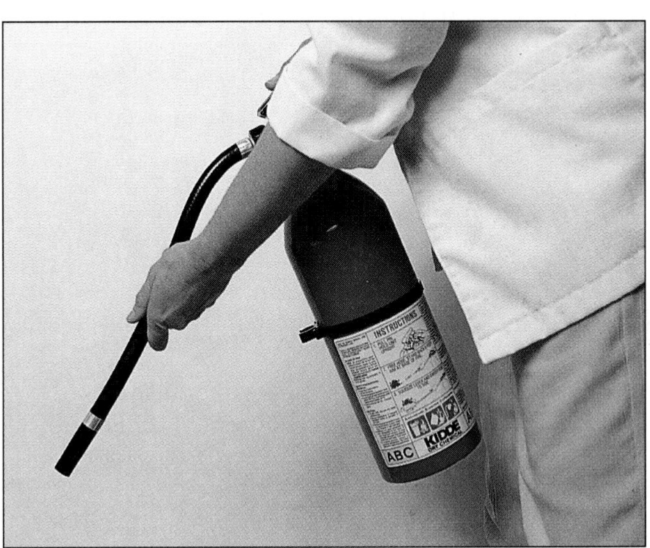

4

Figure 22-9. To use a fire extinguisher, (1) hold it upright, (2) remove the safety pin, (3) push the top handle down, and (4) direct the hose at the base of the fire.

Summary

Preparing the examination and treatment area for doctors and patients is part of your responsibility as a medical assistant. Room readiness involves making sure the room is clean, neat, and orderly and has adequate lighting, heat, and ventilation. You must select the instruments each doctor requires and make sure they are sanitized, disinfected, or sterilized (as appropriate) and ready for use. Room preparation also includes removing obstacles to physical safety, taking safety precautions, and following fire safety guidelines.

Your role in preparing the area is an important one for several reasons. First, you reduce the chance that infections will spread. Second, you help make the examination proceed efficiently. Third, you contribute to the comfort and safety of patients, doctors, and coworkers. Perform these tasks well, and you will inspire patients' confidence in the quality of the medical care provided at the facility.

22 Chapter Review

Discussion Questions

1. Identify steps you should take to ensure the cleanliness of an examination room.
2. Describe steps you should follow in preparing instruments for a general examination.
3. List five situations that might lead to falls or other accidents in the examination room and what you can do to prevent them.

Critical Thinking Questions

1. How does a clean and orderly examination room contribute to patients' psychological well-being?
2. Discuss special steps you would take to prepare the examination room in the following situations: a mother bringing in her 2-year-old son for a checkup; a patient in a wheelchair.
3. What steps could you take to prepare for a power failure in the entire office?

Application Activities

1. Make a checklist of steps for preparing the examination room. List tasks in the following categories: before/after an examination, daily, weekly, and monthly.
2. Working in small groups, prepare a "tip sheet" explaining how a patient could apply methods of infection control in the home. Have everyone in the group contribute at least one idea.
3. Go through the classroom, noting any safety hazards and listing solutions to the problems. Discuss hazards with classmates to make a master list of solutions.

Further Readings

Bloodborne Pathogens and Acute Care Facilities. Washington, DC: U.S. Department of Labor, 1992.

Occupational Exposure to Bloodborne Pathogens. Washington, DC: U.S. Department of Labor, 1993.

Planning Guide for Physicians' Medical Facilities. Chicago: American Medical Association, 1986.

Raloff, Janet. "Sponges and Sinks and Rags, Oh My!" *Science News* 150, no. 11 (14 September 1996): 172–173.

Smela, Diane-Marie. "Interacting With the Hearing Impaired." *The Professional Medical Assistant* 28, no. 3 (May/June 1995): 21–23.

Ward, Deney. "Are Your Gloves Safe?" *The Professional Medical Assistant* 26, no. 6 (November/December 1993): 6.

Williams, Martha R., and Marcia L. Russell. *ADA Handbook: Employment & Construction Issues Affecting Your Business.* Chicago: Real Estate Educators Association, 1993.

Section Two

Understanding the Body and Assisting With Patients

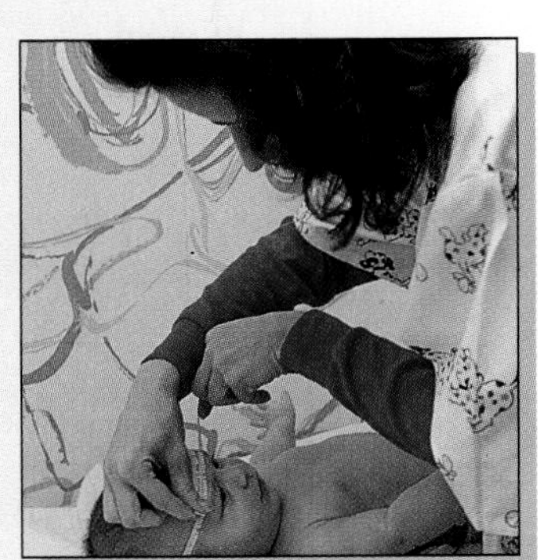

AREAS OF COMPETENCE

1997 ROLE DELINEATION STUDY

ADMINISTRATIVE

- Administrative Procedures

CLINICAL

- Fundamental Principles
- Diagnostic Orders
- Patient Care

GENERAL (Transdisciplinary)

- Communication Skills
- Legal Concepts
- Instruction

CHAPTER LIST

Anatomy and Physiology

CHAPTER OUTLINE

- The Study of the Body
- Organization of the Body
- Identifying the Locations of Body Parts
- Disease Mechanisms
- The Integumentary System (Skin)
- The Skeletal System
- The Muscular System
- The Nervous System
- The Endocrine System
- The Circulatory System
- The Respiratory System
- The Digestive System
- The Urinary System
- The Reproductive System

OBJECTIVES

After completing Chapter 23, you will be able to:

- Describe how the body is organized from simple to more complex levels.
- Label the parts of a cell and list their functions.
- Describe the four types of body tissue.
- Use anatomical position terms to locate specific areas on or in the body.
- Name the body cavities.
- Define disease and list the possible causes of disease.
- Name and describe the structure and function of the following organ systems in the body: integumentary, skeletal, muscular, nervous, endocrine, circulatory, respiratory, digestive, urinary, and reproductive.

AREAS OF COMPETENCE

1997 ROLE DELINEATION STUDY

ADMINISTRATIVE

Administrative Procedures

- Perform medical transcription

GENERAL (Transdisciplinary)

Communication Skills

- Use medical terminology appropriately

Key Terms

abduction
adduction
alveoli
atrium
bronchi
chromosome
dermis
electrolyte
enzyme
epidermis
estrogen
extension
flexion
homeostasis
hormone
insulin
lymph
meiosis
menstruation
metabolism
mitosis
nephron
neuron
nucleus
ova
ovulation
parasympathetic
peristalsis
respiration
semen
spermatozoa
sympathetic
testosterone
ventricle

The Study of the Body

The human body is complex in structure and function. *Anatomy* is the scientific term for the study of body structure. *Physiology* is the term for the study of how the body functions. These areas of study are closely related.

A knowledge of anatomy will help you grasp the meaning of diagnostic and procedural codes. A basic understanding of physiology will make it easier to see how and why certain disease states injure the body. Knowledge of anatomy and physiology will help you understand the clinical procedures you will perform as a medical assistant.

Organization of the Body

Like all living things, the human body is organized from simple levels to more complex levels. Organization begins at the chemical level and proceeds to the cellular, tissue, organ, system, and organism levels. Figure 23-1 illustrates this progressively complex structure.

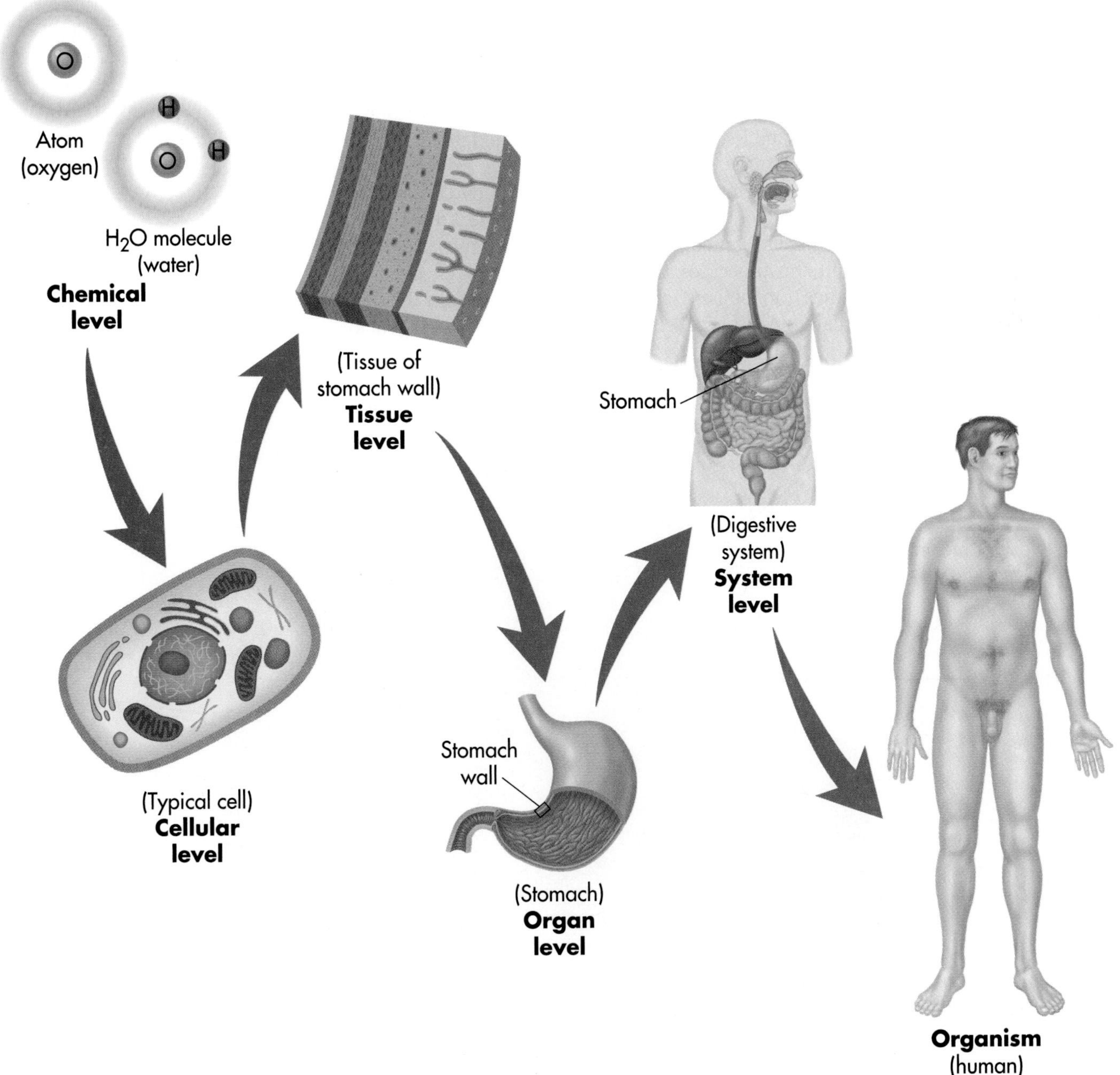

Figure 23-1. The human body is organized in levels, beginning with the chemical level and progressing to the cellular, tissue, organ, system, and organism (whole body) levels.

Chemicals

The lowest level of organization is the chemical level, which includes all the chemical elements that are essential to life. Atoms are the fundamental units that make up these chemical elements.

When two or more atoms are chemically combined, a molecule is formed. Molecules are the basic units of compounds. When two or more atoms of more than one element are combined, a compound is formed. An example of a compound is water, which is composed of two hydrogen atoms and one oxygen atom. Water is critical to both chemical and physical processes in human physiology. Other main types of compounds in the body are carbohydrates, lipids (fats), and proteins.

Compounds that separate into positively and negatively charged parts (ions) when they dissolve are called **electrolytes.** The movement of ions into and out of body structures regulates or triggers many physiologic states and activities in the body. For example, electrolytes are essential to fluid balance, muscle contraction, and nerve impulse conduction. (Very rapid movement of ions triggers the latter two.)

Metabolism is the overall chemical functioning of the body. Metabolism includes all the processes that build small molecules into large ones (anabolism) and break down large molecules into small ones (catabolism).

Cells

Chemicals react to form the complex substances that make up cells, the basic unit of life. The human body has millions of cells. There are many kinds of cells, and each kind has a specific function.

Structure and Function of the Cell. Cells have three main parts: nucleus, cytoplasm, and cell membrane. The **nucleus** is the "brain" of the cell. It is surrounded by the nuclear membrane and contains **chromosomes,** threadlike structures that are made of deoxyribonucleic acid (DNA). DNA consists of long, double chains of chemical bases along a sugar backbone. The pattern of bases provides the hereditary information that directs all cell activities and allows the cell to reproduce. The cytoplasm surrounds the nucleus. Most cellular activity takes place in special structures, or organelles, found in the cytoplasm. The cell membrane surrounds the cytoplasm and allows materials to pass into and out of the cell. Figure 23-2 provides a detailed view of structures found in various kinds of body cells.

One important function of the cell is to produce protein molecules, mainly in the form of **enzymes** (proteins that speed up chemical processes necessary for life). To accomplish this task, DNA molecules direct the synthesis of ribonucleic acid (RNA) molecules. RNA consists of

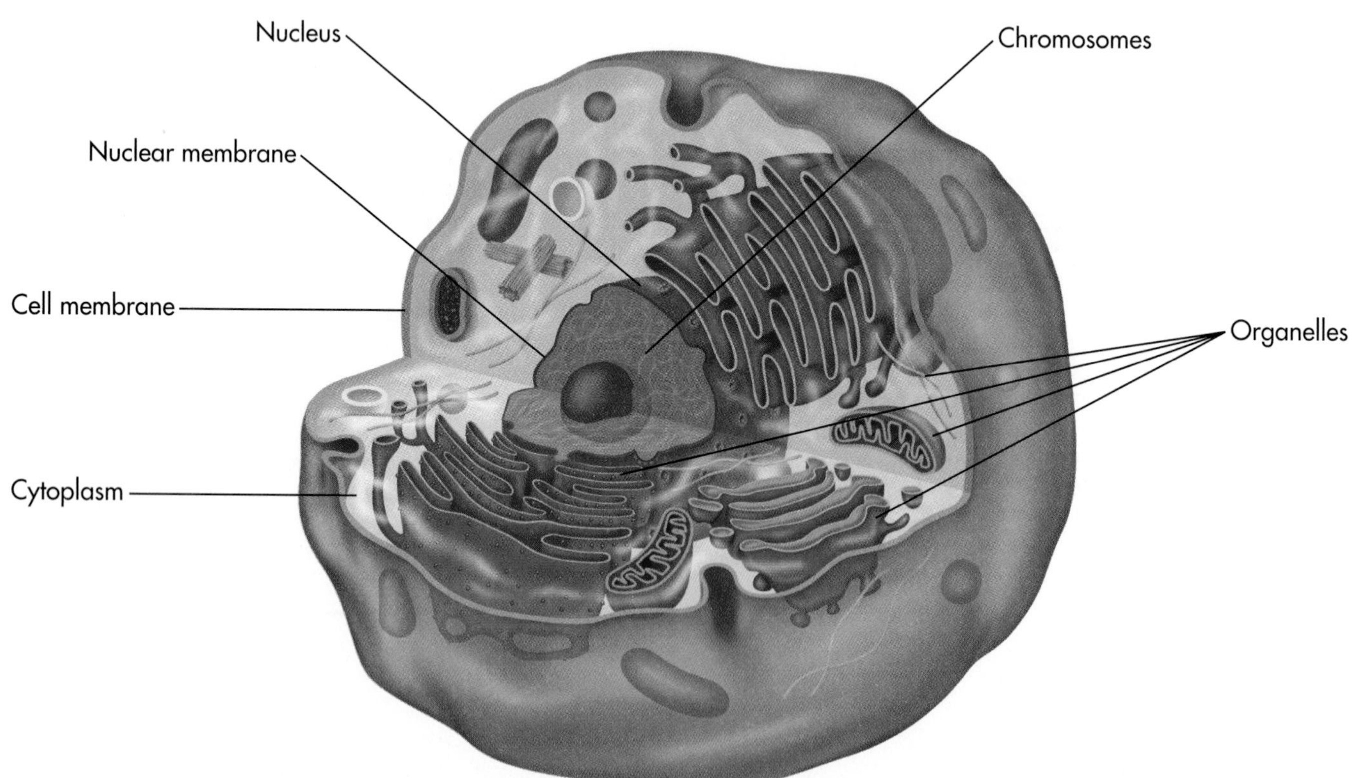

Figure 23-2. The cell is the basic unit of life. The human body has millions of cells of many kinds and functions.

long, single chains of chemical bases along a sugar backbone slightly different from DNA's. RNA molecules are transported from the nucleus into the cytoplasm, where they direct the formation of proteins.

Cell Division. Cells can become damaged, diseased, or worn out, and replacements must be made. New cells are necessary for normal growth. Cells reproduce by cell division, a process that involves splitting the nucleus and cytoplasm. Two types of cell division occur in the body. The types of division differ according to how the nucleus divides.

Somatic Cell Division. Somatic cell division occurs in most cells of the body. The cell divides by a process called **mitosis.** During mitosis the nucleus makes a complete copy of all 23 of its chromosome pairs (46 chromosomes altogether). As the cell divides, each new cell receives a complete set of chromosome pairs. The resultant cells are identical to each other.

Reproductive Cell Division. Reproductive cell division takes place only in the reproductive organs when the male and female sex cells are formed. The cell divides by the process of **meiosis.** During meiosis the nucleus copies all 23 chromosome pairs, but two divisions take place. The four cells that are formed each contain only one of each chromosome pair, or a total of 23 chromosomes. This type of cell division must occur so that when the sex cells combine during fertilization, the resulting cell contains the usual number of chromosomes (46).

Movement of Molecules Across the Cell Membrane. For cells to obtain nutrients and remove waste products, materials must be able to pass through the cell membrane. Some molecules, such as water, can pass naturally through the cell membrane. Other molecules must be actively transported from one side of the cell membrane to the other. This transportation requires energy, special structures in the membrane, and agents that carry molecules across.

Tissues

Tissues are groups of cells that are similar in structure and perform a specific function. The four main types of tissues in the body are epithelial, connective, muscle, and nervous. Examples of these tissue types are shown in Figure 23-3.

Epithelial Tissue (Epithelium). Epithelial tissue forms a protective covering for the body and all its organs and body cavities. Examples of epithelial tissue are the skin and the linings of the respiratory and digestive tracts, or mucous membranes. Epithelial tissue also forms the glands of the body. Glands are organs that produce a variety of substances, such as hormones, sweat, and digestive juices.

Connective Tissue. Connective tissue connects, protects, supports, and forms a framework for all parts of the body. The texture and other qualities of different connective tissues vary widely. Connective tissues include fat, tendons, ligaments, and tissues found under the skin and around blood vessels and organs. Cartilage and bone are hard connective tissues. Connective tissue can even be liquid—for example, blood and lymph. Intervertebral disks are a specific type of connective tissue located between the vertebrae in the spinal column. They act as shock absorbers, helping to form a strong, flexible support for the neck and trunk.

Muscle Tissue. Muscle tissue provides movement, maintains posture, and produces heat. The three types of muscle tissue are skeletal, cardiac, and smooth. Skeletal muscle is attached to bone and provides the body's voluntary movement. Cardiac and smooth muscle provide involuntary movement. Cardiac muscle is found only in the heart; it produces regular contraction of the heart, heard as a heartbeat. Smooth muscle is found in the walls of blood vessels, allowing the inside diameter of blood vessels to enlarge (dilate) and contract. Smooth muscle is also found in organs such as the stomach and intestines, where it helps move food through the digestive tract.

Nervous Tissue. Nervous tissue carries nerve impulses between the brain or spinal cord and other parts of the body. The basic structural unit of nervous tissue is the **neuron,** or nerve cell.

Organs and Systems

Tissues are grouped together to form organs, each of which performs a specific job. Examples of organs are the heart, lungs, and stomach. Organs that work together to perform a particular body function make up a system. Table 23-1 provides an overview of the ten body systems. Keep in mind that organ systems, although studied as individual sections in this chapter, work with each other. All organ systems depend on all others for the maintenance of **homeostasis**—a balanced, stable state within the body.

Identifying the Locations of Body Parts

You will need to precisely describe locations on or in patients' bodies as you perform various tasks as a medical assistant. Recording symptoms in a patient's chart, transcribing an order for an x-ray, and preparing a patient for a clinical procedure all require that you clearly understand and communicate the part of the body involved. You will use many concepts and terms to clarify locations in the body.

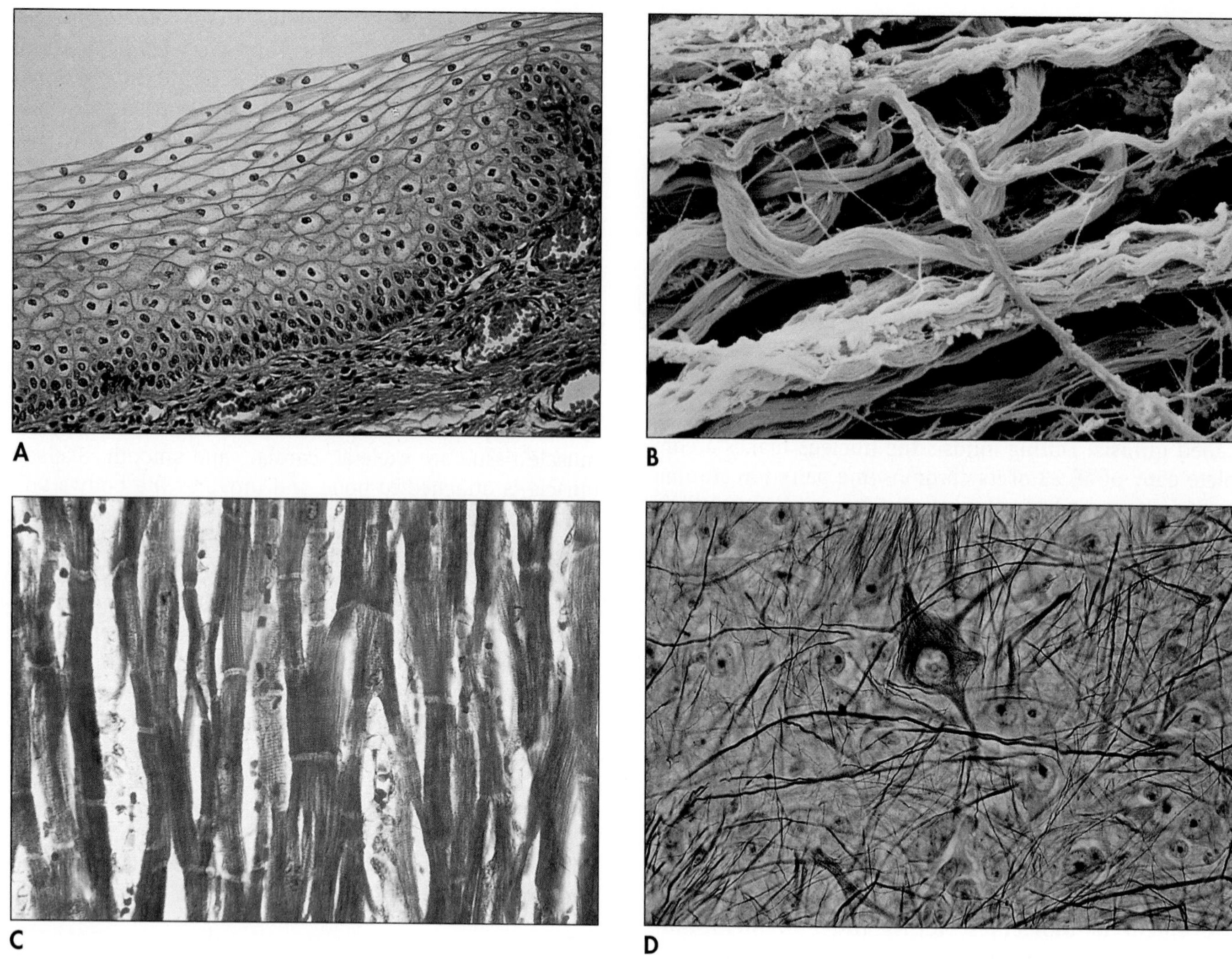

Figure 23-3. There are four main types of tissue in the body: (a) epithelial, (b) connective, (c) muscle, and (d) nervous.

Anatomical Position

Terms have been devised to note specific areas and directions in the body. All the terms refer to the body standing up straight, eyes open, facing forward, feet together, and arms hanging at the sides with palms facing forward. This position is referred to as the anatomical position.

Your proper use of anatomical position terms is essential to the well-being of the patients with whom you deal as a medical assistant. You need mastery of these terms to order or describe various laboratory, pathology, and radiology studies correctly. To write referrals to specialists for follow-up care or to describe a patient's symptoms correctly, you must be fluent and accurate in your use of these terms.

"Caution: Handle With Care" describes and illustrates the anatomical position terms you must master. Some of these terms refer to directional relationships, comparable to north, south, east, and west on a map. Other terms describe spatial relationships, which help provide a three-dimensional map of organ location.

Body Cavities

The body also contains several large spaces, or cavities, which contain various organs (Figure 23-6, p. 400). There are two main body cavities:

- Dorsal cavity
- Ventral cavity

The dorsal cavity, located in the back of the body, is divided into the cranial and spinal cavities, although the two are connected. The cranial cavity contains the brain and nearby blood vessels and nerves; the spinal cavity contains the spinal cord.

The diaphragm separates the ventral cavity, located in the front of the body, into the thoracic and abdominal cavities. The thoracic cavity contains the lungs, heart, major blood vessels, and esophagus. The abdominal cavity is divided into two parts by an imaginary line across the hip bones. The upper part of the abdominal cavity contains the stomach, most of the intestines, the kidneys, liver, gallbladder, pancreas, and spleen. The lower part of the abdominal cavity, called the pelvic cavity, contains

Table 23-1

The Body Systems

System	Functions	Organs
Integumentary	Protection, temperature regulation, defense, excretion, sensory reception	Skin, hair, nails, sweat and oil glands
Skeletal	Support, protection, movement, blood cell production, mineral storage	Bones, joints
Muscular	Movement, posture maintenance, heat production	Muscles, tendons, ligaments
Nervous	Control and coordination of body activities	Brain, spinal cord, nerves
Endocrine	Control and coordination of body functions	Pituitary, thyroid, parathyroid, adrenal (adrenal cortex and adrenal medulla), and pineal glands; pancreas, ovaries, testes, thymus
Circulatory	Nutrient and oxygen transport to cells, waste removal, disease resistance	Heart, arteries, veins, capillaries, blood, lymph vessels, lymph nodes
Respiratory	Oxygen supply for cells, carbon dioxide removal	Nose, pharynx, larynx, trachea, bronchi, lungs
Digestive	Breakdown of food, nutrient absorption, waste removal	Mouth, pharynx, esophagus, stomach, intestines, liver, gallbladder, pancreas, rectum, anus
Urinary	Elimination of wastes from blood and body, maintenance of fluid volume and chemistry	Kidney, ureters, urinary bladder, urethra
Reproductive	Production of new human beings	Male: testes, scrotum, penis, vas deferens, prostate Female: ovaries, fallopian tubes, uterus, vagina, external genitalia, breasts

the urinary bladder, rectum, and internal parts of the reproductive system.

Body membranes are thin layers of epithelial and connective tissue that line the body cavities and cover or separate organs or structures of the body. Mucous membranes line the nasal and oral cavities, serous membranes line the body cavities, and synovial membranes line the joint cavities.

Disease Mechanisms

Disease is defined as a disturbed or abnormal state of the body. Part or all of the body may be incapable of performing its normal functions. The severity of disease can vary from mild to life-threatening. Disease can be caused by the following:

- Disease-producing organisms, such as bacteria, viruses, or fungi
- Malnutrition (lack of essential vitamins, minerals, proteins, or energy sources)
- Physical agents (heat, cold, or injury)
- Toxic chemicals
- Birth defects (inherited or occurring during pregnancy)
- Degenerative processes (breakdown of tissue because of aging or repeated infection or injury)
- Neoplasms ("new growths"; cancerous or noncancerous tumors)

CAUTION

HANDLE WITH CARE

Locating Body Parts by Anatomical Position

You will use anatomical position terms to precisely locate areas on or in the body. Such terms are universally accepted in all areas of medicine, from general practice to specialized fields, so that physicians and surgeons understand information in reports and patients' charts. It is essential that you know how to use anatomical position terms correctly in written documents for which you are responsible. A variety of health-care professionals may rely on the documents' accuracy. Because it may not always be obvious from the outside of a patient's body what is actually wrong, physicians may use the information you provide in diagnosing a patient's condition and prescribing subsequent treatment.

Directional Relationships

Just as we have terms to indicate geographic directions, such as north, south, east, and west, there are terms for indicating certain regions and directions in the body (Figure 23-4). Some of the most common opposite pairs are as follows:

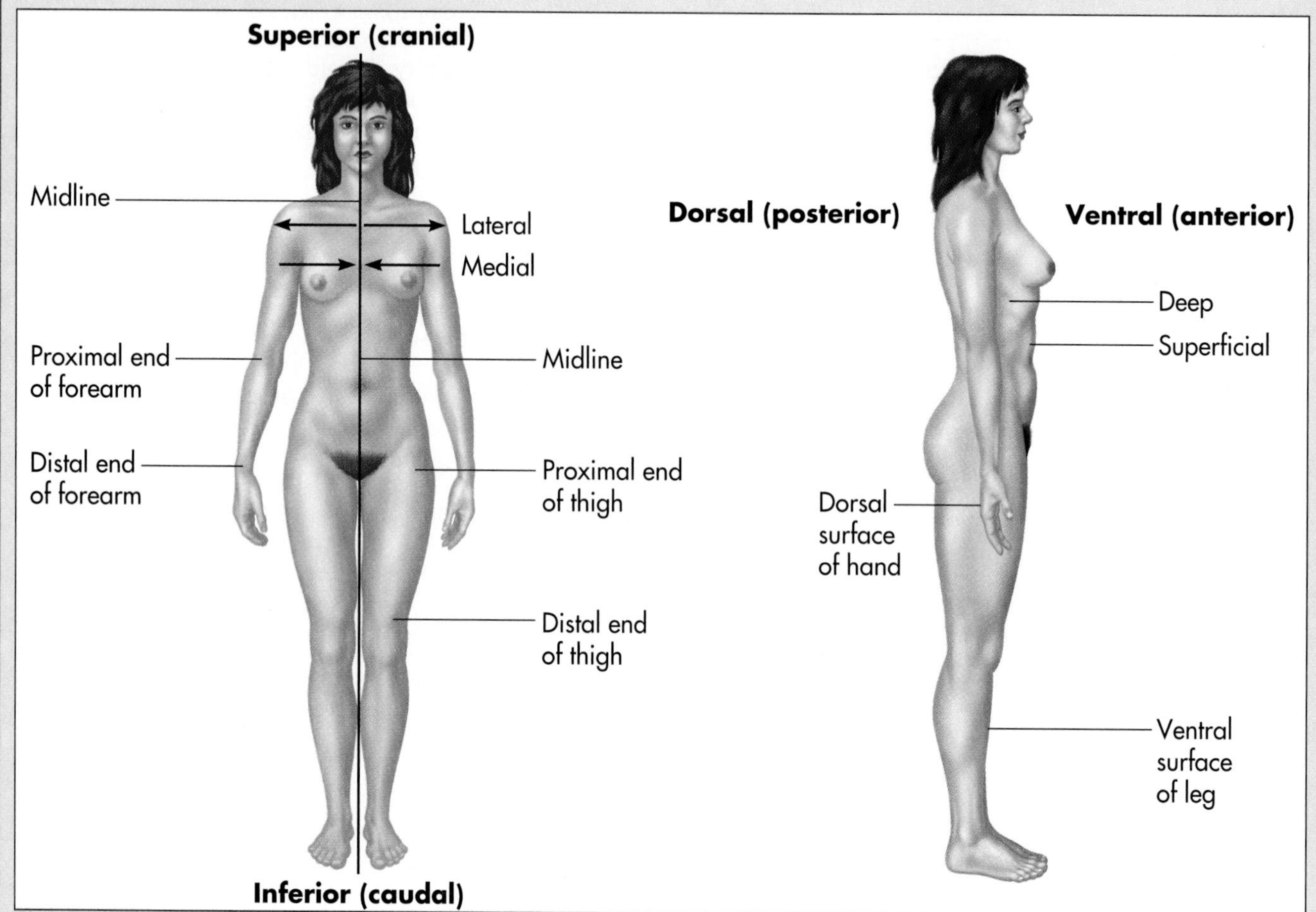

Figure 23-4. Directional terms provide mapping instructions for locating organs and body parts.

continued

The Integumentary System (Skin)

Integumentary means "covering." The skin is referred to as a system because it contains several organs that work together.

Structure and Function of the Skin

The skin consists of the epidermis, dermis, and subcutaneous layer (Figure 23-7). The **epidermis** is the outermost layer; it is made entirely of epithelial cells. The outer surface of the epidermis contains mainly dead ep-

CAUTION

HANDLE WITH CARE

Locating Body Parts by Anatomical Position continued

- Superior (cranial) and inferior (caudal). *Superior* or *cranial* refers to a structure above, or in a higher position than, another (toward the head). *Inferior* or *caudal* means below, or lower (toward the feet or tail region). For example, the lungs are superior to the intestines and inferior to the neck.
- Ventral (anterior) and dorsal (posterior). *Ventral* or *anterior* means toward the front of the body. *Dorsal* or *posterior* means toward the back. For example, the nose is anterior to the ears, and the brain is posterior to the eyes.
- Medial and lateral. *Medial* indicates a position in relation to the midline, an imaginary line passing through the center of the body and dividing it into right and left halves. *Lateral* means away from the middle, toward the side. For example, the bridge of the nose is medial to the eyes, and the ears are lateral to the mouth.
- Proximal and distal. *Proximal* means nearest the origin of a structure, whereas *distal* means the farthest from that point. For example, the shoulder is proximal to the arm, and the foot is distal to the hip.
- Superficial and deep. *Superficial* means near the surface of the body; *deep* means far from the surface. For example, the ribs are more superficial than the lungs and deeper than the skin.

Spatial Relationships

To help visualize the spatial relationships of various internal body structures to one another, the body is divided into a series of imaginary cuts or planes (Figure 23-5). Each plane creates an inside view of the body called a section. The following descriptions of planes explain how you would go about obtaining a particular type of plane or section:

- A sagittal plane. If you were to cut through the body, from front to back and from top to bottom, so that there were left and right sections, each would be a *sagittal* section. A cut made exactly down the midline of the body, for example, would produce two midsagittal sections.
- A frontal plane. Visualize a cut through the body from side to side and from top to bottom (perpendicular to a sagittal plane). Such a cut would create two *frontal* sections.
- A transverse plane. A horizontal cut through the body from front to back, at any level, would divide the body into upper and lower parts and would create two *transverse* sections.

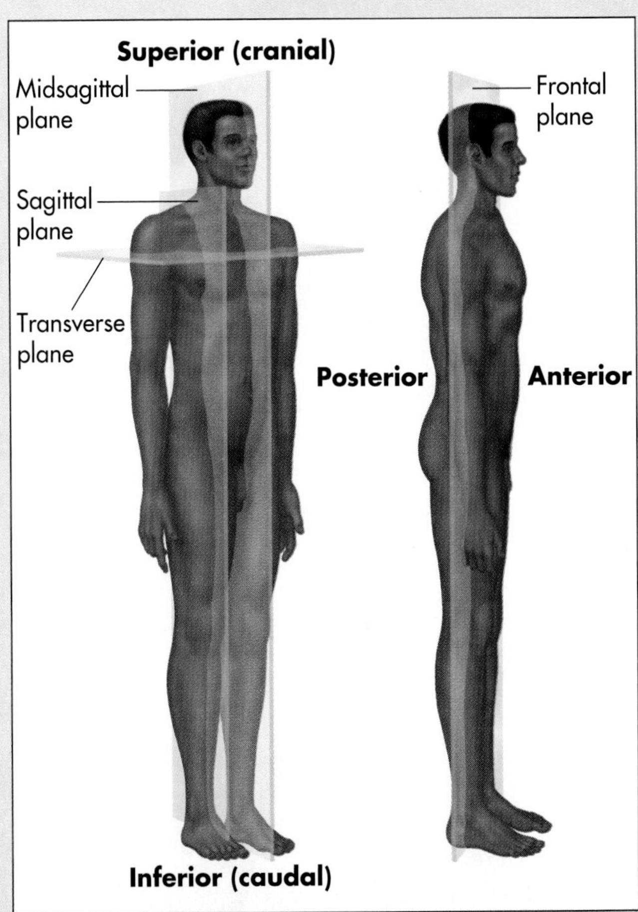

Figure 23-5. Spatial terms are based on imaginary cuts or planes through the body.

ithelial cells that have thickened, forming a protective layer. The **dermis** is the middle layer; it contains connective tissue, nerve endings, and hair follicles (small cavities that contain the hair root). The sweat and oil glands are also located in the dermis. Blood and lymph vessels, fat, and other loose connective tissue are the main components of the innermost, or subcutaneous, layer.

In addition to the sweat and oil glands, the skin contains the hair and nails. The oil (sebaceous) glands

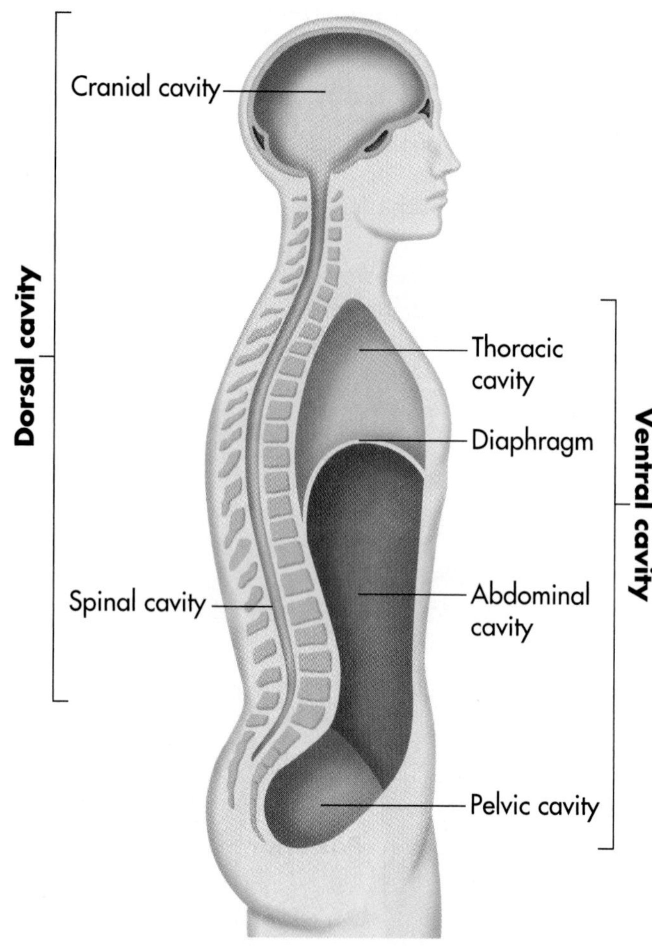

Figure 23-6. The two main body cavities are dorsal and ventral.

produce an oily secretion that helps lubricate the skin and hair and prevents them from drying out.

As the first defense of the body against infection, the skin covers and protects underlying body structures. Fat stored in the subcutaneous layer cushions these structures against injury.

The skin also eliminates some waste products through perspiration and assists in regulating body temperature. Perspiration is secreted by the sweat (sudoriferous) glands. To further cool the body, or to increase heat loss, the blood vessels in the skin expand, or dilate, bringing more heat to the surface. When the blood vessels contract, body heat is retained.

The skin contains nerve endings that send sensory messages of heat, cold, pain, touch, or pressure to the brain. When exposed to sunlight, the skin helps produce vitamin D.

The Skin as a Diagnostic Tool

Skin and nails reveal much about a person's state of health and can even help in the diagnosis of certain disorders. In fact, the first sign of some serious diseases can be a skin problem. Four important aspects of skin are used in diagnosis:

- Color
- Lesions
- Rashes
- Bruises

Skin color is an important indicator of health because many disorders can cause color changes. For example, the skin often appears pale when someone feels faint or

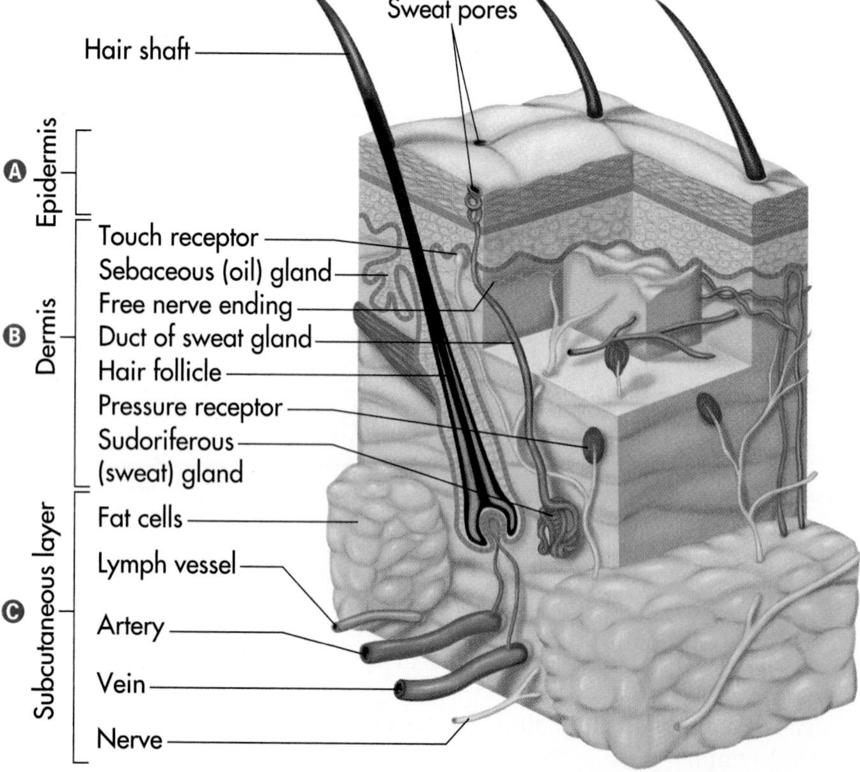

Figure 23-7. The skin consists of three layers. **A.** The epidermis (outer layer) is made entirely of epithelial cells. **B.** The dermis (middle layer) contains connective tissue, nerve endings, hair follicles, and the sweat and oil glands. **C.** The subcutaneous (innermost) layer contains fat cells, loose connective tissue, and blood and lymph vessels.

MULTISKILL FOCUS

Histologic Technician

To gain medical assistant credentials, you must fulfill the requirements of either the American Association of Medical Assistants (for a Certified Medical Assistant) or the American Medical Technologists (for a Registered Medical Assistant). After obtaining your medical assistant certification or registration, you may wish to acquire additional skills in specialty areas through course work or on-the-job training. Although this course work or training may not lead to an additional certification or degree, it will enable you to expand your role in the medical office and advance your career as the demand for multiskilled health professionals increases.

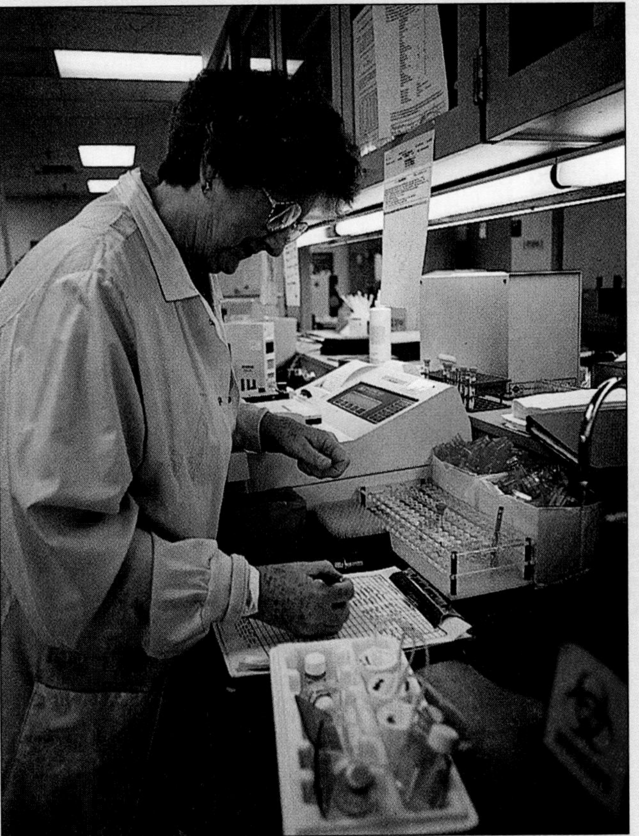

Skills and Duties

A histologic technician processes samples of body tissue to be examined under a microscope by a pathologist. The tissue samples may come from humans or from animals and may be used to diagnose disease, conduct medical research, or teach students. Depending on the planned tests, the histologic technician may freeze, dehydrate, embed, decalcify, or microincinerate the samples. Usually she will fix, section, and stain the tissue before mounting it on a slide. The histologic technician works under the supervision of a histologic technologist, a laboratory manager, or a pathologist.

One of the histologic technician's most important duties is preparing slides for diagnostic purposes. Because this process occasionally takes place while a patient is still in the operating room, the need for care and accuracy is overlaid with the need for rapid results. The technician must freeze and section the tissue sample, mount it, and treat it with a special dye to make cellular details more visible. She also checks for correctness of nuclear and cellular detail, checks the accuracy of the staining process, and corrects any identified problems. The pathologist then examines the slide to diagnose possible dysfunction or malignancy. When the surgeon needs immediate results, a frozen section is used, and the results must be returned within 20 minutes.

The histologic technician must be able to use fragile instruments with precision. For example, she may use a rotary microtome (a sharp blade) for sectioning. She must also operate computerized laboratory equipment, such as a tissue processor, which leaves a specimen in each of several reagents for a specified time.

Workplace Settings

The histologic technician works in a clinical laboratory setting. The laboratory may be part of a hospital, private pathology laboratory, research institution, government agency, or medical examiner's or coroner's office.

Education

A histologic technician must complete an accredited clinical pathology program in histologic techniques. Such a program may be offered at a junior or community college, resulting in an associate degree, or it may be a one-year certification program at a hospital. After completing the program, the technician can take the American Society of Clinical Pathologists' examination to become certified as a histologic technician, HT (ASCP).

Where to Go for More Information

American Medical Technologists
710 Higgins Road
Park Ridge, IL 60068
(708) 823-5169

American Society for Clinical Laboratory Science
7910 Woodmont Avenue, Suite 1301
Bethesda, MD 20814
(301) 657-2768

International Society for Clinical Laboratory Technology
818 Olive Street, Suite 918
St. Louis, MO 63101
(314) 241-1445

National Society for Histotechnology
4201 Northview Drive, Suite 502
Bowie, MD 20716-1073
(301) 262-6221

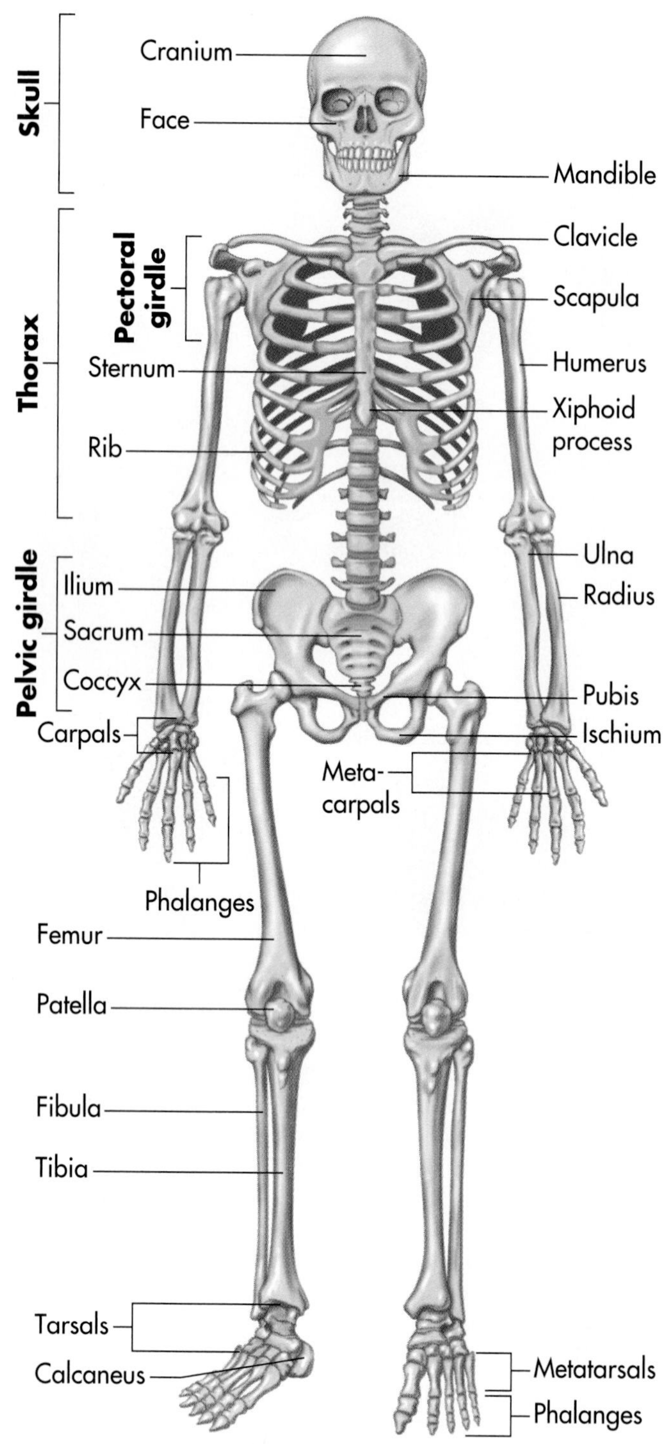

Figure 23-8. The skeletal system is composed of bones, joints, and related connective tissue.

nauseous or has a disorder such as anemia. Jaundice, a yellowing of the skin, can be a symptom of many disorders, including hepatitis, gallbladder disease, and certain blood disorders. In cases of chronic poisoning, the skin may be grayish or brownish. The color of the nails can also indicate a disease state. Bluish color or white spots, for example, may indicate infection.

Lesions are abnormal growths, wounds, or local injuries. The presence of a lesion or areas of redness can indicate an infection, allergy, irritation, or other skin problem. Abnormal growths may be benign (warts or moles) or malignant (skin cancer such as melanoma). Rashes can be caused by certain infectious diseases or allergic reactions. Diseases such as chickenpox and measles are often diagnosed by the appearance of the rash alone. Multiple bruises can be a sign of leukemia or physical abuse.

The Skeletal System

Bones are the framework of the body, giving it structure and support. Bones contain several kinds of tissue, including blood vessels and nerves. Bones are attached to each other at joints. The skeletal system is composed of 206 bones, as well as joints and related connective tissue (Figure 23-8).

The skeleton has two major divisions: the axial skeleton and the appendicular skeleton. The axial skeleton forms the longitudinal axis of the body. It is made up of the skull, vertebral column, sternum, and ribs. The appendicular skeleton is composed of the upper and lower extremities as well as the girdles (encircling structures) that attach the upper and lower appendages to the axial skeleton.

Structure and Function of the Bones

Although bones are hard and seemingly dead, they consist of living tissue. Bones have their own blood supply and network of nerves. Each of the four types of bones in the body has a different shape and purpose. The four types are as follows:

- Long bones
- Short and small bones
- Irregular bones
- Flat bones

The long bones, located in the arms and legs, give shape to the body and support body parts. The short and small bones are found in the fingers, wrists, toes, and ankles. They allow flexibility of body parts. The irregular bones are the vertebrae of the spine. They provide both support and flexibility, as well as protection for the spinal cord. Examples of flat bones are the ribs and skull. They protect soft tissues and vital organs.

In addition to offering support and protection, bones serve other functions. Because muscles attach to them, bones allow movement. The inner part of the bone, called the marrow, is one site where blood cells are made (hematopoiesis). Bones also store vital minerals, such as calcium and phosphorus, that are necessary for certain body functions.

Structure and Function of the Joints

Joints are the areas where bones connect with each other. Many structures make up a joint. Ligaments (tough fibrous bands of tissue) connect bone to bone. In some cases the ligaments completely enclose the joint, forming a capsule. The membrane lining the capsule secretes a thick, transparent liquid called synovial fluid, which lubricates the joint. Tendons (cordlike fibrous tissues) connect muscle to bone. Under the tendons, bursae (small sacs filled with synovial fluid) help eliminate friction.

Joints differ according to how much movement they allow. Some joints, such as those between the bones of the skull, allow no movement. Other joints are slightly movable, such as those between the vertebrae. Most joints, however, such as the knee, shoulder, and hip, are freely movable.

Besides their degree of movement, joints are distinguished by the type of movement they allow. For example, the knee and elbow are called hinge joints because they move like hinges. In addition, the hip is called a ball-and-socket joint, the joint formed by the two vertebrae at the top of the spine is called a pivot joint, and the wrist is called a gliding joint.

The Muscular System

Bones and joints do not themselves produce movement. By alternating between contraction and relaxation, muscles cause bones and supported structures to move. The human body has more than 600 individual muscles. Many are shown in Figure 23-9. Although each muscle is a distinct structure, muscles act in groups to perform particular movements.

Structure of Muscle

As explained earlier, muscle tissue may be skeletal, cardiac, or smooth. Individual muscle cells are often called fibers, because they are long and threadlike. Muscle fibers are held together in bundles by connective tissue. Groups of bundles are in turn held together by more connective tissue, forming the muscle. Muscles are attached to bone by connective tissue, such as tendons.

Function of Muscle

The main function of muscle is to allow movement. Muscle movement is classified as voluntary or involuntary. Skeletal muscles are under voluntary control; an individual can control them and is aware of the resulting movement. People do not, however, have control over cardiac and smooth muscle. The movements of these muscles are described as involuntary.

Most muscle groups function in pairs and act in a coordinated fashion to produce movement. While one muscle contracts, an opposite muscle relaxes. For example, when you bend your elbow, your biceps contracts while your triceps relaxes. This movement is an example of **flexion.** Straightening out your arm is an example of **extension.** Other types of motion include **adduction,** or moving toward the body, and **abduction,** moving away from the body. These movements are illustrated in Chapter 30.

In addition to movement, muscles have other functions. Some muscles steady body parts; others assist other muscles. Muscles help maintain posture, and they produce heat for the body by metabolizing nutrients during movement.

The Nervous System

The nervous system controls all body activity. It senses changes both outside and inside the body and responds to those changes by sending out signals (called impulses) to other nerves and organs.

Structure and Function of the Nerves

As mentioned earlier, the nervous system consists of the brain, spinal cord, and nerves (Figure 23-10). The sensory organs are also part of the nervous system. Nervous tissue is made up of nerve cells, or neurons. A neuron consists of a cell body, a long projection called an axon, and shorter projections called dendrites. Dendrites pick up nervous impulses and conduct them toward the cell body. The axon then conducts the impulses away from the cell body to another neuron, a muscle, or a gland.

Central Nervous System (CNS)

The nervous system is organized into the central nervous system (CNS) and the peripheral nervous system. The central nervous system consists of the brain and the spinal cord.

Brain. The brain is located in the cranial cavity and is protected by the skull bones, membranes, and a cushion of cerebrospinal fluid. The three main areas of the brain are as follows:

- Cerebrum
- Brainstem
- Cerebellum

The cerebrum, the largest part of the brain, is divided into right and left halves called hemispheres. The outer portion of the cerebrum (the cerebral cortex) is the origin of all thought processes, actions, and senses. The central part of the cerebrum contains the thalamus, which sorts impulses and directs them to certain areas of the cerebral cortex, and the hypothalamus, which assists in controlling body temperature, water balance, sleep, appetite, and emotions, such as fear and pleasure. It is also the control center for the body's

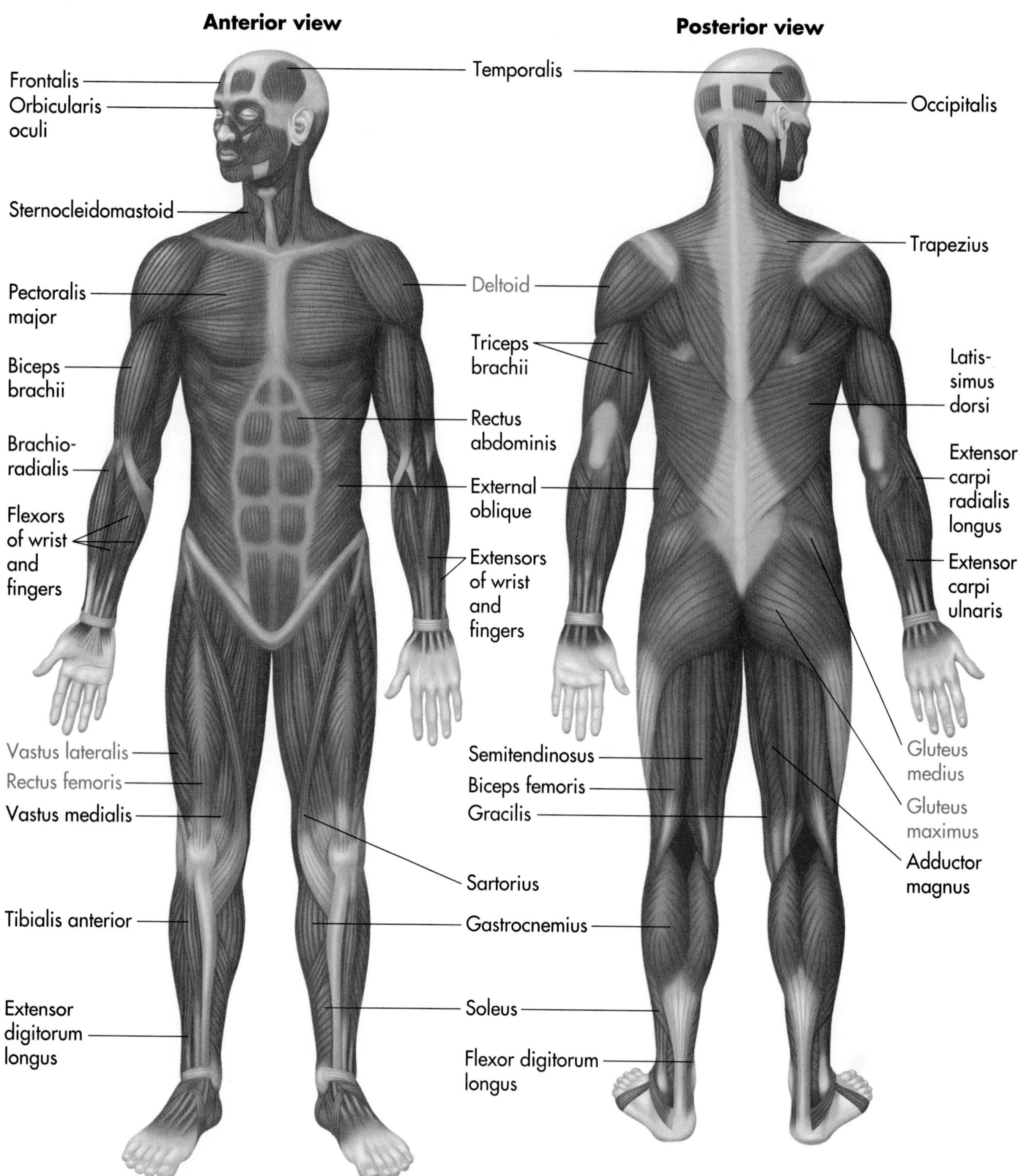

Figure 23-9. Many of the large muscles in the body are visible in these anterior and posterior views. Intramuscular injections are generally given in the highlighted muscles.

involuntary functions—those functions over which a person has no control.

The brainstem is located at the back of the neck at the base of the brain. It connects the cerebrum with the spinal cord. The cerebellum assists in controlling muscles and maintaining balance and muscle tone. It lies at the base of the brain posterior to (behind) the brainstem.

Spinal Cord. The spinal cord conducts sensory impulses from the nerves to the brain in response to pressure, heat, cold, pain, and touch, and it conducts motor impulses from the brain to the nerves. The spinal cord also conducts reflex impulses to and from the nerves, a process that does not involve the brain. The knee jerk is an example of a spinal reflex.

Peripheral Nervous System

The peripheral nervous system consists of all the nerves in the body. These include 12 pairs of cranial nerves and 32 pairs of spinal nerves. The cranial nerves carry sensory messages to the brain and motor impulses to the skeletal and involuntary muscles. The spinal nerves carry similar messages to and from the spinal cord.

Peripheral Autonomic Nervous System

The autonomic nervous system controls the involuntary motor activities of the heart, internal organs, and glands by using the same nerve pathways that control voluntary actions. Thus, the autonomic nervous system, which is largely regulated by the hypothalamus, is actually a part of the peripheral nervous system.

The peripheral autonomic nervous system consists of sympathetic and parasympathetic divisions. The **sympathetic** nervous system responds to body stress in several ways, such as increasing the heart rate, dilating the pupils of the eyes, and increasing hormone production in certain glands. The sympathetic nervous system may also respond by slowing a system that is not directly involved in the response to stress, such as the digestive system. After body stress has passed, the **parasympathetic** nervous system responds by returning the body to its normal state.

The Sensory Organs

The sensory organs and senses are also part of the nervous system. The special senses of vision, hearing, taste, and smell are included, along with the general senses of pressure, heat, cold, pain, touch, and body position. (The anatomy and physiology of the eye and ear are discussed in detail in Chapter 26.)

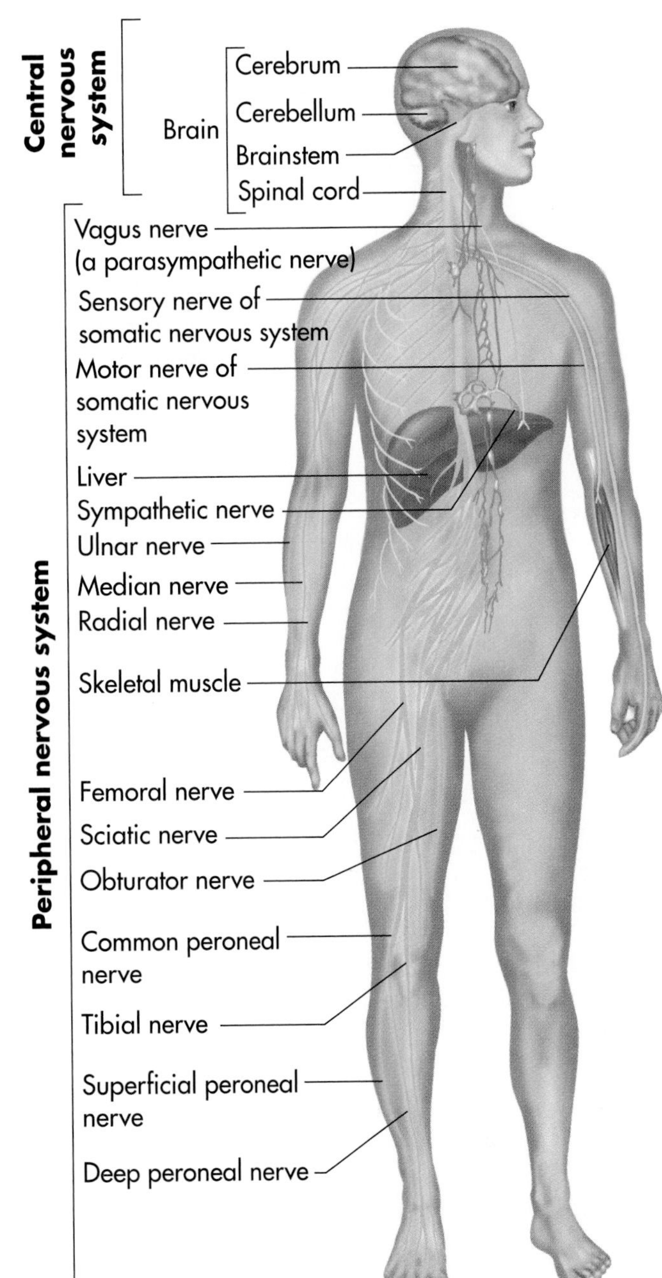

Figure 23-10. The main organs of the nervous system are the brain, the spinal cord, and the nerves. The spinal nerves originate in the spinal cord, whereas the cranial nerves (for example, the vagus nerve) originate in the brain.

The Endocrine System

Along with the nervous system, the endocrine system controls and coordinates many body functions. Although the nervous system responds very quickly to changes inside and outside the body, the endocrine system's response is slower and more prolonged. The endocrine system affects activities such as growth, metabolism, and reproduction.

The glands of the endocrine system act through chemical messengers called **hormones.** Endocrine glands are sometimes referred to as ductless glands because their hormones are released directly into the bloodstream and carried throughout the body. The affected tissues may lie far from where the hormone is produced. In contrast, the exocrine glands, such as sweat glands, release their products through ducts into a body cavity or onto the skin surface.

The glands of the endocrine system (Figure 23-11) include the following:

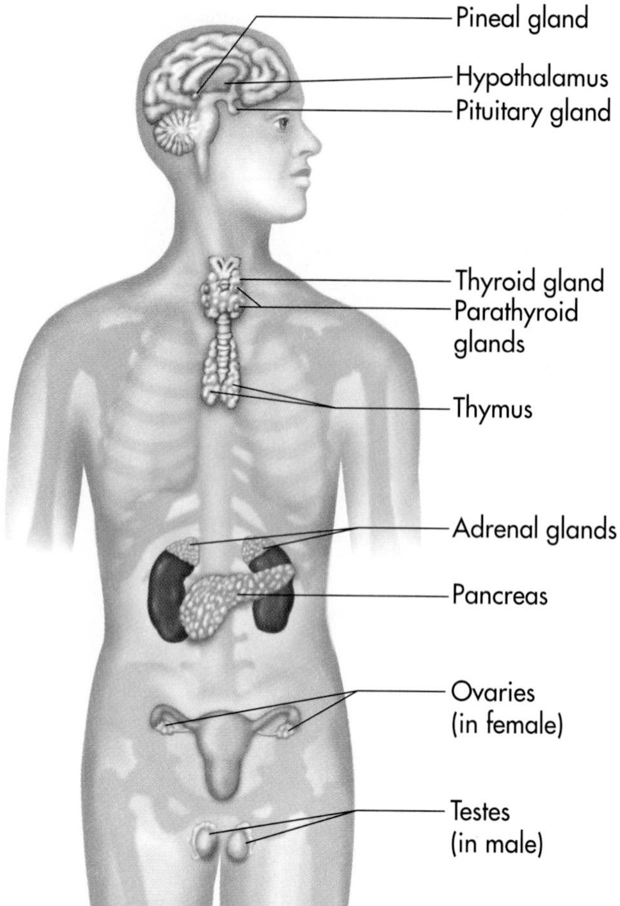

Figure 23-11. The endocrine system produces hormones that affect activities such as growth, metabolism, and reproduction.

- Pituitary gland
- Thyroid and parathyroid glands
- Adrenal glands (adrenal cortex, adrenal medulla)
- Pancreas
- Ovaries and testes
- Thymus
- Pineal gland

The pituitary gland is attached to the hypothalamus. The hypothalamus releases regulating substances called releasing and inhibiting hormones. These substances control the secretions of the pituitary gland. The pituitary gland releases hormones that affect the other endocrine glands, such as the thyroid and adrenal glands and the ovaries, as well as hormones that affect body cells directly. Pituitary hormones regulate metabolism, growth, and physical and mental development. Examples of pituitary hormones include growth hormone (GH), thyroid-stimulating hormone (TSH), luteinizing hormone (LH), and follicle-stimulating hormone (FSH).

The thyroid gland is the largest endocrine gland. It is located in the neck, surrounding the voice box, or larynx. The main function of thyroid hormones is to regulate metabolism for the production of heat and energy in body tissues.

The four parathyroid glands are located within the capsule of the thyroid. The parathyroid glands produce a hormone that works in conjunction with one of the thyroid hormones to regulate the levels of the electrolytes calcium and phosphate in the blood. Calcium and phosphate are important in many body functions, including muscle contraction and conduction of nerve impulses.

The adrenal glands are located directly above the kidneys. Each adrenal gland is an organ made up of two separate endocrine glands, the adrenal cortex and the adrenal medulla. Both glands are involved in the body's response to stress. The adrenal medulla releases epinephrine and norepinephrine when stress stimulates the sympathetic nervous system. Without adrenal hormones, people would not be able to adapt to constant changes in the environment. The functions of the adrenal cortex include maintaining blood pressure; regulating (countering) inflammatory, allergic, and immune responses; and governing sexual characteristics.

The pancreas has both endocrine and exocrine functions. The endocrine portion of the pancreas produces the hormones glucagon, which elevates blood sugar, and insulin. **Insulin** regulates the amount of sugar in the blood by facilitating its entry into the cells. If the pancreas does not produce enough insulin, excess sugar remains in the blood, resulting in the condition known as diabetes mellitus. (In its exocrine role, the pancreas produces digestive enzymes.)

The gonads, or sex glands, in women and men produce the hormones that affect the development and function of the reproductive organs. The female gonads are the ovaries, which produce eggs and the female sex hormones, estrogen and progesterone. The male reproductive organs, the testes, produce sperm and the primary male sex hormone, testosterone. The hormones also affect the expression of secondary sexual characteristics. These characteristics are the sexually distinct features, such as body hair and enlarged genital organs, that develop during puberty.

The thymus is found in the upper part of the chest, above the heart. It plays an important role in the immune system by aiding in the development of certain white blood cells. The thymus is most active before birth and early in life; it is large during childhood but gradually shrinks as a person matures.

The pineal gland is located in the center of the brain, between the two halves of the thalamus. This gland produces the hormone melatonin. Although the exact function of melatonin is not known, it appears to affect sleep and to regulate the production of certain reproductive hormones.

The Circulatory System

The circulatory system is composed of the blood, blood vessels, and heart. The lymphatic system, comprising lymph vessels and nodes, is also considered part of the circulatory system. The blood carries nutrients and oxygen to the cells of the body and carries away waste products. The heart acts as a muscular pump, moving the blood continuously through the blood vessels. This movement of blood is known as its circulation.

The Blood

Blood is a type of connective tissue that contains cellular and liquid components. The cellular components—erythrocytes, leukocytes, and platelets—are manufactured in bone marrow.

Erythrocytes are red blood cells that transport oxygen from the lungs to the body tissues and carbon dioxide from the body tissues to the lungs. The white blood cells that protect the body against infection are called leukocytes. Platelets are cell fragments that are necessary for the clotting of blood.

These solid parts of the blood are suspended in the liquid portion of the blood, the plasma. The blood has several functions, as summarized in Table 23-2.

The Blood Vessels

There are three major types of blood vessels:

- Arteries
- Veins
- Capillaries

The major arteries and veins are shown in Figure 23-12.

Arteries carry blood away from the heart. They have thick walls, because they must withstand the pressure of receiving blood that is pumped from the heart. The largest artery is the aorta, which extends directly from the heart. Arteries decrease in size as they move away from the heart; the smallest arteries are called arterioles.

Veins carry blood back to the heart. Because this blood is under less pressure, the walls of veins are not as thick as those of arteries. The largest veins are the superior vena cava and the inferior vena cava, which empty into the heart. The smallest veins are called venules.

Capillaries, the smallest blood vessels, connect arterioles and venules. They also have the thinnest walls—only one cell layer thick. The thin walls allow free exchange of nutrients and oxygen for wastes and carbon dioxide between the blood and other body tissues.

Blood vessels are also identified as belonging to either the pulmonary or the systemic circulation. Pulmonary blood vessels carry blood back and forth between the heart and the lungs, where carbon dioxide is removed from the blood and oxygen is restored to the red blood cells. Systemic blood vessels carry blood back and forth between the heart and other body tissues, where the blood exchanges nutrients and oxygen for metabolic waste products such as carbon dioxide.

The Heart

The heart is a hollow, muscular organ. It serves as a pump, controlling the flow of blood in the body. The septum, a thick, muscular wall, divides the heart into right and left halves that are completely separate from each

Table 23-2

Functions of the Blood

Category	Body Substances or Conditions Affected
Transportation	Oxygen from lungs to body tissues Carbon dioxide from body tissues to lungs Food from intestines to cells of the body Waste products from cells to kidneys Hormones from endocrine organs to other organs
Regulation	Fluid volume Electrolyte levels in body fluids Body temperature
Resistance	Infection Fluid loss at site of injury

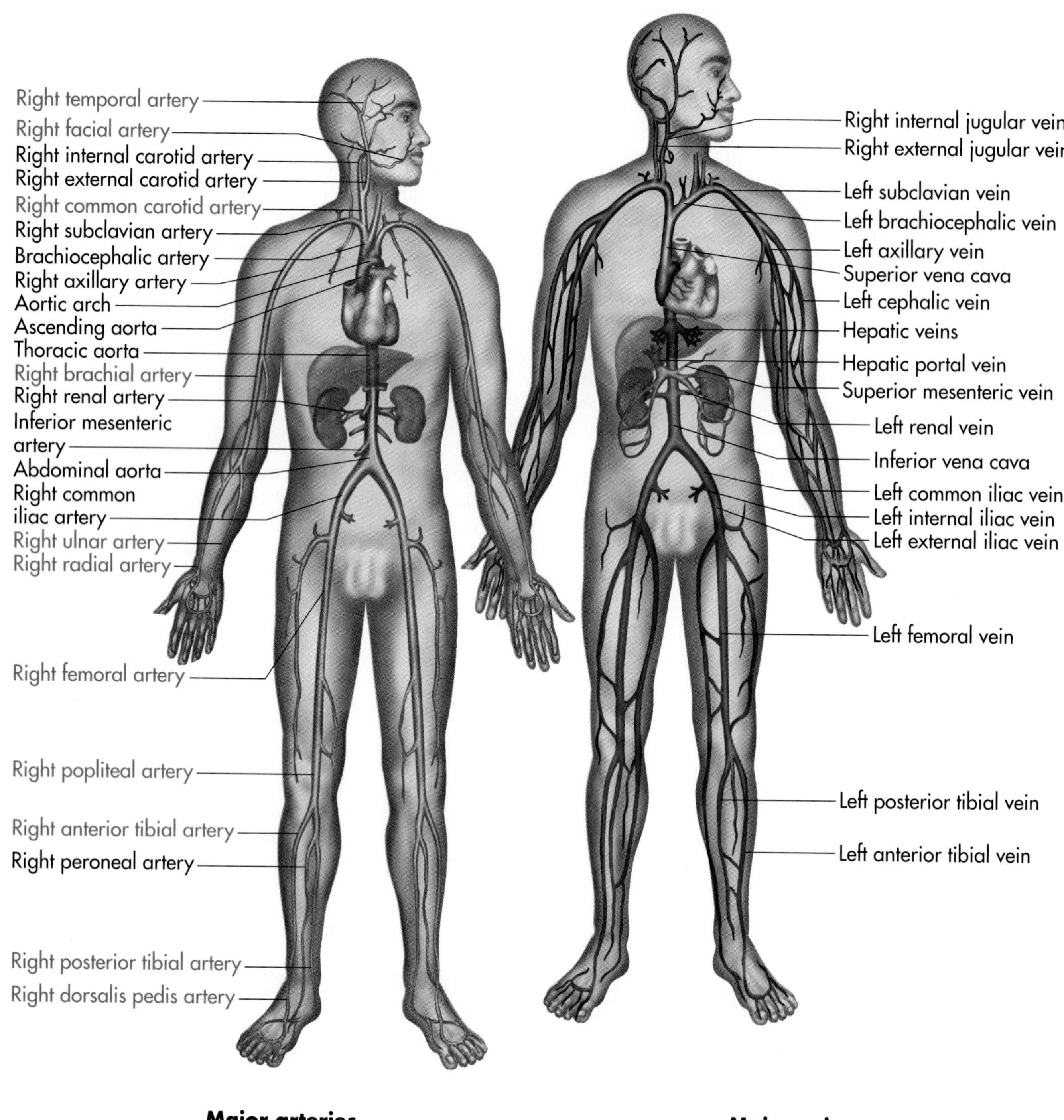

Figure 23-12. Arteries carry blood away from the heart. The pulse is usually measured where the highlighted arteries come close to the surface of the skin. Veins carry blood back to the heart.

other. Each half is again divided into upper and lower quarters, or chambers. Each side of the heart has an upper, receiving chamber, called an **atrium,** and a lower, pumping chamber, called a **ventricle.** Thus, the heart has a total of four chambers.

Blood-Flow Pathway. As shown in Figure 23-13, blood travels through all four chambers. The right atrium receives blood returning from the body tissues (systemic circulation) through the superior vena cava and the inferior vena cava. This blood is carried in the veins and is low in oxygen. From the right atrium, blood flows into the right ventricle through the tricuspid valve. Then the blood is pumped through the pulmonary semilunar valve to the pulmonary artery and on to the lungs, where it exchanges carbon dioxide for oxygen. This blood is now part of the pulmonary circulation.

After leaving the lungs, blood flows through the pulmonary veins to the left atrium of the heart. This blood then flows through the mitral (bicuspid) valve to the left ventricle, from which it is pumped through the aortic semilunar valve to the aorta and from there to the body tissues. Because of the force required to pump blood throughout the entire body, the left ventricle has the thickest walls of the four chambers.

The ventricles have one-way valves at their entrances and exits so that blood goes in the proper direction as the heart pumps. Although separate, the right and left sides of the heart pump in unison.

The heart has its own blood supply from which it obtains oxygen and nutrients. The heart cannot obtain these substances from the blood that passes through it, because only the inner lining of the heart (the endocardium) comes in contact with blood. The coronary arteries supply blood to the heart muscle.

Pulse and Blood Pressure. A pulse point is an area where an artery comes close enough to the skin to be felt with the fingers. When you feel a pulse, you are feeling a wave of increased pressure that began with the contraction of the left ventricle and traveled along the arteries to the point at which you are measuring the pulse. The rate of the increased pressure in the artery where you are measuring the pulse is the same as the heart rate. Heart rate is expressed as beats per minute (bpm).

Systolic blood pressure represents the blood pressure during the contraction of the heart muscle. The diastolic pressure is the pressure during the relaxation of the heart muscle. Blood pressure (BP) is expressed as two numbers, with the systolic number first and the diastolic number second (for example, 120/80 mm Hg [millimeters of mercury]).

The Lymphatic System

Water, dissolved nutrients, and oxygen in the blood pass through the capillary walls into body tissue. Part of this fluid then returns to the capillaries, carrying waste products with it. The **lymph,** the fluid that does not return to the capillaries, drains into lymph vessels for a special

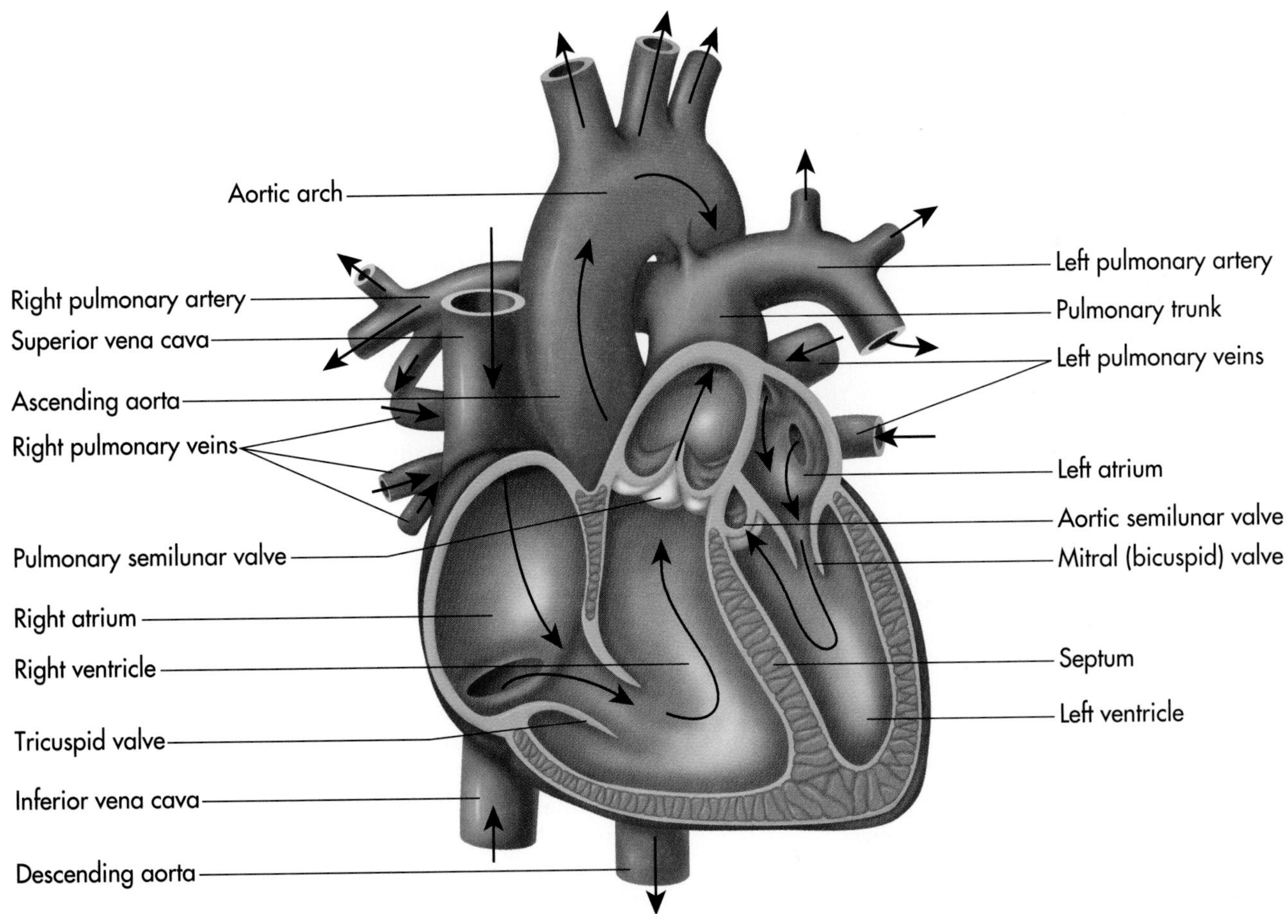

Figure 23-13. The heart has four main chambers: left and right atria and left and right ventricles. This figure shows the pathway of the blood through the heart.

type of maintenance processing before it is returned to the systemic circulation. This special processing involves filtering the fluid through a series of lymph nodes to remove foreign material and bacteria.

Thus, the lymphatic system provides a continuous special cleaning of the fluid portion of blood. This process is essential to the body's resistance to disease. The lymph nodes and organs, such as the spleen, tonsils, and thymus, all contain lymphoid tissue, primarily leukocytes that perform important immune functions. The immune system is discussed in detail in Chapter 19.

The Respiratory System

The respiratory system provides oxygen to cells and removes carbon dioxide, a waste product of metabolism. The process of **respiration** is the exchange of gases between air and blood and between blood and body cells. The respiratory and circulatory systems work together to perform this function.

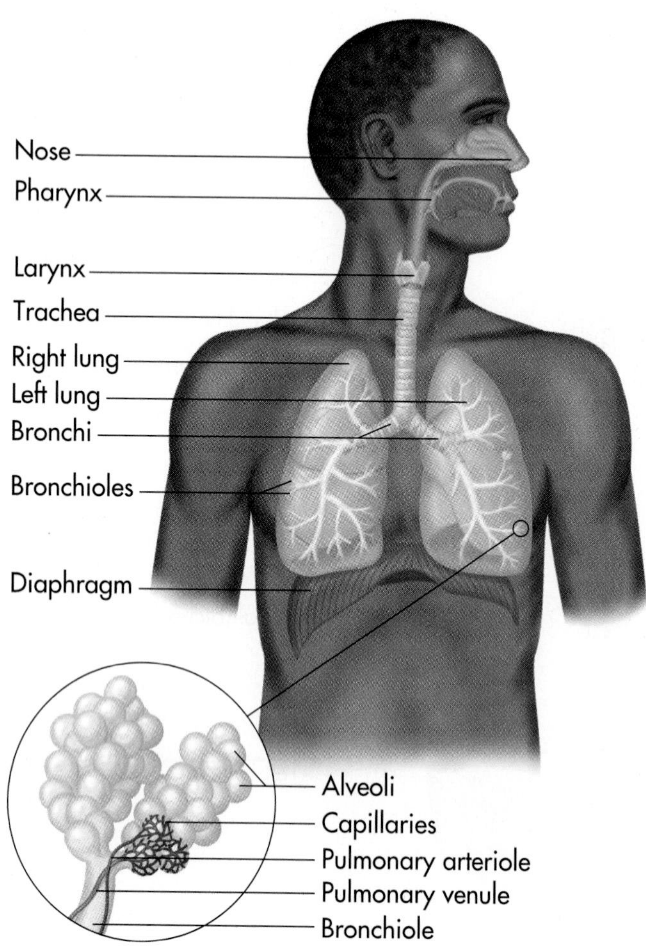

Figure 23-14. The exchange of oxygen for carbon dioxide between the air and blood occurs within the lungs, where the alveoli and the capillaries are in intimate contact.

Respiration involves both external respiration and internal respiration. Breathing, or ventilation, is part of external respiration. Inhalation and exhalation constitute breathing—taking air in and expelling it. External respiration also includes the exchange of gases between air and the blood in the lungs. Internal respiration is the exchange of gases between the blood and body cells.

The organs of the respiratory system include the following:

- Nose
- Pharynx (throat)
- Larynx (voice box)
- Trachea (windpipe)
- Bronchi
- Lungs

The nose, pharynx, larynx, and upper trachea are collectively known as the upper respiratory tract. The lower respiratory tract consists of the lower trachea, the bronchi, and the lungs. Figure 23-14 illustrates the respiratory system in relation to other body structures.

The nose performs several important functions. Hairs and cilia that line the nasal cavity trap particles such as dust and bacteria that are present in the inhaled air, preventing these particles from reaching the lungs. The nose also warms and moistens the air and contains the olfactory receptor cells—neurons involved in the sense of smell. The nasal passages are connected to the sinuses, which are small cavities in some of the bones of the skull that affect the quality of vocal sounds.

After air passes through the nose, it goes through the pharynx. The pharynx also carries food and liquids into the digestive tract. The pharynx branches off into the larynx and the esophagus, the tube leading to the stomach.

The larynx, located between the pharynx and trachea, contains the vocal cords, which vibrate to make speech. The opening of the larynx is covered with a small fold of tissue called the epiglottis. The epiglottis closes over the larynx during swallowing to keep food out of the lungs. The trachea extends downward from the larynx and divides into two branches, called **bronchi,** that enter the lungs.

The lungs are the organs that perform external respiration. After entering the lungs, the bronchi (singular, bronchus) continue to branch out into progressively smaller tubes. The smallest tubes are called bronchioles. At the end of the bronchioles are clusters of air sacs called **alveoli.** The alveoli (singular, alveolus) are surrounded by capillaries. The exchange of gases (oxygen for carbon dioxide) occurs in the alveoli: the blood in the capillaries exchanges carbon dioxide for oxygen from inhaled air in the alveoli, and carbon dioxide is released during exhalation. The oxygenated blood returns to the heart, where it is pumped to the entire body.

Each lung contains a pleural (serous) membrane. This membrane consists of the inner visceral pleura directly on the lung and the parietal pleura lining the wall of the thoracic cavity. The pleural membrane helps keep the lungs moist, aids in the mechanics of breathing, and effectively separates the lungs.

The Digestive System

The functions of the digestive system are to break down food into usable nutrients and to absorb the nutrients for use by the cells. This process is known as digestion. The organs of the digestive system (Figure 23-15) include the following (from top to bottom):

- Mouth
- Pharynx
- Esophagus
- Stomach
- Small and large intestines

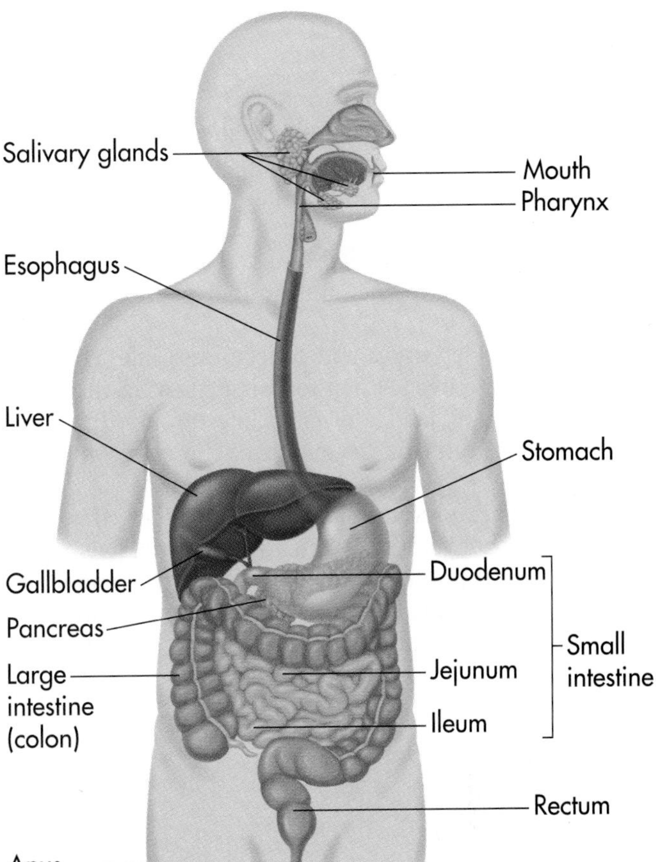

Figure 23-15. The main organs and accessory organs of the digestive system change food into a form the body can use.

Structure and Function of the Digestive Tract

The abdominal cavity is lined with a double membrane that also folds over the abdominal organs. This membrane is called the peritoneum. Fused layers of peritoneum called mesenteries help support the organs of the digestive system and the various blood vessels and nerves that serve the area.

Mechanical and chemical digestion begins in the mouth, where food is chewed into small pieces and is mixed with saliva to form a moist, soft lump called a bolus. Saliva, which moistens food and begins the chemical breakdown of carbohydrates, is produced by salivary glands located along the upper and lower jaws and under the tongue.

Food leaves the mouth when it is swallowed. It enters the pharynx, moves into the esophagus, and then goes into the stomach, by the use of rhythmic muscular contractions. The lower esophageal sphincter, a band of smooth muscle, connects the esophagus to the stomach. It remains contracted except when it opens to allow food and liquids to pass into the stomach. **Peristalsis,** the rhythmic contractions that move food, occurs throughout the digestive tract.

The stomach is a muscular J-shaped organ that stores, churns, and further digests food. The stomach produces strong acids and enzymes that, combined with the churning action, begin the chemical breakdown of proteins in the food. By the time food leaves the stomach and enters the intestines, it is in a semiliquid form called chyme.

The intestines are two long, tubular organs distinguished by the difference in their diameters. The chemical digestion of fats and the final breakdown of carbohydrates and proteins occur in the first intestinal organ along the pathway, the small intestine. Ducts from accessory organs of digestion empty into the duodenum, the first of three portions of the small intestine. The small intestine is the longest part of the digestive tract, approximately four times as long as the large intestine. As chyme proceeds along the length of the small intestine, digestive juices produced in the liver, pancreas, and cells lining the small intestine complete the breakdown of food into its basic components.

Most of the nutrients in food are absorbed in the small intestine. The inner lining of the small intestine is composed of millions of tiny, fingerlike projections called villi. Nutrients are absorbed through the villi into the bloodstream, which carries them throughout the body.

The large intestine, or colon, is responsible for making vitamin K and some B vitamins (produced by colonic bacteria); absorbing water, electrolytes, and vitamins produced in the colon; and storing and eliminating undigested waste. The material the body cannot use makes its way through the large intestine and is excreted from the rectum through the anus as feces.

Accessory Organs of Digestion

Several accessory organs release substances into the digestive tract that are necessary for the digestive process. These organs include the following:

• Liver
• Gallbladder
• Pancreas

The liver, the largest glandular organ, is located in the upper right portion of the abdominal cavity, under the diaphragm. Although the liver has many functions, its main role in the digestive process is the production of bile. Bile helps the body digest and absorb fat. Bile travels down the hepatic duct and up the cystic duct to the gallbladder.

The gallbladder stores and concentrates bile, which is produced by the liver. When food is present in the small intestine, the gallbladder releases bile through the common bile duct into the beginning of the small intestine (duodenum).

The pancreas produces enzymes that digest fats, proteins, and carbohydrates. Pancreatic substances also neutralize the acids produced by the stomach. The endocrine function of the pancreas is to manufacture insulin and glucagon, as discussed previously.

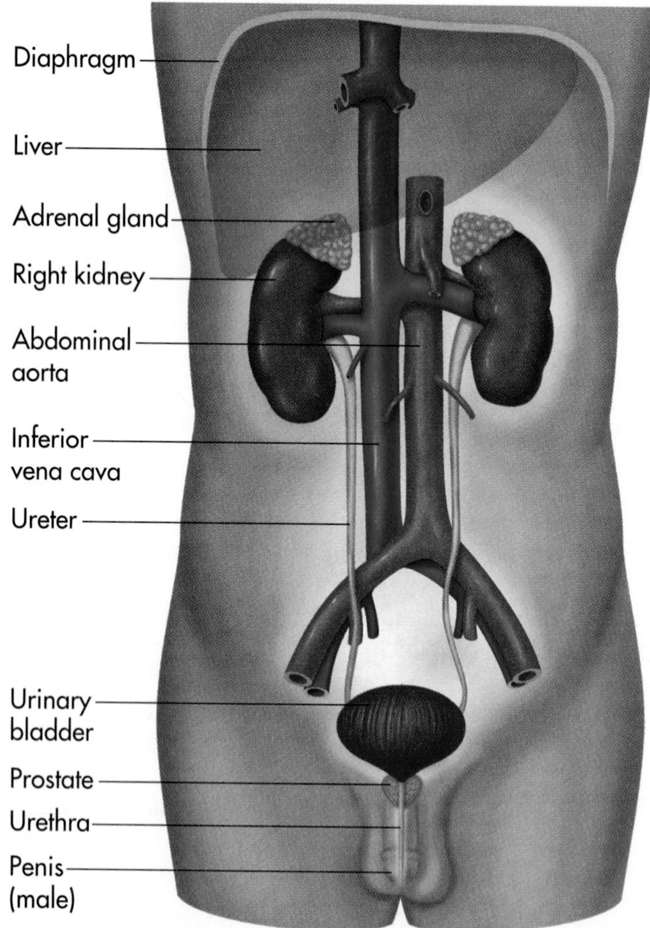

Figure 23-16. The urinary system, also known as the excretory system, removes waste products from the body and maintains the proper balance of body fluids and their chemistry.

The Urinary System

The urinary system is also called the excretory system because its primary function is to remove waste products from the body. Other functions include maintaining the proper balance of body fluids and electrolytes. The organs of the urinary system (Figure 23-16) include the following:

• Kidneys
• Ureters
• Urinary bladder
• Urethra

Structure and Function of the Urinary System

The kidneys are the main functional organs of the urinary system. They lie behind the peritoneum in the abdominal cavity, against the back muscles of the upper abdomen. The lower ribs protect the kidneys. The word *renal* describes kidney-related matters.

The kidneys utilize three processes to produce and modify urine: glomerular filtration, tubular reabsorption, and tubular secretion. During glomerular filtration, **nephrons** (functional units that act independently to make urine) filter water and waste products from the blood. During tubular reabsorption, useful substances, such as water, some salts, and glucose, are returned to the blood to maintain a proper balance. Tubular secretion is the process of selectively secreting waste as urine through the ureters.

The ureters are long, slender tubes that extend from the kidneys to the urinary bladder. The muscles of the ureters move the urine toward the bladder by peristalsis.

The urinary bladder is an expandable organ that temporarily stores urine. As the urinary bladder is filled from the ureters, stretch receptors are stimulated, creating the urge to urinate. Urination is also called voiding the urine and micturition.

Urine leaves the body from the bladder through a tube called the urethra. Muscles in the bladder control urination. The urethra is longer in men than in women because it passes through the penis, an organ that also serves a sexual function.

The Maintenance of Fluid Balance

In addition to removing waste, the kidneys help buffer body fluids and maintain balance in the volume of body fluid and in the levels of the electrolytes potassium, sodium, and chloride. These functions are important because disease can result from even slight variations in fluid volume or chemical characteristics.

The Reproductive System

The primary function of the human reproductive system is to produce new human beings. This function requires that male and female reproductive, or sex, cells be joined. In men, the specialized sex cells are called **spermatozoa,** or sperm. In women, they are called **ova,** or eggs. Reproductive cells have exactly half as many chromosomes as other body cells, because reproductive cells are formed by meiosis rather than mitosis. When the male and female reproductive cells are joined in fertilization, the resulting organism has a full complement of chromosomes.

Structure and Function of the Male Reproductive System

The testes (singular, testis), the primary reproductive organs in men, are a pair of glands located outside the body. They are suspended between the thighs in a sac called the scrotum. The scrotum is located posterior to the penis, the male sex organ. Together, the penis and scrotum are referred to as the external genitalia.

Spermatogenesis, the development of spermatozoa (singular, spermatozoon), takes place in the seminiferous tubules contained in each testis. Between the seminiferous tubules are clusters of endocrine cells, called interstitial cells, that secrete male sex hormones. Sperm travel upward into the body through a duct called the vas deferens. Each duct passes alongside a seminal vesicle and becomes an ejaculatory duct. The ejaculatory ducts pass through the prostate gland and empty into the urethra (Figure 23-17).

The seminal vesicles and prostate are glands that produce various substances that nourish and transport sperm. These substances and sperm are together referred to as **semen.**

Besides producing sperm, the testes produce a hormone called **testosterone.** Testosterone maintains the reproductive structures and male characteristics such as deep voice, body hair, and muscle mass.

Structure and Function of the Female Reproductive System

The ovaries, the primary reproductive organs in women, are the female counterparts of the testes. Other main structures of the female reproductive system (Figure 23-18) include the following:

- Fallopian, or uterine, tubes
- Uterus
- Vagina
- External genitalia

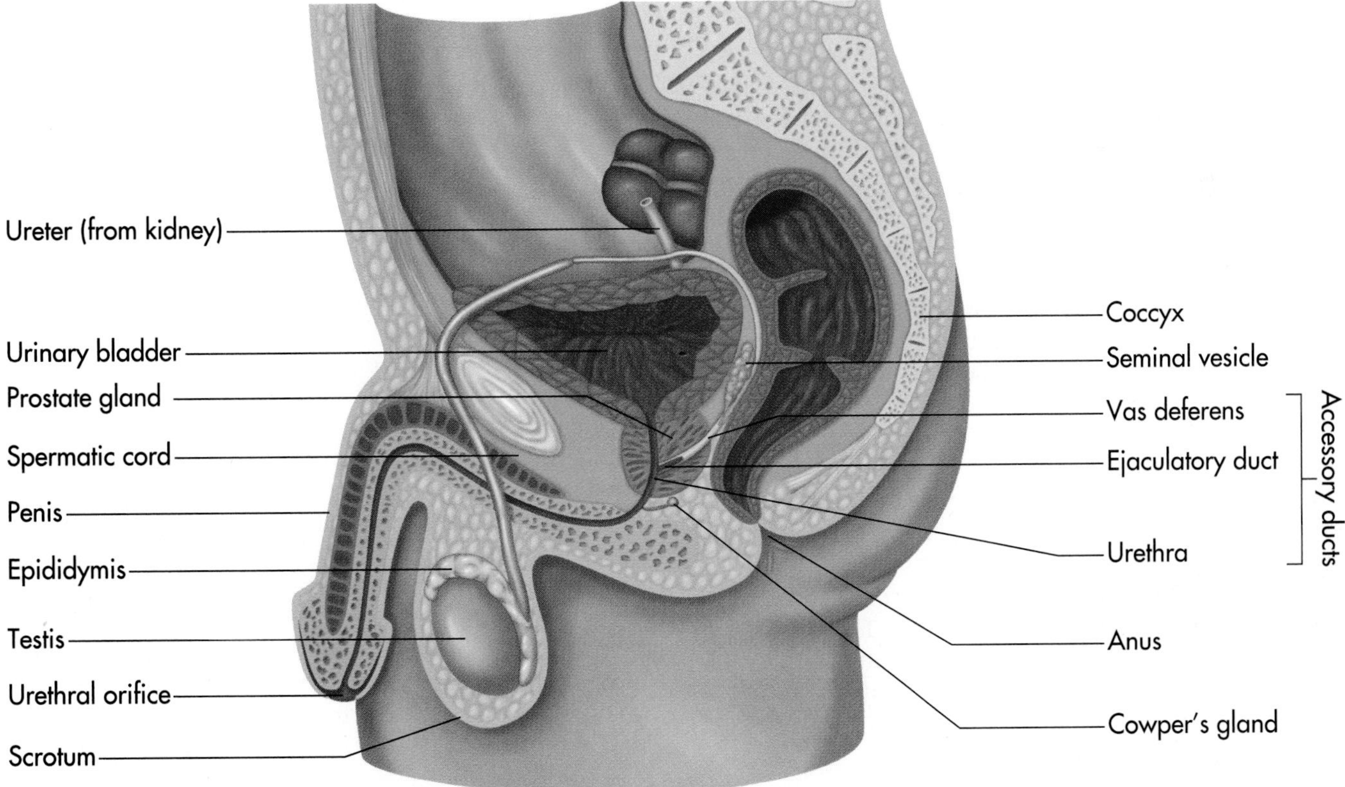

Figure 23-17. The male reproductive system produces sperm and delivers them in a form that keeps them viable long enough to fertilize an egg.

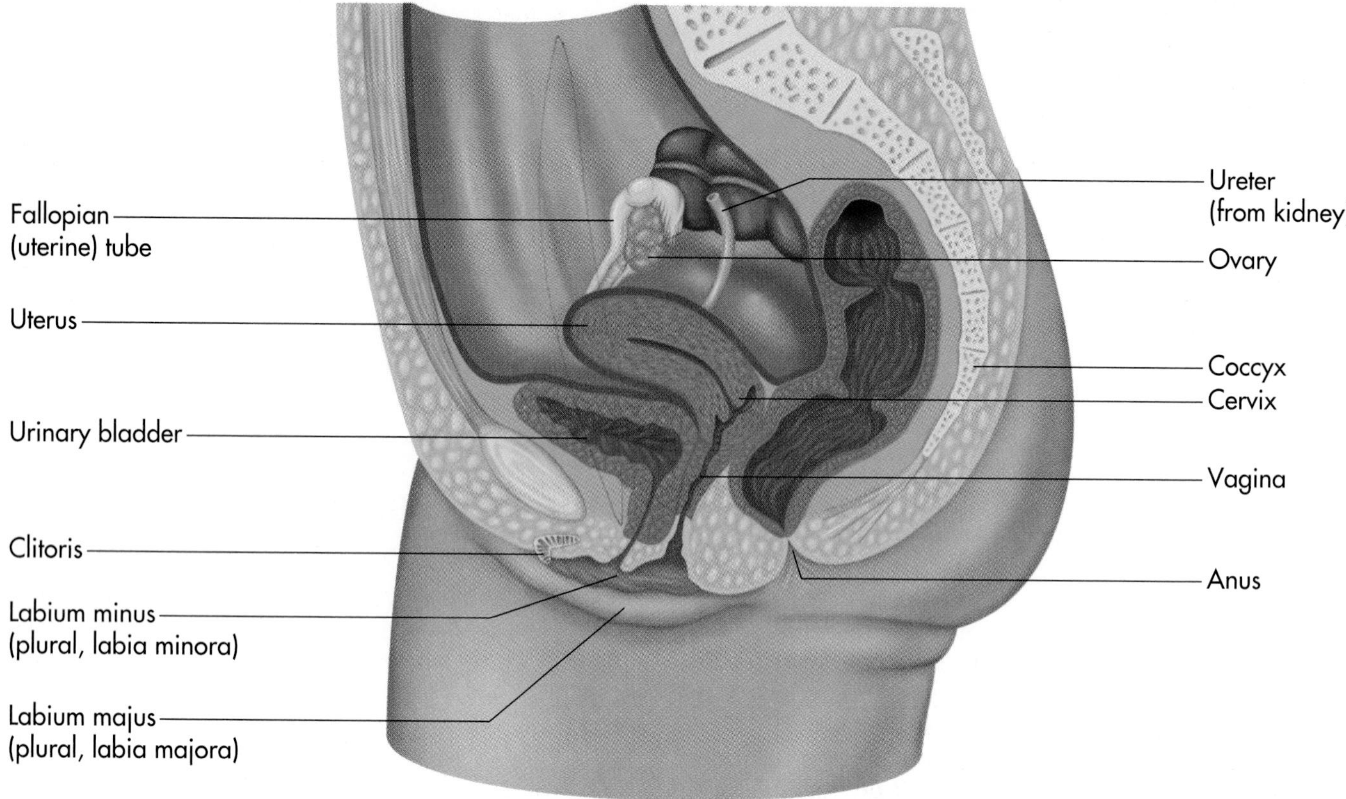

Figure 23-18. The female reproductive system produces eggs for fertilization and provides the place and means for a fertilized egg to develop.

Ova (singular, ovum) are formed in the ovaries. One ovum is released approximately every 28 days in a process called **ovulation.** The female hormone **estrogen** causes a buildup of the lining of the uterus (womb) to prepare it for a possible pregnancy. The egg travels through the fallopian tube to the uterus. If an egg is fertilized by a sperm as the egg moves through the fallopian tube, it implants itself in the wall of the uterus and begins to grow. If fertilization does not occur, the lining of the uterus breaks down and is shed, along with the unfertilized ovum, during **menstruation.**

Below the uterus lies the cervix, which is at the top of the vagina. The vagina, or birth canal, exits the body between the labia minora and posterior to the urethra. The external genitalia include the labia minora, labia majora, and clitoris.

The breasts (mammary glands) are considered accessory parts of the reproductive system. These exocrine glands provide nourishment for a baby after birth. Milk produced in the milk glands travels through a series of ducts that lead to the nipple.

Summary

A basic understanding of anatomy and physiology is pivotal to your work as a medical assistant. Whether interviewing a patient about symptoms of illness, recording diagnostic or procedural codes in a patient's chart, or preparing a patient for a clinical procedure, you need a working knowledge of body structure and function.

Your studies of anatomy and physiology may help you identify particular areas of interest as a medical assistant. If the chemical, cellular, or tissue level of body organization fascinates you, you may lean toward work in a physician's office laboratory or other laboratory facility. Consider working in a specialized medical practice if you find that a single organ or organ system captures your attention as you work to master this material.

Be assured, above all, that you will use this information on a daily basis. A solid understanding of anatomy and physiology will serve you and the patients with whom you work very well indeed.

23 Chapter Review

Discussion Questions

1. Explain the function of the four types of tissue in one of the body systems.
2. How do the pituitary gland and the gonads affect the reproductive system?
3. Explain the interaction between the lymphatic system and the circulation of the blood.

Critical Thinking Questions

1. What symptoms would you expect with a condition that causes degeneration of connective tissues in a joint?
2. If a glandular disorder is primarily affecting body temperature, energy level, and weight, which gland is likely to be involved?
3. What can a medical assistant do to interfere with mechanisms that cause disease?

Application Activities

1. Referring to the figures of the various organ systems and "Caution: Handle With Care," use anatomical position terms to describe the locations of the following organs:
   a. Liver
   b. Uterus
   c. Thyroid
   d. Kidney
   e. Eye
   f. Small intestine
   g. Skin
   h. Larynx
2. Referring to figures in the chapter and "Caution: Handle With Care," name an organ or part of the body that is located:
   a. Distal to the elbow.
   b. Proximal to the ankle.
   c. In the thoracic cavity.
   d. In the pelvic cavity.
3. What organs would you expect to see if you were looking at a transverse plane cut at the level of the umbilicus (navel)?

Further Readings

Brundage, Dorothy J. *Renal Disorders.* St. Louis, MO: Mosby–Year Book, 1992.

Hin, Marcia J. *Skin Disorders.* St. Louis, MO: Mosby–Year Book, 1994.

Memmler, Ruth L., Barbara J. Cohen, and Dena L. Wood. *The Human Body in Health and Disease.* 6th ed. Philadelphia: J. B. Lippincott, 1996.

Monrad, Lena A. *Orthopedic Disorders.* St. Louis, MO: Mosby–Year Book, 1991.

Tortora, Gerard J., and Nicholas P. Anagnostakos. *Principles of Anatomy and Physiology.* 6th ed. New York: Harper & Row, 1990.

Van Wynsberghe, Donna, Charles R. Noback, and Robert Carola. *Human Anatomy & Physiology.* 3d ed. New York: McGraw-Hill, 1995.

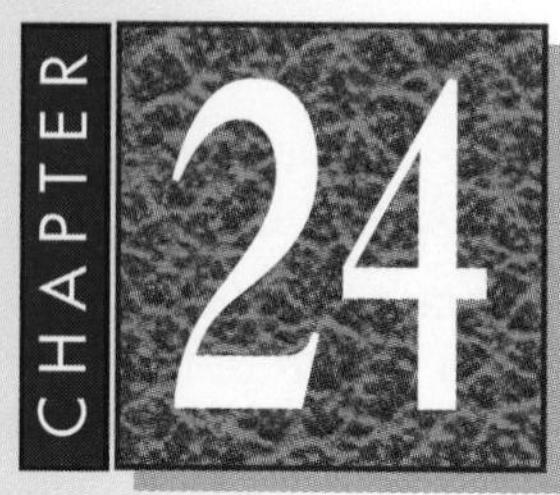

Interviewing the Patient and Taking History and Measurements

CHAPTER OUTLINE

- Conducting the Patient Interview
- Recording the Patient's Medical History
- Your Role as an Observer
- Mensuration
- Vital Signs

OBJECTIVES

After completing Chapter 24, you will be able to:

- List procedures that are typically performed before a general physical examination.
- State the six Cs for writing an accurate patient history.
- Name the skills necessary to conduct a patient interview.
- Explain the procedure for conducting a patient interview.
- Recognize signs of anxiety, depression, and physical, mental, or substance abuse.
- Describe the instruments used to measure weight, height, and vital signs.
- Describe the procedure for measuring the weight and height of adults, children, and infants.
- Describe the methods for measuring temperature, pulse, respiration, and blood pressure.

AREAS OF COMPETENCE

1997 ROLE DELINEATION STUDY

CLINICAL

Patient Care

- Obtain patient history and vital signs

GENERAL (Transdisciplinary)

Communication Skills

- Adapt communications to individual's ability to understand
- Use effective and correct verbal and written communications
- Recognize and respond to verbal and nonverbal communications
- Receive, organize, prioritize, and transmit information

continued

Key Terms

addiction
afebrile
antecubital space
apex
apical
auscultated blood pressure
axilla
brachial artery
calibrate
Celsius (centigrade)
chief complaint
diastolic pressure
dyspnea
Fahrenheit
febrile
hyperpnea
hypertension
hypotension
meniscus
mensuration
palpatory method
radial artery
sphygmomanometer
stethoscope
substance abuse
systolic pressure
tachypnea
tympanic thermometer

AREAS OF COMPETENCE continued

Legal Concepts

- Maintain confidentiality
- Prepare and maintain medical records

Instruction

- Instruct individuals according to their needs

Conducting the Patient Interview

It is your job to prepare the patient and the patient chart before the physician enters the examination room to examine the patient. You are the first contact with the patient in the examination room. How you conduct yourself during those first few moments can make a major difference in the patient's attitude. The patient must cooperate fully to provide the information the physician needs to diagnose and treat the patient successfully.

The first step in the examination process is the patient interview. A well-conducted interview helps establish a beneficial relationship between you and the patient.

When a patient makes an office visit for a medical problem, you will ask the patient (or an attending family member) for specific pieces of information called data. These data include symptoms and the **chief complaint** (a subjective statement made by a patient describing the patient's most significant symptoms or signs of illness). Medicare and most insurers require this information. When a patient makes an office visit for a routine checkup, you will ask the patient about general health and lifestyle and about any changes in health status since the last visit.

The initial interview with the patient in the examining room is more than the process of filling out a standard form. It is an important communication tool that allows an exchange of information. The interview provides far more pertinent information than you and the physician could obtain from the standardized form alone.

The Patient's Bill of Rights

Remember that all data you obtain are subject to legal and ethical considerations. In 1972 the American Hospital Association issued a Patient's Bill of Rights. These guidelines, which were updated in 1992, list several aspects of quality care that should be provided to all patients (Figure 24-1).

An important aspect of the Patient's Bill of Rights is the right to privacy in regard to medical treatment. All communications between you and the patient, as well as all patient records, are confidential. Thus, you must remember to conduct the patient interview discreetly.

The Patient Chart: A Legal Document

Whenever you interview a patient, keep in mind that the patient chart is a legal document. The chart can be used as evidence in a court of law. Therefore, you must meet certain guidelines when recording data.

The Six Cs of Charting. To help ensure that you record patient data accurately, you must follow the six Cs of charting. These guidelines are as follows.

1. *Client's words* must be recorded exactly. The doctor may uncover clues to use in diagnosing the patient's condition.
2. *Clarity* is essential when you describe the patient's condition. You must use medical terminology and precise descriptions.
3. *Completeness* is required on all the forms used in the patient record.
4. *Conciseness* can save time and space when you are recording information.

*Bill of Rights**

1. The patient has the right to considerate and respectful care.
2. The patient has the right to and is encouraged to obtain from physicians and other direct caregivers relevant, current, and understandable information concerning diagnosis, treatment, and prognosis.

   Except in emergencies when the patient lacks decision-making capacity and the need for treatment is urgent, the patient is entitled to the opportunity to discuss and request information related to the specific procedures and/or treatments, the risks involved, the possible length of recuperation, and the medically reasonable alternatives and their accompanying risks and benefits.

   Patients have the right to know the identity of physicians, nurses, and others involved in their care, as well as when those involved are students, residents, or other trainees. The patient also has the right to know the immediate and long-term financial implications of treatment choices, insofar as they are known.
3. The patient has the right to make decisions about the plan of care prior to and during the course of treatment and to refuse a recommended treatment or plan of care to the extent permitted by law and hospital policy and to be informed of the medical consequences of this action. In case of such refusal, the patient is entitled to other appropriate care and services that the hospital provides or transfer to another hospital. The hospital should notify patients of any policy that might affect patient choice within the institution.
4. The patient has the right to have an advance directive (such as a living will, health care proxy, or durable power of attorney for health care) concerning treatment or designating a surrogate decision maker with the expectation that the hospital will honor the intent of that directive to the extent permitted by law and hospital policy.

   Health care institutions must advise patients of their rights under state law and hospital policy to make informed medical choices, ask if the patient has an advance directive, and include that information in patient records. The patient has the right to timely information about hospital policy that may limit its ability to implement fully a legally valid advance directive.
5. The patient has the right to every consideration of privacy. Case discussion, consultation, examination, and treatment should be conducted so as to protect each patient's privacy.
6. The patient has the right to expect that all communications and records pertaining to his/her care will be treated as confidential by the hospital, except in cases such as suspected abuse and public health hazards when reporting is permitted or required by law. The patient has the right to expect that the hospital will emphasize the confidentiality of this information when it releases it to any other parties entitled to review information in these records.
7. The patient has the right to review the records pertaining to his/her medical care and to have the information explained or interpreted as necessary, except when restricted by law.
8. The patient has the right to expect that, within its capacity and policies, a hospital will make reasonable response to the request of a patient for appropriate and medically indicated care and services. The hospital must provide evaluation, service, and/or referral as indicated by the urgency of the case. When medically appropriate and legally permissible, or when a patient has so requested, a patient may be transferred to another facility. The institution to which the patient is to be transferred must first have accepted the patient for transfer. The patient must also have the benefit of complete information and explanation concerning the need for, risks, benefits, and alternatives to such a transfer.
9. The patient has the right to ask and be informed of the existence of business relationships among the hospital, educational institutions, other health care providers, or payers that may influence the patient's treatment and care.
10. The patient has the right to consent to or decline to participate in proposed research studies or human experimentation affecting care and treatment or requiring direct patient involvement, and to have those studies fully explained prior to consent. A patient who declines to participate in research or experimentation is entitled to the most effective care that the hospital can otherwise provide.
11. The patient has the right to expect reasonable continuity of care when appropriate and to be informed by physicians and other caregivers of available and realistic patient care options when hospital care is no longer appropriate.
12. The patient has the right to be informed of hospital policies and practices that relate to patient care, treatment, and responsibilities. The patient has the right to be informed of available resources for resolving disputes, grievances, and conflicts, such as ethics committees, patient representatives, or other mechanisms available in the institution. The patient has the right to be informed of the hospital's charges for services and available payment methods.

* *These rights can be exercised on the patient's behalf by a designated surrogate or proxy decision maker if the patient lacks decision-making capacity, is legally incompetent, or is a minor.*

Figure 24-1. The Patient's Bill of Rights describes the quality of care that should be provided to all patients. (Reprinted with permission of the American Hospital Association, copyright 1992.)

5. *Chronological order* and dates on all entries in patient records are critical in the documentation of patient care. This information can also be used for legal questions regarding medical services.
6. *Confidentiality* is essential to protect the patient's privacy. You cannot discuss a patient's records, forward them to another office, fax them, or show them to anyone except the doctor unless the patient gives you written permission to do so.

Contents of Patient Charts. Each physician's office has its own forms and medical charts. All records, however, must contain the following standard information.

- The patient registration form carries the date of the patient's current visit and generally lists the patient's age, address, Social Security number, medical insurance, occupation, education, racial or ethnic background, marital status, number of children, and nearest relative.
- Patient medical history usually includes the chief complaint, history of the present illness, past medical history (including medical treatment, surgeries, known allergies, and current medications), family history, and social and occupational history (including diet, exercise, smoking, and use of alcohol or drugs). This section may also be used to record the results of a general physical examination.
- Test results include those performed in the office and those received from other physicians, hospitals, or independent laboratories. Physicians may have tests run on a patient's blood, urine, or tissue samples to aid in their diagnoses. Figure 24-2 shows an example of a laboratory report of a panel of chemical tests on blood performed by an outside laboratory.
- Records from other physicians or hospitals are accompanied by a copy of the patient's written authorization to release the records.
- The physician's diagnosis and treatment plan are specific and detailed.
- Operative reports include a record of all procedures, surgeries, follow-up care, and additional notes the physician makes regarding the patient's case. You can use continuation forms for additional information. You may also keep a separate log of telephone calls to and from the patient.
- Informed consent forms verify that the patient has understood the treatment offered and the possible outcomes or side effects of it. The patient signs the consent form but may withdraw consent if she decides to change or discontinue treatment.
- A discharge summary form is used when a patient is hospitalized. This form includes information that summarizes the reason the patient entered the hospital; tests, procedures, or operations performed in the hospital; medications administered; and the disposition, or outcome, of the case.
- Correspondence with or about the patient is marked or stamped with the date the document was received in the physician's office.

When recording information in the patient chart, be careful not only to date every item but also to initial it. This documentation makes it easy to tell which items you entered into the chart and which items others entered. The physician usually initials reports before they are filed to prove that he saw them.

Documenting Information

You will follow a series of steps to document information in medical records (Figure 24-3). These steps are referred to as the SOAP approach to documentation. They are as follows:

1. Subjective data. You obtain subjective data from conversation with the patient or an attending family member. Subjective data include thoughts, feelings, and perceptions, including the chief complaint.
2. Objective data. Objective data are readily apparent and measurable; for example, vital signs or test results and the physician's examination.
3. Assessment. Assessment is the physician's diagnosis or impression of the patient's problem.
4. Plan of action. Options for treatment, the type of treatment chosen, medications, tests, consultations, patient education, and follow-up are included in a plan of action.

Interviewing Skills

To conduct a successful patient interview, you will need to apply a variety of skills, including the following:

- Effective listening
- Being aware of nonverbal clues and body language
- Using a broad knowledge base
- Summarizing to form a general picture

Effective Listening. Listening attentively is one of the most important skills you will need for a successful interview. When you listen to what the patient is saying, you not only listen for details but also try to get an overall view of the patient's situation. As you become more experienced in conducting patient interviews, these skills will improve.

One way to be a good listener is to hear, think about, and respond to what the patient has said. This technique is called active listening. Passive listeners simply sit back and hear. When you are an active listener, you pay attention and provide feedback. For example, you might repeat what the patient says in your own words or ask questions so that you understand details.

Being Aware of Nonverbal Clues and Body Language. Verbal communication is the asking and answering of questions. To conduct a successful interview, you must also be aware of nonverbal communication. The patient's tone of voice, facial expression, and body language are examples of nonverbal communication. These signs often communicate more than words could ever say. For example, a patient who has difficulty making eye contact may

Morris A. Turner, MD

MEDLAB

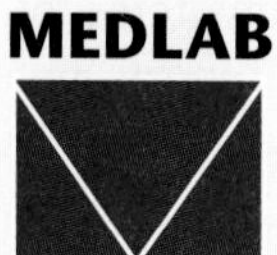

266 Line Road
Montclair, Delaware 00956
800-555-4567

C.L.I.A. #21-1862

Patient Name	Date Drawn	Date Received	Date of Report
WELLS, KARLA	09/12/97	09/12/97	09/13/97

Sex: F — Age: 43

Patient ID/Soc. Sec. Number: 166241809

Lisa W. Clark, MD
22 Landover Lane
Newark, Delaware 00964

ID Number: 23341

Account Number: 67294

Specimen Number: 897211

TEST NAME	RESULT ABNORMAL	RESULT NORMAL	UNITS	REFERENCE RANGE
CHEM-SCREEN PANEL				
GLUCOSE		76.0	MG/DL	65.0-115
SODIUM		139.0	MMOL/L	134-143
POTASSIUM		4.00	MMOL/L	3.60-5.10
CHLORIDE		107.0	MMOL/L	96.0-107
BUN		17.0	MG/DL	6.00-19.0
BUN/CREATININE RATIO		14.2		
URIC ACID		4.30	MG/DL	2.20-6.20
PHOSPHATE		2.40	MG/DL	2.40-4.50
CALCIUM		9.50	MG/DL	8.60-10.0
MAGNESIUM		1.75	MEG/L	1.40-2.00
CHOLESTEROL	237.0		MG/DL	130-200
CHOL. PERCENTILE	90.0		PERCENTILE	1.00-75.0
HDL CHOLESTEROL	41.0		MG/DL	48.0-89.0
CHOL./HDL RATIO		5.80		
LDL CHOL., CALCULATED	175.0		MG/DL	65.5-130
TRIGLYCERIDES		104.0	MG/DL	00.0-200
TOTAL PROTEIN		6.60	GM/DL	6.40-8.00
ALBUMIN		4.10	GM/DL	3.70-4.80
GLOBULIN		2.50	GM/DL	2.20-3.60
ALB/GLOB RATIO		1.64		1.10-2.10
TOTAL BILIRUBIN		0.80	MG/DL	0.20-1.30
DIRECT BILIRUBIN		0.15	MG/DL	0.00-0.20
ALK. PHOSPHATASE		44.0	UNITS/L	25.0-125
G-GLUTAMYL TRANSPEP.		8.00	UNITS/L	1.00-63.0
AST (SGOT)		21.0	IU/L	1.00-40.0
ALT (SGPT)		14.0	IU/L	1.00-50.0
LD		134.0	IU/L	90.0-250
IRON		130.0	MCG/DL	35.0-180

Figure 24-2. Laboratory reports provide physicians with valuable information about patients' health. Test results are accompanied by normal ranges appropriate for the laboratory's testing procedures.

OUTLINE FORMAT PROGRESS NOTES

Patient Name *Hansen* (LAST) *Christopher* (FIRST) *M.* (MIDDLE) Date of Birth *3 / 1 / 65* Chart # *H234*

Prob. No. or Letter	DATE	S Subjective	O Objective	A Assess	P Plans	Page *1*
	6/16/98	*Patient complaining of pain in lower right quadrant. Has been running fever of between 100.5° F and 101.3° F since Sunday morning. Has queasy feeling in stomach and has been unable to eat since yesterday morning.*				
			BP 125/75. Temperature 101.2° F. Abdominal exam revealed rebound tenderness and distension in lower right quadrant.			
				Appendicitis		
					1. Admit to hospital *2. Surgically remove appendix.*	

Start each Progress Note (Subjective, Objective, Assessment, and Plans) at the appropriate shaded column to create an outline form. Write through the intervening columns to the right margin of the page.

PROGRESS NOTES

TO REORDER CALL TOLL FREE: (800)BIBBERO (800 242-2376)
FORM # 26-7215-01

Figure 24-3. When you use the SOAP approach to documenting patient information, start each progress note at the appropriate shaded column to create an outline form. Write through the intervening columns to the right margin of the page.

be embarrassed by some symptoms and may need your extra patience and encouragement to report symptoms fully.

Using a Broad Knowledge Base. To conduct a successful interview, you must have a broad knowledge base so that you can ask questions that will elicit the most meaningful information about the patient. You must take every opportunity to expand your knowledge base by learning more about medical terminology, symptoms, and diseases.

Summarizing to Form a General Picture. You will gather a variety of subjective and objective data as you conduct a patient interview. You must consider the relative importance of each piece of information so that you can summarize the data to formulate a general picture of the patient.

Interviewing Successfully

One of the main goals of the patient interview is to give the patient an opportunity to fully explain in her own words the reason for the current office visit. These eight steps will help you conduct a successful interview.

1. Do your research before the patient interview.
2. Plan the interview.
3. Approach the patient and request the interview.
4. Make the patient feel at ease.
5. Conduct the interview in private without interruptions.
6. Deal with sensitive topics with respect.
7. Do not diagnose or give a diagnostic opinion.
8. Formulate the general picture.

Doing Research Before the Patient Interview. Before the interview review the patient's medical record for history, medications, and chronic problems (for example, diabetes or high blood pressure). Note whether the patient has family problems that might have an impact on health issues.

Planning the Interview. Develop a plan for the interview. Have a general idea of the questions you will ask. Planning the interview helps you maintain your focus and ensures that you will obtain all the necessary information.

Approaching the Patient and Requesting the Interview. Ask the patient whether you may pose some questions about the reason for the visit and the patient's current health situation. You may need to explain that the questions are necessary to plan the most effective care. It is more courteous to seek permission to ask questions than to say that you "need to take a history." Asking permission helps the patient feel more comfortable and emphasizes the importance of the interview process. It also makes the patient feel more like a participant in the medical care being provided.

Making the Patient Feel at Ease. Using certain words or phrases known as icebreakers can help set the stage for the interview. Icebreakers put the patient at ease and create a relaxed atmosphere. Examples of icebreakers include acknowledging the patient's reason for the visit or commenting about the weather. Icebreakers that also convey a sincere and sensitive interest in the patient are asking the patient how she prefers to be addressed or clarifying the pronunciation of a difficult name.

Another way to convey an image of a professional who is sensitive to the patient's needs is to sit with the patient and appear relaxed. By appearing relaxed, you help the patient relax and encourage a more open and comfortable interview.

Conducting the Interview in Private Without Interruptions. After setting the stage for the interview, ensure privacy by showing the patient to a private room or area or by closing the door if the patient is already in a private room. You can then begin to ask relevant questions. Some approaches are more effective than others, as shown in Table 24-1. Listening carefully to the patient's responses may lead you to ask questions other than those in your interview plan.

Developing a rapport with the patient is essential. Keep the atmosphere relaxed, do not rush, maintain eye contact, and use the patient's name in conversation. Avoid interruptions, such as taking phone calls and letting people walk in and out of the room.

Dealing With Sensitive Topics With Respect. Sometimes you will have to ask patients questions about sensitive topics. Such topics may be related to sexuality, lifestyle, or behaviors that put a person at risk for diseases, such as those that are sexually transmitted. You must approach these topics gently so that the patient does not feel threatened by the questioning. You can show respect for the patient's rights and privacy by knowing when to stop. Both verbal and nonverbal clues can guide you in this area.

Avoiding Making a Diagnosis or Giving a Diagnostic Opinion. Only the physician can make a diagnosis, based on the patient's symptoms and complaints. If the patient asks for your opinion about a diagnosis, explain that the physician should be asked about diagnoses. If pressed, you may need to say that it is not your place to give opinions about a diagnosis. Never go beyond the scope of your knowledge.

Formulating the General Picture. Summarize the key points of the interview. Ask the patient whether he has questions or other information to add. You will be most successful with the interview process if you remain alert and organized but flexible. Procedure 24-1 demonstrates the proper approach to an interview.

Recording the Patient's Medical History

A patient's medical history includes pertinent information about the patient and the patient's family. Age, previous illnesses, surgical history, allergies, medication history, and family medical history are key items.

The medical office usually has a standard medical history form that is used for all patients (Figure 24-7, p. 426). Specific arrangement and wording of items vary from office to office.

When recording a patient history, you must do more than fill out the form. You must review the pieces of information, organize them, determine their importance, and document the facts. When you write your first histories, you may find it to be a lengthy process. When you become more experienced, however, you will be able to write histories more quickly.

Your Role as an Observer

During the preexamination stage of the office visit, you will gather most of your information through verbal communication. The nonverbal communication that occurs during the interview and history taking, however, sometimes reveals more about a patient than the patient's words. Listening attentively and observing the patient closely may help you detect a problem that might otherwise go unnoted.

Anxiety

Anxiety is a common emotional response in patients. Some patients respond with anxiety to a specific fear, such as fear of pain. Others simply feel anxious when they are in an unfamiliar situation.

To recognize anxiety, you must understand that its levels vary from mild to severe. A patient with mild anxiety may have a heightened ability to observe and to make connections. A patient with severe anxiety has difficulty focusing on details, feels panicky, and is virtually helpless. A heightened focus or a lack of focus in a patient can hinder your ability to get the information and cooperation you need.

When you observe signs of anxiety in a patient, make every effort to help him relax and release or reduce the anxious feelings. You may be able to help by allowing the patient to describe his feelings. If a patient becomes agitated while discussing a physical complaint, you may need to postpone talking about the matter until the patient is calmer. In either situation, give support in nonverbal ways by trying to make the patient as comfortable as possible.

Depression

Some symptoms of depression are the same as those of many common illnesses. Many patients with major depression develop great skill in hiding depression or are unaware they are suffering from it. Thus, depression may be difficult to recognize. Many patients, especially the elderly, have undiagnosed depression.

To recognize depression, you must be aware of common symptoms associated with the condition. Classic symptoms of depression are profound sadness and fatigue. In addition, a depressed person may have difficulty falling asleep at night or getting up in the morning. The depressed patient may suffer from loss of appetite, loss of energy, or both.

Table 24-1

Methods of Collecting Patient Data

Effective Methods	Characteristics
Asking open-ended questions	Requires more than a yes or no answer; allows the patient to more fully explain the situation, resulting in more relevant data. Instead of asking, "Do you have a cough?" ask, "Can you tell me about your symptoms?"
Asking hypothetical questions	Allows you to determine the patient's knowledge of the situation and whether it is accurate. Ask the patient to describe how he would handle a hypothetical situation.
Mirroring patient's responses and verbalizing the implied	Allows nonthreatening ways for the patient to discuss the situation further and to provide underlying meaning. *Mirroring* means restating what the patient says in your own words. *Verbalizing the implied* means stating what you believe the patient is suggesting by his response.
Focusing on patient	Shows the patient you are really listening to what he is saying. You maintain eye contact (as culturally appropriate), assume a relaxed and open body posture, and use the proper responses.
Encouraging patient to take the lead	Motivates the patient to discuss or describe the situation in his own way. Ask a question such as "Where would you like to begin?"
Encouraging patient to provide additional information	Conveys sincere interest in the patient by continuing to explore topics in more detail when appropriate. You might ask the patient if he has experienced a symptom before or if he associates it with a change in routine.
Encouraging patient to evaluate his situation	Provides an idea of the patient's point of view about the situation; allows you to determine the patient's knowledge of the situation and possible fears. Ask the patient, "What do you think is going on here?"
Ineffective Methods	**Characteristics**
Asking closed-ended questions	Provides little information because closed-ended questions offer the patient little freedom to explain his answers. Closed-ended questions require only yes or no answers.
Asking leading questions	Leading questions suggest a desired response instead of the patient's true response. The patient tends to agree with such statements instead of elaborating on them. An example of a leading question is "You seem to be making progress, don't you agree?" This type of question limits the patient's response.
Challenging patient	The patient may feel you are disagreeing with what he is saying if you ask an emotional question or use a certain tone of voice. The patient may become defensive, which might block further communication.
Probing	Continuing to question a patient after he appears to have finished giving information can make him feel that you are invading his privacy. The patient may become defensive and withhold information.
Agreeing or disagreeing with patient	When you agree or disagree with a patient, it implies that the patient is either "right" or "wrong." This action can block further communication.

Depression seems to occur most frequently during late adolescence, in middle age, and after retirement. It is common in the elderly but is often mistaken for senility. If you observe any signs of depression, indicate them in the patient's chart and alert the physician.

Signs of depression, addiction, and substance abuse in adolescents can be difficult to distinguish. Signs of substance abuse or addiction can be mistaken for depression. The reverse is also true. Sometimes all three conditions exist simultaneously. If you have any clues that point to one of these conditions in an adolescent patient, notify the physician immediately. For symptoms that may be signs of these disorders, see "Caution: Handle With Care."

Physical and Psychological Abuse

Abuse can involve people from all walks of life and of all ages. Abuse can be physical, psychological, or both. As a medical assistant, you are in a unique position to detect abuse in the patients you see. (See Chapter 27 for additional information related to child abuse, domestic violence, and elder abuse.)

Although you must not make hasty judgments, you may suspect abuse when a patient speaks in a guarded way. An unlikely explanation for an injury may also be a sign of abuse. There may be no history of the injury, or the history may be suspicious. In either case the following injuries may be signs of physical abuse:

PROCEDURE 24-1

Using Critical Thinking Skills During an Interview

Objective: To be able to use verbal and nonverbal clues to optimize the process of obtaining data for the patient's chart

OSHA Guidelines: This procedure does not involve exposure to blood, body fluids, or tissues.

Materials: Patient chart, pen with black ink

Method

Example 1: Getting at an Underlying Meaning

1. You are interviewing a female patient with Type II diabetes who has recently started insulin injections. She is in the office for a follow-up visit.
2. You ask her how she is managing her diabetes. (This open-ended questioning allows the patient to explain the situation in her own words and often provides more information than closed-ended questioning.)
3. The patient states that she "just can't get used to the whole idea of injections" (Figure 24-4).
4. To encourage her to verbalize her concerns more clearly, you can mirror her response. For example, you might say, "You seem to be having some difficulty giving yourself injections." (Your response should encourage her to verbalize the specific area in which she is having problems [for example, loading the syringe, injecting herself, finding the time for the injections, and so on].)
5. After you determine the specific problem, you will be able to address it in the interview or note it in the patient's chart for the doctor's attention.

Example 2: Dealing With a Potentially Violent Patient

1. You are interviewing a 24-year-old male patient who is new to the office. He appears agitated. You ask his reason for seeing the doctor today.
2. The patient explains that he does not want to talk to "some assistant" about his problem. He just wants to see the doctor.
3. You say that you respect his wish not to discuss his symptoms but explain that you need to ask him a few questions so that the doctor can provide the proper medical care. (The patient has the right to refuse to answer a question, even if it is a reasonable one.)

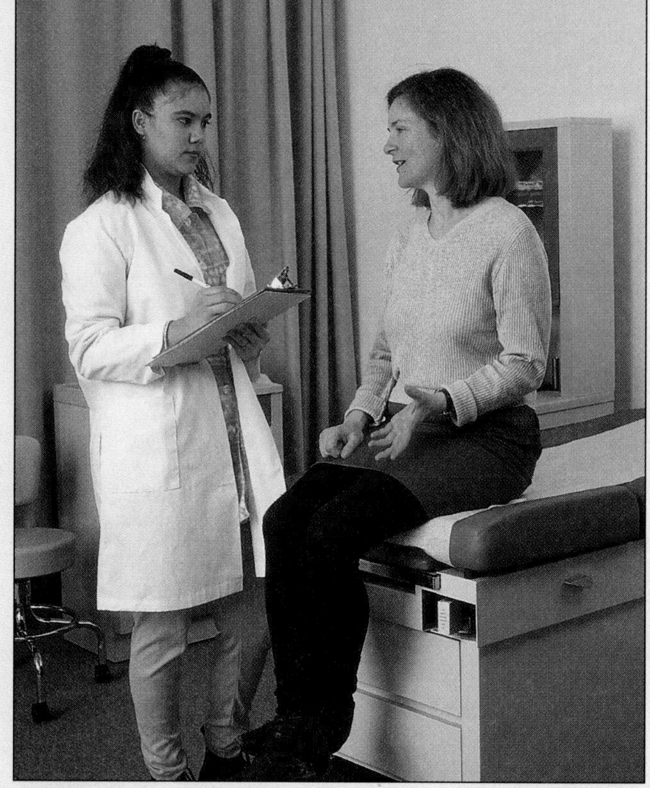

Figure 24-4. Encourage the patient to verbalize her concerns.

- Head injuries and skull fractures
- Burns (especially those that appear to be deliberate, such as from a cigarette or an iron)
- Broken bones
- Bruises (especially multiple bruises, those that are clearly in the shape of an object, and those in various stages of healing)

Although a patient can recover physically from abuse, the emotional and psychological scars may last a lifetime. Other signs of physical abuse (including sexual abuse and neglect) and signs of psychological abuse include the following:

- A child's failure to thrive
- Severe dehydration or underweight
- Delayed medical attention
- Hair loss
- Drug use
- Genital injuries

Battered Women. Women who are abused by their partners may come to the medical office with bruises or other injuries. Often they are afraid to discuss the problem. A woman may fear that her partner will "get even" if she tells anyone about what happened. The woman may not feel strong enough emotionally to leave an abusing partner. If you suspect abuse, bring it to the physician's attention immediately. You or the physician,

4. The patient begins to yell at you, saying he wants to see the doctor and doesn't "want to answer stupid questions" (Figure 24-5).
5. The fact that the patient appears agitated and begins to raise his voice in anger should be a warning to you that he may become violent. It would be best not to handle this patient by yourself.
6. If you are alone with the patient, leave the room and request assistance from another staff member.

Example 3: Gathering Symptom Information About a Child

1. A parent brings a 6-year-old boy to the office because the child is complaining about stomach pain.
2. To gather the pertinent symptom information, ask the child various types of questions. (Talking to the child first allows him to feel that his view of the problem is important.)

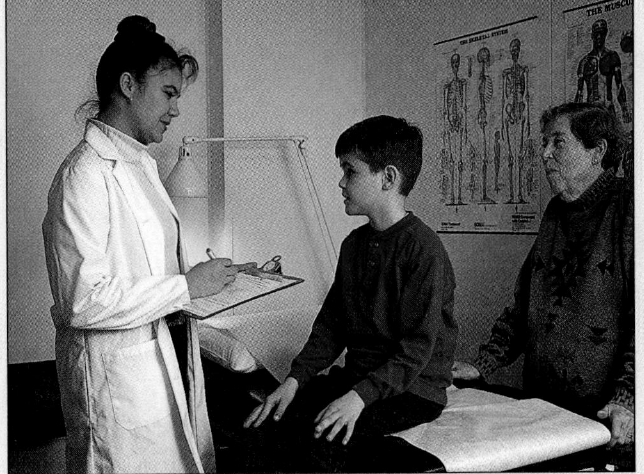

Figure 24-6. Gather any symptom information you can from a child. Then ask the parent or caregiver similar questions.

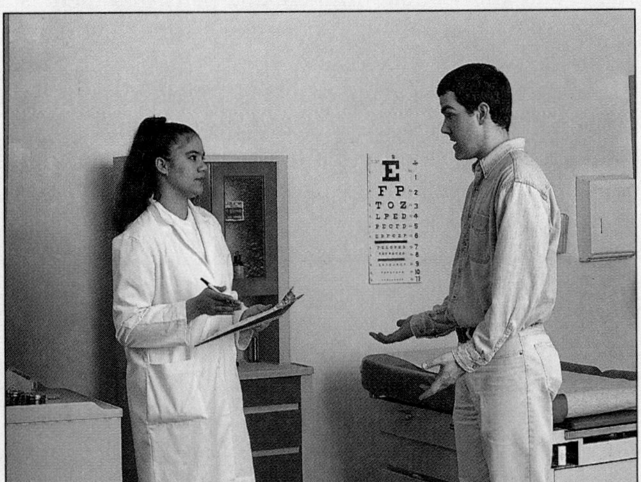

Figure 24-5. Do not try to handle a patient who may become violent by yourself. Ask for help from other staff members.

   a. Can he tell you about the pain? (Open-ended questioning allows him to tell you about his problem in his own words.)
   b. Can he tell you exactly where it hurts (Figure 24-6)?
   c. Is there anything else that hurts?
3. To confirm the child's answers, ask the parent to answer similar questions.
4. You should then ask the parent additional questions. Begin with an open-ended question, as above. Follow up with specific questions such as these.
   a. How long has he had the pain?
   b. Is the pain related to any specific event (such as going to school)?
5. Ask the child to confirm the parent's answers. He may be able to provide additional information at this time.

The Medical Center at Springfield
Medical History

Name | Age | Sex | S M W D
Address | Phone | Date
Occupation | Ref. by
Chief Complaint
Present Illness

History —Military
—Social
—Family
—Marital
—Menstrual | Menarche | Para. | LMP
—Illness | Measles | Pert. | Var. | Pneu. | Pleur. | Typh. | Mal. | Rh. Fev. | Sc. Fev. | Diphth. | Other
—Surgery
—Allergies
—Current Medications

Physical Examination

Temp. | Pulse | Resp. | BP | Ht. | Wt.
General Appearance | Skin | Mucous Membrane
Eyes: | Vision | Pupil | Fundus
Ears:
Nose

Figure 24-7. Your office may have its own patient history form. This is a sample form.

or the two of you together, may be able to convince the patient to seek help. Obtain the battered-woman hot-line number for your area, and have it available for quick reference.

Abused Children. Children are often the targets of violence, much of which occurs in the home. In addition to being physically, emotionally, or sexually abused, children can be abused by being neglected. If you suspect child abuse, you must report it to the proper authorities. Keep the child abuse hot-line number for your area on file.

The Abused Elderly. Physical or mental disabilities can make elderly people dependent on others for care. When such care is perceived as a burden by the caregiver, elder abuse may occur. The disabilities that make an elderly person dependent can also leave him defenseless against abuse. Such a patient may have suspicious injuries or show signs of neglect. Find out whether there is an elder abuse hot-line number for your area, and if so keep it available for quick reference.

Drug and Alcohol Abuse

Substance abuse and addiction to drugs or alcohol are serious social problems. Symptoms of substance abuse or addiction differ from drug to drug, as indicated in Table 24-2. Addiction, however, typically causes a gradual decline in the quality of someone's work or relationships. The patient may behave erratically, have frequent mood changes, suffer from loss of appetite, and be constantly tired.

Someone who is abusing alcohol may have no apparent signs or symptoms at first. As time goes on, however, that person may suffer from blackouts (failure to remember what happened while drinking) or may become secretive and guilty about drinking and deny that there is a problem. She may suffer from bruises, trembling hands, or chronic stomach problems.

Even though the patient may feel she does not have a problem of substance abuse or addiction, members of the health-care team may recognize a problem. Then their job is to try to persuade the patient to seek help.

Mensuration

After you interview the patient and record the medical history, you will obtain certain measurements. **Mensuration** is the general word for the measurement of weight and height. Mensuration of infants also includes measurement of the circumference of the head.

At the first visit these measurements provide baseline (normal) values for a patient's current condition. Thereafter, any abnormal changes may be indicators of possible disease or disorders of metabolism. Metabolism includes the processes that break down food and convert it

CAUTION HANDLE WITH CARE

Signs of Depression, Substance Abuse, and Addiction in Adolescents

Signs of depression, substance abuse, and addiction are often hard to distinguish in adolescents. Part of the difficulty is that adolescents are particularly skilled at hiding signs of all three disorders.

Various signs may indicate depression in an adolescent. One teenager may lose interest in or be unable to enjoy everyday activities. Another may sleep for long periods and have difficulty getting up in the morning, whereas yet another may sleep very little. Chronic fatigue or aches and pains may signal depression, as may trouble with concentration or school absenteeism. These signs may also indicate substance abuse or addiction.

It is important to know the difference between substance abuse and addiction. **Substance abuse** refers to the use of a substance, even an over-the-counter drug, in a way that is not medically approved. Inappropriate use includes such practices as using diet pills to stay awake or consuming large quantities of cough syrup that contain codeine. It also includes taking larger-than-prescribed doses of a medication. Substance abusers are not necessarily addicts, however.

Addiction refers to a physical or psychological dependence on a substance. Addiction usually involves a pattern of behavior that includes an obsessive or compulsive preoccupation with a substance and the security of its supply, as well as a high rate of relapse after withdrawal.

As a medical assistant, you should not try to make a diagnosis. Quite probably an adolescent with one or more of these disorders will be uncooperative and refuse to answer relevant questions. You must be aware, however, of physical signs or behaviors that may be associated with depression, substance abuse, or addiction in an adolescent patient. The following signs or behaviors are important clues that you should report immediately to the doctor.

- The patient complains of altered eating habits or disturbed sleep patterns (either too much or too little sleep).
- The patient's weight has changed drastically (either up or down) since the previous office visit.
- The patient appears lethargic or sullen or exhibits radical mood changes.
- The patient has slurred speech.
- The patient appears to have illogical thought patterns.
- The patient appears to have needle tracks (anywhere on the body, especially on the arms or legs).
- The patient has pinpoint (highly constricted) pupils.

into energy or build it into body tissue. Abnormal changes in weight, height, and body proportions may indicate a metabolic problem.

Weight and height measurements of children and adolescents, taken at each office visit, allow the physician to follow growth and development. Many physicians use growth charts to compare a child's growth with that of other children the same age (Figure 24-8). These charts help physicians recognize possible growth and nutritional problems.

Measurements are also important in determining certain treatment regimens. For example, dosages of certain medications are based on patient weight. These measurements may also be necessary for correct interpretation of certain diagnostic tests, such as electrocardiography. Metric conversions for weight and height measurements are given in Figures 24-9 and 24-10.

Measuring the Weight of Adults

An adult's weight is taken at each office visit. Weight should be listed in the patient's chart to the nearest quarter of a pound. The steps for weighing an adult are described in Procedure 24-2.

Measuring the Weight of Children and Infants

Children and infants are weighed at each office visit. Children (2 years of age and older) may be weighed on an adult scale. If toddlers cannot remain still on an adult scale, weight may be determined by weighing an adult holding the toddler, then subtracting the weight of the adult.

Infants are weighed on infant scales, which typically measure pounds and ounces. Infant scales are sometimes built into a pediatric examination table. The steps for weighing children and infants are described in Procedure 24-2.

Measuring the Height of Adults

The height of an adult should be measured at the patient's initial visit and whenever a complete physical examination is performed. Height should be measured to the nearest quarter of an inch.

Measure the patient's height after weighing the patient. Most office scales have a height bar located in the center of the scale. This bar is calibrated in inches and quarter inches (Figure 24-11). The steps for mea-

Table 24-2

Symptoms Associated With Commonly Abused Drugs

Drug Name/Type	Trade or Other Name	Symptoms, Effects
Amphetamines/stimulants	Benzedrine, Dexedrine, methamphetamine	Altered mental status, from confusion to paranoia; hyperactivity, then exhaustion; insomnia; loss of appetite
Barbiturates/sedatives	Amobarbital, phenobarbital, Butisol, secobarbital	Slowed thinking, slowed reflexes, slowed respiration, loss of anxiety
Benzodiazepines/sedatives	Ativan, diazepam, Librium, Valium	Poor coordination, drowsiness, increased self-confidence
Cocaine/stimulant	Coke, snow, crack	Alternating euphoria and apprehension, intense craving for more of the drug
LSD (lysergic acid diethylamine)/hallucinogen	Acid, microdot	Heightened sense of awareness, grandiose hallucinations, mystical experiences, flashbacks
Marijuana/cannabis	Pot, grass, joint, reefer, weed, bone, buds	Altered thought processes, distorted sense of time and self, impaired short-term memory
Opium, morphine, codeine/ opiate narcotics	Same as list	Decreased level of consciousness, detachment, drowsiness, impaired judgment
PCP (phencyclidine)/ hallucinogen	Angel dust	Decreased awareness of surroundings, hallucinations, poor perception of time and distance, possible overdose and death

suring the height of an adult are described in Procedure 24-2.

Measuring the Height of Children and Infants

The height of children and infants is measured at each office visit. Measure children in the same manner as you measure an adult. Some offices are equipped with height bars or wall charts that are separate from a scale. Use these devices in the same way as those that are attached to a scale.

Measure infants while they are lying down. In this instance you are measuring length instead of height. Some pediatric examination tables have a built-in bar for measuring length. You can also use a tape measure or yardstick. The steps for measuring the height of a child or the length of an infant are described in Procedure 24-2.

Measuring the Head Circumference of Infants

The circumference of an infant's head is an important measure of growth and development. You may be asked to perform this measurement (Figure 24-12) when you measure the infant's length. In some offices you will be asked to assist the doctor with this measurement during the general physical examination. The steps for measuring the circumference of an infant's head are described in Procedure 24-2.

Vital Signs

After obtaining the patient's weight and height measurements, you will take measurements of vital signs—temperature, pulse, respiration, and blood pressure. You usually take these measurements immediately before the doctor examines the patient. They provide the doctor with information about the patient's overall condition. This information helps the doctor make a diagnosis.

Preexamination procedures in some offices are performed in a general area outside the patient examination room. In other offices and in most pediatric offices, these measurements are taken in the examination room. In either case you will usually take the measurements before the patient disrobes. Follow the standard procedure used in your office.

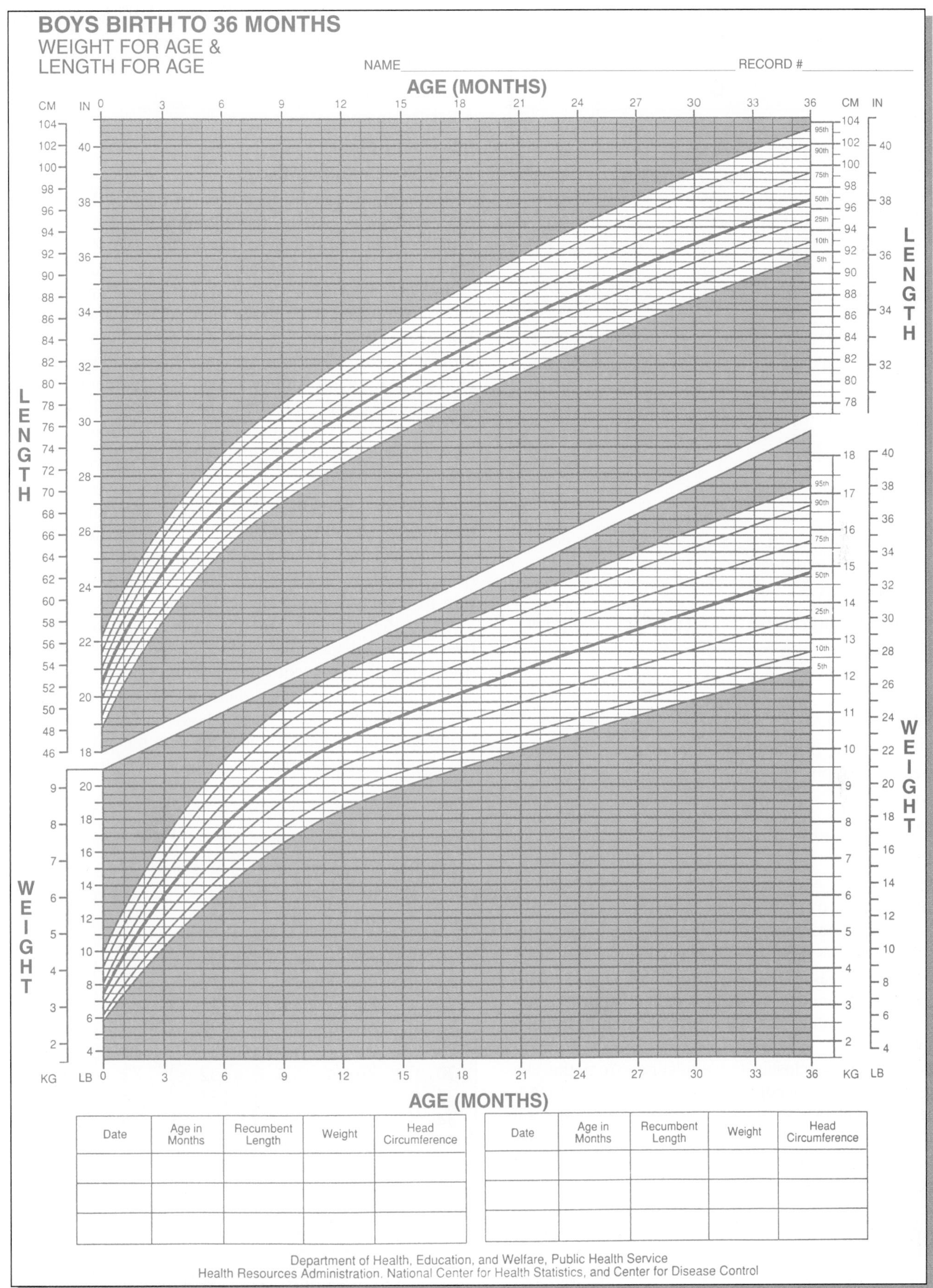

Date	Age in Months	Recumbent Length	Weight	Head Circumference

Date	Age in Months	Recumbent Length	Weight	Head Circumference

Figure 24-8. The curved lines on this growth chart show the normal range of growth for boys from birth to age 36 months.

Metric Conversions for Weight

lb	kg	lb	kg	lb	kg
10	4.5	95	43.1	180	81.7
15	6.8	100	45.4	185	84.0
20	9.1	105	47.7	190	86.3
25	11.4	110	49.9	195	88.5
30	13.6	115	52.2	200	90.8
35	15.9	120	54.5	205	93.1
40	18.2	125	56.8	210	95.3
45	20.4	130	59.0	215	97.6
50	22.7	135	61.3	220	99.9
55	25.0	140	63.6	225	102.2
60	27.2	145	65.8	230	104.4
65	29.5	150	68.1	235	106.7
70	31.8	155	70.4	240	109.0
75	34.1	160	72.6	245	111.2
80	36.3	165	74.9	250	113.5
85	38.6	170	77.2		
90	40.9	175	79.5		

Note: kg = lb x 0.454; lb = kg x 2.205. Conversions are rounded to nearest tenth.

Figure 24-9. Use this chart to convert pounds to kilograms and vice versa.

General Considerations

Vital signs are the primary indicators of a patient's overall general condition. The four vital signs are as follows:

- Temperature
- Pulse
- Respiration
- Blood pressure

Vital signs are usually measured at every office visit. There is a standard range of values for each measurement, as shown in Table 24-3. Each patient has an individual baseline value that is normal for that patient, however. The difference between a patient's current values and normal values can help the physician in making a diagnosis.

You must follow closely the guidelines from the Department of Labor's Occupational Safety and Health Administration (OSHA) for taking measurements of vital signs (Table 24-4). These guidelines are intended to prevent transmission of disease from the patient. They help protect you and keep the workplace safe.

Temperature

When you take a patient's temperature, you will determine whether the patient is **febrile** (has a body temperature above the patient's normal range) or whether the patient is **afebrile** (has a body temperature at about the patient's normal range). A fever is usually a sign of inflammation or infection. You can take a temperature in one of four locations:

- Mouth (oral)
- Ear (tympanic)
- Rectum (rectal)
- Armpit, or **axilla** (axillary)

Temperature can be measured in degrees **Fahrenheit** (°F) or degrees **Celsius** (**centigrade;** °C). Figure 24-13, p. 435, gives equivalent values for the two temperature scales. Normal adult oral temperature is considered to be about 98.6°F or 37.0°C. Rectal and tympanic temperatures are normally 1° higher than an oral temperature. When used properly, the rectal and oral methods usually provide the most accurate temperatures. Axillary temperatures are normally 1° lower than oral temperatures because the area is outside the body and exposed to air.

Temperature is measured with a thermometer. Thermometers may be one of three types: mercury, electronic digital, or disposable.

Mercury Thermometers. A mercury thermometer is a thin glass tube with a mercury-filled bulb at the end. The mercury expands and rises in the tube as the temperature rises. The glass tube is marked for reading the temperature in degrees Fahrenheit or degrees Celsius. Although mercury thermometers are disinfected with alcohol between uses, disposable plastic protective sheaths are used on them to prevent transmission of infection.

The bulb of a mercury thermometer varies in shape with its purpose (see Figure 24-14, p. 435). Oral thermometers have a long, slender tip, and rectal thermometers have a pear-shaped tip. The stubby, or security,

Metric Conversions for Height

in	cm	in	cm	in	cm
20	51	42	107	62	157
22	56	44	112	64	163
24	61	46	117	66	168
26	66	48	122	68	173
28	71	50	127	70	178
30	76	52	132	72	183
32	81	54	137	74	188
34	86	56	142	76	193
36	91	58	147	78	198
38	97	60	152	80	203
40	102				

Note: cm = in x 2.54; in = cm x 0.394. Conversions are rounded to nearest whole number.

Figure 24-10. Use this chart to convert inches to centimeters and vice versa.

thermometer, currently the most popular type of mercury thermometer, can be used to take either oral or rectal temperatures. Security thermometers, which have a short, blunt tip, should be reserved for either the oral or the rectal method.

Electronic Digital Thermometers. Electronic digital thermometers are used in medical offices more frequently now than they were previously. These thermometers provide a digital readout of the patient's temperature (Figure 24-15, p. 436). They are similar to mercury thermometers in accuracy but have certain advantages. They are faster and easier to read, do not need to be shaken down, and are more comfortable for the patient.

One type of electronic thermometer is designed for oral, rectal, or axillary use. This type of thermometer has a battery-powered display unit, a wire cord, and a temperature-sensitive probe covered by a disposable plastic tip. Separate probes and tips are available for oral or rectal use. Most units have an audible indicator, such as a beep, to let you know when the temperature has registered and is displayed.

A newer type of electronic thermometer, the **tympanic thermometer,** is designed for use in the ear, as shown in Figure 24-16, p. 436. This thermometer measures infrared energy emitted from the tympanic membrane (eardrum). This energy is converted into a temperature reading. Because of its speed, ease of use, and comfort for the patient, the tympanic thermometer is popular in pediatric offices. The tip is covered with a disposable sheath.

Disposable Thermometers. Disposable, single-use thermometers are usually made of thin strips of plastic with specially treated dot or strip indicators. The indicators

PROCEDURE 24-2

Mensuration of Adults, Children, and Infants

Objective: To accurately measure weight and height of adults, children, and infants and infant head circumference

OSHA Guidelines

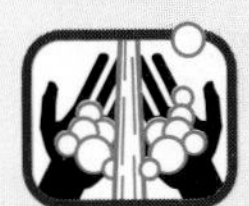

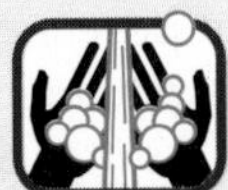

Materials: For an adult or older child, adult scale with height bar, disposable towel; for toddler, adult scale with height bar or height chart, disposable towel; for an infant, pediatric examination table or infant scale, cardboard, pencil, yardstick, tape measure, disposable towel

Method

Adult or Older Child: Weight

1. Identify the patient and introduce yourself.
2. Wash your hands and explain the procedure to the patient.
3. Check to see whether the scale is in balance by moving all the weights to the left side. The indicator should be level with the middle mark. If you are using a scale equipped to measure either kilograms or pounds, check to see that it is set on the desired units and that the upper and lower weights show the same units.
4. Place a disposable towel on the scale.
5. Ask the patient to remove her shoes, if that is the standard office policy. (Use the same procedure for all visits for consistency.)
6. Ask the patient to step on the center of the scale, facing forward. Assist as necessary.
7. Place the lower weight at the highest number that does not cause the balance indicator to drop to the bottom.
8. Move the upper weight slowly to the right until the balance bar is centered at the middle mark, adjusting as necessary.
9. Add the two weights together to get the patient's weight.
10. Record the patient's weight in the chart to the nearest quarter of a pound or tenth of a kilogram.
11. Return the weights to their starting positions on the left side.

Height

12. Raise the height bar well above the patient's head and swing out the extension.
13. Ask the patient to step on the center of the scale and to stand up straight.
14. Gently lower the height bar until the extension rests on the patient's head.
15. Have the patient step off the scale before reading the measurement.
16. If the patient is fewer than 50 inches tall, read the height on the bottom part of the ruler; if the patient is more than 50 inches tall, read the height on the top movable part of the ruler at the point at which it meets the bottom part of the ruler. Note that the numbers increase in opposite directions on the top and bottom parts of the ruler, and read the height in the right direction.
17. Record the patient's height.

continued

Mensuration of Adults, Children, and Infants

18. Have the patient put her shoes back on, if necessary.
19. Properly dispose of the used towel and wash your hands.

Toddler: Weight

1. Identify the patient and obtain permission from the parent to weigh the toddler.
2. Wash your hands and explain the procedure to the parent.
3. Check to see whether the scale is in balance, and place a disposable towel on the scale.
4. Ask the parent to hold the patient and to step on the scale. Follow the procedure for obtaining the weight of an adult (see above).
5. Have the parent put the child down or hand the child to another staff member.
6. Obtain the parent's weight.
7. Subtract the parent's weight from the combined weight to determine the weight of the child.
8. Record the patient's weight in the chart to the nearest quarter of a pound or tenth of a kilogram.

Height

9. Measure the child's height in the same manner as you measure adult height, or have the child stand with the back against the height chart. Measure height at the crown of the head.
10. Record the height in the patient's chart.
11. Properly dispose of the used towel and wash your hands.

Infant: Weight

1. Identify the patient and obtain permission from the parent to weigh the infant.
2. Wash your hands and explain the procedure to the parent.
3. Ask the parent to undress the infant. (The infant's clothing and diaper can affect the results.)
4. Check to see whether the infant scale is in balance, and place a disposable towel on it.
5. Have the parent place the child face up on the scale (or on the examination table if the scale is built into it). Keep one hand over the infant at all times to prevent a fall. (When weighing a male infant, it is a good idea to hold a diaper over the penis to catch any urine the infant might void.)
6. Place the lower weight at the highest number that does not cause the balance indicator to drop to the bottom.
7. Move the upper weight slowly to the right until the balance bar is centered at the middle mark, adjusting as necessary.
8. Add the two weights together to get the patient's weight.
9. Record the patient's weight in the chart in pounds and ounces or to the nearest tenth of a kilogram.
10. Return the weights to their starting positions on the left side.

Length: Scale With Height (Length) Bar

11. If the scale has a height bar, move the infant toward the head of the scale or examination table until her head touches the bar.
12. Have the parent hold the infant by the shoulders in this position.
13. Holding the infant's ankles, gently extend the legs and slide the bottom bar to touch the soles of the feet.
14. Note the length and release the infant's ankles.
15. Record the length in the patient's chart.

Length: Scale or Examination Table Without Height (Length) Bar

11. If neither the scale nor the examination table has a height bar, have the parent position the infant close to the head of the examination table and hold the infant by the shoulders in this position.
12. Place a stiff piece of cardboard against the crown of the infant's head, and mark a line on the towel, or hold a yardstick against the cardboard.
13. Holding the infant's ankles, gently extend the legs and draw a line on the towel to mark the heel, or note the measure on the yardstick.
14. Release the infant's ankles and measure the distance between the two markings on the towel using the yardstick.
15. Record the length in the patient's chart.

Head Circumference

Measurement of head circumference may be performed at the same time as weight and height, or it may be part of the general physical examination.

16. With the infant in a sitting or supine position, place the tape measure around the infant's head at the forehead.
17. Adjust the tape so that it surrounds the infant's head at its largest circumference.
18. Overlap the ends of the tape, and read the measure at the point of overlap.
19. Record the circumference in the patient's chart.
20. Properly dispose of the used towel and wash your hands.

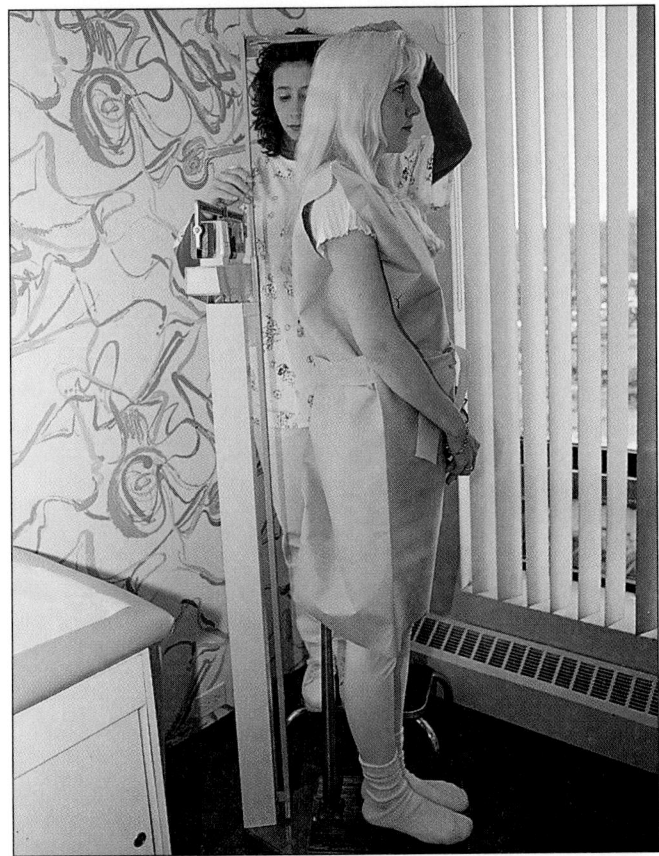

Figure 24-11. The scale with attached height bar is used for measuring the height and weight of children and adults.

change color according to the temperature. This type of thermometer is used most commonly for oral and axillary temperature measurements, particularly in children. Typically, however, it does not give as accurate a reading as other types of thermometers do.

Taking Temperatures

Using the proper instrument and technique provides the most accurate temperature readings. Temperatures can vary according to the location used. Thus, you must be sure to indicate the site (oral, rectal, axillary, tympanic) of the temperature measurement when you enter the reading in the patient's chart. If no site is specified, it is presumed to be oral. All temperature measurements should be recorded to the nearest two-tenths of a degree for mercury thermometers and one-tenth of a degree for digital thermometers.

Using Mercury Thermometers. Before you use a mercury thermometer, you must shake the mercury down. Holding the thermometer securely at the end opposite the insertion tip, use a snap of the wrist to shake the mercury down to a reading between 96.0° and 97.0°F. If you shake down the mercury too far, it may take longer to get an accurate reading. When you shake a mercury thermometer, stand clear of furniture or counters to avoid hitting the thermometer and breaking it.

If you break a mercury thermometer, clean up the spill quickly. Put on rubber gloves, and use two pieces of stiff paper to scoop up the mercury. Place it in a biohazardous waste container. Then use a damp cloth or paper towels to clean up the pieces of broken glass. Place the glass shards and cloth or towels in a biohazardous waste container. Clean the area of the spill with towels and disinfectant, dry it thoroughly, and dispose of the towels and your gloves in a biohazardous waste container.

When taking a patient's temperature, leave a mercury thermometer in place for the time indicated by office policy. The general rule is to leave the thermometer in place for at least 3 minutes for oral temperatures, 5 minutes for rectal temperatures, and 10 to 15 minutes for axillary temperatures.

Using Tympanic Thermometers. Although accurate when used correctly, tympanic thermometers can give incorrect readings if you do not follow the proper technique exactly. For a description of tympanic thermometers and potential problems with their use, see "Caution: Handle With Care."

Although you must follow manufacturers' instructions precisely, these thermometers are easy to use. First remove the thermometer from its recharging cradle, then wait for the indicator light to show that the unit is ready. Attach a disposable sheath, and place the thermometer in the opening of the ear so that the fit is snug. Pull the ear up and back for adults and down and back for children. Press the button, and the result will be displayed within seconds.

Measuring Oral Temperatures. To take an oral temperature, make sure the patient is able to hold the thermometer in the mouth. The patient must also be able to breathe through the nose. Place the thermometer under the tongue in either pocket just off-center in the lower jaw. The patient should hold the thermometer with lips closed. Wait at least 15 minutes after a patient has been eating, drinking, or smoking before taking an oral temperature; otherwise, you may obtain an inaccurate result.

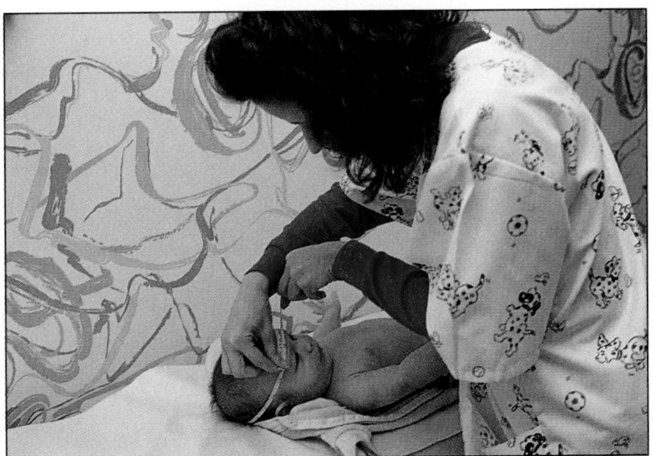

Figure 24-12. The medical assistant uses a flexible tape to measure the circumference of an infant's head.

Table 24-3

Normal Ranges for Vital Signs

Vital Sign	Age					
	0–1 year	1–6 years	6–11 years	11–16 years	Adult	Elderly
Temperature						
Oral (°F)	96–99.5 (less than 4 weeks)	98.5–99.5	97.5–99.6	97.6–99.6	97.6–99.6	97.2–99.6
Rectal (°F)	99.0–100.0	99.0–100.0	98.5–99.6	98.6–100.6	98.6–100.6	—
Pulse (beats per minute)	80–160	75–130	70–115	55–110	60–100	60–100
Respirations (per minute)	26–40	20–30	18–24	16–24	12–20	12–24
Blood Pressure (mm Hg)						
Systolic	74–100	80–112	84–120	94–140	90–140	100–150
Diastolic	50–70	50–80	54–80	62–88	60–90	60–90

Table 24-4

OSHA Guidelines for Taking Measurements of Vital Signs

Situation	OSHA Guidelines
Before and after all patient contact	Examination area cleaned according to OSHA standards Aseptic hand washing (Procedure 19-1 in Chapter 19)
Temperature by oral or rectal route Contact with patient with lesions Contact with patient suspect for infectious disease	Gloves worn Biohazard bags used for disposal of used thermometer sheaths, otoscope tips, alcohol swabs, dressings, and bandages
In presence of patient suspect for airborne infectious disease (particularly sneezing)	Mask worn Patient weighed, measured, and examined in room away from staff and other patients Protective clothing (laboratory coat, gown, or apron) worn Biohazard bags used as above

Measuring Rectal Temperatures. Temperatures are usually measured rectally in infants or in adults in whom an oral temperature cannot be taken. When taking rectal temperatures, you must wear gloves to prevent contamination from microorganisms present in the stool.

To take a rectal temperature, use a mercury thermometer with a lubricated sheath or an electronic thermometer with a rectal probe and disposable rectal tip. The patient should be positioned on one side or on the stomach with the anus exposed. The bulb of the thermometer should be inserted slowly and gently until it is covered or until you feel resistance, at approximately 1 inch. Hold the thermometer in place while taking the temperature.

Measuring Axillary Temperatures. To take an axillary temperature, first have the patient sit down. Place the tip of the thermometer in the middle of the axilla, with the shaft facing forward. The patient's upper arm should be pressed against his side, and his lower arm should be crossed over the stomach to hold the thermometer in place.

Special Considerations in Children. Taking a child's or an infant's temperature can be a challenge. If the infant or child is likely to cry or become agitated, take the temperature last. Measure pulse, respiration, and blood pressure (if ordered) before you take the temperature to avoid having these measurements elevated because of the child's agitation.

Fahrenheit and Celsius Equivalents for Temperature

°F	°C	°F	°C	°F	°C	°F	°C
95.0	35.0	98.4	36.9	101.8	38.8	105.2	40.7
95.2	35.1	98.6	37.0	102.0	38.9	105.4	40.8
95.4	35.2	98.8	37.1	102.2	39.0	105.6	40.9
95.6	35.3	99.0	37.2	102.4	39.1	105.8	41.0
95.8	35.4	99.2	37.3	102.6	39.2	106.0	41.1
96.0	35.6	99.4	37.4	102.8	39.3	106.2	41.2
96.2	35.7	99.6	37.6	103.0	39.4	106.4	41.3
96.4	35.8	99.8	37.7	103.2	39.6	106.6	41.4
96.6	35.9	100.0	37.8	103.4	39.7	106.8	41.6
96.8	36.0	100.2	37.9	103.6	39.8	107.0	41.7
97.0	36.1	100.4	38.0	103.8	39.9	107.2	41.8
97.2	36.2	100.6	38.1	104.0	40.0	107.4	41.9
97.4	36.3	100.8	38.2	104.2	40.1	107.6	42.0
97.6	36.4	101.0	38.3	104.4	40.2	107.8	42.1
97.8	36.6	101.2	38.4	104.6	40.3	108.0	42.2
98.0	36.7	101.4	38.6	104.8	40.4		
98.2	36.8	101.6	38.7	105.0	40.6		

Note: °F = (°C × 9/5) + 32; °C = (°F − 32) × 5/9.

Conversions are rounded to nearest tenth.

Figure 24-13. Use this chart to convert Fahrenheit temperature readings to Celsius and vice versa.

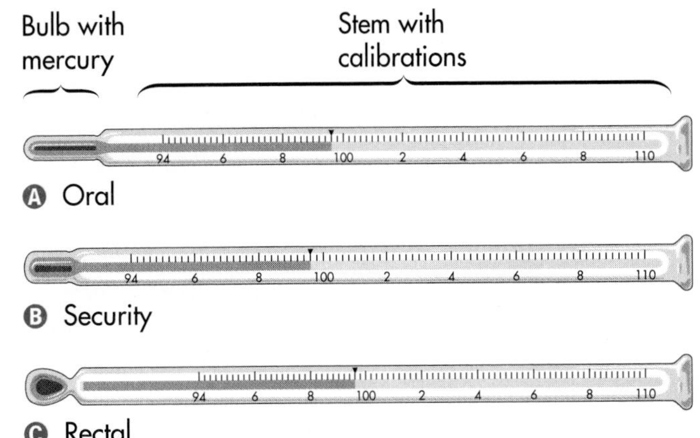

Figure 24-14. There are three types of mercury thermometers. **A.** Oral thermometers have a long, slender tip. **B.** The stubby, or security, thermometer, currently the most popular type of mercury thermometer, has a short, rounded tip and can be used to take either oral or rectal temperatures. **C.** Rectal thermometers have a pear-shaped tip.

Oral thermometers are not appropriate for children under 5 years of age because these children are too young to safely hold the thermometer in their mouths. Instead, take axillary, rectal, or tympanic temperatures. If you use a rectal thermometer, hold it in place until the temperature registers, because the thermometer can be expelled easily. Furthermore, children, especially infants, can injure themselves if they move while having a rectal temperature taken. Tympanic thermometers are especially useful in pediatric offices because of their speed and safety ("Guide to Thermometers," April/May 1994).

Pulse and Respiration

Pulse and respiration are related because the circulatory and respiratory systems work together. Pulse is measured as the number of times the heart beats in 1 minute. Respiration is the number of times a patient breathes in 1 minute. One breath, or respiration, equals one inhalation and one exhalation. Usually if either the pulse or respiration rate is high or low, the other is also. The usual ratio of the pulse rate to the respiration rate is about 4:1.

Pulse. A pulse rate gives information about the patient's cardiovascular system. It is an indirect measurement of the patient's cardiac output. If the pulse is abnormally fast, slow, weak, or irregular, the patient may have a medical problem.

Measure the pulse of adults at the **radial artery,** where it can be felt in the groove on the thumb side of the inner wrist. Pressing lightly on this pulse point and counting the number of beats you feel in 1 minute will yield an accurate pulse. Office policy may direct that

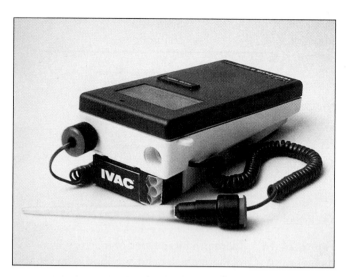

Figure 24-15. The electronic digital thermometer provides a digital readout of the patient's temperature.

you count the pulse for 30 seconds and multiply the results by 2 to obtain the beats per minute. If you take a pulse for less than 1 minute and notice irregularities, you must count for 1 full minute and document the irregularities.

In young children the radial artery may be hard to feel. You may instead take the pulse at the **brachial artery,** which is in the bend of the elbow (the **antecubital space**).

You may not be able to feel the brachial artery in an infant. If you cannot, then take the pulse over the **apex** (the left lower corner) of the heart, where the strongest heart sounds can be heard. Count the **apical** pulse while you listen with a **stethoscope,** an instrument that amplifies body sounds. The apex is located in the fifth intercostal space between the ribs on the left side of the chest, directly below the center of the clavicle. Consult Figure 24-17 for placement of the stethoscope.

You may also use other locations to take a pulse. Figure 24-18 shows the location of common pulse points.

Respiration. Respiration rate indicates how well a patient's body is providing oxygen to tissues. The best way to check respiration is by watching the movement at the patient's chest, stomach, back, or shoulders. If you cannot see the chest movement, then listen for the patient's breathing. You may not be able to see or hear the breathing of some patients. In that case the most reliable method for measuring respiration is with a stethoscope. Place the stethoscope on one side of the spine in the middle of the back to count respirations. You need to do this subtly, however, because once the patient is aware that respiration is being measured, he may unintentionally alter his breathing.

Counting respirations for less than 1 full minute may cause you to miss certain breathing abnormalities. Irregularities such as **dyspnea** (difficult or painful breathing), **tachypnea** (rapid breathing), or **hyperpnea** (deep, rapid breathing) are important indications of possible infection or disease.

Respiration rates are higher in infants and children than in adults. Become familiar with the normal ranges of respiration for each age group, as presented in Table 24-3.

Blood Pressure

Blood pressure (also known as arterial blood pressure) is the force at which blood is pumped against the walls of the arteries. The standard unit for measuring blood pressure is millimeters of mercury (mm Hg). The pressure measured when the left ventricle of the heart contracts is known as the **systolic pressure.** The pressure measured when the heart relaxes is known as the **diastolic pressure.** The diastolic pressure indicates the minimum amount of pressure exerted against the vessel walls at all times.

Adults' systolic pressures normally range from 90 to 140 mm Hg, but these values increase with advancing age. Diastolic pressures normally range from 60 to 90 mm Hg.

Certain disease states may cause blood pressure to rise above or fall below these ranges. Thus, it is important to recognize these abnormalities. **Hypertension,** or high blood pressure, is a major contributor to heart attack and

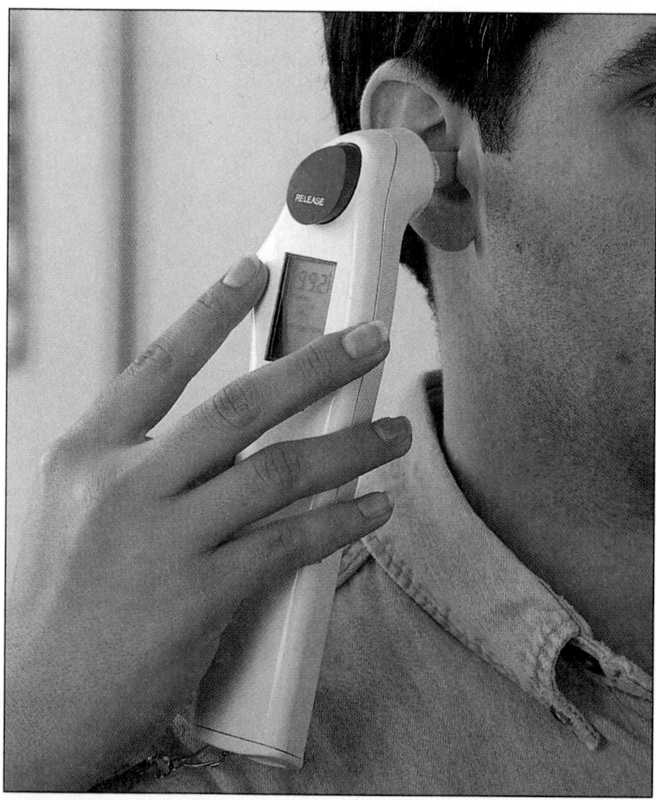

Figure 24-16. The tympanic thermometer measures infrared energy emitted from the tympanic membrane. The result, converted to body temperature, is displayed within seconds of insertion of the shielded tip into the ear.

CAUTION HANDLE WITH CARE

Tympanic Thermometers: What You Need to Know

Tympanic thermometers are becoming popular in medical offices because they are fast and accurate when used correctly. They are also particularly useful with uncooperative pediatric patients and with patients who have been eating, drinking, or smoking, because tympanic temperature readings are not affected by these activities.

If you do not use the proper technique, however, you can get inaccurate temperature readings with a tympanic thermometer. Here is a summary of what you need to know.

Why the Eardrum?

The idea of using the tympanic membrane as a site for temperature measurement originated in the 1960s as a means of measuring temperature in astronauts. The eardrum is an ideal place to measure temperature because it shares the same blood supply with the hypothalamus, the organ that controls body temperature.

How Do Tympanic Thermometers Work?

Tympanic thermometers work by measuring infrared energy, a type of heat energy, emitted from the tympanic membrane (eardrum). The thermometer converts this information into a temperature reading, usually within seconds. Most of the newer tympanic thermometers run on a rechargeable battery that must be recharged between uses.

Where Problems Can Occur

The technique for taking a tympanic temperature may vary slightly, depending on which brand of thermometer you use. You must follow the manufacturer's instructions for your instrument to get accurate results.

Most units have an indicator to let you know when the thermometer is ready for use. Some units require taking the temperature within a certain period after removing the thermometer from its charging base. Read the manufacturer's instructions for specific information.

There can be problems with most units if the outer opening of the ear is not sealed completely when the probe is placed at the ear canal. An improper seal may also mean that the thermometer is not aimed at the eardrum and will give an inaccurate reading. You may need to tug gently on the ear to position the thermometer properly.

If the thermometer has been charging for several hours before use, the initial reading may be inaccurately high. Therefore, some experts believe you should take two measurements on the first patient after charging the unit and record only the second reading.

Even with good technique, errors can sometimes occur. If you do obtain a reading that does not appear to match the patient's general condition, repeat the temperature measurement to be sure.

stroke. The doctor may ask a patient whose blood pressure is elevated to return in 2 months for a checkup. If blood pressure is still elevated at the follow-up visit, the patient may be diagnosed with hypertension. **Hypotension,** or low blood pressure, is not generally a chronic health problem. Slightly low blood pressure may be normal for some patients and does not usually require treatment. Severe hypotension may be present with shock, heart failure, severe burns, and excessive bleeding.

Blood Pressure Measuring Equipment. Blood pressure is measured with an instrument called a **sphygmomanometer.** A sphygmomanometer consists of an inflatable cuff, a pressure bulb for inflating the cuff, and a device (manometer) to read the pressure. The three basic types of sphygmomanometers differ in how the pressure is displayed (Figure 24-19).

Mercury Sphygmomanometers. Like mercury thermometers, mercury sphygmomanometers contain a column of mercury. Instead of rising with temperature, however, the mercury column rises with an increase in pressure as the cuff is inflated. Mercury sphygmomanometers may be wall-mounted units, tabletop units, or free-standing units on wheels. Mercury instruments are the most accurate of the devices used to measure blood pressure.

Aneroid Sphygmomanometers. Aneroid sphygmomanometers have a circular gauge instead of a mercury column for registering pressure. The needle on the gauge rotates as

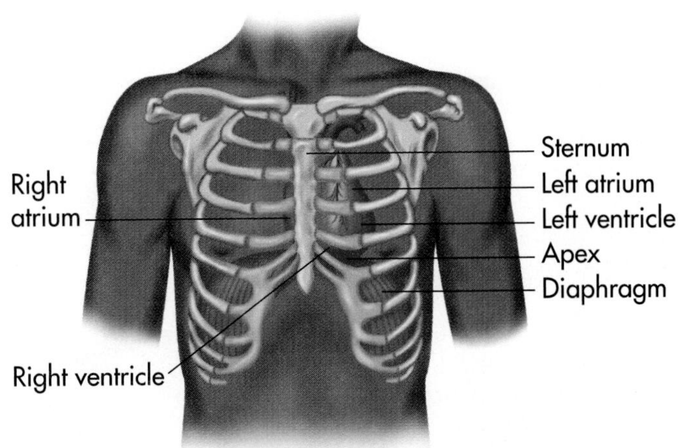

Figure 24-17. A stethoscope is used over the apex of the heart to listen for the pulse in patients in whom pulse is not otherwise detectable.

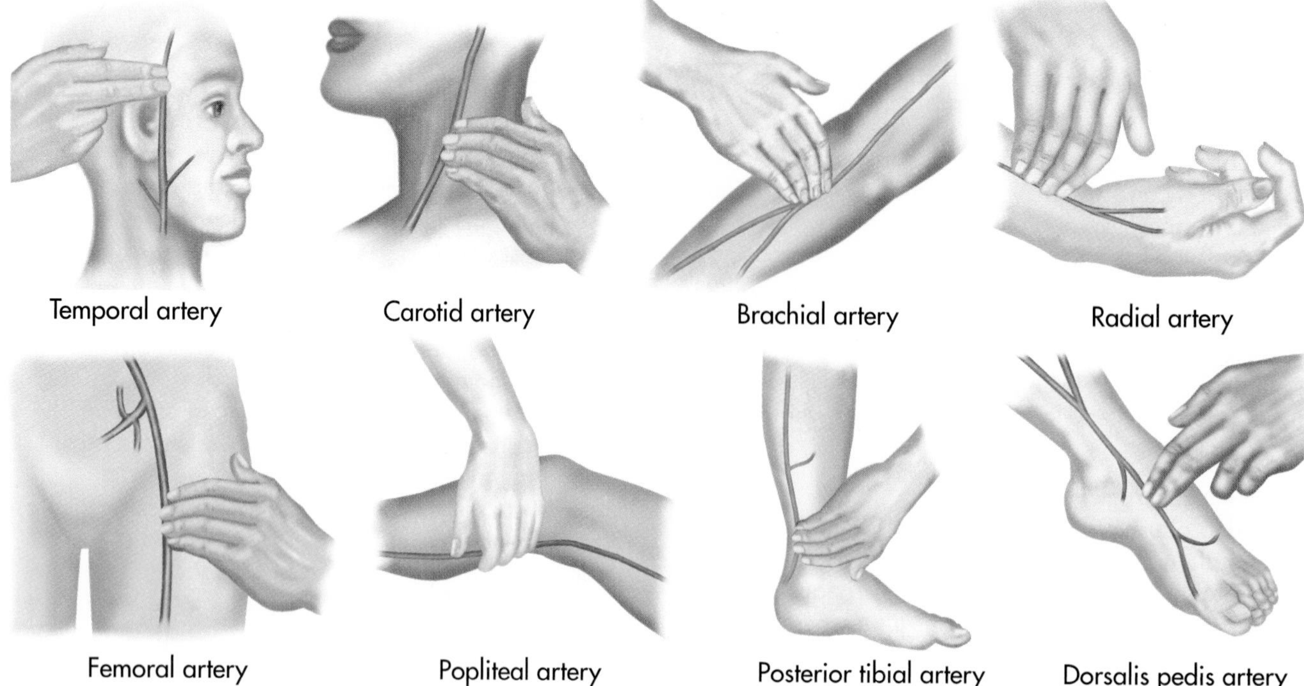

Figure 24-18. There are many locations on the body where major arteries are close enough to the surface to allow a pulse to be felt and counted.

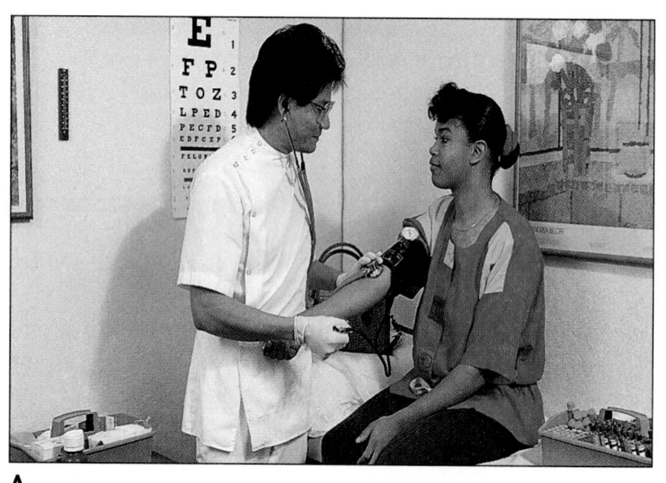

A

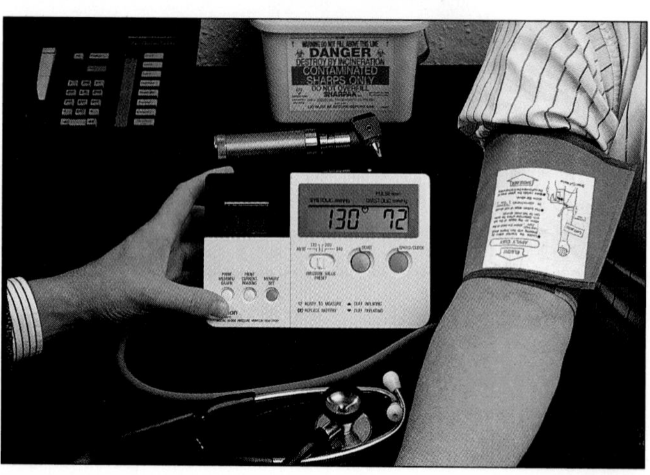

B

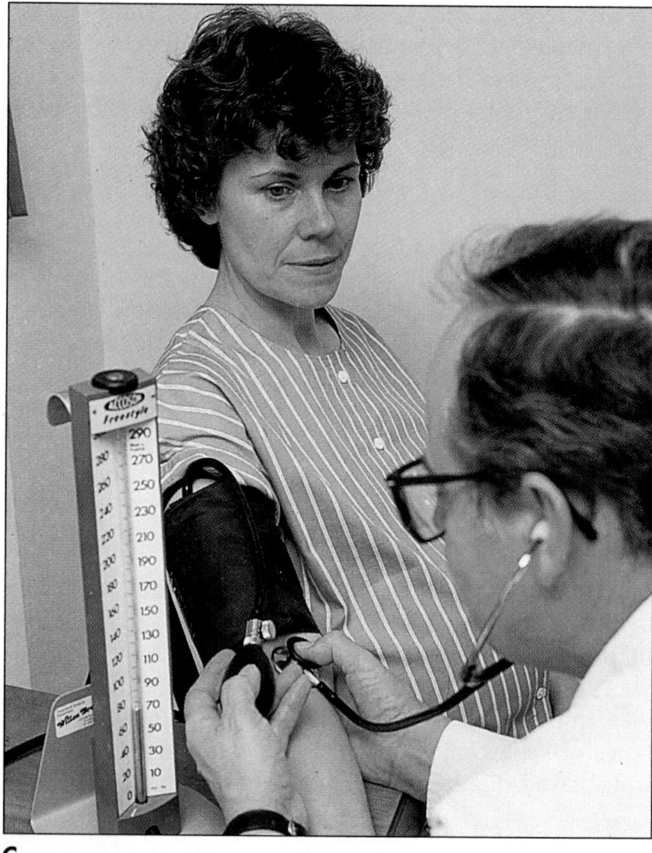

C

Figure 24-19. Pressure readings are displayed differently by each of the three types of sphygmomanometers: (a) aneroid, (b) electronic, and (c) mercury.

pressure rises. This type of sphygmomanometer is very accurate and less awkward than the mercury column.

Electronic Sphygmomanometers. Newer electronic sphygmomanometers provide a digital readout of blood pressure on a lit display. Unlike mercury and aneroid sphygmomanometers, these devices do not require use of a stethoscope to determine blood pressure. Although they are easy to use, electronic sphygmomanometers are very costly and the least likely to give you an accurate reading.

Calibrating the Sphygmomanometer. To ensure that sphygmomanometers are working properly, you or a medical supply dealer must calibrate them regularly. To **calibrate** means to standardize a measuring instrument. Mercury sphygmomanometers must be checked for faults, serviced, and calibrated every 6 to 12 months. Aneroid sphygmomanometers must be checked, serviced, and calibrated every 3 to 6 months. Follow the manufacturer's instructions for an electronic sphygmomanometer.

Each time you use a mercury or aneroid sphygmomanometer, you need to ensure that it is correctly calibrated. To do so, follow these steps.

- For a mercury sphygmomanometer, check that the **meniscus** (curve in the air-to-liquid surface of the specimen in the cylinder) of mercury on the mercury column rests at zero when you view it at eye level.
- For an aneroid sphygmomanometer, check that the recording needle on the dial rests within the small square at the bottom of the dial. To calibrate the dial, use a Y connector to attach the dial to a pressure bulb and a calibrated mercury manometer. Use the pressure bulb to elevate both manometer readings to 250 mm Hg. As you let the pressure fall, record both readings at four different points. The difference between paired readings should not exceed 3 mm Hg.

Do not use a sphygmomanometer that is not correctly calibrated. The patient's blood pressure reading will not be accurate.

The Stethoscope. A stethoscope amplifies body sounds, making them louder. It consists of earpieces, binaurals, rubber or plastic tubing, and a chestpiece (Figure 24-20). For best results the earpieces should fit snugly and comfortably in your ears.

The chestpiece consists of two parts: the diaphragm and the bell. The diaphragm is the larger, flat side of the chestpiece. It is covered by a thin, plastic disk. The diaphragm must be placed firmly against the skin for proper amplification of sound. The diaphragm is best at amplifying high-pitched sounds, such as bowel and lung sounds.

The bell is the cone-shaped side of the stethoscope chestpiece. It must be held lightly against the skin to amplify sound. The bell is best at amplifying low-pitched sounds, such as vascular and heart sounds. With practice you may find you prefer to use one side rather than the other for various purposes.

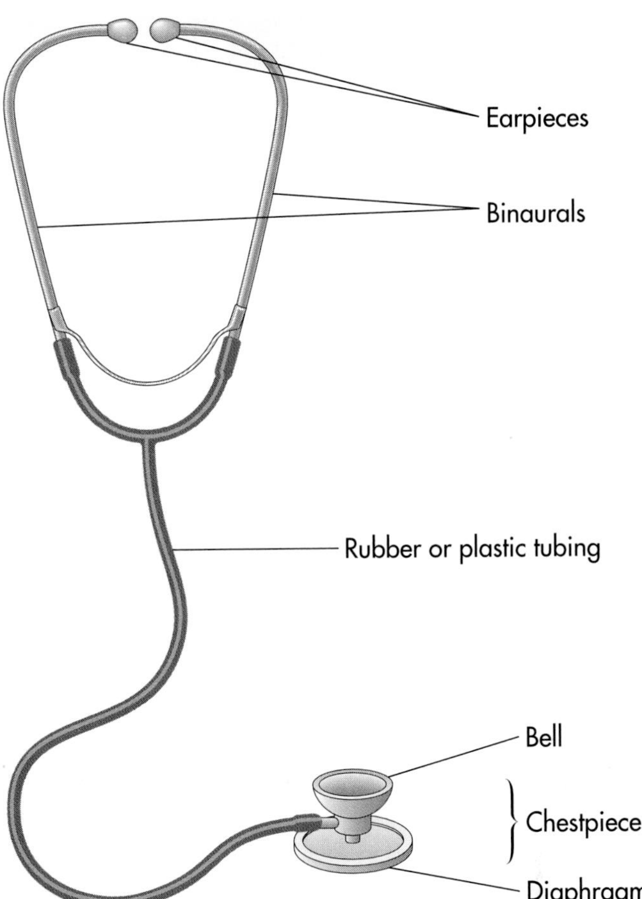

Figure 24-20. The stethoscope amplifies body sounds.

Measuring Blood Pressure. To measure blood pressure, wrap the rubber cuff of the sphygmomanometer around the patient's upper arm, just above the pulse point of the brachial artery. This pulse point is located in the bend of the elbow, or the antecubital space. If the patient has an injury to one arm, then place the cuff on the other arm. Otherwise, palpate the pulse in both arms, and use the one with the stronger pulse. Inflate the cuff to the maximum inflation level. Then while you release the air in the cuff, listen with the stethoscope. You will hear vascular sounds that will change. These sounds are also called Korotkoff sounds. They are produced by the obstruction and release of the arterial blood flow.

The first heartbeat you hear is the systolic pressure. As the pressure in the cuff is released, this strong heartbeat changes to a softer, muffled sound. The point at which the sound disappears is the diastolic pressure. The patient's blood pressure reading is recorded as the numbers registered for the first and last sounds separated by a slash mark, as in BP 120/76. Although only the systolic and diastolic readings are usually recorded for adults, a third number may be included at times. For example, if there is a pressure difference greater than 10 mm Hg between the muffled sound and its disappearance, the blood pressure is recorded with all three sounds noted, such as 120/80/60. The process of taking blood pressure is described in Procedure 24-3.

PROCEDURE 24-3

Taking Blood Pressure (Adults and Older Children)

Objective: To accurately measure blood pressure in adults and older children

OSHA Guidelines

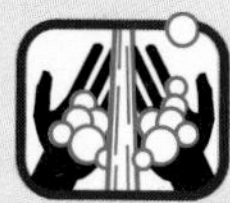
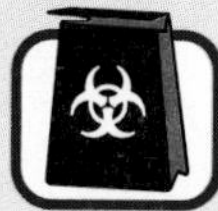
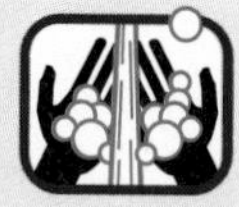

Materials: Mercury or aneroid sphygmomanometer, stethoscope, alcohol gauze squares

Method

1. Identify the patient and introduce yourself.
2. Wash your hands and explain the procedure to the patient.
3. Have the patient sit in a quiet area. If she is wearing long-sleeved clothing, have her loosely roll up one sleeve. If she cannot, have her change into a gown. (A sleeve that is tightly rolled up may restrict the blood flow and give inaccurate readings. The cuff should not be placed over clothing for the same reason.)
4. Have the patient rest her bared arm on a flat surface so that the midpoint of the upper arm is at the same level as the heart.
5. Make sure the sphygmomanometer is in working order and is correctly calibrated.
6. Select a cuff that is the appropriate size for the patient. The bladder inside the cuff should encircle 80% of the arm in adults and 100% of the arm in children under the age of 13. If you are not sure about the size, use a larger cuff.
7. Locate the brachial artery in the antecubital space.
8. Position the cuff so that the midline of the bladder is above the arterial pulsation. Then wrap and secure the cuff snugly around the patient's bare upper arm. The lower edge of the cuff should be 1 inch above the antecubital space, where the head of the stethoscope is to be placed.
9. Place the manometer so that the center of the mercury column or aneroid dial is at eye level and easily visible and so that the tubing from the cuff is unobstructed.
10. Close the valve of the pressure bulb until it is finger-tight.
11. Inflate the cuff rapidly to 70 mm Hg with one hand, and increase this pressure by 10 mm Hg increments while palpating the radial pulse with your other hand. Note the level of pressure at which the pulse disappears and subsequently reappears during deflation. This procedure, the **palpatory method,**

Special Considerations in Adults. Blood pressure is elevated during and just after exercise. If a patient has engaged in strenuous activity before the examination, you should wait 15 minutes before taking blood pressure measurements. This waiting period also applies to patients with ambulatory disabilities, to those who are obese, and to those who have a known blood pressure problem. If you ensure that patients have relaxed for 15 minutes before you measure their blood pressure, you will get an accurate reading.

Blood pressure may also be elevated when a patient is anxious or under extreme stress. If the patient seems stressed, allow him to rest for about 5 minutes before measuring his blood pressure. To help the patient relax, try to engage the person in conversation rather than calling attention to the fact that you are waiting to take his blood pressure. If the patient still appears anxious or under stress, take his blood pressure anyway, and make a notation for the physician (who may want to repeat the measurement later in the visit).

There are certain instances when you should not take a blood pressure measurement on a particular arm. Blood pressure should not be taken on an arm that has an injury, a blocked artery, or a device under the skin (implant) at the site. In such cases use the other arm or the upper leg. Note the measurements and their locations in the patient's chart.

Be sure you use the proper size cuff when taking blood pressure. Although the standard adult cuff can be used for most adults, some may require the larger size. Using an improper size may result in an inaccurate reading.

Sometimes a patient is aware that a blood pressure reading is abnormally high or low. If the patient is upset about a reading, tell him that the physician may take another reading later, perhaps on the other arm.

Special Considerations in Children. Blood pressure in children or infants is not routinely measured at each visit. Instead, the measurement is taken on the order of

provides a necessary preliminary approximation of the systolic blood pressure to ensure an adequate level of inflation when the actual auscultatory measurement is made.

12. Open the valve to release the pressure, deflate the cuff completely, and wait 30 seconds. (If you do not deflate the cuff completely and wait, blood may pool in the artery and give a falsely high reading.)
13. Place the earpieces of the stethoscope in your ear canals, and adjust them to fit snugly and comfortably. Switch the stethoscope head to the low-frequency position (bell). Confirm the setting by listening as you tap the stethoscope head gently.
14. Place the head of the stethoscope over the brachial artery pulsation, just above and medial to the antecubital space but below the lower edge of the cuff. Hold the stethoscope firmly in place, making sure the head is in contact with the skin around its entire circumference. (Do not hold the stethoscope with the thumb, because the pulse of your thumb can interfere with the reading.)
15. Inflate the bladder rapidly and steadily to a pressure 20 to 30 mm Hg above the level previously determined by palpation. Then partially open (unscrew) the valve, and deflate the bladder at 2 mm per second while you listen for the appearance of the Korotkoff sounds.
16. As the pressure in the bladder falls, note the level of pressure on the manometer at the first appearance of repetitive sounds. This reading is the systolic pressure.
17. Continue to deflate the cuff gradually, noting the point at which the sound changes from strong to muffled.
18. Continue to deflate the cuff, and note when the sound disappears. This reading is the diastolic pressure.
19. Deflate the cuff completely, and remove it from the patient's arm.
20. Record the three numbers, separated by slashes, in the patient's chart. (This value is an exact measurement of the **auscultated blood pressure,** meaning that it was determined by listening with a stethoscope.) Remember to indicate the date and time of the measurement, the arm on which the measurement was made, the subject's position, and the cuff size when a nonstandard size is used.
21. Fold the cuff and replace it in the holder.
22. Inform the patient that you have completed the procedure.
23. Disinfect the earpieces and diaphragm of the stethoscope with gauze squares moistened with alcohol.
24. Properly dispose of the used gauze squares and wash your hands.

the doctor. The procedure is the same as that for taking blood pressure in adults, except for these modifications.

1. Ideally, take the patient's blood pressure before performing other tests or procedures that may cause anxiety. In this way you can avoid a falsely high result.
2. Be sure to use the correct cuff size for the child or infant. Remove the adult-size cuff from the sphygmomanometer, and put on the smaller size.
3. Do not attempt to estimate an infant's blood pressure in the manner described in Procedure 24-3—the palpatory method usually cannot be used on an infant.
4. Inflate the pressure cuff to 20 mm Hg above the point at which radial pulse disappears.
5. Deflate the cuff at a rate of 2 mm Hg per second.
6. You may continue to hear a heartbeat on a child or infant until the pressure reaches zero, so note when the strong heartbeat becomes muffled.

Summary

As a medical assistant, you will play a key role in a patient's visit to the physician's office. Because you will begin the examination by interviewing the patient, you will set the tone of the visit. Keep in mind that some patients may be nervous or uncomfortable. It is important to make them feel at ease. Using interviewing skills effectively will help make the interview productive as well as comfortable for the patient.

You will record the patient's medical history and then measure weight, height, and vital signs. Gathering this information is crucial to the outcome of the patient's visit. Remember that the physician relies on these data, as they appear in the patient's chart from visit to visit, when making a diagnosis. Using proper techniques each and every time you measure a patient's weight, height, and vital signs will help you provide information that is precise and accurate.

24 Chapter Review

Discussion Questions

1. Explain the difference between subjective and objective data. Give examples of each type.
2. What are the pros and cons of using growth charts when charting children's growth?
3. Compare and contrast the different types of sphygmomanometers.

Critical Thinking Questions

1. A patient comes into the office with abdominal pain. On her chart is a notation that she is coming in with symptoms of appendicitis. What questions might you ask her to assist the doctor in determining whether her condition is appendicitis?
2. A parent brings in her 3-year-old son, who has chronic diarrhea. You note that the child has a large bruise on the side of his face. He appears very thin and pale. You suspect he may have been abused. What questions might you ask to obtain the information necessary to rule out or confirm abuse? What might you look for when you perform mensuration and take vital signs?
3. Describe how you might obtain height and weight measurements of a patient who is deaf.

Application Activities

1. Have a partner assume the role of a patient who has come into the office with what appears to be the flu. Conduct an interview and take a patient history.
2. Pair up with a classmate, and practice measuring each other's weight and height.
3. Practice measuring vital signs of several classmates.

Further Readings

Baird, Sandra C., Nancy E. White, and Marjorie Basinger. "Can You Rely on Tympanic Thermometers?" *RN,* August 1992, 48–51.

"Guide to Thermometers." *Healthy Kids,* April/May 1994, 30.

McAfee, Robert E. "Violence in America: Making a Difference One Patient at a Time." *The Professional Medical Assistant,* January/February 1996, 5–9.

Monteleone, James A. *Recognition of Child Abuse for the Mandated Reporter.* St. Louis, MO: G. W. Medical Publishing, 1994.

National Committee for Prevention of Child Abuse, Indiana Chapter. *Child Abuse and Neglect Identifying and Reporting for Health Care Providers.* Indianapolis: Indiana State Department of Health, 1995.

Simmers, Louise. *Diversified Health Occupations.* 3d ed. Albany, NY: Delmar, 1993.

White, Nancy, Sandra Baird, and Deborah L. Anderson. "A Comparison of Tympanic Thermometer Readings to Pulmonary Artery Catheter Core Temperature Recordings." *Applied Nursing Research,* November 1994, 165–169.

Assisting With a General Physical Examination

CHAPTER OUTLINE

- The Purpose of a General Physical Examination
- The Role of the Medical Assistant
- Safety Precautions
- Preparing the Patient for an Examination
- Examination Methods
- Components of a General Physical Examination
- Completing the Examination

OBJECTIVES

After completing Chapter 25, you will be able to:

- State the purpose of a general physical examination.
- Describe the role of the medical assistant in a general physical examination.
- Explain safety precautions used during a general physical examination.
- Outline the steps necessary to prepare the patient for an examination.
- Describe how to position and drape a patient in each of the ten common examination positions.
- Explain ways to assist patients from different cultures, patients with disabilities, children, and pregnant women.
- Identify and describe the six examination methods used in a general physical examination.
- List the components of a general physical examination.
- Explain the special needs of the elderly for patient education.
- Identify ways to help a patient follow up on a doctor's recommendations.

Key Terms

clinical diagnosis
culture
differential diagnosis
digital examination
hyperventilation
nasal mucosa
patient compliance
quadrant
scoliosis
symmetry

AREAS OF COMPETENCE

1997 ROLE DELINEATION STUDY

CLINICAL

Fundamental Principles

- Comply with quality assurance practices

Patient Care

- Prepare patient for examinations, procedures, and treatments
- Assist with examinations, procedures, and treatments

The Purpose of a General Physical Examination

Physicians perform general physical examinations for two purposes. The first is to examine a healthy patient to confirm an overall state of health and to provide baseline values for vital signs and mensuration. The second is to examine a patient to diagnose a medical problem.

To confirm a patient's health status, physicians usually perform examinations on a routine basis, such as once a year. Some examinations are done to fulfill a requirement before an individual starts school, begins a new job, or starts an exercise program.

To diagnose medical problems, physicians usually focus on a particular organ system, as indicated by the patient's chief complaint. Because organ systems are so interdependent, however, physicians generally perform an overall physical examination even when a specific medical problem exists.

During a general physical examination, physicians check all the major organs and body systems. They can determine much about a patient's general condition of health from the examination. If appropriate, they also try to make a **clinical diagnosis,** a diagnosis based on the signs and symptoms of a disease.

After forming an initial diagnosis of a patient's problem, physicians may order laboratory or other diagnostic tests. These tests are done to confirm a clinical diagnosis or to rule out other possible disorders. These additional steps are necessary when a patient has symptoms that may indicate more than one condition. Determining the correct diagnosis when two or more diagnoses are possible is called making a **differential diagnosis.**

Laboratory and diagnostic tests may also aid physicians in developing a prognosis, or a forecast of the probable course and outcome of the disorder and the prospects of recovery. In addition, such tests help physicians formulate a treatment plan or appropriate drug therapy. Physicians may ask to have these tests repeated as part of the follow-up evaluation of a patient's progress.

The Role of the Medical Assistant

Your job as a medical assistant is to assist both the doctor and the patient during the general physical examination. Your presence enables the doctor to perform his examination as efficiently and professionally as possible. Patients benefit from your positive and caring attention; you contribute to their confidence in the care they receive.

As described in Chapter 24, the process begins when you first have contact with the patient. You interview the patient, write an accurate history, determine vital signs, and measure weight and height. You then assist the doctor during the examination.

Generally, your responsibilities include ensuring that all instruments and supplies are readily available to the doctor during the examination. You also ensure that the patient is physically and emotionally comfortable during the examination. It is important to observe the patient for signs that indicate distress or the need for assistance. Elderly patients, who may have physical limitations or special needs, often require extra time and attention.

Safety Precautions

As you prepare for and assist with a general physical examination, you will use a variety of safety measures. Some of these are outlined by the Department of Labor's Occupational Safety and Health Administration (OSHA). OSHA standards and guidelines (detailed in Chapter 19) are designed to protect employees and make the workplace safe. The Department of Health and Human Services' Centers for Disease Control and Prevention (CDC) establishes the guidelines intended to protect both patients and health-care professionals in the medical office and the hospital setting. (These guidelines are also discussed in Chapter 19.) Taken together, these safety measures help protect you, the physician, and the patient from disease transmission.

Safety measures that you must take before, during, and after a general physical examination include the following.

1. Perform a thorough hand washing before and after contact with each patient and before and after each procedure. Procedure 19-1 in Chapter 19 describes how to perform aseptic hand washing.
2. Wear gloves whenever there is a possibility that you may come in contact with blood, body fluids, nonintact skin, or moist surfaces (during the examination of the patient or when handling specimens). Refer to Chapter 19 for details on personal protective equipment.
3. Wear a mask in the presence of a patient suspected of having an infectious disease that is transmitted by airborne droplets (Table 25-1).
4. Patients with highly contagious infectious diseases, such as diphtheria or chickenpox, must be examined under isolation precautions, such as in a private room. Wear personal protective equipment during contact. For more information on isolation guidelines, see Chapter 20. (Because infectious diseases are common in children, you are most likely to deal with them in a pediatrician's office.)
5. Discard in biohazardous waste containers all disposable equipment and supplies that come in contact with a patient's blood or body fluids. See Chapter 19 for guidelines on the proper disposal of biohazardous waste.
6. Clean and disinfect the examination room following the examination of each patient. Refer to Chapter 22

Table 25-1

Infectious Diseases Transmitted by Airborne Droplets

Viral Infections	Bacterial Infections
Chickenpox	Epiglottitis (caused by *Haemophilus influenzae* type B)
Diphtheria	Meningitis
Herpes zoster (shingles)	Pertussis (whooping cough)
Meningitis	Pneumonia
Mumps	Tuberculosis
Pneumonia	
Rabies	
Rubella (German measles)	
Rubeola (measles)	

Note: Health-care professionals should use masks when coming in contact with patients suspected of having any of these diseases.

for information on cleanliness in the examination room.

7. Sanitize, disinfect, and sterilize equipment, as appropriate, after the examination of each patient. Chapter 20 describes these procedures in detail.

Preparing the Patient for an Examination

You can help prepare patients for examinations by making sure that they are comfortable and know what to expect. It is easier for the doctor to obtain an accurate assessment of a patient's condition when the patient is emotionally and physically prepared.

Emotional Preparation

To prepare patients, begin by explaining exactly what will occur during the examination. Use simple, direct language that patients can understand. Describe what patients can expect to feel and how their cooperation can contribute to the success of the procedure.

Emotional preparedness is particularly important when dealing with children. They deserve to have the same sort of information and reassurance as adults. To involve children in the examination process, you might allow them to inspect the blunt instruments. Speak to them calmly during the procedure, and praise them when they are cooperative.

Infants and toddlers are likely to be afraid of you because you are a stranger. Approach these children slowly, smile, and use a gentle voice. Children of preschool age are sometimes uncooperative and challenging. In such cases remain calm, perform the procedures quickly, and restrain the child (with assistance from the parent) when appropriate. To prevent children from getting injured, watch them at all times.

If you are a male medical assistant, a female doctor may ask you to remain in the room when she examines a male patient. Likewise, if you are a female medical assistant, a male doctor may ask you to remain in the room when he examines a woman. These measures are for the protection of both the patient and the doctor. Such policies depend on the standard procedures in each medical practice or facility.

Physical Preparation

To ensure that the patient is physically prepared before the doctor enters the examination room, give the patient an opportunity to empty his bladder or bowels. If a urine specimen is needed, it should be collected at this time. That way the patient will be more comfortable during the examination.

When the patient is ready, ask him to disrobe and put on an examination gown or cover himself with a drape. The extent of disrobing depends on the type of examination and the doctor's preference. If the doctor requests a gown for the patient, show the patient how to put on the gown. Include specific instructions on whether the gown should open in the back or front and whether it should be left open or tied. Leave the examination room while the patient disrobes to give him privacy, unless he needs and requests assistance.

Positioning and Draping

During the examination, the patient may need to assume a variety of positions. These positions facilitate the physician's examination of certain areas of the body. The physician will indicate which positions are needed for specific examinations. You will help the patient assume these positions. Some positions are embarrassing or physically uncomfortable for some patients. If you perceive embarrassment, explain the need for the position, and help the patient assume the position when necessary. Help minimize the time a patient spends in any embarrassing position.

If a patient is physically uncomfortable in a position, you may be able to ease the discomfort by using a small pillow to support part of the body. You may have to help the patient maintain a position during the examination. Always try to make the patient as comfortable as possible.

When you need to make changes in the patient's position, do so gradually. If your office is equipped with an examination table that can be adjusted automatically, learn to use the controls efficiently to maximize patient comfort. Always tell the patient what movement to expect.

When patients have assumed the correct position, cover them with an appropriate drape. Drapes vary in size. Make sure you choose one that will help keep the patient warm and maintain privacy. You will position drapes differently depending on the examination position and the parts of the patient's body the physician examines.

Examination Positions

The positions commonly used during a medical examination include the following:

- Sitting
- Supine (recumbent)
- Dorsal recumbent
- Lithotomy
- Trendelenburg's
- Fowler's
- Prone
- Sims'
- Knee-chest
- Proctologic

Sitting. In the sitting position the patient sits at the edge of the examination table without back support (see Figure 25-1a). The physician examines the patient's head, neck, chest, heart, back, and arms. While the patient is in the sitting position, the physician evaluates the patient's ability to fully expand the lungs. She then checks the upper body parts for **symmetry,** the degree to which one side is the same as the other. In this position the drape is placed across the patient's lap for men or across the patient's chest and lap for women.

If a patient is too weak to sit unsupported, another position is necessary. One possible alternative is the supine position.

Supine (Recumbent). In the supine, or recumbent, position, the patient lies flat on the back (Figure 25-1b). (*Supine* means "lying down faceup"; *recumbent* means "lying down." Either term is used to describe this position.) This is the most relaxed position for many patients. A doctor can examine the head, neck, chest, heart, abdomen, arms, and legs when a patient is in the supine position. The patient is normally draped from the neck or underarms down to the feet.

The supine position may not be comfortable for patients who become short of breath easily. Also, patients with a back injury or lower-back pain may find it uncomfortable. You can make these patients more comfortable by placing a pillow under their heads and under their knees. Some patients, however, may need to be placed in the dorsal recumbent position.

Dorsal Recumbent. In the dorsal recumbent position, the patient lies faceup, with his back supporting all his weight. (The term *dorsal* refers to the back.) This position is the same as the supine position, except that the patient's knees are drawn up and the feet are flat on the table, as shown in Figure 25-1c. The physician may examine the head, neck, chest, and heart while a patient is in this position. The patient is normally draped from the neck or underarms down to the feet.

Patients who have leg disabilities may find the dorsal recumbent position uncomfortable or even impossible. On the other hand, patients who are elderly or have painful disorders such as arthritis or back pain may find the dorsal recumbent position more comfortable than the supine position because the knees are bent. This position is sometimes used as an alternative to the lithotomy position when patients have severe arthritis or joint deformities.

Lithotomy. The lithotomy position is used during examination of the female genitalia. In this position the patient lies on her back with her knees bent and her feet in stirrups attached to the end of the examination table. You may need to help the patient place her feet in the stirrups. She should then slide forward to position her buttocks near the edge of the table, as shown in Figure 25-1d.

Many women are embarrassed and physically uncomfortable in this position, so you should not ask a patient to remain in this position any longer than necessary. Use a large drape that covers the patient from the breasts to the ankles.

A patient with severe arthritis or joint deformities in the hips or knees may have difficulty assuming the lithotomy position. She may be able to place only one leg in

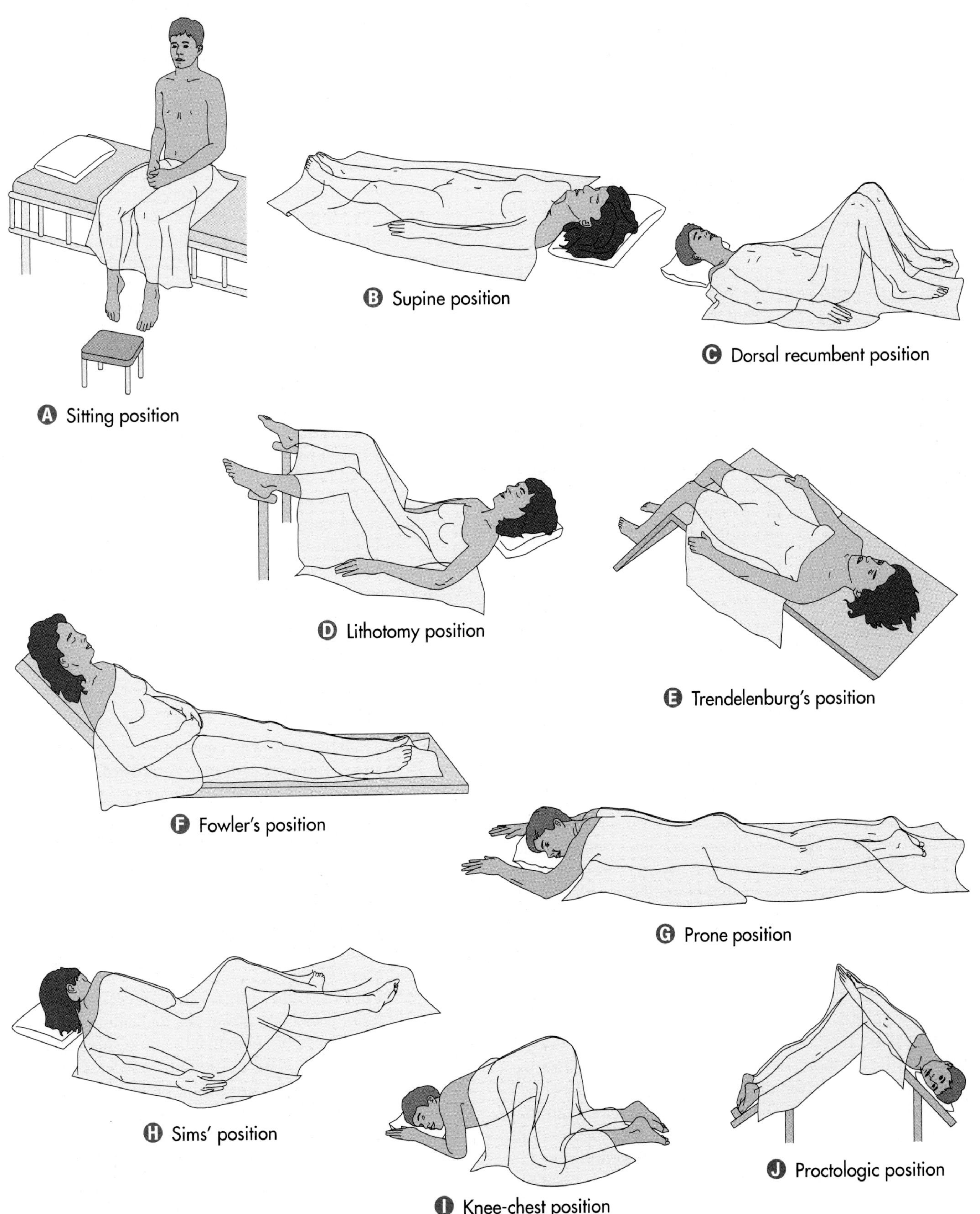

Figure 25-1. These positions may be used during the general physical examination.

the stirrup or she may need your assistance in separating her thighs. An alternative position for such a patient is the dorsal recumbent position. Other patients who may have difficulty with the lithotomy position are those who are obese or in the late stages of pregnancy.

Trendelenburg's. In Trendelenburg's position the patient is supine on a tilted table with the head lower than the legs. Some tables have flexible positioning so that the patient's legs can be bent with the feet lower than the knees, as shown in Figure 25-1e. Although physicians do not generally use this position for physical examinations, they use it in certain surgical procedures. It may also be used for patients with low blood pressure or for those who are in shock. It cannot be used for patients who have a head injury, however. The drape is typically positioned from the neck or underarms down to the knees.

Fowler's. In Fowler's position the patient lies back on an examination table on which the head is elevated, as shown in Figure 25-1f. Although the head of the table can be raised to a 90° angle, the most common position is a 45° angle. The doctor may examine the head, neck, and chest areas while the patient is in this position. The patient is usually draped from the neck or underarms down to the feet.

Fowler's position is one of the best positions for examining patients who are experiencing shortness of breath or individuals with a lower-back injury. The procedure for helping a patient prepare for an examination in Fowler's position is outlined in Procedure 25-1.

Prone. In the prone position the patient is lying flat on the table, facedown. The patient's head is turned to one side, and his arms are placed at his sides or bent at the elbows, as shown in Figure 25-1g. The patient is normally draped from the upper back to the feet.

With the patient in this position, the physician can examine the back, feet, or musculoskeletal system. The prone position is unsuitable for women in advanced stages of pregnancy, obese patients, patients with respiratory difficulties, or the elderly.

Sims'. In Sims' position the patient lies on the left side. The patient's left leg is slightly bent, and the left arm is placed behind the back so that the patient's weight is resting primarily on the chest. The right knee is bent and raised toward the chest, and the right arm is bent toward the head for support, as shown in Figure 25-1h. The patient is draped from the upper back to the feet.

Sims' position is used during anal or rectal examinations and may also be used for perineal and certain pelvic examinations. Patients with joint deformities of the hips and knees may have difficulty assuming this position.

Knee-Chest. In the knee-chest position the patient is lying on the table facedown, supporting the body with the knees and chest. The patient should have the thighs at a 90° angle to the table and slightly separated. The head is turned to one side, and the arms are placed to the side or above the head, as shown in Figure 25-1i. The patient may need your assistance to assume this position correctly and to maintain it during the examination.

The knee-chest position is used during examinations of the anal and perineal areas and during certain proctologic procedures. Some patients—those who are pregnant, obese, or elderly—have difficulty assuming this position. An alternative that puts less strain on the patient and is easier to maintain is the knee-elbow position. This position is the same as the knee-chest position except that the patient supports body weight with the knees and elbows rather than the knees and chest. In either of these two positions, the patient is commonly covered with a fenestrated drape, in which the opening provides access to the area to be examined.

Proctologic. The proctologic position may be used as an alternative to the Sims' or knee-chest position. In the proctologic position, also called the jackknife position, the patient is bent at the hips at a 90° angle. The patient can assume this position by standing next to the examination table and bending at the waist until the chest rests on the table. If an adjustable examination table is available, the patient can assume the position by lying prone on the table, which is then raised in the middle with both ends pointing down. This places the patient at the correct 90° angle, as shown in Figure 25-1j. In either variation of this position, the patient is draped with a fenestrated drape, as in the knee-chest position.

Special Considerations: Patients From Different Cultures

During your career you will come in contact with patients from many different cultures. A **culture,** in this sociological sense, is defined as a pattern of assumptions, beliefs, and practices that shape the way people think and act. Avoid the temptation to stereotype an individual or group on the basis of a single patient's behavior. Stereotyping can lead to incorrect judgments, which may influence the care you provide to patients. Avoid making judgments about patients or cultural groups on the basis of your experience with other patients or with your own family and friends.

Patients from different cultures may never have had a medical examination by a physician and may not know what to expect. These patients may be more modest than other patients and may have a greater need for privacy. They may not want the physician to examine certain areas of their bodies. Procedure 25-2 describes techniques you can use to ensure effective communication with patients from other cultures while meeting their privacy needs.

Special Considerations: Patients With Disabilities

As a medical assistant, you will come in contact with patients with physical disabilities. These patients will have

PROCEDURE 25-1

Helping the Patient Prepare for an Examination in Fowler's Position

Objective: To effectively assist a patient in assuming Fowler's position for a general physical examination

OSHA Guidelines 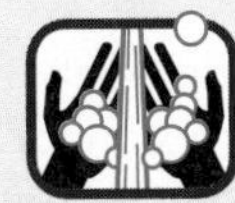

Materials: Adjustable examination table or gynecologic table, step stool, examination gown, drape

Method

1. Identify the patient and introduce yourself.
2. Wash your hands.
3. Explain the procedure to the patient.
4. Provide a gown or drape if the physician has requested one, and instruct the patient in the proper way to wear it after disrobing. Allow the patient privacy while disrobing, and assist only if the patient requests help.
5. Ask the patient to step on the stool or the pullout step of the examination table.

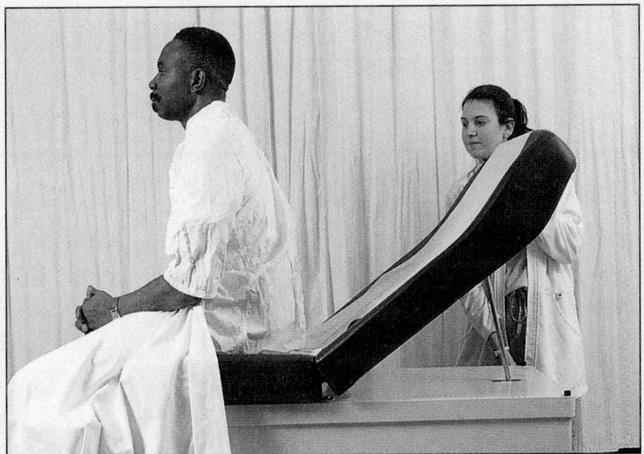

Figure 25-2. Adjust the head of the examination table to a 45° angle.

6. If necessary, assist the patient onto the examination table and into a sitting position, facing the foot of the table.
7. Adjust the head of the table to the desired angle (Figure 25-2). (The most common angle for examination in this position is 45°.)
8. Help the patient move toward the head of the table until the patient's buttocks meet the point at which the head of the table begins to incline upward (Figure 25-3).

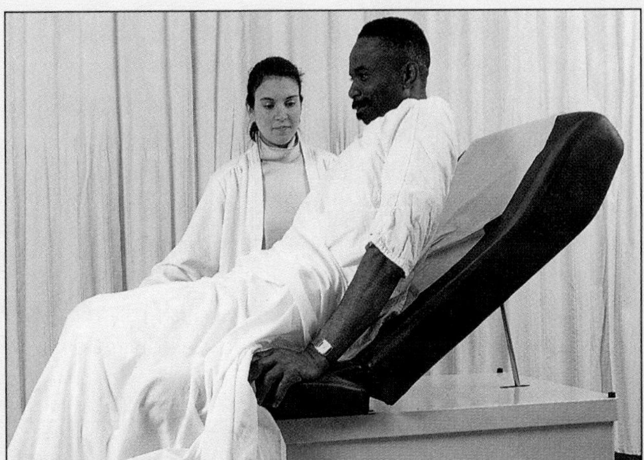

Figure 25-3. Encourage the patient to slide back until the buttocks meet the point at which the head of the table begins to incline upward.

9. Assist the patient in leaning back by supporting the patient's back and cervical spine and encouraging the patient to roll back, starting at the hips.
10. If needed, place a pillow under the patient's knees.
11. Adjust the drape as necessary.

different strengths and weaknesses. They will also vary in their ability to ambulate (move from place to place). Many patients with physical disabilities require the use of devices such as wheelchairs, canes, or walkers or other special equipment that permits or enhances mobility.

Depending on the extent of their disability, these patients may require extra assistance in preparing for a general physical examination. You may need to help them disrobe, move from a mobility device to the examination table, and assume certain positions on or off the examination table. At all times you should ask another staff member for assistance if you are not sure whether you can safely move or lift a patient on your own. Procedure 25-3 describes the steps you would take to transfer a patient from a wheelchair to the examination table.

Special Considerations: Children

No matter what type of office you work in, you will probably deal with children at times. You will base your choice of an examination position for children on each child's age and ability to cooperate. Although young

PROCEDURE 25-2

Communicating Effectively With Patients From Other Cultures and Meeting Their Needs for Privacy

Objective: To ensure effective communication with patients from other cultures while meeting their needs for privacy

OSHA Guidelines: This procedure does not involve exposure to blood, body fluids, or tissues.

Materials: Examination gown, drapes

Method

Effective Communication

1. When it is necessary to use a translator, direct conversation or instruction to the translator.
2. Direct demonstrations of what to do, such as putting on an examination gown, to the patient.
3. Confirm with the translator that the patient has understood the instruction or demonstration.
4. Allow the translator to be present during the examination if that is the patient's preference.
5. If the patient understands some English, speak slowly, use simple language, and demonstrate instructions whenever possible.

Meeting the Need for Privacy

1. Before the procedure, thoroughly explain to the patient or translator the reason for disrobing. Indicate that you will allow the patient privacy and ample time to undress.
2. If the patient is reluctant, reassure him that the physician respects the need for privacy and will look at only what is necessary for the examination.
3. Provide extra drapes if you think doing so will make the patient feel more comfortable.
4. If the patient is still reluctant, discuss the problem with the physician; the physician may be able to negotiate a compromise with the patient.
5. During the procedure, ensure that the patient is undraped only as much as necessary.
6. Whenever possible minimize the amount of time the patient remains undraped.

infants are usually examined on an examination table, older infants and toddlers may need to be examined while held on a parent's lap. Some toddlers may cooperate while standing on the examination table with a parent nearby. Preschool children can usually be placed on the examination table if a parent is nearby. Regardless of their position, watch children at all times to prevent injury.

When examining young children, doctors typically perform percussion and auscultation first, because children are more likely to be calm and quiet at the outset. Doctors always examine painful areas last. Doctors may examine older children's genitalia last, because after a certain age children tend to find such an examination embarrassing.

Special Considerations: Pregnant Women

When a pregnant patient needs a general physical examination, remember that she has several special needs. Some positions (such as the prone position or, in the late stages of pregnancy, the lithotomy position) are not recommended for a pregnant patient. Other positions may be difficult or impossible for a pregnant woman to achieve. Procedure 25-4 outlines steps you can take to ensure that a pregnant woman's needs are addressed during an examination.

Examination Methods

There are six methods for examining a patient during a general physical examination. These methods enable the physician to gather important information about the patient's condition, and they are normally performed in the following sequence:

- Inspection
- Palpation
- Percussion
- Auscultation
- Mensuration
- Manipulation

Inspection

Inspection is the visual examination of the patient's entire body and overall appearance. During inspection the physician assesses posture, mannerisms, and hygiene. The physician also inspects parts of the body for size, shape, color, position, symmetry, and the presence of abnormalities such as rashes or growths. You can help the physician perform the inspection by making sure that good lighting is available and that the patient's body parts are properly exposed.

PROCEDURE 25-3

Transferring a Patient in a Wheelchair and Preparing for an Examination

Objective: To assist a patient in transferring from a wheelchair to the examination table safely and efficiently

OSHA Guidelines 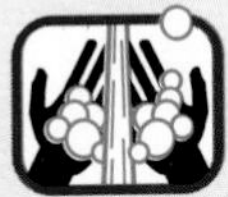

Materials: Adjustable examination table or gynecologic table, step stool (optional), examination gown, drape

Method

Never risk injuring yourself; call for assistance when in doubt. As a rule you should not attempt to lift more than 35% of your body weight.

Preparation Before Transfer

1. Identify the patient and introduce yourself.
2. Wash your hands.
3. Explain the procedure in detail.
4. Position the wheelchair at a right angle to the end of the examination table. This position reduces the distance between the wheelchair and the end of the examination table across which the patient must move.
5. Lock the wheels of the wheelchair to prevent the wheelchair from moving during the transfer.
6. Lift the patient's feet and fold back the foot and leg supports of the wheelchair.
7. Place the patient's feet on the floor, and ensure that the patient will not slip on the floor. (The patient should have shoes or slippers with nonskid soles.) Place your feet in front of the patient's feet to prevent further slipping.
8. If needed, place a step stool in front of the table, and place the patient's feet flat on the stool.

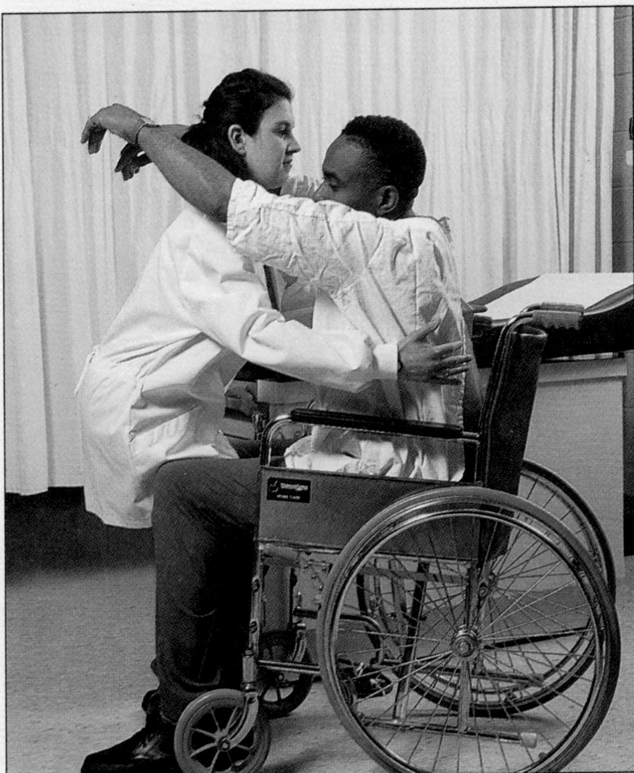

Figure 25-4. Align your knees, slightly bent, with the patient's knees. Have the patient hold on to your shoulders while you place your arms around the patient, under the patient's arms.

Transferring Patient by Yourself

9. Face the patient, spread your feet apart, align your knees with the patient's knees, and bend your knees slightly. (If you lift while bending at the waist instead of bending your knees, you can cause serious injury to your back.)
10. Have the patient hold on to your shoulders.
11. Place your arms around the patient, under the patient's arms (Figure 25-4).
12. Tell the patient that you will lift on the count of 3, and ask the patient to support as much of his own weight as possible (if he is able).
13. At the count of 3, lift the patient.
14. Pivot the patient to bring the back of the patient's knees against the table.
15. Gently lower the patient into a sitting position on the table. If the patient cannot sit unassisted, help him move into a supine position (Figure 25-5).
16. Move the wheelchair out of the way.
17. Assist the patient with disrobing as necessary, providing a gown and drape.

Transferring Patient With Assistance

9. Working with your partner, you both face the patient, spread your feet apart, position yourselves so that one of each of your knees is aligned with the patient's knees, and bend your knees slightly. (If you lift while bending at your waist instead of bending your knees, you can cause serious injury to your back.)
10. Have the patient place one hand on each of your shoulders and hold on.

continued

Transferring a Patient in a Wheelchair and Preparing for an Examination

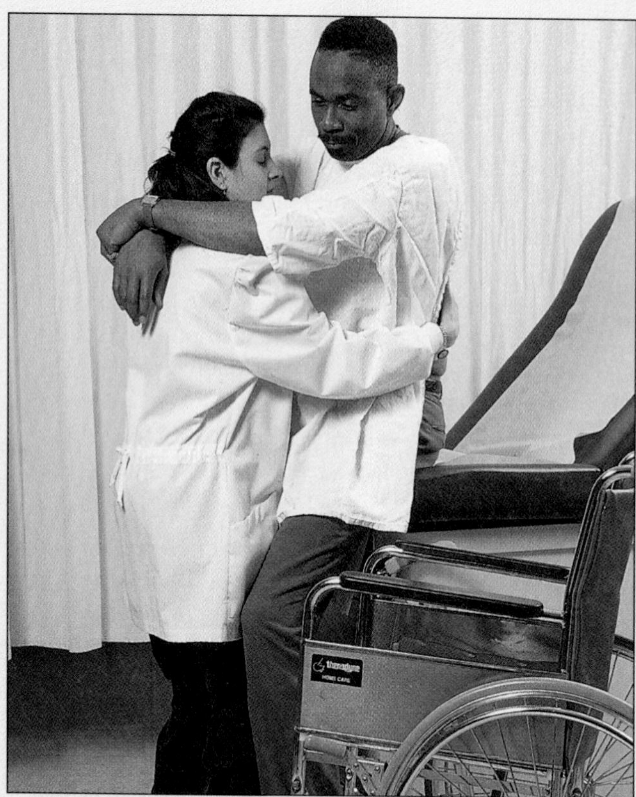

Figure 25-5. When you have lifted the patient, pivot him to bring the back of the knees against the table. Gently lower the patient into a sitting position, or into a supine position if the patient cannot sit unassisted.

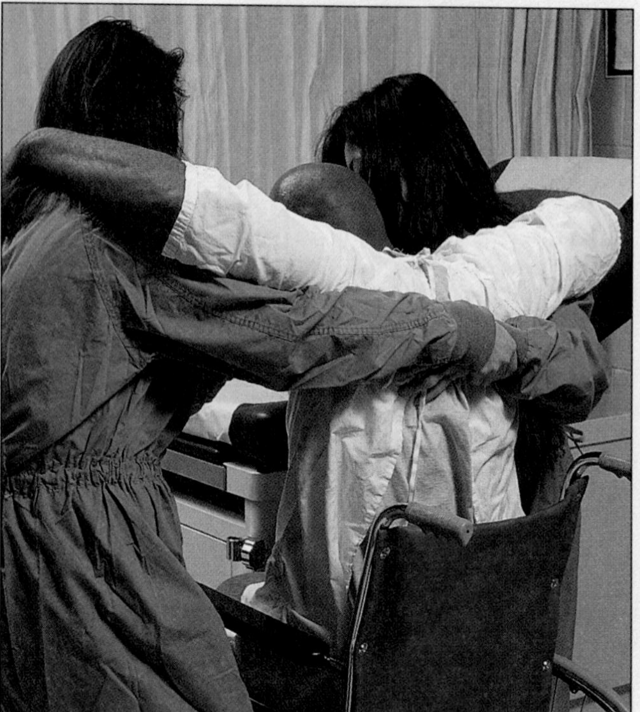

Figure 25-6. If you have an assistant, have the patient place one hand on each of your shoulders. Each of you should place your outermost arm around the patient, under one of the patient's arms. Interlock your wrists and, together, lift the patient.

11. Each of you places your outermost arm around the patient, one under each of the patient's arms. Then interlock your wrists (Figure 25-6).
12. Tell the patient that you will lift on the count of 3, and ask the patient to support as much of his own weight as possible (if he is able).
13. At the count of 3, you should lift the patient together.
14. The stronger of the two of you should pivot the patient to bring the back of the patient's knees against the table.
15. Working together, gently lower the patient into a sitting position on the table. If the patient cannot sit unassisted, help him move into a supine position (Figure 25-7).
16. Move the wheelchair out of the way.
17. Assist the patient with disrobing as necessary, providing a gown and drape.

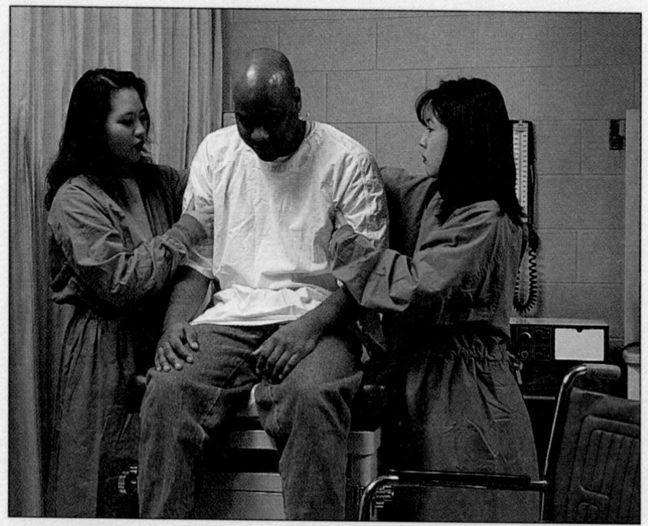

Figure 25-7. The stronger of the two of you should pivot the patient to bring the back of the patient's knees against the table. Gently lower the patient into a sitting position, or a supine position if the patient cannot sit unassisted.

PROCEDURE 25-4

Meeting the Needs of the Pregnant Patient During an Examination

Objective: To meet the special needs of the pregnant woman during the general physical examination

OSHA Guidelines 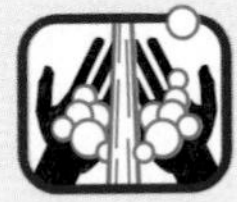

Materials: Patient education materials, examination table, examination gown, drape

Method

Providing Patient Information

1. Identify the patient and introduce yourself.
2. Assess the patient's need for education by asking appropriate questions.
3. Provide any appropriate instructions or materials.
4. Ask the patient whether she has any special concerns or questions about her pregnancy that she might want to discuss with the physician.
5. Communicate the patient's concerns or questions to the physician; include all pertinent background information on the patient.

Ensuring Comfort During the Examination

1. Identify the patient and introduce yourself.
2. Wash your hands.
3. Explain the procedure to the patient.
4. Provide a gown or drape, and instruct the patient in the proper way to wear it after disrobing. (Allow the patient privacy while disrobing, and assist only if she requests help.)
5. Ask the patient to step on the stool or the pullout step of the examination table.
6. Assist the patient onto the examination table.
7. Keeping position restrictions in mind, help the patient into the position requested by the physician.
8. Provide and adjust additional drapes as needed.
9. Keep in mind any difficulties the patient may have in achieving a certain position; suggest alternative positions whenever possible.
10. Minimize the time the patient must spend in uncomfortable positions.
11. If the patient appears to be uncomfortable during the procedure, ask whether she would like to reposition herself or take a break; assist as necessary.
12. To prevent pelvic pooling of blood and subsequent dizziness or hyperventilation, allow the patient time to adjust to sitting before standing after she has been lying on the examination table.

Palpation

The doctor uses palpation (touch) extensively in the general physical examination. During palpation the doctor assesses characteristics such as texture, temperature, shape, and the presence of vibrations or movements. The doctor may palpate superficially (on the skin surface), or she may palpate with additional pressure. She uses extra pressure when assessing characteristics of underlying tissues and organs. Depending on the characteristic the doctor is measuring, she may perform palpation using the fingertips, one hand, two hands (bimanual), or the palm of the hand.

Percussion

Percussion involves tapping or striking the body to hear sounds or feel vibrations. Physicians use percussion to determine the location, size, or density of a body structure or organ under the skin. For example, physicians use percussion to determine whether the lungs contain air or fluid.

The physician may perform percussion by striking the body directly with one or two fingers. More commonly, however, he performs indirect percussion by placing one finger of one hand on the area and striking it with a finger from the other hand.

Auscultation

Auscultation is the process of listening to body sounds. Doctors use auscultation to detect the flow of blood through an artery. Doctors perform auscultation extensively in the general examination to assess sounds from the heart, lungs, and abdominal organs. They use a stethoscope to hear most of these sounds.

Mensuration

Mensuration, the process of measuring, is discussed in Chapter 24 as part of charting the patient. In addition to the measurements you take before the examination—weight and height—you may need to take other measurements during the examination. For example, measurements may be done to monitor the growth of the uterus during pregnancy or to note the length and diameter of an extremity. You will usually use a tape measure or small ruler to take measurements.

Manipulation

Manipulation is the systematic moving of a patient's body parts. Physicians may palpate an area of the body while manipulating it to check for abnormalities that affect movement. Physicians often use manipulation to determine the range of motion of a joint.

Components of a General Physical Examination

Each physician performs the general physical examination in a certain order. Most physicians begin by assessing the patient's overall appearance and the condition of the patient's skin, nails, and hair. They usually then proceed with the examination in the following order, using the examination methods described above:

- Head
- Neck
- Eyes
- Ears
- Nose and sinuses
- Mouth and throat
- Chest and lungs
- Heart
- Breasts
- Abdomen
- Genitalia
- Rectum
- Musculoskeletal system
- Neurological system

Learn the standard order the physicians in your facility follow when performing the general examination. You should also be familiar with the components of the examination and the instruments and supplies needed for each component (Table 25-2). Instruments and supplies are discussed in detail in Chapter 22. Be sure you know how to perform the aspects of the examination for which you are responsible and that you understand the parts of the examination the physician performs.

Part of the medical assistant's role in the general examination is to ensure that the patient is as comfortable as possible. You can do this by helping to protect the patient's modesty as much as possible. For example, when the physician removes a drape or gown to expose an area for inspection, watch the patient for signs of embarrassment. If you notice any such signs, do your best to keep the patient covered as much as possible without hindering the physician's examination.

General Appearance

The physician usually begins the examination by reviewing the patient's general appearance and noting whether the patient appears to be in good health and of an acceptable weight. The physician also notes whether the patient appears to be distressed or in pain and assesses the level of the patient's alertness. Then the physician examines the patient's skin, nails, and hair.

Skin. The physician may prefer to examine all of the patient's skin at one time or to look at certain areas of skin while examining specific body parts. The physician notes the color, texture, moisture level, temperature, and elasticity of the skin. The condition of the skin is a good indicator of overall health. If the physician notices any lesions, she wears gloves to prevent possible transmission of microorganisms. The physician may also request that a specimen be taken from a lesion or wound for later examination to determine the infecting microorganism.

Nails. When the physician examines the patient's nails, he looks at both the nails and the nail beds. The condition of the nails may indicate poor nutrition, disease, infection, or injury. If applicable, remind the patient to remove nail cosmetics prior to the appointment.

Hair. The physician notes the patient's pattern of hair growth and the texture of the hair on the patient's scalp and on the rest of the body. Sudden hair loss or changes in hair growth may be indicators of an underlying disease.

Head

After reviewing the patient's general appearance, the doctor examines the patient's head. He looks for any abnormal condition of the scalp or skin, puffiness around the eyes or lips or in other areas of the face, or any abnormal growths.

Neck

To check the neck, the doctor palpates the patient's lymph nodes, thyroid gland, and major blood vessels. Enlarged lymph nodes may be a sign of infection or a blood cancer. An enlarged thyroid gland may indicate thyroid disease. The doctor also checks the neck for symmetry and range of motion.

Eyes

The physician examines the patient's eyes—particularly the eyelids and conjunctiva—for the presence of disease or abnormalities. She checks eye muscles by observing the patient's ability to follow the movement of a finger. She checks the pupils for their response to light (the pupils should contract—become smaller—when a penlight is directed toward them). Then she uses an ophthalmoscope to examine the patient's retinas and other internal structures of the eyes.

You may be required to perform various vision tests either before or after the general physical examination. (The tests are described in Chapter 26.)

Ears

The doctor checks the patient's outer ears for size, symmetry, and the presence of lesions, redness, or swelling. Using an otoscope, he then examines the inner structures of the patient's ears. The doctor may ask you to assist in

Table 25-2

Components and Materials of a General Physical Examination

Component	Materials Required*
General appearance (skin, nails, hair)	No special materials needed
Head	No special materials needed
Neck	No special materials needed
Eyes and vision**	Penlight, ophthalmoscope, vision charts, color charts
Ears and hearing**	Otoscope, audiometer
Nose and sinuses	Penlight, nasal speculum
Mouth and throat	Gloves, tongue depressor
Chest and lungs	Stethoscope
Heart	Stethoscope
Breasts	No special materials needed
Abdomen	Stethoscope
Genitalia (women)	Gloves, vaginal speculum, lubricant
Genitalia (men)	Gloves
Rectum	Gloves, lubricant
Musculoskeletal system	Tape measure
Neurological system	Reflex hammer, penlight

*Gloves should always be worn if the hands will come in contact with the patient's nonintact skin, blood, body fluids, or moist surfaces or if the patient is suspected of having an infectious disease.

**Procedures performed alone by the medical assistant are described in Chapter 26; all other listed procedures are performed by a physician with help from a medical assistant.

keeping the patient's head still during the otoscopic examination, particularly when the patient is a young child. Although this procedure is usually painless, patients with an ear infection may find it uncomfortable or painful.

The doctor checks the patient's ear canals for redness, drainage, lesions, foreign objects, or the presence of excessive cerumen (a waxy secretion from the ear, also known as earwax). During the most important part of the examination of the ears, the doctor assesses the color, shape, and reflectiveness of the eardrums. If an eardrum bulges outward or reflects light abnormally, the middle ear could be infected.

One of your responsibilities may be to perform various hearing tests either before or after the general physical examination. (These tests are described in Chapter 26.)

Nose and Sinuses

When examining the nose, the physician checks for the presence of infection or allergy. She uses a penlight to view the color of the **nasal mucosa** (lining of the nose) and notes any discharge, lesions, obstructions, swelling, or inflammation. A mucosa that is red or swollen and is accompanied by a yellowish discharge usually indicates an infection. A pale, swollen mucosa accompanied by a clear discharge indicates an allergy. When examining adults, the physician uses the nasal speculum to view the structures of the nose.

The physician may use palpation to check for tenderness in a patient's sinuses. Tenderness is an indication of inflammation or swelling.

Mouth and Throat

The doctor checks the condition of the patient's mouth to get a general impression of overall health and hygiene. Using a tongue depressor to draw back the patient's cheeks, the doctor examines the lining of the cheeks, the underside of the tongue, and the floor of the mouth. Changes in color or any lesions in these areas may indicate possible infection or oral cancer. The doctor also assesses the condition of the teeth and gums. When examining children, she counts the number of teeth. Most doctors leave this part of the examination of infants and toddlers until last, because children of this age tend to resist opening their mouths.

The doctor examines the patient's throat carefully because it is a common site of infection. She uses a tongue depressor to press the patient's tongue down and out of the way while asking the patient to say "ah." This procedure allows the doctor to view the throat and tonsils more clearly while checking them for redness or swelling, which can indicate the presence of infection.

Chest and Lungs

The physician usually assesses the patient's chest and lungs while the patient sits at the end of the examination table. When the patient is examined in this position, the chest can expand to its maximum capacity. Typically, the physician removes the patient's gown or lowers the drape from the waist up. Then he asks the patient to breathe normally or to take deep breaths. If the patient becomes dizzy during deep breathing, she may be hyperventilating. **Hyperventilation** is overly deep breathing that leads to a loss of carbon dioxide in the blood. You can help the patient by having her breathe into a paper bag. With your help the patient should recover quickly.

The physician inspects the patient's chest from the back, side, and front. He checks its shape, symmetry, and postural position and looks for the presence of any type of deformity. Postural abnormalities often occur in the elderly. Frequently, especially in elderly women, these abnormalities are caused by osteoporosis, the loss of bone density.

The physician also palpates the chest and performs percussion to check for the presence of fluid or a foreign mass in the lungs. The physician then uses a stethoscope to auscultate the chest from the back, side, and front. He listens to the lung sounds during both normal and deep breathing. The stethoscope allows him to hear abnormal breathing that may result from such disorders as bronchitis, asthma, or pneumonia.

Heart

The doctor usually examines the patient's heart and vascular system at the same time as, or immediately after, examining the lungs. He may palpate the area first to locate the correct anatomical landmarks for placing the stethoscope. He may use percussion to check the size of the heart. The patient should not speak while the physician auscultates the heart sounds with the stethoscope. The physician notes the rate, rhythm, intensity, and pitch of the heart.

Breasts

During a general physical examination, every woman should have a complete breast examination. Breast cancer is the most common cancer in women. Because growths are also possible in men's breasts, doctors should perform a breast examination on all patients.

The doctor begins the examination with the patient in a sitting position. The doctor asks the patient to hold her arms at her sides while he inspects the breasts for symmetry, contour, masses, and retracted areas. The doctor then asks the patient to raise her arms above her head while he palpates the lymph nodes under her arms.

Next the doctor asks the patient to lie down and place her hand under her head on the first side to be examined. The doctor may ask you to place a small pillow or folded towel under the patient's shoulder blade on the same side. This procedure allows the breast tissue to flatten evenly against the chest wall, permitting easier palpation. The doctor then palpates the breast in a circular, systematic manner to check for lumps, examines the areola and nipple, and then repeats the procedure on the other side.

When examining male patients, the doctor palpates the patient's breasts and lymph nodes in the same manner as he does with his female patients. The doctor also checks the breasts of his male patients for lesions or swelling.

Abdomen

The physician examines the patient's abdomen while the patient is in a supine position with arms down at the sides. The abdominal muscles should be completely relaxed for this part of the examination. The physician may ask you to place a small pillow under the patient's head or knees (or both) to keep the abdomen relaxed. If the patient is wearing a gown, it is raised to just under the breasts. If the patient is draped, the drape must be lowered to just above the genitalia to allow a complete view of the area. A separate drape should be placed to cover a female patient's breasts.

The order of examination methods for examining the abdomen is different from the order for other areas. The physician begins with inspection and auscultation, followed by percussion and palpation. Following this order allows the physician to listen to bowel sounds before palpating the abdominal organs. Palpation of this area can

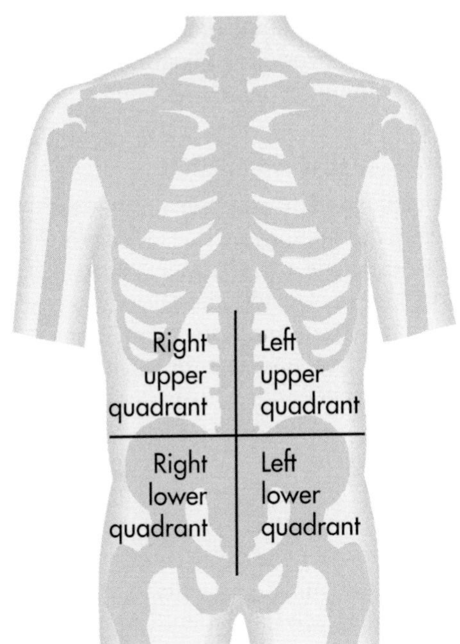

Figure 25-8. The abdomen is typically divided into four equal sections, or quadrants.

change bowel sounds in such a way that the physician could misdiagnose a patient's condition.

The physician must assess the abdomen thoroughly, because there are many organs in the abdominal cavity. The physician describes observations based on a system of landmarks that map out the abdominal region. The abdomen is typically divided into four equal sections, or **quadrants,** as shown in Figure 25-8. Some physicians divide the abdomen into nine sections, similar to a tick-tack-toe board, as shown in Figure 25-9.

If the physician has not assessed the skin in this area already, she begins with an inspection of the abdominal skin's color and surface and follows with an inspection of the shape and symmetry of the abdomen. She then uses auscultation to check bowel and vascular sounds and uses percussion to note the size and position of the organs. Lastly, she uses palpation to check muscle tone and to determine the presence of any tenderness or masses.

Female Genitalia

Female patients may feel self-conscious or anxious in the lithotomy position—which is most commonly used during examination of the genitalia. The medical assistant may help the patient relax during this procedure and may assist patients in maintaining the position.

If the doctor who performs the examination is male, a female medical assistant should always be in the room to protect both the patient and doctor from potential lawsuits. This type of examination may be performed by a specialist or by a primary care physician. (The procedure for a gynecologic examination is described only briefly here; for greater detail, refer to Chapter 27.)

When the patient is in position, the doctor follows these steps.

1. She puts on examination gloves and examines the external genitalia by inspection and palpation. You should position the examination light over the doctor's shoulder to illuminate the area properly.
2. The doctor uses a vaginal speculum to view the internal genitalia. Before you pass the speculum to the doctor, she may request that you warm the speculum blades under warm running water to reduce the patient's discomfort.
3. After the doctor inserts the vaginal speculum and opens the blades, she examines the cervix and obtains material for a Pap smear (Papanicolaou smear). Be prepared to pass a cotton-tipped applicator or other piece of collection equipment to the doctor and to present a properly labeled slide for the application of the endocervical sample.
4. Pass the cervical scraper to the doctor, and present the opposite end of the same slide (or a new, properly labeled slide) for the cervical sample.
5. The doctor then uses the opposite end of the cervical scraper to collect a vaginal sample. This material goes on a separate slide. You must apply fixative to the specimens on each slide.
6. After the doctor removes the speculum, she performs a digital examination to check the position of the internal organs. During a **digital examination,** the doctor inserts two fingers of one hand into the vagina and examines by palpation both internally and externally, with the other hand on the abdomen. This is

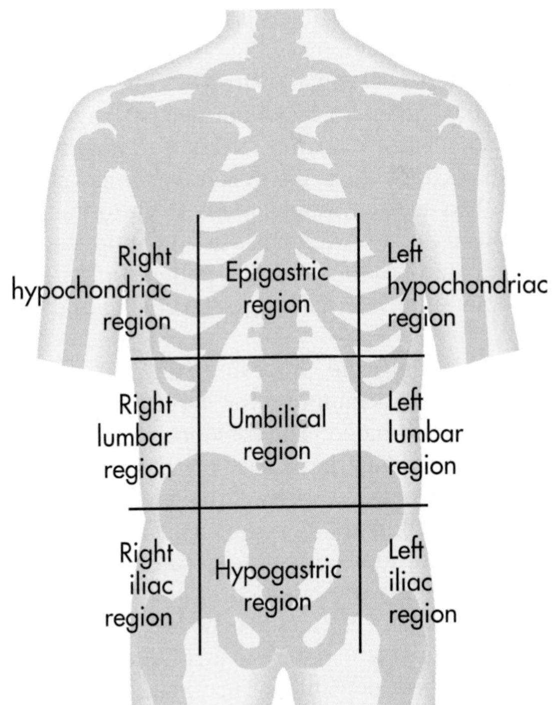

Figure 25-9. Some physicians divide the abdomen into nine sections, similar to a tick-tack-toe board.

referred to as a bimanual examination. You assist by applying lubricant to the doctor's gloved fingers before the examination begins.

7. When the doctor completes the examination, help the patient switch from the lithotomy position into a supine or sitting position. You should also offer the patient the opportunity to clean herself before you adjust the drape.

Male Genitalia

During the examination of the genitalia, men may be just as embarrassed or uncomfortable as women may be. If the physician who is performing the assessment is female, a male medical assistant should be in the room to protect both the patient and physician from potential lawsuits.

The procedure begins with the patient in the supine position. The physician puts on gloves and visually inspects the patient's penis for signs of infection or structural abnormalities, palpating any lesions. The physician then examines the scrotum in the same manner, palpating the testicles for lumps. The patient is asked to stand while the physician checks for any bulges in the groin that may indicate a hernia. At the same time, the physician palpates the local lymph nodes to check for any abnormality.

Rectum

The doctor usually examines the rectum after examining the genitalia. You may need to assist an adult patient into a dorsal recumbent or Sims' position. The doctor normally examines a child when the child is in the prone position and inspects only the external areas of the rectum.

In adults the doctor uses digital examination to palpate the rectum for lesions or irregularities. Doctors recommend that patients older than age 40 have a yearly digital examination for early detection of colorectal cancer. For this examination the doctor puts on a clean pair of gloves. You assist by applying lubricant to the doctor's gloved index finger before the examination begins. As with examination of the genitalia, patients often find digital examination of the rectum embarrassing and uncomfortable.

After performing the procedure, the doctor may request that any stool found on the glove be tested for the presence of occult blood. The presence of occult blood in the stool is a possible indication of colorectal cancer or gastrointestinal bleeding. This test—often called by its brand name, Hemoccult or Seracult test—involves placing a sample of stool on a special cardboard slide. You assist by presenting the slide to the doctor. To produce an accurate test, three consecutive bowel movements are tested; this sample is usually the first. After the examination you may be responsible for instructing the patient on how to collect the additional two samples. The procedure is outlined on the package of the occult blood-testing kit.

After the rectal examination offer the patient the opportunity to clean the anal area before you adjust the drape. Dispose of gloves and soiled materials in a biohazardous waste container.

Musculoskeletal System

If the physician did not examine the patient's back during the chest examination, he does so during the musculoskeletal assessment. The physician checks for good posture from the back and side. He may ask the patient to walk so that he can assess her gait. The physician always asks a child to bend at the waist so that he can check for the presence of **scoliosis,** a lateral curvature of the spine.

During the musculoskeletal assessment the physician determines range of motion, the strength of various muscle groups, and body measurements. The physician also examines the arms, hands, legs, and feet for any lesions, deformities, or circulatory problems.

The physician checks a patient's range of motion to detect joint deformities and to learn whether the patient has any limitations in movement caused by an injury or other conditions, such as arthritis. Checking a patient's range of motion also allows the physician to follow a patient's progress during recovery from an injury or surgery.

As part of the assessment of a child's health, the physician asks the child to perform certain tasks, such as walking a straight line and balancing or hopping on one foot. The physician uses these tasks to evaluate the child's development and coordination and to provide the physician with information about the functioning of the child's neurological system.

Neurological System

The doctor's neurological assessment includes an evaluation of the patient's reflexes, mental and emotional status (including intelligence, speech, and behavior), and sensory and motor functions. The doctor often performs the neurological assessment at the same time as the musculoskeletal assessment because both systems are involved in movement and coordination.

The doctor may incorporate certain aspects of the neurological assessment into other parts of the examination. For example, testing how a patient's pupils react to light is part of an eye examination, but because this test also examines the patient's light reflex, the test includes a neurological assessment as well.

The doctor checks the patient's reflexes to assess both sensory and motor nerve pathways at different areas of the spinal cord. To check reflexes, the doctor uses a reflex hammer to tap tendons in different areas of the patient's body.

Most examinations of children also include an intellectual assessment, in which the doctor asks the child general questions appropriate to the child's age. Doctors may also test the mental status and memory of older adults to detect disorders such as senility and Alzheimer's disease in patients who show signs of confusion or complain of memory loss.

Completing the Examination

After the physician completes the examination, you should help the patient into a sitting position. Then allow the patient to perform any necessary self-hygiene measures.

Additional Tests or Procedures

Before the patient dresses, check to see whether the physician has ordered any additional tests or procedures that are more conveniently performed while the patient is undressed. These tests might include taking body fat measurements or blood samples or preparing the patient for a diagnostic or therapeutic procedure, such as an x-ray or physical therapy session. The physician may also ask you to perform other procedures. Some of these procedures, which are covered in other chapters, include the following:

- Cold or heat therapy (Chapter 30)
- Applying a bandage (Chapter 31)
- Collecting culture specimens (Chapters 33, 34, and 35)
- Administering an injection (Chapter 38)
- Applying a topical medication (Chapter 38)

If the physician has not ordered any additional procedures—or if wearing clothing does not interfere with the procedures ordered—the patient may dress. Help the patient get off the examination table, and allow her to dress in privacy. Make sure she knows you are available to assist if she needs help dressing.

The physician may ask you to perform other tests and procedures that can be done after the patient has dressed, including these procedures, which are discussed in detail where noted:

- Vision and hearing tests (Chapter 26)
- Otic or ophthalmic irrigation (Chapter 26)
- Pulmonary function tests (Chapter 39)
- Administration of certain medications (Chapter 38)

Patient Education

The general physical examination provides you with the opportunity to assess the patient's educational needs. Basing your findings on the patient's interview, history, and examination, you can identify areas in which the patient may benefit from additional education.

Pay special attention to educating patients about risk factors for disease. For example, women are often instructed about the risk factors for breast cancer. These factors include being older than 50 (many physicians recommend that women older than 40 have a mammogram every 2 years and that women older than 50 have one every year), having a family history of breast cancer, having the first child after age 30, never being pregnant, and beginning to menstruate at an early age.

The physician may also request that you teach patients how to perform diagnostic or self-help techniques or how to administer certain medications at home. These procedures may involve collecting samples for occult blood testing or urine testing, applying cold or hot packs, or instilling eyedrops. It is important to teach the patient the correct way to perform a diagnostic test. If a specimen is incorrectly obtained, the test results will be inaccurate.

Regardless of the type of instruction, be sure that you address patients at a language level they can understand without talking down to them. To ensure that they understand fully, ask patients to repeat each instruction and to perform each demonstration as you give it to them. (For patient education tips related to specialty examinations, refer to Chapters 27 and 28.) Give patients written instructions that they can refer to at home.

Special Problems of the Elderly

The elderly often have a greater need for patient education than do younger patients because many diseases are common in older patients. Moreover, the elderly frequently are not aware of these diseases or of advances in their treatment. Here are some common problems of the elderly:

- Incontinence
- Depression
- Lack of information on preventive medicine
- Lack of compliance when taking medications

Incontinence. Physicians estimate that most patients who suffer from incontinence (involuntary leakage of urine) can be helped. Because most people are too embarrassed to ask for help or are unaware of possible solutions, however, only 1 out of 12 persons actually seeks help for the condition.

Depression. Depression is common in the elderly, but many of the symptoms of depression mimic those of other conditions. You can help elderly patients—and their families—recognize the signs of depression. Knowing what to look for may help patients seek help sooner than they otherwise would and receive prompt diagnosis and treatment. See "Diseases and Disorders" for a discussion of symptoms and treatment of depression in the elderly.

Lack of Information on Preventive Medicine. Many of the elderly are still not aware of the concept of preventive medicine (measures taken to prevent illness). Many come from environments in which people went to a doctor only when they were very ill. Thus, they do not realize the importance of preventive measures such as regular checkups and yearly digital rectal examinations to detect colorectal cancer. Older women often do not recognize the need for regular mammograms and Pap smears to detect cancers of the breast and cervix.

DISEASES AND DISORDERS

Helping Elderly Patients With Depression

Depression is a common problem among elderly people. Studies published by the National Institutes of Health (NIH) indicate that at least 5% of elderly people attending primary care clinics suffer from depression. For elderly people in nursing homes, that percentage rises to between 15% and 25%. The NIH also indicates that only about 10% of elderly people who need treatment for depression ever receive it.

One reason for this low rate of treatment is that many older people—and their families—believe that depression is a normal consequence of growing old. After all, people generally experience occasions of profound sadness and have to adjust to many changes in their later years. Older people may experience the deaths of a spouse and siblings; they have to adjust to retirement and, possibly, loneliness. They may have to deal with a relocation. They may suffer economic hardship and are likely to experience a variety of physical ailments.

Recognizing the Symptoms

There is, unfortunately, no specific diagnostic test for depression, so a diagnosis must be made on the basis of symptoms. The symptoms of depression in the elderly are similar to those in other age groups and include the following:

- Decreased ability to enjoy life or to show an interest in activities or people
- Slow thinking, indecisiveness, or difficulty in concentrating
- Increased or decreased appetite
- Increased or decreased time spent sleeping
- Recurrent feelings of worthlessness
- Loss of energy and motivation
- Exaggerated feelings of sadness, hopelessness, or anxiety
- Recurrent thoughts of death or suicide

The failure to realize that symptoms such as these indicate an illness prevents many older people from seeking help. Yet there is evidence that treatment for depression in the elderly can be highly effective.

Treatment for Depression

Treatment for depression generally combines a course of antidepressant drugs with psychotherapy. Older people generally respond to antidepressants more slowly than younger people do, so older people may not experience relief until more than 6 weeks after starting treatment. For this and other reasons, compliance in taking medications for depression is a problem with elderly people. Many of them do not understand depression and the importance of taking medications as prescribed. They may also be frightened by the idea of taking medication for a mental problem.

Psychotherapy aims to help older people talk through their anxieties, develop coping skills, and improve the quality of their lives. Again, compliance is a problem. Many older people are unwilling to admit that they have a mental-health problem and refuse to follow up on referrals to mental-health professionals.

Benefits of Treatment

Elderly people who follow a course of treatment for depression benefit in a number of ways. They gain:

- Relief from many of the symptoms associated with depression.
- Relief from some of the pain and suffering associated with physical ailments.
- Improved physical, mental, and social well-being.

Health-care providers can play a significant role in recognizing symptoms of depression in the elderly and in encouraging them to get the treatment they need.

Use any educational tools available to you to make elderly patients more aware of these disorders and the importance of preventive measures. If you reinforce the doctor's recommendations with education, you increase the chance that patients will heed the advice they are given.

Lack of Compliance When Taking Medications. Some elderly people need several medications, and many of them find it difficult to keep track and take the right medication at the right time. You can help by telling elderly patients about available medication reminder boxes, timers, or medication organizers. These devices can help ensure **patient compliance** (obedience in following the physician's orders). Patient compliance helps patients remain healthier and get well faster.

Follow-up

After the examination, you must help the patient follow up on all of the doctor's recommendations. Follow-up may include these actions:

CAUTION

HANDLE WITH CARE

Helping Patients With Suspected Breast Cancer

If the physician detects a suspicious lump in a patient's breast during the general physical examination, your main concern is to help the patient remain calm. Although most suspicious lumps are not cancerous, the patient is likely to be anxious and upset about the finding. The best thing you can do for her is to schedule her for a mammogram as soon as possible.

Preparing the Patient for a Mammogram

To alleviate some of the patient's fears, explain exactly what a mammogram is. Give the patient the following information.

1. A mammogram is a special type of x-ray of the breast that is used to detect cancer and other abnormalities of the breast.
2. A technician specially trained in performing mammography will position the patient's breast along a flat plastic plate. A second plate will be brought into position and pressure will be applied for about 20 to 30 seconds to flatten the breast (to obtain a clearer x-ray) while the x-ray is taken. This will be done in two directions (planes) for each breast.
3. Mammography is generally not a painful procedure, but some women may find it uncomfortable. Many professionals suggest that patients avoid scheduling a mammogram during the week prior to a menstrual period to reduce potential discomfort.
4. The mammography appointment normally takes no longer than half an hour. The actual mammography takes only about 15 minutes.
5. Because the patient will have to undress from the waist up, she should wear a separate top and slacks or a skirt rather than a dress.
6. The patient should have no creams, powders, or deodorants on her breasts or underarms when the mammography is performed because chemicals in these preparations can produce misleading images in the mammogram.

Answer any questions the patient has, and provide patient education materials related to mammography and breast disease. Reassure her that most lumps are not cancerous.

If your office refers patients to a particular facility that you are familiar with, give the patient an idea of how long she can expect to wait for the results. Ensure her that she will be notified as soon as the physician receives the report. You may want to schedule a follow-up visit at this time, based on when results are expected.

Because this is a difficult time for a patient, you should be as supportive as possible. You can help the patient cope by showing your concern and giving her prompt attention. Tell the patient that if she has any questions at all, she should call the physician.

1. Scheduling the patient for future visits at the office
2. Making outside appointments for certain diagnostic tests—such as mammograms or other radiologic procedures—or for therapeutic procedures—such as physical therapy
3. Helping the patient and the patient's family plan for home nursing care after an illness or a surgical procedure
4. Helping the patient obtain help from community or social service organizations, such as adult day care, counseling, or meal programs

Patient follow-up is particularly crucial for patients suspected of having breast cancer. You have an important responsibility to track patients who have suspicious findings on a breast examination. See "Caution: Handle With Care" for an explanation of the steps you can take to help such patients. Patients may file medical malpractice suits if doctors fail to diagnose breast cancer. In fact, this is currently the most frequent cause of malpractice suits.

Summary

The general physical examination provides substantial information about a patient's overall health status and assists the physician in making a diagnosis, prognosis, and treatment plan. The general physical examination is the cornerstone of medical care.

The physician uses a number of assessment methods to gather information during the examination. Although one common order of examination is presented in this chapter, you should learn the order preferred by the physician(s) you assist. Be aware, too, that a physician may change the order of an examination to accommodate the needs of a particular patient.

During the examination, your first priority as a medical assistant is to address the comfort, privacy, and educational needs of the patient. You must also anticipate the needs of the physician throughout the procedure. In addition, you must be aware of the special needs of children, pregnant women, and the elderly and the areas in which patient education is likely to be needed.

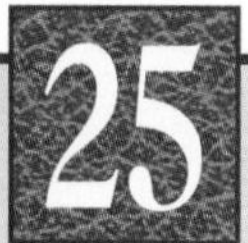

Chapter Review

Discussion Questions

1. How can a medical assistant help prepare a patient emotionally and physically for a general physical examination?
2. In what ways do children and the elderly present special problems during or after a general physical examination?
3. In what ways can medical assistants help in providing patient education after a general physical examination?

Critical Thinking Questions

1. How might the physician change the typical order of the general physical examination for an infant who is suffering from an ear infection and appears agitated?
2. What steps can you take to help ensure that an elderly patient takes her medicine properly?
3. How can you help patients who are on crutches prepare for an examination?

Application Activities

1. With a partner, practice assisting each other in assuming the various examination positions and in placing drapes properly.
2. Interview a physician to find out what order of components she follows when performing a general physical examination. Present your findings to the class.
3. With a partner, practice identifying instruments that are used during each component of a general physical examination.

Further Readings

Buchwald, Dedra, et al. "Caring for Patients in a Multicultural Society." *Patient Care,* 15 June 1994, 105–120.

National Institute on Drug Abuse. *Using Your Medicines Wisely: A Guide for the Elderly.* U.S. Department of Health and Human Services Publication No. (ADM) 92–705, 1992.

NIH Consensus Development Panel on Depression in Late Life. "Diagnosis and Treatment of Depression in Late Life." *Journal of the American Medical Association,* 26 August 1992, 1018–1024.

"A Nurse's Guide to Patient Positioning." *American Journal of Nursing,* March 1996, 35–36.

Plautz, R. "Positioning Can Make the Difference." *Nursing Homes Long Term Care Management* 41, no. 1 (January/February 1992): 30–34.

Sternberg, S. "Colorectal Cancer: To Screen or Not?" *Science News* 150, no. 23 (7 December 1996): 358.

Yeaw, E. M. "How Position Affects Oxygenation: Good Lung Down?" *American Journal of Nursing,* March 1992, 26–29.

Providing Eye and Ear Care

CHAPTER OUTLINE

OBJECTIVES

After completing Chapter 26, you will be able to:

- Describe the anatomy and physiology of the eye.
- State ways that vision changes with age.
- Describe ways to detect vision problems.
- List treatments for eye disorders.
- Identify ways that patients can practice preventive eye care.
- Describe the anatomy and physiology of the ear.
- State ways that hearing changes with age.
- List the types of hearing loss.
- Explain the procedures for screening and diagnosing ear problems.
- Describe treatments for ear and hearing disorders.
- Explain how patients can be educated about preventive ear care.

AREAS OF COMPETENCE

1997 ROLE DELINEATION STUDY

CLINICAL

Diagnostic Orders

- Perform diagnostic tests

Patient Care

- Prepare patient for examinations, procedures, and treatments
- Assist with examinations, procedures, and treatments
- Prepare and administer medications and immunizations
- Maintain medication and immunization records

continued

Key Terms

aqueous humor
audiologist
audiometer
auricle
bone conduction
cerumen
choroid
ciliary body
cochlea
cone
conjunctiva
cornea
decibel
eustachian tube
frequency
incus
iris
labyrinth
lacrimal gland
lens
malleus
ophthalmologist
optometrist
orbit
otologist
pupil
retina
rod
sclera
semicircular canals
stapes
tympanic membrane
vitreous humor

DACUM COMPETENCIES continued

GENERAL (Transdisciplinary)

Communication Skills

- Adapt communications to individual's ability to understand

Instruction

- Instruct individuals according to their needs
- Explain office policies and procedures
- Teach methods of health promotion and disease prevention

The Medical Assistant's Role in Eye and Ear Care

Part of your clinical assisting duties for a general medical practice may involve performing basic tests for vision and hearing. You may also assist the doctor in providing treatment related to the eyes and ears. You will be expected to know the basic structure and function of these organs and to advise patients about general eye and ear care and concerns. Specialized examinations and treatments for the eye and the ear are discussed in Chapter 28 under ophthalmology and otology, respectively.

Vision

A person's visual system consists of the eyes, the optic nerve, which connects the eye to the vision center of the brain, and several accessory structures. If these parts of the system are healthy and normal, the individual is able to see normally.

The Eye

The eye is a complex organ that processes light to produce images. It is made up of three main layers and a number of specialized parts, as shown in Figure 26-1.

The Outer Layer. The white of the eye, called the **sclera,** is the tough, outermost layer of the eye. This layer, through which light cannot pass, covers all except the front of the eye. Here the sclera gives way to the cornea. The **cornea** is a transparent area on the front of the eye that acts as a window to let light into the eye.

The Middle Layer. The **choroid** is the middle layer of the eye, which contains most of the eye's blood vessels. In the anterior part of the choroid are the iris and the ciliary body. The **iris** is the colored part of the eye. It is made of muscular tissue. As this tissue contracts and relaxes, an opening at its center grows larger or smaller. This opening is the **pupil.** The size of the pupil regulates the amount of light that enters the eye. In bright light the pupil becomes smaller. In dim light it becomes larger.

The **ciliary body** is a wedge-shaped thickening in the middle layer of the eyeball. Muscles in the ciliary body control the shape of the lens—making the lens more or less curved for viewing either near or distant objects. The **lens** is a clear, circular disk located just posterior to the iris. Because the lens can change shape, it helps the eye focus images of objects that are near or far away.

The space between the cornea and the lens contains a liquid called **aqueous humor,** which is produced by capillaries in the ciliary body. The part of the eye behind the lens is filled with a jellylike substance called **vitreous humor,** which helps the eye hold its shape.

The Inner Layer. The inner layer of the eye consists of the **retina.** Nerve cells at the posterior of the retina sense light. There are two types of nerve cells, each named for its shape. **Rods** are highly sensitive to light. They function in dim light but do not provide a sharp image or detect color. **Cones** function only in bright light. They are sensitive to color and provide sharp images.

There are three types of cones—one each for detecting red, green, or blue light. A person who completely lacks cones cannot see colors and is said to be color-blind. Someone who lacks one type of cone is partially color-blind and has difficulty telling two or more colors apart.

The Process of Seeing

The eye works much like a camera. Light reflected from an object, or produced by one, enters the eye from the outside and passes through the cornea, pupil, lens, and fluids in the eye. The cornea, lens, and fluids help focus

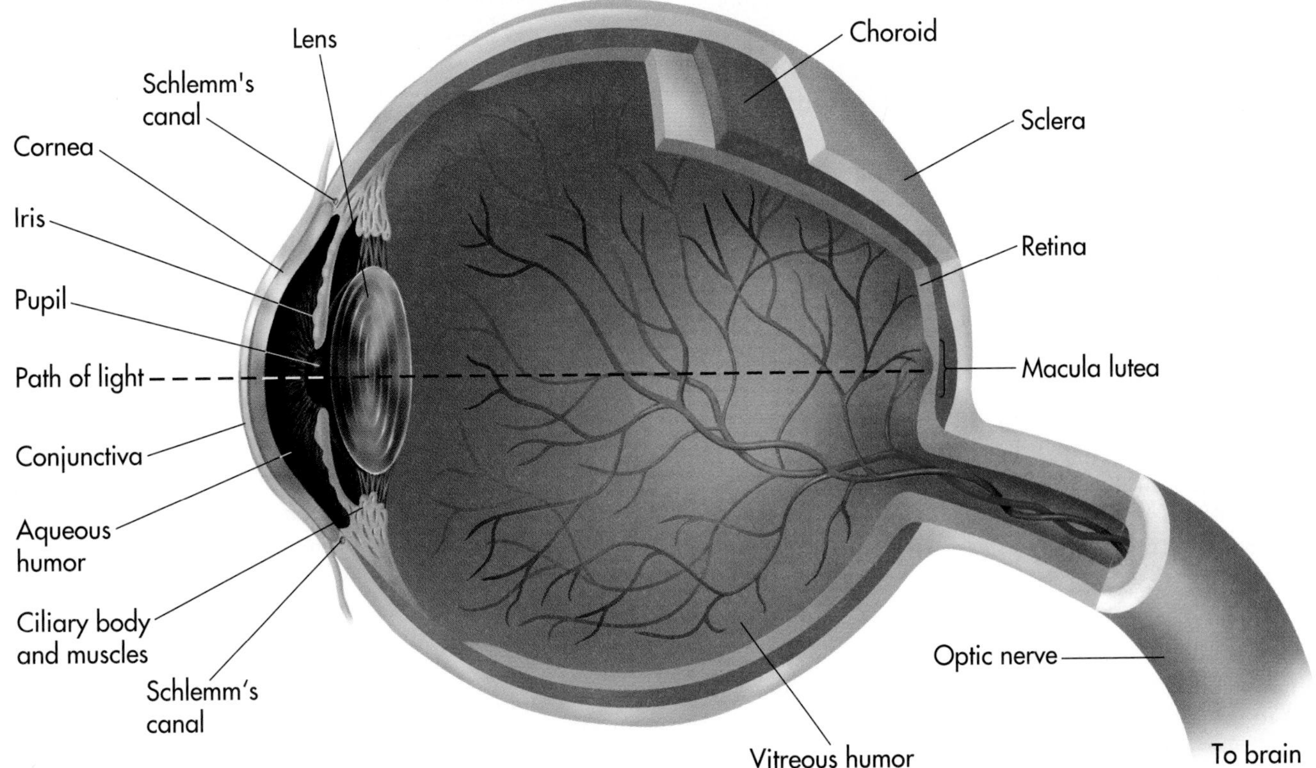

Figure 26-1. The eye is composed of a number of structures that work in harmony to produce vision.

the light onto the retina by bending, or refracting, the light. As in a camera, an image of an object is carried by light patterns. The image is projected upside down—on film in the case of a camera and on the retina in the case of an eye. The retina converts the light into nerve impulses. These impulses are transmitted along the optic nerve to the brain. This nerve, which consists of about a million fibers, serves as a flexible cable connecting the eyeball to the brain. The brain interprets these impulses, turns the image right-side up, and "develops" a picture of the object from which the light originally came.

Accessory Structures

Several structures protect, lubricate, and move the eye, all of which contribute to healthy vision. These structures include the following:

- Eye sockets
- Eyebrows and eyelashes
- Eyelids
- Conjunctiva
- Lacrimal apparatus
- Eye muscles

The eye sockets, or **orbits,** form a protective shell around the eyes. Eyebrows and eyelashes also serve to protect the eyes by reducing the chances that sweat and direct sunlight will enter the eyes. The eyelids are a part of the blinking reflex, which protects the eyes from foreign materials such as dust. Blinking also helps lubricate the eyes by spreading tears over their surface. The protective membrane that lines the eyelids and covers the anterior of the sclera is the **conjunctiva.**

The lacrimal apparatus consists of the **lacrimal gland** (the source of tears) and a drainage system. Tears moisten and lubricate the eye and wash away foreign materials. They also inhibit the growth of bacteria. Excess tears drain from the eye through ducts located in the inner corner of the eye. The ducts empty into the nose.

In addition to the muscles inside the eye, there are six muscles that attach to the outside of each eyeball. These muscles control the movement of the eyes and normally allow both eyes to move in harmony.

The Aging Eye

With age, a number of changes occur in the structure and function of the eye.

- The amount of fat tissue diminishes; this loss may cause the eyelids to droop.
- The quality and quantity of tears decrease.
- The conjunctiva becomes thinner and may be drier because of a decrease in tear production.
- The cornea begins to appear yellow, and a ring of fat deposits appears around it.
- The sclera may develop brown spots.

- Changes in the iris cause the pupil to become smaller, limiting the amount of light entering the eye.
- The lens becomes denser and more rigid; this trend reduces the amount of light that reaches the retina and makes focusing more difficult.
- Yellowing of the lens causes problems in distinguishing colors.
- Changes in the retina may make vision fuzzy.
- The ability of the eye to adapt to changes in light intensities may be reduced; glare can become painful as this ability diminishes.
- Night vision may be impaired.
- Peripheral vision is reduced, limiting the area a person can see and reducing depth perception.
- The vitreous humor breaks down, producing tiny clumps of gel or cellular material that cause floaters—dark spots or lines—that appear in a person's field of vision.
- Rubbing of the vitreous humor on the retina produces flashes of light or "sparks."

Because of changes that impair vision—such as reductions in the field of vision, in depth perception, and in visual clarity—elderly people may fall more often than younger people. See "Educating the Patient" for some tips for preventing such falls.

Vision Testing

When doctors perform complete physical examinations, they usually screen patients for vision problems and for the general health of the eyes. An **ophthalmologist** (a medical doctor who is an eye specialist) usually performs a thorough eye examination (described in Chapter 28). She tests the external as well as internal structures of the eyes, along with eye movement and coordination. The kinds of testing you will perform or help perform will depend on where you work. You will, however, be expected to assist the doctor and ensure that the patient is comfortable.

Types of Vision Screening Tests

Screening tests are used to detect a number of common visual problems. Some problems may involve the ability to see clearly. Others may involve the ability to distinguish shades of gray or colors. When you record the results of vision tests, you will use the following abbreviations:

- O.D.—right eye
- O.S.—left eye
- O.U.—both eyes
- $\overline{cc}$—with correction

EDUCATING THE PATIENT

Preventing Falls in the Elderly

Falls can occur at any age, but in the elderly they can have especially serious consequences. Bones become brittle with age, and falls can cause breaks in major bones, such as the hip. Complications from falls and bone fractures can lead to death in individuals in this age group.

The elderly are prone to falling because of vision problems, possible poor health, slowing reflexes, and changes in the ear that cause equilibrium problems. In addition, medications can increase the risk of falls because they may make the patient less alert. Discuss a safety checklist with elderly patients and their families. Point out that by taking the precautions listed, elderly patients can reduce the risk of falling. Make sure patients and their families understand these instructions.

- Remove reading glasses before getting up and walking around.
- Make sure that potentially hazardous areas, such as stairs and doorway entrances, are well lit.
- Use night-lights in the bedroom and bathroom to help prevent falls at night.
- When getting up from a reclining or recumbent position, sit at the edge of the bed for a few minutes before trying to stand to allow blood flow to adjust.
- Wear well-fitting shoes with low heels and slippers with nonslip soles.
- Use a cane or walker if you are unsteady on your feet.
- Secure rugs and floor coverings to the floor to prevent slippage.
- Attach all electrical cords to the walls or floor moldings.
- Place sturdy banisters along all stairs inside and outside the home.
- Install secure handrails near the bathtub and toilet.
- Use nonslip mats in the bathtub and shower.
- Minimize clutter in the home.
- Store frequently used items within easy reach.

MULTISKILL FOCUS

Ophthalmic Assistant

To gain medical assistant credentials, you must fulfill the requirements of either the American Association of Medical Assistants (for a Certified Medical Assistant) or the American Medical Technologists (for a Registered Medical Assistant). After obtaining your medical assistant certification or registration, you may wish to acquire additional skills in specialty areas through course work or on-the-job training. Although this course work or training may not lead to an additional certification or degree, it will enable you to expand your role in the medical office and advance your career as the demand for multiskilled health professionals increases.

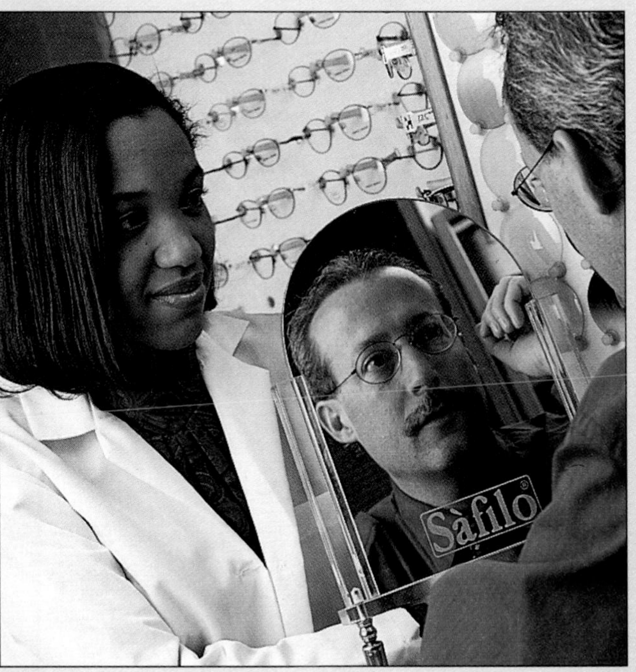

Skills and Duties

An ophthalmic assistant provides administrative and clinical support for an ophthalmologist. The assistant works with patients, assists with surgery, and keeps instruments and equipment in proper working order.

The ophthalmic assistant works with patients in a number of ways. Taking the medical history is basic to the ophthalmic assistant's job. She must gather information about the patient's ocular history, family medical history, past and present systemic illnesses, medications, and allergies. She needs to preserve patient confidentiality and use proper recording techniques.

An ophthalmic assistant may conduct tests that evaluate aspects of vision, such as distance acuity, near acuity, and color perception. She must understand how these tests work and how to run them and be prepared to help patients with special needs as she conducts the tests. Tonometry, the measurement of fluid pressure in the eyeball with a machine called a tonometer, may also be the responsibility of an ophthalmic assistant.

When patients need help with their eyeglasses, the ophthalmic assistant is often the person who records prescriptions, adjusts and repairs damaged frames and lenses, and instructs patients in the care of their eyeglasses. The assistant is trained to administer eye medications to patients in the form of drops, ointments, and irrigating solutions.

The ophthalmic assistant may also assist the ophthalmologist with minor surgery. She prepares the room and instruments, instructs the patient before and after the procedure, and assists the doctor during the surgical procedure.

The operation and care of specialized ophthalmologic instruments, such as ophthalmoscopes, retinoscopes, tonometers, and slitlamps, are often the responsibility of an ophthalmic assistant. She must maintain infection control in the office or operating room, including sanitization, disinfection, and sterilization of instruments and surfaces.

Workplace Settings

The ophthalmic assistant always works under the supervision of an ophthalmologist. She may work in a private office or in a hospital setting.

Education

Certification as an ophthalmic assistant requires a high school diploma or equivalency, followed by a clinical program approved by the Joint Review Committee for Ophthalmic Medical Personnel (JRCOMP). After completing the program, the student must pass an examination that tests seven basic content areas: history taking, basic skills and lensometry, patient services, basic tonometry, instrument maintenance, general medical knowledge, and special studies. She must also provide a current CPR card (such as those issued by the Red Cross or the American Heart Association) and an endorsement from her supervising ophthalmologist. After passing the examination, the student gains the title of Certified Ophthalmic Assistant (COA). Certification must be renewed every 3 years.

Where to Go for More Information

American Academy of Ophthalmology
655 Beach Street
San Francisco, CA 94109
(415) 561-8500

Association of Technical Personnel in Ophthalmology
c/o Norma Garber
50 Lee Road
Chestnut Hill, MA 02167
(617) 232-4433

Joint Commission on Allied Health Personnel in Ophthalmology
2025 Woodlane Drive
St. Paul, MN 55125-2995
(800) 284-3937

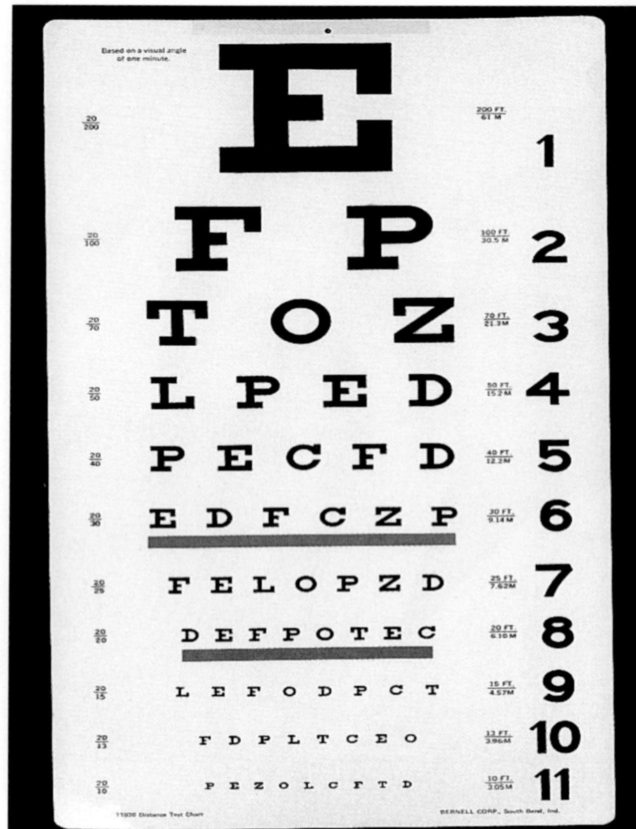

Figure 26-2. The Snellen letter chart is used to test the ability to see objects that are relatively far away.

Distance Vision. To test the distance vision of adults, the Snellen letter chart (Figure 26-2) is commonly used. This chart has several rows of letters of the alphabet. Within each row, letter size is the same, but from row to row, letter size decreases from top to bottom. Patients are asked to read the letters from larger to smaller. A chart such as the Snellen E chart (Figure 26-3a), the Landolt C chart (similar to Snellen E, using the letter C), or a pictorial chart (Figure 26-3b) is used for children and adults who do not know the alphabet.

When distance vision is tested, normal vision is referred to as 20/20. This number means that at the standard testing distance of 20 ft (first number), a patient can see what a person with normal vision can see at 20 ft (second number). A patient who has 20/80 vision can see at 20 ft what a person with normal vision sees at 80 ft. The first number (20) always stays the same because a patient always stands 20 ft away from the chart. The second number, however, changes with a patient's visual acuity. If a patient misses only one or two letters on a line during vision testing, record the results with a minus sign. For example, one letter missed with the right eye would be O.D. 20/30 –1. Two letters would be O.D. 20/30 –2.

Near Vision. To test for near vision, special handheld charts are used. These cards contain letters, numbers, or paragraphs in various sizes of print (Figures 26-4 and 26-5). They may be held and read at a normal reading distance or mounted in a plastic and metal frame and read through optical lenses.

Contrast Sensitivity. To test for the ability to distinguish shades of gray (contrast sensitivity), the Pelli-Robson contrast sensitivity chart, the Vistech Consultants vision contrast test system (Figure 26-6), or another testing system is used. Newer systems use special equipment to provide contrast variations in a projected image. These tests can detect cataracts or problems of the retina even before the sharpness of the patient's vision is impaired.

Color Vision. To test color vision, illustrations such as those of the Ishihara color system or the Richmond pseudoisochromatic color test (Figure 26-7) are used. These illustrations contain numbers or symbols made up of colored dots that appear among other colored dots. The patient is asked to identify what he sees. A patient who is color-blind will not be able to report seeing the numbers or symbols. Color blindness may be inherited; it occurs more commonly in males. Changes in one's ability to see colors, however, may indicate a disease of the retina or optic nerve. For details on how to perform color vision and other vision tests, see Procedure 26-1.

Special Considerations. Certain patients may need special attention when having vision tests. For example, children may be uncooperative or unable to follow directions. To encourage cooperation, show a child the chart you will be using before you begin the test. Point to the symbols and read them aloud once so the child knows the proper term for each symbol. Most physicians use pictorial charts when they start screening a child's vision at the 4-year or 5-year checkup. You can provide assistance during the test by guiding the child through each step in the procedure or by covering the child's eye. Watch the child closely for signs that she is having difficulty seeing the chart. Examples of signs include straining, blinking or watering of the eyes, and puckering of the face.

If a child has difficulty following directions, enlist the parent's or guardian's help. He may be able to explain or interpret information for the child more effectively than you can. Ask the parent if he has ever observed signs of vision problems in his child. For example, does the child rub her eyes frequently, blink a great deal, or hold books very close to her face? Be sure to note the answers in the child's chart so the physician is aware of them.

A patient with Alzheimer's disease may also require special attention during a vision test. Before the test encourage a family member to stay with the patient so he is more comfortable. During the test use simple language to explain the procedure and demonstrate whenever possible. Proceed through the examination slowly, one step at a time. Because the patient's memory and language skills may be impaired, you may need to repeat directions many times and help him name a particular object. If he appears to have trouble with one part of the examination,

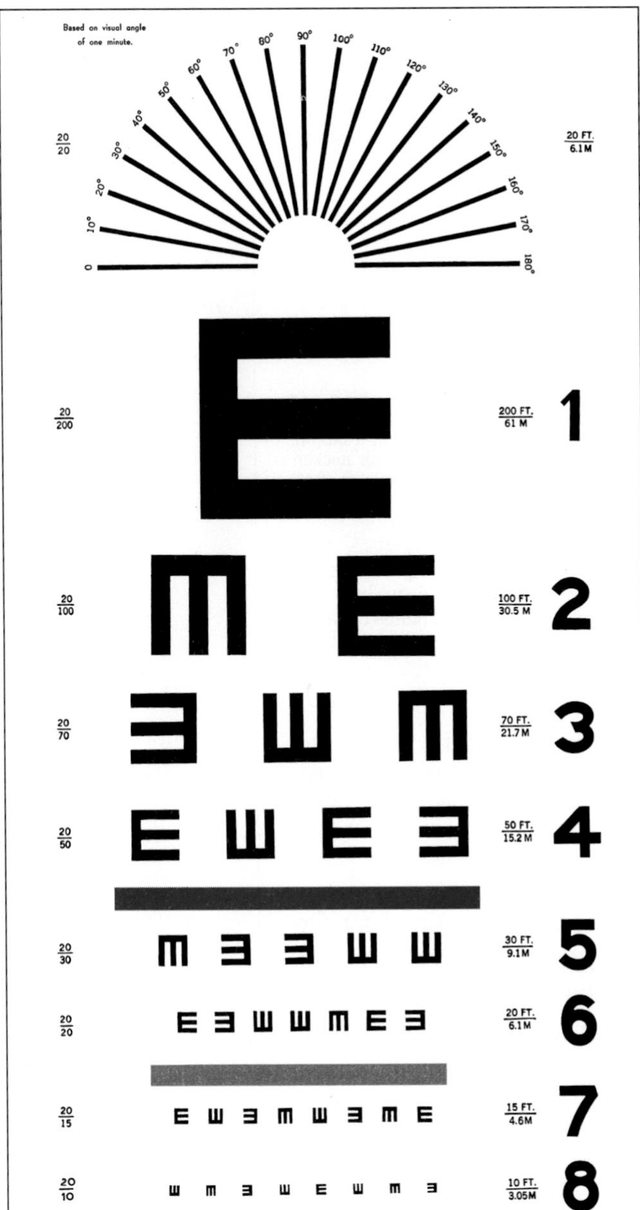

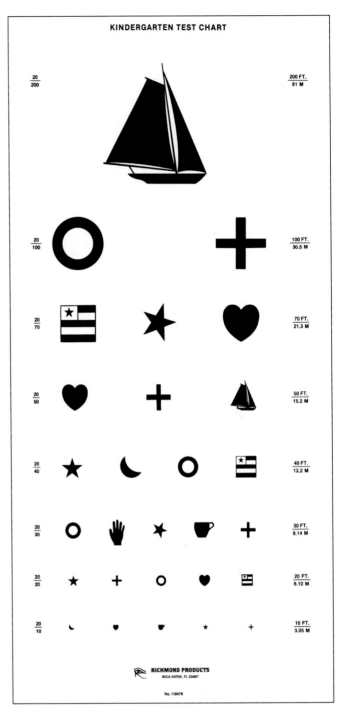

Figure 26-3. The Snellen E eye chart (above) or a pictorial (right) eye chart is used to test the vision of children and nonreading adults. (Richmond International, Inc., Boca Raton, Florida.)

proceed to another part and return later to the part that was difficult for him.

Treating Eye Problems

Some common eye problems include conjunctivitis (inflammation of the conjunctiva), blepharitis (inflammation of the eyelid), and corneal abrasions (scratching of the cornea). The eye is an extremely delicate organ. Even what seems to be a minor injury or infection can have lasting consequences. Therefore, you must use the greatest caution as well as proper techniques when treating a patient's eyes. You should also provide patients with information on how to routinely care for their eyes. See "Educating the Patient" for specific guidelines to follow when presenting preventive eye-care information.

Administration of Medications to the Eye

Your responsibilities as a medical assistant include dispensing medications and explaining their use. Some medications are used to diagnose conditions, whereas

V = .50 D.

The fourteenth of August was the day fixed upon for the sailing of the brig Pilgrim, on her voyage from Boston round Cape Horn, to the western coast of North America. As she was to get under way early in the afternoon, I made my appearance on board at twelve o'clock in full sea-rig, and with my chest, containing an outfit for a two or three years voyage, which I had undertaken from a determination to cure, if possible, by an entire change of life, and by a long absence from books and study, a weakness of the eyes which had obliged me to give up my pursuits, and which no medical aid seemed likely to cure. The change from the tight dress coat, silk cap and kid gloves of an undergraduate at Cambridge, to the

V = .75 D.

loose duck trousers, checked shirt and tarpaulin hat of a sailor, though somewhat of a transformation, was soon made, and I supposed that I should pass very well for a Jack tar. But it is impossible to deceive the practiced eye in these matters; and while I supposed myself to be looking as salt as Neptune himself, I was, no doubt, known for a landsman by every one on board, as soon as I hove in sight. A sailor has a peculiar cut to his clothes, and a way of wear-

V = 1. D.

ing them which a green hand can never get. The trousers, tight around the hips, and thence hanging long and loose around the feet, a superabundance of checked shirt, a low-crowned, well-varnished black hat, worn on the back of the head, with half a fathom of black ribbon hanging over the left eye, and a peculiar tie to the black silk neckerchief, with sundry other *details,* are signs the want of which betray the beginner at once.

V = 1.25 D.

Beside the points in my dress which were out of the way, doubtless my complexion and hands would distinguish me from the regular *salt,* who, with a sun-browned cheek, wide step and rolling gait, swings his bronzed and toughened hands athwartships half open, as though just to ready to grasp a rope. "With all my imperfections

V = 1.50 D.

on my head," I joined the crew, and we hauled out into the stream and came to anchor for the night. The next day we were employed in preparation for sea, reeving and studding-sail gear, crossing royal yards, putting on chafing gear, and taking on board our powder. On the

V = 1.75 D.

following night I stood my first watch. I remained awake nearly all the first part of the night, from fear that I might not hear when I was called; and when I went on deck, so great were my ideas of the importance of my trust, that I

V = 2. D.

walked regularly fore and aft the whole length of the vessel, looking out over the bows and taffrail at each turn, and was not a little surprised at the unconcerned manner in which the billows turned up their

Your glasses are of value to you only as they accurately interpret your prescription and this only as they are fitted and serviced in accordance with these needs. They are a therapeutic device.

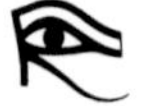

RICHMOND PRODUCTS
BOCA RATON, FL 33487

No. 11974 R

Figure 26-4. This near-vision chart is used to test the ability to see objects at a normal reading distance. (Richmond International, Inc.)

others are used to treat conditions. Only medications for ophthalmic use should be used in the eye. You should teach patients to check medication labels carefully before administering them at home. *Optic* medications for use in the eye could easily be confused with *otic* medications for the ear. Medications other than optic medications may be too concentrated or may contain substances that will injure sensitive eye tissue.

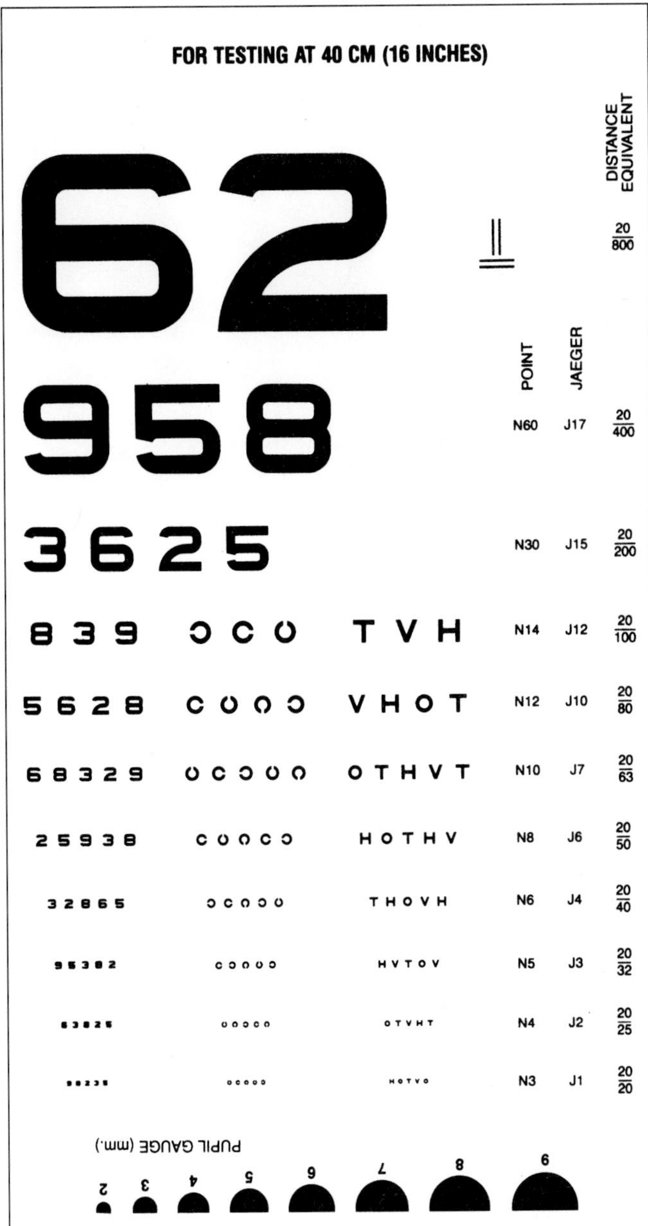

Figure 26-5. The Richmond pocket vision screener is also used to test the ability to see close objects. (Richmond International, Inc.)

If you administer eye medications as part of your job, avoid touching a dropper or ointment tube tip to the eye. Such touching can injure the eye, cause an infection, and contaminate the medication. Procedure 26-2 describes the proper technique for administering eye medications.

Eye Irrigation

When foreign materials enter the eye, they must be flushed out. Flushing (or irrigation) should be done with a sterile solution especially formulated for this purpose. Someone's eye may also need to be irrigated to relieve discomfort from irritating substances, such as smog, pollen, chemicals, or chlorinated water. The steps involved in irrigating the eye are outlined in Procedure 26-3.

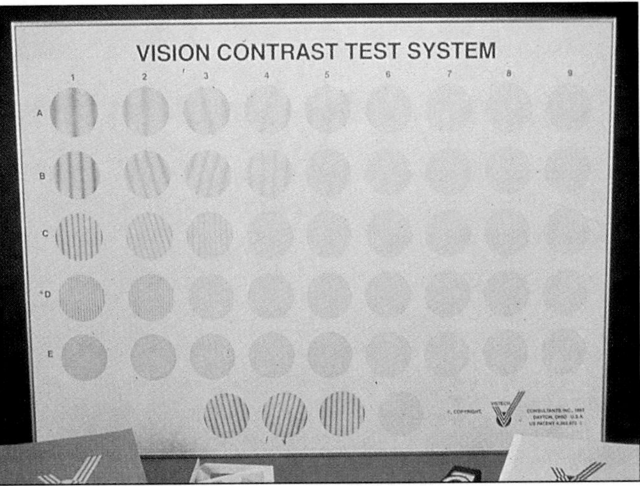

Figure 26-6. The Vistech Consultants vision contrast test system is used to test the ability to differentiate various shades of gray.

Vision Aids

Vision screening tests may indicate that a patient has a vision problem. Common refractive disorders, such as myopia, hyperopia, presbyopia, and astigmatism, are discussed in detail in Chapter 28. Most of these vision problems are corrected with eyeglasses or contact lenses.

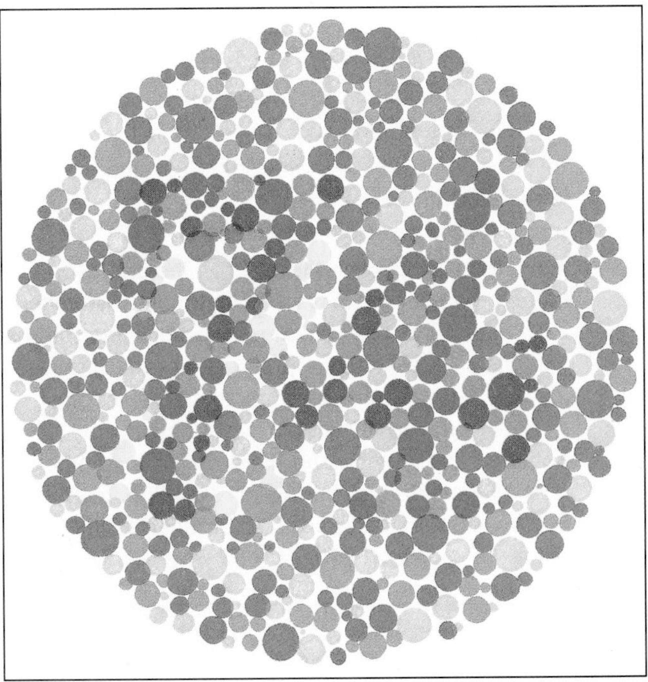

Figure 26-7. The Richmond pseudoisochromatic color chart is used to test a person's ability to see colors. (Richmond International, Inc.)

PROCEDURE 26-1

Performing Vision Screening Tests

Objectives: To screen a patient's ability to see distant or close objects, to determine contrast sensitivity, or to detect color blindness

OSHA Guidelines

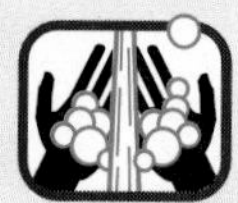  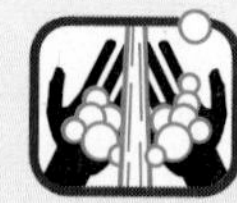

Materials: Occluder or card, alcohol, gauze squares, appropriate vision charts to test for distance vision, near vision, contrast sensitivity, and color blindness

Method

Distance Vision

1. Wash your hands, identify the patient, introduce yourself, and explain the procedure.
2. Mount one of the following eye charts at eye level: Snellen letter or similar chart (for patients who can read); Snellen E, Landolt C, pictorial, or similar chart (for patients who cannot read). If using the Snellen letter chart, verify that the patient knows the letters of the alphabet. With children or nonreading adults, use demonstration cards to verify that they can identify the pictures or direction of the letters.
3. Make a mark on the floor 20 ft away from the chart.
4. Have the patient stand with the heels at the 20-ft mark or sit with the back of the chair at the mark.
5. Instruct the patient to keep both eyes open and not to squint or lean forward during the test.
6. Test both eyes first, then the right eye, and then the left eye. (Different offices may test in a different order. Follow your office policy.)
7. Have the patient read the lines on the chart (or identify the picture/direction), beginning with the 20-ft line. If the patient cannot read this line, begin with the smallest line the patient can read (Figure 26-8). (Some offices use a pointer to select one symbol at a time in random order to prevent patients from memorizing the order. It is common to start with children at the 40- or 30-ft line, or larger if low vision is suspected, and proceed to the 20-ft line.)

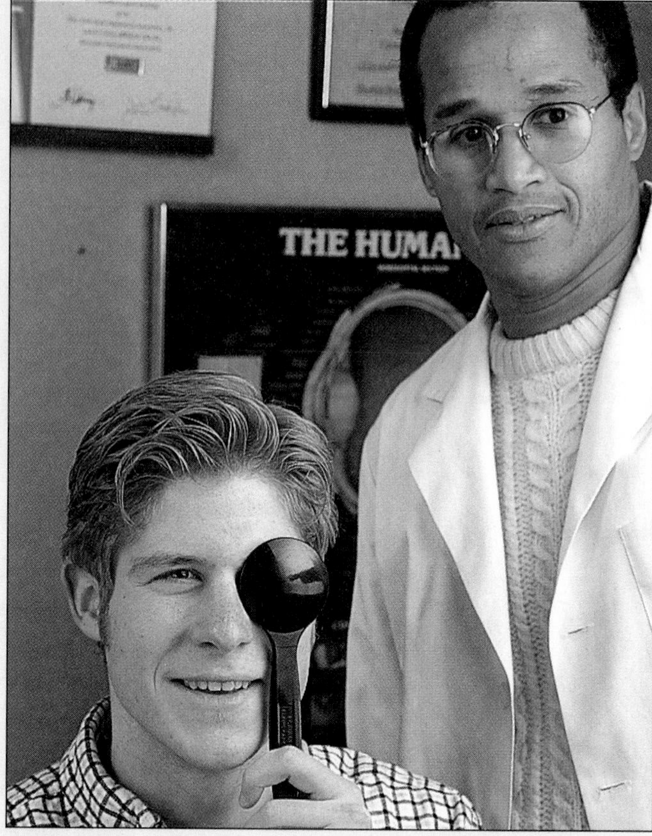

Figure 26-8. Have the patient cover the left eye with the occluder. The patient should keep both eyes open and not squint.

8. Note the smallest line the patient can read or identify. (When testing children, note the smallest line on which they can identify three out of four or four out of six symbols correctly.)
9. Record the results as a fraction (for example, O.U. 20/40 –1 if the patient misses one letter on a line or O.U. 20/40 –2 if the patient misses two letters on a line).
10. Show the patient how to cover the left eye with the occluder or card. Again instruct the patient to keep both eyes open and not to squint or lean forward during the test.
11. Have the patient read the lines on the chart.

These corrective aids are usually prescribed by an ophthalmologist or an **optometrist** (a trained and licensed vision specialist who is not a physician). You may be asked to provide patients who have vision problems with information on eye-care and vision specialists or to make appointments for them.

Hearing

The ability to hear depends on the normal functioning of a number of structures in the ear. It also depends on the normal transmission of nerve impulses from the ear to the brain.

12. Record the results of the right eye (for example, O.D. 20/30).
13. Have the patient cover the right eye and read the lines on the chart.
14. Record the results of the left eye (for example, O.S. 20/20).
15. If the patient wears corrective lenses, record the results using $\overline{cc}$ (if your office uses this abbreviation for "with correction") in front of the abbreviation (for example, $\overline{cc}$ O.U. 20/20).
16. Note and record any observations of squinting, head tilting, or excessive blinking or tearing.
17. Ask the patient to keep both eyes open and to identify the two colored bars, and record the results in the patient's chart.
18. Clean the occluder with a gauze square dampened with alcohol.
19. Properly dispose of the gauze square and wash your hands.

Near Vision

1. Wash your hands, identify the patient, introduce yourself, and explain the procedure.
2. Have the patient hold one of the following at normal reading distance (approximately 14 to 16 inches): Jaeger, Richmond pocket, or similar chart or card.
3. Ask the patient to keep both eyes open and to read or identify the letters, symbols, or paragraphs.
4. Record the smallest line read without error.
5. If the card is laminated, clean it with a gauze square dampened with alcohol.
6. Properly dispose of the gauze square and wash your hands.

Contrast Sensitivity

1. Wash your hands, identify the patient, introduce yourself, and explain the procedure.
2. Mount a contrast sensitivity chart at eye level. (The following steps apply to use of the Vistech Consultants vision contrast test system. The procedures for using other contrast sensitivity charts vary slightly.)
3. Make a mark on the floor 10 ft from the chart.
4. Have the patient stand with the heels at the mark or sit with the back of the chair at the mark.
5. Test both eyes first.
6. Beginning with circle A1, have the patient identify the direction of the stripes in each circle in row A—left, right, up and down, or blank.
7. In column A on the answer grid that accompanies the chart, mark the point for the last circle for which the patient can correctly identify the direction of the stripes. (If the point falls within the shaded area, the patient's vision is within the normal range.)
8. Repeat steps 6 and 7 for rows B through E.
9. Have the patient cover his left eye with an occluder or card, and repeat steps 6 through 8 for the right eye.
10. Have the patient cover his right eye, and repeat steps 6 though 8 for the left eye.
11. Clean the occluder or card with a gauze square dipped in alcohol.
12. Properly dispose of the used gauze square and wash your hands.

Color Vision

1. Wash your hands, identify the patient, introduce yourself, and explain the procedure.
2. Hold one of the following color charts or books at the patient's normal reading distance (approximately 14 to 16 inches): Ishihara, Richmond pseudoisochromatic, or similar color-testing system.
3. Ask the patient to tell you the number or symbol within the colored dots on each chart or page.
4. Proceed through all the charts or pages.
5. Record the number correctly identified and failed with a slash between them (for example, 13 passed/1 failed).
6. If the charts are laminated, clean them with a gauze square dampened with alcohol.
7. Properly dispose of the gauze square and wash your hands.

The Ear

The ear is the organ that enables people to hear. It also helps people maintain balance. As shown in Figure 26-13, the ear is divided into three parts:

- External ear
- Middle ear
- Inner ear

The External Ear. The external, or outer, ear is made up of the outer part of the ear, or **auricle,** and the ear canal. The auricle is made of cartilage and is covered

EDUCATING THE PATIENT

Preventive Eye-Care Tips

You can help patients take care of their eyes and protect their vision by providing them with guidelines to follow. Go over each item slowly and carefully. Ask whether the patients have questions before moving on to the next item. Answer all the patients' questions and make sure they understand the answers. Eye-care tips include the following.

1. Get regular health checkups. Patients may not appreciate the connection between their general health and their eyes. Point out that high blood pressure and diabetes can cause eye problems.
2. Get regular eye examinations. Most people need eye examinations every 1 to 2 years. Patients with diabetes should see their eye-care specialists more frequently.
3. Be alert for the warning signs of eye disease. Tell patients to call their eye-care specialist immediately if they experience any of these signs:
   - Eye pain
   - Loss of vision
   - Double or blurred vision
   - Headache with blurred vision
   - Redness of the eye or eyelid
   - A gritty or sticky feeling around the eye
   - Excessive tearing
   - Difficulty seeing in the dark
   - Flashes of light
   - Halos around lights
   - Sensitivity to light
   - Loss of color perception
4. Wear sunglasses with ultraviolet protection to shield the eyes from bright sunlight, even in the winter. Recommend that patients ask to have ultraviolet protection added when purchasing new distance prescription glasses. Explain to patients that the cornea can get sunburned, which can be painful and damaging. Also tell patients that excessive exposure to the sun is a contributing factor in malignant melanoma of the eye—a dangerous type of skin cancer that may spread through the bloodstream or lymphatic system.
5. Wear protective eye equipment to prevent eye injury. Indicate to patients that they should wear protective eyewear every time they participate in sports, work with chemicals, or encounter a situation in which they may be exposed to flying debris.
6. Use nonprescription eye medications properly. Show patients how to use eyedrops; emphasize that the tip of the dropper should never touch the eye. Explain to patients that medications should be used only as indicated on the label and discarded after the condition has cleared up.

with skin. The ear canal is lined with skin that contains hairs and glands that produce **cerumen,** a waxlike substance also called earwax. The eardrum, or **tympanic membrane,** is a fibrous partition located at the inner end of the canal. The eardrum separates the external ear from the middle ear.

The Middle Ear. The middle ear is a small, air-filled cavity between the eardrum and the inner ear. It contains three small bones: the hammer, the anvil, and the stirrup. The **malleus,** or hammer, is attached to the eardrum, and the **stapes,** or stirrup, is attached to the inner ear. The **incus,** or anvil, lies between them. An opening in the middle ear, the **eustachian tube,** leads to the back of the throat. The eustachian tube helps equalize air pressure on both sides of the eardrum.

The Inner Ear. The inner ear, or **labyrinth,** contains a number of important structures. Among these are the **cochlea,** a spiral-shaped canal that contains the hearing receptors, and three **semicircular canals,** which help a person maintain balance.

The Hearing Process

A sound consists of waves of different frequencies that move through the air. The external ear initiates sound conduction when it collects these waves and channels them to the eardrum. There the waves make the eardrum vibrate. The vibrations, in turn, are amplified by the bones of the middle ear. The amplified waves enter the inner ear and the cochlea. These waves cause tiny hairs that line the cochlea to bend. Movements of the hairs trigger nerve impulses. The impulses are transmitted by the auditory nerve to the brain, where they are perceived as sound.

Sound waves are also conducted through the bones of the skull directly to the inner ear, a process called **bone conduction.** This alternative pathway for sound bypasses the external and middle ears. When you hear your own voice, the sound has reached your inner ear mainly through bone conduction. By comparing a person's ability to sense sounds by bone conduction and through the entire ear, doctors can often identify what part of the ear is causing a hearing problem. For

PROCEDURE 26-2

Administering Eye Medications

Objective: To instill medication into the eye for treatment of certain eye disorders

OSHA Guidelines

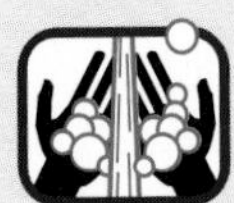
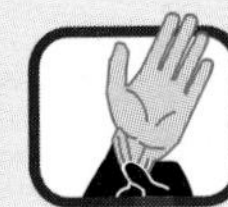

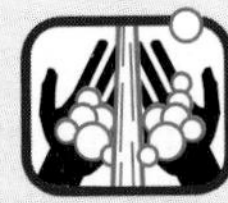

Materials: Medication (drops, cream, or ointment), tissues, eye patch (if applicable)

Method

1. Identify the patient, introduce yourself, and explain the procedure.
2. Review the doctor's medication order. This should include the patient's name, drug name, concentration, number of drops (if a liquid), into which eye(s) the medication is to be administered, and the frequency of administration.

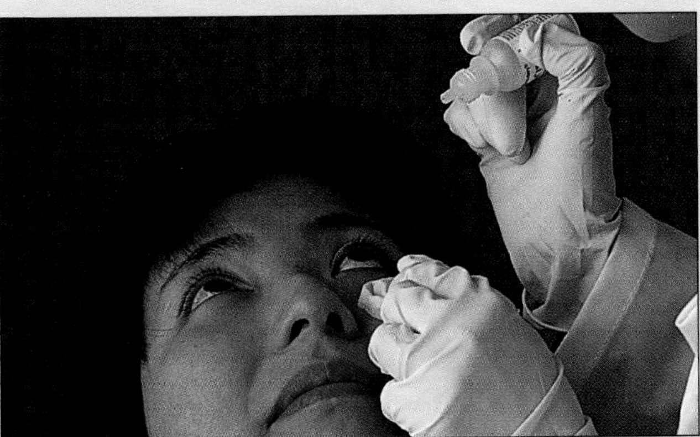

Figure 26-9. Use a tissue to press down on the patient's cheekbone just below the eyelid, opening up a pocket of space between the eyelid and the eye.

3. Compare the drug with the medication order three times.
4. Ask whether the patient has any known allergies to eye medications.
5. Wash your hands and put on gloves.
6. Assemble supplies.
7. Ask the patient to lie down or to sit back in a chair with the head tilted back.
8. Give the patient a tissue to blot excess medication as needed.
9. Remove an eye patch, if present.
10. Ask the patient to look at the ceiling. Instruct the patient to keep both eyes open during the procedure.
11. With a tissue, gently pull the lower eyelid down by pressing downward on the patient's cheekbone just below the eyelid with your nondominant hand. This pressure will open a pocket of space between the eyelid and the eye (Figure 26-9).

Eyedrops

12. Resting your dominant hand on the patient's forehead, hold the filled eyedropper or bottle approximately ½ inch from the conjunctiva (Figure 26-10).
13. Drop the prescribed number of drops into the pocket. If any drops land outside the eye, repeat instilling the drops that missed the eye.

Creams or Ointments

12. Rest your dominant hand on the patient's forehead, and hold the tube or applicator above the conjunctiva.
13. Evenly apply a thin ribbon of cream or ointment along the inside edge of the lower eyelid on the conjunctiva, working from the medial (inner) to the lateral (outer) side (Figure 26-11).

All Medications

14. Release the lower lid and instruct the patient to gently close the eyes.
15. Repeat the procedure for the other eye as necessary.
16. Remove any excess medication by wiping each eyelid gently with a fresh tissue from the medial to the lateral side (Figure 26-12).

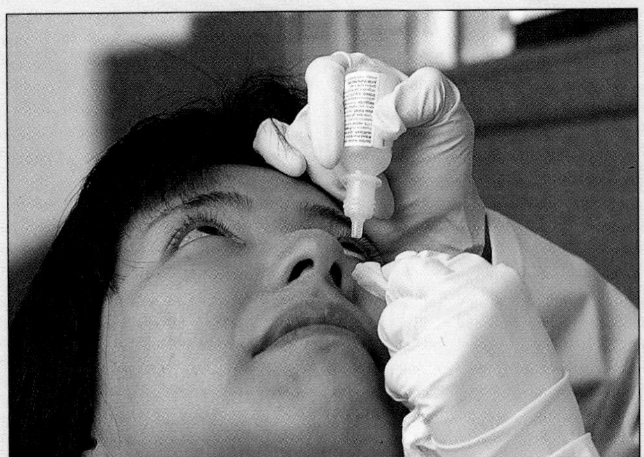

Figure 26-10. The bottle should be approximately ½ inch from the conjunctiva as you prepare to instill drops in the patient's eye.

continued

Administering Eye Medications

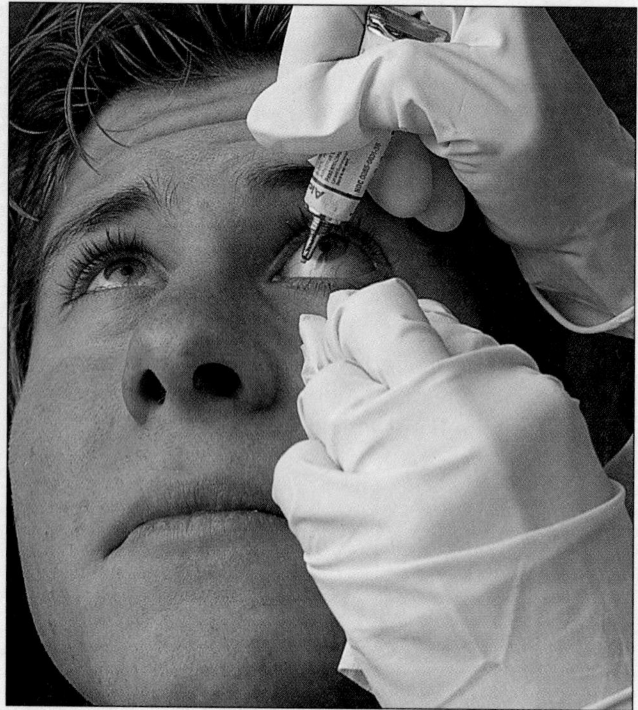

Figure 26-11. Apply a thin ribbon of cream or ointment along the inside of the lower eyelid on the conjunctiva.

17. Apply a clean eye patch to cover the entire eye as necessary.
18. Ask whether the patient felt any discomfort, and observe for any adverse reactions. Notify the doctor as necessary.
19. Instruct the patient on self-administration of medication and patch application as necessary.
20. Ask the patient to repeat the instructions.
21. Provide written instructions.
22. Properly dispose of used disposable materials.
23. Remove gloves and wash your hands.
24. Document administration in the patient's chart. Include the drug, concentration, number of drops, time of administration, and which eye(s) received the medication.

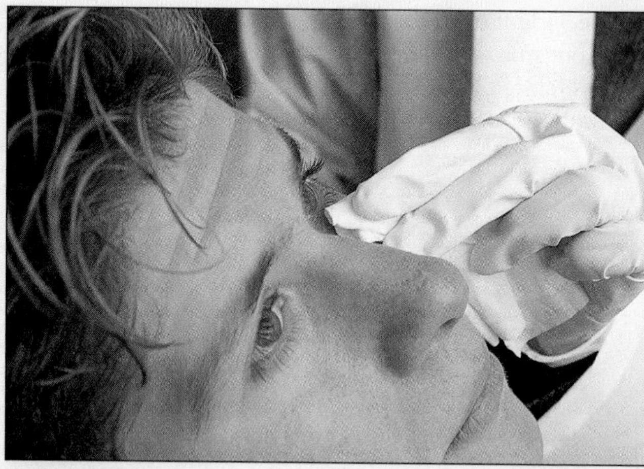

Figure 26-12. Use a tissue to remove excess medication from the eyelid.

example, if bone conduction is normal, a hearing problem likely involves the middle or external ear rather than the inner ear.

The Ear and Balance

The brain constantly monitors the position of one's body on the basis of information it receives from the semicircular canals, eyes, and muscles. Each canal is at a right angle to the other two. In other words, each is oriented in a different dimension or plane: height, depth, and width. Together they detect any change in the position of the body. Such information is passed on to the brain along with data from the eyes and muscles. The brain then uses the information to maintain balance.

The Aging Ear

As a person grows older, a number of changes occur in the ear. The external ear appears larger because of continued growth of cartilage and the loss of skin elasticity. The ear lobe gets longer and may have a wrinkled appearance. The glands that produce cerumen become less efficient, producing earwax that is much drier. The ear canal also becomes narrower.

In the middle ear, changes in the eardrum cause it to shrink and appear dull and gray. The joints between the bones of the middle ear degenerate, so they do not move as freely. In the inner ear, the semicircular canals become less sensitive to changes in position, and this reduced sensitivity affects balance.

PROCEDURE 26-3

Performing Eye Irrigation

Objective: To flush the eye to remove foreign particles or relieve eye irritation

OSHA Guidelines

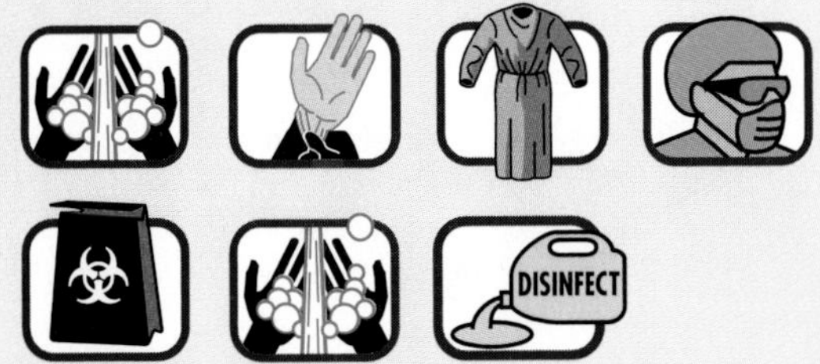

Materials: Sterile irrigating solution, sterile basin, sterile irrigating syringe and kidney-shaped basin, tissues

Method

1. Identify the patient, introduce yourself, and explain the procedure.
2. Review the physician's order. This should include the patient's name, irrigating solution, volume of solution, and for which eye(s) the irrigation is to be performed.
3. Compare the solution with the instructions three times.
4. Wash your hands and put on gloves, a gown, and a face shield (splashing is possible when a syringe is used).
5. Assemble supplies.
6. Ask the patient to lie down or to sit with the head tilted back and to the side that is being irrigated. The solution should not spill over into the other eye.
7. Place a towel over the patient's shoulder (or under the head and shoulder, if the patient is lying down). Have the patient hold the kidney-shaped basin at the side of the head next to the eye to be irrigated.
8. Pour the solution into the sterile basin.
9. Fill the irrigating syringe with solution (approximately 50 mL).
10. Hold a tissue on the patient's cheekbone below the lower eyelid with your nondominant hand, and press downward to expose the eye socket.
11. Holding the tip of the syringe ½ inch away from the eye, direct the solution onto the lower conjunctiva from the inner to the outer aspect of the eye. (Avoid directing the solution against the cornea because it is sensitive; do not use excessive force.)
12. Refill the syringe and continue irrigation until the prescribed volume of solution is used or until the solution is used up.
13. Dry the area around the eye with tissues.
14. Properly dispose of used disposable materials.
15. Remove gloves, gown, and face shield, and wash your hands.
16. Record the procedure, the amount of solution used, time of administration, and eye(s) irrigated in the patient's chart.
17. Put on gloves and clean the equipment and room according to OSHA guidelines.

Problems with equilibrium make the elderly prone to falls. Some ear disorders are also more common in older individuals.

Hearing Loss

Hearing loss is actually a symptom of a disease, not a disease in itself. Contrary to what most people believe, hearing loss is not a normal part of the aging process and should always be evaluated for proper treatment.

Types of Hearing Loss

There are two types of hearing loss, conductive and sensorineural. The two types differ in the point at which the hearing process is interrupted.

A conductive hearing loss is caused by an interruption in the transmission of sound waves to the inner ear. Conditions that can cause conductive hearing loss include obstruction of the ear canal, infection of the middle ear, and reduced movement of the stirrup.

A sensorineural hearing loss occurs when there is damage to the inner ear, to the nerve that leads from the ear to the brain, or to the brain itself. In this kind of loss, sound waves reach the inner ear, but the brain does not perceive them as sound. This type of hearing loss can be hereditary, can be caused by loud noises or viral infections, or can occur as a side effect of medications.

Sensorineural hearing loss can be differentiated from conductive hearing loss by hearing tests. It is possible for both types of hearing loss to occur together.

Noise Pollution

Prolonged exposure to loud noises is a common cause of hearing loss because of damage to the sensitive cells in the cochlea. People who work around noisy equipment, including construction workers, aircraft personnel, and machine operators, are likely to suffer from this type of

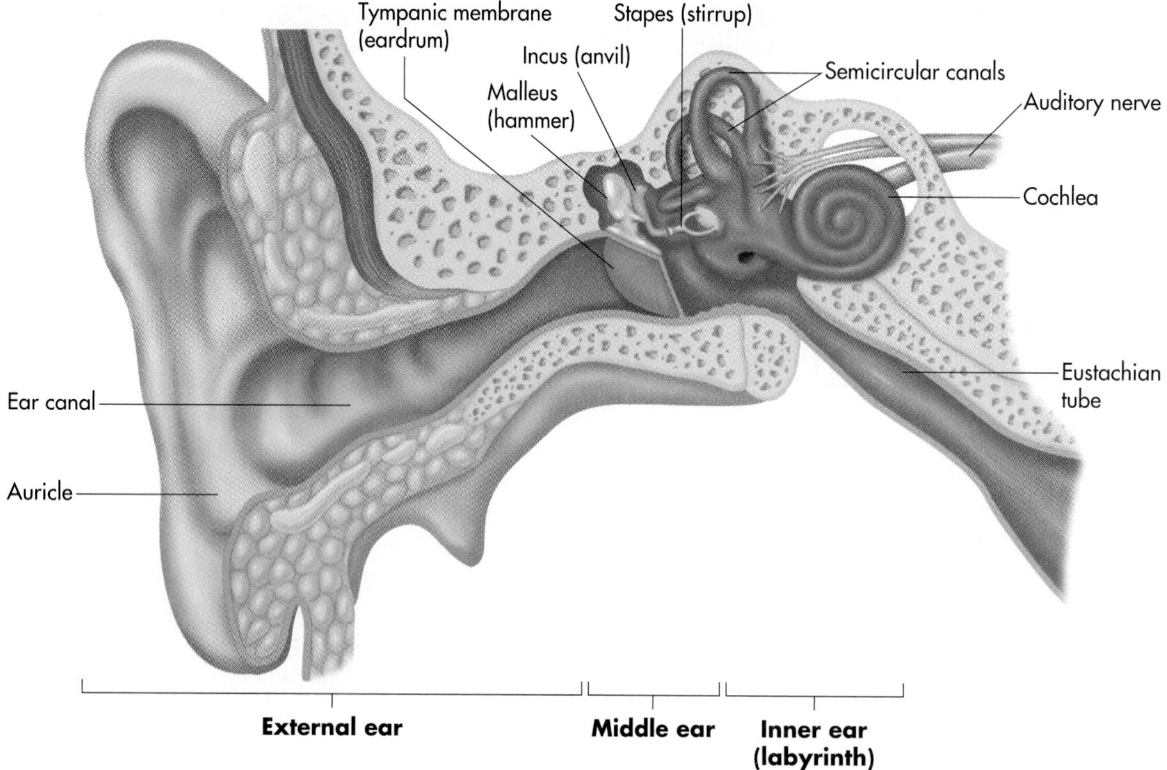

Figure 26-13. The ear is composed of a number of structures that work in harmony to produce hearing and a sense of balance.

hearing loss unless they protect their ears (see Figure 26-14). Repeatedly listening to loud music from a personal stereo set at too high a volume can also damage the ears.

Working With Patients With a Hearing Impairment

You may come in contact with patients of all ages who have hearing impairments. Many patients wear hearing aids to amplify normal speech. Some patients, however, may not admit they have a problem—out of fear, vanity, or misinformation. It is estimated that one-third of patients between the ages of 65 and 74 and one-half of those between the ages of 75 and 79 suffer from some loss of hearing.

To improve communication with a patient whose hearing is impaired, you can do the following:

1. Speak at a reasonable volume. Do not shout. Shouting can actually make your words harder to understand. A hearing aid filters out loud sounds, so the patient may not hear everything you say if you shout.
2. Speak in clear, low-pitched tones. Elderly patients lose the ability to hear high-pitched sounds first.
3. Avoid speaking directly into the patient's ear. Stand 3 to 6 ft away, and face the patient so she can see your lip movements and facial expressions. Avoid covering your mouth with your hands. Speak at a normal rate.
4. Avoid overemphasizing your lip movements, which makes lipreading difficult.

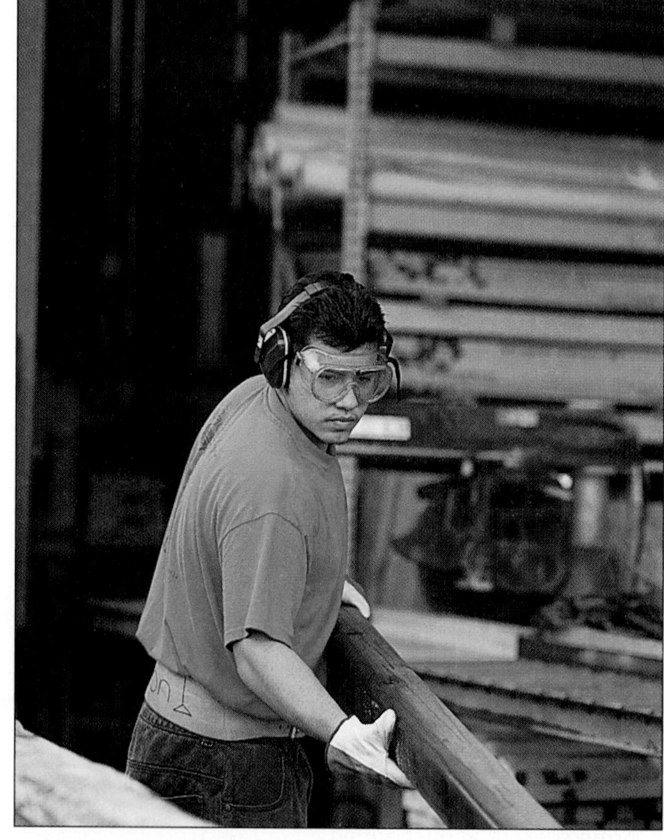

Figure 26-14. Loud noises, such as those produced by a jet engine, can damage hearing unless appropriate ear protectors are worn.

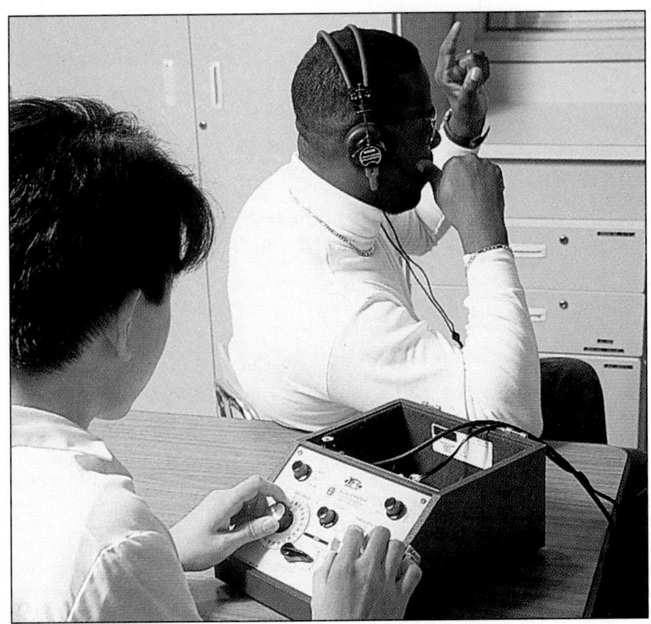

Figure 26-15. An audiometer is used to test hearing.

5. Avoid hand gestures unless they are appropriate.
6. If the patient does not understand what you say, restate the message in short, simple sentences. Have the patient repeat the message to verify that your words were understood.
7. Treat patients who have a hearing impairment with patience and respect.

Hearing and Diagnostic Tests

Various tests are performed to find out whether a person hears normally. If the tests reveal a problem, follow-up tests are performed to determine the cause of the problem.

Hearing Tests

As part of a general examination, physicians may perform a simple hearing test with one or more tuning forks. Physicians use the tuning forks to determine whether there is a hearing loss. Tuning forks can also be helpful in differentiating conductive from sensorineural hearing loss.

If you have the necessary training, you may help perform a test that uses an audiometer, as shown in Figure 26-15. An **audiometer** is an electronic device that measures hearing acuity by producing sounds in specific frequencies and intensities. A **frequency** is the number of complete fluctuations of energy per second in the form of waves. The audiometer allows a physician or other health practitioner to test a person's hearing and to determine the nature and extent of a person's hearing loss.

Many types of audiometers are available. Some machines automatically generate the various tones at different **decibels** (units for measuring the relative intensity of sounds on a scale from 0 to 130) and print out the patient's responses. Others must be manually adjusted and the results charted by hand, as shown in Figure 26-16.

During the test the patient wears a headset to hear the sounds produced by the audiometer. Depending on the particular unit, the patient indicates hearing a sound by raising a finger or by pushing a button. In the former case the person administering the test records the response. In the latter case the response may be recorded automatically or by the test giver.

Adults and children who can understand directions and respond appropriately can be screened in this manner. If you work in a pediatrician's office, you may also help check an infant's response to sounds. These tests require special techniques because infants cannot understand directions. The general steps involved in performing hearing tests on different age groups are outlined in Procedure 26-4.

Diagnostic Testing

A diagnostic test called tympanometry measures the eardrum's ability to move and thus gauges pressure in the middle ear. Tympanometry is used to detect diseases and abnormalities of the middle ear.

To perform the test, a small, soft-rubber cuff is placed over the external ear canal, producing an airtight seal. The tympanometer then automatically measures air pressure and prints out a graph of the results.

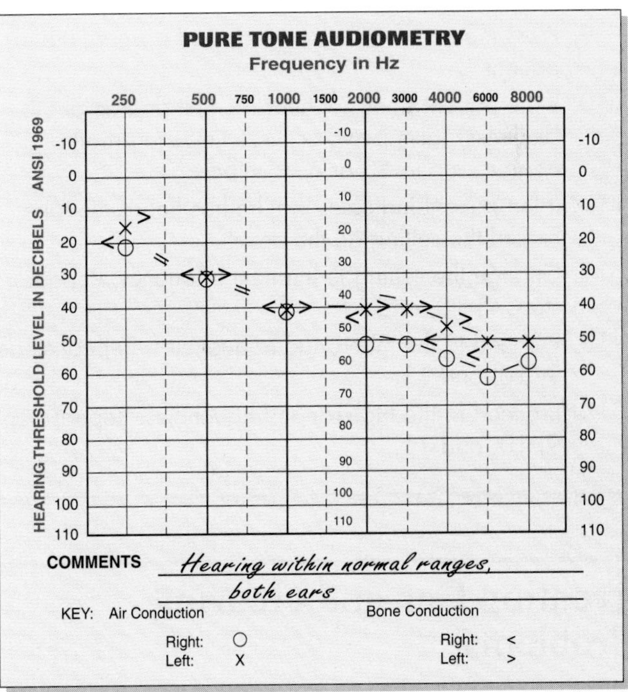

Figure 26-16. The results of an audiometer test are displayed on a graph that indicates the response of each ear to various sounds conducted through air and bone.

PROCEDURE 26-4

Measuring Auditory Acuity

Objective: To determine how well a patient hears

OSHA Guidelines

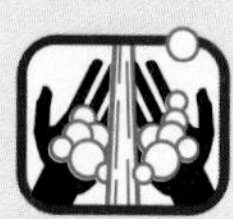 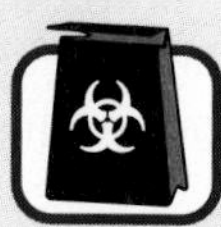 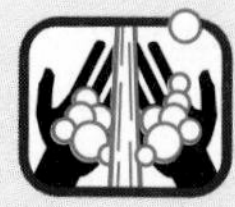

Materials: Audiometer, headset, graph pad (if applicable), alcohol, gauze squares

Method

Adults and Children

1. Wash your hands, identify the patient, introduce yourself, and explain the procedure.
2. Clean the earpieces of the headset with a gauze square dampened with alcohol.
3. Have the patient sit with his back to you.
4. Assist the patient in putting on the headset, and adjust it until it is comfortable.
5. Tell the patient he will hear tones in the right ear.
6. Tell the patient to raise his finger or press the indicator button when he hears a tone.
7. Set the audiometer for the right ear.
8. Set the audiometer for the lowest range of frequencies and the first degree of loudness (usually 15 decibels). (When using automated audiometers, follow the instructions printed in the user's manual.)
9. Press the tone button or switch and observe the patient.
10. If the patient does not hear the first degree of loudness, raise it two or three times to greater degrees, up to 50 or 60 decibels.
11. If the patient indicates that he has heard the tone, record the setting on the graph.
12. Change the setting to the next frequency. Repeat steps 9, 10, and 11.
13. Proceed to the mid-range frequencies. Repeat steps 9, 10, and 11.
14. Proceed to the high-range frequencies. Repeat steps 9, 10, and 11.
15. Set the audiometer for the left ear.
16. Tell the patient that he will hear tones in the left ear, and ask him to indicate when he hears a tone as noted in step 6.
17. Repeat steps 8 through 14.
18. Set the audiometer for both ears.
19. Ask the patient to listen with both ears and to indicate when he hears a tone as noted in step 6.
20. Repeat steps 8 through 14.
21. Have the patient remove the headset.
22. Clean the earpieces with a gauze square dampened with alcohol.
23. Properly dispose of the used gauze square and wash your hands.

Infants and Toddlers

1. Identify the patient and introduce yourself.
2. Wash your hands.
3. Pick a quiet location.
4. The patient can be sitting, lying down, or held by the parent.
5. Instruct the parent to be silent during the procedure.
6. Position yourself so your hands are behind the child's right ear and out of sight.
7. Clap your hands loudly. Observe the child's response. (Never clap directly in front of the ear since this can damage the eardrum. As an alternative to clapping, use special devices, such as rattles or clickers, that may be available in the office to generate sounds of varying loudness.)
8. Record the child's response as positive or negative for loud noise.
9. Position one hand behind the child's right ear, as before.
10. Snap your fingers. Observe the child's response.
11. Record the response as positive or negative for moderate noise.
12. Repeat steps 6 through 11 for the left ear.

Treating Ear and Hearing Problems

Some common ear problems you may encounter in the physician's office include cerumen impaction (a buildup of earwax in the ear canal), rupture of the eardrum, and otitis media (inflammation of the middle ear). Physicians use various approaches and techniques with each problem to restore the health of a patient's ears. For a detailed description of the techniques used for patients with otitis media, see "Diseases and Disorders."

Physicians also employ special techniques and devices to improve patients' hearing and maintain the health of their ears. As a medical assistant, you can provide pa-

DISEASES AND DISORDERS

Otitis Media: The Common Ear Infection

Otitis media, commonly referred to as an ear infection, affects almost all children by age 6. This inflammation of the middle ear accounts for 24.5 million doctor visits each year—second only to upper respiratory infections.

Ear infections typically start when fluid becomes trapped in the middle ear. The lining of the middle ear and eustachian tube is blanketed with a layer of fluid similar to that found in the nose. The normal flow of this fluid from the ear into the back of the nose helps keep the middle ear and the eustachian tube free of bacteria. When a child gets a cold or flu, the lining of the eustachian tube and middle ear can become inflamed and trap the fluid. The child can develop one of the following four types of otitis media.

- Acute otitis media typically refers to a bacterial infection of the middle ear that comes on suddenly. This type is common in children and typically follows an upper respiratory tract infection. The symptoms include pain, a feeling of fullness in the ear, some loss of hearing, and possible fever. In severe cases the eardrum may rupture because of the fluid pressure. Acute infections are usually treated with oral antibiotics. If not treated, this type of otitis media can cause permanent hearing loss.
- Recurrent otitis media is diagnosed when a child contracts acute otitis media again and again, perhaps once or twice every month.
- Otitis media with effusion, also known as OME, involves an accumulation of fluid in the middle ear. Children with OME do not exhibit any symptoms, and they may not experience any discomfort.
- Chronic otitis media is diagnosed when fluid is present in the ear and fails to clear up after 3 months or more. Infection may or may not be present. Without treatment the undrained fluid thickens, resulting in possible changes in the shape of the eardrum. These changes may cause temporary hearing loss. Antibiotics and reconstructive surgery may be used to treat chronic otitis media.

If a child suffers from recurrent or chronic otitis media, myringotomy, or the surgical insertion of tubes, may be recommended to keep the fluid draining continuously. This procedure usually removes enough fluid so the infection clears up. Depending on the type of tube, it falls out on its own within 3 to 18 months of insertion.

Ear infections may be difficult to identify, especially in a young child who cannot talk. The following symptoms may be indications of a possible ear infection, particularly if more than one is present:

- Tugging or rubbing the ear
- Fever ranging from 100° to 104°F
- Difficulty balancing
- Excessive crankiness
- Difficulty hearing or speaking
- An unwillingness to lie down (The pain may become more severe in a reclining position because of increased pressure against the eardrum.)

tients with information on preventive ear-care techniques, as described in "Educating the Patient."

Ear Medications and Irrigation

Part of your job may be to administer ear medications to patients. You may also teach patients how to administer ear medications at home. The proper procedure for administering eardrops is described in Procedure 26-5.

Irrigating the ear may relieve inflammation or irritation of the ear canal and may help loosen and remove impacted cerumen (earwax) or a foreign body. This procedure is performed in the physician's office. The steps used to irrigate the ear are described in Procedure 26-6.

Hearing Aids

Hearing aids may be worn inside or outside the ear. If worn outside, they may be located behind the ear, mounted on eyeglasses, or worn on the body. Hearing aids consist of the following parts:

- A tiny microphone to pick up sounds
- An amplifier to increase the volume of sounds
- A tiny speaker to transmit sounds to the ear

You may need to teach patients how to obtain a hearing aid. You can also pass along tips to patients to help them take proper care of their hearing aids and to troubleshoot problems.

Obtaining a Hearing Aid. A patient with signs of hearing loss should be referred to an **otologist,** a medical doctor specializing in the health of the ear, or an **audiologist,** a specialist who focuses on evaluating and correcting hearing problems. Audiologists are not medical doctors and do not treat diseases of the ear. Instead, they evaluate the patient's hearing, fit hearing aids, give instruction in the use of hearing aids, and provide service for hearing aids if necessary. It is important for hearing aids to fit properly. If they do not, sounds may not be transmitted well into the ear.

EDUCATING THE PATIENT

Preventive Ear-Care Tips

You can help patients protect their ears and take care of their hearing by providing them with guidelines to follow. As with any patient education, go over items slowly, ask patients whether they have questions before moving on, and answer questions completely. Ear-care tips include the following.

1. Get routine hearing examinations. Screening for hearing problems is often part of a comprehensive physical examination. Encourage patients who have not had their hearing screened or who suspect they have hearing problems to arrange for testing by their doctor. Older patients, who may not admit they have a problem, may need special encouragement.
2. Avoid injury when cleaning the ears. Instruct patients in proper ear care. Point out that they should not put objects in the ear that might injure the eardrum or ear canal.
3. Avoid injury from nonprescription ear-care products. Tell patients to check with a doctor before using nonprescription products for softening earwax.
4. Use proper ear protection. Urge patients to wear ear protectors around loud work equipment and to avoid listening to loud music. It is especially important to keep the volume at a reasonable level when listening through earphones.
5. Use all medications properly. Show patients how to use eardrops; emphasize that they must follow instructions precisely. Explain to patients that following instructions applies to all medications because many, including aspirin and some antibiotics, may cause hearing loss if used improperly.
6. Be alert for warning signs. Tell patients to call their doctor immediately if they experience any of these signs of ear problems:
   - Ear pain
   - Stuffiness
   - Discharge from the ear
   - Vertigo (dizziness)

Also have patients notify the doctor if they have any of these signs of hearing problems:

- Tinnitus (ringing)
- Hearing others' speech as mumbled sounds
- Speaking in a very loud voice without being aware of it

Care and Use of Hearing Aids. Hearing aids run on batteries that typically last about 2 weeks. Therefore, the patient must keep a fresh supply of batteries on hand. The hearing aid itself must be routinely cleaned, or the microphone, switches, or dials may not work properly. Moisture can damage the aid, so it must not get wet. Hair sprays can clog hearing aid openings or interfere with the operation of moving parts. For these reasons spray should be applied before a hearing aid is inserted. Cerumen often builds up behind hearing aids that are worn in the ear. Wax buildup reduces sound transmission. If buildup occurs, the earwax plug can be removed by ear irrigation.

Other Devices and Strategies

People whose hearing cannot be substantially improved by hearing aids may need to use other devices or strategies to overcome the problem. These devices include appliances that light up as well as ring, such as telephones, doorbells, smoke detectors, alarm clocks, and burglar alarms. Patients can purchase amplifiers for the telephone, television set, and radio. Many closed-captioned television programs are also available. To benefit from closed captioning, the patient must have a television set with a decoder that translates the captioning and displays the captions on the screen.

Summary

You can help prevent, detect, and treat eye and ear problems in your work as a medical assistant. Because conditions that affect the eyes and ears can have an impact on vision, hearing, and balance, these conditions affect a patient's quality of life. Vision and hearing provide people with information about the world around them; balance allows people to move securely and effectively through their environment.

A basic understanding of the anatomy and physiology of the eyes and ears will help you provide good eye and ear care to patients. You must also become familiar with many health, medication, safety, and hygiene concerns to teach patients to care for their own eyes and ears properly. Take time to comprehend and master the various

PROCEDURE 26-5

Administering Eardrops

Objective: To instill medication into the ear to treat certain ear disorders

OSHA Guidelines

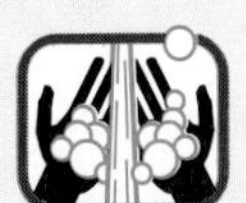
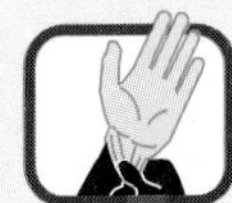
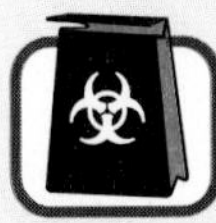
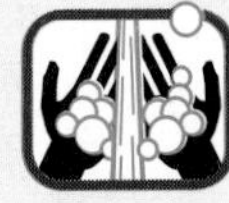

Materials: Liquid medication, cotton balls

Method

1. Identify the patient, introduce yourself, and explain the procedure.
2. Check the physician's medication order. It should include the patient's name, drug name, concentration, number of drops, into which ear(s) the medication is to be administered, and the frequency of administration.
3. Compare the drug with the instructions three times.
4. Ask whether the patient has any allergies to ear medications.
5. Wash your hands and put on gloves.

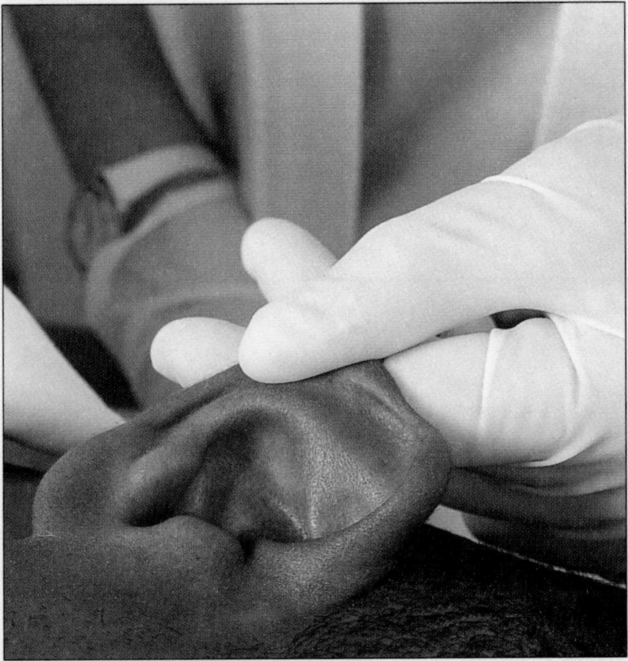

Figure 26-17. Straighten an adult's ear canal by pulling the auricle upward and outward.

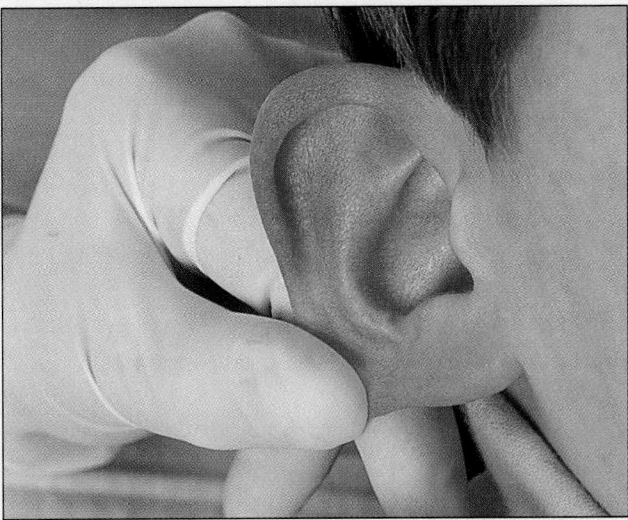

Figure 26-18. Straighten an infant's or a child's ear canal by pulling the auricle downward and back.

6. Assemble supplies.
7. If the medication is cold, warm it to room temperature with your hands or by placing the bottle in a pan of warm water. **Warning:** Internal ear structures are very sensitive to extreme heat or cold. Administration of cold medications can result in vertigo (dizziness) or nausea.
8. Have the patient lie on the side with the ear to be treated facing up.
9. Straighten the ear canal by pulling the auricle upward and outward for adults (Figure 26-17), down and back for infants and children (Figure 26-18).
10. Hold the dropper ½ inch above the ear canal.

continued

PROCEDURE 26-5 continued

Administering Eardrops

11. Gently squeeze the bottle or dropper bulb to administer the correct number of drops (Figure 26-19).
12. Have the patient remain in this position for 10 minutes.
13. If ordered, loosely place a small wad of cotton in the outermost part of the ear canal.
14. Note any adverse reaction, notifying the physician as necessary.
15. Repeat the procedure for the other ear if ordered.
16. Instruct the patient on how to administer the drops at home.
17. Ask the patient to repeat the instructions.
18. Provide written instructions.
19. Remove the cotton after 15 minutes.
20. Properly dispose of used disposable materials.
21. Remove gloves and wash your hands.
22. Record the medication, concentration, number of drops, time of administration, and which ear(s) received the medication in the patient's chart.

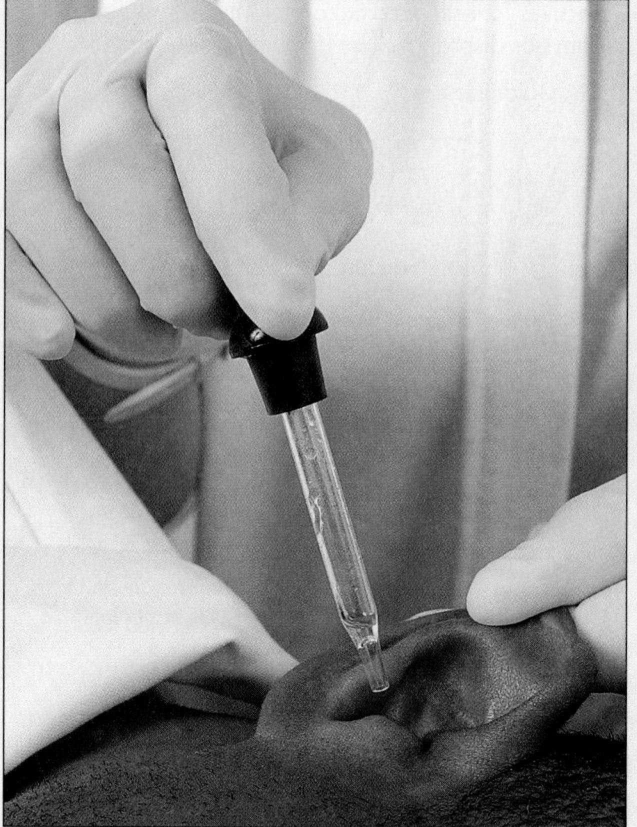

Figure 26-19. Apply slow, gentle pressure to the dropper bulb so you can count the drops and administer the prescribed number.

tests of vision and hearing so you can provide accurate information to the physician about each patient's performance on each test.

Be sensitive to the needs of individual patients as you care for their eyes and ears. Learn all you can about how to meet the special needs of children, elderly patients, and patients with conditions that make preventing, detecting, and treating eye and ear problems a challenge. Practice the administration of eye and ear medications until it becomes second nature to provide the prescribed treatment calmly, accurately, and with the least discomfort to the patient.

The more knowledgeable and proficient you become, the better the eye and ear care you will provide. Knowing just what you are doing and why will make your assistance to the patient and the physician a valuable asset to the office.

PROCEDURE 26-6

Performing Ear Irrigation

Objective: To wash out the ear canal to remove impacted cerumen, relieve inflammation, or remove a foreign body

OSHA Guidelines

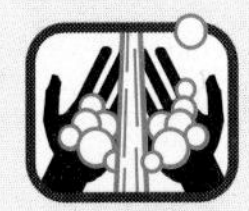
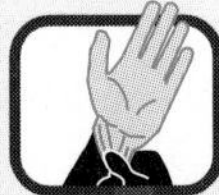
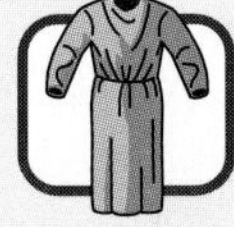

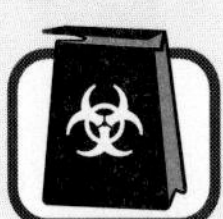
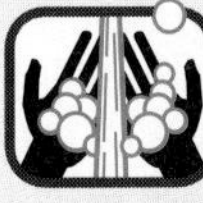
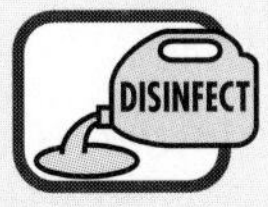

Materials: Fresh irrigating solution, clean basin, clean irrigating syringe, towel or absorbent pad, kidney-shaped basin, cotton balls

Method

1. Identify the patient, introduce yourself, and explain the procedure.
2. Check the doctor's order. It should include the patient's name, irrigating solution, volume of solution, and for which ear(s) the irrigation is to be performed. If the doctor has not specified the volume of solution, use the amount needed to remove the wax.
3. Compare the solution with the instructions three times.
4. Wash your hands and put on gloves, a gown, and a face shield (splashing is possible when a syringe is used).
5. Look into the patient's ear if cerumen or a foreign body needs to be removed so you will know when you have completed the irrigation.
6. Assemble the supplies.
7. If the solution is cold, warm it to room temperature by placing the bottle in a pan of warm water. **Warning:** Internal ear structures are very sensitive to extreme heat or cold. Administration of cold liquids can result in vertigo or nausea.
8. Have the patient sit or lie on her back with the ear to be treated facing you.
9. Place a towel over the patient's shoulder (or under the head and shoulder if she is lying down), and have her hold the kidney-shaped basin under her ear.
10. Pour the solution into the other basin.
11. If necessary, gently clean the external ear with cotton moistened with the solution.
12. Fill the irrigating syringe with solution (approximately 50 mL).
13. Straighten the ear canal by pulling the auricle upward and outward for adults, down and back for infants and children.
14. Holding the tip of the syringe ½ inch above the opening of the ear, slowly instill the solution into the ear. Allow the fluid to drain out during the process.
15. Refill the syringe and continue irrigation until the canal is cleaned or the solution is used up.
16. Dry the external ear with a cotton ball, and leave a clean cotton ball loosely in place for 5 to 10 minutes.
17. If the patient becomes dizzy or nauseated, allow her time to regain balance before standing up. Then assist her as needed.
18. Properly dispose of used disposable materials.
19. Remove gloves, gown, and face shield, and wash your hands.
20. Record the procedure and result, amount of solution used, time of administration, and ear(s) irrigated in the patient's chart.
21. Put on gloves and clean the equipment and room according to OSHA guidelines.

26 Chapter Review

Discussion Questions

1. How can you help elderly patients cope with the changes that occur in the eyes and ears as a result of aging?
2. Which common warning signs of eye problems and of ear problems might people tend to ignore and why?
3. Discuss the difference between sensorineural and conductive hearing loss, and give an example of how each might be caused.

Critical Thinking Questions

1. What questions might you ask as you interview an 80-year-old patient who comes to the office for an eye examination?
2. What types of questions might you ask as you interview a patient who comes into the office complaining of poor hearing?
3. What questions would you ask, in order, of a patient who comes into the office complaining that her hearing aid does not seem to be working properly?

Application Activities

1. Research a procedure, such as radial keratotomy, used to help restore people's vision. Present an oral report to the class in which you describe the procedure, its results, and the characteristics of good candidates for the procedure.
2. Practice conducting vision tests with your classmates.
3. Shop around for a hearing aid. Find out how much aids cost, what sizes are available, the cost of a fitting, and how to change batteries and clean a hearing aid properly. Present your findings in a written report. Remark on the service you received and whether you would recommend the place or places where you shopped.

Further Readings

Aston, Sheree J., and Joseph H. Maino. *Clinical Geriatric Eyecare.* Boston: Butterworth-Heinemann, 1993.

Clayman, Charles B. *The American Medical Association Family Medical Guide.* 3d ed. New York: Random House, 1994.

"Interacting With the Hearing Impaired." *The Professional Medical Assistant,* May/June 1995, 21–23.

Perry, Anne G., and Patricia A. Potter. *Clinical Nursing Skills and Techniques.* 3d ed. St. Louis, MO: Mosby–Year Book, 1994.

Sataloff, Robert Thayer, and Joseph Sataloff. *Hearing Loss.* 3d ed. New York: Marcel Dekker, 1993.

Wong, Donna L. *Wong and Whaley's Clinical Manual of Pediatric Nursing.* 4th ed. St. Louis, MO: Mosby–Year Book, 1996.

Section Three

Specialty Practices and Medical Emergencies

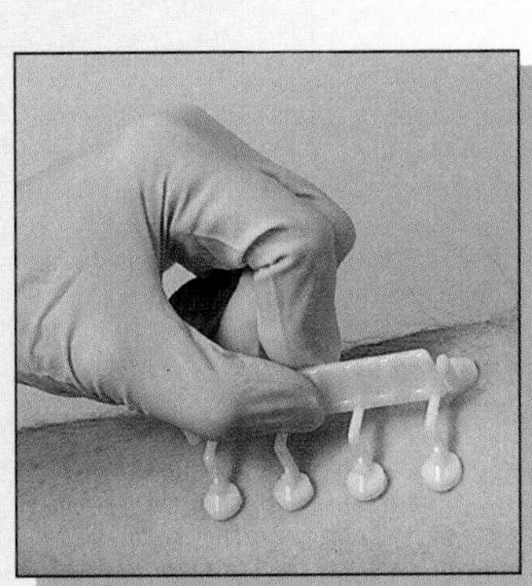

AREAS OF COMPETENCE

1997 ROLE DELINEATION STUDY

ADMINISTRATIVE

- Administrative Procedures

CLINICAL

- Fundamental Principles
- Diagnostic Orders
- Patient Care

GENERAL (Transdisciplinary)

- Professionalism
- Communication Skills
- Legal Concepts
- Instruction

CHAPTER LIST

Assisting With Examinations in the Basic Specialties

CHAPTER OUTLINE

- The Medical Assistant's Role in Specialty Examinations
- Internal Medicine
- Pediatrics
- Obstetrics and Gynecology

OBJECTIVES

After completing Chapter 27, you will be able to:

- Briefly describe the medical specialties of internal medicine, pediatrics, and obstetrics and gynecology.
- Describe the types of examinations and diagnostic tests performed in each of these specialties and the medical assistant's role in them.
- List and describe some common diseases and disorders seen in these medical specialties and typical treatments for them.
- Explain the medical assistant's duties in assessing for chronic fatigue syndrome.
- Identify common signs of domestic violence and child abuse.
- Describe the medical assistant's responsibilities in performing a scoliosis examination.
- Describe the medical assistant's role in assisting with a cervical biopsy.

Key Terms

acute
arterial blood gases
atherosclerosis
chronic
colposcopy
embolism
osteoporosis
puberty
speculum
thrombus

AREAS OF COMPETENCE

1997 ROLE DELINEATION STUDY

CLINICAL

Patient Care

- Obtain patient history and vital signs
- Prepare patient for examinations, procedures, and treatments
- Assist with examinations, procedures, and treatments

GENERAL (Transdisciplinary)

Communication Skills

- Treat all patients with compassion and empathy
- Adapt communications to individual's ability to understand

continued

AREAS OF COMPETENCE continued

Legal Concepts

- Practice within the scope of education, training, and personal capabilities
- Follow federal, state, and local legal guidelines

Instruction

- Instruct individuals according to their needs
- Teach methods of health promotion and disease prevention

The Medical Assistant's Role in Specialty Examinations

Every state has a medical practice act, or law, that defines the exact duties permitted by law for medical assistants and other health-care workers. This act determines the ways that you can assist in examinations, procedures, and diagnostic tests. It also determines which of these tasks you can perform alone. Because state laws vary, you will need to know the scope of practice for medical assistants in the state where you work.

Specialists are physicians, such as pediatricians and gynecologists, who have taken additional training beyond medical school and their required residencies to become board-certified in their respective specialties. Physicians who wish to become board-certified must pass rigorous examinations in their chosen specialty and be elected by the board for that specialty.

If you work for a specialist, she may have her own rules regarding examinations, procedures, and diagnostic tests with which she permits assistance. The physician may want to perform some procedures alone, with only minimal assistance from you. She may need more assistance with other procedures. She may ask you to perform some procedures on your own.

You must have a thorough understanding of basic anatomy and physiology of various body systems (see Chapter 23) to perform procedures alone and to communicate effectively with patients. You must also be familiar with the specific examinations and steps for the procedures in the specialty in which you are employed. Acquiring this knowledge will help you become a valuable member of your practice.

Providing Emotional Support

You will often deal with a variety of diseases and disorders in a specialty setting. Patients' illnesses may be acute, chronic, or both. **Acute** means that a disease's onset and progress is rapid, as in acute appendicitis. An illness that lasts a long time or recurs frequently is referred to as **chronic,** such as chronic osteoarthritis. Patients may have strong reactions to acute or chronic illness, including fear, defensive behavior, and frustration with physical limitations. Your empathy and support will help patients identify and cope with their feelings and behaviors.

Providing Patient Education

Patients do not generally visit specialists as frequently as they do a general practitioner, and they may have more questions than during a general physical examination. Consequently, communicating effectively with patients and providing educational materials will be one of your primary responsibilities. You will explain the functioning of the appropriate body system and the purpose of and preparation for specific examination procedures and tests. You will also teach patients how to perform prescribed home-care regimens.

Internal Medicine

Internal medicine is the specialty of an internist, who diagnoses and treats disorders and diseases of the body's internal organs. The internist is often the first doctor to see a patient with a complaint. Internists treat medical problems with medicine, either alone or in combination with other modalities (therapeutic agents). In some cases an internist refers the patient to a doctor in one of the internal medicine subspecialties.

Assisting With the Physical Examination

An internist's physical examination is usually conducted in the same way as is the general physical examination described in Chapter 25. As you gather information and prepare a patient for a physical examination, you may be expected to assess for chronic fatigue syndrome. You may also use this opportunity to detect possible substance abuse, domestic violence, or elder abuse. These topics were introduced in Chapter 24.

Assessing for Chronic Fatigue Syndrome. Chronic fatigue syndrome (CFS) is an accumulation of symptoms, the most noticeable of which is incapacitating, profound

PROCEDURE 27-1

Performing an Assessment for Chronic Fatigue Syndrome

Objective: To assess a patient for possible chronic fatigue syndrome

OSHA Guidelines: This procedure does not involve exposure to blood, body fluids, or tissues.

Materials: Patient chart, pen

Method

When a patient makes an office visit for fatigue, be alert to the possibility that the patient may have chronic fatigue syndrome. You can give a more accurate report to the physician if you work from a checklist of symptoms.

1. Identify the patient and introduce yourself.
2. Question the patient (Figure 27-1) about the following:
   - Persistent, overwhelming fatigue (that does not go away even with rest) for at least 6 months
   - Lingering fatigue after levels of exercise that would normally be easily tolerated
   - Frequent headaches
   - Sore throat and swollen lymph nodes in neck or armpits
   - Low-grade fever
   - Unexplainable muscle weakness or pains
   - Pain in joints without swelling
   - Forgetfulness or confusion
   - Irritability
   - Depression
   - Sensitivity to light
   - Impaired vision
   - Sleep disturbances
   - Inability to concentrate or perform mental tasks such as arithmetic
   - Numbness or tingling sensations
3. Document any of these symptoms in the patient's chart, and report them to the internist, who will follow up with appropriate diagnostic tests.

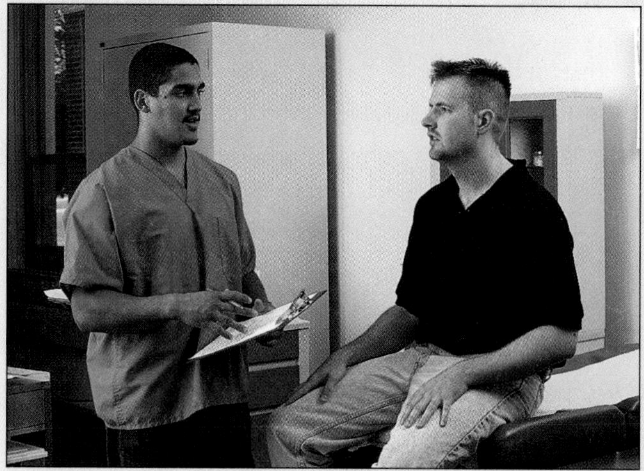

Figure 27-1. During the patient interview you can use your interviewing skills to help determine whether CFS may be the cause of fatigue.

fatigue. Because there is no test for CFS, physicians diagnose it by ruling out other diseases with similar symptoms, such as acquired immunodeficiency syndrome (AIDS), thyroid problems, anemia, and hepatitis. Another complicating factor when diagnosing CFS is that one of the most common reasons for patients to visit a physician is fatigue, which might also be caused by stress or depression.

Symptoms of CFS can begin suddenly but may continue for 3 to 4 years. The cause of CFS is unknown. Some researchers theorize, however, that it results from a genetic predisposition. Others believe that CFS may be caused by a virus or an immune system breakdown. Patients with CFS are treated for the symptoms as needed. Treatments may include an antidepressant for severe depression.

Because you check vital signs, take history, and chart, you are in a position to notice the symptoms for this disorder. Procedure 27-1 explains how to assess for CFS.

Detecting Substance Abuse. You should be alert for signs of substance abuse when you assist with an examination. Signs of substance abuse vary, depending on the type of drug and the individual's response to it. In general, signs you can observe are as follows:

- Alcohol: depressed pulse rate, respiration, and blood pressure; slurred speech; odor of alcohol on breath; reduced coordination and reflexes; poor vision and depth perception
- Cocaine and amphetamines: excitation, increased pulse rate and blood pressure, increased respiration and body temperature, dilated pupils, loss of appetite
- Hallucinogens such as LSD and angel dust: hallucinations, poor perception of time and distance, severe panic, violent and bizarre behavior
- Inhalants such as nitrous oxide and household solvents: muscle weakness, hearing loss, changes in heart rate, nausea, dizziness

- Marijuana: reddening of the eyes, increased heart rate, heightened appetite, muscular weakness
- Narcotics such as codeine and morphine: drowsiness, depressed respiration, constricted pupils, nausea, vomiting, constipation
- Sedatives such as barbiturates: nausea, slurred speech, drunken behavior without odor of alcohol

If you see any of these signs of substance abuse in a patient, inform the physician. Also inform the physician if you find such indications in someone who works in your office. If your state requires reporting suspected substance abuse by health-care workers, be sure you know the procedure for doing so.

Detecting Domestic Violence. During a physical examination you and the internist are in a position to detect signs of domestic violence. It is crucial that you bring to the doctor's attention any clues you notice during the initial interview. The doctor can then use your observations to examine and question the patient for possible internal injuries. See "Caution: Handle With Care" for guidelines on dealing with this issue.

Detecting Elder Abuse. It is difficult to detect elder abuse. There is no uniform and comprehensive definition of this type of abuse, and bruises from falls and other accidents can be mistaken for abuse. Also, the signs of neglect can be similar to the signs of some chronic medical conditions.

The three types of elder abuse are physical, psychological, and material (which includes financial). More than one type of abuse can occur simultaneously. Elder abuse occurs in all racial, socioeconomic, and religious groups. Risk factors include the following:

- History of alcoholism, drug abuse, or violence in the family
- History of mental illness in the abuser or victim
- Isolation of the victim from family members and friends other than the abuser
- Recent stressful events affecting the abuser or victim

You can assist the doctor by taking a careful history. Ask the patient about living arrangements, social contact, and emotional stress. Try to note the interaction between caregiver and patient. If you suspect abuse, inform the doctor. He will then be able to direct the physical examination toward possible internal injuries, malnutrition, or lack of cognitive ability. Signs of neglect include the following:

- Foul odor from the patient's body
- Poor skin color
- Inappropriate clothing for the season
- Soiled clothing
- Extreme concern about money

You can increase your awareness by consulting the guidelines for diagnosis and treatment of elder abuse and neglect published by the American Medical Association (AMA). Most states require doctors who suspect elder abuse or neglect to report their concerns to a designated office. Early intervention usually results in better living arrangements for both the patient and the caregiver.

Diagnostic Testing

Based on a patient's physical examination, an internist may order a number of diagnostic tests. As a medical assistant in an internist's office, you must be familiar with commonly ordered tests. They include urine and blood tests, radiologic tests, bacterial cultures, electrocardiograms (ECGs), and pulmonary function tests, all of which are discussed in later chapters. Descriptions of a few specific diagnostic tests follow.

CAUTION

HANDLE WITH CARE

Domestic Violence Detection

Physicians and medical assistants are in a position to detect signs of domestic violence. These signs can be seen in unusual bruising. They may also be evident in other injuries the patient may try to hide or excuse. You may hear signs in a patient's tone of voice or choice of words during a conversation in the office or over the telephone.

You play an important role in noticing these signs, and you must inform the physician of any signs that you detect. You must also create a supportive office environment where the patient can seek help. Encourage the physician to join the American Medical Association's Physicians' Coalition Against Family Violence, if she is not already a member. This organization provides posters, which often help patients feel encouraged to discuss domestic violence, in addition to pamphlets and other information.

Reporting suspected domestic violence is mandatory in some states. You should have a folder that contains lists of the phone numbers for domestic violence hot lines, women's shelters, and other helpful resources. You can offer the following general guidelines to women.

- Ignoring the problem never works—silence does not help anyone.
- Understand that abusive family members may not be able to help themselves.
- Call for help if a physical threat exists.

Measurement of Arterial Blood Gases. The internist may order measurement of **arterial blood gases** to determine the exchange of oxygen and carbon dioxide in the lungs and to monitor blood chemistry. Blood is drawn from an artery (instead of a vein) for this test, which is usually performed by a respiratory therapist. The oxygen measurement for arterial blood (partial pressure of oxygen) indicates how well the lungs are providing oxygen to body tissues. The carbon dioxide measurement for arterial blood (partial pressure of carbon dioxide) evaluates how well the lungs are eliminating carbon dioxide. These measurements help one diagnose and monitor conditions such as central nervous system (CNS) depression, pulmonary disorders, and kidney diseases.

Radiologic Tests. The physician orders a radiologic test to confirm or rule out a diagnosis. The choice of radiologic procedure depends on the suspected problem. Internists order plain films (roentgenograms or x-rays), computed tomography (CT) scans, magnetic resonance imaging (MRI), ultrasound, and radionuclide imaging (also known as nuclear imaging). Radiologic procedures are discussed in detail in Chapter 40.

Although you will not perform radiologic procedures, the physician will expect you to set up appointments and explain procedures to the patient. You may need to explain what kinds of preparations the patient must make prior to the test. Be sure to ask the radiologic facility about the requirements for the specific type of test.

Chest X-Ray. Internists may order a chest x-ray, which can reveal respiratory and cardiac disorders such as pneumonia, tuberculosis, or cardiomegaly (enlarged heart). It may also reveal abnormal masses in the upper thoracic region.

Venography and Venous Ultrasonography. Venography and venous ultrasonography are tests used to rule out deep-vein thrombosis (DVT). A patient has DVT when there is a **thrombus,** or blood clot, in the veins. If the thrombus becomes dislodged and travels in the bloodstream, it is known as an embolus. This moving blood clot can obstruct a blood vessel, causing an **embolism.** An embolism can be fatal, depending on its location. Risk factors for DVTs are generally poor circulation, vein injury, prolonged bed rest, recent surgery or childbirth, irregular blood coagulation, and use of oral contraceptives.

For a venogram a contrast medium is injected into a vein, and x-rays are taken of the veins. Venous ultrasonography uses inaudible sound waves that bounce off liquid (in this case blood) to form a two-dimensional image. Internists generally prefer venous ultrasonography to venography because it is noninvasive.

Diseases and Disorders

Internists treat a variety of diseases and disorders. Some of the most common include diseases of aging, infectious diseases, and sexually transmitted diseases.

Diseases of Aging. The elderly constitute a large percentage of patients in an internal medicine practice. Many of the serious disorders frequently seen in the elderly are discussed in Chapter 28. They include hypertension, coronary artery disease, and diabetes mellitus. Other disorders, such as constipation, diarrhea, and osteoporosis—while not serious for young and middle-aged adults—can create major problems for the elderly.

Constipation-Diarrhea Cycle. The cycle of constipation followed by diarrhea occurs when people's diets lack the fiber and liquids to maintain healthy bowel function and they use harsh laxatives to treat their constipation. The patient then complains of diarrhea and asks for antidiarrheal medication, which in turn causes constipation again. Encourage elderly patients to eat more high-fiber foods, such as cereals, fruits, and vegetables, and to increase their fluid intake.

Hyperlipidemia. Hyperlipidemia is a condition in which cholesterol levels are above normal. It is not just a disease of the elderly, but it can cause serious problems for older people. High cholesterol levels can lead to **atherosclerosis,** the accumulation of fatty deposits along the inner walls of arteries. These deposits, along with other substances in the blood, can form an atherosclerotic plaque. This plaque can narrow the opening in an artery to the point of obstructing blood flow. Atherosclerosis is a primary cause of cardiovascular disease, including stroke.

Your role as a patient educator is vital to helping those with high cholesterol levels. Take every opportunity to teach patients about eating foods with lower amounts of cholesterol (see Chapter 36). Provide patients with printed materials on cholesterol, available from the AMA and other sources. The doctor may also prescribe medication to lower cholesterol in patients when diet modification and exercise are not adequate.

Osteoporosis. **Osteoporosis** is an endocrine and metabolic disorder of the musculoskeletal system. The condition is prevalent in the elderly and is more common in women than men. It is characterized by hunched-over posture (Figure 27-2). The disorder may be caused by inadequate calcium consumption, estrogen deficiency, or alcoholism. Prevention methods include regular exercise, a diet high in calcium (perhaps including supplemental calcium), and hormone replacement therapy in women who are menopausal or postmenopausal.

Alzheimer's Disease. Alzheimer's disease is a severely debilitating brain disorder. Warning signs include changes in personality, mood, or behavior; recent memory loss and an increase in forgetfulness; decreased ability to perform familiar tasks; difficulty with use of language and abstract thinking; decreased powers of judgment; and disorientation to time or place. Because there is no cure, the primary role of caregivers is to provide comfort and safety to the patient.

Infectious Diseases. An internist is usually the primary physician for treating infectious diseases. Most of the infectious diseases discussed in Chapters 20 and 21 are treated by either an internist or a pediatrician. Descrip-

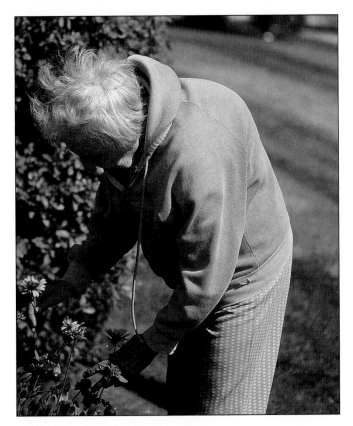

Figure 27-2. Osteoporosis is most prevalent in elderly women.

tions of other common infectious diseases follow.

Infectious Mononucleosis. Infectious mononucleosis is caused by either the cytomegalovirus (CMV) or the Epstein-Barr virus (EBV). Unexplained fever, fatigue, and sore throat are usually the dominant symptoms. If patients have these symptoms without any apparent cause, the doctor orders blood tests to rule out mononucleosis. Other symptoms may include weakness, headache, and swollen lymph nodes. With proper rest, nutrition, and antibiotics to prevent secondary infections, patients usually recover from acute symptoms in 7 to 10 days. Complete recovery may take as long as a month or more.

Lyme Disease. Lyme disease is a serious infection caused by a spirochete bacterium carried by the deer tick. When the condition is diagnosed early, treatment with antibiotics is effective. Diagnosis is difficult, however, because symptoms can occur in any order or overlap.

The first symptom of Lyme disease is often the appearance of a raised, red dot at the site of the tick bite. A circular rash may surround the bite (Figure 27-3). In many cases, however, the bite goes unnoticed. Headache, fever, and fatigue develop, followed by muscle aches and inflammation of the joints. Left untreated, the disease can progress to arthritis and heart and neurological problems.

When a patient calls with a reported tick bite, ask whether the tick was saved. If it was, tell the patient to place it in a plastic bag and take it to a U.S. Department of Agriculture Extension Office for identification. A tick identified as a deer tick should be tested for the presence of the spirochete bacterium. Even if the tick tests positive for Lyme disease bacteria, the risk of the patient contracting the disease is not great if the tick was removed from the patient within 24 hours. Your main role in dealing with Lyme disease is patient education. Many doctors' offices display pamphlets or posters to show patients how to prevent Lyme disease.

Pneumonia. Pneumonia is an acute infection of the lung tissue caused by bacteria or viruses. It often occurs in conjunction with a chronic weakening illness. Symptoms range from coughing, sputum production, and chest pain to chills and fever. It is treated with bed rest, antibiotics, adequate fluids, respiratory support measures, and pain medication.

Rabies. Rabies is a virus transmitted to humans by a bite from a mammal, such as a dog, rat, or bat. A patient who has been bitten by an animal that may be rabid should receive a rabies vaccination, which is a series of injections. Dogs, cats, and people who are at risk for exposure to the virus should have the vaccination at regular intervals. Patients must be vaccinated during the incubation period, before symptoms appear. Symptoms are nonspecific at onset and include malaise, fatigue, anxiety, or insomnia. Later there are neurological symptoms. After symptoms have occurred, nearly 100% of people who are infected with rabies die.

Staphylococcal and Streptococcal Infections (Staph and Strep). Staphylococci and streptococci are common bacteria, with many species occurring naturally in the body. When the body's resistance is low, however, these bacteria can cause infections, such as strep throat, skin abscess, impetigo, and pneumonia. Antibiotics are the standard treatment for staphylococcal and streptococcal infections. Because these organisms become resistant to antibiotics, however, researchers are constantly working to develop effective new drugs. Always stress to patients the importance of finishing the entire course of prescribed medication. Otherwise the patient will not receive enough of the drug to kill the organism, and the organism will build up a tolerance to the antibiotic.

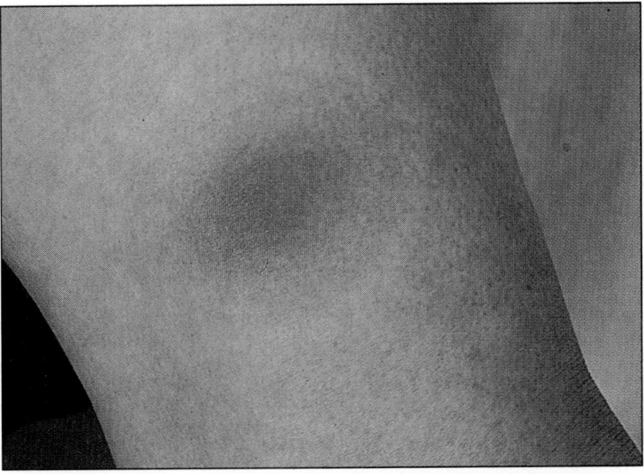

Figure 27-3. A bull's-eye rash is a symptom of the first stage of Lyme disease.

Sexually Transmitted Diseases. Sexually transmitted diseases (STDs)—diseases acquired through sexual contact with an infected person—are also infectious diseases. The number and severity of these diseases, their high incidence, and the great amount of misinformation about them warrant a discussion apart from other infectious diseases. (AIDS is discussed in Chapter 21.) Internists, infectious disease specialists, pediatricians, urologists, and gynecologists are all involved in the diagnosis and treatment of STDs.

Patient Education About STDs. Your role as an educator is vital in dealing with patients who have STDs. Some patients may be hesitant to ask for information. Providing materials in the office waiting room and examination room will help answer their questions and put them at ease. Placement in the examination room is especially appropriate when materials deal with sensitive or embarrassing topics. Printed materials are available from several medical agencies (Figure 27-4). In addition, you must educate patients about prevention and treatment of STDs. "Educating the Patient" provides more information on this topic.

Common Types of STDs. Your role in assisting the doctor in the treatment of STDs will involve emphasizing to the patient the importance of completing the course of therapy and avoiding sexual contact while the infection is still active. Sexual partners must also be treated to avoid reinfection. Several types of STDs are fairly common.

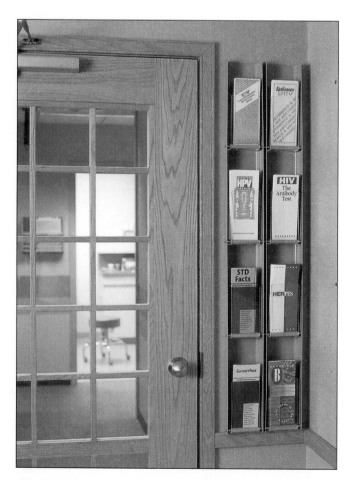

Figure 27-4. An important part of patient education is providing printed materials about STDs.

Candidiasis is a yeast infection. It is not a true STD but is included with the STDs because the infection can be transmitted between sexual partners. Symptoms include severe genital itching, redness and swelling of the vaginal or vulval tissue, light yellow or white patches (usually cheesy or curdlike) on the vagina, and vaginal discharge. The infection is treated with an antimycotic (antifungal) drug.

Chlamydia usually produces symptoms of discharge and uncomfortable urination, although it may be asymptomatic, particularly in women. Untreated, the disease can cause scarring of the fallopian tubes and eventual infertility. Diagnosis is made by aspirating pus from the urethra of men, the endocervix of women, or other infected tissue and having it examined in a laboratory. Chlamydia is treated with antibiotics.

Genital herpes is a type of herpes virus. Symptoms include blisterlike sores on the genitalia, difficult urination, swelling of the legs, fatigue, and a general ill feeling. Because this disease is cyclical, symptoms disappear and reappear periodically. Although there is no cure for genital herpes, an antiviral drug can reduce or suppress the symptoms. Herpes may be transmitted to the fetus during pregnancy or delivery. It is often fatal to an infant.

Genital warts and human papilloma virus (HPV) are found on or in men and women. Patients may generally be asymptomatic, but some have burning and itching in the genital area. There appears to be an increased risk of cancer of the vulva, vagina, and cervix in women with genital warts. Although there is no treatment for the virus, it usually disappears within 6 to 18 months in a person with a normal immune system.

Gonorrhea causes inflammation of the genitalia, with a greenish yellow discharge from the cervix, sore throat, anal discharge, swollen glands, and lower abdominal pain. Treatment is with antibiotics such as penicillin or tetracycline.

Trichomoniasis symptoms in women include inflammation of the genital area and an abundant white or yellow vaginal discharge with a foul odor. (It is usually asymptomatic in men.) The infection is diagnosed by inspecting a specimen of the discharge under the microscope. The condition is usually treated with a course of antibiotics.

Other Diseases and Disorders. Internists may diagnose and treat other diseases and disorders, including anemia, appendicitis, arthritis, gout, and peptic ulcer (see Table 27-1). They may also refer patients to a physician in one of the highly specialized areas.

Pediatrics

A pediatrician specializes in the health care of children, monitoring their development and diagnosing and treating their illnesses. Just as with internal medicine, there are subspecialties of pediatrics, such as surgery and oncology.

EDUCATING THE PATIENT

Teaching Patients About Sexually Transmitted Diseases

You must provide complete and detailed information with a nonjudgmental and supportive attitude when you teach patients about sexually transmitted diseases. Begin with the principle that all STDs are preventable. The key to prevention is avoiding sexual activities in which blood, semen, or vaginal secretions pass from one person to another.

There are various levels of protection in connection with STDs. The only absolute methods of "safe sex" are abstinence (no sex) and masturbation (self-stimulation). The next level is mutual monogamy, in which partners have sex only with each other. Emphasize that monogamy provides protection from STDs only if neither partner has an STD when the relationship begins. A final level of prevention applies to people who do not practice abstinence or mutual monogamy but wish to protect themselves and others from STDs. The following measures provide some protection.

- Use a latex condom and spermicide for every act of intercourse. (Use a latex condom during oral sex.)
- Know all your sexual partners, and discuss STD prevention with them.
- Have a physician regularly screen you for STDs because many people have no signs when they are infected.
- Consult a physician if any signs of STDs develop, such as a blister, sore, discharge, rash, or abdominal pain.

Encourage patients to ask questions and discuss any concerns they have. Explain the need to make follow-up appointments with a physician if appropriate.

Teaching a patient who has been diagnosed with an STD how to treat or manage the disease is especially important. Make sure the patient understands all directions and the necessity for treatment. Bacterial infections such as chlamydia, gonorrhea, and syphilis can be cured with antibiotics as long as the patient takes all the medication in the prescribed manner. Viral infections such as AIDS, genital herpes, and genital warts cannot be cured, although they can be treated and managed to differing degrees.

Emphasize to patients with an STD that they should avoid all sexual contact until the infection has been treated completely. Many STDs can be spread through any type of genital contact, including vaginal intercourse, anal sex, and oral sex. Herpes can be spread through kissing if there are herpes sores in the mouth. Encourage patients to inform each person with whom they had sexual contact that they have contracted an STD. Explain that unless all sexual partners are treated successfully, the disease will pass back and forth indefinitely.

You can reinforce your education efforts by providing patients with materials on the prevention and treatment of STDs. Keep a variety of pamphlets, books, and videotapes in your office to help patients cope with and manage STDs.

To be a good pediatric medical assistant, you must first like children of all ages. If you do, you will be better able to relate to them and to communicate with them effectively.

Parent or caregiver education, adherence to immunization schedules (see Chapter 20), and child abuse detection are primary areas of responsibility for medical assistants who work in pediatrics. You will also assist with the physical examination and treatment of the pediatric patient. Your role as liaison in these areas between caregiver and physician will be an important one.

Assisting With a Pediatric Physical Examination

Many of the examination procedures for a pediatric patient are the same as those for an adult. While you prepare the child or adolescent for examination, you might discuss with the parent, caregiver, or child such topics as eating habits, sleep patterns, daily activities, immunization schedules, and toilet training. This discussion will provide important clues to possible abnormal mental, physical, emotional, or social development. Topics such as STDs and drugs and alcohol may be appropriate for you to discuss with an adolescent. Point out potential problems to the doctor.

Be mindful of adolescents' sensitivity toward rapid growth and physical, sexual, and social development when you prepare them for examination. Adolescents and preadolescents often feel awkward and self-conscious about being examined. They may also prefer to dress alone and to be alone with the doctor.

Some children are afraid of going to the doctor's office. You can help relieve a child's fear by calmly explaining procedures before they occur, giving the reason for each procedure, and being cheerful and mindful of a child's feelings. Allowing a child to examine some of the instruments may also alleviate fear (Figure 27-5). If a patient is physically resistant to examination, you may need to call for assistance from the doctor or caregiver, or the child may need to be restrained.

Try to speak in terms aimed at the child's age level, and kneel if necessary to make eye contact with the child. Treat the child with respect and provide positive

Table 27-1

Common Diseases and Disorders Treated by Internists

Condition	Description	Treatment
Anemia	Results from deficiency of iron or vitamins, such as folic acid and vitamin B_{12}; can also result from loss of blood (acute blood loss anemia); body's cells do not get enough oxygen, resulting in fatigue, listlessness, pallor, inability to concentrate, difficulty breathing on exertion	Oral supplements of appropriate vitamin or iron; if caused by acute blood loss, blood transfusion
Appendicitis	Acute inflammation of appendix as result of serious infection, blood clotting, or tissue destruction, which can lead to rupture or perforation of appendix; ruptured appendix can be fatal; symptoms include general abdominal pain and tenderness often starting at the umbilical area and radiating to lower right quadrant (McBurney's point), fever, loss of appetite, gastrointestinal (GI) distress	Surgical removal of appendix
Arthritis	Chronic inflammatory disease of tissues of joints; symptoms include pain and stiffness in joints	Medication to reduce inflammation and pain, surgery in severe cases
Gout	Metabolic disease involving acute joint pain, most commonly in the big toe at night; caused by overproduction or retention of uric acid	Medication and diet restrictions to decrease production of uric acid and promote its excretion
Peptic ulcer	Lesion of mucous membrane of esophagus, stomach, or duodenum (first section of small intestine); symptoms include heartburn, vomiting, and dull, gnawing pain or burning sensation in area	Medication and diet restrictions to reduce amount and acidity of gastric juices, stress reduction, surgery in severe cases

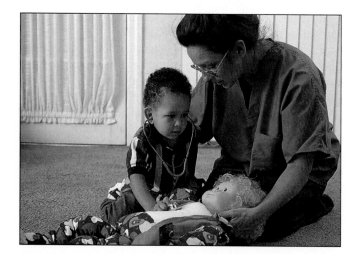

Figure 27-5. Providing a pediatric patient with a diversion may help alleviate the child's fear.

reinforcement when a child is cooperative. Avoid making light of crying or pain. Make a game out of some aspect of a procedure, and provide a small token reward at the end of a visit. For infants a gentle approach, such as talking quietly and holding them comfortingly, is helpful.

Examining the Well Child. Parents should bring their infants and children to the pediatrician for regular checkups and growth monitoring. The American Academy of Pediatrics recommends the following frequency.

- Infants need seven well-baby examinations during their first year, at these intervals: 2 weeks, 1 month, 2 months, 4 months, 6 months, 9 months, 1 year.
- Children in the second year of life should have checkups at 15 and 18 months.
- From the age of 2, children should have checkups every year.

Follow Universal Precautions and prepare for the physical examination the same way you would for an adult, except for draping and positioning. Ask the parent of an infant or toddler to remove all the child's clothing except the diaper because the child should be nude for the examination. Then keep the child covered until the physician enters the examining room.

An infant or toddler may be crying during the examination. To assist the physician in hearing chest sounds with a stethoscope, ask the parent to allow the child to suck on a pacifier to quiet the crying. Feeding the child during the examination is not encouraged because stomach sounds interfere with clear auscultation.

Parents play a more active role during the examination of infants and toddlers than they play during the examination of older children. You or the parent may assist the child into position during the examination, or the physician may allow the parent to hold the child. Distracting infants and toddlers with mobiles, shiny surfaces, or toys may help the examination go more smoothly.

Examining for Scoliosis. One examination performed frequently in the pediatric office is that for scoliosis, an abnormal lateral curving of the spine into an S curve. It can appear in a child of any age but is more common in adolescent girls during their growth spurt. This condition is undetectable when the child is young. As she grows, however, it can be detected in an examination. Procedure 27-2 explains how to perform a scoliosis examination.

Report any symptoms that you notice during your examination to the pediatrician. If the pediatrician confirms

PROCEDURE 27-2

Performing the Scoliosis Examination

Objective: To assess a patient for possible scoliosis

OSHA Guidelines: This procedure does not involve exposure to blood, body fluids, or tissues.

Materials: Patient chart, pen

Method

Scoliosis is an abnormal, lateral curving of the spine into an S shape (Figure 27-6). It results from rotation of the spinal column, with the thorax usually curving to the right and the lumbar spine to the left. The two forms of scoliosis are functional, caused by poor posture or uneven leg lengths, and structural, resulting from vertebral deformities.

Genetic scoliosis, a type of structural scoliosis, is seldom apparent before the age of 10. It is most noticeable at the beginning of the preadolescent growth spurt. It is seven times more common in girls than in boys. Screening for scoliosis by school nurses is routine in most schools. It can be detected in an examination. You can perform a scoliosis examination on a child as follows.

1. Identify the patient and introduce yourself.
2. Explain the procedure.
3. Have the child remove his shirt and stand up straight. Look to see whether one shoulder is higher than the other or one shoulder blade is more prominent.
4. With the child's arms hanging loosely at his sides, check whether one arm swings away from the body more than the other, whether one hip is higher or more prominent than the other, and whether the child seems to tilt to one side.
5. Have the child bend forward, with arms hanging down and palms together at knee level. Check to see whether there is a hump on the back at the ribs or near the waist.
6. Document your findings in the patient's chart, and report them to the doctor.

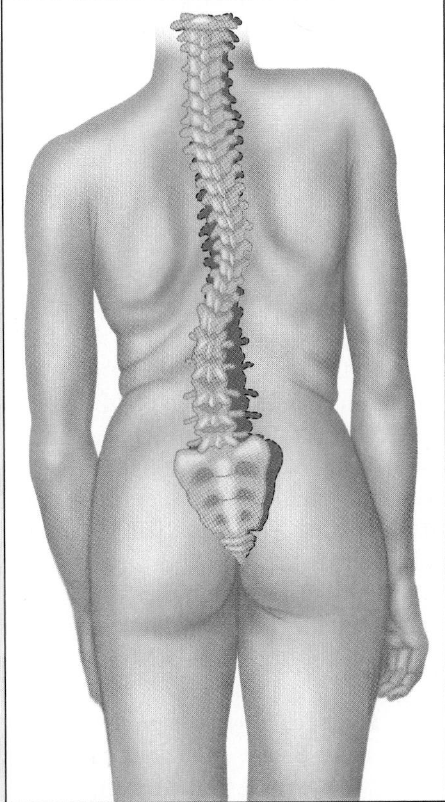

Figure 27-6. Scoliosis causes the spine to curve into an S shape.

scoliosis, she may recommend exercises, a Milwaukee brace, surgical rod implantation, or a combination of therapies.

Your role as educator in regard to scoliosis is important. Untreated scoliosis can cause debilitating symptoms as the patient matures to adulthood. Encourage parents to bring older children and adolescents to the office annually for routine screening. If the Milwaukee brace is prescribed, the adolescent may need encouragement from you and the physician to wear the brace as directed.

Detecting Child Abuse or Neglect. Child abuse is an all-too-common and potentially fatal problem. Whenever a child comes to the office, you should watch for any signs of serious problems in the relationship between the parent or caregiver and the child. Also notice any signs of physical injury, such as unexplained bruises or burns. Any suspicious lesion on a child's genitalia should prompt an investigation of sexual abuse. Possible signs of neglect include dirty or neglected appearance, hunger, extreme sadness or fear, and an inability to communicate. Note any suspicions in the chart, and report them to the doctor before he sees the patient. The doctor will respond to your information by examining the child for clues to indicate the following:

- Internal injuries: tenderness when palpated or auscultated
- Malnutrition: tooth discoloration, unhealthy gums or skin color
- Lack of cognitive ability: dulled neurological responses

Studies show that certain risk factors are usually present in parents who abuse their children. Some risk factors are stress, single parenthood, inadequate knowledge of normal developmental expectations, lack of family support, family hostility, financial problems, and mental health problems. Other risk factors include prolonged separation of parent and child, ambivalent feelings toward the child, and a mother younger than 16 years. Additional risk factors include an unhealthy or unsafe home environment, inappropriate supervision, substance abuse, a parental crime record, a negative attitude toward pregnancy, and a history of parents having been abused.

Intervention, such as home visits by nurses, can significantly lower the rate of child abuse. Managed care systems may provide this service as part of their postpartum program. These nurses provide information on normal child growth and development and routine health needs, serve as informational support persons, and refer families to appropriate services when they require assistance.

You are legally responsible for reporting suspected child abuse or neglect. Contact the child protection agency in your community. Post the appropriate telephone number in your office.

Examining for Growth Abnormalities. Pediatricians look for any sign of growth abnormality during routine well-child visits. Physicians compare a child's physical, intellectual, and social signs to charts showing national averages. In general, physicians look for signs that the child is in the appropriate stage of growth for her age. Growth can be divided into five stages.

Stages One and Two: The First and Second Years. Infancy, the first year of life, is marked by the development of strength and coordination of the trunk, head, and limbs. Intellectual growth primarily involves receiving information through the senses and performing motor (physical) functions in response to the environment. In the second year of life, the child develops fine motor skills (involving control of smaller muscles, such as those in the fingers) and manual dexterity. Sociologically, the child develops some independence and begins to test parental limits.

Stage Three: Ages 3 to 5 Years. During ages 3 to 5 years, the child develops physical skills of muscle coordination and both large motor skills (involving control of larger muscles, such as those in the arms and legs) and fine motor skills. Intellectually, the child observes and copies older children and adults without fully understanding them. The child also learns to initiate play with others and begins to make requests of family members.

Stage Four: Age 6 Years to Puberty. The fourth stage occurs from approximately age 6 to **puberty,** the period of adolescence when a person begins to develop sexual traits. Muscle coordination and fine motor and large motor skills develop further. The child begins to get involved in scholastic and extracurricular activities. The child also develops an identity, based partially on both intellectual and physical skills, and learns how to achieve goals in the environment.

Stage Five: Adolescence. Physical growth and development in the teenage years are centered on normal sexual change. Girls usually begin puberty between 8 and 14 years of age; boys begin between 9½ and 16, on average. Menarche, the onset of menstruation, usually occurs about 2½ years after the onset of puberty. The beginning of nocturnal emissions of seminal fluid signals sexual maturation in boys. This awareness of sexuality is accompanied by concern with body image. Intellectually, adolescents are able to understand abstract concepts and think about themselves in terms of the past and future. The process of developing independence, a personal identity, and future plans is also important during this time of life.

General Eye Examination. As part of the general examination, the pediatrician examines the interior of the child's eyes with an ophthalmoscope. You will probably perform the visual acuity test (Figure 27-7). Make a game of covering the child's eye if the child resists this part of the procedure. Watch for signs of visual difficulty during the test, such as tilting the head in a certain direction, blinking, squinting, or frowning. If the caregiver brought the child in specifically for a vision test, record in the child's chart whatever symptoms the caregiver mentions.

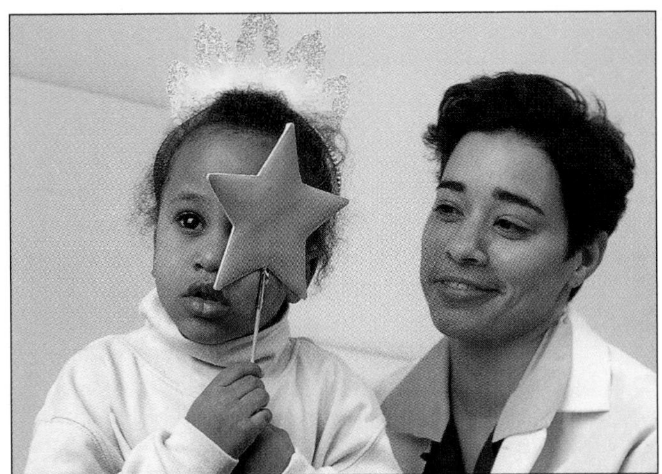

Figure 27-7. Making a game out of the visual acuity test helps put a child at ease.

General Ear Examination. A pediatric ear examination is important because so many children have ear infections or upper respiratory infections involving the ear. Because children's eustachian tubes are more horizontal than those of adults, fluid collects more easily in the tubes and can promote bacterial growth. The tubes are also short and connected to the throat. Any upper respiratory infections can easily travel to the ear. (The ear examination is described in Chapter 26.)

Diagnostic Testing

Many adult diagnostic procedures are also used for children. The pediatrician uses the same laboratory tests and radiologic tests. He performs some diagnostic tests in the office.

Because streptococcal infection can be especially serious in a child, some pediatricians perform a rapid test for the presence of streptococcal bacteria so they can immediately start the appropriate medical treatment. If the test is positive, the physician begins treatment with antibiotics specifically for this type of bacteria.

Some physicians believe the rapid strep test is not always reliable. To confirm a negative test result, these physicians also do a throat culture. A throat culture can determine which of the streptococcal bacteria is present or whether other organisms are causing the symptoms. The results can indicate a possible change in medication. The method for obtaining a throat culture is outlined in Chapter 35.

Immunizations

Immunizations are usually given during routine office visits (Figure 27-8). Public health authorities recommend a schedule (see Chapter 20) for immunizing children against diseases such as hepatitis B, diphtheria, tetanus, pertussis (whooping cough), poliomyelitis, measles, mumps, rubella (German measles), chickenpox, and *Haemophilus influenzae* type B (Hib). Many vaccines have largely eliminated the threat of these once-prevalent, life-threatening diseases.

The first vaccine, for hepatitis B, is given to a newborn the day after birth. Some vaccines require a series of doses to give immunity. Booster doses may be required for a particular vaccine at a later age. The patient must not have an illness or fever at the time of immunization. If these conditions exist, reschedule the appointment.

Pediatric Diseases and Disorders

If you work in a pediatric office, you should know the signs and symptoms of common childhood diseases. Some diseases, including chickenpox, influenza, measles, mumps, rubella, scarlet fever, and tetanus, are described in Chapter 20. Other common diseases are outlined in Table 27-2. Many common disorders found in children are not specific diseases. Upper respiratory infections, including colds and viral influenza, occur frequently among children.

It is important not to make assumptions regarding diagnosis or treatment. When reported symptoms include fever, sore throat, runny nose, and earache, any number of conditions could be the cause. Encourage the parent to bring the child to the office. You should, however, tell the doctor as soon as possible when a child has an extremely high fever. The doctor may want the child to go to an emergency room. Do not recommend aspirin for fever in children. The use of aspirin in children has been associated with Reye's syndrome, a potentially fatal disease of the central nervous system and liver. Acetaminophen (Tylenol) is preferred for treating fever in children.

Other diseases and disorders found in children are not considered common. You need to be aware of the basic symptoms and treatments for these disorders.

AIDS. Most childhood cases of human immunodeficiency virus (HIV) infection are transmitted from a mother to her infant. When a woman is HIV-positive, her baby has a 15% to 30% chance of being infected. All babies born to HIV-positive mothers have HIV antibodies that are

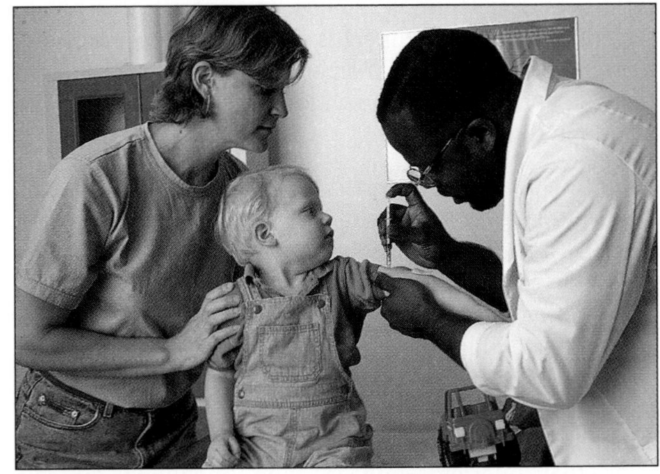

Figure 27-8. Immunizations are part of routine well-child visits in a pediatric practice.

Table 27-2

Common Pediatric Diseases and Disorders

Condition	Description	Treatment
Head lice	Small insects easily spread among children by head-to-head contact and sharing objects such as combs and hairbrushes; lice live on scalp and lay eggs strongly attached to hair shafts; symptoms include itchy scalp; identify by locating crawling lice or nits (eggs) attached to hair; examine parted hair carefully at scalp and bottom of hair strands	Antilice shampoo or 1% permethrin cream rinse; removal of eggs with fine-tooth comb; disinfection of clothing, bedding, and washable toys by machine washing and drying in hot cycles or by dry cleaning; tight bagging for 30 days of items that cannot be washed; disinfection of combs and brushes by washing in shampoo used for hair
Herpes simplex virus (HSV)	In children virus causes cold-sore blisters on or near mouth; diagnosis made by inspecting lesions; first stage (2–12 days before appearance of blister) involves tingling and itching sensations; later blister ruptures and forms yellow crust; outbreak takes about 3 weeks to heal completely	Application of ice cube to blister, which may promote faster healing; ointments to alleviate cracking and discomfort; avoidance of sun exposure because it may trigger outbreak
Impetigo	Highly contagious dermatologic disease caused by staphylococcal, sometimes streptococcal, bacteria; transmitted by direct contact; causes inflammation and pustules, small lymph-filled bumps, which rupture and become encrusted before healing; frequently seen around mouth and nostrils	Avoidance of scratching lesions and sharing utensils, towels, bed linens, or bath or pool water that could cause further transmission; careful washing of affected areas two to three times per day to keep lesions clean and dry; topical antibacterial cream
Infectious conjunctivitis ("pink eye")	Highly contagious streptococcal or staphylococcal bacterial infection of conjunctiva of eye; transmitted by direct contact; causes redness, pain, swelling, discharge; usually begins in one eye and spreads to other	Avoidance of scratching eyes and sharing utensils, towels, or bed linens that could cause further transmission; warm compresses to relieve discomfort; antibiotic drops or ointment

continued

detectable through testing at birth. The antibodies persist for a period of 15 to 18 months, but not all such babies remain permanently infected. AIDS has no cure, but treating the pregnant woman and newborn child with antiviral agents has been shown to lower the rate of HIV infection in the child.

Attention Deficit Hyperactivity Disorder and Learning Disabilities. Attention deficit hyperactivity disorder (ADHD) and learning disabilities (LD) are found in children, adolescents, and adults. These disorders can cause gross motor disability, inability to read or write, hyperactivity, distractibility, impulsiveness, and generally disruptive behavior. ADHD encompasses all conditions formerly identified as hyperactivity, or hyperkinesis, and attention deficit. LD encompasses a wide range of conditions that interfere with learning, including dyslexia (reading problems), dysgraphia (writing problems), and dyscalculia (math problems).

ADHD is among the most misunderstood, misdiagnosed, and overdiagnosed problems in children. Some physicians fail to recognize ADHD as a cause of academic, social, and emotional problems. Others are quick to attribute too many such problems to ADHD. When ADHD is the correct diagnosis, methylphenidate hydrochloride (Ritalin) and other drugs may alleviate the symptoms but not without risk of adverse effects, such as insomnia, increased heart rate and blood pressure, and interference with growth rate. Successful treatment usually requires a combination of drug and behavioral therapies and educational, psychological, and emotional support tailored to the child.

Cerebral Palsy. Cerebral palsy, a birth-related disorder of the nerves and muscles, is the most frequent crippling disease in children. It is caused by brain damage that occurs before, during, or shortly after birth or in early childhood. Signs of spastic cerebral palsy (the

Table 27-2 continued

Common Pediatric Diseases and Disorders

Condition	Description	Treatment
Pinworms	Parasites transmitted by swallowing worm eggs, by touching something that infected person has touched, or by putting infested sand or dirt into mouth; when eggs hatch in body, worms attach to intestinal lining; mature females travel to areas just outside rectum to lay eggs, which causes itching	Medication usually given to whole family to treat and prevent further infestation
Ringworm	Contagious fungal infection involving scalp, groin, feet, or other areas of body, causing flat, dry, and scaly or moist and crusty lesions; lesions develop into clear center with outer ring; when scalp is affected, may cause bald patches	Oral and topical antifungal medication; isolation to prevent spreading; frequent changing of towels, bedding, with no sharing with others in family; caution that child not use others' combs or brushes
Streptococcal sore throat ("strep throat")	Contagious disease caused by streptococcal bacteria and spread by droplet; complications include progression to rheumatic fever (with arthritis, nephritis, and inflammation of endocardium, or inner lining of heart); symptoms include headache, high fever, vomiting, and extremely painful, swollen, and red or white sore throat; causes difficulty swallowing	Streptococci-specific antibiotics given as soon as possible; because of potential complications, empiric therapy usually given without confirmed diagnosis from throat culture; antibiotic adjusted as necessary with confirmation of infecting organism; possible hospitalization in acute cases

most common form) include hyperactive tendon reflexes, rapid alteration between muscular contraction and relaxation, permanent muscle shortening, and underdevelopment of extremities. Among people who have this disease, 40% are mentally retarded, 25% have seizures, and 80% have impaired speech. There is no known cure, but the effects of the disorder can be alleviated with physical therapy, speech therapy, orthopedic surgery, splints, skeletal muscle relaxants, and anticonvulsant medication.

Congenital Heart Disease. Congenital heart disease is caused by a cardiovascular malformation in the fetus before birth. If the fetus survives, the newborn is usually small. The defect may be so small, however, that it may not be recognized until days, months, or even years later. Some patients have such a mild case of the disease that no treatment is necessary. Others require only low-risk surgery. In still others major high-risk surgery is necessary. Many patients diagnosed with the problem are treated with antibiotics to avoid secondary infections.

A cardiovascular defect can be caused by genetic mutations (changes in the genes), maternal infections (such as rubella or cytomegalovirus), maternal alcoholism, or maternal insulin-dependent diabetes. Blue lips and fingernails, signs of cyanosis in a newborn, are obvious indications of a cardiac defect.

Down Syndrome. Down syndrome is a genetic disorder resulting from one extra chromosome in each of the millions of cells formed during development of the fetus. It is the most common chromosomal abnormality in humans. Down syndrome is not caused by any parental behavior, such as diet or activity. The estimated risk for a Down syndrome birth increases, however, as maternal age increases. Down syndrome is characterized by low muscle tone, which can be alleviated with physical therapy. Characteristic facial features are also evident

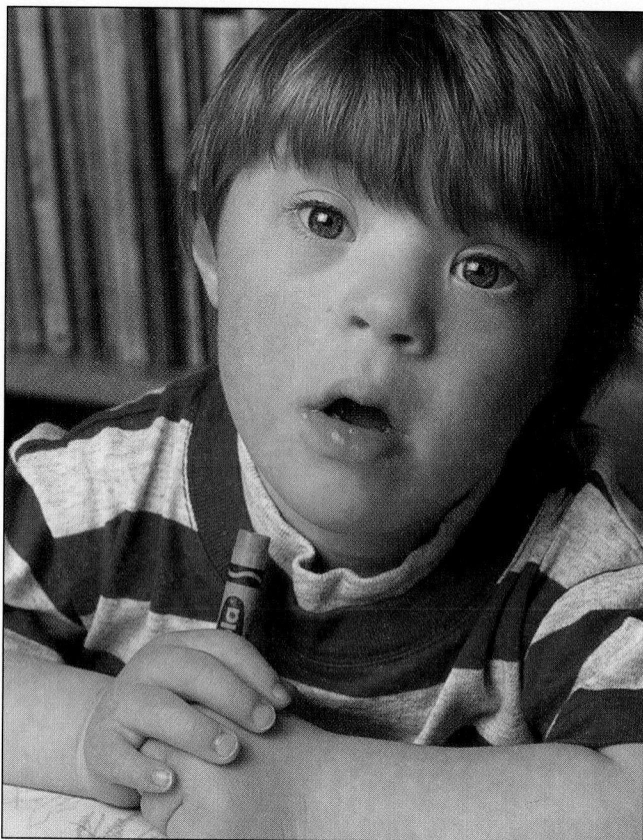

Figure 27-9. A child with Down syndrome usually has distinct facial features.

(Figure 27-9). These include broad face, flattened nasal bridge, narrow nasal passages (increasing the risk of congestion), slanting eyes (vision problems are common), and small teeth and ears. Mental retardation, which can range from mild to severe, is also a characteristic of Down syndrome.

Hepatitis B. Infection with the hepatitis B virus (HBV) can lead to a serious and chronic infection of the liver. A child can carry the virus for years and only later develop liver failure or liver cancer. The virus can be transmitted across the placenta or during birth if the mother is infected. The disease may also be transmitted sexually, by blood transfusion, or by direct contact. It is frequently seen among drug abusers who share needles. Immunization is available, and children should be immunized starting the day after birth. Children who have not been immunized should begin to receive the series of immunizations for protection from infection.

Respiratory Syncytial Virus. The respiratory syncytial virus (RSV) is a major cause of lower respiratory disease in infants and young children. RSV is seen yearly in the winter and spring outbreaks of pneumonia, bronchiolitis, and tracheobronchitis. It is highly contagious and reinfection is common. Treatment is difficult because the infection is viral rather than bacterial. Antibiotics are thus effective for treating only the possible secondary infections that develop during or after contracting RSV.

Sudden Infant Death Syndrome. Sudden infant death syndrome (SIDS)—formerly known as crib death—is the sudden death of an infant that remains unexplained after all other possible causes have been carefully ruled out. Most SIDS cases occur before the infant is 6 months of age. Victims appear to be healthy and are more likely to be male than female. SIDS occurs during sleep. Some factors that may put babies between the ages of 1 week and 1 year at high risk have been identified:

- Being exposed to smoke in utero and to secondhand smoke after birth
- Being overheated when ill
- Being exclusively bottle-fed
- Being born prematurely
- Receiving little or no prenatal care

The National Sudden Infant Death Foundation has local chapters for parents whose babies have died of the syndrome. Counseling and information are available through local health organizations.

Spina Bifida. Spina bifida is a defect of spinal development that results when tissues fail to close properly around the spinal cord during the first trimester of pregnancy. Neurological symptoms are common because the spinal cord is not fully protected by the bony and connective tissues of the spine. These symptoms may vary with the severity of the defect, ranging from foot weakness and bladder or bowel problems to paralysis of the lower extremities and mental retardation. The skin over the spinal cord often has a depression, tuft of hair, or port wine stain when the defect is not readily apparent.

The treatment and outcome of spina bifida are based on the extent of damage. Surgical closure or implants are sometimes required. Unfortunately, the neurological conditions cannot be reversed.

Viral Gastroenteritis. Gastroenteritis is an inflammation of the stomach and intestines. Gastroenteritis caused by a virus may be called the flu, traveler's diarrhea, or food poisoning. Viral gastroenteritis usually subsides within 1 to 2 days. It can be serious in young children, however, because it can cause extreme fluid loss that results in dehydration and electrolyte imbalances.

Symptoms include fever, nausea, abdominal cramping, diarrhea, and vomiting. Gastroenteritis is treated with bed rest, increased fluid intake, dietary modifications (usually only clear liquids), and medication for vomiting and diarrhea if necessary. Antibiotics may be prescribed if evidence of bacterial involvement is present.

Patient and Caregiver Education for Pediatric Patients

Patients and caregivers in a pediatrician's office usually have many questions. You will be able to answer some of the questions yourself, sparing valuable time for the pediatrician. Helpful brochures and booklets are available from the American Academy of Pediatrics. You should obtain the current list of publications and encourage your employer to order what the office needs.

Obstetrics and Gynecology

An obstetrician/gynecologist (OB/GYN) specializes in the female reproductive system. Physicians who focus on caring for women during pregnancy and childbirth are called obstetricians. Physicians who treat other conditions of the female reproductive system are called gynecologists.

As a medical assistant in an OB/GYN office, you will need to be familiar with the female reproductive system and its functions, including pregnancy, fertility, and menopause. You need to know about the common diagnostic tests and procedures performed in this specialty. You must also be familiar with the common diseases and disorders in obstetrics and gynecology, be prepared to answer patients' questions, and provide patient education materials.

Assisting With the Gynecologic Physical Examination

An annual gynecologic examination is recommended for all women age 18 and older. The examination is intended to provide an overview of a woman's health and to provide the opportunity for important cancer-screening examinations and tests. A female medical assistant should be in the examining room during the physical examination to assist a male doctor and to provide legal protection. Your role during the examination is similar to that for the general physical examination.

Ask the patient to empty her bladder; if a urine specimen is needed, it should be collected at this time. Provide the patient with a gown before the examination, and give her privacy while she changes. When you interview her, discuss her gynecologic and general health, and inquire about any changes in appetite, weight, or emotional status. Also find out the date of her last menstrual period. Then have her sit on the examining table while you check her vital signs.

The Physician's Interview. The gynecologic physical examination is more than an internal pelvic examination. It is an evaluation of the patient's total health and a review of factors that could be an indication of possible cancer or STDs. The physician asks questions about the patient's menstrual cycle and about any abnormal discharge or discomfort during sexual intercourse. The physician also listens to the patient's heart and lungs before beginning the gynecologic examination.

Breast Examination. The physician examines the patient's breasts and underarm areas to check for abnormal lumps that could be cancerous. Your role as patient

EDUCATING THE PATIENT

How to Perform a Breast Self-Examination

You may be responsible for reinforcing patient education about monthly breast self-examination (BSE), which can be instrumental in the early detection of breast cancer. Figure 27-10 shows the steps suggested by the National Cancer Institute for performing this procedure.

Check the office policy to see which of several methods it recommends for teaching BSE. One approach uses the following steps.

1. Explain the purpose of BSE.
2. Assist the patient to the standing position, and instruct her to use a large mirror to view the breasts during this part of the procedure.
3. Explain to the patient what she should look for when inspecting her breasts while standing.
4. Demonstrate the positioning of arms and hands for this visual inspection: first, her arms at her sides; then, her arms raised and her hands clasped behind her head; finally, her arms lowered with her hands on her hips.
5. Demonstrate, on the patient's breast, how to perform the small rotary motions with the flat pads of the fingers from the outer rim (including the armpit and collarbone area) toward the nipple. (Synthetic breast models are available that may be helpful in teaching the proper technique.)
6. Demonstrate how to inspect the nipples.
7. Ask the patient to practice the procedure.
8. Observe the patient's self-examination technique. (If the patient is reluctant to examine herself in front of you, have her repeat the highlights of the procedure.)
9. Assist the patient to lie down, with a small pillow or folded towel under the shoulder on the side to be examined.
10. Repeat steps 5 through 8.
11. Suggest that the patient mark her calendar for a monthly reminder to perform the examination 1 week after the onset of menses.
12. Give the patient educational materials that explain how to perform BSE.

Make sure the patient knows that she should perform BSE around the same date of each month—after her period ends, if she is still menstruating. (At this time the breasts are most normal and least swollen and lumpy.) You must also emphasize that BSE is not a substitute for mammograms or regular breast examination by a doctor. Early cancer detection depends on the performance of all three types of breast examination.

continued

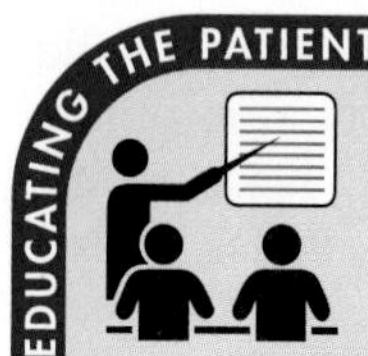

How to Perform a Breast Self-Examination continued

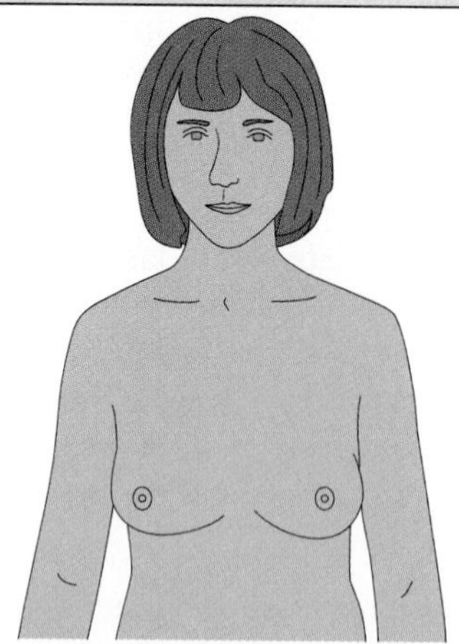

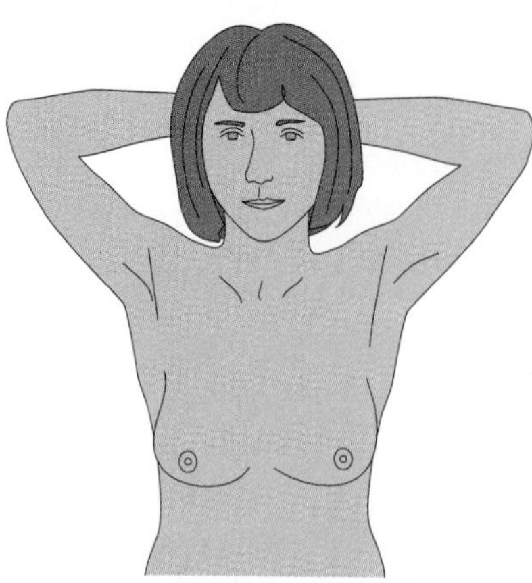

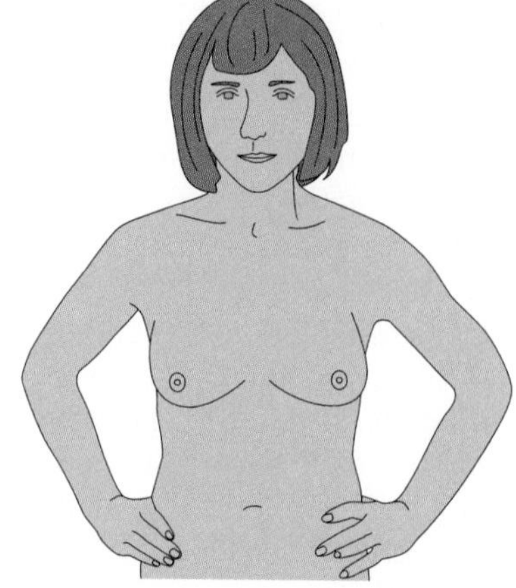

❶ Stand before a mirror. Inspect both breasts for anything unusual such as any discharge from the nipples or puckering, dimpling, or scaling of the skin.

The next two steps are designed to emphasize any change in the shape or contour of your breasts. As you do them, you should be able to feel your chest muscles tighten.

❷ Watching closely in the mirror, clasp your hands behind your head, and press your hands forward.

❸ Next, press your hands firmly on your hips, and bow slightly toward your mirror as you pull your shoulders and elbows forward.

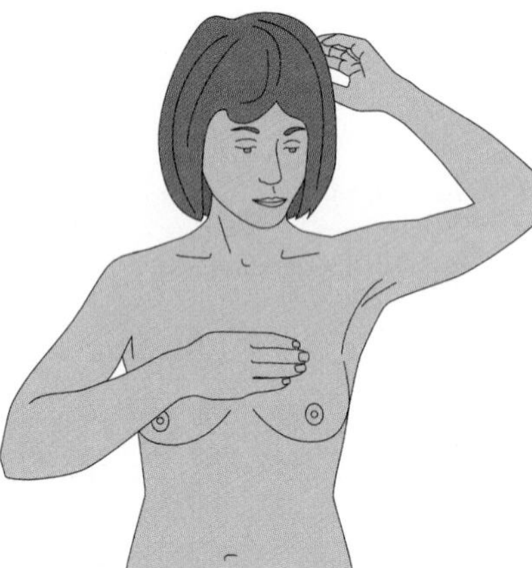

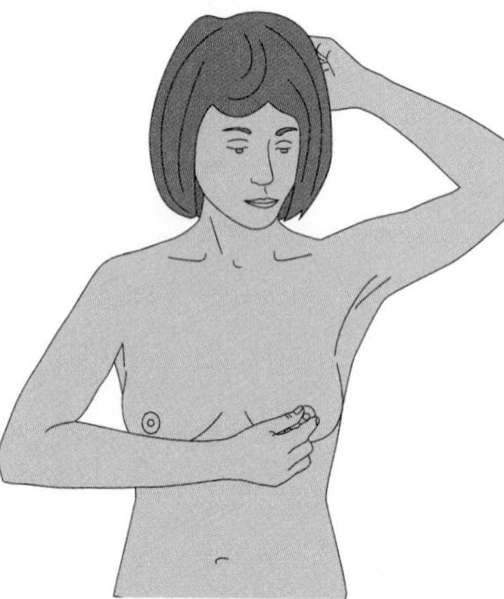

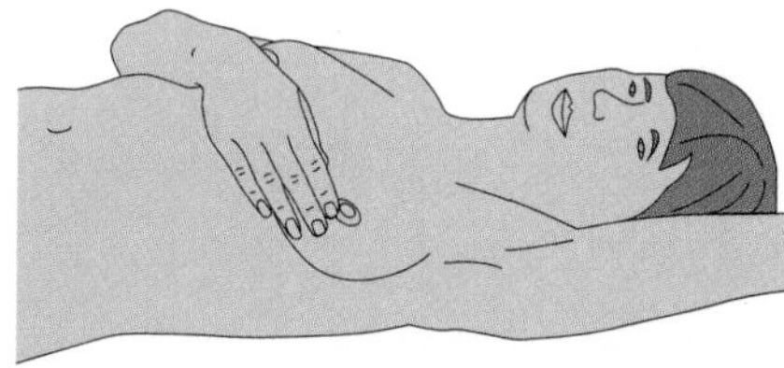

Some women do the next part of the exam in the shower because fingers glide over soapy skin, making it easy to concentrate on the texture underneath.

❹ Raise your left arm. Use three or four fingers of your right hand to explore your left breast firmly, carefully, and thoroughly. Beginning at the outer edge, press the flat part of your fingers in small circles, moving the circles slowly around the breast. and the underarm, including the underarm itself. Feel for any unusual lump or mass under the skin.

❺ Gently squeeze the nipple and look for a discharge. (If you have any discharge during the month—whether or not it is during BSE—see your doctor.) Repeat steps 4 and 5 on your right breast.

❻ Steps 4 and 5 should be repeated lying down. Lie flat on your back with your left arm over your head and a pillow or folded towel under your left shoulder. This position flattens the breast and makes it easier to examine. Use the same circular motion described earlier. Repeat the examination on your right breast.

Figure 27-10. The National Cancer Institute includes these instructions and illustrations in the brochure *Breast Exams: What You Should Know* (NIH Publication No. 90-2000).

educator is crucial. Patients must understand the need for regular breast examinations. When interviewing the patient and after the examination, emphasize the National Cancer Institute's three-point breast cancer detection program.

1. Beginning at age 40, all women should be encouraged to have a mammogram every 1 to 2 years until age 50. Mammography should be done annually after age 50.
2. Women should have breast examinations during their annual routine checkups.
3. Women should do breast self-examination (BSE) monthly.

While reviewing the patient's chart, the physician checks to see when the last mammogram was performed. He may also ask the patient whether she knows how to perform a BSE and whether she is performing it monthly. If needed, he may ask you to instruct the patient in performing the BSE. For BSE teaching techniques, see "Educating the Patient."

Pelvic Examination. During the pelvic examination the doctor checks the external genitalia, cervix, vaginal wall, internal reproductive organs, and rectum. Examination methods include palpation and inspection with a **speculum,** an instrument that expands the vaginal opening to permit viewing of the vagina and cervix. The doctor wears gloves and uses a lubricant for patient comfort.

Your role is to assist the patient into position, with her feet in the stirrups of the examining table and her buttocks at the end of the table. Drape her so that only the area between the thighs is exposed. Assist the doctor by having gloves and instruments ready for use and by applying lubricant to the doctor's gloved fingers. You may also warm the speculum for the patient's comfort. Be prepared to provide reassurance and explanation to a patient who appears to be uncomfortable or nervous. Encourage her to breathe deeply to help relax the pelvic muscles and reduce discomfort.

After checking the vagina and cervix and while the speculum is still in place, the doctor will most likely take a Pap smear (Papanicolaou smear) (Figure 27-11). The doctor then removes the speculum and begins the bimanual phase of the examination. She will ask for your assistance in removing the examining gloves, putting on new gloves, and lubricating two fingers. Placing those fingers in the vagina and using the other hand to palpate the abdomen, the doctor assesses the position of the uterus. She may then place a lubricated finger in the rectum and palpate for abnormal growths with the other hand by pressing on the lower abdomen.

When the doctor completes the examination, she usually asks the patient if she has any questions or concerns. Ask the patient whether she has additional questions after the doctor leaves the examining room. You may need to provide written information in addition to answering the patient's questions orally.

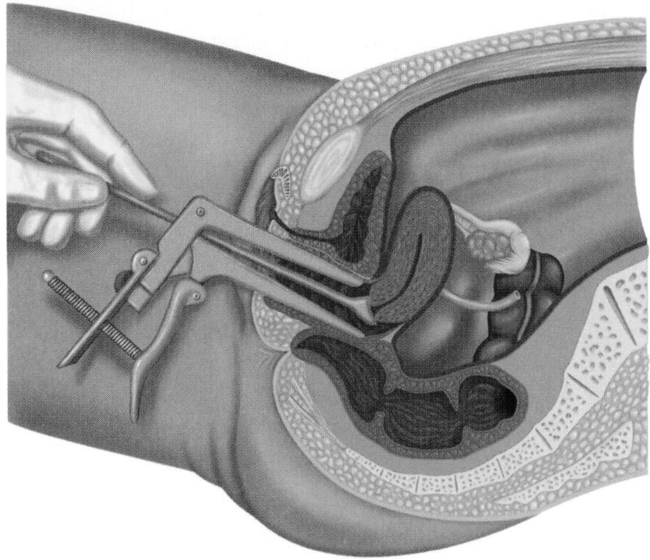

Figure 27-11. A speculum is used to expand the vaginal opening to help view the vagina and cervix.

The medical assistant in many OB/GYN offices provides calendar reminders for noting the last menstrual period and the suggested time for a BSE. Many offices also provide handouts describing female anatomy. Printed materials are available from a variety of sources, including the AMA, government agencies, and pharmaceutical companies.

Life Cycle Changes

Women experience physical changes as a result of maturation. The two distinct changes that occur as part of the life cycle involve menstruation and menopause.

Menstruation. Menstruation is a woman's normal cycle of preparation for conception (the union of egg and sperm that initiates pregnancy). The normal age range of menarche, the beginning of menstruation, is 10 to 15 years of age. Each month (averaging every 28 days) the endometrium, which lines the uterus, is shed in vaginal bleeding. If the woman becomes pregnant, this shedding does not occur, and the woman misses her menstrual period. Note the last menstrual period (LMP) for each patient in her chart at each visit. A period lasts an average of 5 days, with durations of 3 to 7 days considered normal. Menstrual cycles are prompted by changes in hormonal (estrogen and progesterone) levels.

Menopause. Menopause is the cessation of the menstrual cycle. Menopause is a natural occurrence, not a disease or disorder. Several stages surround menopause. Premenopause is the time period before menopause, during which the menstrual periods may be irregular. The time just before and after menopause is called perimenopause. During perimenopause a woman may experience irregular periods, hot flashes, and vaginal dryness, all caused by changing levels of estrogen. Because hormonal change is occurring, the woman may experience mood swings or other psychological changes.

Menopause can also be brought on by the surgical removal of the uterus and ovaries (see the discussion of hysterectomy in this chapter). The symptoms and treatment are the same as those of naturally occurring menopause.

A woman entering menopause may feel embarrassed to discuss her symptoms with you. Reassure her not only that it is a natural occurrence but also that there are ways to make menopause more comfortable. Hormone replacement therapy may be recommended for menopausal comfort and as a preventive treatment for osteoporosis.

Diagnostic Tests and Procedures

The physician uses a number of diagnostic tests, including urine and blood tests (described in Chapters 33 and 34). Many OB/GYN offices have their own small laboratories for immediate results, especially for pregnancy-related tests.

Pregnancy Test. Pregnancy tests are done on a specimen of blood or urine (the patient's first urine of the morning). These tests detect whether or not the hormone human chorionic gonadotropin (HCG), which is produced during pregnancy, is present. A variety of testing kits are available, including over-the-counter urine self-test kits that the patient can use at home.

These tests are not foolproof; false positives and false negatives do occur. An abnormal pregnancy can result in a lower level of HCG, not detectable by the tests. Urine specimens that contain blood, protein, or drugs can also give a false positive result. False negatives may result from testing too early or from a urine specimen that is too dilute. The tests are also subject to human error. The physician confirms pregnancy after taking the patient's history, performing an examination, and ordering a pregnancy test.

Tests for STDs. The doctor diagnoses and treats STDs by taking bacterial and tissue cultures, examining lesions, ordering blood tests, and discussing the patient's history, as appropriate for the specific disease. Some facilities do not permit the release of these results, even to the parents of a minor, without the patient's written consent. Be sure you are familiar with your state's regulations regarding the reporting of STDs to the state epidemiology department.

Radiologic Tests. Several radiologic tests are used in obstetrics and gynecology. The gynecologist uses x-ray, ultrasonography, CT scan, and MRI. X-rays are avoided when a patient is pregnant. If it is crucial for a pregnant woman to have an x-ray, a lead apron must cover her abdomen, and she must be made aware that the x-ray could possibly cause an abnormality in the fetus. You will usually schedule the appointment for radiologic tests. Tell the patient when and where to go for the test, and answer her questions about the procedure. Medical assistants need further training to assist with x-ray procedures.

Hysterosalpingography. Hysterosalpingography is an x-ray examination of the fallopian, or uterine, tubes and the uterus that uses a contrast medium, such as dye or air. Because the procedure is quite uncomfortable, the physician may prescribe a sedative.

Mammogram. A mammogram is a low-dose x-ray of the breast, taken with a special mammogram camera. It can detect cancer about 2 years before it can be palpated with BSE. A first, or baseline, mammogram is taken when a woman is between the ages of 35 and 40 for later comparison.

A patient should schedule mammography for the week after her menstrual period, when the breasts are most normal and least swollen. The procedure involves compressing the breast to obtain a clear x-ray (see Figure 27-12). Tell the patient that although the procedure is uncomfortable, it is usually not painful. The patient should avoid wearing perfume, deodorant, or body powders on the day of the examination because they can cause false readings.

Fetal Screening. Tests for determining the health of an unborn child are performed on many women. Some, such as an ultrasound, may be performed routinely. Other tests are used only for women whose unborn babies are at high risk of having birth defects. Fetal screening tests can indicate the presence of several birth defects, including Down syndrome and spina bifida.

The results of a pregnancy test can provide an early indication of abnormality in the level of HCG. (Some abnormalities produce low levels of HCG, whereas others produce high levels.) This is not definitive, however, and the doctor will probably order other tests. The doctor will

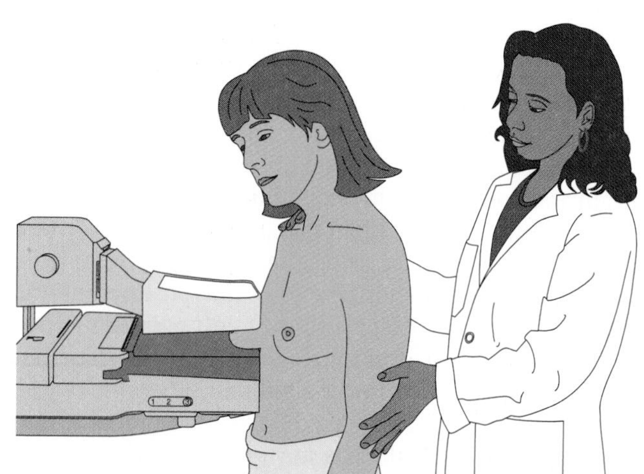

Figure 27-12. Mammography consists of two views of each breast and is achieved by compressing the breast between the radiography plates.

also consider the patient's age and medical history and the age of the unborn baby.

Alpha Fetoprotein. Alpha fetoprotein (AFP) is a protein produced by the unborn child that normally passes into the blood of the mother. A blood test determines whether the AFP level in the blood is normal. Too little or too much AFP in the blood can indicate a fetal abnormality. AFP is also measured in amniotic fluid collected by amniocentesis.

Ultrasound. Ultrasound translates the echoes of sound waves into a picture of an internal part of the body. The picture or image is called a sonogram, and it can help identify and diagnose cysts and tumors in the abdominal cavity or obstructions of the urinary tract. Ultrasound is painless and safe to use on pregnant women to determine fetal size and position. It is also used to guide a physician in performing amniocentesis.

A patient who is going to have an ultrasound examination during early pregnancy should be instructed not to urinate before the test, because a full bladder allows a better view of the uterus. The patient is asked to lie on an examining table, and a gel or lotion is applied to enhance sound wave conduction and reduce friction of the transducer on the skin (Figure 27-13).

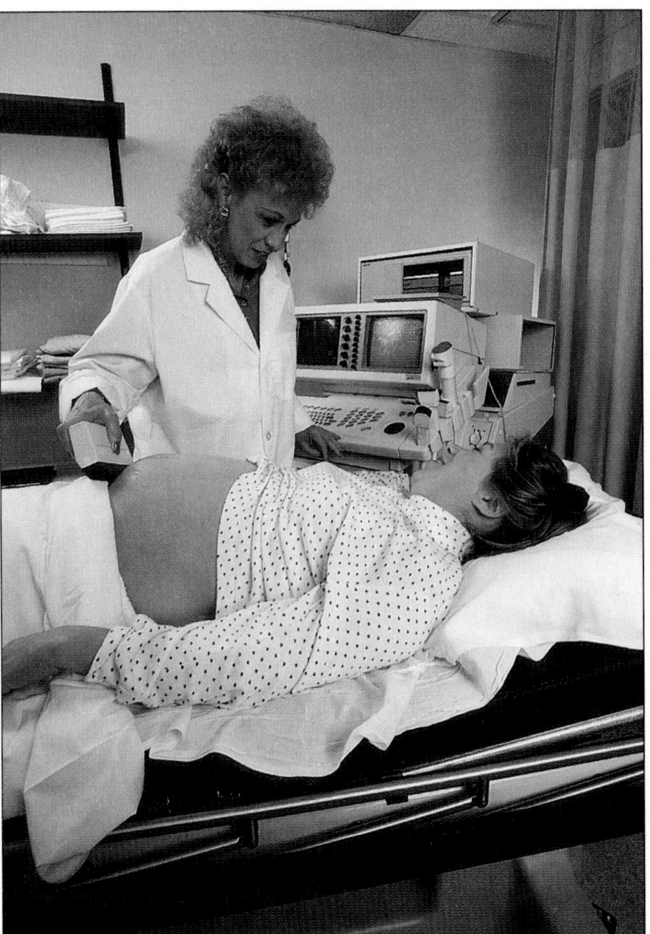

Figure 27-13. An ultrasound technician lightly rubs the transducer over a pregnant woman's abdomen to reveal the anatomy of her fetus.

Diagnostic and Therapeutic Procedures. Many surgical OB/GYN procedures require the use of needles or other instruments to obtain tissue or amniotic fluid samples. Some procedures are used for obstetric reasons only; others may be used gynecologically and obstetrically.

Amniocentesis. Amniocentesis is a procedure performed when a genetic or metabolic defect is suspected in a fetus. The test involves removing a small amount of amniotic fluid, which surrounds the fetus, from the uterus. The doctor inserts a needle, which is guided with ultrasonography, through the anesthetized lower abdominal wall. Fetal skin cells obtained from the fluid are then grown in a culture and examined for chromosomal abnormalities. The level of AFP may also be measured in amniotic fluid.

Biopsy. Biopsy is the surgical removal of tissue for later microscopic examination. It is the most accurate and, in some cases, the only way to diagnose breast and other cancers. Biopsy of the endometrium, which is the mucous membrane lining the uterus, may help the doctor diagnose uterine cancer and show whether ovulation is occurring. It may also indicate whether infection, polyps, or abnormal cells are present. If a patient's Pap smear indicates abnormal cells, a cervical or endocervical biopsy may be performed to rule out or diagnose cervical cancer. Procedure 27-3 explains how to assist with a cervical biopsy.

To assist with these biopsies, you must have knowledge of the female anatomy, the order of procedure, and the instruments used. You will also need to instruct patients about having an escort, appropriate clothing, and any special dietary restrictions. A careful medical history must be obtained to screen for problems such as possible allergic reactions. The day before the biopsy, you might call the patient to confirm the appointment and address any concerns.

Assisting with a biopsy is assisting with minor surgery and consequently requires observance of Universal Precautions and sterile technique. Depending on the extent and site of the biopsy, the patient may be given sedation or local anesthesia. During the procedure you may be responsible for clipping excess material from sutures (stitches) and any other special assistance the doctor requests. You must place the biopsy specimen in a sterile solution-filled container provided by the laboratory. You may assist with or perform the cleaning and bandaging of the site after the procedure.

Colposcopy. **Colposcopy** is the examination of the vagina and cervix with an instrument called a colposcope. Assisting with the colposcopy procedure is similar to assisting with a cervical biopsy. The physician first cleanses the cervix with saline solution. She then cleanses the cervix with acetic acid, which makes abnormal tissue appear white. The physician inserts the colposcope into the vagina and uses the attached magnifying lens to identify abnormal cells, such as cancerous or precancerous cells.

PROCEDURE 27-3

Assisting With a Cervical Biopsy

Objective: To assist the physician in obtaining a sample of cervical tissue for analysis

OSHA Guidelines

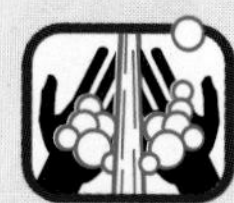 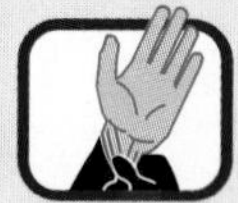 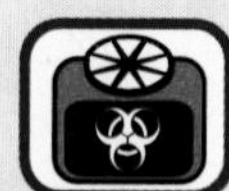

 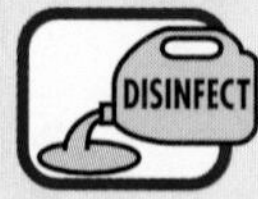

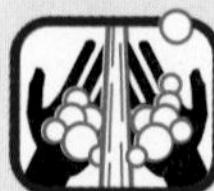

Materials: Gown and drape, tray or Mayo stand, disposable cervical biopsy kit (disposable forceps, curette, and spatula in a sterile pack), transfer forceps, vaginal speculum, biopsy specimen container, clean basin, sterile cotton balls, sterile gauze squares, sanitary napkin

Method

1. Identify the patient and introduce yourself.
2. Look at the patient's chart, and ask the patient to confirm information or explain any changes. Specific patient information you need to ask about and note in the chart includes the following:
   - Date of birth and Social Security number (verify that you have the correct chart for the correct patient)
   - Date of last menstrual period
   - Method of contraception if any
   - Previous gynecologic surgery
   - Use of hormone replacement therapy or other steroids
3. Describe the biopsy procedure to the patient, noting that a piece of tissue will be removed to diagnose the cause of her problem. Explain that it may be painful but only for the brief moment during which tissue is taken.
4. Give the patient a gown, if needed, and a drape. Direct her to undress from the waist down and to wrap the drape around herself. Tell her to sit at the end of the examining table.
5. Wash your hands and put on examination gloves.
6. Using sterile method, open the sterile pack to create a sterile field on the tray or Mayo stand, and arrange the instruments with transfer forceps. Add the vaginal speculum and sterile supplies to the sterile field.
7. When the physician arrives in the examining room, ask the patient to lie back, place her heels in the stirrups of the table, and move her buttocks to the edge of the table.
8. Assist the physician by arranging the drape so that only the genitalia are exposed, and place the light so that the genitalia are illuminated.
9. Use transfer forceps to hand instruments and supplies to the physician as he requests them. When he is ready to obtain the biopsy, tell the patient that it may hurt. If she seems particularly fearful, instruct her to take a deep breath and let it out slowly.
10. When the physician hands you the instrument with the tissue specimen, place the specimen in the specimen container and discard the instrument in the appropriate container.
11. Label the specimen container with the patient's name, the date and time, cervical or endocervical (as indicated by the physician), the physician's name, and your initials.
12. Place the container and the cytology laboratory requisition form in the envelope or bag provided by the laboratory.
13. When the physician has removed the vaginal speculum, place it in the clean basin for later sanitization, disinfection, and sterilization. Properly dispose of used supplies and disposable instruments.
14. Remove the gloves and wash your hands.
15. Tell the patient that she may get dressed. Inform her that she may have some vaginal bleeding for a couple of days, and provide her with a sanitary napkin. Instruct her not to take tub baths or have intercourse and not to use tampons for 2 days. Encourage her to call the office if she experiences problems or has questions.

This procedure is often performed prior to a biopsy after results of a Pap smear show the presence of abnormal cells. The abnormal cells may not be cancerous but caused by infection or medication.

Dilation and Curettage (D & C). A D & C consists of widening the opening of the cervix (dilation) and scraping the uterine lining (curettage). Reasons for the D & C procedure include assessing the size and shape of the uterus, removing polyps and fibroids from the endometrium, obtaining endometrial specimens for biopsy, performing an abortion, and completing an incomplete miscarriage. Other diagnoses for which a D & C may be performed include abnormal uterine bleeding, abnormal menstrual bleeding, postcoital bleeding, spotting between periods, postmenopausal bleeding, and an imbedded intrauterine device (IUD).

The procedure is usually performed in a hospital or outpatient surgical facility. Tell the patient she will need to have someone take her to and from the facility. Inform the patient that she will have anesthesia before the doctor performs a routine pelvic examination. The doctor then swabs the vagina with an antiseptic and inserts a speculum. After dilating the cervix, the doctor uses a curette to remove a portion of the endometrium to assess the texture. Both cervical and endometrial tissue may be sent to a laboratory for examination. Exploration of the uterine cavity and removal of any abnormal growths complete the procedure.

Instruct the patient not to have intercourse, take tub baths, or use tampons for 1 week after the procedure. She should also avoid strenuous activity.

Fine-Needle Aspiration. During fine-needle aspiration the physician uses a fine needle to remove by vacuum a sample of tissue from a cyst, lump, or tumor of the breast. This procedure may be used instead of mammography to diagnose breast disorders in pregnant patients, thus avoiding the use of radiation. Patients with fibrocystic breast disease (involving multiple cystic lumps within the breast tissue) may have needle aspiration of a cyst followed by replacement of the cystic fluid with a steroid to prevent recurrence.

Hysterectomy. A hysterectomy is the surgical removal of the uterus. If surgery includes removal of one or both fallopian tubes, it is called a hysterosalpingectomy. Surgical removal of the uterus, the fallopian tubes, and the ovaries is called a hysterosalpingo-oophorectomy. A hysterectomy or a related surgery may be performed for the following reasons: cervical or endometrial cancer; severe endometriosis; unusual bleeding; a leiomyoma, or fibroid; defects of pelvic supports; pregnancy-related problems; and pelvic adhesions or other causes of uterine pain not controllable by other methods.

Inform the patient that a procedure of this type is major surgery that requires hospitalization. It also requires preadmission urine and blood tests, cleansing enemas, and shaving of the pelvic area. Normal activities, including sexual intercourse, can usually be resumed within a few weeks.

Premenopausal women who have hysterectomies or hysterosalpingectomies may begin menopause sooner than they otherwise would have. Premenopausal women who have hysterosalpingo-oophorectomies will experience menopause immediately after the surgery. The doctor may prescribe hormone replacement therapy to help alleviate menopausal symptoms.

Laparoscopy. A laparoscope is a long tubular instrument. It contains fiberoptic fibers that illuminate the organs and a lens that resembles a small telescope. A physician can use the laparoscope to view the internal female organs. Laparoscopy is used to help determine the cause of infertility, to obtain tissue samples, to remove abnormal growths, and to surgically sterilize a patient. It is also used in the treatment of ectopic pregnancies, endometriosis, and laparoscopy-assisted hysterectomy.

The patient is anesthetized before a tube is inserted into a small incision in or near the navel. Carbon dioxide or another gas is pumped into the abdomen to spread the organs apart and thereby make them easier to see. The patient's body is then tilted with her head lower than her hips to allow the intestines to move away from the lower abdomen. This positioning permits a clearer view of the ovaries, uterus, and fallopian tubes.

Pap Smear. A Pap smear is used to determine the presence of abnormal or precancerous cells. During a pelvic examination, cells from the cervix, endocervix, and vagina are smeared on a special, properly labeled slide. They are then sprayed with a fixative and sent to a laboratory for microscopic analysis. The test results are classified according to level of abnormality, using the standardized Bethesda system (Figure 27-14):

- Within normal limits: no abnormal cells
- Atypical cells: no evidence of malignant cells; slight abnormal cellular changes noted (these changes are often associated with inflammatory conditions and frequently return to normal after appropriate treatment)
- Low-grade lesion: cellular abnormalities consistent with a potentially precancerous condition
- High-grade lesion: cellular abnormalities suspicious for early noninvasive cancer
- Malignancy: cellular abnormalities consistent with an invasive cancerous condition

Pregnancy

Pregnancy progresses in three stages. These stages are referred to as trimesters, and each lasts for 3 months. Figure 27-15 shows the developing fetus during each stage of growth.

First Trimester. After conception the resulting cell begins to divide. This cluster of cells, the embryo, is implanted in the uterine wall about 36 hours after fertilization. Implantation initiates the embryonic period, during which most of the organ systems develop. The embryonic period lasts 8 weeks, after which the embryo is called a fetus. Week 12 marks the end of the first trimester, or one-third of the pregnancy.

Second Trimester. Fine, soft hair (lanugo) appears on the shoulders, back, and head of the fetus during the fourth month. By the twentieth week fetal movement may be felt, and the pregnant woman begins to show fullness in the abdomen. There are identifiable periods of fetal sleep and wakefulness as the second trimester ends at the completion of the sixth month.

Third Trimester. The last trimester encompasses the most noticeable period of growth, both in the fetus and

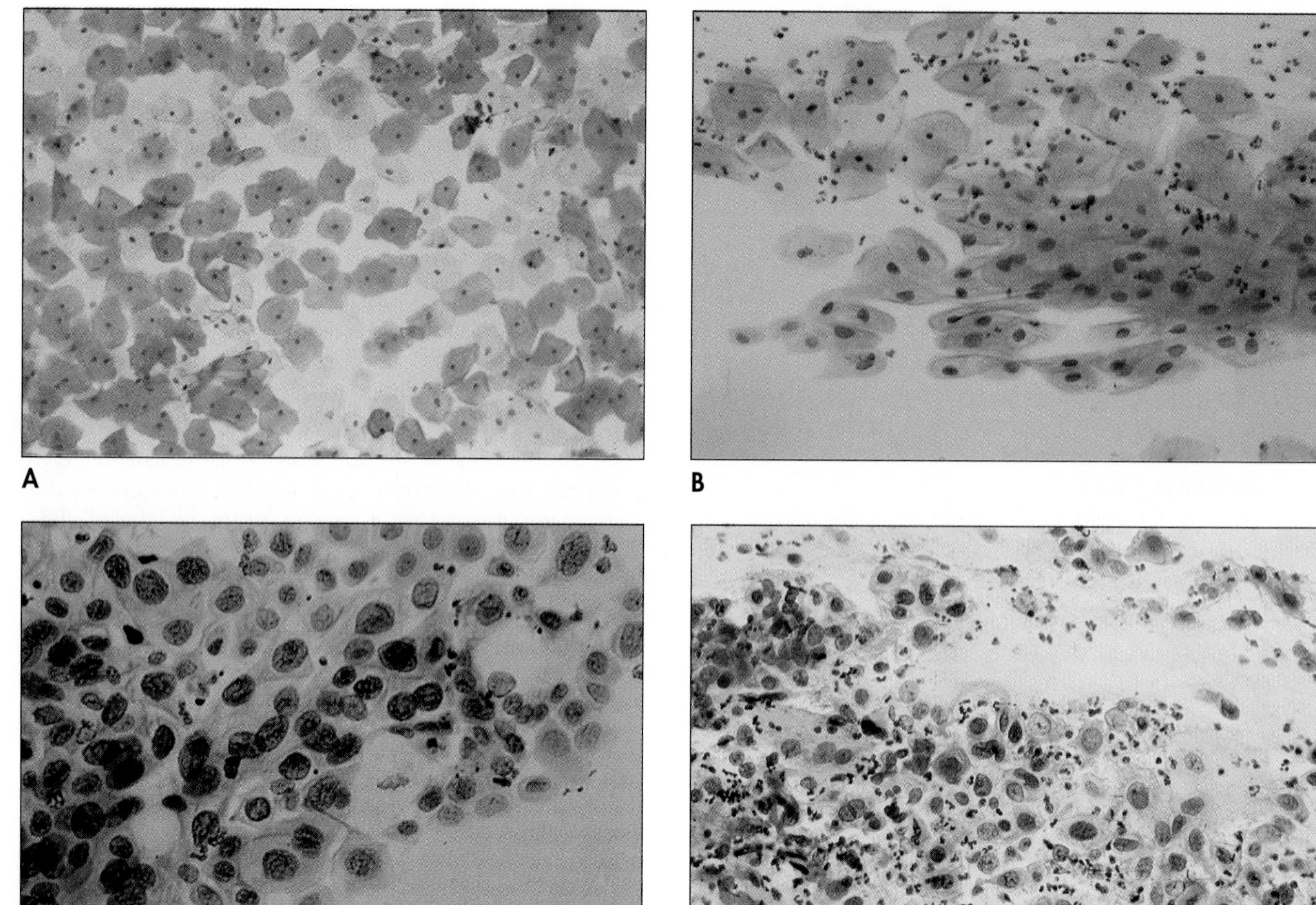

Figure 27-14. Upon treatment with Papanicolaou stain and microscopic evaluation, cervical and vaginal cells may indicate normal variations, as shown in (a); one of three levels of increasingly abnormal changes, as shown in (b), (c), and (d); or malignancy, as shown in (e). The abnormal changes include variations in size and shape, increasing nucleus-to-cytoplasm ratios, and invasiveness.

in the mother. By the end of 30 weeks, the fetus has assumed a head-down position and has a 50% chance of survival if it is born at this time. The fetus is said to have come full term after it is approximately 9 months (40 weeks) old.

Nägele's Rule. To estimate the delivery date for a pregnant woman, most doctors use Nägele's rule. Begin with the first day of the patient's last menstrual period, subtract 3 months, and add 7 days plus 1 year. If, for example, the first day of the last menstrual period was June 30, 1998, subtracting 3 months would give you March 30, 1998. After the addition of 7 days plus 1 year, April 6, 1999, would be the estimated delivery date.

Prenatal Care. Pregnant women need to be particularly attentive to nutrition, exercise, medical monitoring, and childbirth classes. They should avoid using tobacco, alco-

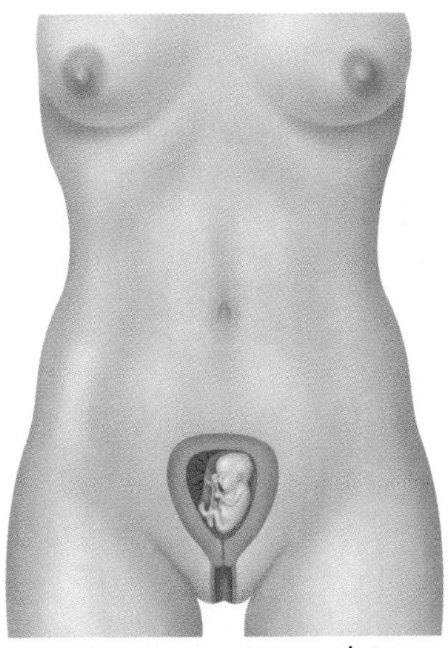
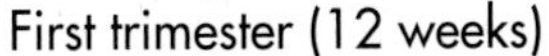
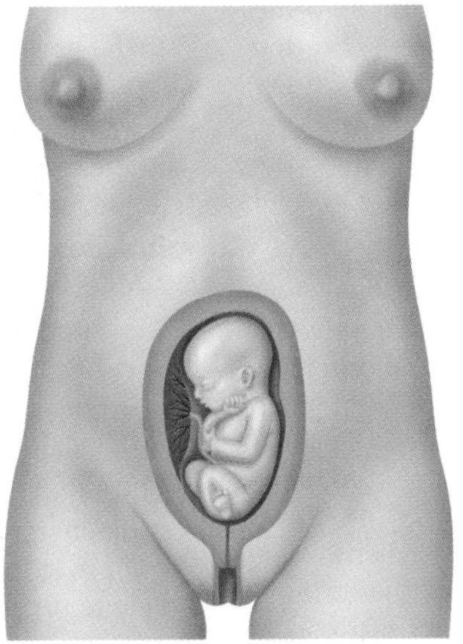
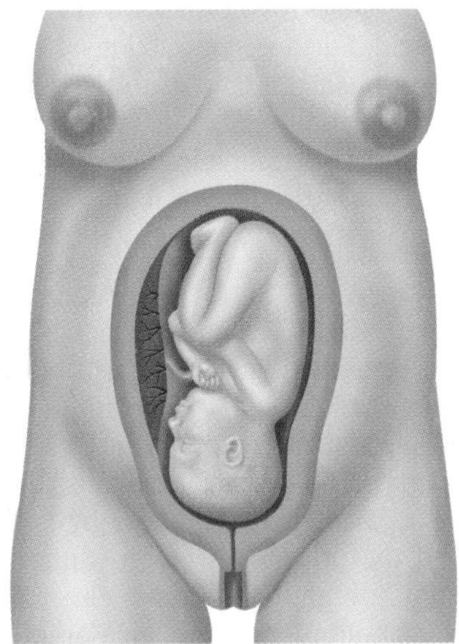

First trimester (12 weeks) Second trimester (24 weeks) Third trimester (38 weeks)

Figure 27-15. The fetus develops over the course of three trimesters.

hol, and drugs. Normal manifestations during pregnancy include morning sickness (usually in the first trimester), weight gain, urinary frequency, fatigue, depression, constipation, and swollen hands and feet.

You may perform or assist with routine tests for pregnant women, or you may send them to an outside laboratory. These tests may include the complete blood count (CBC), Rh-antibody determination, blood typing, Pap smear, urinalysis, and hematocrit. Others may include tests for syphilis, hepatitis B antibodies, HIV, and chlamydia.

Assisting With Prenatal Care. You will play an important role in encouraging the obstetric patient to have regular checkups and to take proper care of herself. You will also help teach and support both parents throughout the pregnancy. You must document all information given to or taken from the patient.

Providing information on the effects of using drugs or alcohol during pregnancy is particularly important. Alcohol, for example, crosses the placental barrier and directly affects fetal development. Drinking alcohol during pregnancy can cause fetal alcohol syndrome (FAS). This syndrome may include fetal growth deficiencies, mental retardation or learning disabilities, heart defects, cleft palate, a small head, a small brain, and deformed limbs. There is no known safe level of alcohol consumption during pregnancy. You can help prevent FAS by teaching all pregnant patients about the potential effects of alcohol on their unborn babies. If a pregnant patient who is an alcoholic expresses a desire to stop drinking, inform the physician, who may wish to discuss admission to an alcoholic rehabilitation program with her. You may also refer the patient to Alcoholics Anonymous or a similar community group for assistance. Drug use during pregnancy poses similar problems for a woman's developing fetus.

When assisting with routine prenatal patient visits, you may:

1. Ask the patient about any problems and record any symptoms she reports.
2. Ask the patient to empty her bladder and obtain a urine specimen in the cup you provide.
3. Weigh the patient and note her weight in the chart.
4. Perform the reagent urine test (chemical analysis) and note the results in her chart.
5. Give the patient a drape and ask her to undress from the waist down if the physician will be performing an internal examination.
6. Assist the patient to the examining table. Take her vital signs. Record them in her chart.
7. Assist the physician as needed with the examination. Provide the flexible centimeter tape measure and Doppler, an instrument used to listen to fetal heartbeat.
8. Assist the patient from the examining table after the examination.

Prenatal Care by the Doctor. The doctor carefully monitors the progress of a pregnancy. She watches blood pressure, weight changes, and urinalysis results for possible signs of preeclampsia. Increased blood pressure (hypertension), unusual weight gain due to edema, and protein in the urine are signs of this serious complication of pregnancy. The doctor examines urine specimens for possible urinary tract infections and occasionally asks for other laboratory tests, such as a complete blood count. She may prescribe special vitamins and iron as dietary supplements.

Labor. Changes occur in the mother's body chemistry when the fetus is ready to be born. These changes signal the release of the hormone oxytocin, which initiates labor. The first stage of labor is marked by regular contractions and cervical dilation. The second stage is characterized by complete cervical dilation and the entrance of the head (or buttocks if it is a breech birth) into the vagina. Further contractions and the mother's bearing down push the baby into the birth canal and out of the mother's body. The last contractions push out the placenta and its membranes (afterbirth), attached to the baby with the umbilical cord. This is the third and final stage of labor.

Delivery. At birth a newborn's average weight and length are 7.5 lb and 20 inches. The baby's mouth and nose are suctioned to clear them of mucus. Crying indicates that the baby is breathing on her own. The lungs inflate and the color of the skin changes from bluish to normal. The physician clamps, ties, and cuts the umbilical cord and presents the baby to the mother.

If the pregnant woman cannot deliver the baby vaginally, the physician may deliver the baby by performing an operation known as a cesarean section. Several conditions may require a cesarean section, such as a large baby in a breech position. To perform a cesarean section, the physician makes a series of incisions. First the skin, underlying muscles, and abdomen are opened. Then the uterus is opened, and the infant is removed.

Newborn Function Testing. The newborn is assessed at 1 and 5 minutes after delivery for neurological function. The tests are repeated until the infant's condition stabilizes. With the Apgar test, the baby's heart rate, respiratory effort, muscle tone, reflex irritability, and color are each evaluated with a score of 0, 1, or 2. The best possible Apgar rating is 10 (five evaluations with a score of 2). A score of 7 to 9 is adequate; 4 to 6 indicates that treatment and close observation are warranted; below 4 requires immediate treatment.

Breast-Feeding. Human milk is the preferred form of nutrition for an infant. Colostrum, the first milk the mother produces after delivery, is rich in antibodies that provide passive natural immunity to the baby as well. Breast-feeding is economical and convenient. There is no need to buy or make formula or wash bottles and nipples. Breast milk is always available to the baby at the correct temperature.

A woman's success at breast-feeding depends largely on her desire to breast-feed, her satisfaction with it, and her available support systems. You can support patients who choose to breast-feed by providing them with pamphlets and other written materials. Emphasize how essential the mother's nutritional intake is, and explain that she needs to follow a high-protein, high-calorie diet. You may also refer patients who need help to lactation consultants or support groups such as the La Leche League.

Contraception

Couples who want to prevent pregnancy practice contraception. The type of contraception chosen is based on variables such as price, convenience, effectiveness, and side effects. The only method that is 100% effective is abstinence. Contraceptive methods include the following.

- The birth control pill is a daily oral contraceptive. Synthetic hormones in the pills inhibit ovulation.
- Subdermal implants consist of six capsules of synthetic hormone that are surgically implanted under the skin of the arm. They provide 5 years of contraception and are reversible.
- Injection is a method in which a synthetic hormone is administered every 3 months to inhibit ovulation.
- A condom is worn on the penis to serve as a barrier to sperm.
- Spermicidal foam, cream, jelly, and vaginal suppositories contain spermicides (sperm-killing chemicals). They are inserted into the woman's vagina.
- A diaphragm is a dome-shaped rubber cup prescribed to fit over the patient's cervix and used with spermicide to provide a barrier to sperm.
- A cervical cap is similar to a diaphragm, except that it covers a smaller area of the woman's cervix.
- An IUD is a small piece of plastic or metal that fits inside the uterus and inhibits fertilization or implantation. Insertion of an IUD is performed by a doctor.
- Sterilization is a surgical procedure. A man can have a vasectomy, in which the doctor removes a section of each tube that carries sperm from each testicle to the penis. A female can have her fallopian tubes cut or blocked.
- Periodic abstinence (sometimes called the rhythm method) involves refraining from sexual intercourse when a woman is fertile and likely to become pregnant.
- Withdrawal consists of withdrawing the penis from the vagina before ejaculation occurs.
- Mifepristone, formerly known as RU-486, is a postcoital pill taken to prevent implantation of the embryo in the uterus. This controversial drug was approved for use in the United States in 1996.

Infertility

Infertility is the inability of a couple to conceive a child. Physicians usually test both the man and woman for infertility. Depending on the cause of the problem, the physician may treat the man, the woman, or both.

If you work in an OB/GYN office, the physicians may test couples for fertility and provide them with treatments or options so they can have children. In such an office you should be familiar with basic infertility tests and treatments. You may need to explain procedures to couples, assist with tests or treatments, and provide emotional support and encouragement.

Tests to determine the cause of infertility in a woman examine whether ovulation occurs, whether the fallopian tubes are clear of obstruction, whether the uterus is healthy enough to support the implantation and growth of a fetus, and whether the woman is healthy enough to maintain pregnancy. Tests to determine the cause of infertility in a man examine whether the sperm are healthy and numerous enough to fertilize an egg.

Treatments for possible abnormal conditions include hormone injections, microsurgery, "washing" of the sperm to remove antibodies, ovulation induction, and artificial insemination. If the treatments are not successful, the couple may accept infertility and decide to adopt a child or remain childless, or they may not accept infertility and decide to use assisted reproductive technologies. Such technologies provide infertile couples with options. The procedures include in vitro fertilization and embryo replacement (IVF-ER) and variations of that procedure.

Diseases and Disorders

Many of the diseases and disorders encountered in the OB/GYN practice have been mentioned in the context of the procedures above. Table 27-3 outlines common obstetric and gynecologic diseases and disorders.

Summary

Many specialties provide you with opportunities for rewarding and challenging work as a medical assistant. You might enjoy working in the specialty of internal medicine, assisting doctors who diagnose and treat disorders and diseases of the body's internal organs. In such a practice you might assess patients for chronic fatigue syndrome or help detect possible substance abuse. You could perform or assist with diagnostic testing such as urine and blood tests and bacterial cultures. You might educate patients on diseases of aging, infectious diseases, and sexually transmitted diseases.

Pediatrics might provide interesting and satisfying work, especially if you like working with children. Your primary responsibilities would involve educating parents or caregivers, preparing children for examination, and detecting child abuse. Specific duties might include performing a scoliosis examination, assisting in regular checkups, and performing a throat culture to test for strep. Your role as an educator could involve providing facts on sudden infant death syndrome to parents or giving pamphlets on learning disabilities to caregivers.

Obstetricians and gynecologists are specialists who treat conditions of the female reproductive system, care for pregnant women, and deliver babies. Assisting in this specialty might involve preparing women for a pelvic examination, assisting with a cervical biopsy, and providing support to infertile couples. You would also be responsible for providing information to pregnant women about prenatal care.

Medical assisting positions in the basic specialties usually involve a wide range of responsibilities and tasks. You will find many opportunities to develop your skills and interests if you work in one of these medical specialties.

Table 27-3

Common Obstetric and Gynecologic Diseases and Disorders

Condition	Description	Treatment
Cancer	Common occurrence in cervix, endometrium (uterus), ovaries; cells divide uncontrollably, eventually forming tumor or other growth of abnormal tissue; most often seen in women between ages of 50 and 60; symptoms differ for each type of cancer	Surgery (hysterectomy), radiation, chemotherapy, hormones; for ovarian cancer, surgical removal of all reproductive organs, affected lymph nodes, appendix, and some muscle tissue, followed by chemotherapy (to extend survival time)
Ectopic pregnancy	Fertilized egg unable to move out of fallopian tube into uterus for implantation; patient experiences pain within a few weeks of conception; can be fatal	Surgery to remove embryo from fallopian tube before tube ruptures
Endometriosis	Endometrial tissue present outside uterus, usually in pelvic area; not life-threatening but may cause sterility; symptoms include abnormal menstruation and pain (sometimes severe) in lower abdominal area and back	Hormone therapy, hysterectomy for severe cases, endometrial ablation (1-day surgery, alternative to hysterectomy), leuprolide acetate injection
Fibroids, or leiomyomas	Common, benign, smooth tumors of muscle cells (not fibrous tissue) grouped in uterus; symptoms include excessive menstruation and bloating; diagnosis by bimanual examination and ultrasound	Surgery for severe cases

continued

Table 27-3 continued

Common Obstetric and Gynecologic Diseases and Disorders

Condition	Description	Treatment
Fibrocystic breast disease	Benign, fluid-filled cysts or nodules in breast; sometimes confused with malignant growths in breast until complete diagnostic tests performed; symptoms include pain and tenderness	Depending on severity, vitamin E supplements, hormones, compresses, analgesics, aspiration, biopsy; restricted caffeine intake
Menstrual disturbances	May be (1) amenorrhea (absence of menstruation), (2) dysmenorrhea (painful menstruation), (3) menorrhagia (excessive amount of menstrual flow or prolonged period of menstruation), or (4) metrorrhagia (bleeding between menstrual periods)	Treatment according to symptoms; analgesics; possibly D & C; for severe cases, hysterectomy
Ovarian cysts	Sacs of fluid or semisolid material, usually benign and without symptoms; occur anytime between puberty and menopause; extensive ovarian cysts may cause pelvic discomfort, lower back pain, and abnormal bleeding	Analgesics and bed rest if severe pain; hormone therapy; surgery, usually reserved for cysts that rupture or are large enough to put pressure on surrounding organs
Pelvic inflammatory disease (PID)	Acute, chronic infection of reproductive tract; causes include untreated STDs, such as gonorrhea and chlamydia, and organisms such as staphylococci and streptococci; symptoms include vaginal discharge, fever, and general discomfort	Antibiotics
Pelvic support problems	Abnormal weakening of vaginal tissue, unusual increase in abdominal pressure, congenital weakening (weakness since birth); symptoms include urine leakage, pelvic heaviness ("bottom falling out"), pain or discomfort in pelvic area, pulling or aching feeling in lower back, abdomen, or groin	Kegel or perineal exercises to strengthen muscles, insertion of pessary (device to hold pelvic organs in place), surgery to repair muscles
Polyps	Red, soft, and fragile growths, with slender stem attachment, sometimes found on mucous membranes of cervix or endometrium; may cause pain	Depending on size and shape, may be removed in office or hospital
Premenstrual syndrome (PMS)	Symptoms include swelling, bloating, weight gain, breast tenderness, headaches, and mood shifts 1 week to 10 days before menstruation	Vitamins, diuretics, hormones, oral contraceptives, tranquilizers, other medications; stress-reduction methods as needed; restricted intake of dietary sodium, alcohol, and caffeine
Sexual function disorders	Interruption or lack of sexual response cycle (excitement, plateau, orgasm, and resolution); unhealthy view of one's feelings about oneself as a woman and feelings toward sex; sometimes caused by painful intercourse, abusive partner, unrealistic demands on oneself, or menopause	Counseling (for both woman and partner) to teach relaxation, effective communication, and identification of cycle stages and natural responses
Vaginitis	Inflammation of vagina caused by bacteria, viruses, yeasts, or chemicals in sprays, douches, or tampons; symptoms include itching, redness, pain, swelling	Treatment prescribed according to cause; avoiding douches, tampons, tight pants, wiping from back to front; sometimes avoiding sex during treatment

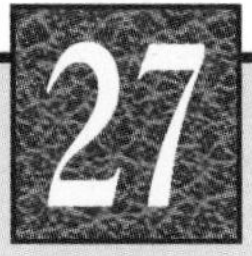

Chapter Review

Discussion Questions

1. Suppose you are the medical assistant to an internist. As you are preparing a patient for an examination, the patient describes some symptoms that sound as if they could be part of an STD. What should you say? What should you not say?
2. What would you say to a child who is afraid to go into the examination room? How could you make her more comfortable?
3. How can a woman take responsibility for the health of her reproductive system? How can you help a patient do this?

Critical Thinking Questions

1. A patient calls because he has found a small tick behind his son's ear. What would you advise him to do?
2. While preparing a woman for a gynecologic examination, you notice several cuts and bruises. What would you say or do?
3. A patient comes in with slurred speech and behavior that suggests intoxication. What types of substances might this patient be abusing? How might you differentiate between them?

Application Activities

1. Find out the scope of practice for medical assistants in the state where you live. Write a brief report in which you describe the ways medical assistants are permitted to assist in examinations, procedures, and diagnostic testing and which of them medical assistants are permitted to perform alone.
2. Instruct another student in how to prevent STDs. Be sure to encourage the student to ask questions. Then ask the student to evaluate your teaching technique.
3. Create a list of potential subjects to discuss with a patient who comes in for a routine examination with a gynecologist—first for a 16-year-old girl and then for a middle-aged woman.

Further Readings

Brody, Jane E. "Strep Throat: Heading Off a Vicious Circle of Infection." *New York Times,* 20 March 1996, sec. C, p. 13.

DiCowden, Marie. "Pediatric Rehabilitation: Special Patients, Special Needs." *Journal of Rehabilitation,* July 1990, 13.

Feil, Sarah J. "Chronic Fatigue Syndrome: A Real and Debilitating Illness." *The Professional Medical Assistant,* July/August 1993, 19–23.

Juckett, Gregory. "Common Intestinal Helminths." *American Family Physician,* 15 November 1995, 2039.

McAfee, Robert E. "Violence in America: Making a Difference One Patient at a Time." *The Professional Medical Assistant,* January/February 1996, 5–9.

Neergaard, Joyce A. "A Proposal for a Foster Grandmother Intervention Program to Prevent Child Abuse." *Public Health Reports,* January 1990, 89.

Pellman, Harry. "Infestations That Itch: Head Lice and Scabies." *Pediatrics for Parents,* March 1994, 4.

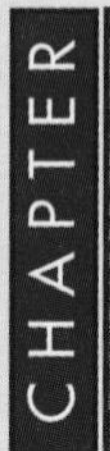
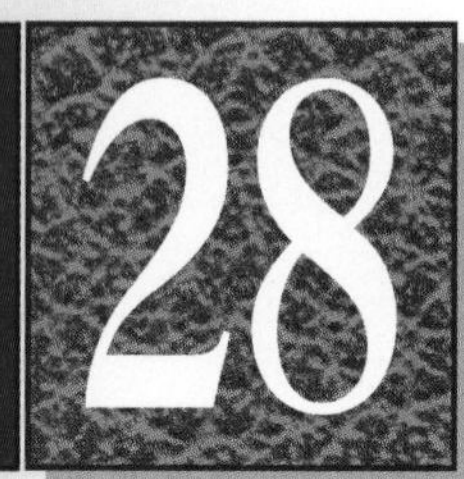

Assisting With Highly Specialized Examinations

CHAPTER OUTLINE

- The Medical Assistant's Role in Specialty Examinations
- Allergy
- Cardiology
- Dermatology
- Endocrinology
- Gastroenterology
- Neurology
- Oncology
- Ophthalmology
- Orthopedics
- Otology
- Surgery
- Urology

OBJECTIVES

After completing Chapter 28, you will be able to:

- Briefly describe the medical specialties of allergy, cardiology, dermatology, endocrinology, gastroenterology, neurology, oncology, ophthalmology, orthopedics, otology, surgery, and urology.
- Describe the types of examinations and diagnostic tests performed in each of these specialties and the medical assistant's role in these examinations and tests.
- Identify and describe the most common diseases and disorders seen in these medical specialties and typical treatments for them.
- Describe the medical assistant's duties in performing a scratch test.
- Describe the medical assistant's role in assisting with a sigmoidoscopy.
- Outline the medical assistant's responsibilities in preparing the ophthalmoscope for use.
- Describe the medical assistant's role in assisting with a needle biopsy.

AREAS OF COMPETENCE

1997 ROLE DELINEATION STUDY

CLINICAL

Diagnostic Orders

- Collect and process specimens
- Perform diagnostic tests

Patient Care

- Prepare patient for examinations, procedures, and treatments

continued

Key Terms

anaphylaxis
angiography
arthroscopy
cardiac catheterization
cholecystography
colonoscopy
computed tomography
diabetes mellitus
echocardiography
electroencephalography
electromyography
endoscopy
fracture
intradermal test
magnetic resonance imaging
metastasis
myelography
ophthalmoscope
patch test
proctoscopy
refraction examination
scratch test
sigmoidoscopy
slitlamp
stress test
vasectomy
whole-body skin examination
Wood's light examination

AREAS OF COMPETENCE continued

GENERAL (Transdisciplinary)

Instruction
- Explain office policies and procedures
- Teach methods of health promotion and disease prevention

The Medical Assistant's Role in Specialty Examinations

You learned about examinations in a number of basic medical specialties in Chapter 27. This chapter discusses examinations that are highly specialized. Physicians working in these areas focus on one body system (such as the skin) or even on a single type of disease (such as cancer) or medical intervention (such as surgery).

Although the examinations and procedures differ from specialty to specialty, as a medical assistant you will be expected to perform certain tasks wherever you are employed. You will, for example, perform general administrative and clinical tasks. You will assist with examinations and procedures and perform certain procedures on your own. It is important that you understand the anatomy and physiology of various body systems as well as the specific examination and procedural steps for each specialty area.

Another responsibility will be communicating with and educating patients. Certain concerns and questions are common to patients within a specialty area. Being prepared to address these concerns and questions will allow you to help patients effectively and fulfill a vital role on the medical team.

Allergy

An allergist specializes in diagnosing and treating allergies. Allergies involve inappropriate immune system responses to substances that are normally harmless. During an allergic reaction, inflammation and tissue damage occur. The substances that cause allergic reactions are called allergens. Common allergens include certain foods (such as eggs and nuts), pollens, medications, insect venom, and animal saliva or dander. Allergic reactions may show themselves locally—with a skin rash or nasal congestion—or may manifest themselves throughout the body.

The most severe kind of allergic reaction is **anaphylaxis,** or anaphylactic shock, which is life-threatening. Symptoms of anaphylaxis include respiratory distress, difficulty in swallowing, pallor, and a drastic drop in blood pressure that can lead to circulatory collapse. When anaphylaxis occurs, immediate medical intervention is needed to save the patient's life. Chapter 31 addresses emergency medical intervention in anaphylaxis.

Allergy Examinations

An allergy examination involves a medical history and, usually, several diagnostic tests. You may assist with these tests or perform them yourself under a physician's supervision. Skin tests, for example, involve introducing solutions containing suspected allergens onto or just below the skin. Any reaction is observed and assessed.

As an allergist's medical assistant, you will need to understand the function of the immune system and how allergies are commonly treated. Allergy treatments include allergen avoidance, medications, and desensitization to a substance by means of injections. Part of your job will be to encourage patients to make necessary lifestyle changes to avoid allergens. You will also help them adhere to regimens of injections or medication.

PROCEDURE 28-1

Performing a Scratch Test

Objective: To determine substances to which a patient has an allergic reaction

OSHA Guidelines

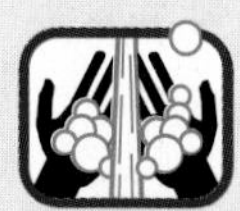
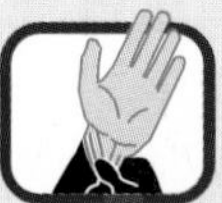
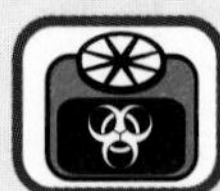

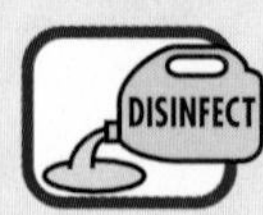

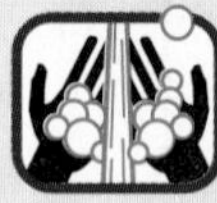

Materials: Disposable sterile needles or lancets, allergen extracts, control solution, cotton balls, alcohol, timer, adhesive tape, ruler, cold packs or ice bag

Method

1. Wash your hands and assemble the necessary materials.
2. Identify the patient and introduce yourself.
3. Show the patient into the treatment area. Explain the procedure and discuss any concerns.
4. Put on examination gloves and assist the patient into a comfortable position.
5. Swab the test site, usually the upper arm or back, with an alcohol-soaked cotton ball. Allow the test site to air-dry.
6. Apply small drops of the allergen extracts and control solution onto the test site at evenly spaced intervals, about 1.5 to 2.0 inches apart.
7. Identify the sites (if more than one) with adhesive-tape labels (see Figure 28-1).
8. Open the package containing the first needle or lancet, making sure you do not contaminate the instrument.
9. Using a new sterile needle or lancet for each site, scratch the skin beneath each drop of allergen, no more than ⅛ inch deep.

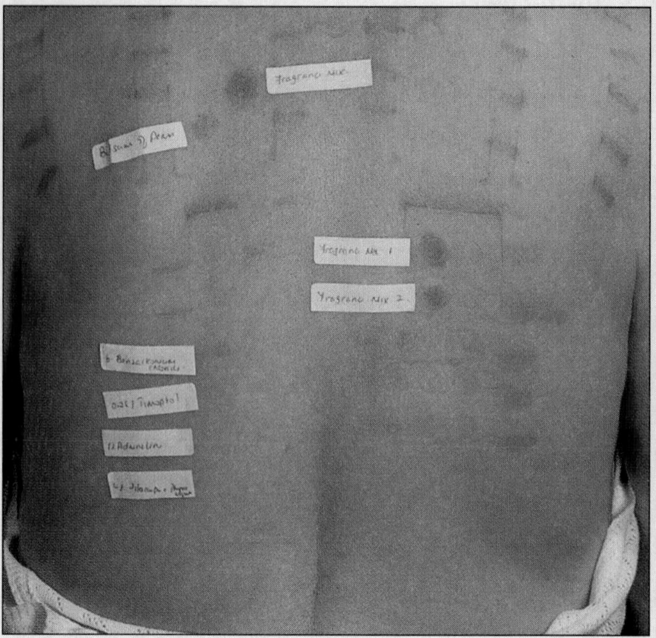

Figure 28-1. Label each site with the name of the allergen or an accepted abbreviation.

10. Start the timer for the 20-minute reaction period.
11. After the reaction time has passed, cleanse each site with an alcohol-soaked cotton ball. (Do not remove identifying labels until the doctor has checked the patient.)
12. Examine and measure the sites (see Figure 28-2).
13. Apply cold packs or an ice bag to sites as needed to relieve itching.
14. Record the test results in the patient's chart, and initial your entries.
15. Properly dispose of used materials and instruments.
16. Clean and disinfect the area according to OSHA guidelines.
17. Remove the gloves and wash your hands.

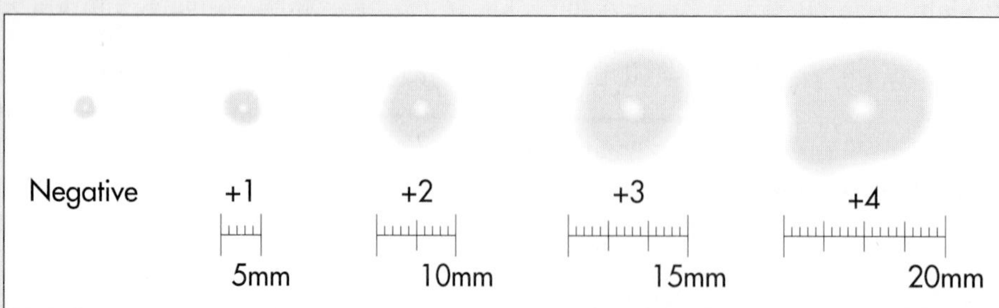

Figure 28-2. Physicians classify skin reactions as either negative (no greater than the reaction to the control) or positive. Positive reactions are rated on a scale of +1 to +4, depending on the size of the wheal.

Allergy Testing

Three tests are commonly performed in the allergist's office. They are the scratch test, the intradermal test, and the patch test. The radioallergosorbent test is performed in a laboratory.

Scratch Test. A **scratch test** is performed to test the patient for specific allergies. Extracts of suspected allergens are applied to the patient's skin, usually on the arms or back. One site is always a negative control—a solution like that used to carry the allergens but containing no allergen is applied. Then the skin is scratched to allow the extracts to penetrate. Procedure 28-1 describes how to perform a scratch test using sterile needles or lancets. Some allergists prefer to use multiple applicators that allow the tester to apply allergens to and puncture the skin in several places at once, as shown in Figure 28-3.

Be sure to let the patient know that the procedure may cause some discomfort and that itching afterward can be relieved with cold packs. The doctor interprets the test results. Because a delayed reaction is possible, the doctor may wish to recheck the scratch sites in 24 hours. When the results of the scratch test are inconclusive, another test, such as an intradermal test, may be ordered.

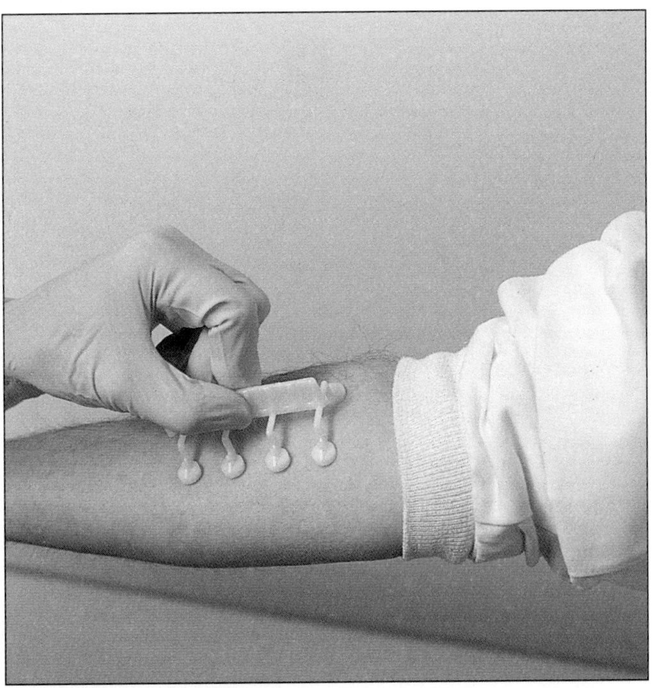

Figure 28-3. A multiple applicator allows the medical assistant to apply several allergens at one time.

Intradermal Test. An allergist performs an **intradermal test** by introducing dilute solutions of allergens into the skin of the inner forearm or upper back with a fine-gauge needle. The intradermal test is more sensitive than the scratch test. A small blister, filled with the introduced fluid, appears on the skin over the injection site. The allergic reaction time is about 15 to 30 minutes, although some substances may cause delayed reactions. If no reaction appears, the test can be repeated with a more concentrated solution to confirm the result. If a severe reaction occurs, the doctor will order epinephrine to be administered.

The tuberculin test, or purified protein derivative (PPD) test, is a type of intradermal skin test. In most offices today it is administered with a needle and syringe. (In the past this test was administered using a disposable device consisting of a disk with tines and was called a tine test.) An extract from the tubercle bacillus is injected into the skin. The results are read in 48 to 72 hours. Raising and hardening of the skin around the area (induration), rather than redness alone, indicate a positive reaction.

Patch Test. You perform a **patch test** by placing a linen or paper patch on uninvolved skin and then using a dropper to soak the patch with the suspected allergen (see Figure 28-4). Cellophane or another occlusive, usually covered with an adhesive patch, is then applied over the linen or paper patch. The test is used to discover the cause of contact dermatitis.

Radioallergosorbent Test (RAST). The RAST measures blood levels of antibodies to particular allergens. You obtain a blood sample from the patient and send it to a laboratory. There the blood serum is exposed to suspected allergens, and the levels of antibodies are measured. This test usually provides more information than skin testing but is more expensive.

Cardiology

A physician specializing in heart diseases and disorders is called a cardiologist. To assist a cardiologist, you must be familiar with the structure of the cardiovascular system and the typical examinations and measurements associated with it. You also need to know about common heart diseases and their treatments.

Many of the diagnostic tests performed in this specialty, including electrocardiography and stress testing, are described in detail in Chapter 39. Imaging techniques, such as x-rays and echocardiography, may also be employed. You will assist with or perform some of these tests. Because caring for a heart condition often involves many lifestyle changes, your role in educating the patient about topics such as diet and exercise will be especially important. You will also provide emotional support to patients with serious illnesses.

Cardiology Examinations

A general cardiovascular examination usually begins with cardiac auscultation to obtain a blood pressure reading and an evaluation of overall cardiac health. The cardiologist also palpates the heart and chest wall and the vessels in the extremities to detect abnormal vibrations, pulses,

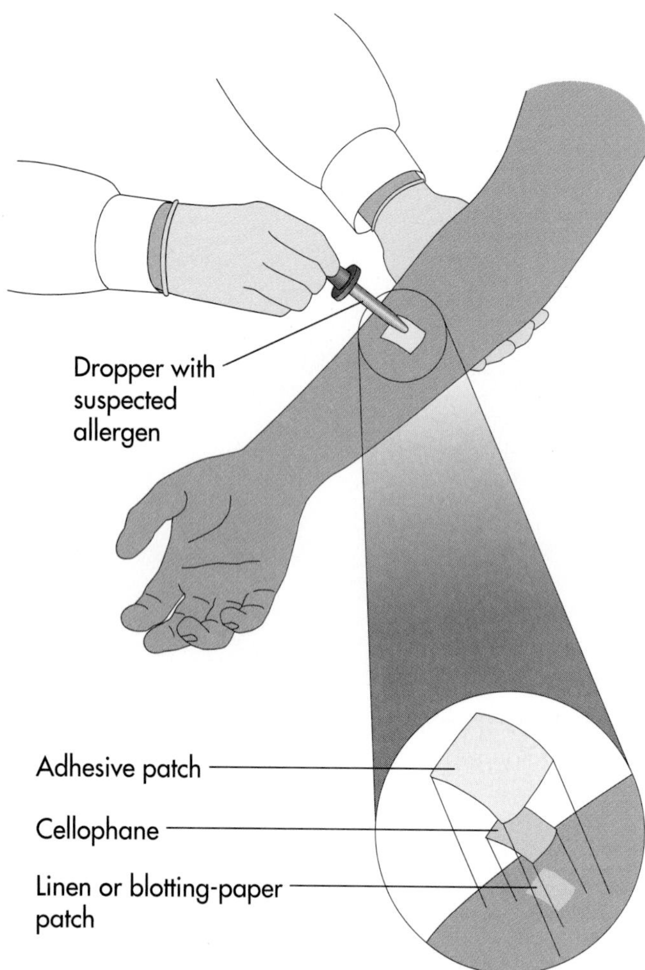

Figure 28-4. A patch test is usually done on the arm and is read in 48 hours.

swelling, or temperature. In addition, an electrocardiogram may be obtained.

Electrocardiogram. An electrocardiogram (abbreviated ECG or EKG) provides a measurement of the electrical activity of the heart. Electrocardiography is a painless, safe diagnostic test that is a routine part of a cardiovascular examination. Electrodes are placed on the skin in particular areas of the chest and limbs. The heart's electrical activity is shown as a tracing on a strip of graph paper.

Stress Test. An ECG is usually obtained in one of two ways. A resting ECG is performed while the patient is lying down. A **stress test** involves recording an ECG while the patient is exercising on a stationary bicycle, treadmill, or stair-stepping ergometer. This test measures the patient's response to a constant or increasing workload. Part of your job may involve keeping the equipment properly maintained and calibrated. You may also be responsible for administering the test itself. A doctor should always be present, however, because of the risk of cardiac crisis.

Before the test the patient has a screening appointment with the doctor, during which you take a careful medical history and explain pretest requirements. On the day of the test, be sure the patient has followed pretest directions, such as abstaining from smoking or consuming alcohol, and has signed the proper consent form.

The patient is prepared as for an ECG by having the electrodes attached to the skin. Show the patient how to use the ergometric device. If the device is a treadmill, show the patient how to step on and off it and how to use the metal railing for balance. (Exercise electrocardiography, or stress testing, is further described in Chapter 39.)

A type of stress test called the stress thallium ECG is performed by injecting the radioisotope thallium (^{201}Tl) into the patient's veins at the time of peak stress. The patient is checked several minutes later to find out how much thallium has been taken up by the heart. Damaged areas do not take up the thallium as rapidly as healthy areas do.

Holter Monitor. The Holter monitor is an ECG device that includes a small cassette recorder, allowing readings to be taken over a period of time. Electrodes are attached to the patient's chest wall in the physician's office. The patient wears a recording device on a belt or sling (see Figure 28-5). The patient returns home, and the device monitors heart activity for 24 hours. (Ambulatory electrocardiography, or Holter monitoring, is fully described in Chapter 39.)

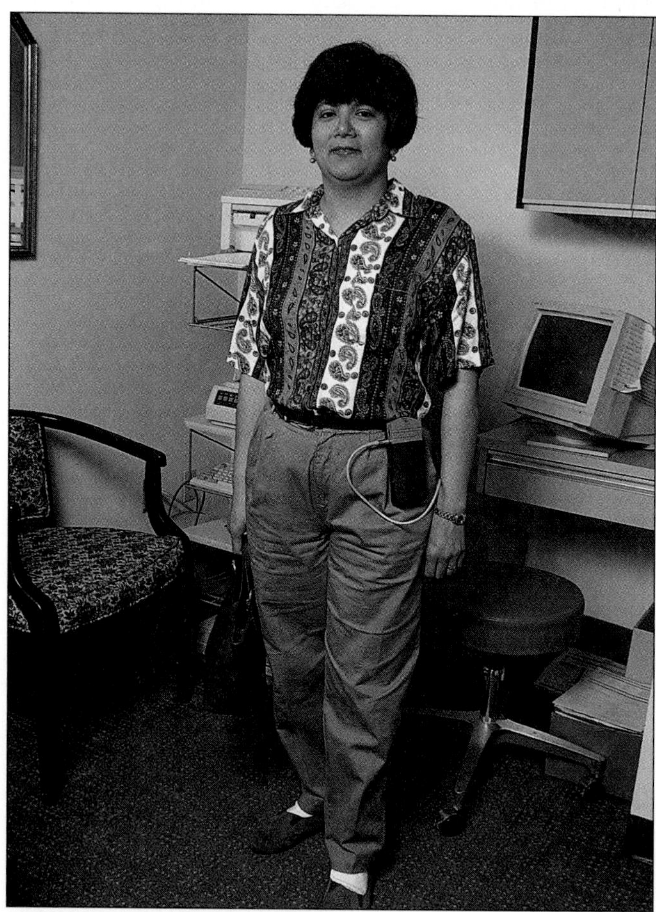

Figure 28-5. A Holter monitor allows the doctor to assess heart function during periods of normal activity.

MULTISKILL FOCUS

Doppler and Stress Testing

To gain medical assistant credentials, you must fulfill the requirements of either the American Association of Medical Assistants (for a Certified Medical Assistant) or the American Medical Technologists (for a Registered Medical Assistant). After obtaining your medical assistant certification or registration, you may wish to acquire additional skills in specialty areas through course work or on-the-job training. Although this course work or training may not lead to an additional certification or degree, it will enable you to expand your role in the medical office and advance your career as the demand for multiskilled health professionals increases.

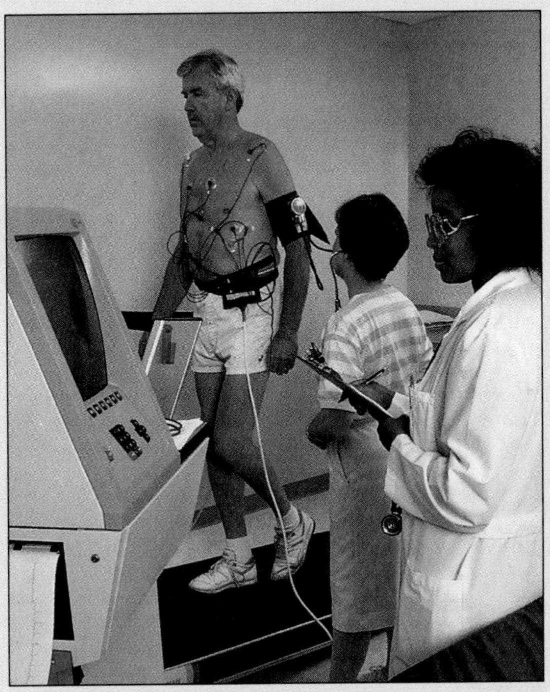

Skills and Duties

Doppler and stress testing are two procedures that help physicians diagnose cardiac problems. The Doppler test uses an ultrasound transducer, a device that emits and receives ultrasonic waves, to provide a sound wave image of blood flow. The stress test monitors the effect of physical activity on a person's heart. Both procedures can be performed by a medical assistant with appropriate training.

The Doppler test takes between 5 and 10 minutes. The medical assistant applies a special gel to the patient's chest. The gel facilitates the transmission of sound waves. The medical assistant then moves the transducer across the patient's chest, producing a picture on the Doppler screen. This picture can be videotaped or copied in still photographs for later viewing. The assistant records the results of the session and reports them to the physician.

To perform a stress test, the medical assistant uses an electrocardiograph, a machine that monitors the electrical activity of the heart and records the activity as an electrocardiogram (ECG) on special graph paper. The medical assistant attaches metal electrodes (sensors) from the electrocardiograph to the patient's chest, arms, and legs. She then gets a baseline ECG of the patient's heartbeat at rest.

The patient then exercises on a treadmill or bicycle, with the level of difficulty increasing every 2 to 3 minutes. The medical assistant monitors the patient's blood pressure and ECG and stops the test as soon as the patient experiences fatigue, breathlessness, chest pain, or unusual ECG readings. (A physician is always present during a stress test to deal with cardiac emergencies.) After the test is completed, the assistant records the patient's vital signs. Medical assistants who specialize in Doppler and stress testing may also maintain the equipment, schedule appointments, type test results and physician instructions, and maintain patient files.

Workplace Settings

Most medical assistants who perform Doppler and stress tests work in a hospital or cardiologist's office. Some medical assistants may perform these tests in clinics, rehabilitation centers, and managed care facilities.

Education

Medical assistants interested in Doppler and stress testing must, at minimum, have a high school diploma. Many medical assistants who specialize in stress testing are trained on the job, a process that takes between 8 and 16 weeks. In addition, some colleges and hospitals offer a 1-year certificate program for stress testing.

To perform Doppler testing, medical assistants must receive additional education. Many colleges offer 2-year programs specializing in noninvasive technology, which features tests such as the Doppler.

Although the job outlook for this area is good, the demand for a technician who performs only these tests may not be high. Health-care professionals who have other skills in addition to training in Doppler and stress testing will find the greatest demand for their services.

Where to Go for More Information

American College of Cardiology
9111 Old Georgetown Road
Bethesda, MD 20814
(301) 897-5400

American Medical Association
Division of Allied Health Education and Accreditation
515 North State Street
Chicago, IL 60610
(312) 464-5000

American Society for Cardiovascular Professionals
120 Falcon Drive, Unit 3
Fredericksburg, VA 22408
(540) 891-0079

Radiography Techniques

Various radiography techniques are used in cardiology. Chest x-rays can reveal conditions such as cardiac enlargement. In radionuclide studies, the patient ingests or is injected with a radioactive contrast medium, often referred to as a dye. X-rays are then taken. For example, fluoroscopy studies are x-ray examinations in which a contrast medium is injected and pictures of the heart in motion are projected onto a closed-circuit television screen. A venogram allows evaluation of the deep veins of the legs. **Angiography** is an x-ray examination of a blood vessel after the injection of a contrast medium. The test, performed in a hospital, usually evaluates the function and structure of one or more arteries.

Ultrasound, a noninvasive diagnostic method, is also used in cardiology. Doppler ultrasonography tests the body's main blood vessels for conditions such as weaknesses in vessel walls or blocked arteries. With the use of a handheld probe, sound waves are transmitted through the skin and are reflected by the blood cells moving through the blood vessels.

Echocardiography tests the structure and function of the heart through the use of reflected sound waves, or echoes. Sound waves of an extremely high frequency are projected through the chest wall into the heart and are reflected back through a mechanical device. The echoes, which are recorded on paper, can indicate conditions such as structural defects and fluid accumulation (see Figure 28-6).

Cardiac catheterization is a diagnostic method in which a catheter (a slender, hollow tube) is inserted into a vein or artery in the right or left arm or leg and passed through the blood vessels into the heart. The cardiologist can use this method to take blood samples for analysis, measure the pressure in the heart's chambers, and view the heart's motions with the aid of fluoroscopy. The procedure is performed in the hospital and is often combined with angiography.

Cardiac Diseases and Disorders

All of these diagnostic tests are used to reveal heart diseases and disorders. Table 28-1 lists the types of diseases and disorders you will encounter in a cardiologist's office.

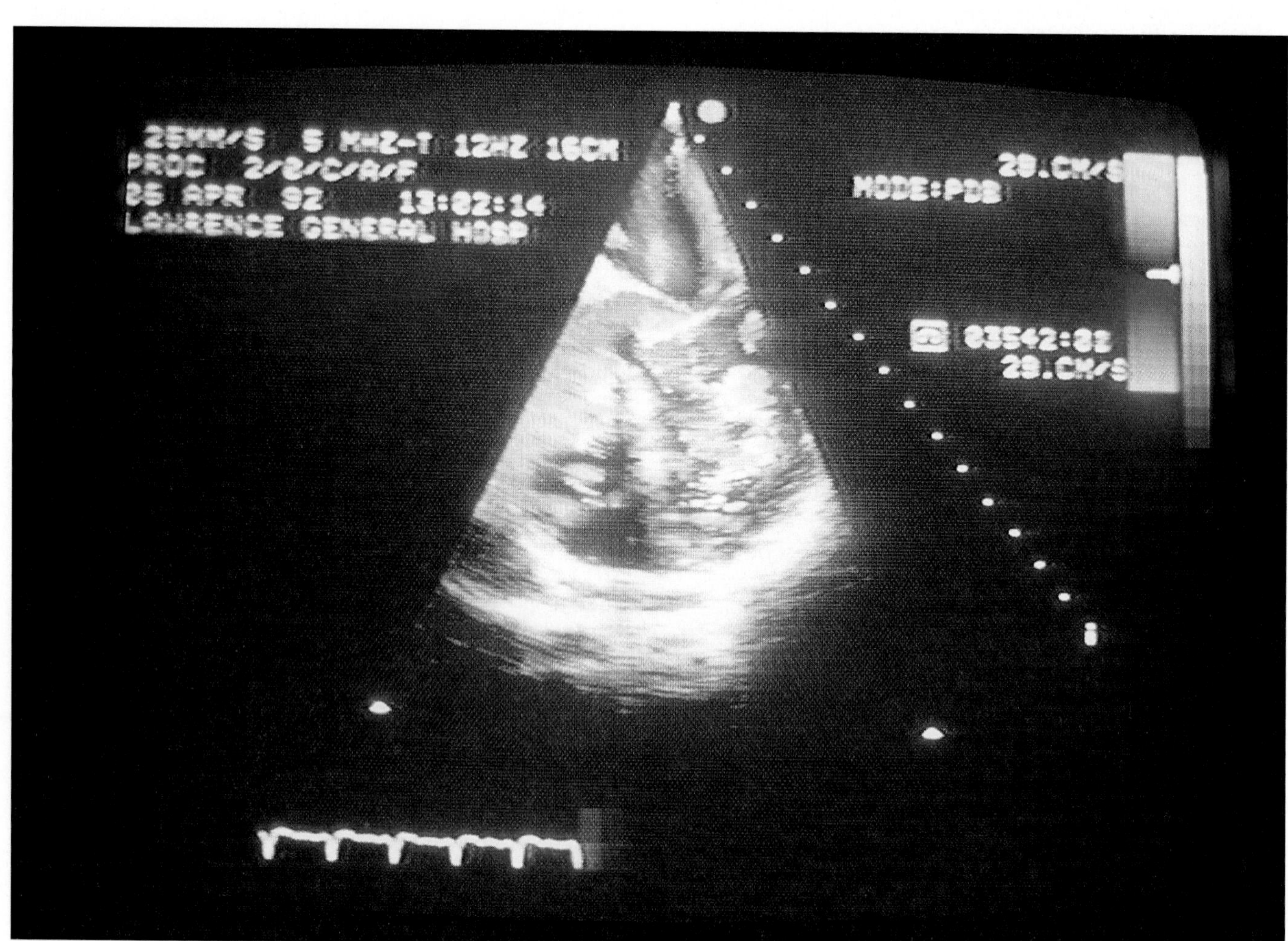

Figure 28-6. An echocardiograph shows the structures and function of the heart.

Dermatology

Dermatologists diagnose and treat skin diseases and disorders such as acne, eczema, and skin cancer. Some skin conditions involve only the skin itself; others are a sign of disease elsewhere in the body.

To assist in a dermatologist's office, you must understand the basic elements of dermatologic examinations and procedures. You should develop familiarity with skin disorders and their treatments. You also need to understand the terminology used to describe skin lesions, as outlined in Table 28-2.

Assisting with positioning and draping during a skin examination and taking skin scrapings or wound cultures might be among your duties in a dermatologist's office. You might also perform procedures such as administering sunlamp treatments and applying topical medications. You will also instruct patients about caring for a skin condition or wound site at home.

Dermatology Examinations

During a **whole-body skin examination,** the dermatologist examines the visible top layer of the entire surface of the skin, including the scalp, the genital area, and the areas between the toes. The physician uses a magnifying lens and a bright light to look for lesions, especially suspicious moles or precancerous growths. The physician may photograph or sketch a lesion to aid in detecting future changes.

Your role in this examination includes preparing patients and helping them into the proper position before examination of each skin area. During the examination, drape patients to protect their privacy as much as possible while exposing the area to be examined. The physi-

Table 28-1

Types of Cardiovascular Diseases and Disorders

Category of Disease/Disorder	Common Conditions	Treatment
Arterial/vascular disorders	*Aneurysms:* abnormal dilation of artery wall caused by area of weakness	Medication, surgery
	Arteriosclerosis: thickening or hardening of arterial wall	Medication, lifestyle and diet management, surgery
	Atherosclerosis: accumulation of deposits along inner walls of arteries, obstructing blood flow	Medication, lifestyle and diet management, surgery
	Hypertension: persistent high blood pressure; systolic pressure greater than 140 mm Hg, diastolic pressure greater than 90 mm Hg	Medication, lifestyle and diet management, stress management
	Varicose veins: distended veins in the legs caused by weakening of vein walls and failure of one-way valves inside veins	Wearing of elastic stockings, weight loss, elevation of legs, weight control, surgery
Cardiomyopathy: disease of heart muscle causing fatigue, breathing problems, and leading to heart failure	*Dilated cardiomyopathy:* dilated heart chambers	Medication, heart transplant surgery
	Hypertrophic cardiomyopathy: thickening of heart walls and narrowing of chambers	Medication, heart transplant surgery
	Restrictive cardiomyopathy: decrease in elasticity and narrowing of heart chambers	Medication, heart transplant surgery
Coronary artery disease: condition involving partial or complete blockage of major coronary arteries that surround heart	*Angina pectoris:* disorder caused by reduced blood supply to heart muscle	Medication, rest, lifestyle management
	Myocardial infarction: death of heart tissue because of oxygen deprivation	Medication, oxygen administration, rest, lifestyle management

continued

Table 28-1 continued

Types of Cardiovascular Diseases and Disorders

Category of Disease/Disorder	Common Conditions	Treatment
Dysrhythmias: disorders of heartbeat	*Atrial fibrillation:* uncoordinated atrial contractions, resulting in diminished cardiac output	Medication, cardioversion (delivery of electric shock to myocardium, or heart muscle)
	Conduction delays or blocks: problems with transmission of electrical impulses in heart	Medication, implantation of pacemaker
	Tachycardia: rapid heartbeat (more than 100 beats per minute)	Medication, diet management
Heart failure	*Congestive heart failure:* inability of heart to pump blood effectively, causing fluid to build up in tissues and lungs	Medication, diet management, rest
Inflammations: infections of heart tissue, often caused by systemic infections	*Endocarditis:* inflammation of heart lining, including valves	Medication, surgery to repair or replace valves
	Myocarditis: inflammation of myocardium, or heart muscle	Specific treatment for underlying cause, medication, rest
	Pericarditis: inflammation of pericardium (tissue sac covering heart)	Medication, rest
Valvular diseases: disorders in which heart valves do not open or close fully	*Aortic stenosis:* narrowing of aortic valve opening, restricting blood flow	Surgical replacement of valve
	Mitral stenosis: narrowing of mitral valve opening, restricting blood flow	Medication, rest, surgical repair or replacement of valve
	Mitral valve prolapse: condition in which a portion of mitral valve falls into left atrium during systole	Medication (usually antibiotic prophylaxis to prevent subacute bacterial endocarditis)

cian may also ask you to take photographs or make sketches of lesions.

Another type of dermatologic examination is the **Wood's light examination,** in which the physician inspects the patient's skin under an ultraviolet lamp in a darkened room. This examination highlights certain abnormal skin characteristics and aids in diagnosis. The dermatologist may also perform more limited, focused examinations to evaluate specific skin conditions or disorders.

Dermatologic Conditions and Disorders

The condition of the skin plays a large part in a person's appearance. Patients with skin disorders, therefore, may worry about their attractiveness to and acceptance by others. Allow patients to express their anxieties; in return, provide encouragement about the course and outcome of their treatment.

Acne Vulgaris. Acne vulgaris, also called acne, is an inflammation of the follicles of the skin's sebaceous (oil) glands. It causes skin eruptions of pimples, blackheads, and cysts, mainly on the face but sometimes on the back or other areas. Acne occurs most frequently in adolescents but can affect adults as well. Its ultimate cause is unknown, but it is thought to involve a hormonal dysfunction that creates excess skin oil (sebum). The sebum hardens at the follicle openings, closing off the flow of skin secretions and causing eruptions.

Treatments may be topical or oral. Topical treatments include antibacterial medications, antibiotics, benzoyl peroxide, and vitamin A products. More severe cases may be treated with oral antibiotics or retinoic acid. Retinoic acid cannot be used by patients who are pregnant or likely to become pregnant, because retinoic acid damages the fetus.

Patients need to understand the prescribed treatment regimen and its requirements, such as avoiding sun overexposure if vitamin A products are being used. You may also be asked to instruct patients in proper skin cleansing and care.

Contact Dermatitis. Contact dermatitis is a skin inflammation that can be caused by irritants as diverse as rough fabrics, cosmetics, pollen, or plants such as poison

Table 28-2

Skin Lesions

Type of Lesion	Appearance	Type of Lesion	Appearance
Macule: flat, discolored spot on skin (less than 1 cm in diameter), such as freckle or flat mole	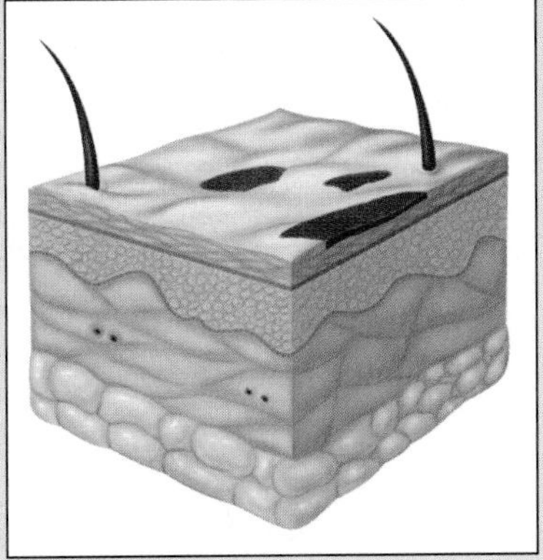	Bulla: large vesicle (more than 1 cm in diameter), such as burn blister	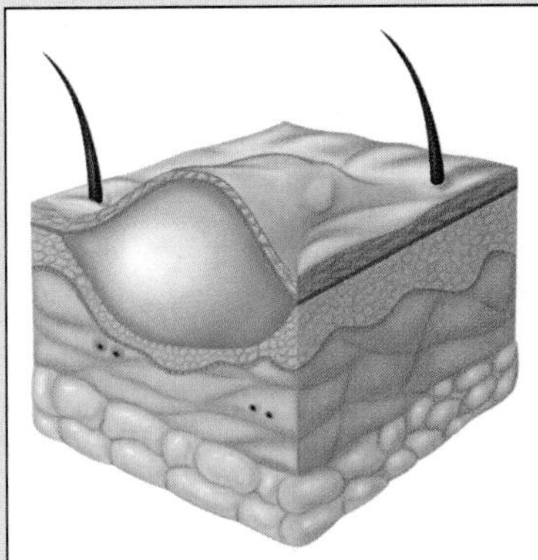
Papule: firm, raised lesion (less than 1 cm in diameter), such as wart or raised mole	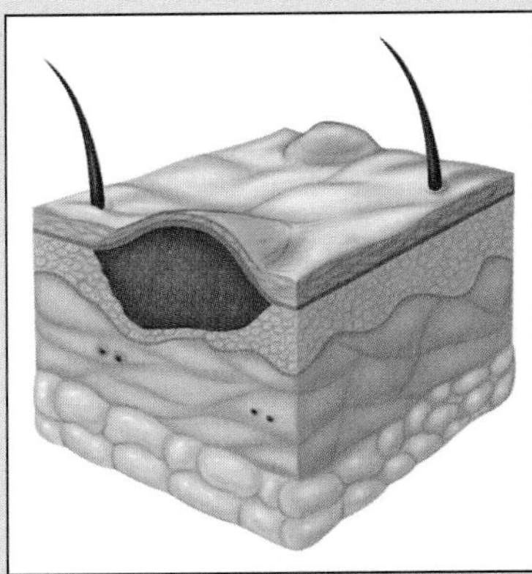	Pustule: raised lesion containing pus, such as acne or impetigo pustule	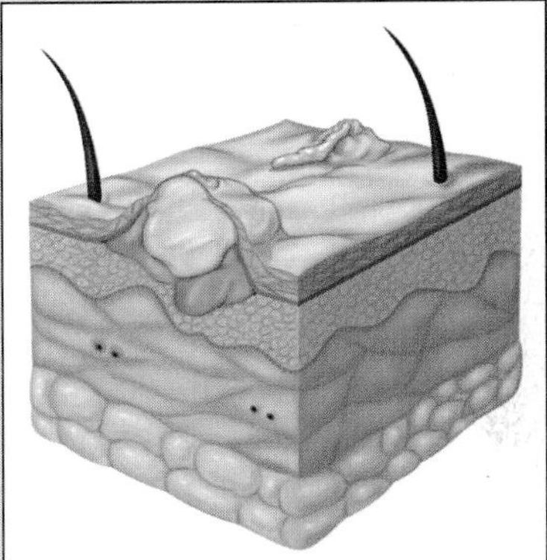
Nodule: raised, firm lesion larger and deeper than papule, such as sebaceous cyst	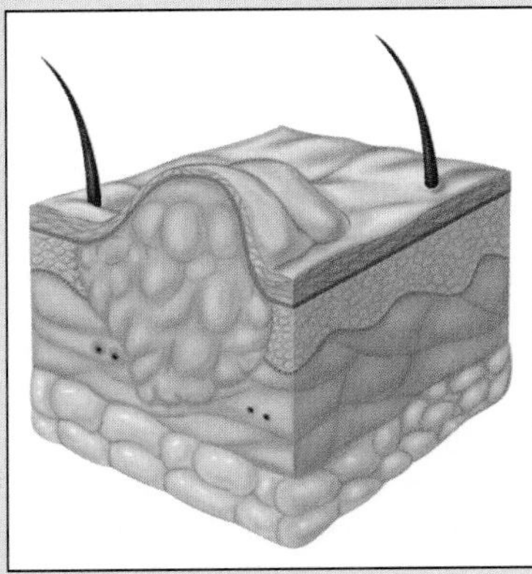	Ulcer: depression in skin formed when skin layers are destroyed, such as pressure sore	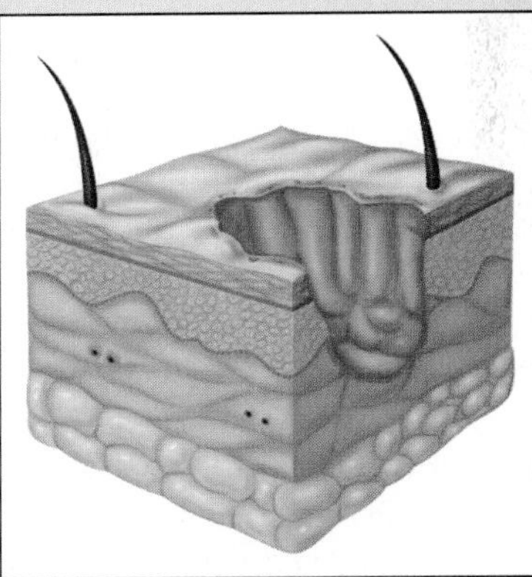
Vesicle: small skin elevation (less than 1 cm in diameter) filled with clear fluid, such as blister	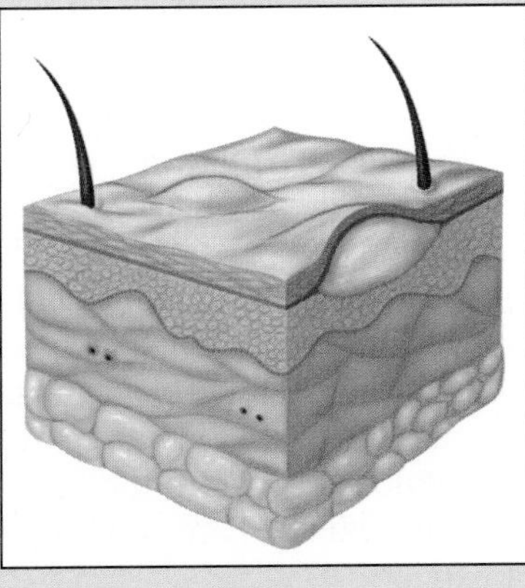	Tumor: solid abnormal mass of cells larger than 1 cm	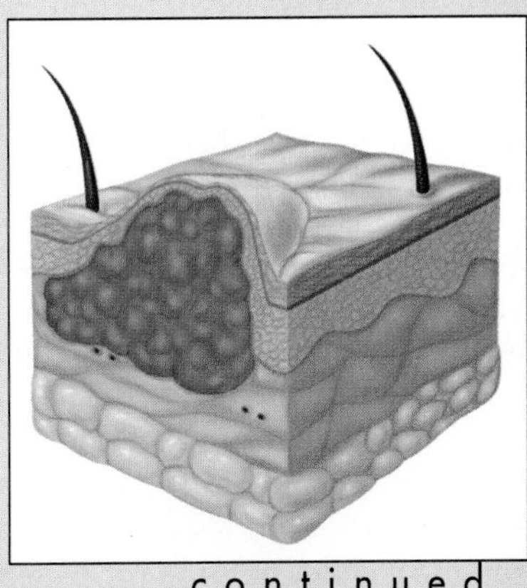

continued

Table 28-2 continued

Skin Lesions

Type of Lesion	Appearance	Type of Lesion	Appearance
Wheal: temporary elevation of skin caused by swelling, as with hives or insect bites, or by administration of an intradermal injection		Fissure: crack in skin, such as fissure caused by athlete's foot	

ivy or poison oak. Symptoms include redness, itching, edema, and lesions.

Treatment of contact dermatitis depends on the cause and type of lesions. Anti-inflammatory medications may be applied to the skin, or antihistamines may be taken internally. Corticosteroids are prescribed for severe inflammation. The dermatologist may wish to use a patch test to determine whether a condition is caused by a specific allergen. If such a cause is found, the patient should be taught how to avoid that substance and what to do after accidental exposure.

Ringworm. Ringworm, or tinea, is a term for various fungal infections that most often affect the feet (athlete's foot, or tinea pedis), groin (jock itch, or tinea cruris), and scalp (tinea capitis). Ringworm produces flat lesions on the body that are dry and scaly or moist and crusty. These lesions eventually develop a clear center with an outer ring, for which these infections are named. When ringworm appears on the scalp, it creates small lesions and scaly bald patches.

Ringworm is treated with topical antifungal medications and, when an infection is well established, oral medications. Ringworm is contagious, so instruct the infected individual in how to prevent contamination. The person should not share bedding, combs, towels, or other personal items with anyone until the infection is gone.

Moles. A mole (nevus) is a raised or unraised brown, black, or tan spot on the skin, with even coloring, a round or oval shape, and clear borders. It is usually less than 6 mm in diameter. It may be present at birth, but most appear during childhood or adolescence. Most moles are harmless; in fact, everyone has some. Because moles have the potential to become malignant, however, they must be monitored for bleeding, itching, or changes in color, size, shape, or texture. Some people choose to have a harmless mole removed because it is cosmetically unappealing or because it is in a place especially vulnerable to injury.

Skin Cancer. One of the most serious conditions treated in a dermatologist's office is skin cancer. Skin cancer can appear in the form of basal cell carcinomas, squamous cell carcinomas, and malignant melanomas. Overexposure to the sun is a risk factor for all these types of skin cancer. Other triggers include x-rays, irritants, various chemical carcinogens, and the presence of premalignant lesions. The following people have a higher-than-average risk of developing skin cancer: those who have had severe, blistering sunburns in their teens or 20s; those who have fair skin and hair and light-colored eyes; and those who work outdoors.

Basal cell carcinomas are malignant lesions that occur most often on areas exposed to the sun, such as the face and neck. Basal cell carcinomas are the most common malignant tumor in Caucasians. The lesions look like small, waxy craters with rolled borders (see Figure 28-7).

Squamous cell carcinomas also appear on sun-exposed areas. The lesions often look ulcerated or have a crust (see Figure 28-8). They invade deeper into the skin and have a greater tendency to spread to other areas of the body than do basal cell carcinomas.

Malignant melanomas, which originate in cells that produce the pigment melanin, are the most dangerous type of skin cancer (see Figure 28-9). Malignant cells may spread through the bloodstream or lymphatic system to the liver, lungs, and other parts of the body. A sudden or continuous change in the appearance of a mole may signal melanoma. Early diagnosis is critical for successful treatment.

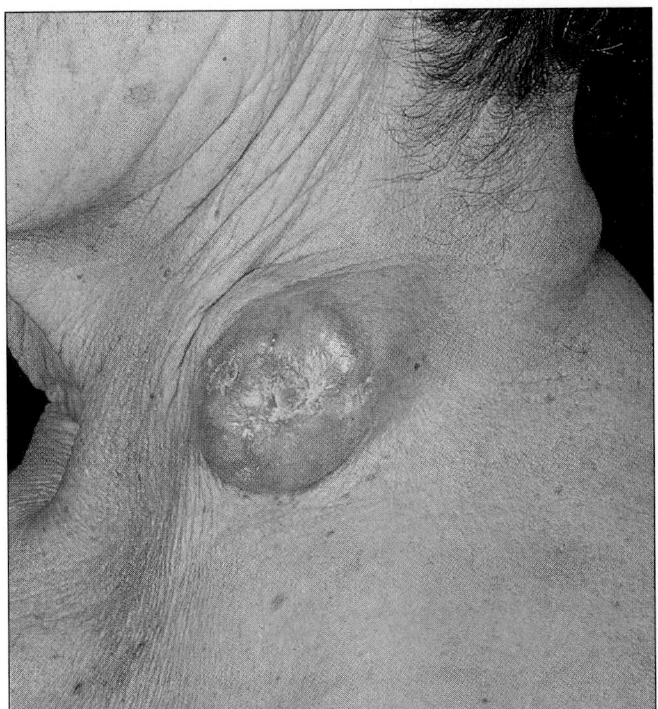

Figure 28-7. Left untreated, basal cell carcinomas can damage bones or blood vessels.

Treatments for skin cancer vary with the type of cancer and its extent. Treatments include surgery, electrosurgery, cryosurgery, radiation therapy, and chemotherapy.

Warts. Warts (verrucae) are benign skin tumors that result from a viral skin infection. If a wart is scratched open, the virus may spread by contact to another part of the body or to another person. There are several kinds of warts. Common warts are raised, rounded, flesh-colored lesions that usually occur on the hands and fingers. Plantar warts appear on the soles of the feet. Venereal warts appear on the genitalia and anus and are transmitted through sexual contact.

Treatment depends on the type of wart. Some warts go away without treatment. Physicians often remove warts by burning or freezing the wart tissue. Instruct the patient to keep the wart removal site clean and dry until a scab forms or the wart falls off in a few days.

Other Conditions and Disorders. The following conditions may also be diagnosed and treated in a dermatologist's office:

- Eczema: skin inflammation that may be an allergic response to allergens, such as chemicals or foods
- Impetigo: highly contagious bacterial skin infection
- Psoriasis: chronic noninfectious disease that manifests itself in itching lesions covered with scales
- Herpes zoster: acute viral infection of nerves under the skin, often called shingles; causes painful skin eruptions
- Scabies: contagious skin disease caused by a mite; causes intense itching

Endocrinology

Endocrinologists treat diseases and disorders of the endocrine system, which includes glands that regulate and coordinate the systems of the body. Hormonal imbalances can affect the basic processes of growth, metabolism, and reproduction. In the endocrinologist's office you will assist with examinations as well as collect specimens for analysis.

Endocrine Examinations

Before an examination you will take a thorough medical history. The physician will assess the patient's skin condition, weight, and cardiac functioning for clues about illness. Most of the endocrine glands are located deep within the body; only the thyroid, the testes and, to some extent, the ovaries can be examined with palpation or auscultation. Therefore, diagnostic urine and blood tests are essential. You may be asked to collect a urine specimen or draw blood (see Chapters 33 and 34). Other diagnostic tools used in endocrinology include radiologic tests such as x-rays and iodine scans.

An endocrinologist will perform a complete physical examination, including palpation of the thyroid gland. In a thyroid scan the patient receives an oral or intravenous (IV) dose of radioactive iodine, and the thyroid is x-rayed as the material is absorbed. Ultrasound can also be employed to view glands or detect tumors. Urine and blood may be tested for the presence of glucose or hormones.

Endocrine Diseases and Disorders

An endocrine disorder commonly treated by endocrinologists is **diabetes mellitus.** This name is used for several related disorders characterized by hyperglycemia, an elevated level of glucose in the blood. When blood sugar is abnormally low, the condition is called hypoglycemia. Normally, the glucose level is regulated by insulin, a

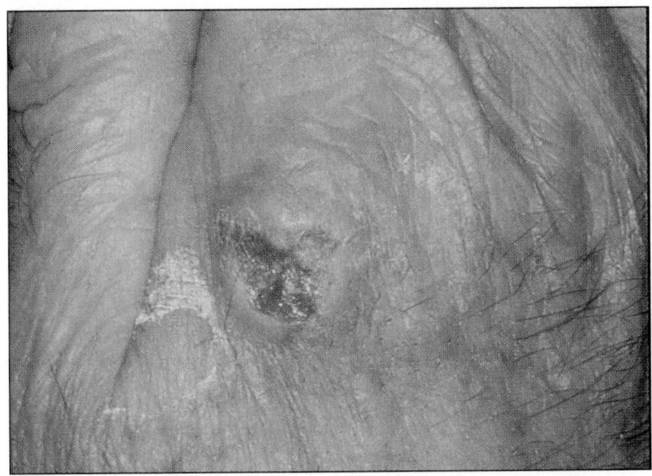

Figure 28-8. Repeated injury to an area, as well as sun exposure, is a risk factor for squamous cell carcinoma.

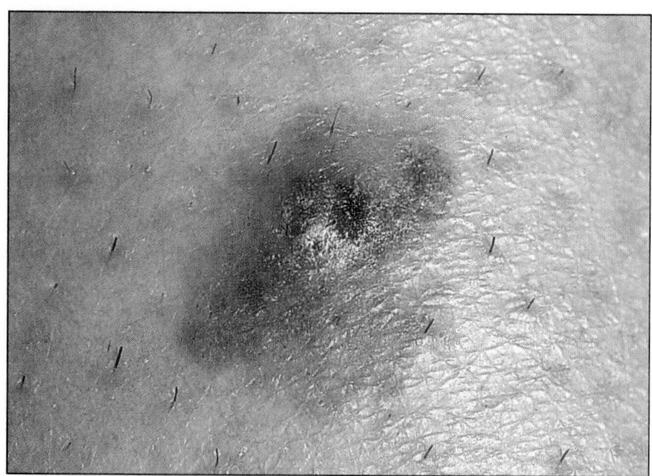

Figure 28-9. Early diagnosis is critical in successfully treating malignant melanoma.

hormone secreted by the pancreas. A deficiency of insulin interferes with the metabolism of carbohydrates, proteins, and fats, raising the glucose level in the blood.

One form of diabetes, insulin-dependent diabetes mellitus (IDDM), usually appears before age 30. Non-insulin-dependent diabetes mellitus (NIDDM) usually appears after age 40. Other forms of diabetes can occur during pregnancy (gestational diabetes) or as a result of other disorders. Symptoms include excessive thirst, hunger, excessive urination, and fatigue. Diabetes is treated through diet and weight control, oral medications, and insulin injections. Special, thorough patient education is necessary for the patient to cope successfully with the blood glucose monitoring, dietary restrictions, and self-care measures associated with this disorder (see Figure 28-10). Physicians must pay special attention to certain secondary conditions, such as eye and foot problems, in patients with diabetes.

Thyroid Gland Dysfunctions. Several of the most common endocrine system disorders occur when there is a dysfunction of the thyroid gland. These disorders include hypothyroidism, hyperthyroidism, and goiter.

Hypothyroidism. Hypothyroidism is characterized by decreased activity of the thyroid gland and underproduction of the hormone thyroxine. This shortage can cause cretinism in children, with resulting mental and physical retardation. Underproduction of thyroxine in adults results in myxedema. Patients with this condition have fatigue, low blood pressure, dry skin and hair, and facial puffiness. Treatment for hypothyroidism consists of thyroid hormone supplements.

Hyperthyroidism. Hyperthyroidism, also called Graves' disease, is characterized by increased thyroid gland activity. Too much thyroxine is produced, and the patient has anxiety, irritability, elevated heart rate and blood pressure, tremors, and weight loss despite an increased appetite. Sometimes this condition causes the patient's eyes to protrude. Treatment includes the administration of radioactive iodine, antithyroid drugs, or surgery to remove part or all of the thyroid gland.

Goiter. An enlarged thyroid gland, commonly called a goiter, is usually caused by a deficiency of iodine in the diet. Iodine is found in seafood, iodized salt, and vegetables grown in soil containing iodine. Without this mineral the thyroid gland enlarges in an attempt to produce more thyroid hormones. Treatment usually involves the administration of iodine.

Cushing's Syndrome. Cushing's syndrome results from overproduction of hormones by the adrenal cortex. This overproduction may be caused by a tumor of the pituitary gland or adrenal cortex. Symptoms include high blood pressure, muscle weakness, easily bruised skin with purple streaks, a rounded face, a fatty hump between the shoulders, and rapidly deposited fat that causes obesity in the trunk while the arms and legs remain slender. Some diabetic symptoms, such as hyperglycemia, may also appear. Treatments include medications to suppress adrenal function and surgical removal of tumors causing the disorder.

Gastroenterology

Gastroenterologists diagnose and treat disorders of the entire gastrointestinal (GI) tract, from the mouth to the anus, as well as the liver and pancreas. (Proctologists treat disorders of the rectum and anus only.)

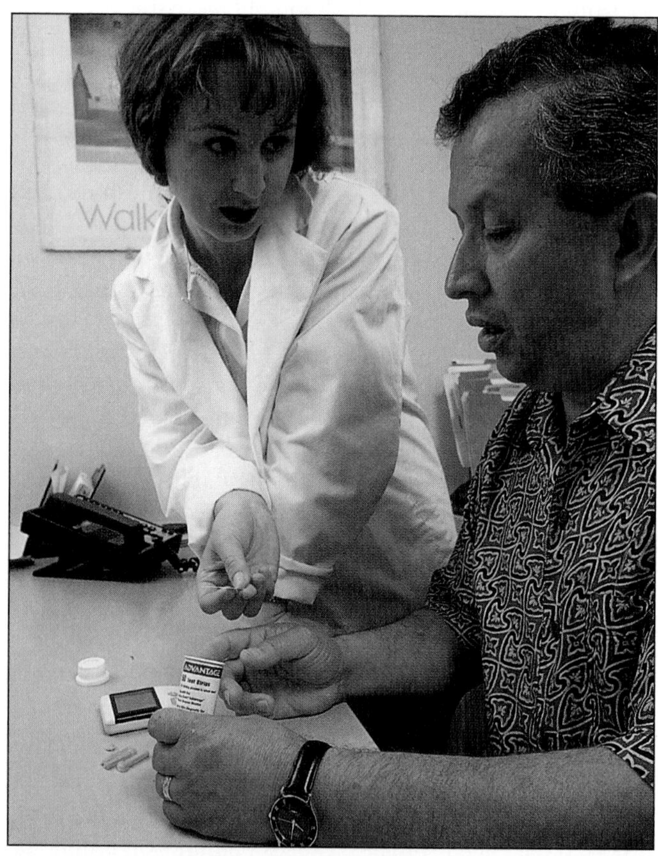

Figure 28-10. Patients with diabetes can use a glucometer to monitor their own blood glucose levels.

A patient who sees a GI specialist has usually been referred by a family doctor, internist, or pediatrician who suspects a GI problem requiring additional expertise. You will need to understand the basic elements of GI examinations and procedures to assist in a gastroenterologist's office. You must also be familiar with common GI disorders, their treatments, and the terminology used to describe them.

In a gastroenterologist's office you will tell patients how to prepare for examinations, whether in the office, a radiology facility, or a hospital. You will order informational brochures and make them available to patients. You will also be prepared to answer patient questions.

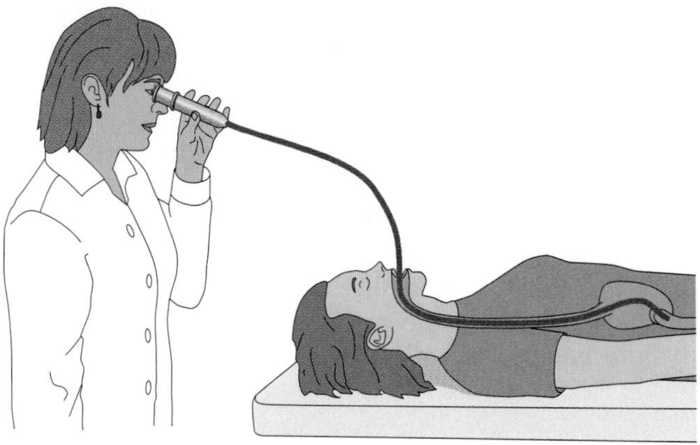

Figure 28-11. To perform peroral endoscopy, the physician inserts a scope into the patient's mouth.

Gastrointestinal Examinations

The gastroenterologist's examination of the patient's GI tract covers the mouth (lips, oral cavity, and tongue), the abdomen and lower thorax, the lower sigmoid colon, the rectum, and the anus. Your role as a medical assistant will be to prepare the equipment and the patient.

Depending on the patient's symptoms, the physician may perform an invasive examination procedure during the patient's first visit. Formerly, such procedures were performed only in hospitals or special medical facilities. Now many GI specialists' offices are equipped for these procedures and the management of possible resulting emergencies.

You must provide reassurance during examinations and help patients be as comfortable as possible. Your duties during the procedures will vary according to your state's scope of practice and the physician for whom you work. Instruct patients in advance to arrange for someone to drive them to and from the examination. After a procedure in which patients have had a local anesthetic at the back of the throat, caution them to avoid eating until the drug has been eliminated from the body. Otherwise, they could choke or aspirate food particles into the trachea.

Gastric Lavage. Gastric lavage involves obtaining a sample of stomach contents by inserting an orogastric tube into the mouth (or nasogastric tube through the nose) and passing it down through the esophagus into the stomach. The patient is usually sedated. You will spray the back of the throat with a local anesthetic to inhibit the gag reflex. The patient should be awake, however, to assist in swallowing the tube. The gastric sample is suctioned up through the tube and sent to a laboratory for analysis.

Endoscopy. **Endoscopy** generally refers to any procedure in which a scope is used to visually inspect a canal or cavity within the body. Several endoscopic examinations are performed with a flexible fiber-optic tube that has a lighted instrument on the end. These examinations provide direct visualization of a body cavity and provide a means for collecting tissue biopsies and removing polyps, as in the colon. Endoscopy helps diagnose tumors, ulcers, structural abnormalities, and other problems. It is particularly useful in performing procedures that formerly would have required an incision, such as removing stones from the bile duct.

Peroral Endoscopy. Peroral endoscopy involves inserting the scope by way of the mouth (Figure 28-11). The patient is sedated, and the gag reflex is inhibited with a local anesthetic. The peroral endoscopic procedures include panendoscopy (esophagus, stomach, and duodenum), esophagoscopy (esophagus only), gastroscopy (stomach only), and duodenoscopy (duodenum only).

Colonoscopy. **Colonoscopy,** which is performed by inserting a colonoscope through the anus, can provide direct visualization of the large intestine. The gastroenterologist uses this procedure to determine the cause of diarrhea, constipation, bleeding, or lower abdominal pain.

Patient preparation is designed to clear the colon of fecal material so that the colon can be seen clearly. Instruct patients to follow a liquid diet for 24 to 48 hours before the procedure. Patients should take a prescribed cathartic on the two evenings prior to the colonoscopy. Instruct patients to use one or more prepackaged enema preparations on the night before and the day of the procedure. (Alternatively, provide patients with 4 L of a prepared electrolyte solution to consume over a 2- to 4-hour period. During this time patients should keep a record of their intake, output, and symptoms. Tell patients to expect diarrhea and possibly mild cramps.)

Immediately before the procedure instruct patients to empty the bladder. Patients should be given a sedative or an analgesic before undergoing the procedure. Patients lie in the Sims' position as the scope is guided through the large intestine. The doctor may manipulate the abdomen to facilitate passage of the scope.

Proctoscopy. **Proctoscopy** is an examination of the lower rectum and anal canal. After an initial digital examination, the proctoscopy is performed with a 3-inch instrument called a proctoscope. This examination can detect hemorrhoids, polyps, fissures, fistulas, and abscesses.

Sigmoidoscopy. **Sigmoidoscopy** is similar to colonoscopy, except that only the sigmoid area of the large intestine (the S-shaped segment between the descending colon and the rectum) is examined. Sigmoidoscopy is an important part of many complete physical examinations and is performed by many general practitioners and internists. It aids in diagnosing colon cancer, ulcerations, polyps, tumors, bleeding, and other lower intestinal problems.

Patient preparation involves using one or two prepackaged enemas either the night before or the morning of the procedure, depending on the doctor's instructions. The method for assisting the doctor during a sigmoidoscopy is described in Procedure 28-2. The sigmoidoscope, a lighted instrument with a magnifying lens, allows the doctor to see and to examine the mucous membrane of the sigmoid colon.

Diagnostic Testing

Common diagnostic tests in this specialty include analysis of the contents of the stomach, analysis of a stool specimen, and urine and blood tests. Gastroenterologists sometimes use imaging techniques, such as x-rays, ultrasound, radionuclide imaging, computed tomography, and magnetic resonance imaging.

Laboratory Tests. A GI specialist may order laboratory analysis of stomach contents (obtained by gastric lavage) to determine the presence of bacteria or gastric bleeding. The physician may also request blood or urine tests. Another important test for GI specialists is the occult blood test, in which the feces are analyzed for occult, or hidden, bleeding from the intestinal tract. (This test is discussed in Chapter 25.)

Radiologic Examinations. Most GI radiologic examinations are not performed in an office, but you should know enough about them to answer patients' questions. Generally, these examinations are performed in a hospital x-ray laboratory or an outpatient facility. You may be responsible for scheduling tests at such facilities for patients. You can help prepare the patient in general terms for these examinations; however, the patient should discuss specific preparation with personnel from the radiologic facility.

PROCEDURE 28-2

Assisting With Sigmoidoscopy

Objective: To assist the doctor during the examination of the rectum, anus, and sigmoid colon using a sigmoidoscope

OSHA Guidelines

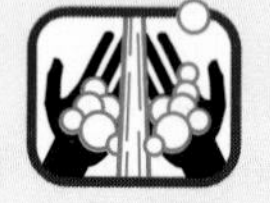
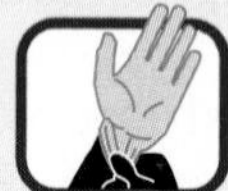
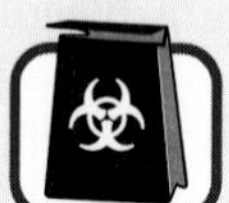
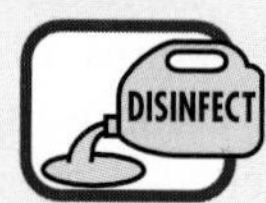

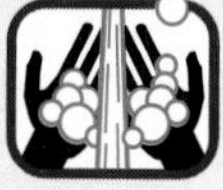

Materials: Sigmoidoscope, suction pump, lubricating jelly, drape, patient gown, tissues

Method

1. Wash your hands and assemble and position materials and equipment according to the preference of the doctor.
2. Test the suction pump.
3. Identify the patient and introduce yourself.
4. Show the patient into the treatment room. Explain the procedure and discuss any concerns the patient may have.
5. Instruct the patient to empty the bladder, take off all clothing from the waist down, and put on the gown with the opening in the back.
6. Put on examination gloves and assist the patient into the knee-chest or Sims' position. Immediately cover the patient with a drape.
7. Use warm water to bring the sigmoidoscope to slightly above body temperature; lubricate the tip.
8. Assist as needed, including handing the doctor the necessary instruments and equipment.
9. Monitor the patient's reactions during the procedure, and relay any signs of pain to the doctor.
10. Clean the anal area with tissues after the examination.
11. Properly dispose of used materials and disposable instruments.
12. Remove the gloves and wash your hands.
13. Help the patient gradually assume a comfortable position.
14. Instruct the patient to dress.
15. Put on clean gloves.
16. Sanitize reusable instruments and prepare them for disinfection and/or sterilization, as necessary.
17. Clean and disinfect the equipment and the room according to OSHA guidelines.
18. Remove the gloves and wash your hands.

Cholecystography. **Cholecystography** is a gallbladder function test performed by x-ray with a contrast agent. The patient swallows tablets of the contrast agent the night before the test. X-rays taken 12 to 14 hours later should show the contrast agent in the gallbladder. The patient then swallows a substance high in fat, which should make the gallbladder contract and empty the contrast agent into the duodenum. If the contrast agent is not taken up by the gallbladder or if the gallbladder does not contract properly, the doctor can determine whether there is bile duct obstruction or gallstones.

Ultrasound. Ultrasound is used commonly for diagnosing problems in the gallbladder, pancreas, spleen, and liver. The patient should have nothing to eat or drink after midnight of the night before and on the morning of the examination. Some gastroenterologists may perform ultrasound examinations in the office.

Barium Swallow. The barium swallow (also called an upper GI series) is used to detect abnormalities in the esophagus, stomach, and small intestine. The patient swallows a liquid containing barium, an insoluble contrast agent. This material is viewed using fluoroscopy (moving x-ray images) as the liquid is swallowed and passes into the stomach. X-ray films are taken at frequent intervals to record the diagnostic images. The patient is asked to move into various positions while the barium is tracked through the small intestine. To prepare for this test, the patient should have nothing to eat or drink after midnight of the night before and on the morning of the procedure.

Barium Enema. A barium enema (also called a lower GI series) is used to detect abnormalities in the large intestine. Barium is given as an enema in this test. A balloon-like tube is inflated in the rectum during the x-ray, and the patient is asked to move into various positions to ensure that the barium is distributed completely (Figure 28-12).

Patients must eat no meats or vegetables for 1 to 3 days before the test to avoid incorrect indications on the x-ray. For 24 hours before the test, they must also follow a liquid diet, which includes drinking special liquid laxative preparations and more than a quart of water. The staff at the facility performing the test instructs patients about the specific steps, but the intent is to cleanse the colon completely.

Radionuclide Imaging. Radiology subspecialists who are trained in nuclear medicine perform nuclear medicine studies with radionuclide imaging. The patient is first injected with a radioactive substance, then waits a prescribed length of time for the radioactive substance to be taken up by the body part that is being imaged. The patient is scanned or photographed with a special gamma camera, which can read the radioactive areas to determine abnormalities in their composition. This technique is commonly used for liver, spleen, thyroid, and bone scans.

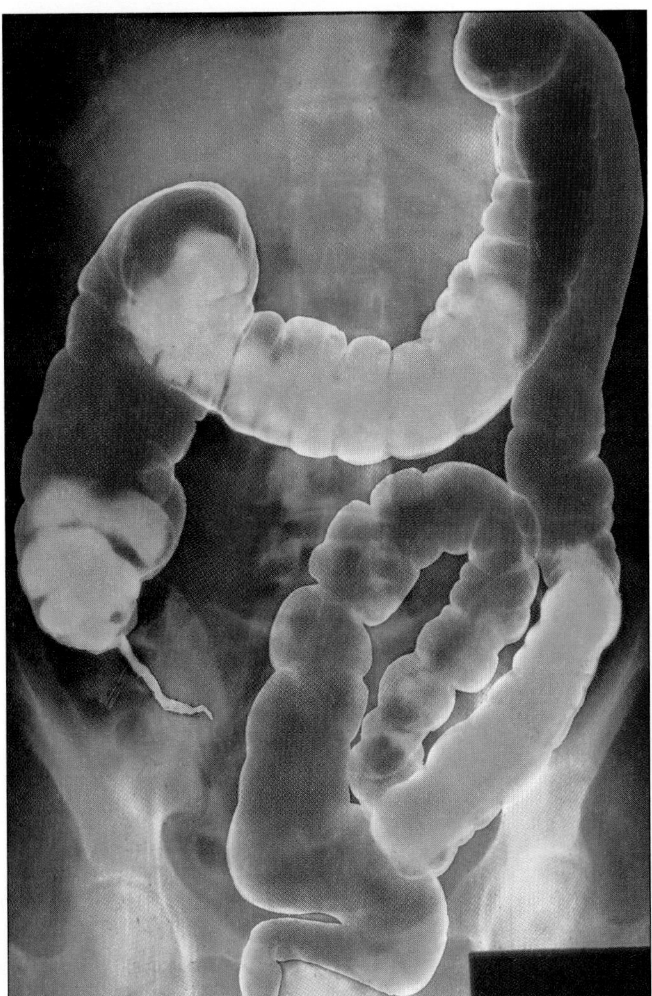

Figure 28-12. During a barium enema the barium is tracked on x-rays.

Gastrointestinal Diseases and Disorders

The level of discomfort from GI disorders can be misleading in relation to severity. There may be severe pain with intestinal gas, which is not serious, whereas there is virtually no pain in the initial stage of appendicitis, which is potentially life-threatening. Be sure that your notes are accurate and complete when a patient reports GI symptoms. Note the level of the patient's pain and whether over-the-counter drugs have been administered. Common diseases and disorders treated by a GI specialist are outlined in Table 28-3.

Neurology

Neurologists diagnose and treat diseases and disorders of the central nervous system and associated systems. Nervous system injuries or diseases can result in loss of sensation, loss or impairment of voluntary movement, seizures, or mental confusion.

Table 28-3

Common Gastrointestinal Diseases and Disorders

Condition	Description	Treatment
Abdominal hernia	Weakness of abdominal wall muscle with outpouching, caused by heavy lifting; exacerbated by general lack of muscle tone; usually asymptomatic except for outpouching; severe pain may indicate complication of strangulated hernia, causing lack of blood supply	Surgery to repair muscle
Anal fissure	Ulcer in anal wall; symptoms include painful defecation with burning; may develop into fistula (abnormal duct to rectum)	Dependent on extent, may include surgery to repair
Cholecystitis	Inflammation of gallbladder; may be caused by intolerance to fatty foods, gallstones, or bacterial infection; symptoms include pain, nausea, diarrhea	Avoidance of fatty foods for intolerance; lithotripsy (noninvasive shock waves) to break up stones; antibiotic for bacterial infection
Cholelithiasis	Formation of gallstones from cholesterol in bile; symptoms include pain, nausea, diarrhea; complications include secondary bacterial infection	Lithotripsy, antibiotics to prevent secondary infection
Colitis	Inflammation of colon caused by bacteria, food intolerance, anxiety, or emotional disorder; symptoms include cramping, pain, diarrhea or bloody diarrhea with mucus or pus, fever, malaise, weight loss, nausea; complications include life-threatening infection or blood poisoning, liver damage, hemorrhoids, anemia, arthritis	Diet modification (clear liquid for acute phase), medication, psychotherapy, fluid replacement, surgery for severe cases; surgery may include insertion of elimination tube (colostomy tube) for temporary or permanent elimination of solid waste
Constipation	Hard feces or stools, decrease in frequency of or ability to have bowel movements, complication of fecal impaction	Diet modification, stool-softener medication, enemas, surgery if necessary for impaction

continued

Your duties in a neurologist's office include assisting with examinations by readying equipment for use, positioning the patient, and handing the doctor tools and other items. You may be asked to perform parts of these examinations, such as visual acuity tests or audiometry. You may also assist with certain diagnostic tests, such as electroencephalography. Your responsibilities will include instructing and educating patients and their families about procedures, disorders, and treatments.

Neurological Examinations

The neurologist evaluates five categories of neurological function in a complete examination:

1. Cognitive function (mental status)
2. Cranial nerves
3. Motor system
4. Reflexes
5. Sensory system

Cognitive function can be assessed by observing general appearance and grooming as well as by asking patients specific questions. The neurologist also determines the status of the cranial nerves, which affect smell and taste, eye movements, hearing, voice quality, facial expression, and facial mobility. The physician may, for example, ask patients to close their eyes and then identify familiar smells. The neurologist observes patients' faces for symmetry of movement and tests visual and auditory acuity. The physician assesses motor ability by testing coordination, observing gait, and determining muscle strength. Finally, the neurologist tests patients' reflexes

Table 28-3 continued

Common Gastrointestinal Diseases and Disorders

Condition	Description	Treatment
Diarrhea	Abnormally frequent and watery bowel movements caused by bacterial or viral infection or food poisoning, complication of dehydration with fluid-electrolyte imbalance	Diet modification, antibiotics for bacterial infection, medication to prevent dehydration
Diverticulitis	Inflammation of diverticulum, usually in colon; symptoms may be absent, may include abdominal pain	Diet modification, surgery possible for severe cases
Gastritis	Inflammation of stomach lining, causing excess secretion of gastric acids and bloating; numerous causes	Diet modification, drug therapy
Gastroesophageal reflux	Gastric acid rising into esophagus due to abnormal valve function; causes heartburn; symptoms may be similar to those of angina, dysphagia (inability to swallow)	Diet modification (including eating small meals), antacids, upright eating, remaining upright for several hours after eating, surgery (rarely)
Hemorrhoids	Enlargement of veins in rectal or anal area, may protrude from anus; symptoms include itching, pain, red blood with defecation	Diet modification, surgery
Hiatal hernia	Protrusion of stomach through diaphragm defect into thorax; symptoms similar to those of gastroesophageal reflux plus pain	Diet therapy with small and frequent meals, exercise, upright eating, medication
Stomatitis (canker sores)	Sore gums or other oral areas caused by herpes virus or acidic body chemistry; exacerbated by emotional distress, foods high in acid; symptoms include ulcerations (canker sores) with burning, sometimes swelling	Bland diet, avoidance of stress, medicated mouth rinses, topical anesthetic

and examines the function of the sensory system in areas of tactile sensation, pain and temperature sensitivity, and awareness of vibration. You are likely to assist the physician in completing these examinations, and you may perform certain components yourself.

Diagnostic Testing

Common diagnostic tests in neurology include electroencephalography and various radiologic tests. You may assist in performing these tests. Many tests are done at a site apart from the physician's office. In such cases you will need to schedule the procedures, instruct patients about pretest preparations, and educate them about the procedure and what to expect.

Electroencephalography. Electroencephalography records the electrical activity of the brain on a strip of graph paper. The tracing is an electroencephalogram (EEG). Electrodes are attached to the patient's scalp, and readings are taken while the patient is at rest and engaged in specific activities (see Figure 28-13). An EEG can be used to detect or examine conditions such as tumors, seizure disorders, or brain injury. You may assist with electrode placement or, after training, obtain the EEG on your own.

Imaging Procedures. Several imaging techniques are used as neurological diagnostic tools. Types of procedures include angiograms, brain scans, computed tomography, magnetic resonance imaging, myelography, and skull x-rays.

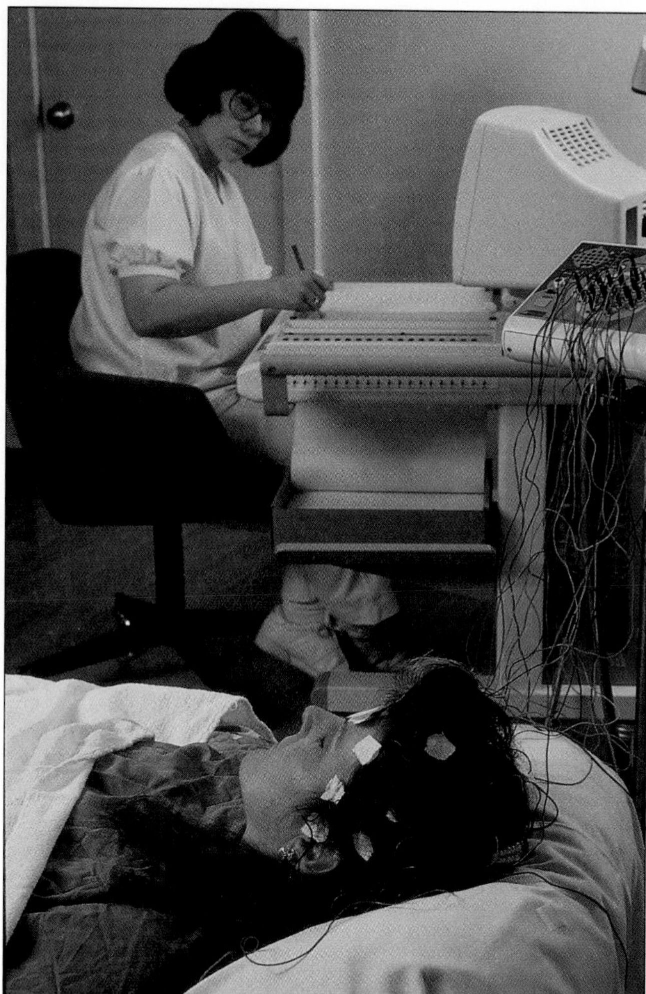

Figure 28-13. EEG readings are taken first while the patient is at rest and then while the patient is breathing deeply or observing a flashing light.

Cerebral Angiography. Cerebral angiography (or angiogram) is a radiologic study of the cerebral blood vessels. After a contrast medium is injected into an artery, x-rays are taken to visualize the cerebral blood vessels.

Brain Scan. A brain scan is performed by injecting the patient with radioisotopes and, after a period of time, using a scanner to detect the material. The radioisotopes tend to gather in areas of abnormality, such as tumors or abscesses.

Computed Tomography. **Computed tomography,** often called a CT scan, is a radiographic examination that produces a three-dimensional, cross-sectional view of the brain. Often one scan is done without a contrast medium. Then a contrast medium is injected for greater clarity. CT scans can help diagnose a wide range of conditions, including tumors, blood clots, and brain swelling.

Magnetic Resonance Imaging. **Magnetic resonance imaging** (MRI) is a viewing technique that enables physicians to see areas inside the body without exposing the patient to x-rays or surgery. The procedure, which takes 30 to 60 minutes, requires the patient to lie still on a padded table that is moved into a tunnellike structure (see Figure 28-14). A powerful magnetic field produces an image of internal body structures.

Myelography. **Myelography** is an x-ray visualization of the spinal cord after the injection of a radioactive contrast medium or air into the spinal subarachnoid space (between the second and innermost of three membranes that cover the spinal cord). This test can reveal tumors, cysts, spinal stenosis, or herniated disks.

Skull X-Ray. Skull x-rays may be used to detect breaks in the skull. They can also be used to locate tumors.

Other Tests. Other diagnostic tests do not involve imaging techniques. They include lumbar puncture and electromyography. A lumbar puncture, or spinal tap, involves collecting a sample of cerebrospinal fluid. A needle is inserted between two lumbar vertebrae and into the subarachnoid space. The collected fluid is sent to a laboratory for analysis. This test is used to diagnose infection, to measure cerebrospinal fluid pressure, and to check for blood cells and proteins in the fluid.

Electromyography is used to detect neuromuscular disorders or nerve damage. Needle electrodes are inserted into some of the patient's skeletal muscles. When the muscles contract, a monitor records the nerve impulses and measures conduction time.

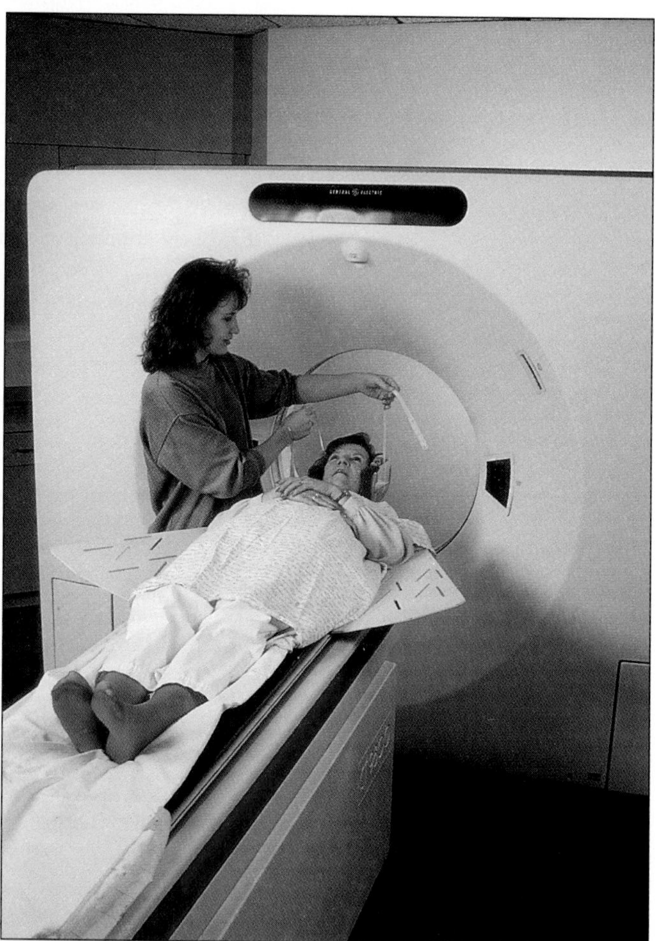

Figure 28-14. Magnetic resonance imaging is used to diagnose disorders in many specialties.

Table 28-4

Common Diseases of the Neurological System

Condition	Description	Treatment
Alzheimer's disease	Disabling disease that usually affects elderly people; involves dementia and deterioration of physical function	Frequent stimulation to possibly help slow deterioration, medications that may slow progression of some symptoms
Bell's palsy	Suddenly occurring cranial nerve disease that causes weakness or paralysis on one side of face	Usually resolves without treatment in 1 to 8 weeks
Encephalitis	Inflammation of brain tissue usually caused by viral infection; symptoms include fever, headache, vomiting, stiff neck, drowsiness	Medication, rest
Epilepsy	Disease caused by misfiring of nerve groups in brain, resulting in seizures	Medication
Herpes zoster	Disease caused by virus that causes chickenpox; symptoms include painful blisters that form along path of one or more nerves	Medication to relieve pain
Meningitis	Inflammation of meninges (membranes covering brain and spinal cord) caused by bacterial or viral infection; symptoms include fever, chills, stiff neck, headache, vomiting	Medication such as antibiotics and drugs to reduce swelling
Migraine headaches	Severe headaches caused by vascular disturbance and characterized by pain, nausea, and sometimes visual disturbances	Medication
Multiple sclerosis	Degenerative disease of central nervous system that results in visual problems, muscle weakness, paralysis	Anti-inflammatory medications used during attacks
Neuritis	Inflammation of one or more nerves; symptoms include severe pain and discomfort or paralysis of affected area	Medication and rest
Parkinson's disease	Progressive neurological disease, causing symptoms of muscular rigidity and tremors	Medication to relieve symptoms
Sciatica	Inflammation of sciatic nerve causing pain in back of thigh and down leg	Medication to relieve pain, rest, heat applications

Neurological Diseases and Disorders

Common diseases of the neurological system are described in Table 28-4. Trauma can also cause damage to the nervous system. Traumatic injuries can result in loss of sensation and voluntary motion. Paralysis on one side of the body, as a result of damage to the opposite side of the brain, is called hemiplegia. Paraplegia involves motor or sensory loss in the lower extremities. Paralysis of the arms, legs, and muscles below the place where the spinal cord is damaged is called quadriplegia.

Patients with acquired immunodeficiency syndrome (AIDS) may exhibit specific neurological symptoms related to their disease. These include:

- Meningitis caused by a fungal infection.
- Encephalopathy (degenerative effect on the brain), resulting in headaches, difficulty concentrating, and apathy.
- Peripheral neuropathies (disorders of the peripheral nerves) that result in pain or changes in gait.

Table 28-5

Common Cancers by Body System

Body System	Symptoms	Treatment
Skeletal System		
Osteosarcoma: malignant lesion, usually in femur, tibia, or humerus	Pain and swelling, central hardened portion with softer edges, possible pathologic fracture	Radiation and chemotherapy to minimize tumor, surgery
Chondrosarcomas: malignant tumors of cartilage	Dull pain and swelling	Radiation and chemotherapy to minimize tumor, surgery
Nervous System		
Malignant gliomas: tumors of brain and brainstem	Headache, vomiting, changes in sensation or personality	Surgery, radiation, chemotherapy
Endocrine System		
Thyroid cancer	Nodules on thyroid gland	Surgery, radiation
Pancreatic cancer	Weight loss, abdominal pain, jaundice; very lethal form of cancer	Surgery, chemotherapy with radiation
Circulatory System		
Leukemia: several diseases involving abnormal overproduction of cells in bone marrow	Fatigue, paleness, repeated infections	Chemotherapy, bone marrow transplants
Lymphoma: cancers of lymph system; divided into Hodgkin's lymphoma and non-Hodgkin's lymphoma	Enlarged lymph nodes, itching, fever, weight loss	Chemotherapy, radiation
Respiratory System		
Lung cancer	Cough, repeated lung infections	Surgery, radiation, chemotherapy
Digestive System		
Oral cancer: cancer of mouth or throat	May begin with painless sore or mass; later, difficulty chewing or swallowing	Surgery, radiation, chemotherapy

continued

Oncology

An oncologist specializes in the detection and treatment of tumors and cancerous growths. *Cancer* refers to a number of oncologic diseases that affect different body systems. All cancers are characterized by the uncontrolled growth and spread of abnormal cells.

A tumor is a lump of abnormal cells. Tumors are classified as benign or malignant. Benign tumors contain abnormal cells, but the cells do not invade and actively destroy surrounding tissue. Malignant tumors contain cells that grow uncontrollably, invading and actively destroying the tissue around them. Malignant, or cancerous, growths are capable of **metastasis,** the transfer of abnormal cells to body sites far removed from the original tumor. When cells become malignant, the process is called carcinogenesis.

You will encounter patients with a variety of medical conditions in an oncologist's office. You must be aware of the various types of cancer, what their symptoms are, and how they are treated (see Table 28-5). Part of your job will involve preparing patients for the side effects of

Table 28-5 continued

Common Cancers by Body System

Body System	Symptoms	Treatment
Esophageal cancer	Often no early symptoms; later, difficulty swallowing, regurgitation of food	Surgery, radiation, chemotherapy
Stomach cancer	Indigestion, weight loss, nausea	Surgery, chemotherapy
Liver cancer	Abdominal pain, fatigue, jaundice	Surgery, liver transplant
Colorectal cancer	Changes in bowel habits, blood in stools, rectal or abdominal pain	Surgery combined with radiation or chemotherapy
Urinary System		
Bladder cancer	Urinary frequency or urgency, blood in urine	Surgery, chemotherapy
Kidney cancer	Back or abdominal pain, blood in urine	Surgery, radiation, chemotherapy
Reproductive System		
Cervical cancer	Usually none, possible painless vaginal bleeding; abnormal Pap smear (Papanicolaou smear)	Surgery, radiation, chemotherapy
Endometrial cancer: cancer of uterine lining	Postmenopausal bleeding	Surgery, radiation, chemotherapy
Ovarian cancer	Usually none, possible abdominal pain	Surgery, radiation, chemotherapy
Breast cancer	Lump or thickening in breast, changed appearance, discharge	Surgery, radiation, chemotherapy
Prostate cancer	Often none; possible difficult, frequent, or painful urination	Surgery, radiation, chemotherapy
Testicular cancer	Lump in testicle	Surgery, radiation, chemotherapy

cancer treatment and helping patients deal with them. Patient and family education and support are essential.

Diagnostic Testing

Cancer is detected and diagnosed through a variety of procedures. You will schedule some of these tests and provide pretest instructions and explanations to patients. You may obtain blood specimens for some tests and assist in other diagnostic procedures, including these:

- X-rays
- CT scan
- MRI
- Blood tests, especially those to detect tumor markers, such as carcinoembryonic antigen (CEA) (increased levels of CEA indicate a variety of cancers)
- Ultrasonography
- Biopsy, the removal of a sample of fluid or tissue from a growth (see the discussion of surgery as a medical specialty later in this chapter)

Cancer Treatment

Cancer treatments fall into three general categories: surgery, radiation therapy, and chemotherapy. Often a combination of these treatment methods is used. All methods damage healthy as well as cancerous cells. The success of treatment depends on many factors, and recovery varies greatly from patient to patient.

Surgery. Surgical removal of all or part of the tumor and some surrounding tissue is one method of cancer treatment. It is most effective when the tumor appears to be contained within a particular organ or is localized in an area of the skin. Surgery is usually followed, however, by either radiation therapy or chemotherapy.

Radiation Therapy. Radiation therapy uses radiation to kill and stop the growth of tumor cells. It is often used in conjunction with surgery or chemotherapy. Radiation therapy is effective because radiation has the most damaging effect on cells that are undergoing rapid division, such as cancer cells.

Chemotherapy. Chemotherapy is also used in conjunction with other therapies. Chemotherapy uses strong anticancer drugs to kill malignant cells. As with radiation therapy, rapidly dividing cells, such as cancer cells, are most strongly affected by these medications. Although it is unlikely that you will prepare or administer anticancer drugs, you need to be aware that they are highly toxic. General protective guidelines must be followed whenever there is risk of contact with the drugs or patients' body fluids. Measures include wearing complete personal protective equipment and properly handling and disposing of materials contaminated with body fluids.

Ophthalmology

An ophthalmologist treats the eyes and related tissues. Chapter 26 covers the anatomy of the eye and the types of eye examinations and procedures that might be dealt with in a general physician's office. Some of these examinations and procedures will also be performed in an ophthalmologist's office. The most common eye disorders an ophthalmologist treats are visual defects, which are often correctable with eyeglasses or contact lenses. Ophthalmologists also treat eye injuries and remove foreign bodies from the eye. More serious disorders, such as cataracts and glaucoma, require medication or surgery. In an ophthalmologist's office you may perform some of the procedures that involve measuring various aspects and functions of the eye, such as visual acuity, color vision, and intraocular pressure.

Ophthalmic Examinations

An ophthalmologist performs an eye examination by inspecting the interior of the patient's eyes, including the retina, optic nerve, and blood vessels. The physician uses an **ophthalmoscope,** a handheld instrument with a light, to view the inner eye structures. You will maintain and prepare this instrument for the physician's use, as described in Procedure 28-3.

An ophthalmologist also tests the patient's visual fields. The visual field is the entire area visible to the eye when

PROCEDURE 28-3

Preparing the Ophthalmoscope for Use

Objective: To ensure that the ophthalmoscope is ready for use during an eye examination

OSHA Guidelines: This procedure does not involve exposure to blood, body fluids, or tissues.

Materials: Ophthalmoscope, lens, spare bulb, spare battery

Method

1. Wash your hands.
2. Take the ophthalmoscope out of its battery charger. In a darkened room turn on the ophthalmoscope light.
3. Shine the large beam of white light on the back of your hand to check that the instrument's tiny lightbulb is providing strong enough light (Figure 28-15).
4. Replace the bulb or battery if necessary. (The battery is located in the ophthalmoscope's handle.)
5. Make sure the instrument's lens is screwed into the handle. If it is not, attach the lens.

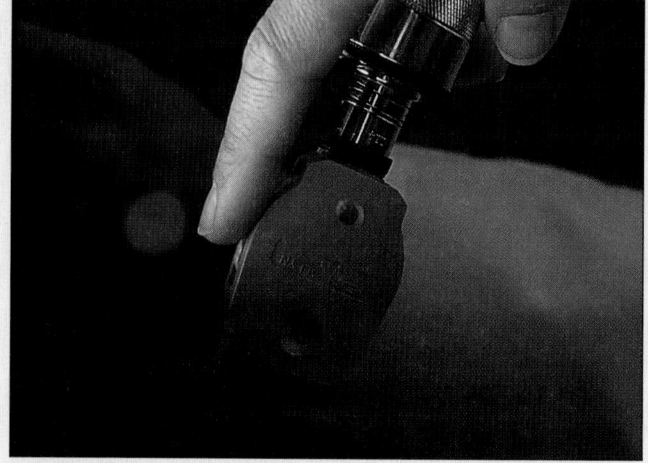

Figure 28-15. Shine the ophthalmoscope light on your hand to check the strength of the beam.

the patient looks at an object straight ahead. Visual fields are assessed by the confrontation method. The doctor stands or sits about 2 ft in front of the patient. The patient covers one eye, and the doctor closes her own opposite eye. (This makes the visual fields of the two individuals roughly the same.) Then the doctor moves a pencil or other object into the patient's horizontal or vertical visual field, asking the patient to say "Now" when the object comes into view. Defects in field of vision are noted. Convergence of the eyes is tested by bringing the handheld object to the patient's nose as the eyes focus on it.

The ophthalmologist also routinely tests for glaucoma, with the aid of a tonometer (see Figure 28-16). The tonometer measures intraocular pressure, shown by the eyeball's resistance to indentation. Your role is to explain the procedure to the patient, instill anesthetizing eyedrops into the patient's eyes when required, assist the patient into position, and hand the doctor the instruments.

The eye examination may also include a **refraction examination** to verify the need for corrective lenses. Normally, the lens and other parts of the eye work together to focus images on the retina. When errors of refraction exist, images are focused incorrectly, causing conditions such as farsightedness and nearsightedness. A refraction examination is performed with a retinoscope or a Phoroptor, the trademark name for a device that contains many different lenses. The doctor has the patient look through a succession of lens combinations to find out which one creates the clearest image (see Figure 28-17).

Another instrument the ophthalmologist may use during the examination is the **slitlamp.** This instrument consists of a magnifying lens combined with a light source. It is used to provide a minute examination of the eye's anatomy. Patients rest their chin on the device's chin rest and stare straight ahead while the doctor shines a narrow beam (slit) of light into the eye and looks at the eye through the instrument's lens.

Eye Diseases and Disorders

An ophthalmologist treats a wide range of eye diseases and disorders. Some, such as a sty or conjunctivitis, do not greatly affect vision and may be treated by a general practitioner. Others affect the internal workings of the eye and require the attention of a specialist.

Disorders of External Eye Structures. Some disorders affect external eye structures. These structures include the eyelid and the eyelashes.

Blepharitis. Blepharitis is a chronic inflammation of the edges of the eyelid, more common in older individuals

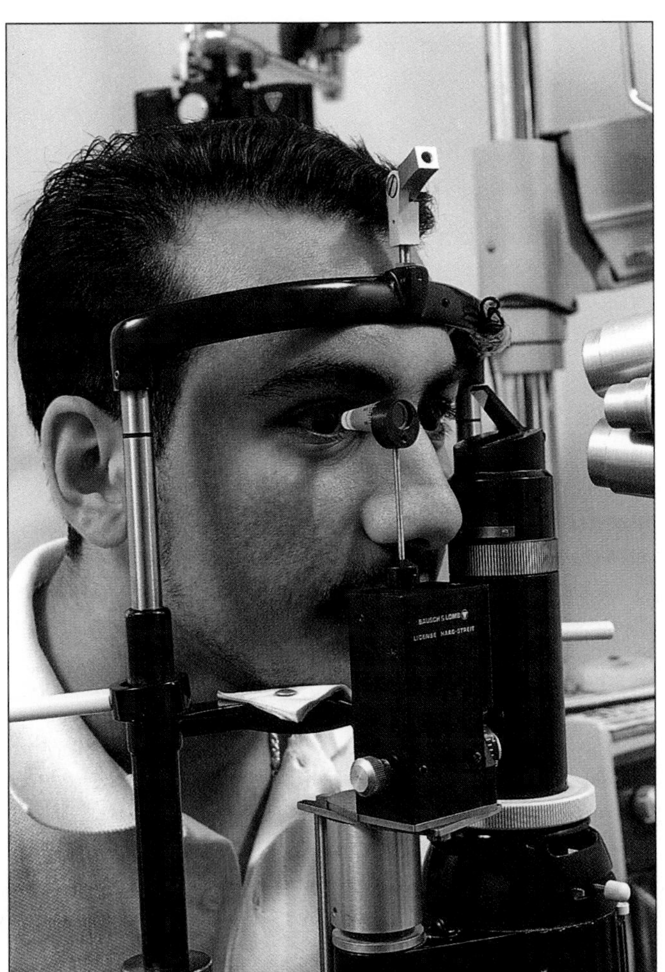

A

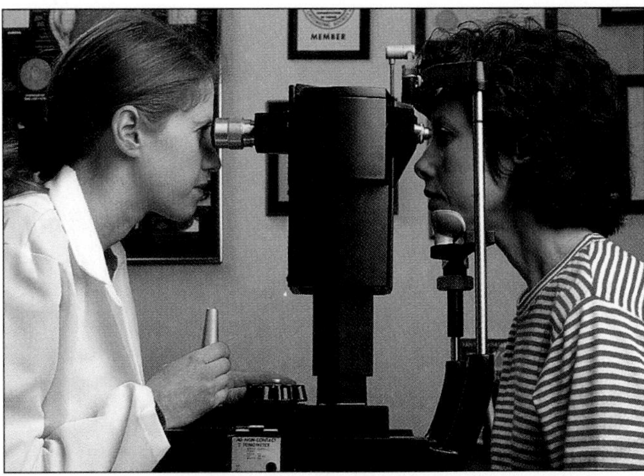

B

Figure 28-16. The two types of tonometers are (a) the applanation tonometer, which actually touches the eyeball during assessment, and (b) the noncontact, or air-puff, tonometer, which directs a puff of air at the cornea.

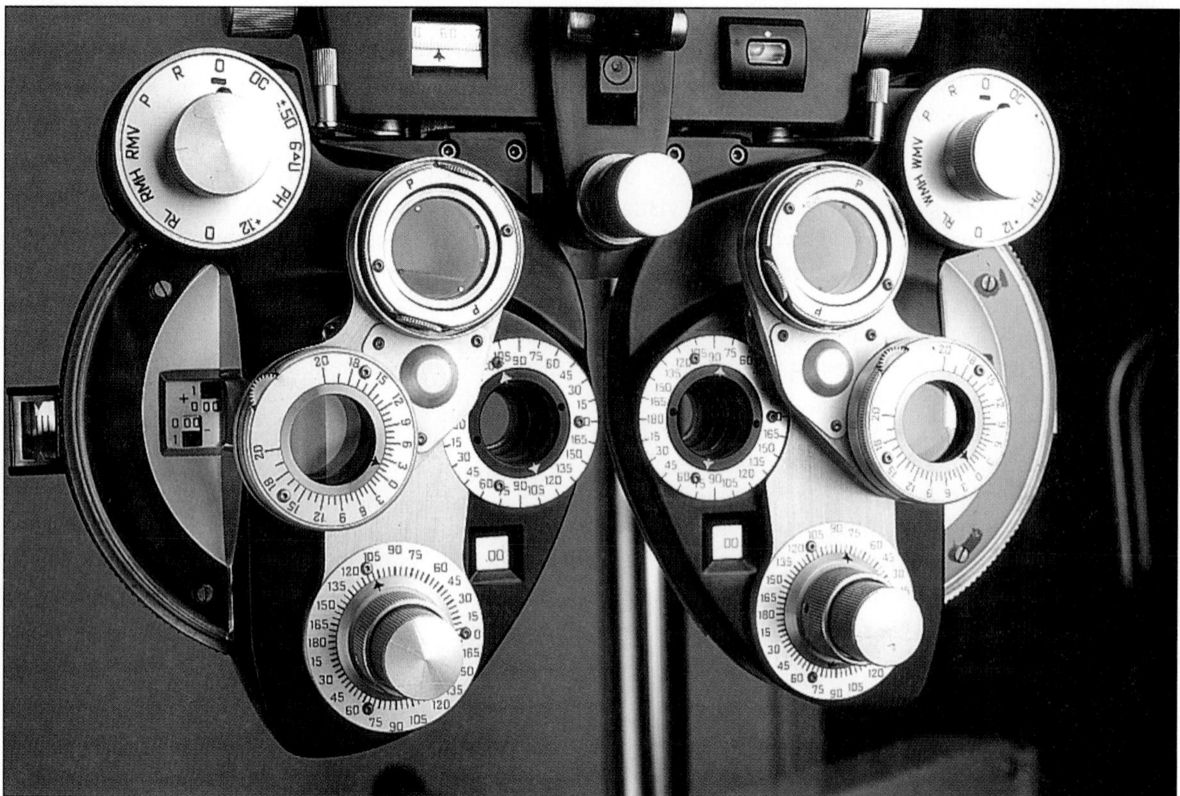

Figure 28-17. The Phoroptor helps the ophthalmologist assess errors of refraction.

than in younger people. It can be caused by infection or by the same skin condition that causes dandruff. Symptoms include red, swollen eyelids with scaling or crusting of skin at the edges. The patient's eyes may be irritated and itchy. Proper eye care and hygiene often clear up the condition successfully. Antibiotic creams may be necessary in severe cases.

Ptosis. Ptosis is a drooping of the upper eyelid in which the lid partially or completely covers the eye. It is caused by weakness of or damage to the muscle that raises the eyelid or by problems with the nerve that controls the muscle. Often no treatment is required, although surgery may be performed if the condition interferes with vision or if the patient is concerned about appearance.

Sty. A sty is the result of an infection of an eyelash follicle. A red, painful swelling appears on the edge of the eye and typically forms a white head of pus. The head bursts and drains before it heals in about a week. Applying warm, moist compresses to the sty may help it drain sooner.

Disorders of Structures at the Front of the Eye. Another group of disorders affects structures at the front of the eye. These structures include the conjunctiva and the cornea.

Conjunctivitis. Conjunctivitis, or pinkeye, is an inflammation of the conjunctiva caused by allergy, an irritant, or infection. It is a common disorder that is annoying but normally not serious.

Allergic conjunctivitis occurs when a person has an allergic reaction to pollen, makeup, or other substance. The symptoms are itchy, red eyes. The doctor may prescribe medication to relieve troublesome symptoms and suggest avoidance of the trigger whenever possible. Conjunctivitis may also be caused by irritants such as dust, smoke, wind, pollutants, and excessive glare.

Infectious conjunctivitis can be caused by either a bacterial or a viral infection. Both forms are easily spread and have symptoms including redness and a gritty feeling in the eye. Bacterial infections typically produce pus, which may form a crust on the eye during sleep. Viral infections usually produce a watery discharge. Although eye irrigation or saline drops may be used to soothe eyes affected by either type of infection, only bacterial infections are treated with antibiotic drops or ointment.

Because you may not know the cause of a patient's conjunctivitis (allergies, irritants, bacteria, viruses), take precautions to avoid spreading infection. As with any potentially infectious disease, use Universal Precautions in medical settings. Wear appropriate personal protective equipment when dealing with any patient who has conjunctivitis.

Corneal Ulcers and Abrasions. Ulcers (lesions) on the cornea may be the result of injury, infection, or both. An injury such as an abrasion (scratch) on the cornea can become infected with bacteria, viruses, or fungi. The symptoms of a corneal ulcer include pain or discomfort and unclear vision. Treatment consists of antibiotic eyedrops or ointments and use of an eye patch.

Disorders Involving Internal Eye Structures. Another group of disorders affects structures inside the eye. Cataracts, for example, affect the lens. Glaucoma can damage several internal eye structures.

Cataracts. Cataracts are cloudy or opaque areas in the normally clear lens of the eye. Cataracts develop gradually, blocking the passage of light through the eye. The result is a progressive loss of vision in one or both eyes. In severe cases you can actually see the cloudy lens through the pupil of the eye (see Figure 28-18).

Cataracts are more common in the elderly than in younger people because the lens deteriorates with aging. Cataracts can also be caused by iritis, injury, ultraviolet radiation, or diabetes. Some cataracts are congenital. Cataracts are treated by surgically removing the lens and using an artificial lens in its place. The artificial lens may be in the form of special eyeglasses, special contact lenses, or an intraocular lens inserted at the time of cataract surgery.

Glaucoma. Glaucoma is a condition in which fluid pressure builds up inside the eye. This pressure damages the internal structures of the eye and gradually destroys vision. Glaucoma is the second leading cause of blindness in the United States and the first cause among African Americans.

Aqueous humor is produced by capillaries in the ciliary body. This fluid circulates between the lens and the cornea. The fluid drains out of this area through the angle formed by the iris and the cornea. The aqueous humor diffuses into a vascular channel (Schlemm's canal) that encircles the cornea where it meets the sclera (see Figure 26-1 in Chapter 26). The aqueous humor then returns to the systemic circulation (the circulation of the blood to body tissues).

In the case of glaucoma, the fluid drains out of the eye too slowly or fails to drain at all. The result is a buildup of intraocular pressure. Retinal nerve fibers are damaged, and blood vessels are destroyed, leading to loss of vision and possible blindness.

Glaucoma is treated with medication that reduces pressure in the eye. Drops, pills, or both may be prescribed to reduce the production of aqueous humor. A procedure called an iridotomy is sometimes performed. This procedure is a type of laser surgery in which a small hole is created in the iris that allows the excess fluid to drain. If the surgery is not effective, an iridectomy (removal of part of the iris) is done to create a larger opening in the iris to allow drainage.

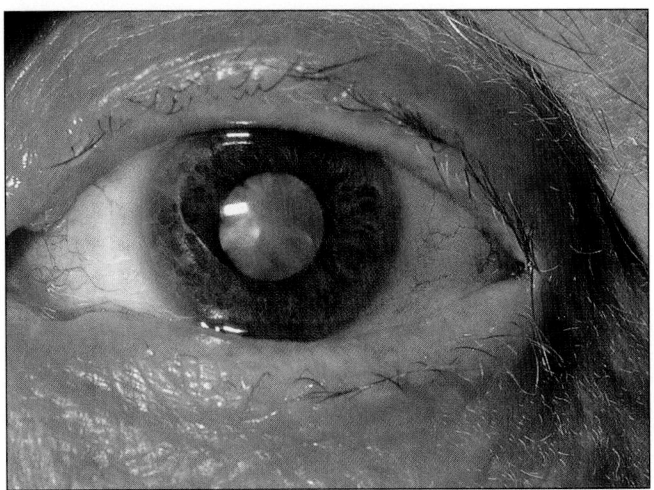

Figure 28-18. The lens of an eye with a cataract has a clouded appearance.

Iritis. Iritis, also known as uveitis, is an inflammation of the iris and sometimes the ciliary body. White blood cells from the inflamed area and protein that leaks from small blood vessels float in the aqueous humor. The symptoms of iritis are pain or discomfort in one or both eyes; pain may be worse in bright light. The eye is red, and loss of vision may occur. Left untreated, iritis can lead to other complications, such as glaucoma and cataracts. Iritis is treated with anti-inflammatory drops or ointment.

Disorders of the Retina. Several serious disorders affect the retina, the internal layer of the back of the eye. These disorders include retinal detachment, diabetic retinopathy, and macular degeneration.

Retinal Detachment. Retinal detachment occurs when the retina separates from the underlying choroid layer. When this separation occurs, vision is damaged.

Retinal detachment is rare; however, it is more common as people age. Early symptoms of detachment include flashes of light or floating black shapes, both of which can occur as the hole in the retina forms. Peripheral vision is lost as the retina detaches. Vision becomes progressively blurred as detachment continues.

When detected early, a hole can be "sealed" so that the retina does not detach. If the retina has already detached, some vision can often be restored with new surgical and laser treatments.

Diabetic Retinopathy. Diabetic retinopathy is a complication of diabetes. People who have had diabetes for a long time or who do not keep their condition under control experience damage to small blood vessels that supply the retina. The vessels initially leak fluid, which distorts vision. As the disease progresses, fragile new blood vessels grow on the retina and bleed into the vitreous humor. Scar tissue may also form on the retina. The result is loss of vision. The damage usually cannot be repaired, but the disorder can be controlled to prevent further loss of vision.

Macular Degeneration. The macula is the area of the retina responsible for the central area of a person's visual field. For unknown reasons the macula begins to deteriorate as some individuals age. Macular degeneration causes loss of vision in the center of an image; peripheral vision remains intact. Macular degeneration is the leading cause of blindness among the elderly in the United States.

Loss of sharp vision occurs very gradually and without pain. One of the first signs is difficulty in reading. The loss of vision often appears as a dark spot in the center of the field of vision. If macular degeneration is detected early, laser surgery may restore some vision or prevent further loss.

Disorders Involving Eye Movement. Normally, both eyes move together when people look at objects. Strabismus is the name for a deviation of one eye. Strabismus in young children is caused by misaligned or unbalanced eye muscles. A condition called amblyopia may occur as the misaligned eye becomes "lazy." The brain tends to ignore what the lazy eye sees; if the condition is not treated, vision will be affected in this eye. Treatment involves putting a patch over the fully working eye to force the child to use the other eye. Eyeglasses may be used along with the patch. In some cases surgery on the eye muscle is required.

Strabismus in adults usually results from problems with the nerves connecting the brain and the eye muscles or with the muscles themselves. Conditions that can cause such problems include diabetes, high blood pressure, brain injury, muscular dystrophy, and inflammation of certain cerebral arteries. Treatment depends on the cause of the condition.

Refractive Disorders. Refraction refers to the way light from objects is focused through the eye to form an image on the retina. The normal eye focuses light exactly at the retina, producing a clear image (see Figure 28-19). In some people the eye focuses light either in front of or behind the retina, so the image is not clear. The problem may be due to abnormal shape of the eye or to abnormal focusing of the light by the cornea and lens. The four most common refractive disorders are nearsightedness, farsightedness, presbyopia, and astigmatism.

Myopia (Nearsightedness). Myopia is the condition in which images of distant objects come into focus in front of the retina and are blurred (see Figure 28-19). This condition occurs if the eye is too long or if the cornea and lens

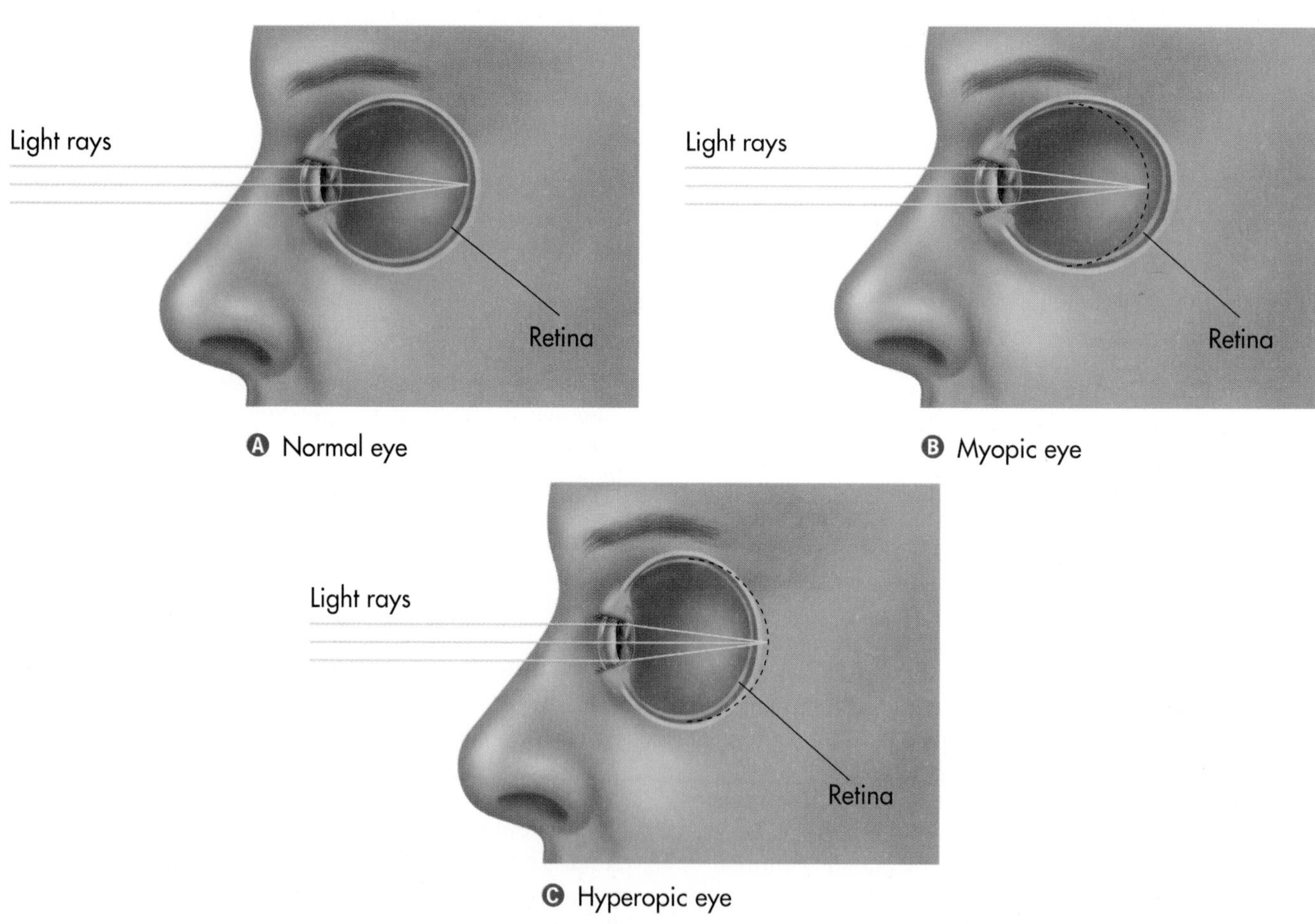

Figure 28-19. A. In the normal eye light rays are focused directly on the retina. **B.** With myopia an elongated eyeball causes light rays to be focused in front of the retina. **C.** With hyperopia a shortened eyeball causes light rays to be focused behind the retina.

bend light rays more than normally. Nearby objects are usually seen clearly, but objects far away are unclear.

Nearsightedness is corrected with eyeglasses or contact lenses that have inwardly curving (concave) lenses. The lenses correct the bending of light rays so that they focus on the retina. Surgical and laser techniques are also used to correct myopia by changing the shape of the cornea.

Hyperopia (Farsightedness) and Presbyopia. Hyperopia, or hypermetropia, causes images to come into focus behind the retina (see Figure 28-19). The eyeball may be too short, or the cornea and lens may bend light rays less than normally. Faraway objects are usually seen clearly, but nearby objects are unclear. Young eyes can compensate for the problem by a process known as accommodation. The ciliary muscles contract during accommodation, thickening the lens and increasing its convexity. These changes allow the image to come into focus on the retina.

Patients with mild farsightedness may have no symptoms or may have blurred vision. They may have symptoms of eyestrain (an aching in the eye) because the ciliary muscles are overworked. Farsightedness is corrected with eyeglasses or contact lenses that have outwardly turning (convex) lenses. Aging usually causes the ciliary muscles to weaken, so a person may need stronger eyeglasses over time.

Presbyopia is a condition that most commonly affects people starting in their mid-40s. Older eyes tend to lose the ability to accommodate because the lens becomes more rigid. As a result images come into focus behind the retina, as they do with farsightedness. Individuals find they must hold reading materials farther away to see them clearly. Corrective lenses are used to treat this condition.

Astigmatism. Sometimes vision is distorted because the cornea is unevenly curved. This condition is called astigmatism. Astigmatism may cause vertical or horizontal lines to appear out of focus. It can occur along with either nearsightedness or farsightedness. Astigmatism is treated with lenses that correct the unevenness of the cornea.

A surgical vision-correcting treatment for myopia and astigmatism is radial keratotomy. The procedure, which is done on an outpatient basis under local anesthesia, involves making corneal incisions in a wheel-spoke configuration. The incisions allow the eye to return to a normal or almost normal shape. This procedure has been very successful for some patients. Others, however, have experienced complications, including worsening of vision. Other techniques that use lasers to correct vision are still under development.

Orthopedics

Orthopedics is the medical specialty focusing on disorders, injuries, and diseases of the muscular and skeletal systems. The two systems are so interdependent that they are sometimes referred to as the musculoskeletal system, especially by orthopedists. In the office of an orthopedist, you will be asked to assist with general examinations. Other responsibilities may include assisting with x-rays, helping with casting, applying hot or cold treatments (discussed in Chapter 30), and educating patients about therapy regimens. You must be knowledgeable about the musculoskeletal system and its common disorders and treatments.

Orthopedic Examinations

An orthopedist uses inspection, palpation, and a variety of diagnostic tests to assess the structure and function of the musculoskeletal system. The patient is asked to stand, walk, and perform several range-of-motion exercises. In these maneuvers the patient moves a joint in a variety of ways; the doctor usually measures the degree of mobility with a device called a goniometer. A complete examination takes some time, and you may need to help drape, position, or physically support the patient, especially if the patient is elderly or incapacitated. You may also be responsible for instructing the patient about care for a musculoskeletal condition, including how to perform therapeutic exercises.

Orthopedists use a variety of diagnostic tests. As in most other specialties, x-rays play a vital role in diagnosis. They are especially useful in determining the nature and extent of a bone injury. Other common radiographic examinations in the orthopedic specialty include the following:

- CT scan
- MRI
- Angiography (for affected vascular structures)
- Myelography (for spinal disorders)
- Diskography (for intervertebral disk disorders)
- Arthrography (for joint disorders)
- Bone scans

Arthroscopy enables the orthopedist to see inside a joint, usually the knee or shoulder, with an arthroscope. This tubular instrument includes an optical system; when the tube is inserted into the joint, it can be visualized (see Figure 28-20). Arthroscopy is used

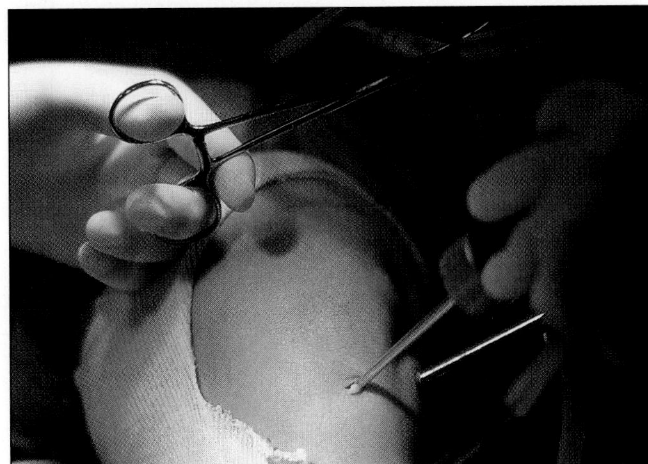

Figure 28-20. Arthroscopy can be used for diagnosis as well as biopsy and surgical repair.

Table 28-6

Common Diseases and Disorders of the Musculoskeletal System

Condition	Description	Treatment
Arthritis	Inflammation of joints—rheumatoid or degenerative (osteoarthritis); rheumatoid arthritis causes joint stiffness and soreness, pain, and swelling and may lead to deformity; osteoarthritis produces pain, stiffness, and possible enlargement of bones, without deformity	Anti-inflammatory medications, application of heat, rest, exercise, occupational and physical therapy, surgery such as joint replacement (arthroplasty)
Bursitis	Inflammation of one or more bursae (sacs surrounding joints); symptoms include pain (especially upon movement), restricted motion, and swelling	Anti-inflammatory medications
Carpal tunnel syndrome	Compression of median nerve, causing wrist pain and numbness	Rest and occupational adjustments, splinting of wrists, injection of corticosteroids, surgical decompression of nerve
Dislocation	Displacement of bones at joint so that parts that are supposed to make contact no longer come together; occurs most often to fingers, shoulder, knee, and hip	Relocation, or shifting bones back into place; anti-inflammatory medications
Herniated intervertebral disk (HID)	Protruding contents of disk compress nerve roots and cause severe pain	Rest, traction, physical therapy, muscle relaxants, surgery
Osteomyelitis	Infection of bone; principal symptom is pain	Antibiotics and analgesics, surgery
Osteoporosis	Metabolic disorder that causes decreased bone mass; bones become brittle and fracture easily	Exercise, dietary supplements, hormone therapy, drug therapy (alendronate)
Paget's disease	Chronic condition that causes bone deformities and affects 2% to 3% of people over age 50	Exercise, dietary supplements, hormone therapy, drug therapy (alendronate)
Scoliosis	Abnormal curving of spine	Back brace, surgery
Sprain	Injury to ligament caused by joint overextension; symptoms include pain, swelling, and discoloration	Rest, support, application of cold, anti-inflammatory medications
Tendonitis	Inflammation of tendon	Rest, support, anti-inflammatory medications

to get a closer look at conditions, such as injuries and degenerative joint diseases, and to guide surgical procedures.

Bone and muscle biopsies may be performed to detect disorders such as bone infection and muscle atrophy. Electromyography is another diagnostic tool used in this specialty. An orthopedist may also order urine and blood tests to detect levels of substances such as calcium or phosphorus.

Orthopedic Diseases and Disorders

Table 28-6 lists many of the diseases and disorders you will encounter in an orthopedic specialty. Back pain, especially lower-back pain, is a common disorder. It can have many causes, including muscle strain, osteoarthritis, and the presence of a tumor. The orthopedist determines the nature of the problem based on the symptoms and diagnostic x-rays and CT scans. Treatments include the application of heat, administration of analgesics or muscle relaxants, exercise therapy, special braces, and traction.

Another condition that is commonly encountered in the orthopedist's office is a **fracture,** or break in a bone. Fractures and their treatment are discussed in Chapter 31.

Otology

An otologist treats diseases and disorders of the ears. Procedures common to this specialty are sometimes performed by other physicians as well, especially general practitioners, internists, and allergists. Chapter 26 covers the anatomy of the ear and the types of ear examinations and procedures that might be done in a general practitioner's office. Some of these are performed in an otologist's office too. You may assist with or perform auditory screening, and you may help with diagnostic tests such as tympanometry. Otology specialists whose practices include problems affecting the nose and throat are called otorhinolaryngologists.

Common Disorders of the Outer Ear

Several disorders affect the external parts of the ear. These include cerumen impaction, otitis externa, and pruritus.

Cerumen Impaction. A condition called cerumen impaction occurs when the ear canal becomes blocked by a buildup of cerumen (earwax). The symptoms include a feeling that the ear is stopped up, partial hearing loss, ringing in the ear and, occasionally, pain. The wax can be softened with special eardrops, and irrigation can be performed to remove the wax.

Otitis Externa. Otitis externa is an infection of the outer ear, usually caused by bacteria or fungi. The infection can be localized, as with a boil or abscess, or the entire ear canal lining can be affected. Fungal infections are common in swimmers because of persistent moisture in the ear canal.

Symptoms of otitis externa include itching, pain, and pus in the ear. This infection is sometimes treated with a combination of antibiotic or antifungal agent and an anti-inflammatory medication.

Pruritus. A common problem in the elderly is pruritus, or itching, of the ear canal. Because the sebaceous glands produce less wax with aging, the ear becomes dry and itchy. Dryness can be overcome by a regular routine of lubricating the ear canal with a few drops of mineral oil.

Common Disorders of the Middle Ear

Middle ear disorders involve the eardrum and the chamber behind it. They include otitis media, mastoiditis, otosclerosis, and ruptured eardrum.

Otitis Media. Otitis media is an inflammation of the middle ear characterized by a buildup of fluid. It is most commonly referred to as an ear infection. For detailed information on otitis media, see Chapter 26.

Mastoiditis. The mastoid bone is located just behind the ear. It is connected to the middle ear by air cells, or sinuses, in the bone. Sometimes, if left untreated, an infection in the middle ear can spread to the mastoid bone through these air cells. Although mastoiditis is fairly rare, it may be serious because the mastoid air cells are close to the organs of hearing, important nerves, the covering of the brain, and the jugular vein. Severe cases of mastoiditis may require removal of the affected bone.

Otosclerosis. Otosclerosis occurs when bone tissue grows abnormally around the stapes, or stirrup (the innermost of the three tiny bones that connect the eardrum and the inner ear). This overgrowth of tissue prevents the stapes from transmitting sound vibrations to the inner ear. The result is hearing loss that involves one or both ears. The condition is often hereditary.

Symptoms of otosclerosis include gradual loss of hearing and tinnitus (described later in the chapter). Surgery to replace the stapes can restore or improve hearing in almost 90% of patients with otosclerosis. Alternatively, a hearing aid may improve hearing for some patients.

Ruptured Eardrum. The eardrum may become ruptured in several ways: by a sharp object, an explosion, a blow to the ear, or a severe middle ear infection. Sometimes the eardrum is ruptured by a sudden change in air pressure, as might occur when flying in an airplane or diving. Symptoms include pain, partial hearing loss, and a slight discharge or bleeding. The symptoms typically last only a few hours. A ruptured eardrum usually heals on its own in 1 to 2 weeks, but the doctor may prescribe an antibiotic or the use of a temporary patch to prevent infection.

Common Disorders of the Inner Ear

Disorders of the inner ear, or labyrinth, affect the cochlea and the semicircular canals. They include labyrinthitis, Ménière's disease, presbycusis, and tinnitus.

Labyrinthitis. Labyrinthitis is an infection of the labyrinth, most commonly caused by a virus. Because the labyrinth includes the semicircular canals, which are involved in balance, this infection causes symptoms of dizziness or vertigo. The room may appear to spin, and any movement exacerbates the sensation, sometimes to the point of nausea and vomiting. Although disturbing, labyrinthitis disappears on its own within 1 to 3 weeks. The patient may need to rest in bed for a few days, and medication can be given for symptoms.

Ménière's Disease. Ménière's disease is caused by increased fluid in the labyrinth. The pressure of the fluid disturbs the sense of balance and may even rupture the labyrinth wall or damage the cochlea with its hearing receptors. One or both ears may be affected. Symptoms of this disorder include vertigo, nausea, vomiting, distorted hearing, and tinnitus. Some people may suffer hearing loss ranging from mild to severe. Medications may be used to combat vertigo, nausea, and vomiting. Other

PROCEDURE 28-4

Assisting With a Needle Biopsy

Objective: To remove tissue from a patient's body so that it can be examined in a laboratory

OSHA Guidelines

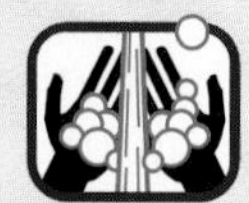
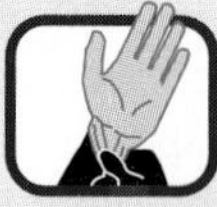
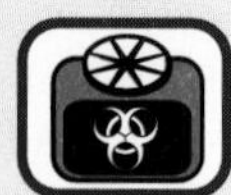
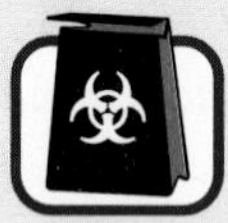
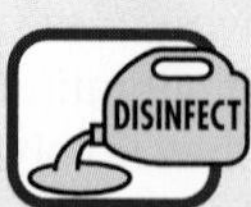

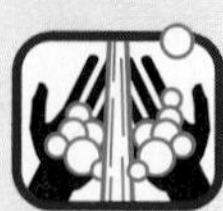

Materials: Sterile drapes, tray or Mayo stand, antiseptic solution, cotton balls, local anesthetic, disposable sterile biopsy needle or disposable sterile syringe and needle, sterile sponges, specimen bottle with fixative solution, laboratory packaging, sterile wound-dressing materials

Method

1. Identify the patient and introduce yourself; instruct the patient as needed.
2. Wash your hands and assemble the necessary materials.
3. Prepare the sterile field and instruments.
4. Put on examination gloves.
5. Cleanse the biopsy site. Prepare the patient's skin.
6. Remove the gloves, wash your hands, and put on clean examination gloves.
7. Assist the doctor as she injects anesthetic.
8. During the procedure help drape and position the patient.
9. If you will be handing the doctor the instruments, remove the gloves, perform a surgical scrub, and put on sterile gloves.
10. Place the sample in a properly labeled specimen bottle, complete the laboratory requisition form, and package the specimen for immediate transport to the laboratory.
11. Dress the patient's wound site.
12. Properly dispose of used supplies and instruments.
13. Clean and disinfect the room according to OSHA guidelines.
14. Remove the gloves and wash your hands.

treatments that help some people include using diuretics and following a low-sodium diet.

Presbycusis. Presbycusis is a type of sensorineural hearing loss. This disorder involves a gradual deterioration of the sensory receptors in the cochlea, leading to gradual loss of hearing. It is the most common form of hearing loss in older adults, affecting about 25% of people by the age of 60 or 70. Men are affected more often than women. Typically both ears are affected, and the patient has difficulty hearing high-pitched tones as well as normal conversation. Presbycusis is thought to be caused by factors such as prolonged exposure to loud noise, infection, injury, certain medications, and some diseases. Hearing loss can be treated effectively, however, with a hearing aid.

Tinnitus. Tinnitus is more commonly called a ringing in the ears. It can, however, take several forms, including a buzzing, whistling, or hissing sound. The most common causes of tinnitus are damage to the hearing receptors from noise or toxins, age-related changes in the organs of the ear, and use of aspirin. Tinnitus can affect people at any age but is more common as people get older. If tinnitus becomes chronic, the patient may find relief by listening to music or other distracting sounds or by using a device similar to a hearing aid that masks the noise with more pleasant sounds.

Surgery

Surgery is used to treat a variety of diseases and disorders. Surgery may be performed to repair wounds and broken bones or to repair or remove diseased or injured tissues, organs, and limbs. Some surgeons specialize in one field, such as ophthalmology or cardiology, and others are general surgeons.

Assisting a general or specialty surgeon requires familiarity with body systems. You should also understand presurgical procedures such as patient education, operating room preparation, and skin preparation; surgical assisting procedures such as maintaining asepsis; and postsurgical responsibilities such as decontaminating the operating room and dressing wounds.

A relatively simple surgical procedure is a tissue biopsy. There are several types of biopsies. A surgeon performs an incisional, or open, biopsy by making an incision and removing a piece of tissue. A needle biopsy is performed by removing tissue with a needle inserted into the growth or area through the skin. A surgeon performs needle aspiration by removing fluid from a lump or cyst with a needle. You may be asked to assist during these types of surgery. Procedure 28-4 describes the steps in assisting with a needle biopsy.

During a biopsy, Universal Precautions and sterile technique must be maintained. Always place the specimen in a prepared, labeled container provided by the laboratory. Transport it according to laboratory instructions, attaching the proper accompanying forms. After the biopsy you might assist with or perform the cleaning and bandaging of the site.

Urology

A urologist diagnoses and treats disorders and diseases of the urinary system in both males and females as well as of the male reproductive system. Urologists also perform surgical procedures such as hernia repairs and vasectomies. A **vasectomy** is a sterilization procedure for men in which a section of each of the vas deferens is removed.

In a urologist's office, you would assist with general examinations; collect and process urine, blood, and other specimens; obtain cultures; and participate in patient education about conditions as well as about presurgical and postsurgical care. You must understand the urinary system and the diseases and disorders you are likely to encounter.

Urology Examinations

You must be thorough when you take a patient's history for a urologist. Much information about urinary problems is obtained by questioning the patient about changes in frequency or urgency of urination, difficulty or pain with urination (dysuria), and incontinence. The physical examination usually includes palpation of the kidneys and bladder and visual inspection of the external genitalia. Women are examined in the lithotomy position, and men are usually seated when the examination begins.

During examination of the male reproductive system, the urologist inspects and palpates the patient's penis and scrotum. The genitalia are usually examined with the patient standing and the chest and abdomen draped. The doctor usually examines the inguinal region for a hernia and, in men over 40, checks the prostate gland. This gland is examined by digital insertion into the rectum.

The doctor instructs the patient as needed in performing regular testicular self-examination (TSE). This instruction, discussed in "Educating the Patient," may also be your responsibility.

Diagnostic Testing

Urologists sometimes use imaging techniques, such as CT scans and MRIs. Pyelography is an x-ray of the kidney area with an iodine-based contrast agent. It is used to diagnose renal (kidney-related) disorders. Urologists also use several other diagnostic techniques.

Urine and Blood Tests. Urinalysis is the most common test ordered in a urology practice. Urine can be tested for the presence of bacteria, blood, and other substances. Blood testing is also done for a variety of reasons, including monitoring for dysfunctions of the prostate gland and for certain sexually transmitted diseases (STDs). The Leydig's cell test is a blood test used to assess testosterone levels.

EDUCATING THE PATIENT

Testicular Self-Examination

Testicular cancer is rare, but when it occurs, it usually affects men between the ages of 29 and 35. The American Cancer Society recommends that all men perform a monthly testicular self-examination (TSE) from age 15 onward to increase the chances of early detection. Although testicular cancer is one of the most curable cancers, early detection is vital to its treatment.

A man who perceives an abnormality during TSE should be examined by a physician right away. TSE should be performed after a warm shower or bath, when scrotal skin is relaxed.

1. The man first observes the testes for changes in appearance, such as swelling. He then manually examines each testicle, gently rolling it between the fingers and thumbs of both hands to feel for hard lumps (see Figure 28-21).
2. After examining each testicle, the man should locate the area of the epididymis and spermatic cord. This area can be felt as a cordlike structure originating at the top back of each testicle.

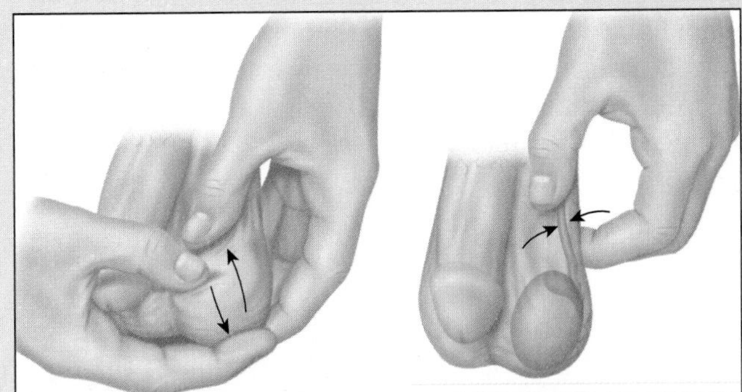

Figure 28-21. Males from age 15 onward should perform a monthly testicular self-examination.

Warning signs of testicular cancer include a heavy or dragging feeling in the groin, enlargement of one testicle, and a dull ache in the groin.

Semen Analysis and Smears. Semen samples may be obtained to determine fertility or to evaluate the success of a vasectomy. The patient usually collects these samples at home, but you may be required to provide a container, written instructions, and laboratory paperwork. Smears are used in diagnosing infections.

Cystometry. Cystometry is used to measure urinary bladder capacity and pressure. Using a catheter passed through the urethra, the doctor fills the bladder with carbon dioxide gas. The test results are examined to diagnose disorders of bladder function.

Cystoscopy. In cystoscopy the physician examines the walls of the bladder and urethra by visualization and inspection. A special viewing instrument, called a cystoscope, is used for this procedure. The cystoscope is inserted into the bladder through the urethra.

Testicular Biopsy. Testicular biopsy, a hospital procedure, involves obtaining a tissue sample of a mass for laboratory examination. The patient will need your support because he will most likely be very anxious about the nature of the lump.

Urologic Diseases and Disorders

Diagnostic tests are used to identify a variety of urologic diseases and disorders. If you work in a urologist's office, you will probably encounter many of these conditions.

Cystitis. Cystitis is an inflammation of the urinary bladder resulting from a bacterial infection. Among women, who are more prone to this disorder than are men, the most common cause is the bacterium *Escherichia coli.* In men the infection is usually related to a separate condition such as prostatitis or epididymitis. The symptoms of cystitis are bladder spasms, fever, nausea and vomiting, chills, lower-back pain, and pain on voiding (dysuria). Diagnosis of cystitis is confirmed through urinalysis, and the condition is treated with antibiotics. Female patients should be taught to wipe and cleanse the perineal area from front to back to prevent bacteria from the rectum from infecting the urethra.

Epididymitis. Epididymitis is a bacterial infection of the epididymis. It causes pain, swelling, and sometimes fever. It is treated with rest and antibiotic medications.

Hydrocele. Hydrocele is the name for excess fluid in the scrotum. It is usually caused by infection of the epididymis or testes. In other cases it results from a congenital defect or occurs after injury. The fluid may be aspirated to relieve discomfort.

Impotence. Impotence is the inability either to achieve or to maintain an erection. The cause may be physical, as when it results from cardiovascular or endocrine disease, or it may be a side effect of some medication such as certain diuretics and chemotherapy agents. The cause may also be psychological or emotional. In at least half the cases, a combination of physical and emotional factors is involved. Treatment depends on the cause or causes and may include medication, counseling, or surgical procedures.

Kidney Stones. Kidney stones occur when chemical substances in the urine form crystals in the kidney, ureter, or bladder. If kidney stones cannot pass through the ureter, they can cause excruciating pain. Although some stones pass, large stones often must be removed surgically or broken up by means of sound waves (lithotripsy) or laser techniques.

Prostatic Hypertrophy. Prostatic hypertrophy, or enlargement of the prostate gland, occurs most commonly in men over 50. Hypertrophy may constrict the urethra, causing difficulty in urinating and repeated urinary infections. Medications to reduce the hypertrophy and surgery are common treatments.

Prostatitis. Prostatitis is an inflammation of the prostate, usually bacterial. Symptoms are pain on urination and, often, fever. Patients are instructed to avoid sitting for long periods. Treatments include antibiotic medications and sitz baths.

Prostate Cancer. Prostate cancer is the most common type of cancer among men. Often no symptoms are evident. Sometimes a nodule may be felt upon palpation of the prostate; if the growth is large enough, problems with urination may occur. Treatment options include radiation therapy and removal of the prostate.

STDs. Urologists also diagnose and treat STDs. These diseases are discussed in Chapter 27.

Urethritis. Urethritis is an inflammation of the urethra. Like cystitis, it is usually caused by bacterial infection and requires similar, if not the same, treatment. Urethritis frequently accompanies cystitis.

Summary

As a medical assistant, you will find interesting and stimulating work in a specialty medical practice. Each specialty has precise requirements for knowledge and skills that are particular to that field of practice. All medical specialties require that you have a firm foundation in and understanding of basic principles and procedures.

You will need to familiarize yourself with the anatomy and physiology relevant to the specialty in which you work. You will assist with highly specialized examinations, diagnostic testing, and modes of treatment. By working to understand the diseases and disorders common to the specialty you choose, you will develop the ability to better educate patients and respond to their concerns.

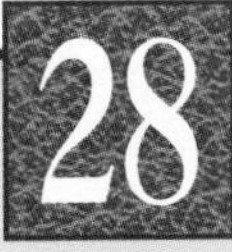

Chapter Review

Discussion Questions

1. Describe the symptoms of anaphylactic shock.
2. Explain three imaging techniques and how they might be used in different specialties.
3. Describe the three basic methods of cancer treatment.

Critical Thinking Questions

1. In the specialty practices of dermatology, endocrinology, ophthalmology, and orthopedics, what concerns might you encounter from an adolescent who is self-conscious about his appearance?
2. How would you counsel a patient who finds out she is allergic to one of her favorite foods?
3. A patient has been told he has a degenerative neurological disease. He begins to exhibit signs of extreme depression and talks about wanting to end his life. What should you do?

Application Activities

1. Using a gauze square that you moisten with water, perform the patch test procedure on another student. Have the other student critique your technique.
2. Demonstrate to another student how you would check an ophthalmoscope and prepare it for use. Ask the other student for suggestions for improvement.
3. Gather information and make a presentation to the class on resources available in your community to help families and patients affected by one of the following diseases: Alzheimer's disease, breast cancer, multiple sclerosis, rheumatoid arthritis, or AIDS.

Further Readings

"Answers to Questions About Hemorrhoids." *The Professional Medical Assistant,* May/June 1995, 13–14.

Ledford, Janice K. "Dry Eye: Something to Cry About?" *The Professional Medical Assistant,* May/June 1996, 14–15.

Leffell, David J., and Douglas E. Brash. "Sunlight and Skin Cancer." *Scientific American,* July 1996, 52–59.

"Migraine Diagnosis and Treatment." *The Professional Medical Assistant,* September/October 1996, 18–19.

Orlowski, Susan A. "Handling Injection Reactions in a Medical Office." *The Professional Medical Assistant,* January/February 1997, 5–7.

"Parkinson's Disease." *The Professional Medical Assistant,* January/February 1997, 17–24; March/April 1997, 15–24.

Zeballos, R. Jorge, and Idelle M. Weisman. "Behind the Scenes of Cardiopulmonary Exercise Testing." *Clinics in Chest Medicine,* June 1994.

Assisting With Minor Surgery

CHAPTER OUTLINE

- The Medical Assistant's Role in Minor Surgery
- Surgery in the Physician's Office
- Instruments Used in Minor Surgery
- Asepsis
- Preoperative Procedures
- Intraoperative Procedures
- Postoperative Procedures

OBJECTIVES

After completing Chapter 29, you will be able to:

- Define the medical assistant's role in minor surgical procedures.
- Describe types of wounds and explain how they heal.
- Describe special surgical procedures performed in an office setting.
- List the instruments used in minor surgery and describe their functions.
- Describe and contrast the procedures for medical and sterile asepsis in minor surgery.
- Describe the medical assistant's duties in preparing to assist in minor surgery.
- Describe the medical assistant's duties in preparing a patient for surgery.
- Describe the types of local anesthetics for minor surgery and the medical assistant's role in their administration.
- Describe the duties of the medical assistant as a floater and as a sterile scrub assistant.
- Describe the medical assistant's duties in the postoperative period.

AREAS OF COMPETENCE

1997 ROLE DELINEATION STUDY

CLINICAL

Fundamental Principles

- Apply principles of aseptic technique and infection control

Patient Care

- Obtain patient history and vital signs
- Prepare and maintain examination and treatment areas
- Prepare patient for examinations, procedures, and treatments
- Assist with examinations, procedures, and treatments

continued

Key Terms

abscess
anesthesia
anesthetic
approximate
biopsy specimen
cryosurgery
debridement
dressing
electrocauterization
fenestrated drape
floater
formalin
incision
intraoperative
laceration
lag phase
ligature
maturation phase
Mayo stand
medical asepsis
needle biopsy
onychectomy
postoperative
preoperative
proliferation phase
puncture wound
sterile field
sterile scrub assistant
surgical asepsis
suture
topical
vial

AREAS OF COMPETENCE continued

GENERAL (Transdisciplinary)

Legal Concepts

- Document accurately

The Medical Assistant's Role in Minor Surgery

Medical assistants play an important role in all aspects of minor surgical procedures. You will perform administrative tasks prior to the patient's surgery, including completing forms for insurance, obtaining signed informed consent forms from the patient, and explaining all aspects of the surgical procedure to the patient. Answering the patient's questions and making sure the doctor is informed about all medications (both prescription and over-the-counter) the patient is currently taking are administrative tasks as well. You will also make sure the patient knows how to follow the appropriate presurgical instructions for diet and fluid intake.

You will perform many tasks directly related to the surgical procedure itself. You will make sure the surgical room is clean, neat, and properly lit. You will see that all the equipment, instruments, and supplies the doctor will use are clean, disinfected, or sterilized, as appropriate, and properly arranged. You may also function as an unsterile assistant, ensuring the safety and comfort of the patient during the procedure and performing other duties. At other times you may directly assist with the surgical procedure in a sterile capacity.

Following the surgical procedure you will help dress the wound and perform other postoperative patient care, making sure the patient is not experiencing ill effects from the surgery or local anesthetic. You will educate the patient about wound care and proper procedures to follow after surgery and make sure the patient has safe transportation home. You will also clean the room and prepare it for the next patient.

Surgery in the Physician's Office

Minor surgical procedures are those that can be safely performed in the physician's office or clinic without general anesthesia. **Anesthesia** is a loss of sensation, particularly the feeling of pain. An **anesthetic** is a medication that causes anesthesia. A general anesthetic affects the entire body, whereas a local anesthetic affects only a particular area. Minor surgical procedures typically involve the use of a local anesthetic in the form of an injection or a cream applied to the skin.

Minor surgical procedures are performed for many reasons. Sometimes the purpose is to diagnose an illness or to repair an injury. Other procedures may be elective, or optional. Removal of a wart, skin tag (a small outgrowth of skin, occurring frequently on the neck as people get older), or other small growth for cosmetic reasons is an elective procedure. Some of the common minor surgical procedures you may assist the doctor with include the following:

- Repair of a laceration
- Irrigation and cleaning of a puncture wound
- Wound debridement
- Removal of foreign bodies
- Removal of small growths
- Removal of a nail or part of a nail
- Drainage of an abscess
- Collection of a biopsy specimen
- Cryosurgery
- Laser surgery
- Electrocauterization

MULTISKILL FOCUS

Surgical Technologist

To gain medical assistant credentials, you must fulfill the requirements of either the American Association of Medical Assistants (for a Certified Medical Assistant) or the American Medical Technologists (for a Registered Medical Assistant). After obtaining your medical assistant certification or registration, you may wish to acquire additional skills in specialty areas through course work or on-the-job training. Although this course work or training may not lead to an additional certification or degree, it will enable you to expand your role in the medical office and advance your career as the demand for multiskilled health professionals increases.

Skills and Duties

The surgical technologist, sometimes called a surgical technician or operating room technician, is a vital member of the surgical team. He assists surgeons, nurses, and other surgical staff before, during, and after an operation.

Prior to an operation the technologist sets up the operating room. He sterilizes and prepares instruments and supplies and arranges them for the surgical staff. He also checks all operating room equipment to make sure the machines are fully functional.

The surgical technologist also prepares the patient for surgery. He washes the surgical site and shaves the area if necessary. He then transports the patient to the operating room and lifts her to position her on the table, requesting assistance if needed. He may apply antiseptic to the incision site and arrange sterile drapes around the site to create a sterile field. He may also help surgeons, nurses, and staff scrub up and dress in their gowns, gloves, and masks.

During the operation the surgical technologist observes vital signs, checks charts, and passes instruments and supplies to nurses and surgeons. He wears a mask and other personal protective equipment during the operation. He also may operate the lights, suction machines, or diagnostic equipment and help prepare specimens for transport to the laboratory or apply dressings to the patient's wound.

Following the operation the technologist lifts and transfers the patient to the recovery room, requesting assistance if needed. He then cleans and disinfects the operating room, restocking supplies as needed.

Workplace Settings

Surgical technologists typically work in hospital operating rooms. Some surgical technologists also work in clinics, surgery centers, or physicians' and dentists' offices where outpatient surgery is performed. A few are employed privately by surgeons who use their own surgical teams for specialized work.

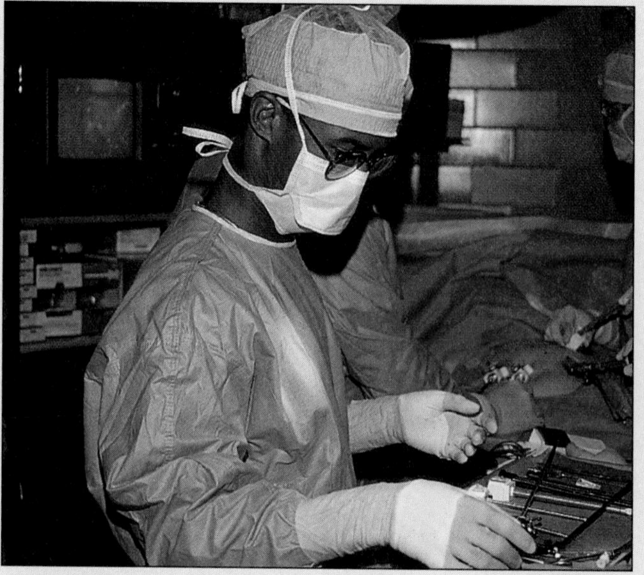

Surgical technologists usually work a standard 40-hour week. They may also be placed on call for emergencies during nights and weekends.

Education

The Committee on Allied Health Education and Accreditation of the American Medical Association recognizes 130 programs for surgical technologists. Programs are offered by colleges and universities, hospitals, vocational schools, and the military. They range from 9 months to 2 years in duration and offer the graduate a certificate, diploma, or associate degree.

After graduating from a program, surgical technologists may voluntarily take an examination to receive professional certification from the Liaison Council on Certification for the Surgical Technologist. Certification must be renewed every 6 years.

Where to Go for More Information

American Hospital Association
One North Franklin
Chicago, IL 60606
(312) 422-3000

Association of Surgical Technologists
7108-C South Alton Way
Englewood, CO 80112
(303) 694-9130

Common Surgical Procedures

Many surgical procedures are routinely performed in a doctor's office. You may perform some of these procedures on your own. For example, you may change dressings for surgical wounds, and under doctor's orders you may remove sutures (commonly called stitches) or staples after wounds have healed. Any procedure that requires an **incision** (a surgical wound made by cutting into body tissue) must be performed by a doctor.

Draining an Abscess. An **abscess** is a collection of pus (white blood cells, bacteria, and dead skin cells) that forms as a result of infection. A protective lining can form around an abscess and prevent it from healing. In such a case the physician may make an incision in the lining of the abscess. The physician may allow the abscess to drain on its own or insert a drainage tube.

Obtaining a Biopsy Specimen. A **biopsy specimen** is a small amount of tissue removed from the body for examination under a microscope. The specimen must be placed in a preservative, most commonly a 10% **formalin** solution (a dilute solution of formaldehyde), to prevent changes in the tissue. Most biopsies involve cutting the tissue. A **needle biopsy** uses a needle and syringe to aspirate (withdraw by suction) fluid or tissue cells. (Procedure 28-4 in Chapter 28 describes how to assist with a needle biopsy.) Preservation concerns apply to all specimens whether obtained by cutting or by aspiration using a needle and syringe.

Caring for Wounds. A wound is any break in the skin. The break may be accidental or intentional, as from a surgical procedure. There are several types of accidental wounds. A **laceration** is a jagged, open wound in the skin that can extend down into the underlying tissue. The jagged edges may have to be cut away before the wound is closed. A **puncture wound** is a deep wound caused by a sharp object. (See Chapter 31 for further information on types and care of accidental wounds.) Both surgical and accidental wounds require special care to prevent infection. Proper wound care that promotes healing without infection is discussed in "Caution: Handle With Care."

Cleaning a Wound. The first step in preventing a nonsurgical wound from becoming infected is careful cleansing. The wound must be thoroughly cleaned with soap and water. Then it must be irrigated with sterile saline solution or sterile water that is applied with a syringe and needle. **Debridement,** the surgical removal of debris or dead tissue from the wound, may be necessary to expose healthy tissue.

Closing a Wound. It is important to know how a wound heals so that you can care for it properly. A wound heals in three phases: lag phase, proliferation phase, and maturation phase. During the initial phase, or **lag phase,** bleeding is reduced as blood vessels in the affected area constrict. White blood cells and blood components play an important role in this phase. They seal the wound, clot the blood that has seeped into the area, and remove bacteria and debris from the wound. The wound contracts under the clot or scab that forms.

During the second phase, or **proliferation phase,** new tissue forms. Skin cells at the edges of the wound begin to move together to close off the wound. The scab that often forms over a wound actually slows down this movement of skin cells. The edges of the wound do eventually come together and form a continuous layer, closing off the wound.

The **maturation phase** (the third phase) involves the formation of scar tissue. Scar tissue is important for closing large, gaping, or jagged wounds. The continuous layer of skin cells formed during the second phase becomes thicker and pushes off the scab, leaving a scar. Scar tissue contains no nerves or blood vessels and lacks the resilience of skin.

The proliferation phase is sped up if the edges of an incision or nonsurgical wound are **approximated**—brought together so the tissue surfaces are close. This intervention protects the area from further contamination and minimizes scab and scar formation. Small wounds can be held together with butterfly closures or sterile strips. Larger wounds or those subject to strain may require suturing or stapling.

Sutures are surgical stitches used to close a wound. Suture materials, or **ligature,** can be either absorbable or nonabsorbable. The body breaks down absorbable sutures, so they do not require removal after the wound has healed. They are typically made of catgut (a sterile strand made of collagen fibers usually obtained from sheep or cow intestines). If a wound is particularly deep, the doctor may need to suture in layers, from inside to outside. In this case absorbable sutures are used for the inner suturing. Removable (nonabsorbable) sutures are generally used for the outside layer. Nonabsorbable ligature must be removed after wound healing is well under way. Nonabsorbable sutures may be made of silk, nylon, or polyester. Suture materials come in thicknesses ranging from size 11-0 (smallest) to size 7 (largest). The needle is already attached to most prepackaged ligature.

Staples may be used to bring the edges of a wound together if there is considerable stress on the incision. For example, a long and deep surgical wound or a wound across the leg would have a strong tendency to gape open if not firmly secured. Surgical staples look somewhat like ordinary staples. They are inserted into the skin with a disposable staple unit.

Special Minor Surgical Procedures

Some types of minor surgical procedures require special surgical instruments. These procedures include laser surgery, cryosurgery, and electrocauterization. They all remove excess or abnormal tissue, as in the case of warts or skin lesions. These procedures usually require surgical aseptic technique because they break the integrity of the skin.

CAUTION HANDLE WITH CARE

Conditions That Interfere With Fast, Effective Wound Healing

The goals for treating both surgical and nonsurgical wounds are similar: they are to heal the wound without infection and to preserve normal skin function and appearance. Nonsurgical wounds often involve conditions that do not promote fast, effective healing. In these cases the wound requires special attention to ensure good results.

Many types of nonsurgical wounds may contain foreign material that can lead to infection. For example, a child may have a deep laceration from landing on a dirty, broken bottle when falling off a bicycle. These types of wounds always need vigorous cleaning. Some need debridement, or the surgical removal of dead tissue or foreign material.

Wounds heal better when the edges are brought closely together, or approximated. Jagged edges in a laceration, as in the example above, make approximation harder. It is also difficult to approximate crushed tissue, as you would see with fingers closed in a car door. Crushing disrupts a tissue's blood supply by rupturing blood vessels throughout the affected area. A physician might debride this type of wound with a scalpel to remove severely damaged tissue and achieve a clean wound edge before suturing.

After a surgical or nonsurgical wound is closed and sutured, it is essential to keep the wound clean and dry. Maintaining this condition serves a number of purposes. Most important is the prevention of infection. Infection delays the healing process and can have other serious consequences.

A sutured wound heals more quickly and smoothly when no scab forms because the migrating skin cells encounter no barrier to their movement. Proper postoperative care, including daily cleaning with soap and water or a mild antiseptic, keeps a wound scab-free. Although skin cells migrate across the space of a wound more easily in a somewhat moist environment, a wet wound offers the ideal conditions for bacteria to grow and cause infection. Covering a wound with antiseptic ointment and a clean, dry dressing keeps the wound slightly moist, yet helps prevent infection.

Wound healing may be delayed in a number of instances not directly related to the surgery or injury. The presence of any of the following conditions can put a patient at risk for wound-healing problems. Wounds in such patients may require extra attention and care.

- Poor circulation: This condition results in inadequate supplies of nutrients, blood cells, and oxygen to the wound, all of which delay the healing process.
- Aging: Physiologic changes that occur with age can decrease a person's resistance to infection.
- Diabetes: Patients with diabetes experience changes in the walls of their arteries that result in poor circulation to peripheral tissues. These patients may also have a decreased resistance to infection.
- Poor nutrition: Patients who are undernourished, particularly those who are deficient in protein or vitamin C, do not have the physiologic resources for vigorous healing.
- High levels of stress: An increase in stress-related hormones can decrease resistance to infection.
- Weakened immune system: Patients who are on certain medications or who have certain chronic diseases may have weakened immune systems, putting them at increased risk of infection.
- Obesity: When someone is obese, the circulation directly under the skin is often poor, leading to slow healing.
- Smoking: Nicotine constricts the blood vessels in the skin, reducing circulation to the area of the wound and slowing healing.

Laser Surgery. A laser emits an intense beam of light that is used to cut away tissue. Laser surgery is sometimes preferred over conventional surgery because it causes less damage to surrounding healthy tissue than does conventional surgery. Laser surgery also promotes quick healing and helps prevent infection.

When a laser is used in an office setting, close blinds and shades to keep out stray light. Remove any items that could catch fire if they came in contact with the laser beam. Cover any shiny or reflective surfaces. Make sure that everyone in the room, including the patient, wears special safety goggles to protect the eyes. Post a standard laser warning placard in the entryway to the room, per Occupational Safety and Health Administration (OSHA) regulations.

Position, drape, and prepare the patient as you would for conventional surgery. Place gauze around the surgical site, and assist the physician with administration of a local anesthetic if requested. The physician uses the laser to vaporize the unwanted tissue; vaporized tissue is cleared away by the vacuum hose portion of the unit (see Figure 29-1). You may be asked to apply pressure to control any bleeding. Clean the wound with an antiseptic, and apply a sterile dressing. Give the patient the normal instructions on wound care, including the recommendation to protect the site from exposure to the sun.

Cryosurgery. The use of extreme cold to destroy unwanted tissue is called **cryosurgery.** Cryosurgery is often used to remove skin lesions and lesions on the cervix.

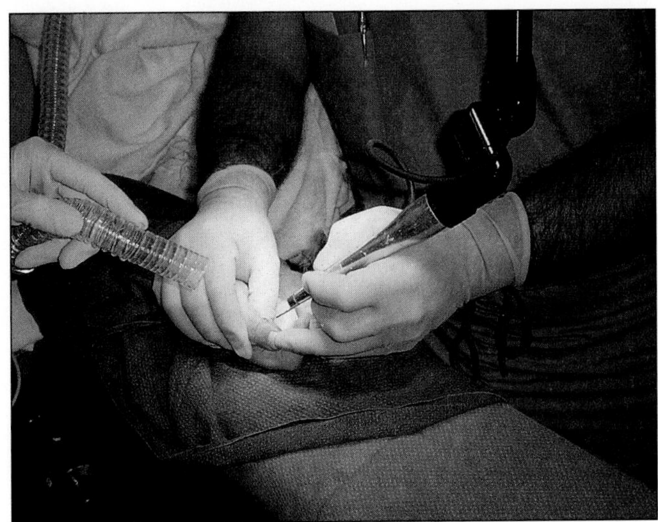

Figure 29-1. Suction eliminates vaporized tissue as a physician uses a laser to remove a wart from a patient's hand.

Before cryosurgery inform the patient that an initial sensation of cold will be followed by a burning sensation. Instruct the patient to remain as still as possible to prevent damage of nearby tissue.

The doctor may freeze the tissue by touching it with a cotton-tipped applicator dipped in liquid nitrogen or by spraying it with liquid nitrogen from a pressurized can. Sometimes a special cryosurgical instrument is used, most often during surgery on the cervix.

Make the patient aware that more than one freezing cycle may be necessary. A local anesthetic is usually not required because the cold itself reduces sensation in the area. After the procedure the area is cleaned with an antiseptic, and a sterile dressing may be applied. An ice pack may be applied to reduce swelling, and pain relievers may be given for pain.

Reassure the patient that some pain, swelling, or redness is normal after a cryosurgical procedure. Encourage the patient to use ice and pain relievers as necessary. Let the patient know that a large, painful, bloody blister may form. Left undisturbed, the blister usually ruptures in about 2 weeks. It should be left intact to promote healing and prevent infection. The patient should call the doctor if a blister becomes too painful. Be sure to provide the patient with complete wound-care instructions.

Electrocauterization. **Electrocauterization** is a technique whereby a needle, probe, or loop heated by electric current destroys the target tissue. A physician may use this technique to remove growths such as warts, to stop bleeding, and to control nosebleeds that either will not subside or continually recur.

Several types of electrocautery units are in use. Some are small, often handheld, units powered by battery or by ordinary household electric current. Other, larger units are designed for countertop placement or for mounting on a wall. Some units use disposable probes, whereas others employ reusable ones.

With certain units a grounding pad or plate is placed somewhere on the patient's body (or under it) during the procedure. This grounding completes the circuit and prevents electric shock to the patient, the physician, and staff members. Reassure the patient that grounding causes no discomfort.

A local anesthetic may be administered before the procedure. A scab or crust generally forms over the area. Healing may take 2 to 3 weeks. General wound-care instructions are appropriate for this procedure, except that a dressing may be omitted to keep the area drier.

Instruments Used in Minor Surgery

The type of minor surgical procedure determines which surgical instruments are used. Surgical instruments have specific purposes and may be classified by function.

Cutting and Dissecting Instruments

Cutting and dissecting instruments have sharp edges and are used to cut, or incise, skin and tissue. Figure 29-2 illustrates some of the basic cutting and dissecting instru-

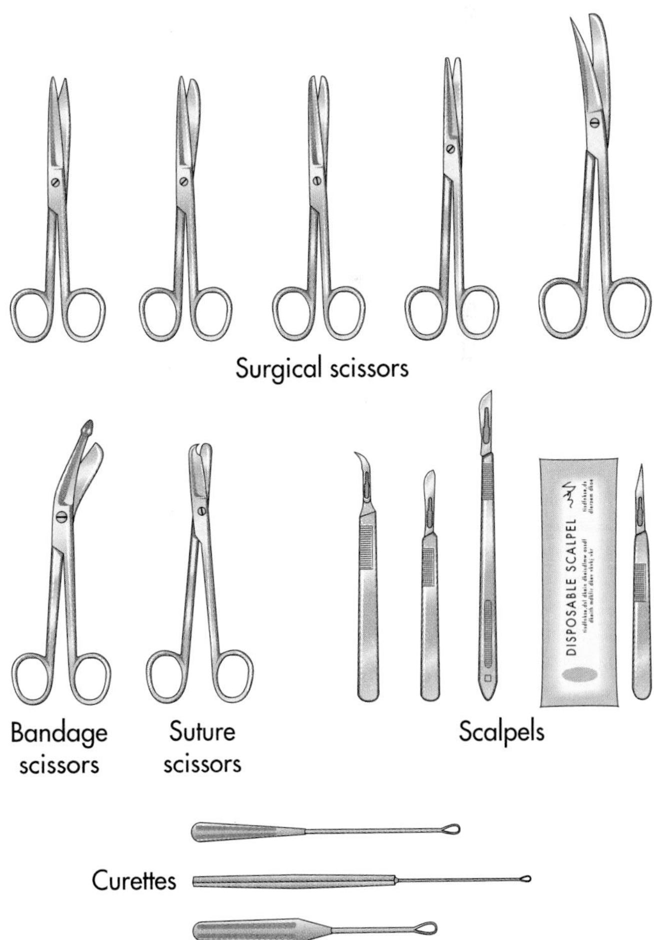

Figure 29-2. These are typical cutting and dissecting instruments used in minor surgical procedures.

ments you will encounter. You must be careful when cleaning, sterilizing, and storing these instruments to avoid injuring yourself and to protect the instruments' sharp edges.

Scalpels. A scalpel consists of a handle that holds a disposable blade. Scalpel handles are either reusable or disposable and vary in width and length. A scalpel's specific use determines the shape and size of its blade. General-purpose scalpels have wide blades and a straight cutting surface. A no. 15 blade is the most common one for performing minor procedures.

Scissors. Surgical scissors come in various sizes. They may be straight or curved and have either blunt or pointed tips. Tissue scissors must be sharp enough to cut without damaging or ripping surrounding tissue. Suture scissors have blunt points and a curved lower blade. The lower blade is inserted under the suture material to cut it. Bandage scissors are used to remove dressings. They have a blunt lower blade so that the skin next to the dressing is not injured. Clippers are scissorlike instruments used for cutting nails or thick materials.

Curettes. The doctor uses a curette for scraping tissue. Curettes come in a variety of shapes and sizes. They consist of a circular blade—actually a loop—attached to a rod-shaped handle. The blade is blunt on the outside and sharp on the inside. The inner part of the blade may also be serrated. Serrated blades may be used to take Pap smears (Papanicolaou smears) and to perform ear irrigations where a large amount of cerumen has accumulated.

Grasping and Clamping Instruments

Special instruments are used for grasping and clamping tissue. Grasping instruments are used to hold surgical materials or to remove foreign objects, such as splinters, from the body. Clamping instruments are used to apply pressure and close off blood vessels. They are also used to hold tissue and other materials in position. Figure 29-3 shows some common grasping and clamping instruments.

Forceps. Forceps are instruments that are most often used to grasp or hold objects. Grasping types are usually shaped like tweezers and include thumb forceps and tissue forceps. Thumb forceps, also called smooth forceps, vary in shape and size. The blades of thumb forceps are tapered to a point and have small grooves at the tip. Tissue forceps (serrated forceps) have one or more fine teeth at the tips of the blades. When closed, these forceps hold tissue firmly. Holding forceps have handles

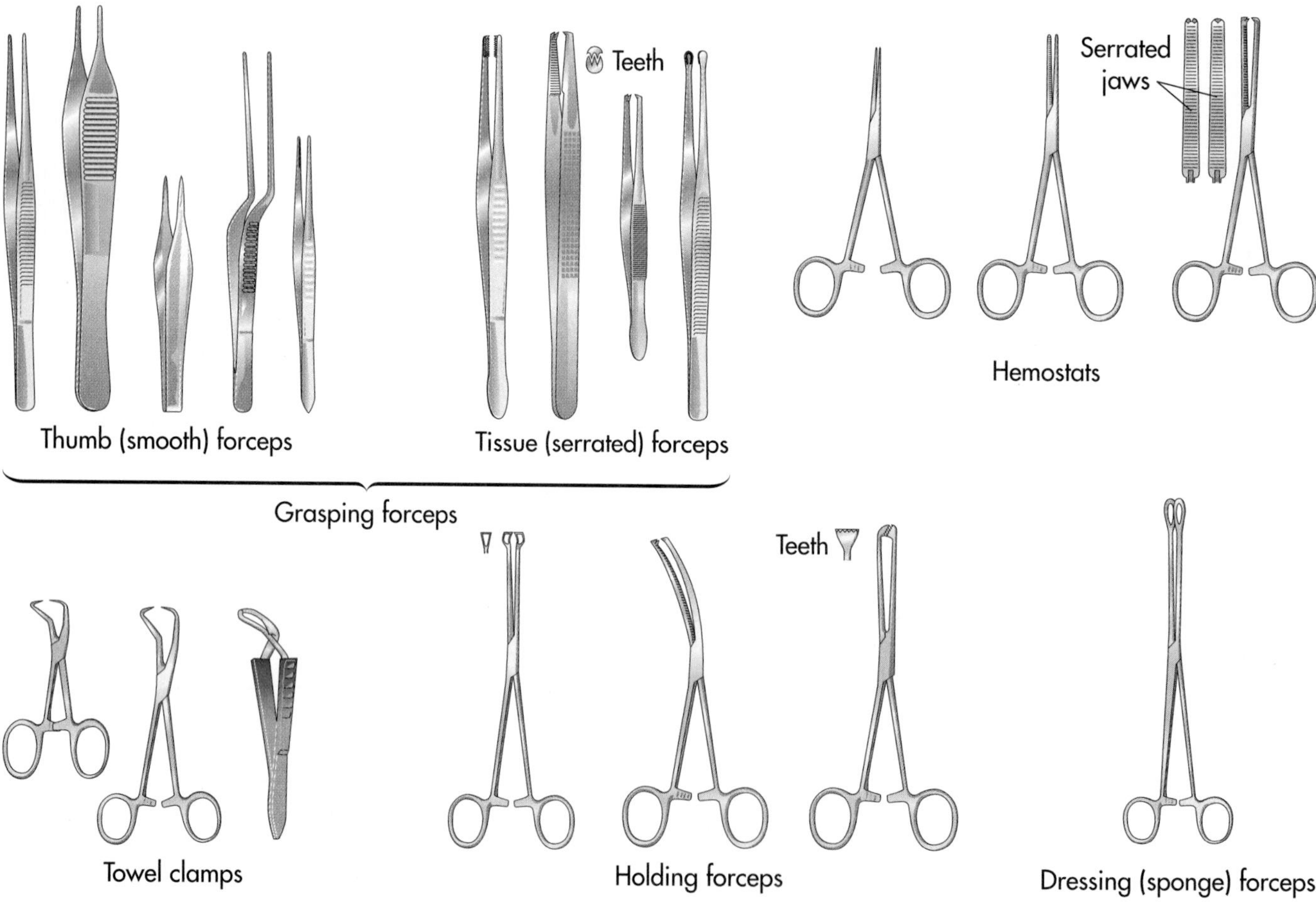

Figure 29-3. These are typical grasping and clamping instruments used in minor surgical procedures.

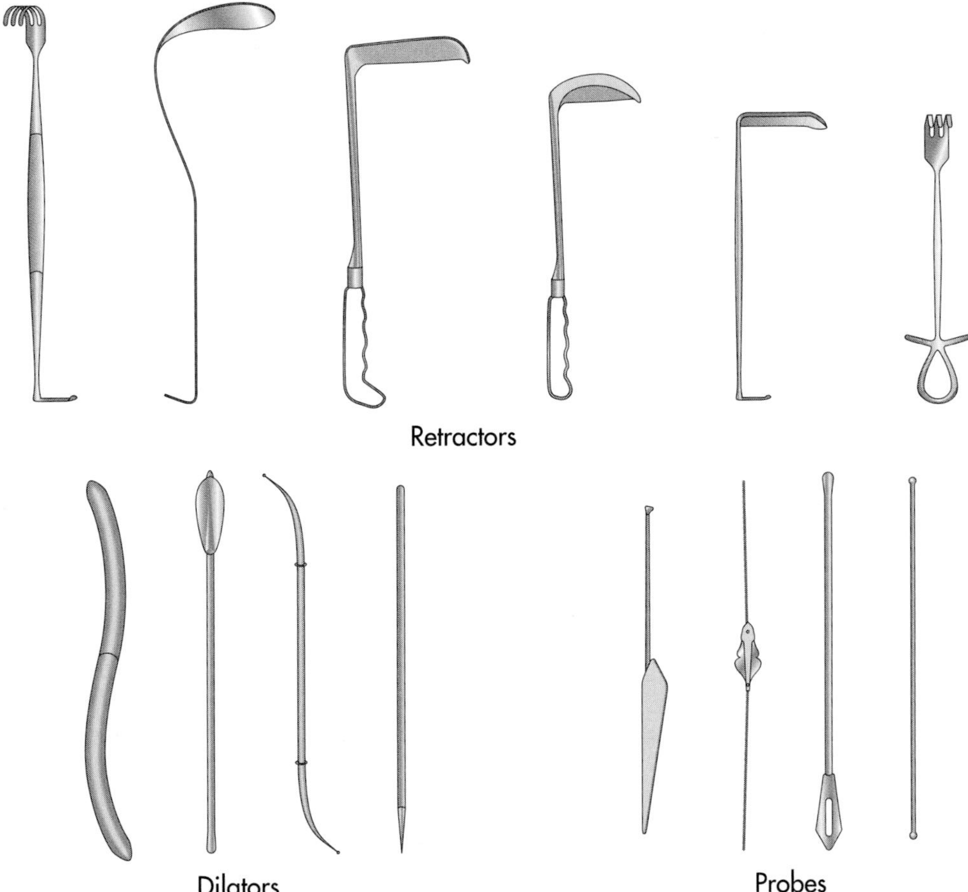

Figure 29-4. These are typical retracting, dilating, and probing instruments used in minor surgical procedures.

with ratchets that lock the teeth in a closed position. Dressing, or sponge, forceps have ridges to hold a sponge or gauze when it is used to absorb body fluids.

Hemostats. The most commonly used surgical instruments are hemostats. These surgical clamps vary in size and shape. Hemostats are typically used to close off blood vessels. The serrated jaws of hemostats taper to a point. Like holding forceps, hemostats have handles that lock on ratchets, holding the jaws securely closed.

Towel Clamps. Towel clamps are used to keep towels in place during a surgical procedure. This stability is important in maintaining a sterile field.

Retracting, Dilating, and Probing Instruments

Retracting instruments are used to hold back the sides of a wound or incision. Dilating and probing instruments may be used to enlarge, examine, or clear body openings, body cavities, or wounds. The shapes of these instruments vary with their functions. Some typical retracting, dilating, and probing instruments are shown in Figure 29-4.

Retractors. The use of retractors allows greater access to and a better view of a surgical site. Some retractors must be held open by hand, whereas others have ratchets or locks to keep them open.

Dilators. Dilators are slender, pointed instruments. They are used to enlarge a body opening, such as a tear duct.

Probes. A surgical probe is a slender rod with a blunt tip shaped like a bulb. Probes are used to explore wounds or body cavities and to locate or clear blockages.

Suturing Instruments

Suturing instruments are used to introduce suture materials into and retrieve them from a wound. Some carry the suture material, whereas others manipulate the suture carriers. Examples of suturing instruments are shown in Figure 29-5.

Suture Needles. Surgical suture needles carry suture material, also called ligature, through the tissue being sutured. They are either pointed or blunt at one end. They may have an eye at the other end to hold suture materials. Ligature often comes prepackaged with the needle already connected. Prepackaged suture needles with attached ligature have no eye and produce less trauma to the tissue being sutured than do suture needles with eyes.

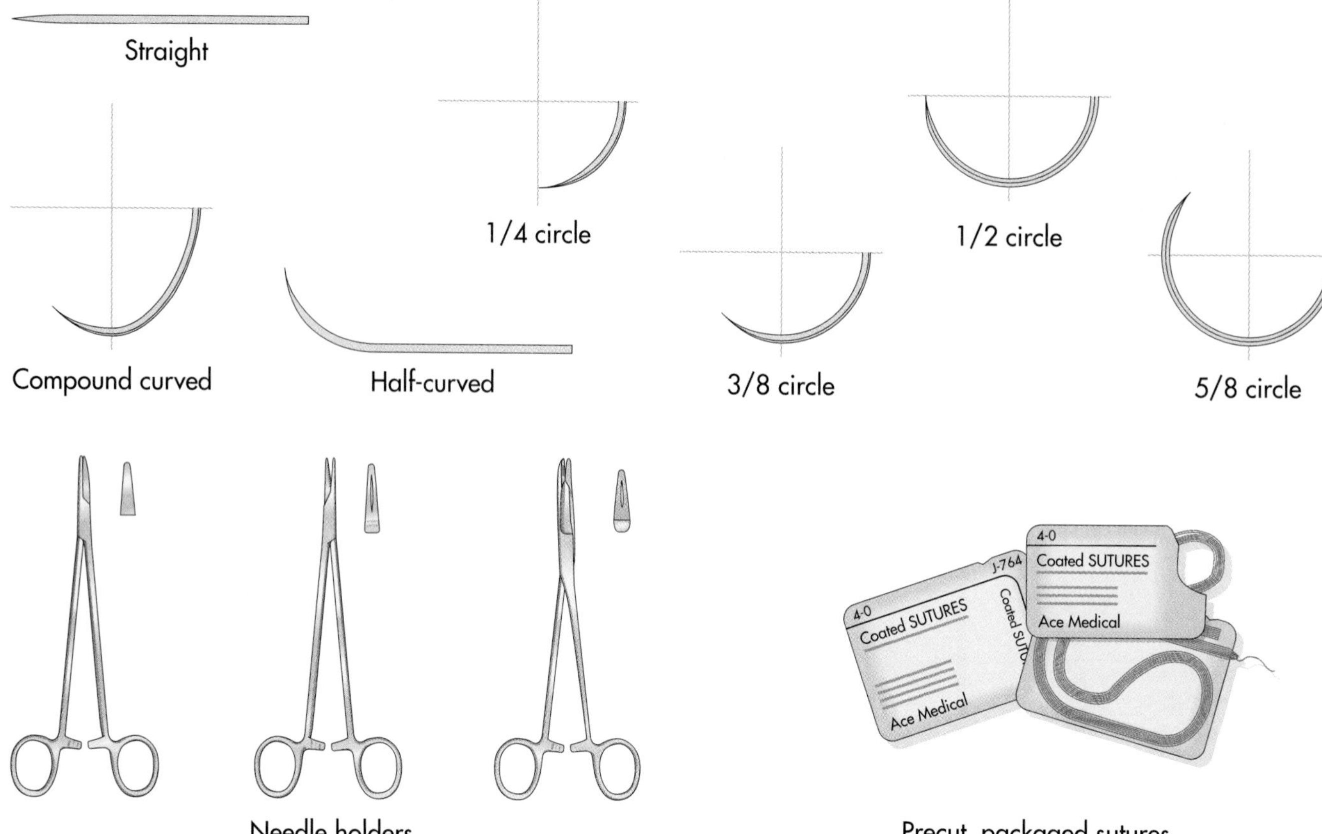

Figure 29-5. These are typical suturing instruments.

Suture needles may be straight, or they may be curved to allow deeper placement of sutures. Taper point needles (needles that taper into a sharp point) are used to suture tissues that are easily penetrated. They create only very small holes, thus minimizing leakage of tissue fluids. Cutting needles (needles that have at least two sharpened edges) are used on tough tissues that are not easily penetrated, such as skin.

Several measurements are used to determine the size of a surgical needle. Needle length is the distance from the tip to the end, measuring along the body of the needle. Chord length is the straight-line distance from the tip to the end of the needle. (Chord length is not the same as needle length in curved needles.) The radius of a curved needle is determined by mentally continuing the curve of the needle into a full circle and finding the distance from the center of the circle to the needle body. The diameter is the thickness of the needle. Needle size generally corresponds to the size of suture material used. Smaller needles are used for delicate procedures, such as eye surgery or repairing a facial laceration. Larger needles are used for suturing wounds of less delicate parts of the body, such as the hands or legs.

Needle Holders. Curved suture needles require special instruments to hold, insert, and retrieve them during suturing. Most needle holders look like hemostats with short, sturdy jaws.

Syringes and Needles

Sterile syringes and needles are used to inject anesthetic solutions, withdraw fluids, or obtain biopsy specimens. The size of the syringe and needle varies with the intended use. For example, a needle used to perform a biopsy is generally larger than needles used for most injections. (Syringes and needles used for injections are discussed and illustrated in Chapter 38.) Both syringes and needles are provided in individual sterile envelopes.

Instrument Trays and Packs

All the surgical instruments needed for a specific procedure are usually assembled beforehand. They are then sterilized together in a pack. Certain surgical supplies necessary for the procedure (such as gauze) are included in the pack because they, too, must be sterile. Surgical trays can be quickly set up with these instrument packs. Individually wrapped items may also be added as needed.

These are common types of instrument trays:

- Laceration repair tray (see Figure 29-6)
- Laceration repair with debridement tray
- Incision and drainage tray
- Foreign body or growth removal tray
- **Onychectomy** (nail removal) tray

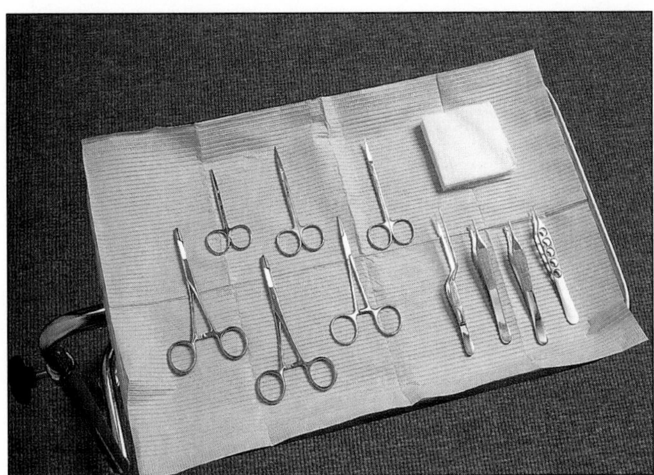

Figure 29-6. This laceration tray contains scissors, several pairs of forceps, a needle holder, suture material, and sterile gauze.

- Vasectomy (male sterilization procedure) tray
- Suture removal tray
- Staple removal tray

Asepsis

Maintaining asepsis during surgical procedures is always a priority. It is critical to the health and safety of both the patient and the health-care professional. The two levels of aseptic technique are medical asepsis (clean technique) and surgical asepsis (sterile technique). Chapter 19 describes in detail the two types of asepsis. You will use both levels of asepsis when assisting with minor surgery.

Medical Asepsis

Medical asepsis involves procedures to reduce the number of microorganisms and thus prevent the spread of disease. These procedures do not necessarily eliminate microorganisms. Hand washing is always the first line of defense against spreading disease. The use of antimicrobial agents (agents that kill microorganisms or suppress their growth) and personal protective equipment are also part of medical asepsis. Other practices include proper handling and disposal of sharps and biohazardous materials.

Personal Protective Equipment. Personal protective equipment, or PPE, includes all items used as a barrier between the wearer and potentially infectious or hazardous medical materials. PPE includes gloves, gowns, and masks and protective eyewear or face shields (Figure 29-7). OSHA regulations regarding PPE are discussed in detail in Chapter 19.

Gloves are of particular importance during surgical procedures. You should wear properly sized latex or vinyl gloves during any procedure that might expose you to potentially infectious or hazardous materials. (Gloves that are too big can catch on instruments or equipment and cause accidents.) When you wear gloves, you also protect the patient from any infectious organisms on your hands.

Both vinyl and latex gloves can prevent contamination of the hands with bacteria. It has been shown, however, that latex gloves prevent contamination to a greater degree (Olsen, 1993). Latex gloves have also been shown to leak less often than do vinyl gloves. As a result, many health-care institutions now prefer latex gloves.

As exposure to latex has increased, however, the incidence of latex allergy among health-care professionals has also grown. Allergic reactions to latex can range from a skin rash to shock and even death. Many health-care institutions are switching to less allergenic latex gloves, such as low-powder and powderless varieties. The powder in the gloves, which makes them easier to put on, is one of the primary sources of latex allergy. The latex protein that causes the allergy mixes with the powder. When the gloves are removed, the powder containing the latex protein becomes airborne and is inhaled (Robbins, 1997).

Other steps to prevent latex allergy include changing gloves frequently, thoroughly drying hands after washing, and frequently applying lotion to the hands. If you notice symptoms of a latex allergy, you should consider consulting an allergist. You should also discuss your symptoms with your supervisor, who may recommend simply switching to hypoallergenic gloves.

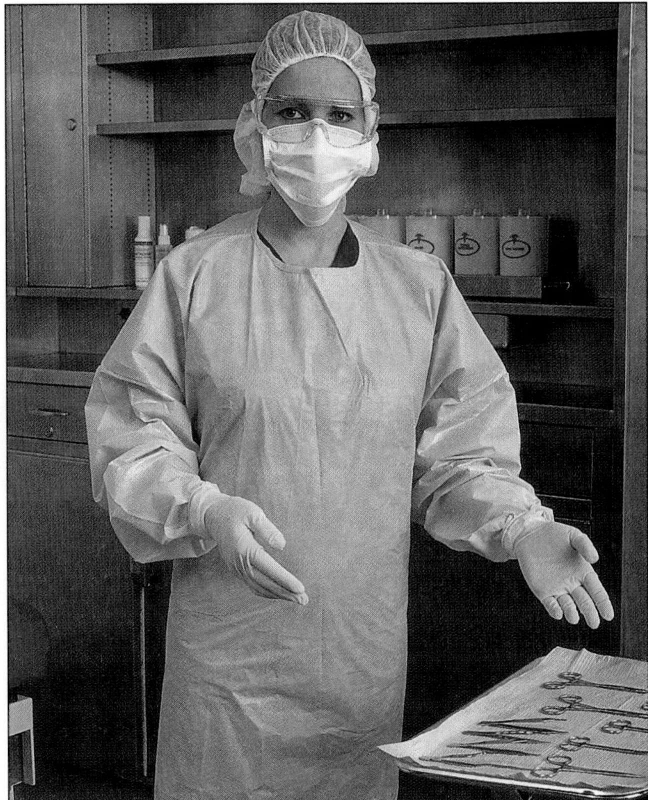

Figure 29-7. Personal protective equipment provides a barrier between infectious or hazardous medical materials and the wearer.

PROCEDURE 29-1

Using a Sterile Instrument Pack to Create a Sterile Field

Objective: To create a sterile field for a minor surgical procedure

OSHA Guidelines: This procedure does not involve exposure to blood, body fluids, or tissues.

Materials: Tray or Mayo stand, sterile instrument pack, sterile transfer forceps

Method

1. Clean and disinfect the tray or Mayo stand.
2. Wash your hands and assemble the necessary materials.
3. Check the label on the instrument pack to make sure it is the correct pack for the procedure (Figure 29-8).
4. Check the date and sterilization indicator on the instrument pack to make sure the pack is still sterile.
5. Place the sterile pack on the tray or stand, and unfold the outermost fold away from yourself.
6. Unfold the sides of the pack outward, touching only the areas that will become the underside of the sterile field.
7. Open the final flap toward yourself (Figure 29-9).
8. Arrange the instruments using sterile transfer forceps.

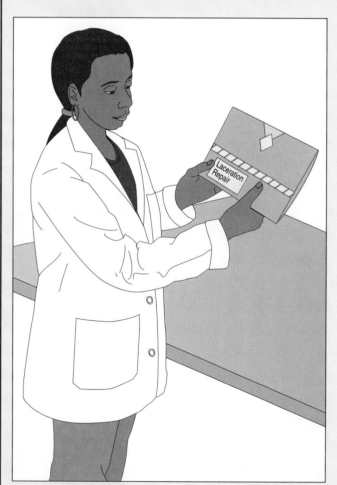

Figure 29-8. Confirm that you have the correct instrument pack before you open it.

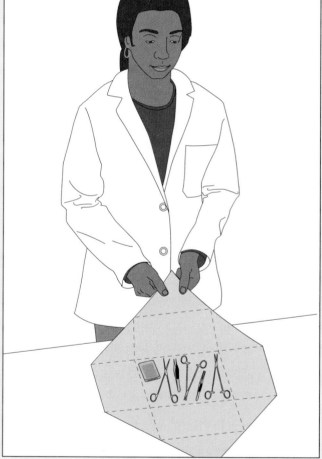

Figure 29-9. The fully open instrument pack constitutes a sterile field.

Sharps and Biohazardous Waste Handling and Disposal. Sharp medical and surgical instruments have great potential for transmitting infection through cuts and puncture wounds. Used scalpels, needles, syringes, and other sharp objects should be disposed of in a puncture-resistant sharps container.

All items other than sharps that have come in contact with tissue, blood, or body fluids must be disposed of in a leakproof plastic bag or container. The container must either be red or be labeled with the orange-red biohazard symbol. The proper procedure for handling and disposing of sharps and biohazardous waste is discussed in detail in Chapter 19.

Surgical Asepsis

In contrast to medical asepsis, the purpose of **surgical asepsis** is to eliminate all microorganisms. Surgical asepsis does not just reduce the quantity of microorganisms but completely eliminates them.

Common procedures involving sterile technique that you will be expected to perform include the following:

- Creating a sterile field
- Adding sterile items to the sterile field
- Performing a surgical scrub
- Putting on sterile gloves
- Sanitizing, disinfecting, and sterilizing equipment

Creating a Sterile Field. A **sterile field** is an area free of microorganisms that will be used as a work area during a surgical procedure. Always be aware that the sterile field is considered to become contaminated and must be redone in the following instances.

- An unsterile item touches the field.
- Someone reaches across the field.
- The field becomes wet.

The sterile field is often set up on a **Mayo stand,** a movable stainless steel instrument tray on a stand. You should adjust the stand so the tray is above waist level. Remember, items placed below waist level are considered contaminated. Before beginning, disinfect the Mayo stand with 70% isopropyl alcohol, and allow it to dry.

To create the sterile field, cover the stand with two layers of sterile material. This material can be sterile disposable drapes, separately sterilized muslin towels, or the muslin towels that the surgical instruments are wrapped in before autoclaving to produce office-sterilized sterile instrument packs. Commercially prepared sterile instrument packs, usually with disposable paper wrappings, are also used to create a sterile field. Procedure 29-1 describes the method for using a sterile instrument pack for this purpose.

When assembling the necessary supplies, place all unsterile items that may be used during the procedure outside the sterile field. Unsterile items include items that are sterile on the inside but not on the outside, such as a sterile gauze pack. Unsterile supplies should be arranged on a counter away from the sterile field. A typical arrangement of unsterile items used in surgery is shown in Figure 29-10. If you place an unsterile item within the sterile field, the field is no longer sterile, and you must repeat the entire process.

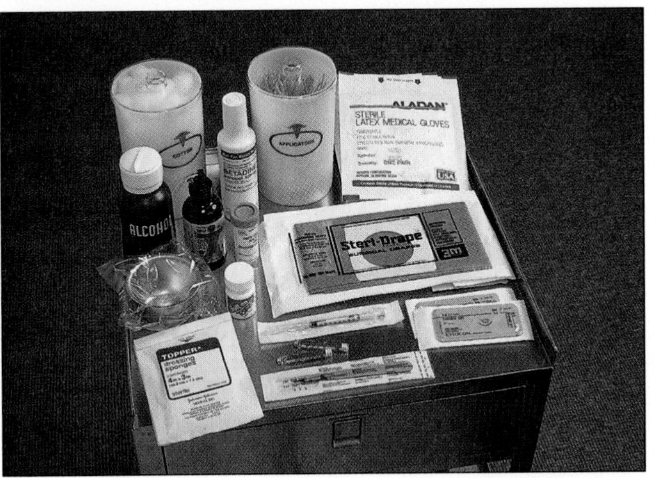

Figure 29-10. For each surgical procedure, unsterile surgical supplies must be gathered and arranged in an area separate from the sterile field.

Adding Sterile Items to the Sterile Field. The outer 1 inch of the sterile field is considered contaminated. Therefore, before you add sterile items to the sterile field, carefully plan where you will place the instruments so that they are within the sterile field.

Instruments and Supplies. If you have used sterile disposable drapes or separately sterilized muslin towels to create the sterile field, you will need to add the necessary instruments. Stand away from the sterile field, and open the sterile instrument pack in the manner described in Procedure 29-1. Place the pack on a counter or hold it open in your hand. Transfer and arrange the instruments on the sterile field with sterile transfer forceps (Figure 29-11). Avoid reaching across the sterile field.

If you must add other items to the field, open them using the same method. Stand away from the sterile field. As you unwrap the item, gather the corners of the wrapping beneath it. You can place the contents on the sterile field using sterile transfer forceps or using the sterile inside of the wrapping to prevent your hands from touching the item. Place basins or bowls near the edge of the sterile field so you can pour liquids without reaching over the field.

Some instruments are sterilized individually in autoclave bags, and sterile supplies are often prepackaged. Stand away from the sterile field as you open an individual bag or package. You can pull the flaps of the packaging partway apart, then snap (remove from position by a sudden movement) the item onto the sterile field from a distance of 8 to 12 inches. Alternatively, you can use sterile forceps to grasp and place the items in the sterile field.

Pouring Sterile Solutions. Sterile solutions are often required during the surgical procedure to rinse or wash the

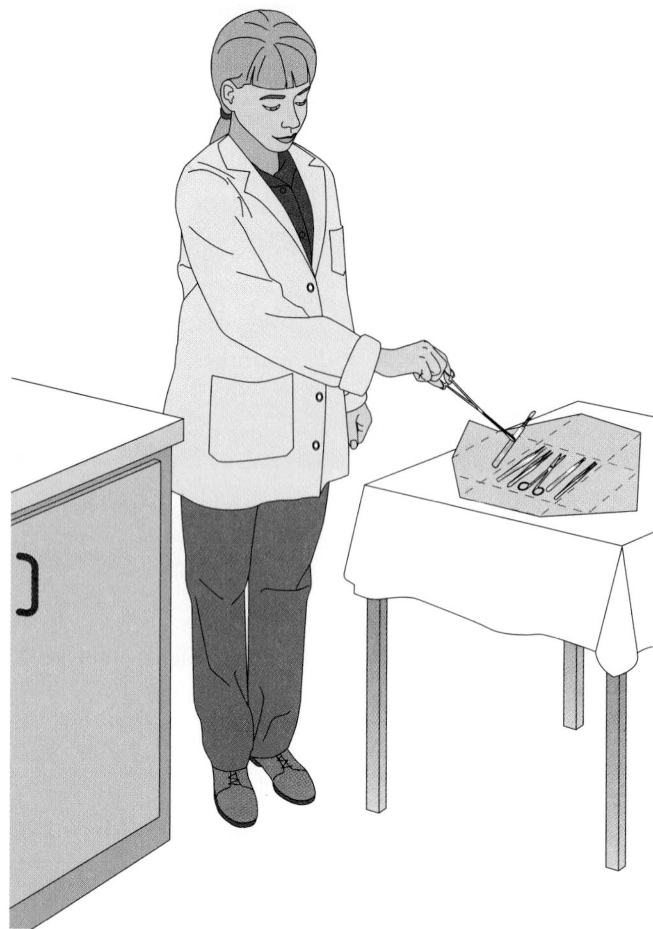

Figure 29-11. You can place sterile items on the sterile field by using transfer forceps.

wound. Sterile solutions can be added to the sterile field after the sterile instruments. Several sterile solutions are commonly used during minor surgical procedures. These include sterile water and physiological saline (0.9% sodium chloride).

Bottles of these sterile solutions come in a variety of sizes. You should choose the smallest size that will meet the solutions needed during the procedure. Using the smallest size possible minimizes the cost because unused solutions must be discarded.

When pouring a solution, cover the label on the bottle with the palm of your hand to keep the label dry. Pour a small amount of the liquid into a liquid waste receptacle to clean the lip of the bottle. As you pour the solution into a sterile bowl on the field, hold the bottle at an angle so that you do not reach over the sterile area (see Figure 29-12). Hold the bottle fairly close to the bowl without touching it. Pour the contents slowly to avoid splashing the drape, which would contaminate the field.

When a sterile solution bottle is opened and may be used again during the procedure, do not let any unsterile object touch the inside of its cap. To accomplish this, place the cap in the same position it was in on the bottle (the sterile inside of the cap facing down).

Performing a Surgical Scrub and Donning Sterile Gloves. If you assist in a surgical procedure, you must perform a surgical scrub and wear sterile surgical gloves. You may wonder why a surgical scrub is necessary if you are planning to wear sterile gloves. The answer is that there is always the possibility that a glove may be punctured. If the skin is as clean as possible, the risk of contamination from a punctured glove is minimized. Nevertheless, if a glove is damaged during a sterile procedure, you must consider anything touched by that glove to be contaminated. Contaminated items must be resterilized or replaced before you continue.

A surgical scrub removes microorganisms more effectively than does routine hand washing. Routine hand washing removes bacteria present on the skin's surface, whereas the surgical scrub removes bacteria in deeper layers of the skin—where the hair follicles and oil-producing glands are. Procedure 29-2 describes the process.

Sterile gloves are required for many procedures. You don sterile gloves after you perform the surgical scrub. The process is described in Procedure 29-3.

Remember that once you are wearing sterile gloves, you may touch only the items in the sterile field. There-

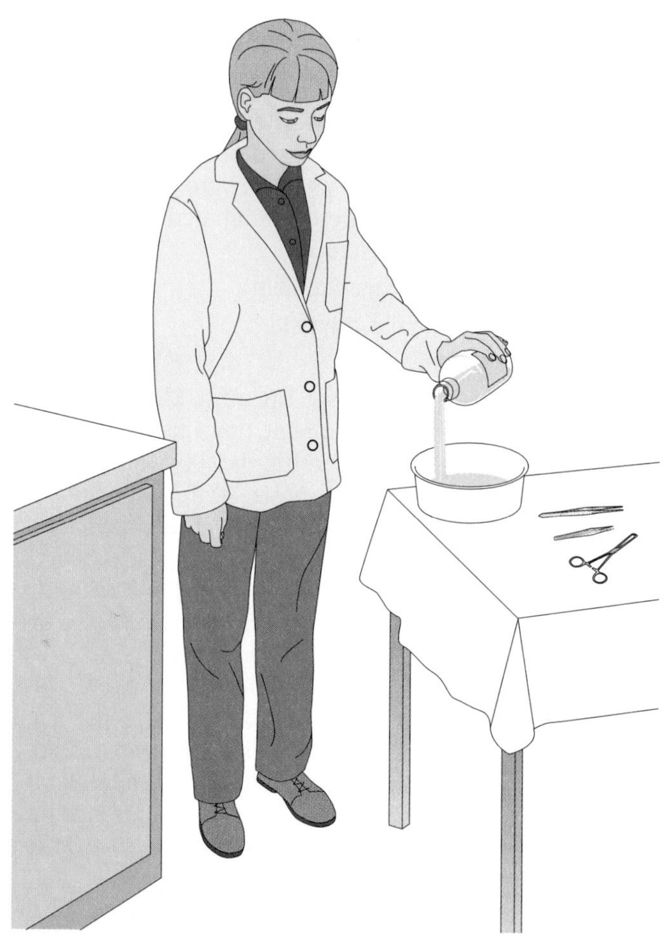

Figure 29-12. Pour a sterile solution into a sterile bowl near the edge of the sterile field without touching the rim of the bowl, splashing the solution, or reaching over the field.

PROCEDURE 29-2

Performing a Surgical Scrub

Objective: To remove dirt and microorganisms from under the fingernails and from the surface of the skin, hair follicles, and oil glands of the hands and forearms

OSHA Guidelines: This procedure does not involve exposure to blood, body fluids, or tissues.

Materials: Dispenser with surgical soap, sterile surgical scrub brush, orange stick, sterile towels

Method

1. Remove all jewelry and roll up your sleeves to above the elbow.
2. Assemble the necessary materials.
3. Turn the water on and adjust it so that it is warm.
4. Wet your hands from the fingertips to the elbows. You must keep your hands higher than your elbows to prevent water from running down your arms and contaminating the washed area.
5. Apply surgical soap and for 2 minutes scrub your hands, fingers, areas between the fingers, wrists, and forearms with the scrub brush, using a firm circular motion (Figure 29-13).
6. Rinse from fingers to elbows, always keeping your hands higher than your elbows (Figure 29-14).
7. Use the orange stick to clean under your fingernails, and rinse your hands again.
8. Apply more surgical soap, and again use the brush to completely scrub your hands, fingers, areas between the fingers, wrists, and forearms. Scrub for at least 3 minutes, and then rinse from fingers to elbows again.
9. Thoroughly dry your hands and forearms with sterile towels, working from the hands to the elbows (Figure 29-15).
10. Turn off the faucet with a clean towel (or foot pedal).

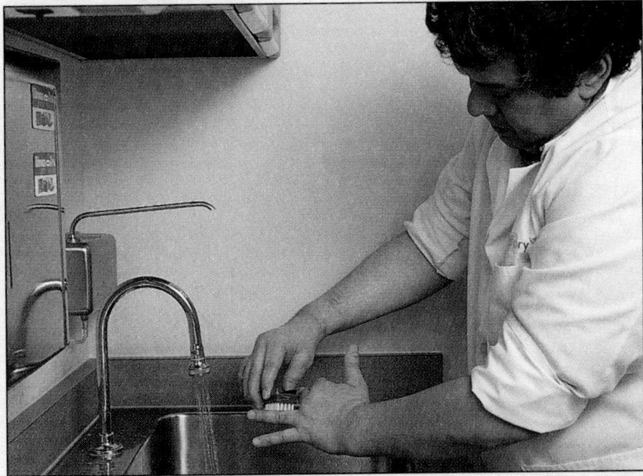

Figure 29-13. Use the scrub brush to work the surgical soap into your fingers, then your wrists, and then your forearms with a firm circular motion.

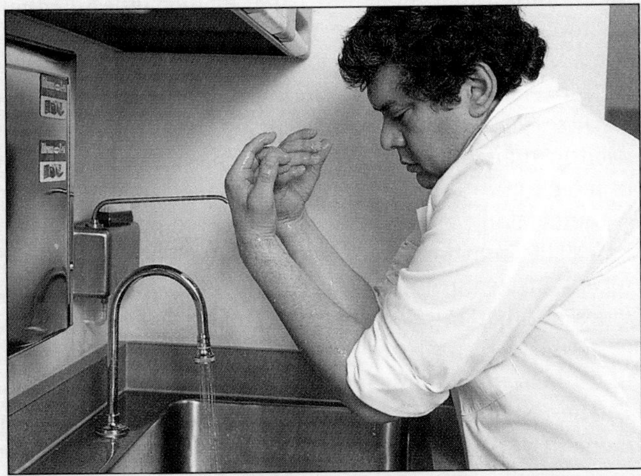

Figure 29-14. Keep your hands above your elbows while rinsing from fingertips to elbows.

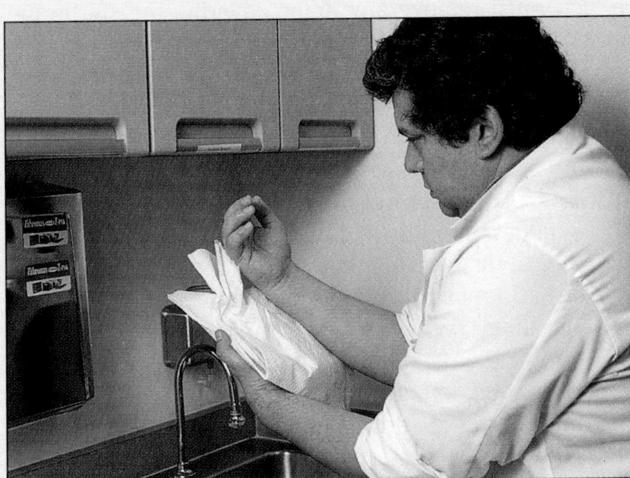

Figure 29-15. Dry your hands thoroughly before carefully drying your forearms.

PROCEDURE 29-3

Donning Sterile Gloves

Objective: To don sterile gloves without compromising the sterility of the outer surface of the gloves

OSHA Guidelines: This procedure does not involve exposure to blood, body fluids, or tissues.

Materials: Prepackaged, double-wrapped sterile gloves

Method

1. Peel open the outer wrapper from the gloves, and place the inner wrapper on a clean surface that is above waist level.
2. Carefully open the inner wrapper, touching only the flaps. Follow any instructions concerning the order in which to open the flaps. If there are no instructions, follow the order described in the procedure for using a sterile instrument pack to create a sterile field. Make sure the cuffs of the gloves are closest to your body, with the fingers pointing away (Figure 29-16), and avoid reaching across the sterile inner surface of the wrap.

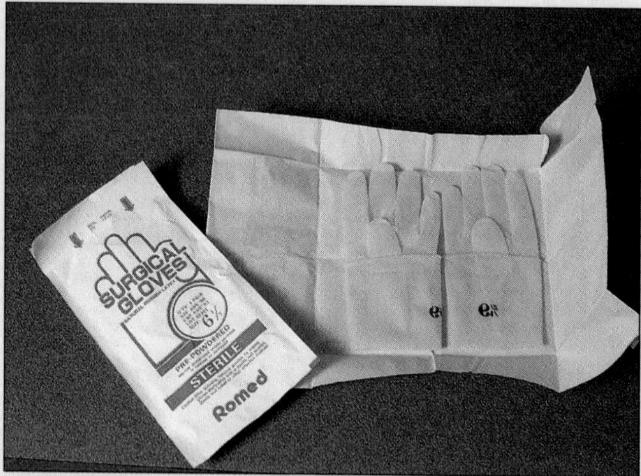

Figure 29-16. You can put these sterile gloves on without reaching across the sterile surfaces of the gloves or the sterile inner wrap of the pack.

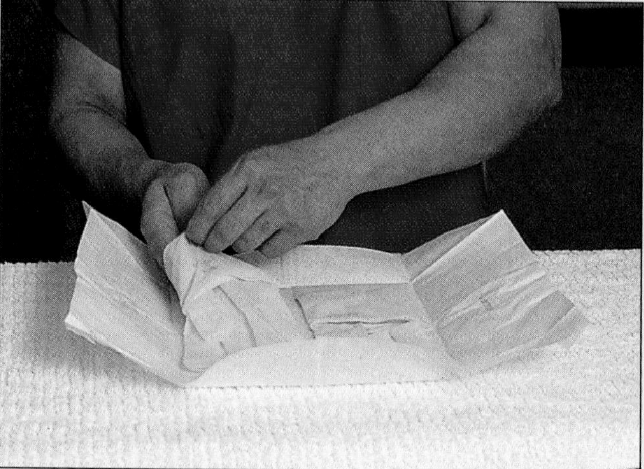

Figure 29-17. Your palm should face up as you slide your dominant hand into the first glove.

fore, you must remove any drape covering the sterile instrument tray before you glove. Sterile gloves provide a small margin of safety in preventing contamination. You must keep your movements controlled and precise to work within that margin to protect the sterile area.

Sanitizing, Disinfecting, and Sterilizing Equipment. Many supplies used in a doctor's office are disposable. Most surgical instruments, however, are made of steel and are reusable. Preparing surgical instruments for reuse involves cleaning them with soap and water (a process called sanitization), then disinfecting and/or sterilizing them, depending on how the equipment will be used. (These procedures are described more fully in Chapter 20.)

Wearing gloves, first clean surgical instruments with soap and water to remove dirt and debris. Then rinse and dry them. After you have sanitized the instruments, disinfect them. If you cannot wash surgical instruments immediately after use, place them directly in disinfectant.

The most common disinfecting agents are chemicals and boiling water. Remember that disinfection kills many microorganisms but does not kill bacterial spores and some viruses. For this reason instruments used in surgical procedures are always sterilized. It is also common to sterilize surgical instruments, even when they will be used in nonsurgical procedures, to reduce the possibility of infection.

Autoclaving is the most common method of sterilization. The autoclave kills microorganisms and spores by means of steam under pressure. The dry heat oven provides another method of sterilization. This technique is preferred for sterilizing sharp instruments, because the moist heat in the autoclave may damage cutting edges.

The Chemiclave is a newer type of sterilization equipment. It uses alcohol under pressure rather than steam. Cold sterilization methods involve lengthy periods of soaking in sterilizing chemicals. Gas sterilization with ethylene oxide is sometimes used for equipment that might be damaged by heat or moisture. The drawback with ethylene oxide gas is that it is highly toxic to hu-

3. The gloves are often labeled "right" and "left." Use your nondominant hand to grasp the opposite glove, touching only the folded edge of its cuff. (A right-handed person would use the left hand to pick up the right glove.)
4. Holding the glove at arm's length and at waist level, slip your dominant hand inside the glove, palm facing up (Figure 29-17).
5. Slide your gloved fingers into the folded cuff of the remaining glove, and slip the glove over the other hand (Figure 29-18).
6. Adjust either glove by sliding the gloved fingers of the other hand under the cuff and pulling the glove taut.
7. Using the technique for adjusting the gloves, unfold each cuff over the arm (Figure 29-19). The maximum sterile surface of the gloves is now exposed.

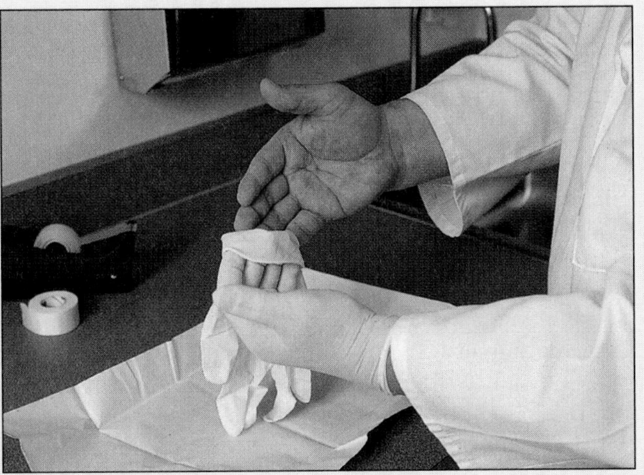

Figure 29-18. Your gloved fingers secure the remaining glove while you slip it over your nondominant hand.

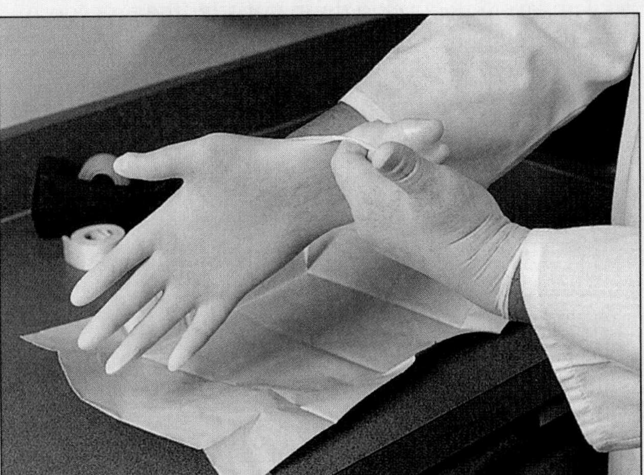

Figure 29-19. Unfold the cuff over your arm while touching only the sterile surface of the glove.

mans and the environment. Because of this potential danger, gas sterilization is generally used only in hospital and manufacturing environments.

Preoperative Procedures

You must complete a number of steps before a surgical procedure. The steps include performing various preliminary duties, preparing the surgical room, and physically preparing the patient for surgery.

Preliminary Duties

You will perform several preliminary tasks before the surgery. They include providing **preoperative** (prior to surgery or "preop") instructions to the patient, completing various administrative tasks, and easing the patient's fears.

Preoperative Instructions. When a patient is scheduled for a minor surgical procedure in the doctor's office, you must explain the preoperative instructions. You should also be prepared to answer the patient's questions about the procedure and about possible risks. The patient may ask you, rather than the doctor, such questions or may need clarification of information provided by the doctor.

A patient may need to follow certain dietary and fluid restrictions before a minor surgical procedure. Not eating or drinking for a specific period of time is a common restriction. There may also be restrictions on what medications a patient may take, because of the administration of an anesthetic during the procedure. You will need to tell non-English-speaking patients to bring along a family member or other interpreter who can help them understand the forms they must sign and their instructions.

You should instruct the patient to wear either comfortable, loose-fitting clothes that will not interfere with the procedure or clothing that can be removed easily. In most cases patients also need to arrange for someone to drive them home after a procedure.

Administrative and Legal Tasks. You must ensure that all the necessary paperwork is completed before surgery. Routine administrative tasks include completing the required insurance forms and obtaining prior authorization from the patient's insurance company.

Make absolutely certain that the patient reads, understands, and signs the surgical consent form. The patient needs a clear understanding of what to expect during and after the surgery to give informed consent as required by law. Sometimes surgery is performed on a child or a patient with limited understanding of legal documents. In such cases the consent form must be signed by the patient's parent or legal guardian.

Failure to obtain the necessary paperwork prior to a surgical procedure can cause serious legal problems. The doctor and other staff members could be held legally liable if problems were to develop during or after the procedure.

It is common practice to call the patient the day before the surgery to confirm the appointment. This call also provides a chance to ensure that the patient follows the preoperative instructions. You may be responsible for making this call.

Easing the Patient's Fears. Knowing what to expect during and after a surgical procedure will ease patients' fears. This information allows them to plan their daily activities and, if necessary, to arrange for help at home during the recovery period.

Some offices may have educational materials such as brochures, fact sheets, or videotapes about minor surgery or the particular procedure the patient will undergo. The availability of such materials varies with the practice specialty and the frequency with which the procedure is performed. You may assist in preparing or acquiring these materials if your office's policy includes such participation for medical assistants. This type of information is extremely helpful to the patient. It may increase patient compliance with the pre- and postoperative instructions.

Much of a patient's fear about a surgical procedure can be overcome if you spend sufficient time before the procedure explaining what to expect. Be prepared to answer the patient's questions honestly, calmly, and confidently. Your calm and knowledgeable manner will reassure the patient. If the answer to a question requires experience or knowledge beyond your own, pass the question on to the doctor.

Preparing the Surgical Room

Prior to surgery the doctor should inform you of specific instructions concerning patient preparation. He will also tell you what special equipment or supplies are necessary for the procedure.

Because patients are likely to feel anxious before a procedure, it is best to have everything ready in the surgical room before you escort the patient into the room. Make sure the room is clean, neat, and free of waste from previous procedures. The examining table should have been cleaned and disinfected, and surface barriers (table paper and pillow covers) should have been changed.

Check to see that there is adequate lighting. Make sure that all equipment and supplies necessary for the procedure are available. Check the date and sterilization indicator on sterilized packs and supplies. Sterile packs are typically considered unsterile if more than 1 month has passed since they were originally sterilized.

You will then wash your hands, put on examination gloves, and prepare the sterile field as outlined in Procedure 29-1. The sterile field and the instruments should be draped with a sterile towel.

Preparing the Patient

Just before the surgery various concerns must be addressed and procedures completed in sequence. The initial tasks are followed by gowning and positioning the patient and preparing the patient's skin for surgery.

Initial Tasks. Before leading the patient into the surgical room, find out whether he has followed the presurgical instructions. Restrictions on food and fluid intake are of particular concern. It is also important to ask what medications the patient is taking and whether or not he has taken that day's dosage.

Measure the patient's vital signs. Ask if there are any symptoms or problems the doctor should know about before the surgery. If any unusual signs or symptoms are present, notify the doctor. The doctor will want to examine the patient before proceeding.

Check the chart for medication orders, such as pain medication or a tranquilizer to calm the patient. Medications should be administered at this time so that they will take effect before surgery.

Gowning and Positioning the Patient. Some procedures require the patient to disrobe and put on a gown to expose the surgical site. If this is the case, you should offer to assist, if appropriate, or leave the room while the patient changes. You should then help the patient onto the table and into the position required for the procedure. You may use one or more small pillows to make the patient as comfortable as possible. Then adequately drape the patient to retain body heat and preserve personal dignity.

Sterile drapes are also used to create a sterile field on a patient's body around the surgical site. Drapes come in a variety of sizes and styles. A **fenestrated drape** has a round or slitlike opening cut out in the center to provide access to the surgical site.

Surgical Skin Preparation. Proper preparation of the patient's skin before surgery reduces the number of microorganisms and the risk of infection. The prepared area should extend 2 inches beyond the surgical field—the area exposed in the center of the fenestrated drape. This extra margin allows for draping without contaminating the field.

Cleaning the Area. Before proceeding with the surgical skin preparation, wash your hands and put on examination gloves. Place a plastic-backed drape under the surgical site to absorb any liquids. Clean the site first with antiseptic soap and sterile water, using forceps and gauze sponges dipped in the solution. Begin at the center of the surgical site, and work outward in a firm, circular motion. Discard the gauze sponge after each complete pass. Clean in concentric circles until you cover the full preparation area. Continue the process, repeating as necessary, for at least 2 minutes or the amount of time specified in the office's procedure manual. Cleaning takes more time if a wound is dirty or contains foreign materials. When procedures are performed on a hand or foot, clean the entire hand or foot.

Shaving the Area. Depending on office policy, you may be required to shave the surgical site to remove hair. Shaving often causes many small wounds on the skin, however, and may increase the risk of infection. Because of this fact some experts feel that hair should not be removed unless it is thick enough to interfere with surgery. Alternatively, hair may be trimmed with scissors or smoothed out of the way.

When shaving is indicated, use a disposable razor and soap for lubrication. Shave in the direction in which the hair grows, and include the same area you cleaned beforehand. When you finish, rinse the area with sterile water and allow it to air-dry. You may also pat the area dry with sterile gauze, starting at the surgical site and moving outward in a circular motion.

Applying the Antiseptic. Next apply antiseptic solution to the area. Antiseptics are agents that are applied to the skin to limit the growth of microorganisms and to help prevent infection. Povidone iodine (Betadine) is most commonly used, but chlorhexidine gluconate (Hibiclens) or benzalkonium chloride (Zephiran Chloride) may also be used, particularly if the patient is allergic to iodine. Swab an area 2 inches larger than the surgical field with the antiseptic solution in a circular outward motion, starting at the surgical site. For surgery on a hand or foot, swab the entire hand or foot. Allow the antiseptic to air-dry; do not pat it dry—that would remove some of the solution's antiseptic properties.

When the area is dry, treat it as a sterile field. Instruct the patient not to touch the area. Cover the area with a sterile fenestrated drape, from front to back. Avoid reaching over the field.

At this point notify the physician that the patient is ready. Then prepare yourself to assist with the surgery.

Intraoperative Procedures

Intraoperative procedures are procedures that take place during surgery. You may be asked to perform a wide variety of unsterile and sterile tasks during surgery, such as preparing local anesthetic for the doctor, monitoring the patient, processing specimens, and handing instruments to the doctor. The doctor may also ask you to explain to the patient step-by-step what will be done next during the procedure.

Administering a Local Anesthetic

Before beginning the surgical procedure, the physician will administer a local anesthetic. Some local anesthetics are injected. An injected anesthetic is packaged in a sterile **vial** (a small glass bottle with a self-sealing rubber stopper). Other local anesthetics come in a cream, gel, or spray form. These anesthetics are **topical** (applied directly to the skin) and affect only the area to which they are applied.

Lidocaine (Xylocaine) is the most commonly used anesthetic. It is often used as a topical gel anesthetic. Tetracaine hydrochloride (Pontocaine), a long-acting anesthetic, is injected.

The physician administers the local anesthetic by injection or by applying it directly to the skin. The choice of administration methods depends on how invasive or painful the procedure is likely to be.

Topical Application. Anesthetic gels, creams, and sprays may be used topically in certain surgical procedures. A topical anesthetic is useful when the pain will be mild or when only the upper layers of the skin are affected. It is common to use such agents to anesthetize the area of a small laceration prior to suturing. Sometimes an anesthetic cream is applied before a local anesthetic is injected. This application reduces or eliminates the pain caused by the injection. A topical anesthetic must usually remain on the skin for 10 to 15 minutes for the area to become sufficiently anesthetized.

Injections. If a local anesthetic is to be injected, it is typically administered after the skin is prepared but before the patient is draped. In some cases, however, the anesthetic is injected prior to skin preparation to allow time for it to take effect. In either case it is important to note the time of anesthetic administration in the patient's chart.

If the doctor is already wearing sterile gloves, you may be asked to assist in administering the anesthetic. Administering anesthetic is an unsterile task because the outside of the vial is unsterile. When performing this task, follow proper procedure to protect the sterility of the doctor's gloves and the anesthetic solution.

First check the label of the anesthetic vial three times to confirm that it is the correct solution. Clean the vial's rubber stopper with 70% isopropyl alcohol, and leave the cotton or gauze on top of the stopper. Present the requested needle and syringe to the doctor by peeling half the outer wrapper away and allowing the doctor to remove them from the wrapper.

Remove the cotton or gauze from the rubber stopper, and hold the vial so the doctor can verify that it is the proper medication. Turn the vial upside down, and hold it securely around the base, without touching the sterile stopper. Be sure to hold the vial in front of you at shoulder height. Because significant force will be necessary to

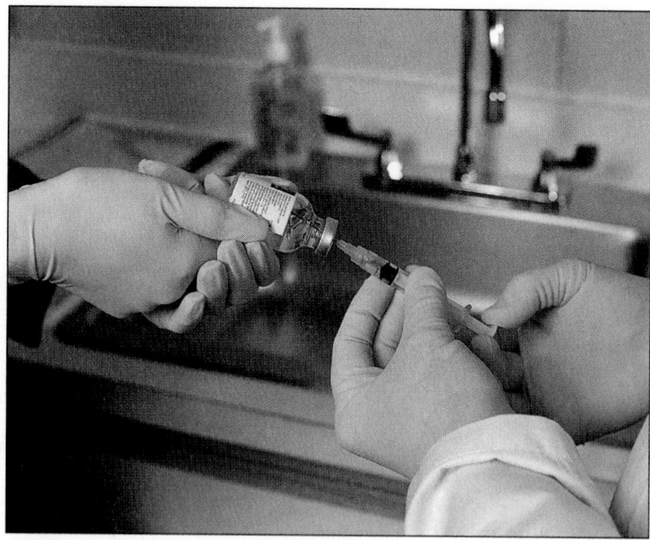

Figure 29-20. You must hold the anesthetic vial firmly to allow the physician to puncture the rubber stopper with the needle.

push the needle through the rubber stopper, you should brace the wrist of the hand holding the vial with your free hand. Hold the vial firmly so the doctor can withdraw the anesthetic from it (Figure 29-20).

Potential Side Effects of the Anesthetic. You should inform the patient of possible reactions to the anesthetic medication. Although rare, reactions may include dizziness, loss of consciousness, seizures, or cardiac arrest. Adverse reactions can occur if the anesthetic dose is too high or if it is absorbed too quickly. They can also occur if the patient is taking other medications that should not be mixed with the anesthetic. It is vital to document all medications (including over-the-counter ones) the patient is taking at the time of the surgery.

Use of Epinephrine. Epinephrine is a sterile solution that is sometimes injected along with an anesthetic. Epinephrine constricts the blood vessels, making them narrower. This constriction reduces bleeding and prolongs the action of the local anesthetic. Epinephrine is used if the site of surgery is an area with many small blood vessels that are expected to bleed profusely (such as the head). Reducing bleeding makes it easier to see and to repair the wound. (Epinephrine should be used with caution, however, in patients with heart disease or respiratory disease.)

When epinephrine is combined with the anesthetic to reduce bleeding, it prolongs the anesthesia because epinephrine slows the rate at which anesthetic spreads into the tissue. This effect may or may not be desirable. Epinephrine should not be used in areas such as the fingers, toes, nose, or ears, where it could also compromise the local blood supply. There is some concern that epinephrine may increase wound infection rates (Boriskin, 1994).

Assisting the Physician During Surgery

Your role in surgical assisting depends on the type of surgery and the physician's preference. You may assist the physician in one of two capacities. You may serve as a **floater,** an unsterile assistant who is free to move about the room and attend to unsterile needs. Alternatively, you may serve as a **sterile scrub assistant,** who assists in handling sterile equipment during the procedure. The duties are different for the two functions. Procedure 29-4 outlines the tasks performed by both sterile and unsterile assistants.

The Floater. First the surgical room is set up and the patient is prepared. If you are assisting as a floater (sometimes called a circulator), you will perform a routine scrub and put on examination gloves. Remember that you cannot touch sterile items in the sterile field because you have not performed a surgical scrub and are not wearing sterile gloves.

Monitoring and Recording. One of the most important duties of a floater is to monitor the patient during the procedure. You must measure vital signs regularly and observe the patient for reactions to the anesthetic. Record all observations in the patient's chart. Also write down any information or notes the doctor requests. You must keep a record of time, including when the anesthetic is administered, when the procedure begins, and when the procedure is completed.

Processing Specimens. When you serve as a floater during surgery, the doctor may ask you to receive and process specimens for laboratory examination. Most tissues are placed in a 10% formalin solution to preserve them before they are sent to the laboratory. Half-fill the specimen container with the formalin solution ahead of time. Remove the lid of the specimen container without touching the rim. Hold the container out toward the doctor so she can place the tissue directly into it without contaminating the sample (Figure 29-21).

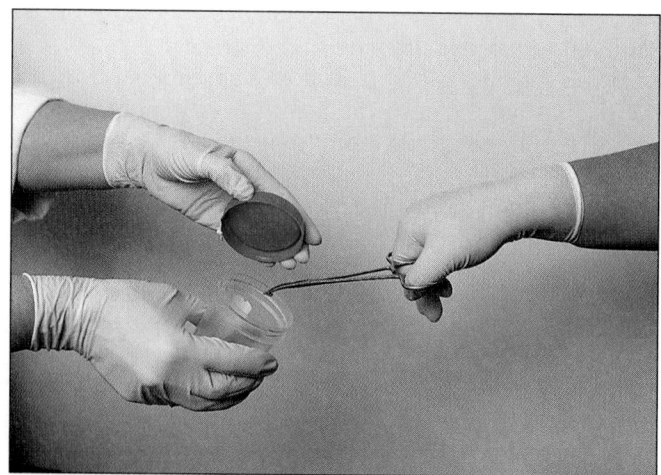

Figure 29-21. Be sure to hold the specimen container so that the doctor can place the tissue in it without touching the rim or the outside of the container with the tissue.

PROCEDURE 29-4

General Assisting Procedures for Minor Surgery

Objective: To provide assistance to the doctor during minor surgery while maintaining clean or sterile technique as appropriate

OSHA Guidelines

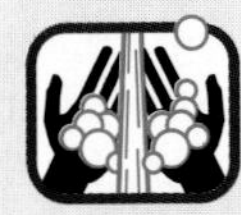
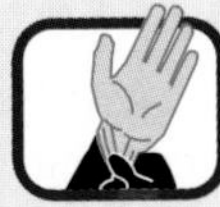

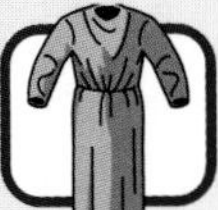
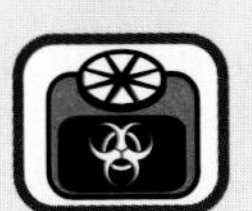
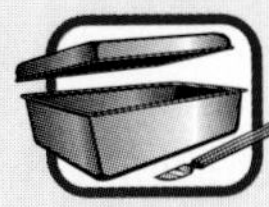
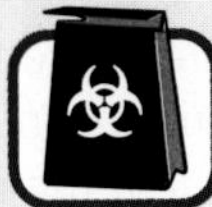
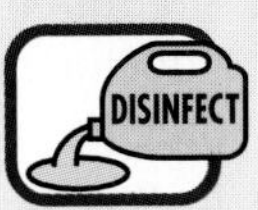

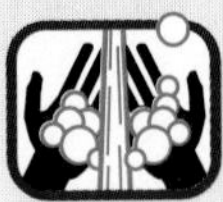

Materials: Sterile towel, tray or Mayo stand, appropriate instrument pack(s), needles and syringes, anesthetic, antiseptic, sterile water or physiological saline, small sterile bowl, sterile gauze squares or cotton balls, specimen containers half-filled with preservative, suture materials, sterile dressings and tape

Method

Floater (Unsterile Assistant)

1. Perform routine hand washing and put on examination gloves.
2. Monitor the patient during the procedure; record the results in the patient's chart.
3. During the surgery assist as needed.
4. Add sterile items to the tray as necessary.
5. Pour sterile solution into a sterile bowl as needed.
6. Assist in administering additional anesthetic.
   a. Check the medication vial three times.
   b. Clean the rubber stopper with alcohol (write the date opened when using a new bottle); leave cotton or gauze on top.
   c. Present the needle and syringe to the doctor.
   d. Remove the cotton or gauze from the vial, and show the label to the doctor.
   e. Hold the vial upside down, and grasp the lower edge firmly; brace your wrist with your free hand. (This firmly supports the vial to sustain the force of the needle being inserted into the rubber stopper.)
   f. Allow the doctor to fill the syringe.
7. Receive specimens for laboratory examination.
   a. Uncap the specimen container; present it to the doctor for the introduction of the specimen.
   b. Replace the cap and label the container.
   c. Treat all specimens as infectious.
   d. Place the specimen container in a transport bag or other container.
   e. Complete the requisition form to send the specimen to the laboratory.

Sterile Scrub Assistant

1. Perform a surgical scrub and put on sterile gloves. (Remember to remove the sterile towel covering the sterile field and instruments before gloving.)
2. Close and arrange the surgical instruments on the tray.
3. Prepare for swabbing by inserting gauze squares into the sterile dressing forceps.
4. Pass the instruments as necessary.
5. Swab the wound as requested.
6. Retract the wound as requested.
7. Cut the sutures as requested.

Floater or Sterile Scrub Assistant (After Surgery)

1. Monitor the patient.
2. Put on clean examination gloves, and clean the wound with antiseptic.
3. Dress the wound.
4. Remove the gloves and wash your hands.
5. Give the patient oral postoperative instructions in addition to the release packet.
6. Discharge the patient.
7. Put on clean examination gloves.
8. Properly dispose of used materials and disposable instruments.
9. Sanitize reusable instruments and prepare them for disinfection and/or sterilization as needed.
10. Clean equipment and the examination room according to OSHA guidelines.
11. Remove the gloves and wash your hands.

The container should be labeled with the following information:

- The patient's name and the doctor's name
- The date and time of collection
- The body site from which the specimen was obtained
- Your initials

If more than one specimen is obtained from a patient, place each specimen in a separate container. Label each container with the necessary information, along with a number to indicate the order in which the specimens are obtained (no. 1, no. 2, and so on). You will also fill out a laboratory requisition slip to send along with the specimen(s). Specimen containers should be red in color or labeled with the biohazard symbol. Specimen containers should be placed in specially designed bags for transport.

Other Duties. As a floater you may also be asked to perform a number of other duties, including these:

- Assisting with the injection of additional anesthetic
- Adding additional sterile items to the sterile tray
- Pouring sterile solutions
- Keeping the surgical area clean and neat during the procedure
- Repositioning the patient as necessary
- Adjusting lighting

The Sterile Scrub Assistant. When you serve as a sterile scrub assistant, you perform a surgical scrub and wear sterile gloves. You may be asked to perform a variety of tasks under sterile conditions. Remember not to touch unsterile items after putting on sterile gloves.

Handling Instruments. Your first duty as a sterile scrub assistant is, typically, to close the instruments on the sterile tray because they are normally left in the open position during sterilization. Your next duty is to rearrange the instruments on the tray. Instruments should be arranged in the order in which they will be used or according to the doctor's preference. Instruments are generally used in the following sequence:

- Cutting instruments
- Grasping instruments
- Retractors
- Probes
- Suture materials
- Needle holders and scissors

Prepare for swabbing by placing several sterile gauze squares in the dressing forceps. They will then be ready when needed. As the sterile scrub assistant, you will be asked to pass instruments to the doctor during the procedure. You must hold instruments so that the doctor can grasp them securely and will not need to reposition them in her hands. At the same time, the instruments must be handled properly to maintain their sterility.

When passing scissors and clamps, hold them by the hinge (Figure 29-22). You will have a clear view of the tip of the instrument, and the doctor will have full use of the handles. Firmly slap the instrument handles into the doctor's extended palm. The doctor's hand will close around the handles as a reflex action to the slapping. This technique reduces the risk of dropping an instrument. If the scissors or clamp is curved, the curve should follow the same curve as the doctor's hand.

When passing a scalpel, hold it above and just behind the cutting edge of the blade so the doctor can grasp the entire handle (Figure 29-23). Pass a needle holder with suture material so that the needle is pointing up, and hold the end of the suture material with your other hand to prevent the material from becoming tangled in the handles.

Other Duties. As a sterile scrub assistant, you may also be asked to swab fluids from a wound or to retract the edges of a wound to help the doctor view the area. While the doctor is closing the wound, you may be required to cut the suture material after each stitch. The doctor may not verbalize every request to you. With practice and after experience with a particular doctor, you will learn how to respond to the doctor's actions.

When cutting suture materials, leave ⅛ inch of the material above the knot. This excess material prevents the suture from coming untied. It also leaves the material short enough so that it does not bother the patient.

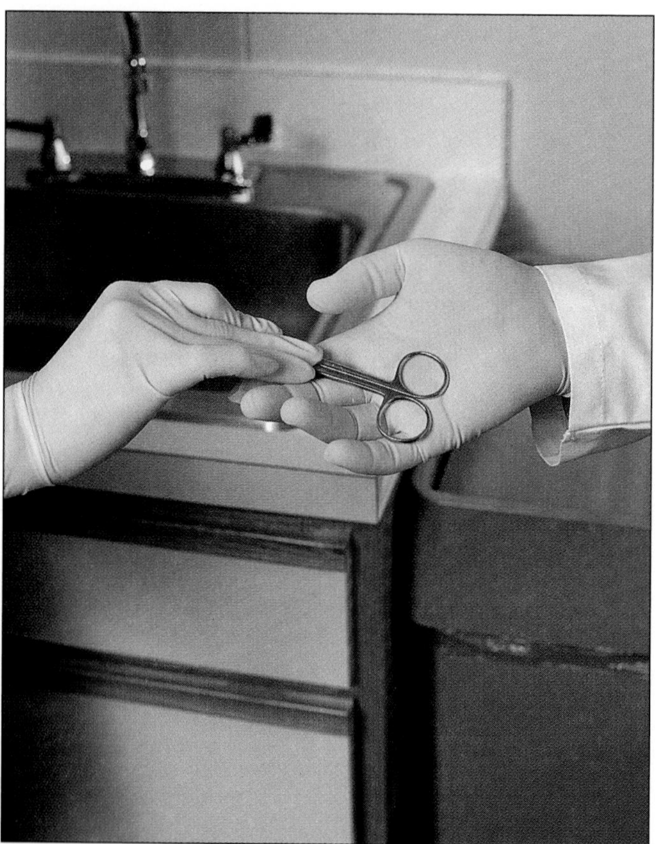

Figure 29-22. Holding the scissors by the hinge, slap the handles into the doctor's hand.

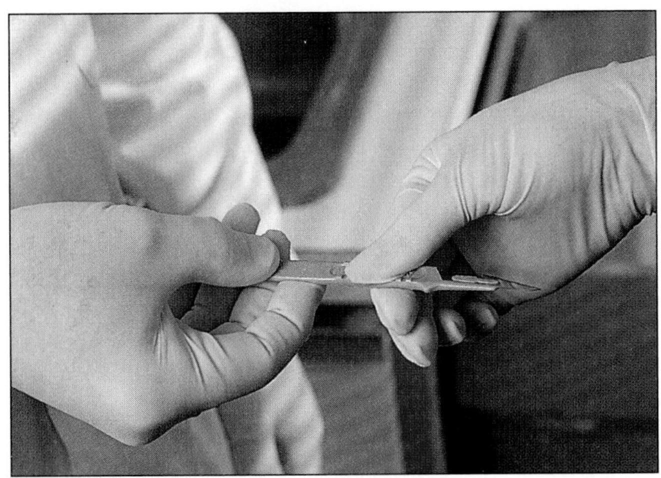

Figure 29-23. Hold a scalpel above and just behind the cutting edge as you pass the handle into the palm of the doctor's hand.

Postoperative Procedures

You will be responsible for the patient's **postoperative** ("postop") follow-up after the surgical procedure. Your duties may include immediate care of the patient, proper cleaning of the surgical room, and follow-up care of the patient.

Immediate Patient Care

Patient care is your top priority as a medical assistant. Except for intravenous medications, you will administer postoperative medications the physician requests for the patient. You will also ensure that the patient remains lying down on the examining table for the prescribed length of time after the procedure. During this period continue to monitor the patient's vital signs, and watch for adverse reactions. It is important to document your observations in the patient's chart.

Dressing the Wound. You may also dress the wound during the monitoring period. **Dressings** are sterile materials used to cover an incision. They serve a number of functions. They protect the wound from further injury and keep the wound clean, thus preventing infection. Dressings also reduce bleeding, absorb fluid drainage, reduce discomfort to the patient, speed healing, and reduce the possibility of scarring. Gauze dressings are the most common type of dressings and come in a variety of sizes and shapes.

Before dressing the wound, put on clean examination gloves. Clean the site with povidone iodine (Betadine), and allow it to dry. If ordered by the physician, apply antibiotic ointment over the wound. Place the sterile dressing over the site, and secure it appropriately.

Bandaging the Wound. It may be necessary to apply a bandage (a clean strip of gauze or elastic material) over the dressing to help hold it in place (Figure 29-24). Bandages may also be used to improve circulation, to provide support or reduce tension on a wound or suture and prevent it from reopening, or to prevent movement of that area of the body. Adhesive tape may also be used for these purposes. Some patients are allergic to the adhesive, but most tapes are now hypoallergenic. The patient is usually more comfortable after a bandage or adhesive tape has been applied.

Postoperative Instructions. After the procedure provide oral postoperative instructions to the patient. You may do this during the monitoring part of the postoperative period or afterward. These instructions include guidelines for pain management and instructions for wound care. Postoperative information also includes dietary or activity restrictions, if any, and when to come in for a follow-up appointment. It is a good idea to ask patients to repeat what you say so that you know they understand the information.

Instructions are often also provided in writing and may be part of a complete postoperative information packet. You may be asked to help prepare or update packet materials, especially if you routinely assist

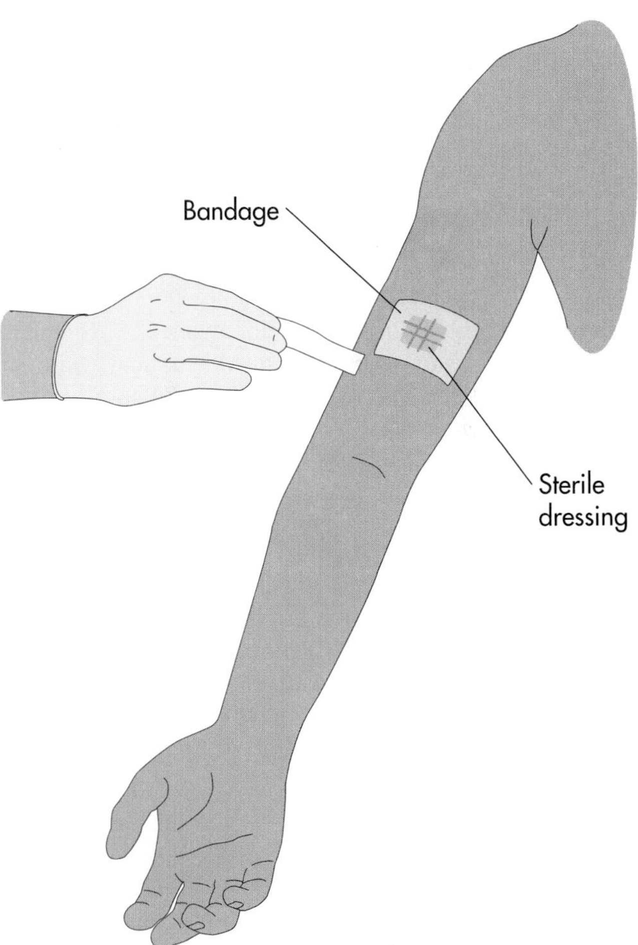

Figure 29-24. A bandage helps keep a sterile dressing in place.

patients as they recover from minor surgery. A postoperative information packet might include the following information:

- Proper wound-care instructions
- Suggestions for pain relief and reduction of swelling, such as medications and hot or cold packs
- Dietary restrictions
- Activity restrictions
- Timing for a follow-up appointment or an appointment card

Wound-care instructions include details on dressing changes, which will vary depending on the depth and size of the wound. Generally a patient should clean the wound daily with soap and water or dilute hydrogen peroxide (3%) and allow it to air-dry. The patient should then apply an antibiotic cream and place a dry, sterile dressing over the wound. Except when cleansing the wound, the patient should keep it dry. The dressing should be replaced if it gets wet. Although cleansing aids wound healing, a wet dressing provides bacteria and other contaminants with access to the wound.

Descriptions, and often illustrations, of normal and infected incisions are an important part of wound-care instructions. The patient should call the physician if any signs of infection are noted. The instructions should also encourage the patient to protect the incision from exposure to the sun. This guideline is advisable for as long as 3 to 6 months to prevent the incision line from becoming darker than surrounding skin (Boriskin, 1994).

The length of time it takes for a wound to heal varies with the site, the patient's age, and the severity of the wound. Each patient therefore needs specific instructions on how long to continue with the dressings and when to return for suture or staple removal.

Patient Release. Notify the doctor when the patient is stabilized and ready to leave. The doctor may want to further observe and instruct the patient. Be sure to offer assistance if the patient needs help getting dressed.

Then help the patient check out. Schedule the next appointment for the patient. Make sure the patient has the correct discharge packet. Confirm arrangements to transport the patient home. Finally, assist the patient to the car or other transport if this is part of office procedure.

If a patient insists on driving himself home, enter this information on the chart. Indicate the time and have the patient initial the entry. This documentation is important for legal reasons. It would clarify liability should an accident occur as a result of a reaction to the surgery or the anesthetic.

Surgical Room Cleanup

If there is time during the monitoring period, begin to clean up the surgical area. If time is not available then, perform the cleanup routine after the patient has been released.

Until the reusable instruments can be cleaned, place them in a disinfectant soak that has anticoagulant properties. A reusable sharps container is generally used for this purpose for surgical instruments. Place disposable waste in the sharps or biohazardous waste container. Clean the counters, examining table, and trays according to OSHA guidelines by disinfecting them. A 10% chlorine bleach solution, which is one part household bleach to nine parts water, is commonly used. Disinfect small pieces of nonsurgical equipment (stethoscopes, thermometers, and so on) with 70% isopropyl alcohol. Replace paper table and pillow covers at this time, along with necessary supplies.

Follow-Up Care

During a follow-up appointment the physician examines the patient's surgical wound. You may be asked to change the dressing or remove the wound closures.

Typically, suture or staple removal takes place 5 to 10 days after minor surgery. The sutures or staples are ready for removal when a clean, unbroken suture line is observed. There should be no scabs, no seepage from the wound, and no visible opening. Any of these signs may indicate unhealed areas. Suture removal is described in Procedure 29-5. Staple removal is similar, except that staple removal forceps, rather than forceps and scissors, are used to remove the staples.

Summary

As the doctor's assistant in minor surgical procedures, you perform many functions. Your responsibilities during the patient's preoperative and postoperative care, however, are just as important.

Before surgery you provide the patient with preoperative instructions, make sure the necessary administrative and legal forms are completed, help prepare the patient emotionally, and set up the surgical room. You then confirm that the patient has followed all preoperative instructions and physically prepare the patient for surgery.

During the procedure you follow proper medical and surgical aseptic techniques. Your actual responsibilities vary with the role you play as a floater or a sterile scrub assistant for a particular surgery. At all times you ensure the safety and comfort of the patient and are knowledgeable enough to function as the doctor's "right hand" during the procedure.

After the surgery you provide the postoperative patient care and instruction that will help ensure prompt healing. Then you clean the surgical room and prepare it for the next procedure.

PROCEDURE 29-5

Suture Removal

Objective: To remove sutures from a healing wound while maintaining sterile technique and protecting the integrity of the closed wound

OSHA Guidelines

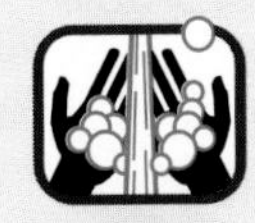
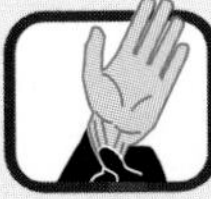
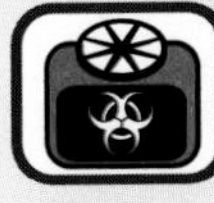
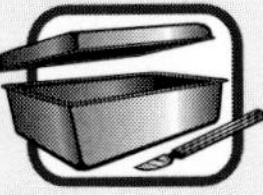
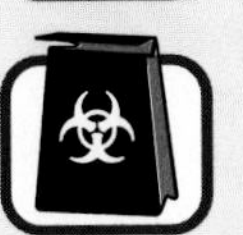
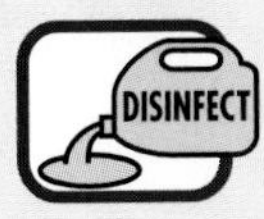

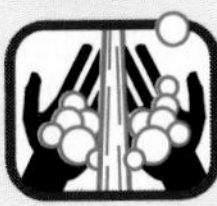

Materials: Tray or Mayo stand, suture removal pack (suture scissors and thumb forceps), sterile towel, antiseptic solution, hydrogen peroxide (3%), two small sterile bowls, sterile gauze squares, sterile strips or butterfly closures, sterile dressings and tape

Method

1. Clean and disinfect the tray or Mayo stand.
2. Wash your hands and assemble the necessary materials.
3. Check the date and sterilization indicator on the suture removal pack.
4. Unwrap the suture removal pack, and place it on the tray or stand to create a sterile field.
5. Unwrap the sterile bowls and add them to the sterile field.
6. Pour a small amount of antiseptic solution into one bowl, and pour a small amount of hydrogen peroxide into the other bowl.
7. Cover the tray with a sterile towel to protect the sterile field while you are out of the room.
8. Escort the patient to the examination room and explain the procedure.
9. Perform a routine scrub, remove the towel from the tray, and put on examination gloves.
10. Remove the old dressing.
    a. Lift the tape toward the middle of the dressing to avoid pulling on the wound.
    b. If the dressing adheres to the wound, cover the dressing with gauze squares soaked in hydrogen peroxide. Leave the wet gauze in place for several seconds to loosen the dressing.
    c. Save the old dressing for the doctor to inspect.
11. Inspect the wound for signs of infection.

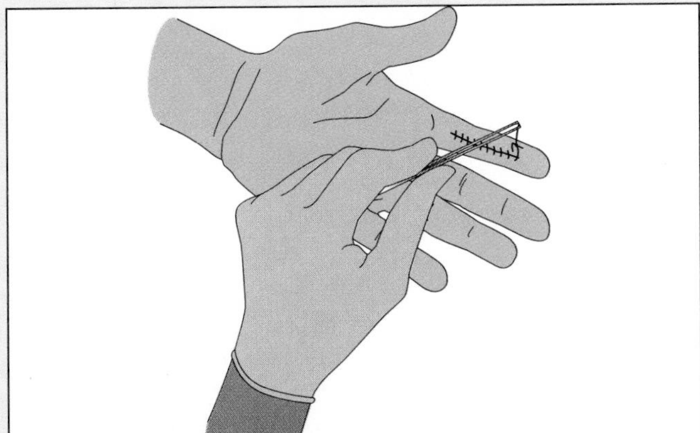

Figure 29-25. Without pulling on the wound, lift the suture knot away from the skin to make room for the suture scissors.

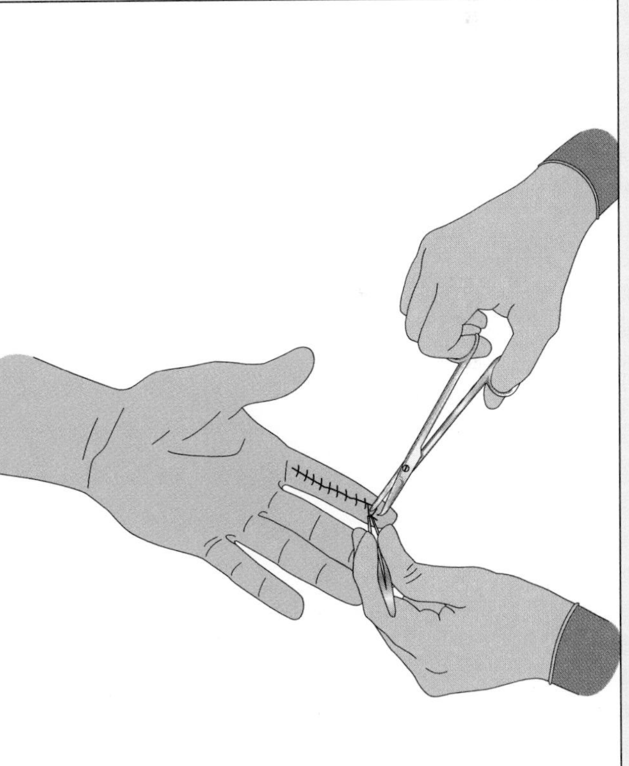

Figure 29-26. Cut the suture material as close as possible to its entry point in the skin.

continued

PROCEDURE 29-5 continued

Suture Removal

12. Clean the wound with gauze pads soaked in antiseptic, and pat it dry with clean gauze pads.
13. Remove the gloves and wash your hands.
14. Notify the doctor that the wound is ready for examination.
15. Once the doctor indicates that the wound is sufficiently healed to proceed, put on clean examination gloves.
16. Place a square of gauze next to the wound for collecting the sutures as they are removed.
17. Grasp the first suture knot with forceps.
18. Gently lift the knot away from the skin to allow room for the suture scissors (Figure 29-25).
19. Slide the suture scissors under the suture material, and cut the suture where it enters the skin (Figure 29-26).
20. Gently lift the knot up and toward the wound to remove the suture without opening the wound (Figure 29-27).
21. Place the suture on the gauze pad, and inspect to ensure the entire suture is present.
22. Repeat the removal process until all sutures have been removed.
23. Count the sutures and compare the number with the number indicated in the patient's record (Figure 29-28).
24. Clean the wound with antiseptic, and allow the wound to air-dry.
25. Dress the wound as ordered, or notify the doctor if the sterile strips or butterfly closures are to be applied.
26. Observe the patient for signs of distress, such as wincing or grimacing.
27. Properly dispose of used materials and disposable instruments.
28. Remove the gloves and wash your hands.
29. Instruct the patient on wound care.
30. In the patient's chart, record pertinent information, such as the condition of the wound and the type of closures used, if any.
31. Escort the patient to the checkout area.
32. Put on clean gloves.
33. Sanitize resuable instruments and prepare them for disinfection and/or sterilization as needed.
34. Clean the equipment and examination room according to OSHA guidelines.
35. Remove the gloves and wash your hands.

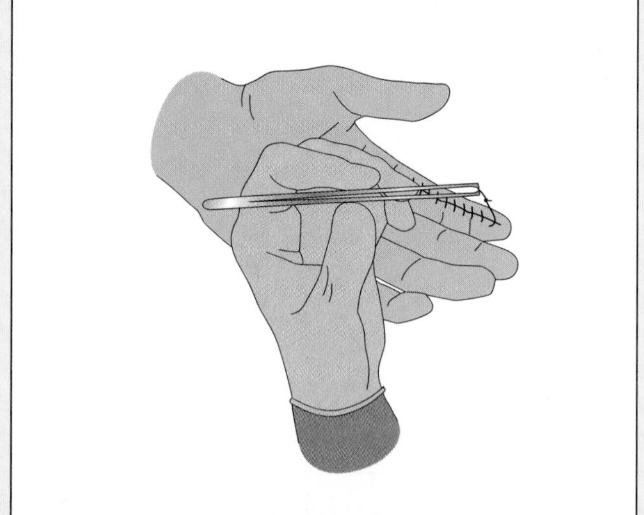

Figure 29-27. Remove the suture by lifting the knot up and toward the wound.

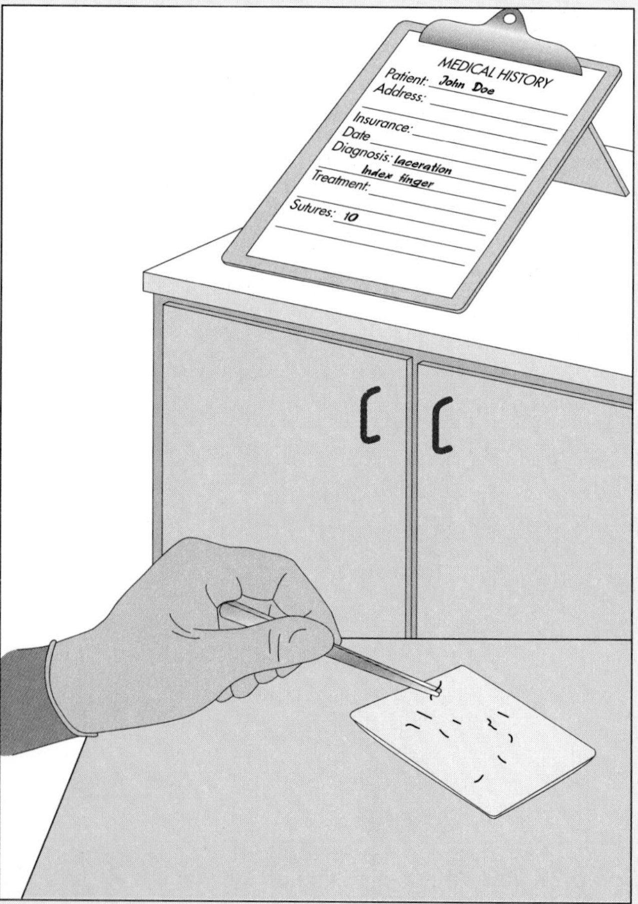
MEDICAL HISTORY
Patient: John Doe
Address:
Insurance:
Date
Diagnosis: laceration
Index finger
Treatment:
Sutures: 10

Figure 29-28. Compare the number of sutures removed with the recorded number of sutures placed.

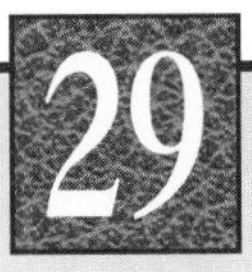

Chapter Review

Discussion Questions

1. Explain the difference between medical and surgical asepsis, and list three procedures that use each technique.
2. List five different categories of surgical instruments by function, give an example of each, and describe how instruments in each category are used.
3. List three minor surgical procedures you may assist with in the doctor's office. Name one procedure you may perform on your own.

Critical Thinking Questions

1. What might you say to ease the fears of an anxious patient who is about to undergo a laceration repair?
2. Explain the procedure you would follow if you were functioning as a sterile scrub assistant and your glove was punctured while you were handling instruments during a surgical procedure.
3. Explain how to make sure that a patient has understood the postoperative instructions for wound care.

Application Activities

1. Using instrument flash cards or actual instruments, choose and list the types of instruments you would need during a procedure to clean and repair a laceration.
2. Working with one or two classmates, practice opening a sterile pack and creating a sterile field. Practice adding additional instruments and a sterile bowl to the sterile field. Offer suggestions to each other for improving your techniques.
3. With a partner, practice handing surgical instruments to each other. The receiver should look the other way while receiving the instrument. This approach simulates actual conditions in which the doctor may be concentrating on a procedure rather than looking at the instrument. This approach also tests the ability of the person handing the instrument to use proper technique.

Further Readings

Atkinson, Lucy J. *Berry & Kohn's Operating Room Technique.* 7th ed. St. Louis, MO: Mosby–Year Book, 1992.

Boriskin, Mitchell I. "Primary Care Management of Wounds." *Nurse Practitioner,* November 1994, 38–58.

Fabian, Denise. "Handling Laboratory Specimens in a Medical Office." *The Professional Medical Assistant,* January/February 1991, 6–7.

Griffith, H. Winter. *Complete Guide to Symptoms, Illness and Surgery.* 3d ed. New York: The Body Press/Perigee Books, 1995.

Olsen, Robin J. "Examination Gloves as Barriers to Hand Contamination in Clinical Practice." *Journal of the American Medical Association,* 21 July 1993, 350–354.

Robbins, Jim. "Rubber Gloves: Peril for Some." *New York Times,* 29 January 1997, sec. C, p. 7.

Swearingen, Pamela L. *Photo Atlas of Nursing Procedures.* 2d ed. Redwood City, CA: Addison-Wesley Nursing, 1991.

Timby, Barbara K., and LuVerne W. Lewis. *Fundamental Skills and Concepts in Patient Care.* 5th ed. Philadelphia: J. B. Lippincott, 1992.

Assisting With Cold and Heat Therapy and Ambulation

CHAPTER OUTLINE

- General Principles of Physical Therapy
- Cryotherapy and Thermotherapy
- Hydrotherapy
- Exercise Therapy
- Massage
- Traction
- Mobility Aids
- Referral to a Physical Therapist

OBJECTIVES

After completing Chapter 30, you will be able to:

- Explain how medical assistants might assist with some forms of physical therapy.
- Describe ways to test joint mobility, muscle strength, gait, and posture.
- Discuss the benefits of cold and heat therapies.
- List contraindications to cold and heat therapies.
- Identify various cold and heat therapies.
- Describe hydrotherapy methods.
- Identify several methods of exercise therapy.
- Describe common massage techniques.
- Compare different methods of traction.
- Demonstrate how to teach a patient to use a cane, a walker, crutches, and a wheelchair.

Key Terms

cryotherapy
diathermy
edema
erythema
fluidotherapy
gait
goniometer
hydrotherapy
mobility aid
physical therapy
posture
range of motion (ROM)
therapeutic team
thermotherapy
traction

AREAS OF COMPETENCE

1997 ROLE DELINEATION STUDY

ADMINISTRATIVE

Administrative Procedures

- Schedule, coordinate, and monitor appointments
- Schedule inpatient/outpatient admissions and procedures

CLINICAL

Fundamental Principles

- Screen and follow up patient test results

GENERAL (Transdisciplinary)

Professionalism

- Work as a team member

continued

AREAS OF COMPETENCE continued

Communication Skills

- Serve as liaison

Instruction

- Instruct individuals according to their needs
- Explain office policies and procedures

General Principles of Physical Therapy

Applying cold and heat therapy and assisting patients with ambulation are common responsibilities of a medical assistant. You may also receive special training to perform additional duties related to physical therapy. **Physical therapy** is a medical specialty for the treatment of musculoskeletal, nervous, and cardiopulmonary disorders. A physical therapist uses a variety of treatments, including cold, heat, water, exercise, massage, and traction. Some physical therapy regimens combine two or more treatments. Exercising in a pool, for example, combines the use of water and exercise. In addition, the physical therapist actively promotes patient education and rehabilitation programs.

Physical therapy benefits patients in several ways. It restores and improves muscle function, builds strength, increases joint mobility, relieves pain, and increases circulation. Physical therapy is used to treat various disorders, including arthritis, stroke, lower-back pain, muscle spasms, muscle injuries or diseases, pressure sores, skin disorders, and burns.

Assisting With Physical Therapy

For a full program of physical therapy, a physician generally refers a patient to a licensed physical therapist. A physician may, however, request that you assist with some forms of physical therapy, including the following:

- Applying cold or heat
- Teaching basic exercises
- Preparing patients for massage therapy
- Demonstrating how to use a cane, walker, or crutches
- Demonstrating how to use a wheelchair
- Discussing with the patient specific therapies for use at home

Assisting Within a Therapeutic Team

Many people who require physical therapy are recovering from traumatic injuries or dealing with chronic illnesses. They may therefore be receiving therapeutic attention from several different specialists. Physicians, nurses, medical assistants, and other specialists who work with patients dealing with chronic illness or recovery from major injuries make up a **therapeutic team.** When you work with such patients, your responsibilities may include:

- Coordinating the patient's schedule of sessions with different specialists.
- Making referrals, as directed by the physician.
- Explaining a specialist's treatment approach to the patient.
- Communicating the physician's findings to the specialist.
- Documenting the specialist's treatments and findings for the physician.
- Reinforcing the specialist's instructions for the patient.
- Answering the patient's questions.

To fulfill these responsibilities, you must have a working knowledge of therapy techniques. If, for example, the physician refers a patient to an art therapist, you would set up an art therapy appointment and explain in general terms what the patient can expect. "Educating the Patient" offers basic information on art therapy and other specialized therapies.

Besides learning the basic information you need to know about physical therapy, you will want to keep up to date on emerging techniques. You may want to become proficient in some of these new techniques. By expanding your knowledge and skills, you increase your value as a member of the therapeutic team.

Assisting With Patient Assessment

Before the doctor prescribes physical therapy, she assesses the patient's physical abilities and condition. She inspects and palpates the patient's joints and muscles and tests the patient's joint mobility, muscle strength, gait, and posture. You will typically assist with these tests. In some cases the doctor may direct you to perform them.

Joint Mobility Testing. People usually assume that their joints are mobile until stiffness or injury limits them. When a patient complains of these difficulties, the doctor may ask you to assist in testing range of motion. **Range of motion (ROM)** is the degree to which a joint is able to move, measured in degrees with a protractor

EDUCATING THE PATIENT

Art Therapy and Other Specialized Therapies

Health-care professionals are beginning to recognize the contribution of art and other specialized therapies to a patient's recovery. Because many people do not know about these specialized therapies, you may be called on to explain them to patients. For example, you can educate patients about the following potential advantages of the use of art therapy:

- Aids both physical and mental healing
- Provides a recreational outlet
- Improves mobility and fine motor coordination
- Provides an outlet for expressing fears or other emotions that patients may be unaware of or unable or unwilling to express verbally
- Helps relieve anxiety
- Allows patients to focus on something other than their physical condition
- Encourages patients to take better care of themselves

As with any therapy or procedure, patients will be more at ease if they know what to expect. You can help by explaining what the art therapist does:

- Organizes group or one-on-one sessions
- Directs patients to express themselves visually through drawing, painting, or sculpture
- Analyzes patients' use of colors, themes, and patterns, which can provide clues to patients' emotional states
- Helps patients understand the visual results of artistic expression and what it can indicate about patients' feelings and states of mind
- Consults with a psychotherapist, who can follow up on the art therapist's findings about patients

To aid in the art therapy process, encourage patients to relax and give this approach time to work. Although the benefits of art therapy may be evident immediately, they are just as likely to be perceived only after the course of therapy is well under way.

Other specialized therapies can also provide insight about patients and aid in their healing.

- In music therapy patients listen to and create music to calm themselves and to alleviate anxiety. This therapy is often used with surgical patients and patients with chronic pain.
- In dance therapy patients participate in dance to improve balance, flexibility, strength, and the quality of life.
- In poetry or other writing therapy, patients express themselves through a chosen form of writing.
- In crafts therapy patients express themselves by using a variety of media to create handiworks.
- In pet therapy patients play with, groom, or walk a pet. Pets provide companionship and the opportunity to nurture.
- In aquatic therapy patients swim in a therapeutic pool equipped with a ramp and a lift so that it is accessible to all. Many patients who cannot walk when on land can move their legs remarkably well in water.
- In horticultural therapy patients work with plants and flowers to bring beauty into their daily lives and to help improve their balance, strength, memory, and socialization skills.
- In equestrian therapy patients ride horses to help develop strength, coordination, and muscle tone and to improve balance.

device called a universal **goniometer** (see Figure 30-1). The measurement of joint mobility is known as goniometry, a noninvasive test that is frequently performed in doctors' offices and that requires the patient to move each major joint in various ways. The specific movements that are evaluated are described in Table 30-1.

The doctor may ask you to assist with or to perform goniometry. Procedure 30-1 explains how to use goniometry to measure ROM in a patient, beginning at the head and working down to the feet. You will compare each joint measurement with a standard measurement (in degrees of movement) for that joint.

Muscle Strength Testing. The physician tests muscle strength to determine the amount of force the patient is able to exert with a muscle or group of muscles. This test is usually done at the same time as ROM testing. It may be performed by the physician with your assistance, or the physician may ask you to perform it yourself. Procedure 30-2 describes the steps used in muscle strength testing.

Like the ROM test, the muscle strength test is usually done from head to foot. The patient is asked to resist the pressure that you or the physician applies to each muscle or group of muscles (usually near a joint). Strength is rated according to a five-point scale, as shown in Table 30-2.

Typically, a patient can move a joint a certain distance and can easily resist the pressure you apply. The patient usually has equal strength on both sides of the body. If the patient has weakness, however, a medical problem may be indicated. Report any weakness to the physician so that he can use this information to develop a treatment plan.

Gait Testing. **Gait** is the way a person walks. A normal gait has two phases: stance and swing (see Figure 30-4).

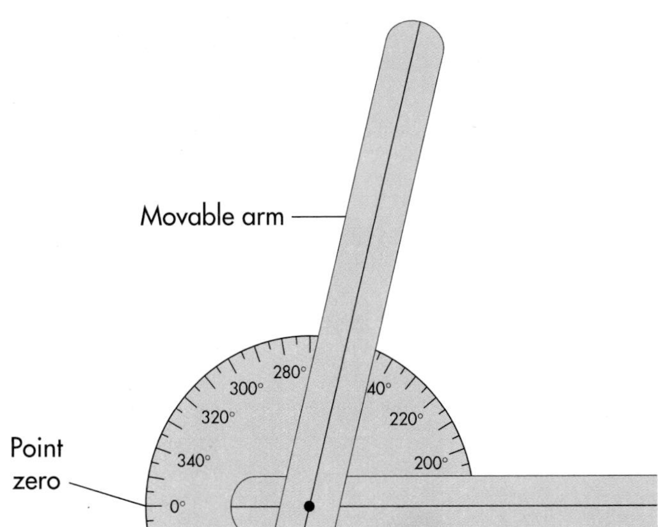

Figure 30-1. A universal goniometer is a protractor with a movable pointer that measures degrees of joint movement.

A typical stance phase begins with the right heel strike (when the patient's right heel meets the floor). As the foot rocks forward and the toes meet the floor, the right foot flattens and bears the body's weight. In midstance the patient lifts the left foot. Then the right foot begins to push off by flexing the toes and lifting the heel off the floor.

The swing phase begins with the right foot poised to begin the swing as the left heel strikes the floor. Then the right foot clears the floor and swings forward. In midswing it passes the left foot. At the end of the swing, the right foot slows, and heel strike occurs again.

Generally, a physician or physical therapist assesses a patient's gait. To do so, the physician asks the patient to walk away, turn around, and walk back. Assessment of gait includes an appraisal of the patient's length of stride, balance, coordination, direction of knees (inward or outward), and direction of feet (inward or outward).

Posture Testing. **Posture** is body position and alignment. The doctor assesses posture by looking at the patient's spinal curve from the sides, back, and front. Normally, the thoracic spine has a convex (outward) curve, and the lumbar spine has a concave (inward) curve. The doctor also notes the symmetry of alignment of the shoulders, knees, and hips.

To assess alignment and degree of straightness of the spine, the doctor asks the patient to bend at the waist and let the arms dangle freely. To assess knee position, the doctor asks the patient to stand with both feet together to determine whether the knees are at the same height, facing forward, and symmetrical.

Cryotherapy and Thermotherapy

Applying cold to a patient's body for therapeutic reasons is called **cryotherapy.** This type of therapy can be administered in a number of ways. Treatments may be dry or wet, and they may be chemical or natural. Examples of dry cold applications are ice bags and ice packs. Wet cold applications include cold compresses and ice massage.

Applying heat to a patient's body for therapeutic reasons is called **thermotherapy.** As with cryotherapy, thermotherapy can be administered in a variety of ways. Examples of devices used in dry heat treatments are electric heating pads, hot-water bottles, and heat lamps. Moist heat treatments include hot soaks and the use of hot compresses and hot packs.

The therapeutic effect of cryotherapy and thermotherapy is based on the body's natural response to temperature. Cold constricts the blood vessels and causes involuntary contraction of some muscles. Heat dilates (expands) the blood vessels and causes muscles to relax.

Factors Affecting the Use of Cryotherapy and Thermotherapy

To choose a cold or heat therapy for a patient, the physician considers the therapy's purpose, the location and condition of the affected area, and the patient's age and general health. After choosing a therapy, the physician may direct you to apply the cold or heat treatment and to teach the patient and family how to continue the therapy at home.

Performed correctly, cold and heat therapies generally promote healing. These therapies can, however, cause side effects in some patients. Therefore, you need to exercise caution when applying the therapies. You also need to be aware of conditions that contraindicate (make inadvisable) cold or heat therapies. Table 30-3 summarizes circumstances that warrant precautions or contraindications for the therapies, as well as possible side effects. When performing any cold or heat therapy, you should consider the age of the patient, treatment location, patient problems with circulation or sensation, and individual temperature tolerance.

Age. Age is an important consideration because young children and elderly patients usually are more sensitive than others to cold and heat. When administering cryotherapy or thermotherapy, stay with the patient during its application to check the patient's skin frequently for excessive paleness or redness.

Treatment Location. Thin-skinned areas that are usually covered with clothing (such as the back, chest, and abdomen) are more sensitive to cold and heat therapies than other areas, such as the face and hands. Use caution around any broken skin (as with a wound), because it is susceptible to further tissue damage from cryotherapy or thermotherapy.

Circulation or Sensation Impairment. Patients with diabetes or cardiovascular disease may have impaired circulation or sensory perception. These impairments may prevent such patients from sensing that a treatment is too

Table 30-1

Movements Measured by Goniometry

Term	Description	Example
Abduction	Movement away from midline of body or movement away from axis of limb	Raising arm straight out to side
Adduction (opposite of abduction)	Movement toward midline of body or movement toward axis of limb	Lowering raised arm down to side
Circumduction	Circular movement of body part	Performing arm circles
Dorsiflexion	Upward or backward movement of body part	Flexing foot—toes pointing upward
Eversion	Outward movement of body part	Moving ankle—sole of foot turning outward
Extension	Movement that spreads apart two body parts or that opens joint	Straightening leg after being in bent-knee position
Flexion (opposite of extension)	Movement that brings together two body parts or that closes joint	Bending leg at knee
Inversion (opposite of eversion)	Inward movement of body part	Moving ankle—sole of foot turning inward
Plantar flexion (opposite of dorsiflexion)	Downward movement of body part	Flexing foot—toes pointing downward
Pronation	Twisting movement that brings palm face down	Turning wrist so palm faces down
Rotation	Movement of body part around axis	Turning head from side to side
Supination (opposite of pronation)	Rotating movement that brings palm facing upward	Turning wrist so that palm faces upward

cold or too hot. These patients require close monitoring during cryotherapy or thermotherapy. Carefully observe their skin to determine the treatment's therapeutic effect.

Temperature Tolerance. Tolerance of temperature extremes varies greatly from person to person. Some people are unusually sensitive to cold or to heat. Listen carefully to patients for any indication of temperature intolerance during treatment. Cases of intolerance should be reported to the physician, who may decide to change the treatment.

Administering Cryotherapy and Thermotherapy

Cryotherapy and thermotherapy have procedural similarities. The steps discussed in Procedure 30-3 can be applied to both therapies.

Principles of Cryotherapy

The application of cryotherapy causes blood vessels to constrict and involuntary muscles of the skin to contract. These physiologic responses can have the following results:

- Prevention of swelling by limiting **edema,** or fluid accumulation in body tissue
- Control of bleeding by constricting blood vessels
- Reduction of inflammation by slowing blood and fluid movement in the affected area
- Provision of an anesthetic effect for pain by reducing inflammation
- Reduction of pus formation by inhibiting microorganism activity
- Lowering of body temperature

PROCEDURE 30-1

Measuring Range of Motion Using a Goniometer

Objective: To use a universal goniometer to measure joint range of motion in a patient

OSHA Guidelines: This procedure does not involve exposure to blood, body fluids, or tissues.

Materials: Universal goniometer, drapes

Method

Instruct the patient to move each body part as specified below. As the patient moves each joint, measure the range of motion (ROM) with the goniometer. Use Figure 30-2 as a guide for positioning the goniometer to measure degrees of movement. Record each measurement in the patient's chart.

1. Measure flexion as the patient touches his chin to his chest. Measure hyperextension as he tilts his head backward (Figure 30-2a).
2. Measure lateral flexion as the patient tries to touch his right ear to his right shoulder and then his left ear to his left shoulder (Figure 30-2b).
3. Measure rotation as the patient turns his head from side to side as far as possible (Figure 30-2c).
4. Measure flexion as the patient lifts both arms straight forward and up. Measure extension as he lowers them down and to the back (Figure 30-2d).
5. Measure abduction as the patient raises his arms straight out to the sides. Measure adduction as he moves each arm down and across his body (Figure 30-2e).
6. As the patient bends an arm at the elbow, measure external rotation as he raises the arm over his head. Measure internal rotation as he lowers the bent arm so that the hand is behind the small of his back (Figure 30-2f).
7. Measure flexion as the patient bends each arm at the elbow so that the hand moves toward the shoulder. Measure extension as he straightens the arm as much as possible (Figure 30-2g).
8. Measure pronation as the patient rotates each arm so that the palm faces the floor. Measure supination as he rotates each arm so that the palm faces the ceiling (Figure 30-2h).
9. Measure flexion as the patient bends his wrist downward. Measure dorsiflexion as he bends the wrist upward (Figure 30-2i).
10. Measure flexion as the patient bends all joints in his fingers toward the palm. Measure dorsiflexion as he straightens and lifts the fingers as much as possible (Figure 30-2j).
11. Measure abduction as the patient moves his hand (with the fingers together) in the direction of the thumb. Measure adduction as he moves his hand in the direction of the pinky (Figure 30-2k).
12. Measure abduction as the patient spreads his fingers as wide as possible. Measure adduction as he brings the fingers together again (Figure 30-2l).
13. Measure flexion as the standing patient bends forward from the waist. Measure hyperextension as he straightens and bends as far back as possible (Figure 30-2m).
14. Measure lateral flexion as the patient bends from the waist, first leaning to the left and then to the right (Figure 30-2n).
15. Measure rotation as the patient turns his upper body from side to side as far as possible (Figure 30-2o).
16. Measure flexion as the patient bends one knee and brings it up to his chest. Measure hyperextension as he straightens the leg and then swings it back (Figure 30-2p). Repeat on the other leg.
17. Measure abduction as the patient moves one straight leg away from his body, and measure adduction as he moves the leg back across his body (Figure 30-2q).
18. Measure internal rotation as the patient bends his knee and moves it inward (toward the other knee), and measure external rotation as he moves his knee outward (away from the other knee) (Figure 30-2r).
19. Measure flexion as the standing patient bends one knee and tries to touch his buttock with the heel of that foot (Figure 30-2s). Repeat on the other leg.
20. Measure plantar flexion as the patient points his foot downward, and measure dorsiflexion as he moves the foot upward toward the knee (Figure 30-2t).
21. Measure inversion as the patient turns the sole of one foot inward (toward the other foot), and measure eversion as he moves the sole of the foot outward (away from the other foot) (Figure 30-2u).
22. Measure abduction as the patient moves one foot outward (away from the other foot), and measure adduction as he moves the foot inward (toward the other foot) (Figure 30-2v).
23. Measure flexion as the patient curls his toes under. Measure hyperextension as he straightens and lifts the toes as high as possible (Figure 30-2w).

continued

Measuring Range of Motion Using a Goniometer

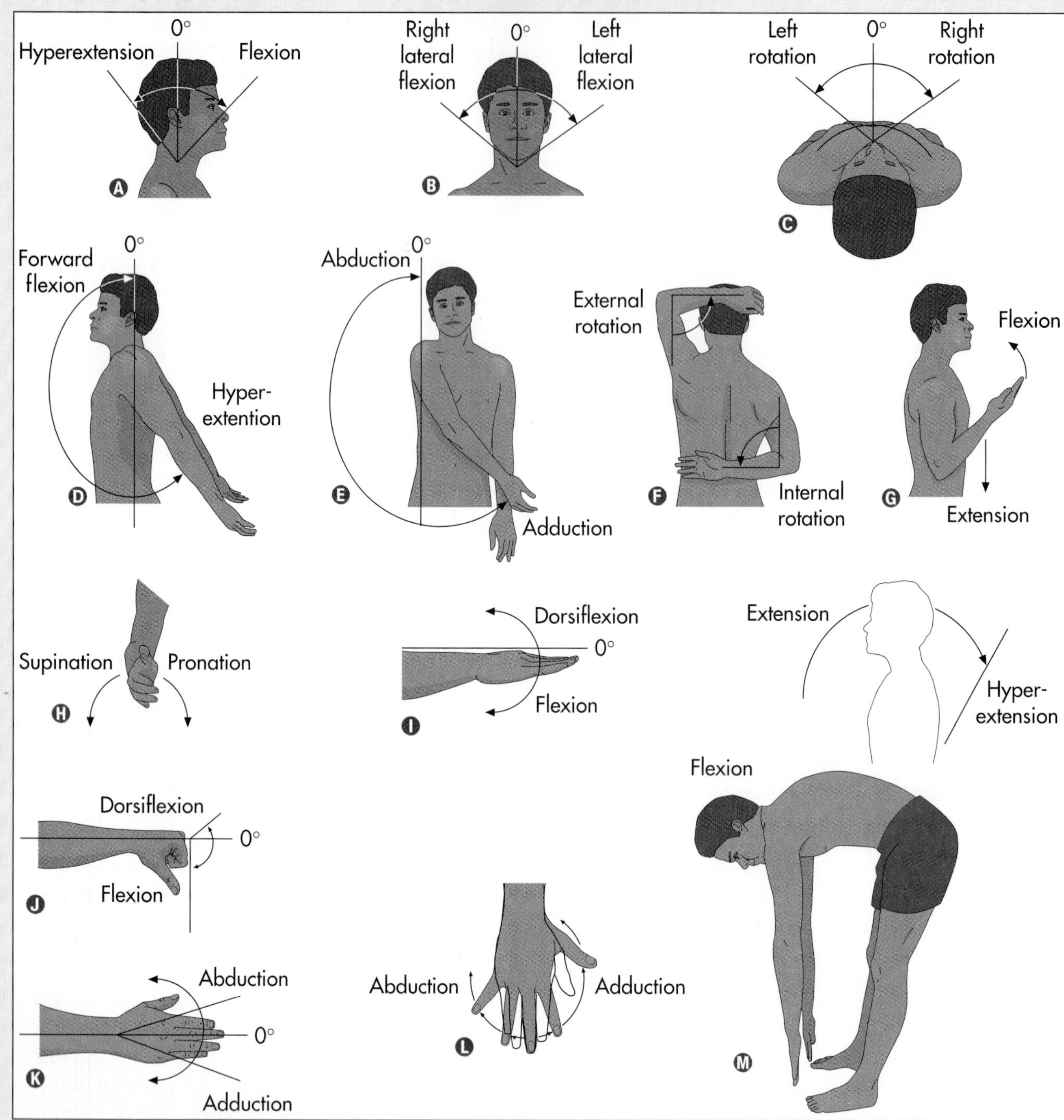

Figure 30-2. When you measure joint ROM, begin at the head and work down to the feet.

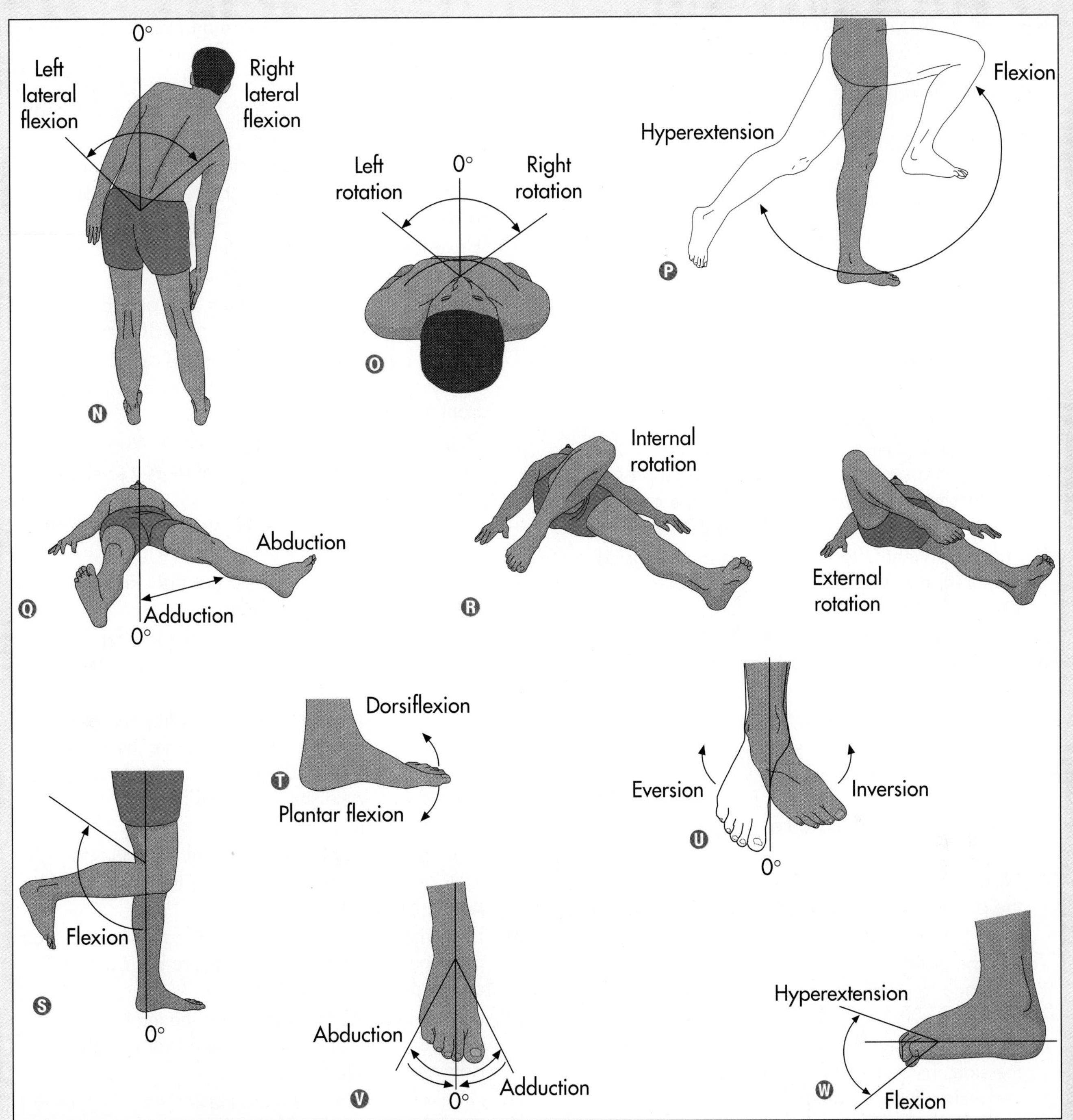

Figure 30-2. (continued)

PROCEDURE 30-2

Performing Muscle Strength Assessment

Objective: To assess the strength of various muscle groups

OSHA Guidelines

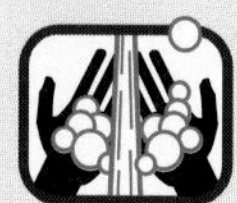 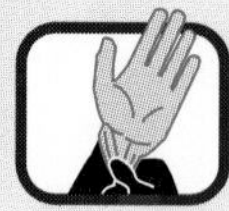 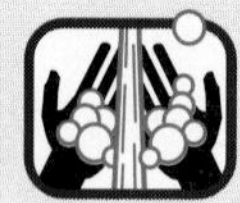

Materials: No special materials are needed.

Method

Evaluate the patient's response to each muscle-testing step, using the rating system indicated in Table 30-2. Record each response in the patient's chart.

1. Wash your hands. Put on examination gloves if the patient has any skin lesions.
2. Begin by checking neck muscle strength. With the patient in a supine position, apply slight pressure on her forehead with your hand. Have the patient try to touch her chin to her chest (Figure 30-3a).
3. Ask the patient to turn over into a prone position, with her head straight. Now apply pressure to the back of her head while asking her to push up against your hand (Figure 30-3b).
4. Help the patient sit up. With your hand on one side of her face, ask her to turn her head against your hand. Repeat on the other side (Figure 30-3c).
5. Next test shoulder muscle strength. Without applying any pressure, place your hands on the patient's shoulders and have her shrug once. Then apply pressure and have her shrug again (Figure 30-3d).
6. Now test the strength of the upper-arm muscles. Ask the patient to try to straighten her right arm while you try to flex it (Figure 30-3e).
7. Ask the patient to hold her right arm with the elbow bent and to resist while you try to straighten it (Figure 30-3f).
8. Have the patient hold her right arm out straight to the side. Try to push down on the right arm while she resists (Figure 30-3g).
9. Repeat steps 6 through 8 on the left arm. Compare your findings from one arm with those from the other arm.
10. Then test wrist and hand strength. Have the patient squeeze the first two fingers of your hand with her right hand (Figure 30-3h).
11. With the patient's right fist in a flexed position, have her resist as you try to straighten it (Figure 30-3i).
12. With the patient's right fist in an extended position, have her resist as you try to flex it (Figure 30-3j).
13. Repeat steps 10 through 12 on the left hand. Compare your findings from one hand with those from the other hand.
14. Next test hip muscle strength with the patient lying prone. Ask her to lift her right leg as you apply downward pressure (Figure 30-3k).
15. Have the patient lie on her left side and lift her right leg while you push down (Figure 30-3l).
16. Have the patient lie on her left side and lower her right leg while you push up (Figure 30-3m).
17. Repeat steps 14 through 16 on the opposite side. Compare your findings from one side with those from the other side.
18. Help the patient to a sitting position. Ask her to raise her right knee to her chest as you push down (Figure 30-3n).
19. Have the patient try to straighten her right leg as you hold it in a bent-knee position (Figure 30-3o).
20. Have the patient try to bend her right knee as you hold it straight (Figure 30-3p).
21. Repeat steps 18 through 20 on the left leg. Compare your findings from one leg with those from the other leg.
22. Now test ankle muscle strength. With one hand, hold the patient's right leg just above the ankle. Place your other hand on top of her right foot, and press down while she tries to lift her right foot (Figure 30-3q).
23. Move your hand to the bottom of the patient's right foot, and push up while she tries to press the foot down (Figure 30-3r).
24. Have the patient move her right foot inward as you press out, and then have her move her right foot outward as you press in (Figure 30-3s).
25. Repeat steps 22 through 24 on the left foot. Compare your findings from one foot with those from the other foot.
26. Finally, assess toe strength. Have the patient try to point the toes on her right foot down as you push them up (Figure 30-3t).
27. Then ask the patient to try to point her toes up as you press them down (Figure 30-3u).
28. Repeat steps 26 and 27 on the toes on the left foot. Compare your findings from one foot with those from the other foot.
29. Remove the gloves, if used, and wash your hands.

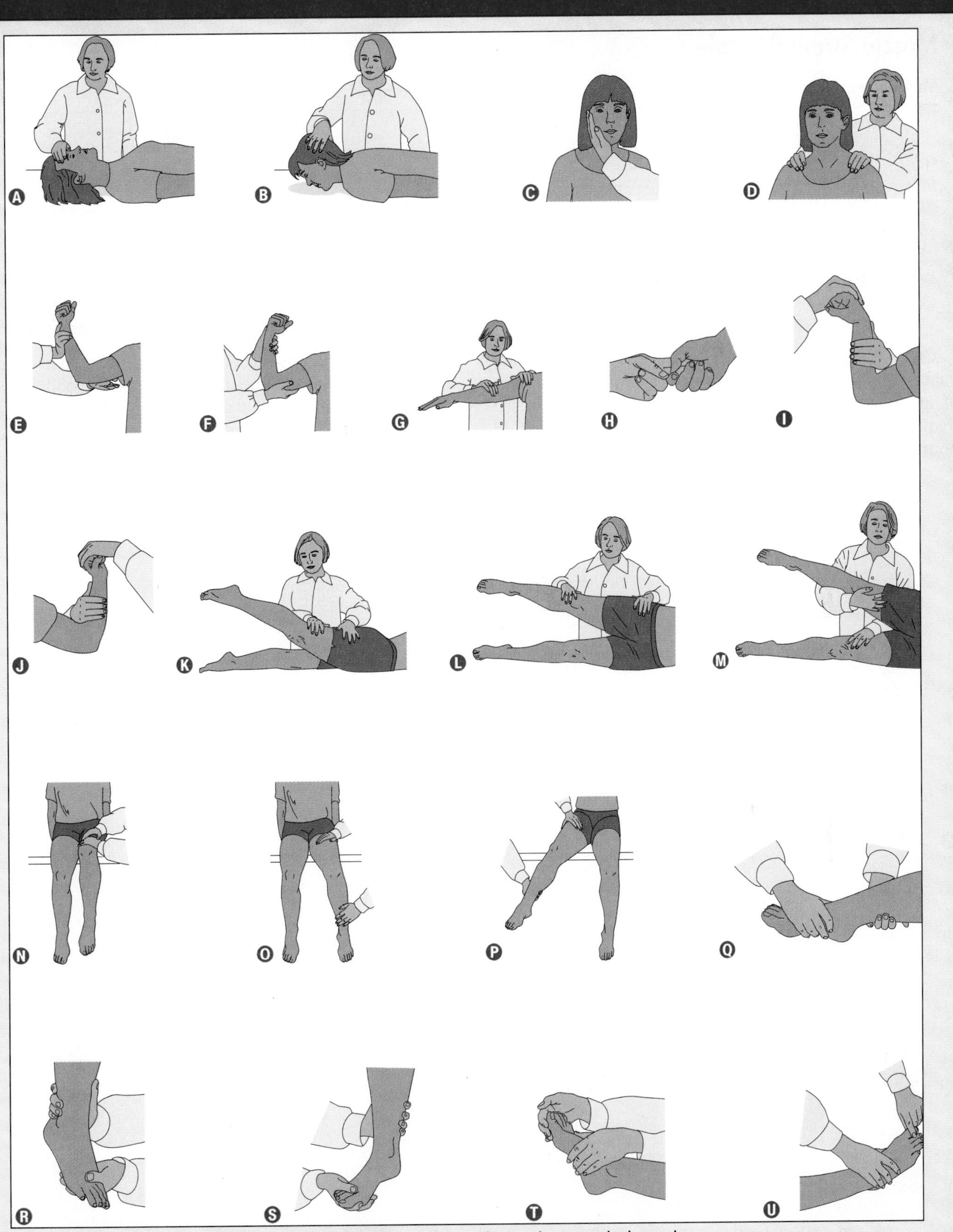

Figure 30-3. Muscle strength testing begins with neck muscles and proceeds through muscles of the shoulders, arms, wrists, hands, hips, legs, ankles, feet, and toes.

Table 30-2

Muscle Strength Scale

Muscle Response	Rating	Meaning
No response	0	Paralysis
Slight contraction felt	1	Severe weakness
Passive ROM when resistance is removed	2	Moderate weakness
Active ROM against gravity or light resistance	3 or 4	Mild weakness
Active ROM against heavy resistance	5	Normal

Cryotherapy is highly effective in alleviating swelling, pain, inflammation, and bleeding caused by various types of injuries. For best results, cryotherapy should be used frequently (about 20 minutes every hour) for the first 48 hours after an injury. As cold is applied, the skin becomes cool and pale, because blood vessels constrict, decreasing the blood supply to the area. The decreased blood supply also reduces tissue metabolism, oxygen use, and waste accumulation. The types of cryotherapy and the ways that they are administered are outlined in Procedure 30-4.

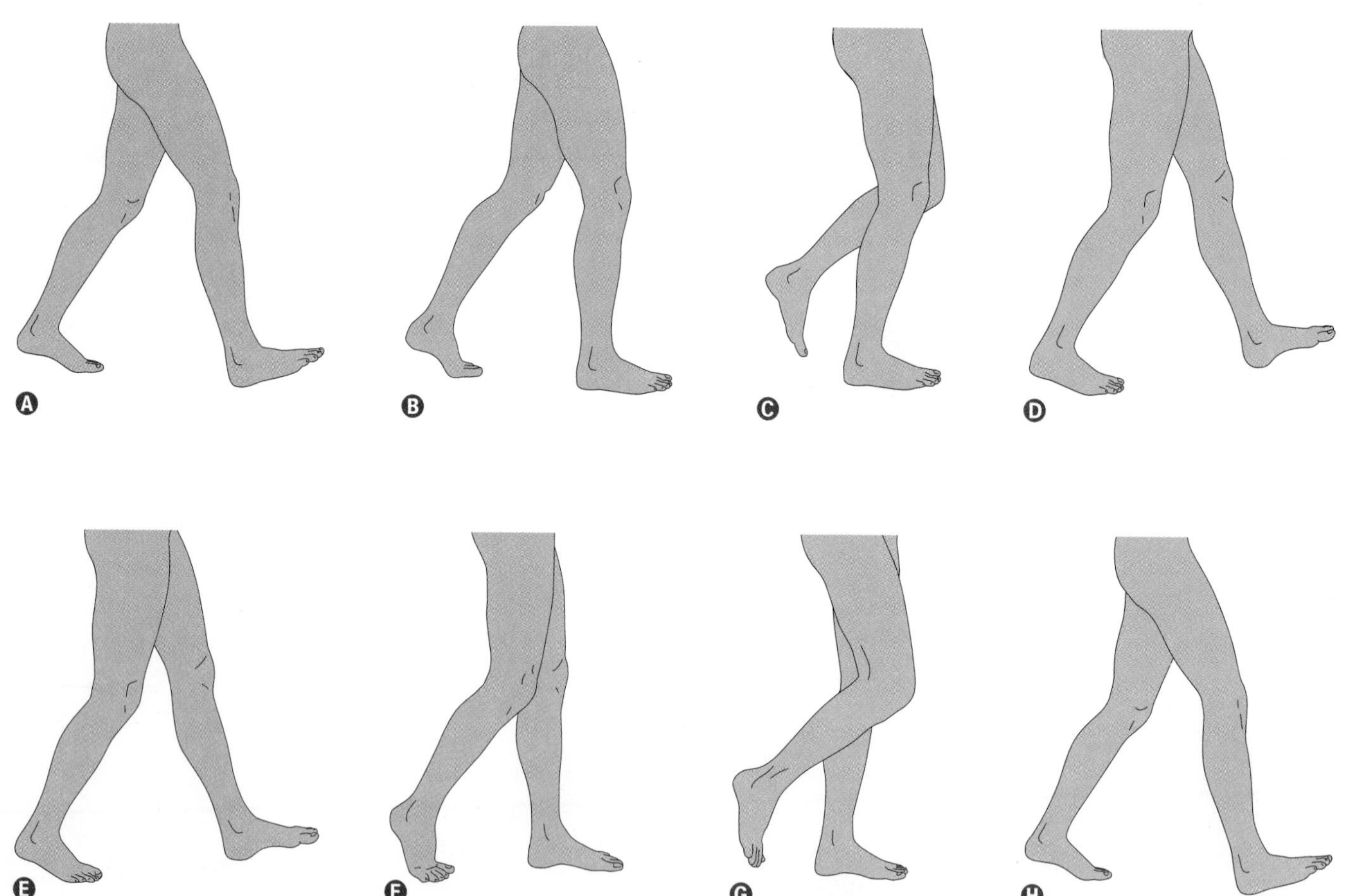

Figure 30-4. These are the two phases of gait. Illustrations (a) through (d) show the movements of the stance phase; illustrations (e) through (h) show the movements of the swing phase: (a) right heel strike, (b) flat right foot, (c) midstance, (d) push off with right foot, (e) right foot poised, (f) left heel strike, (g) midswing, (h) right heel strike.

Table 30-3

Contraindications, Precautions, and Side Effects Related to Cold and Heat

Therapy	Precautions	Contraindications	Side Effects
Dry and moist cold applications	Poor circulation, extreme age or youth, arthritis, impaired sensation (insensitivity to cold)	Inability to tolerate weight of device, pain caused by application (more common with moist cold)	Numbness, pain, very pale or bluish skin, blood clots (rare)
Dry and moist heat applications	Impaired kidney, heart, or lung function; arteriosclerosis and atherosclerosis; impaired sensation (insensitivity to heat); extreme age or youth; pregnancy	Possibility of hemorrhage; malignancy; acute inflammation, such as appendicitis; severe circulation problems; pain caused by weight of device	Burns (especially with heat lamps), increased respiratory rate, lowered blood pressure

Dry Cold Applications. Dry cold applications include ice bags, ice collars, and chemical ice packs. An ice bag is a rubber or plastic bag with a locking lid. An ice collar is a rubber or plastic kidney-shaped bag that is specially curved to fit around the back of the neck.

A chemical ice pack is usually a flat plastic bag containing a semifluid chemical. Ice packs come in various sizes and types. Some are disposable whereas others can be stored in a freezer and reused. The chemical prevents them from freezing solid, allowing them to be molded to the area to be treated. Chemical ice packs may require squeezing or shaking to activate the cooling action. Most packs remain cold for 30 to 60 minutes. Some ice packs come with a soft covering; others must be wrapped in a cloth before they are applied to the skin.

Wet Cold Applications. Wet cold applications include cold compresses and ice massage. A cold compress is a cloth or gauze pad moistened with ice water. It may be used to treat the pain associated with a toothache, tooth extraction, eye injury, or headache. The ice used in ice massage may be a cube wrapped in a plastic bag or water frozen in a paper cup. The combination of the cold temperature and the motion of the massage can provide therapeutic relief for the localized pain resulting from a sprain or strain. Although cold causes muscles to contract, the pain-relieving effect can help a patient relax.

Principles of Thermotherapy

Heat therapies cause blood vessels to dilate (expand), which increases the blood supply to—and tissue metabolism in—the area. Increased metabolism brings oxygen and nutrients to cells and carries toxins and wastes away from the cells, and this process can promote healing. During thermotherapy the treated skin becomes warm and develops **erythema** (redness) as the capillaries in the deeper layers of the skin fill with blood.

Thermotherapy can be used to help relieve pain, congestion, muscle spasms, and inflammation and to promote muscle relaxation. By increasing the blood supply to an area, heat increases fluid absorption from the tissues. This increased absorption reduces swelling from edema.

If heat is applied for too long, however, it may increase skin secretions that soften the skin and lower resistance. Heat that is too extreme can burn the skin or increase edema. Always monitor patients receiving thermotherapy, particularly children and elderly patients. The three basic types of thermotherapy are dry heat, moist heat, and diathermy.

Dry Heat Therapies. There are several types of dry heat therapy. They include the use of chemical hot packs, heating pads, hot-water bottles, heat lamps with infrared or ultraviolet bulbs, and fluidotherapy.

Chemical Hot Pack. A chemical hot pack is a disposable, flexible pack of chemicals that becomes hot when you activate it by kneading or slapping it. After activating the pack, cover it with a cloth, and place it on the patient's skin in the area being treated. Chemical hot packs are pliable and conform to body contours. For best results, follow the manufacturer's directions.

Heating Pad. A heating pad is a flat pad with electrical coils between layers of soft fabric. When turned on, the coils provide localized heat. The physician should specify the heating pad temperature (low, medium, or high) and the length of time the pad should be applied.

Before applying a heating pad, cover it with a pillowcase or towel, check to be sure the cord is not frayed, and plug it into an electrical outlet. Make sure the patient's skin is dry. Then turn on the pad, and set the temperature selector switch to the specified temperature. The patient should never lie on top of a heating pad.

Hot-Water Bottle. A hot-water bottle is a flat, flexible, plastic or rubber bottle with a stopper. Fill the bottle with

PROCEDURE 30-3

Following General Rules for Administering Cryotherapy and Thermotherapy

Objective: To administer cryotherapy or thermotherapy safely, following the general rules for both

OSHA Guidelines

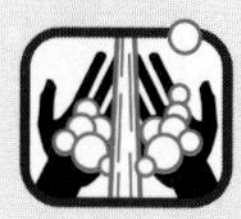 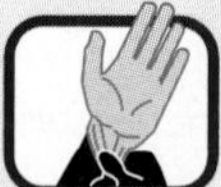 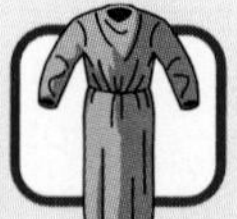  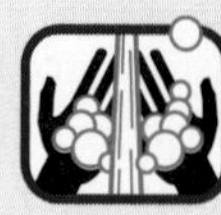

Materials: Cold or hot applications as ordered by the physician, drapes, sterile dressing (if needed)

Method

Follow these steps for both cryotherapy and thermotherapy.

1. Double-check the physician's order. Be sure you know where to apply therapy on the body, the proper temperature for the application, and how long it should remain in place.
2. Wash your hands and put on examination or utility gloves, as appropriate for the temperatures involved, and a laboratory coat.
3. Gather the supplies and equipment. Put them where you can reach them easily without danger of accidental burns or spillage of any hot or cold liquids.
4. Check the temperature of all applications before and during the treatment. Remember that ice packs and hot compresses may return to room temperature quickly. As necessary, cool or reheat devices or solutions that provide therapeutic temperatures, then reapply them.
5. Identify the patient, introduce yourself, and clearly explain the procedure, its purpose, and its effects.
6. Have the patient undress and put on a gown, if required; provide privacy or assistance as needed.
7. Position and drape the patient properly.
8. If the patient has a dressing covering the area to be treated, remove the dressing and discard it in a biohazardous waste container. (Replace the dressing with a new dressing after the treatment is completed.)
9. Carry out the procedure while timing it carefully. Be sure to check the skin frequently. Ask the patient to inform you of any pain or discomfort.
10. During any heat therapy, remember that dilated blood vessels cause heat loss from the skin and that this heat loss may make the patient feel chilled. Be prepared to cover the patient with sheets or blankets.
11. Remove the application and observe the area that was treated.
12. Help the patient dress, if needed.
13. Remove equipment and supplies, properly discarding used disposable materials and arranging for the appropriate sanitization, disinfection, and/or sterilization of reusable equipment and materials as needed.
14. Remove the gloves and wash your hands.
15. Record the treatment and the results in the patient's chart.

hot water, using a thermometer to make sure the water temperature does not exceed 125°F. For children under the age of 2 years and for elderly patients, the temperature should range from 105° to 115°F. For older children, a safe temperature is 115° to 125°F. Fill the bottle halfway; then compress it to expel air. The half-filled bottle can conform to the area to be treated. A half-filled bottle is also lighter than a full one and therefore more comfortable for the patient. Cover the bottle with a cloth or pillowcase before you apply it.

After you apply the hot-water bottle, check with the patient to make sure the temperature is not too hot. Check the temperature frequently, and replace the hot water as needed. Each time you remove the bottle, check the patient's skin to make sure that it is merely warm to the touch.

Heat Lamp. A heat lamp uses an infrared or ultraviolet bulb to provide heat. When the lamp is turned on, infrared rays heat and penetrate the skin's surface to a depth of 3 to 5 mm. To avoid burning the skin, place an infrared heat lamp 2 to 4 ft from the area being treated. Treatment usually lasts for 20 to 30 minutes or as directed by the physician.

Although ultraviolet rays produce little heat, they can burn the skin and damage the eyes. They are used to kill bacteria and to promote vitamin D formation. Ultraviolet rays stimulate epithelial cells and cause blood vessels to overfill, increasing the skin's defenses against bacterial infections. Ultraviolet lamps are used to treat acne, psoriasis, pressure sores, and wound infections.

Before recommending the use of an ultraviolet lamp, the physician assesses the patient's sensitivity and determines the treatment duration. Treatments typically range from 30 seconds to a few minutes. The duration is usually increased in 10-second intervals. Because ultraviolet rays can burn the skin, monitor the patient closely. Do not leave the room during the treatment. Both you and the patient must wear goggles to prevent harm to the eyes.

Fluidotherapy. **Fluidotherapy** is a relatively new technique for stimulating healing, particularly in the hands and feet. The patient places the affected body part in a container of glass beads that are heated and agitated with hot air. Although the therapy is dry, its effect is similar to that of a therapy using water.

Moist Heat Applications. Moist heat is often used to soften dried, crusted exudates (discharges from body tissues) for easy removal. Moist heat applications include hot soak, hot compress, hot pack, and paraffin bath.

Hot Soak. With hot-soak therapy, the patient places the affected body part—usually an arm or leg—in a container of plain or medicated water that has been heated to no more than 110°F. A hot soak should last about 15 minutes.

Hot Compress. A compress is a piece of gauze or cloth suitable for covering a small area. After soaking the compress in hot water, wring it out and apply it to the area to be treated. Keep the compress warm either by placing a hot-water bottle on top of it or by frequently rewarming the compress in hot water.

Hot Pack. A hot pack is a large canvas bag filled with heat-retaining gel that is used on a large body area. Like a hot compress, a hot pack retains heat after being placed in hot water.

Paraffin Bath. A paraffin bath is a receptacle of heated wax and mineral oil. It is used to reduce pain, muscle spasms, and stiffness in patients with arthritis and similar disorders. The patient's affected area is dipped repeatedly into the mixture until the area is covered with a thick coat of wax. The wax remains on the area for about 30 minutes and then is peeled off. Particularly useful for joints, the paraffin bath has the added benefit of leaving the skin warm, flexible, and soft. Some erythema may result.

Diathermy. **Diathermy** is a type of heat therapy in

PROCEDURE 30-4

Administering Different Types of Cryotherapy

Objective: To use cryotherapy to reduce pain and prevent swelling

OSHA Guidelines

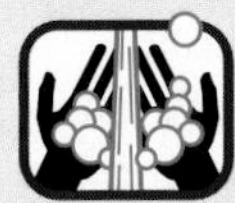
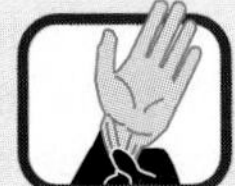
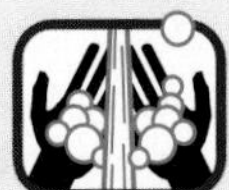

Materials: Ice bag, ice collar, or chemical cold pack; towel; basin; washcloth or gauze squares (for cold compress); ice (or other materials appropriate to cryotherapy)

Method

1. Wash your hands, put on examination gloves, and gather the supplies needed.
2. Explain the procedure and its purpose. Ask whether the patient has any questions.

If you are using an ice bag or ice collar:

3. Check the ice bag or collar for leaks.
4. Place ice chips or small ice cubes in the ice bag or collar. (Using small pieces of ice helps the device conform to the patient's body and to conduct the cold better.) Fill the container two-thirds full. Then compress the container to expel air, and close it.
5. Dry the bag or collar completely, and cover it with a towel to absorb moisture and provide comfort.

If you are using a chemical ice pack:

3. Check the pack for leaks.
4. Shake or squeeze the pack to activate the chemicals.
5. Cover the pack with a towel.

If you are using a cold compress:

3. Place large ice cubes and a small amount of water in the basin. Large pieces of ice do not melt as quickly as smaller ones, so they should last the length of the procedure.
4. Place the washcloth or gauze squares in the basin.
5. Moisten and wring them out.

For all cryotherapy procedures:

6. Place the cryotherapy device on the patient's affected body part. If you are using a compress, place an ice bag on it, if desired, to keep it colder longer.
7. Ask the patient how the device feels. Explain that the cold is of great benefit, although it may be somewhat uncomfortable.
8. Leave the device in place for the length of time ordered by the physician. Periodically check the skin for color, feeling, and pain. If the area becomes excessively pale or blue, numb, or painful, remove the device and have the physician examine the area.
9. After the treatment check for reduced swelling, redness, and pain.
10. Remove the gloves and wash your hands.
11. Document the treatment and your observations in the patient's chart. If you teach the patient or the patient's family how to use the device, document your instructions.

MULTISKILL FOCUS

Physical Therapist Assistant

To gain medical assistant credentials, you must fulfill the requirements of either the American Association of Medical Assistants (for a Certified Medical Assistant) or the American Medical Technologists (for a Registered Medical Assistant). After obtaining your medical assistant certification or registration, you may wish to acquire additional skills in specialty areas through course work or on-the-job training. Although this course work or training may not lead to an additional certification or degree, it will enable you to expand your role in the medical office and advance your career as the demand for multiskilled health professionals increases.

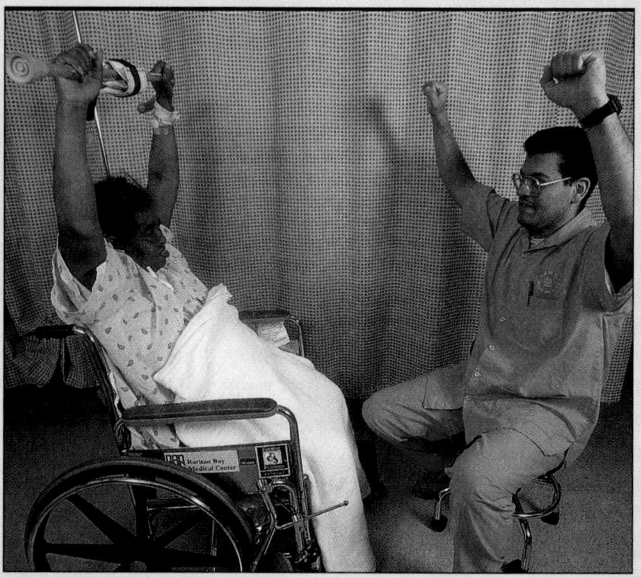

Skills and Duties

A relatively new profession, physical therapist assisting was first developed in the late 1960s because of the overwhelming interest in the potential of physical therapy in rehabilitation. The goal of physical therapy is to restore or increase physical movement and strength. A physical therapist assistant helps patients improve their physical function when it has been impaired by injury, disease, birth defects, or other causes. Physical therapist assistants often work as part of a team of therapeutic specialists, which may include physicians, physical therapists, occupational therapists, and sometimes social workers.

Working under the supervision of a physical therapist, the assistant carries out the treatments and exercises prescribed by the therapist. She may administer cold and heat therapy, massage, or ultraviolet light to decrease pain and relax muscles. In addition, she helps the patient perform physical exercises to build muscle strength and stamina and to increase mobility. When helping patients exercise, the physical therapist assistant often works in swimming pools or with gym equipment, such as stationary bicycles, weights, and parallel bars. She may take measurements, such as vital signs or range of motion, to help evaluate patients' progress.

The physical therapist assistant may also fit patients who have lost limbs or need mobility training with assistive devices. She routinely teaches them how to use and care for wheelchairs, walkers, braces, and artificial arms and legs. In all cases she records patients' progress for the physical therapist to evaluate. In addition, the physical therapist assistant may perform administrative office work, such as scheduling therapy sessions and maintaining records, and prepare both equipment and patients for therapy.

Because the job can be physically demanding, people entering this career should be physically fit. Good communication skills are also important.

Workplace Settings

Physical therapist assistants most often work in hospitals and rehabilitation centers. They may also work in nursing homes, physicians' offices, or clinics. Most work 40-hour weeks, although some are employed part-time.

Education

A physical therapist assistant requires less education than a physical therapist. In most states she must complete an accredited 2-year associate degree program at a junior or community college. In 36 states physical therapist assistants must also become licensed by passing a written examination. License renewal differs from state to state.

Where to Go for More Information

American Physical Therapy Association/Foundation for Physical Therapy
1111 North Fairfax Street
Alexandria, VA 22314
(703) 684-2782

National Rehabilitation Association
633 South Washington Street
Alexandria, VA 22314
(703) 836-0850

which a machine produces high-frequency waves that achieve deep heat penetration in muscle tissue. The heat helps decrease joint stiffness, dilate blood vessels, relieve muscle spasms, and reduce discomfort from sprains and strains. Three types of diathermy are ultrasound, shortwave, and microwave. Equipment for these therapies is continually being improved. Be sure to familiarize yourself with the manufacturer's instructions regarding the specific equipment in your office.

Ultrasound. Ultrasound is the most common type of diathermy. It projects high-frequency sound waves that are converted to heat in muscle tissue. This type of diathermy is used to treat sprains, strains, and other acute ailments.

Ultrasound diathermy may be administered by rubbing a gel-covered transducer over the skin in circular patterns. It may also be administered to a body part under water. Do not use ultrasound in areas where bones are near the skin's surface, because it could cause bone damage.

Shortwave. Shortwave diathermy uses radio waves that travel through the body between two condenser plates and are converted to heat in the tissues. This type of diathermy is used to treat acute, subacute, and chronic inflammation. Treatment duration typically ranges from 20 to 30 minutes. Do not use shortwave diathermy on a patient who has a pacemaker.

Microwave. Microwave diathermy uses microwaves to provide heat deep in body tissues. Contraindications include use on patients with pacemakers, use in combination with wet dressings, or use in high dosages on patients with swollen tissue. Also, never use microwave diathermy near metal implants, because the reaction between metal and microwaves could cause burns.

Hydrotherapy

Hydrotherapy is the use of water to treat physical problems. It is typically performed in the physical therapy department of a hospital, in an outpatient clinic, or at home. Common forms of hydrotherapy include the use of whirlpools and contrast baths and underwater exercises.

Whirlpools

Whirlpools are tanks in which water is agitated by jets of air under pressure. Whirlpools vary in size from small (capable of accommodating only one body part) to very large (capable of accommodating a wheelchair or full-body submersion). The action of the agitated water in a whirlpool generates a hydromassage, which relaxes muscles and increases circulation. Whirlpools are also used to cleanse and debride (remove foreign matter and dead tissue from) the skin of patients with wounds, ulcers, or burns.

Contrast Baths

Contrast baths are separate baths, one filled with hot water and the other with cold water. The patient alternately moves the treated body part quickly from one bath to the other. This treatment induces relaxation, stimulates improved circulation (which speeds up healing), and results in greater mobility.

Underwater Exercises

Underwater exercises are usually performed in a warm swimming pool. They are prescribed for patients with joint injuries, burns, and arthritis. Because the water's buoyancy takes pressure off the joints, underwater exercises are particularly useful for patients with painful or limited movement. Combined with the movement of the water around the body, the exercises promote relaxation and increased circulation.

Exercise Therapy

For many patients, exercise is as important as medications or other treatments. Exercise offers both preventive and therapeutic benefits. As a patient ages, exercise helps promote flexibility, mobility, muscle tone, and strength. Exercise is a primary treatment for fractures, arthritis, and some respiratory disorders; it can minimize symptoms or help slow disease progression. For patients who have had surgery, stroke, burns, or amputation, regular exercise therapy can help prevent problems caused by inactivity.

A doctor orders exercise therapy for many reasons. Exercise improves or restores general health and is especially therapeutic when a patient is weak from illness. Explain to patients that exercise will help them to:

- Improve muscle tone and strength.
- Regain range of motion (ROM) after an injury.
- Prevent ROM from diminishing in chronic conditions.
- Prevent or correct physical deformities.
- Promote neuromuscular coordination.
- Improve circulation.
- Relieve stress.
- Lower cholesterol levels.
- Aid in the resumption of normal daily activities.

Exercise therapy is commonly used for treating sports injuries. Exercise therapy for injured athletes is described in "Educating the Patient." This type of therapy focuses primarily on regaining muscle strength and flexibility in the injured area.

Role of the Medical Assistant

As a medical assistant, you may have several roles in exercise therapy. As an information resource for the patient and family, you must understand various types of exercise programs and the patient's specific treatment plan. You may also serve as a source of support and encouragement when exercise programs are long and difficult. You may, for example, assist with ROM exercises and

EDUCATING THE PATIENT

The Injured Athlete

The risk of injury is associated with most sports, but some sports carry a greater risk of serious injury than others. Many sports-related injuries affect joints—in the neck, shoulders, elbows, wrists, hands, knees, ankles, and feet.

You may be called on to educate injured athletes and to start them on the road to recovery. To do so, you need to understand the mind of the athlete. Why do many athletes get injured in the first place? Here are some reasons.

- The sport they participate in has a high injury rate.
- They return to a sport before their injuries are completely healed.
- They become impatient with a physical therapy regimen.
- They do not work at gradual muscle strengthening.

When does your job begin? After diagnosing the injury, the physician will probably refer the athlete to a sports medicine center or other physical therapy setting, where an individualized program will be set up. As a medical assistant, you will often be responsible for counseling an athlete about the physical therapy program she will be entering. Here are some basic rules that you can communicate.

- Follow the physical therapy regimen set up by the physician or physical therapist—even if it is tedious or time-consuming.
- Use only the equipment specified by the therapist: free weights, weight-training equipment, stationary bike, other aerobic equipment, or swimming pool.
- Do not rush the therapy in an attempt to recover more quickly.
- Work slowly to strengthen muscles and improve flexibility.
- Continue exercises at home as instructed.
- Be patient.

Explain to the athlete how the physical therapy program will be presented. Knowing what to expect from the physical therapist can improve the athlete's compliance. Here are some explanations you might offer.

- The therapist will demonstrate exercises and then watch you perform them.
- The therapist may increase the number of repetitions or the amount of resistance (weight) but probably not both at the same time.
- The therapist will provide handouts illustrating the exercises, along with instructions on how to perform them.
- The therapist may provide an activity log to help you chart your progress.

An athlete who is impatient with a physical therapy regimen and returns to a sport before an injury has completely healed has an increased risk of repeated injury. Impress on the athlete the importance of the physical therapy process. Emphasize the need for gradual strengthening and healing over a period of time. To help the athlete in the long run, focus on recovery from injury and on the need to prevent recurrent injury.

teach the patient and family how to perform them at home.

When teaching patients about exercises, give them illustrations of the exercises. Include with each illustration written instructions on the number of times to perform the exercise, as prescribed by the doctor.

After demonstrating each exercise, have patients perform it while you watch and give direction. Patients are more likely to perform exercises properly at home if they can perform them correctly in your presence. It is also helpful for patients' caregivers or family members to watch and perform the exercises to become familiar with them.

Types of Exercise

Before a patient begins an exercise program, the doctor evaluates the patient's heart and lung function and overall physical condition. The doctor adjusts the level of exercise accordingly and may prescribe other forms of physical therapy, such as cryotherapy, thermotherapy, or hydrotherapy. Careful preparation by the doctor and patient before beginning a program of exercise therapy helps prevent injuries. Some measures to prevent and treat common exercise therapy problems are outlined in Table 30-4. A doctor may also refer a patient to a physical therapist, who will develop an exercise program specifically for that patient. Types of exercises in therapeutic programs include active mobility, passive mobility, aided mobility, active resistance, isometric, and ROM.

Active Mobility Exercises. Active mobility exercises are self-directed exercises the patient performs without assistance. Their purpose is to increase muscle strength and function. They often require equipment such as a stationary bicycle or a treadmill.

Passive Mobility Exercises. In passive mobility exercises the physical therapist or a machine moves a patient's body part. The patient does not actively assist in these exercises. Patients who require passive mobility exercises may have neuromuscular disability or weakness. Passive mobility exercises can help retain patients' ROM and improve their circulation.

Table 30-4

Preventing and Treating Common Problems of Exercise Therapy

Problem	Prevention Methods	Treatment
Muscle strain	Beginning with gentle warm-up exercises	Rest and application of ice followed by heat
Muscle aches	Keeping track of number of repetitions and amount of weight (resistance), if used; increasing number of repetitions or amount of weight slowly	Rest, soaking in hot bath to relieve aches
Impatience with slowness of progress	Discussing expectations with patient; setting realistic goals with patient; stressing necessity of avoiding recurrent injury, which would prolong recovery	Creation of goal sheet, noting small successes as therapy progresses

Aided Mobility Exercises. Aided mobility exercises are self-directed exercises. The patient performs them with the aid of a device such as an exercise machine or a therapy pool.

Active Resistance Exercises. In active resistance exercises the patient works against resistance (counterpressure). Resistance is provided manually by the therapist or mechanically by an exercise machine. These exercises increase the patient's muscle strength.

Isometric Exercises. During isometric exercises the patient relaxes and then contracts the muscles of a body part while in a fixed position. Isometric exercises can maintain the patient's muscle strength when a joint is temporarily or permanently immobilized.

ROM Exercises. ROM exercises move each joint through its full range of motion. These exercises should be done slowly and gently. Doing them too quickly or too soon after an injury can cause pain, fracture, or bleeding into the joint. For this reason a physical therapist assesses the patient and determines a recommended regimen of ROM exercises. You may be asked to educate the patient and caregiver or family about the regimen.

ROM exercises are typically prescribed after a joint injury. The physical therapist may recommend that the joint be moved in its full range of motion three times, twice a day. ROM exercises are also recommended for elderly people, to improve circulation and muscle function. The therapist will prescribe one of two types of ROM exercises for patients:

- Active range-of-motion exercises: performed by the patient without assistance
- Passive range-of-motion exercises: performed by the patient with the help of another person or a machine

Active and passive ROM exercises do not build muscle strength but do improve flexibility and mobility. Typical ROM exercises are illustrated in Figure 30-5.

Electrical Stimulation

Electrical stimulators deliver controlled amounts of low-voltage electric current to motor and sensory nerves to stimulate muscles. Electrical stimulation helps prevent atrophy in muscles that cannot move voluntarily by causing the muscles to contract involuntarily (on impulse) and relax. Frequent and regular electrical stimulation also aids in healing injured joints and in revitalizing muscles.

Electrical stimulation can help retrain a patient to use injured muscles by creating a perceivable connection between the stimulus (muscle movement) and the area of the brain that controls those muscles. If a limb does not function because of injury or disease, this therapy can give the patient hope that injured muscles are not dead. Hope often encourages a patient to work harder and to cooperate in the physical therapy regimen, which can be long and arduous. Electrical stimulation units that patients can wear are being developed for people with spinal cord injuries to help them retrain affected muscles.

Massage

Massage is one of the oldest methods of promoting healing. It is used to treat strains, bruises, muscle soreness or tightness, lower-back pain, and dislocations. It can also relieve muscle spasms, restore motion and function to a body part, and decrease swelling from edema.

Role of the Medical Assistant

To prepare patients properly for massage therapy, you must understand the basics of this type of treatment. Explain to patients that the massage therapist may recommend breathing exercises and play gentle music before and during the massage to help them relax. Reassure

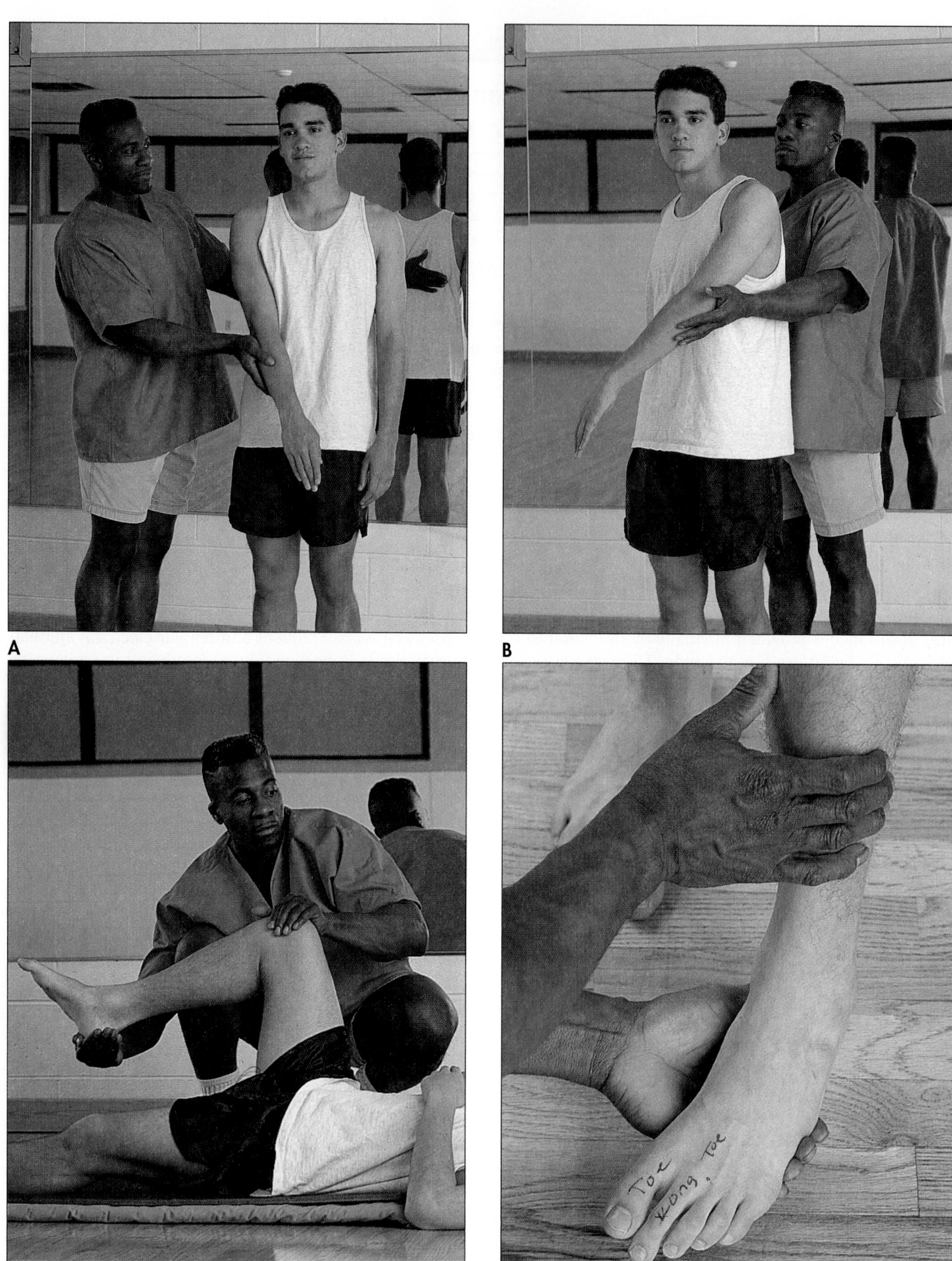

Figure 30-5. A medical assistant helps a patient perform typical ROM exercises: (a) shoulder abduction; (b) back rotation; (c) hip flexion; (d) toe abduction.

patients that only the parts of the body being massaged will be exposed. Explain that an oil or cream may be used to lubricate the skin and to allow for smooth, effective massage movements.

Massage Techniques

Massage promotes muscle and full-body relaxation and increases circulation. Increasing circulation helps remove blood and waste products from injured tissues and brings fresh blood and nutrients to the area to speed healing. Common massage techniques include the following:

- Effleurage: using the fingertips to make long, circular, light or firm strokes over the skin, especially on the back
- Friction: deep rubbing and stroking
- Percussion or tapotement: rhythmic and rapid tapping—with the fingertips, sides of hands, or cupped hands—in alternating patterns
- Petrissage: rolling and kneading while pressing on soft tissues

Traction

Traction is the pulling or stretching of the musculoskeletal system to treat fractured bones and dislocated, arthritic, or other diseased joints. It is traditionally performed by a therapist in a specially equipped setting. A physical therapist may set up traction in the patient's home and visit regularly to ensure that the equipment is used and maintained properly. Traction may be used to:

- Create and maintain proper bone alignment.
- Reduce or prevent joint stiffening and abnormal muscle shortening.
- Correct deformities.
- Relieve compression of vertebral joints.
- Reduce or relieve muscle spasms.

Although you will not be setting up or performing traction, you should know about its types and uses. This information will prepare you to answer basic questions from patients and family members.

Manual Traction

The physical therapist performs manual traction by using his hands to pull a patient's limb or head gently. Pulling stretches the muscles and separates the joints, allowing for greater motion and less stiffening. Manual traction is used with patients who have muscle spasms, stiffness, and arthritis.

Static Traction

To perform static traction (also called weight traction), the therapist places a patient's limb, pelvis, or chin in a harness. The harness is then attached to weights through a system of pulleys. This type of traction is commonly used to relieve muscle spasms.

Skin Traction

During skin traction, the therapist wraps foam rubber or other types of pads around both sides of a limb and then attaches the pads to pulleys and weights. Elastic bandages are used to secure the foam. This type of traction uses limited weight to prevent injury to the skin while decreasing painful muscle spasms. It may be set up in a patient's home or an inpatient facility.

Skeletal Traction

Skeletal traction is performed in inpatient facilities on patients whose injuries require long traction time and heavy weights. During surgery a surgeon inserts pins, wires, or tongs into bones. After surgery the pins, wires, or tongs are attached to pulleys and weights to provide continuous traction.

Mechanical Traction

Mechanical traction uses a special device that pulls and relaxes intermittently. The therapist sets the time intervals between contractions and relaxations. Mechanical traction is used to promote relaxation.

Mobility Aids

Mobility aids (also called mobility assistive devices) include canes, walkers, crutches, and wheelchairs. These devices are designed to improve patients' ability to ambulate, or move from one place to another.

The appropriate aid depends on the patient's disability, muscle coordination, strength, and age. The patient may need a device temporarily—perhaps crutches after a sprain—or permanently—such as a wheelchair in the case of permanent paralysis.

Canes

Canes come in several styles, including standard, tripod, and quad-base. All styles are lightweight, made of wood or aluminum, and have a rubber tip or tips at the bottom. They provide support and help patients maintain balance. Canes are especially useful for patients with weaknesses on one side of the body (possibly due to a stroke), joint disability, or neuromuscular defect.

A standard cane is best for a patient who needs only a small amount of support. Its curved handle is convenient, allowing the patient to hang it from a pocket or a doorknob. When the patient uses a standard cane, however, the curved handle concentrates most of the patient's weight in one small area of the hand. To avoid stressing the hand in this way, some standard canes have a T-shaped handle, which distributes pressure on the hand more evenly.

Tripod canes have three legs, and quad-base canes have four. The multiple legs create a wide base of support, making them more stable than a standard cane. Tripod and quad-base canes can stand alone, freeing up the patient's hands when she sits down. These canes are bulkier

and more difficult to pick up and put down than a standard cane, however. Both styles have T-shaped handles.

After determining the most suitable cane for the patient, the physical therapist adjusts the cane's height. When the cane is the correct height, the patient's elbow is flexed at 20° to 25°, and the patient stands tall while using the cane (instead of leaning on it for support). The therapist makes sure that the handle is the right size for the patient's hand and instructs the patient on how to use the cane. If directed, you may do the teaching or reinforce it, as discussed in Procedure 30-5.

Walkers

A walker is an aluminum frame that is open on one side and has four widely placed legs with rubber tips. The legs are adjustable for various heights. Some models are designed to fold up for storage. To use a walker, the patient stands within the frame and leans on the upper bar, which has a handgrip on each side. The frame is lightweight, so it is easy for most patients to use.

Typically, a walker is used by older patients who are too weak to walk unassisted or who have balance problems. The walker is designed to give these patients a sense of stability as they ambulate. In tight spaces or in areas with throw rugs, however, a walker may be difficult to manage. A patient who is too weak to pick up the walker may use a walker on wheels. Wheeled walkers have brakes for safety.

A physical therapist selects a walker that suits the patient's abilities and height. A walker should reach the patient's hipbone. Although the physical therapist usually trains the patient in the use of a walker, you may be asked to do this, or you may need to reinforce the information presented in Procedure 30-6.

Crutches

Crutches allow a patient to walk without putting weight on the feet or legs by transferring that weight to the arms. Crutches are made of aluminum or wood. Aluminum crutches are lighter and usually more expensive

PROCEDURE 30-5

Teaching a Patient How to Use a Cane

Objective: To teach a patient how to use a cane safely

OSHA Guidelines: This procedure does not involve exposure to blood, body fluids, or tissues.

Materials: Cane suited to the patient's needs

Method

Standing From a Sitting Position

1. Instruct the patient to slide his buttocks to the edge of the chair.
2. Tell the patient to place his right foot against the right front leg of the chair and his left foot against the left front leg of the chair. (This provides him with a wide, stable stance.)
3. Instruct the patient to lean forward and use the armrests of the chair to push upward. Caution the patient not to lean on the cane.
4. Have the patient position the cane for support on the strong side of his body.

Walking

1. Teach the patient to hold the cane on the strong side of her body with the tip(s) of the cane 4 to 6 inches from the side of her strong foot. Remind the patient to make sure the tip is flat on the ground.
2. Have the patient move the cane forward approximately 12 inches and then move her affected foot forward, parallel to the cane.
3. Next have the patient move her strong leg forward past the cane and her weak leg.
4. Observe as the patient repeats this process.

Ascending Stairs

1. Instruct the patient to always start with his strong leg when going up stairs.
2. Advise the patient to keep the cane on the strong side of his body and to use the wall or rail for support on the weak side.
3. After the patient steps on the strong leg, instruct him to bring up his weak leg and then the cane.
4. Remind the patient not to rush.

Descending Stairs

1. Instruct the patient to always start with her weak leg when going down stairs.
2. Advise the patient to keep the cane on the strong side of her body and to use the wall or rail for support on the weak side.
3. Have the patient use the strong leg and wall or rail to support her body, bending the strong leg as she lowers the weak leg and cane to the next step. She can move the cane and weak leg simultaneously, or she can move the cane first, followed by the weak leg.
4. Instruct the patient to step down with the strong leg.

Walking on Snow or Ice

Suggest that the patient try a metal ice-gripping cane or a ski pole. These can be dug into the snow or ice to prevent slipping.

PROCEDURE 30-6

Teaching a Patient How to Use a Walker

Objective: To teach a patient how to use a walker safely

OSHA Guidelines: This procedure does not involve exposure to blood, body fluids, or tissues.

Materials: Walker suited to the patient's needs

Method

Walking

1. Instruct the patient to step into the walker.
2. Tell the patient to place her hands on the handgrips on the sides of the walker.
3. Make sure the patient's feet are far enough apart so that she feels balanced.
4. Instruct the patient to pick up the walker and move it forward about 6 inches.
5. Have the patient move one foot forward and then the other foot.
6. Instruct the patient to pick up the walker again and to move it forward. If the patient is strong enough, explain that she may advance the walker after moving each leg rather than waiting until she has moved both legs.

Sitting

1. Teach the patient to turn his back to the chair or bed.
2. Instruct the patient to take small, careful steps and to back up until he feels the chair or bed at the back of his legs.
3. Instruct the patient to keep the walker in front of himself, let go of the walker, and place both his hands on the arms of the chair or on the bed.
4. Teach the patient to balance himself on his arms while lowering himself slowly to the chair or bed.

Ascending and Descending Stairs

1. Teach the patient not to use a walker when going up or down stairs.
2. Tell the patient to use the railing and a small quad-base cane instead of the walker.
3. Instruct the patient to ask her caregiver to place the walker at the top or bottom of the stairs as appropriate. It will then be ready for the patient to use after she has gone up or down the stairs.

than those made of wood. Pediatric crutches are available for children. The two basic types of crutches are axillary and Lofstrand.

Axillary crutches reach from the ground to the armpit. Each crutch has a rubber tip on the bottom to prevent slipping. This type of crutch is designed for short-term use by patients with such injuries as a sprained ankle.

Lofstrand, or Canadian, crutches reach from the ground to the forearm, and each one has a rubber tip on the bottom to prevent slipping. For additional support, this type has a handgrip extension attached at a 90° angle and a metal cuff that fits securely around the patient's forearm. Lofstrand crutches are geared for long-term use by patients with such disorders as paraplegia.

Measuring the Patient for Crutches. To prevent back pain and nerve injury to the armpits and palms, crutches must be measured to fit each patient. Axillary crutches that are too long can put pressure on nerves in the armpit, causing a condition called crutch palsy (muscle weakness in the forearm, wrist, and hand). They can also force the patient's shoulders forward, causing strain on the back and making ambulation difficult. Crutches that are too short force the patient to bend forward during ambulation, causing back pain or imbalance, which can lead to falls.

Before a patient who uses crutches leaves the office, make sure the crutches fit properly and that the patient is comfortable walking with them. To confirm that the fit is correct, check for the following conditions.

1. The patient is wearing the type of shoes he will wear when walking.
2. The patient is standing erect with feet slightly apart.
3. The crutch tips are positioned 2 inches in front of the patient's feet and 4 to 6 inches to the side of each foot.
4. The axillary supports allow 2 to 3 finger-widths between supports and armpits. (Use wing nuts and bolts to adjust crutches.)
5. The handgrips are positioned to create 30° flexion at the elbows. (Use wing nuts and bolts to adjust; use a goniometer to check flexion.)

Teaching Patients to Use Crutches. Elderly patients or patients with muscle weakness may have difficulty using crutches. Teach these patients muscle strength exercises for the arms to encourage them to use the crutches properly and for long periods. Give all patients the following general information about using crutches.

- Report to the physician any tingling or numbness in arms, hands, or shoulders.
- Support body weight with the hands.

- Always stand erect to prevent muscle strain.
- Look straight ahead when walking.
- Generally, move the crutches no more than 6 inches at a time to maintain good balance.
- Check the crutch tips regularly for wear; replace the tips as needed.
- Check the crutch tips for wetness; dry the tips if they are wet.
- Check all wing nuts and bolts for tightness.
- Wear flat, well-fitting, nonskid shoes.
- Remove throw rugs and other unsecured articles from traffic areas.
- To elevate an injured leg when sitting, use a crutch to support the thigh.
- To support the body when fatigued, place the back against a wall, and divide weight between the back and the strong leg and foot.
- Report any unusual pain in the affected leg.

Crutch Gaits. To teach a patient how to stand and walk with crutches, you must learn the crutch gaits, or walks. First show the patient the standing, or tripod, position. To do this, have the patient stand erect and look straight ahead. The patient should place the crutch tips 4 to 6 inches in front of her feet and 4 to 6 inches away from the side of each foot.

To determine the proper gait for a patient, you will make a preteaching assessment of the patient's muscle coordination and physical condition. In general, instruct a patient to use a slow gait in crowded areas or when feeling tired. The patient can use a faster gait in open places or when feeling more energetic. Using various gaits and speeds enables the patient to exercise different muscle groups and improve overall conditioning.

Four-Point Gait. The four-point gait is a slow gait used only when a patient can bear weight on both legs. Because this gait has three points of contact with the ground at all times, it is stable and safe. It is especially useful for patients with leg muscle weakness, spasticity, or poor balance or coordination. To teach this gait, have the patient start in the tripod position. Then outline the following steps, as illustrated in Figure 30-6.

- Move the right crutch forward.
- Move the left foot forward to the level of the left crutch.
- Move the left crutch forward.
- Move the right foot forward to level of the right crutch.

Three-Point Gait. The three-point gait is used when a patient cannot bear weight on one leg but can bear full weight on the unaffected leg. This gait allows the patient's weight to be carried alternately by the crutches and by the unaffected leg. It is appropriate for amputees, patients with tissue or musculoskeletal trauma (such as a fractured or sprained leg), and those recovering from leg surgery. The patient must have good muscle coordination and arm strength, however. To teach this gait, have the patient start in the tripod position. Then give the patient the following instructions, as illustrated in Figure 30-6.

- Move both crutches and the affected leg forward.
- Move the unaffected leg forward while weight is balanced on both crutches.

Two-Point Gait. The two-point gait is faster than the four-point gait and is used by patients who can bear some weight on both feet and have good muscle coordination and balance. To teach this gait, have the patient start in the tripod position. Then outline the following steps, as illustrated in Figure 30-6.

- Move the left crutch and the right foot forward at the same time.
- Move the right crutch and the left foot forward at the same time.

Swing Gaits. Patients with severe disabilities, such as leg paralysis or deformity, may use one of two swing gaits: the swing-to gait or the swing-through gait (Figure 30-7). To teach the swing-to gait, have the patient start in the tripod position. Then outline the following steps.

- Move both crutches forward at the same time.
- Lift the body and swing to the crutches.
- End with the tripod position again.

To teach the swing-through gait, have the patient start in the tripod position. Then go over the following steps.

- Move both crutches forward.
- Move the body and swing past the crutches.

Wheelchairs

Wheelchairs range from small, folding models to large, motorized ones. Depending on the patient's disability and the length of time the wheelchair will be needed, the physical therapist will select an appropriate wheelchair.

When patients come to the medical office in a wheelchair, the doctor may not be able to examine them adequately if they remain in their wheelchair. If this is the case, you will be responsible for transferring the patients from the wheelchair to the examining table and back to the wheelchair after the examination. To ensure their safety and yours, follow the steps in Procedure 25-3 in Chapter 25. Some reminders on preventing injury follow.

- Ask for help if the patient is weak, heavy, or unstable.
- Explain to the patient the steps of transfer you will use.
- Before starting the transfer, make sure that the wheelchair is in the locked position and that the patient is sitting at the front of the wheelchair seat.
- Use the large muscles in your thighs, which are stronger than your back muscles, when you lift.
- When lifting, bend from the knees and keep your back straight.
- Count to 3 and enlist the patient's help on the count of 3.

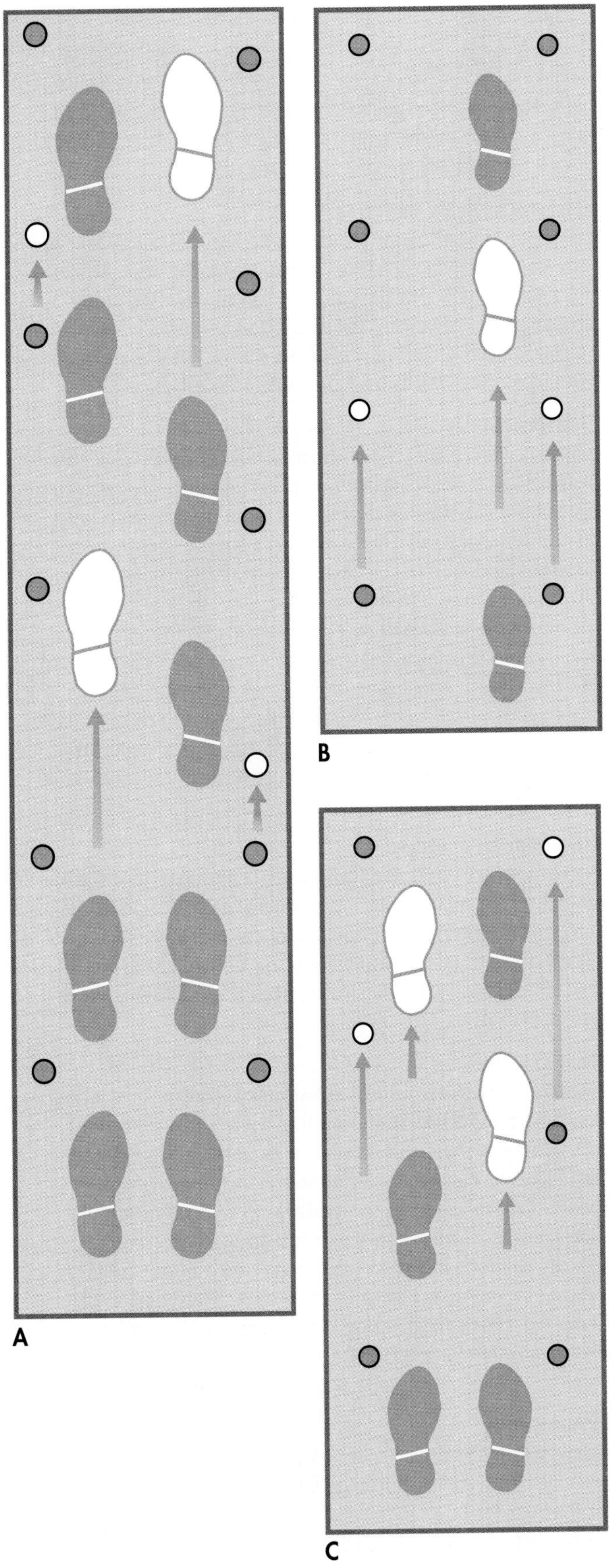

A

B

C

Figure 30-6. Crutch gaits include (a) four-point gait, (b) three-point gait, and (c) two-point gait.

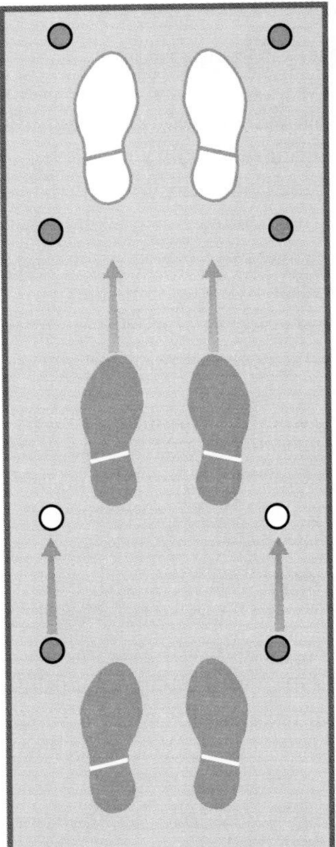

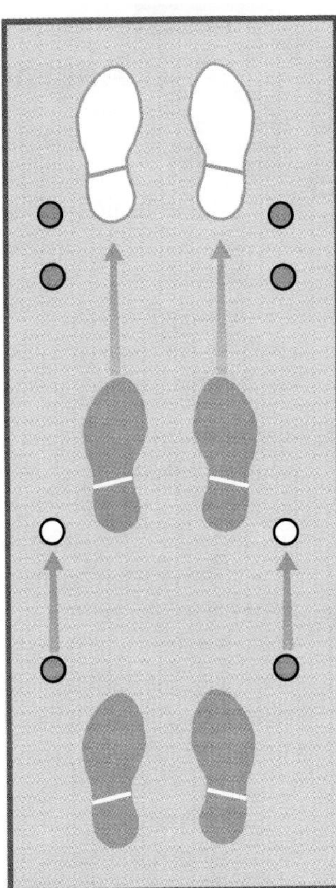

Figure 30-7. The swing gaits for walking with crutches are used by patients with severe disabilities.

Referral to a Physical Therapist

If the doctor refers the patient to a physical therapist or other specialist, you may be asked to contact the specialist directly or to give the patient a written order and information about contacting the specialist. Keep a file with information about the therapists your office uses. In the file note the forms and information each therapist requires. If you speak to the therapist, be sure to inform the doctor and to document the referral in the patient's chart. The therapist may be an independent practitioner or may be employed by a hospital, clinic, or home health-care agency.

In addition to physical therapy, some patients may decide to try alternative therapies, such as acupuncture, chiropractic, or biofeedback training. Although some doctors believe that alternative therapies provide some benefits, such as pain relief, many doctors do not. See "Educating the Patient" for information on a variety of alternative therapies.

Summary

Physical therapy is a medical specialty that helps patients with musculoskeletal and neurological disorders. It produces therapeutic effects through physical and mechanical

EDUCATING THE PATIENT

Alternative Therapies

Some patients will choose to consult alternative practitioners for pain relief, for help with chronic problems, and for improvement of overall health. If a patient shows interest in an alternative therapy, encourage the patient to view it as a complementary therapy to the doctor's primary medical treatment. Be aware that some doctors consider alternative therapies incompatible with conventional medicine.

Acupuncture
Acupuncture originated in China more than 5000 years ago, but it was not introduced in the United States until the early 1970s. Acupuncture is a system of healing that uses special needles inserted into points on the body to alleviate pain, to increase energy and balance, and to treat diseases of the heart, muscles, nerves, and eyes. Many people believe that acupuncture can aid the digestive and reproductive systems, treat chemical addictions, and take the place of anesthesia for certain surgical procedures.

Inform patients considering acupuncture that licensing varies from state to state. Some states have no licensing, while others stipulate that only medical doctors and chiropractors may practice acupuncture. You will want to caution patients considering acupuncture to be sure that the practitioner has graduated from an approved school and, if required, has passed a state licensing examination.

Aromatherapy
Aromatherapy uses essential oils from plants and herbs, such as peppermint, eucalyptus, chamomile, rosemary, and lavender. It is used to relieve pain, to induce sleep, and to treat stress, skin conditions, digestive disorders, and a variety of other conditions.

Aromatherapy actually is not limited to aroma, because many of the oils are readily absorbed through the skin. You will want to caution patients considering aromatherapy that some practitioners recommend internal application of the oils. This practice is not sanctioned in the United States. In general, medical doctors have not incorporated aromatherapy into their treatments.

Biofeedback Training
Biofeedback training uses simple electronic devices that measure selected changes in the body, such as muscle activity, brain wave activity, and cardiovascular activity. A trained expert views a readout of the patient's responses during relaxation and during stress. The readout is a scan of electronic information on paper.

Biofeedback training teaches the patient to control breathing, heart rate, and blood pressure. The purpose of the training is to improve the patient's responses to stress or pain and to alleviate other problems, such as muscular dysfunctions, back pain, sleep disorders, hyperactivity, gastrointestinal disorders, headaches, and fatigue. Counsel the patient who is considering biofeedback to find a practitioner who is certified.

Bodywork
Bodywork includes massage, deep-tissue manipulation, movement therapies, shiatsu, acupressure, and reflexology. All forms of bodywork aim to improve the body's structure and function. Patients often seek bodywork to help soothe injured muscles and joints, reduce pain, stimulate circulation, and promote relaxation.

Chiropractic
Chiropractic is a holistic approach to health that treats disease by manipulating the spinal column. The philosophy of chiropractic is that the nervous system can help the body heal itself. Some patients seek out chiropractors for relief of musculoskeletal problems, including misalignment of the spine. Inform patients that chiropractic is becoming increasingly accepted in the medical community and that more chiropractors are on staff at hospitals and becoming involved in sports medicine than there were in the past. You will also want to tell patients, however, that some physicians do not agree with the philosophy of chiropractic for treatment of musculoskeletal conditions.

Craniosacral Therapy
In craniosacral therapy the bones of the skull are manipulated through rhythmic motions that shift the pressure of the cerebrospinal fluid. Craniosacral therapy is used to treat headaches and ear infections as well as more serious conditions, such as stroke, spinal cord injury, and cerebral palsy.

Homeopathy
Homeopathy uses natural substances from plants, minerals, and animals to stimulate the body's physical healing. Homeopathic remedies are based on the principle that "like cures like," which means that the same substance that in large doses causes an illness, in minute doses cures it. Because these substances are often greatly diluted, many people consider homeopathy to be a safe, nontoxic form of medicine. The Food and Drug Administration recognizes homeopathic substances and regulates their production and dispensation to the public.

Naturopathy
Naturopathy treats conditions by using the body's natural mechanisms of healing. Diet, herbs, and preventive techniques are its hallmarks. Naturopathy advocates changing one's lifestyle, reducing stress, participating in regular exercise, and consuming a high-fiber diet.

processes, patient education, and rehabilitation programs.

Before prescribing physical therapy, the physician must assess a patient's joint mobility, muscle strength, gait, and posture. Depending on the patient's needs, the physician may decide to include cryotherapy, thermotherapy, or hydrotherapy in the physical therapy program. The physician or physical therapist may also recommend exercise therapy, massage, or traction. If the patient has difficulty with ambulation, a cane, a walker, crutches, or a wheelchair may be indicated as a mobility aid.

As a medical assistant, you may be asked to help a patient with cryotherapy or thermotherapy, range-of-motion (ROM) exercises, hydrotherapy, and other treatments. You may also need to teach a patient how to use mobility aids. Working directly with patients to help alleviate their pain and improve their mobility will reward you with immediate and long-term satisfaction.

30 Chapter Review

Discussion Questions

1. Identify three conditions that can be treated with cryotherapy, and give two examples of dry cold applications and two examples of wet cold applications.
2. Identify three conditions that can be treated with thermotherapy. Give two examples of dry heat applications and two examples of moist heat applications.
3. Explain how to teach a patient the four-point, three-point, and two-point crutch gaits.

Critical Thinking Questions

1. Your patient's physical therapist has prescribed hydrotherapy three times a week. Although the patient can drive, he tells you that he cannot keep his appointments because his wife has Alzheimer's disease and should not be left alone. How could you help solve this problem?
2. When teaching patients how to use a walker, what changes to their home environment would you suggest to ensure their safety?
3. Describe how you can improve your skills in applying physical therapy and how you can keep informed about new therapies and techniques.

Application Activities

1. Prepare an ice bag and apply it to a classmate's elbow. Ask your classmate to evaluate your technique in cold application. Exchange roles and evaluate your classmate's technique.
2. Teach a classmate how to use a cane to walk up and down stairs. Ask the classmate to critique your instructions. Exchange roles and critique your classmate's instructions.
3. Measure crutches for three different classmates. Teach each one a different gait. Then have a classmate measure crutches for you and teach you a gait.

Further Readings

Glasgow, G., et al. "Exercise Therapy: Physiological Aspects." *American Journal of Sports Medicine,* March/April 1993, 243–246.

Peck, David M. "Apophyseal Injuries in the Young Athlete." *American Family Physician,* June 1995, 1891–1897.

Pryor, Sally R. *Getting Back on Your Feet.* Post Mills, VT: Chelsea Green, 1991.

Rhodes, Maura. "Complementary Exercise: Five Mind-Body Workouts, Five Sports, Five New Ways of Thinking About Training." *Women's Sports and Fitness,* January/February 1995, 45.

Strohecker, James, ed. *Alternative Medicine: The Definitive Guide.* Puyallup, WA: Future Medicine, 1994.

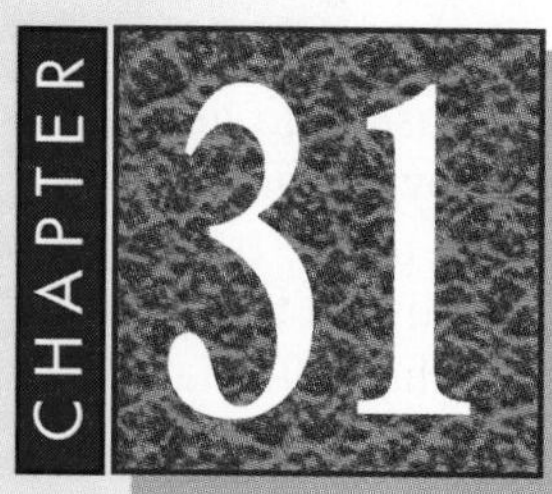

Medical Emergencies and First Aid

CHAPTER OUTLINE

- Understanding Medical Emergencies
- Preparing for Medical Emergencies
- Accidental Injuries
- Common Illnesses
- Less Common Illnesses
- Common Psychosocial Emergencies
- The Patient Under Stress
- Educating the Patient
- Disasters

OBJECTIVES

After completing Chapter 31, you will be able to:

- Discuss the importance of first aid during a medical emergency.
- Describe the purpose of the emergency medical services (EMS) system and explain how to contact it.
- List items found on a crash cart or first-aid tray.
- List general guidelines to follow in emergencies.
- Compare various degrees of burns and their treatments.
- Demonstrate how to help a choking victim.
- Demonstrate cardiopulmonary resuscitation (CPR).
- Demonstrate four ways to control bleeding.
- List the symptoms of heart attack, shock, and stroke.
- Explain how to calm a patient who is under extreme stress.
- Describe your role in responding to natural disasters and those caused by humans.

Key Terms

botulism
cast
chain of custody
concussion
contusion
crash cart
dehydration
dislocation
epistaxis
hematemesis
hematoma
hyperglycemia
hypoglycemia
hypovolemic shock
myocardial infarction
palpitations
seizure
septic shock
splint
sprain
strain
tachycardia
xiphoid process

AREAS OF COMPETENCE

1997 ROLE DELINEATION STUDY

CLINICAL

Patient Care

- Adhere to established triage procedures
- Obtain patient history and vital signs
- Recognize and respond to emergencies

continued

AREAS OF COMPETENCE continued

GENERAL (Transdisciplinary)

Professionalism

- Prioritize and perform multiple tasks

Instruction

- Teach methods of health promotion and disease prevention
- Locate community resources and disseminate information

Understanding Medical Emergencies

A medical emergency is any situation in which a person suddenly becomes ill or sustains an injury that requires immediate help by a health-care professional. Your prompt action in a medical emergency could prevent permanent disability or even death.

You may see life-threatening medical emergencies in the health-care setting. For example, a patient in the waiting room may have chest pains that could indicate a heart attack is imminent. You may see emergencies that are not life-threatening, such as a coworker sustaining a minor injury on the job. You may also encounter emergencies outside the office. For example, a family member might cut a finger while using a kitchen knife, or a patron in a restaurant might choke on a piece of food. Your quick response is vital in all of these situations.

In or out of the office, a medical emergency may require you to perform first aid. First aid is the immediate care given to someone who is injured or suddenly becomes ill, before complete medical care can be obtained. Prompt and appropriate first aid can:

- Save a life.
- Reduce pain.
- Prevent further injury.
- Reduce the risk of permanent disability.
- Increase the chance of early recovery.

Because most emergencies do not occur in a medical office, your role in patient education is critical. The more you teach patients about first aid and the proper way to respond to emergencies, the better equipped they will be to handle accidental injuries and illnesses.

Preparing for Medical Emergencies

How well prepared you are for an emergency can mean the difference between life and death for a patient. You must be able to perform procedures quickly and correctly. Keeping your skills up to date will enable you to handle medical emergencies effectively.

Just as important is your ability to ensure that the medical office where you work is ready to handle whatever emergencies arise. This preparedness will depend on your own organizational skills and knowledge of community resources.

Preparing the Office

You must first establish with the doctor which duties are expected of you and of other office personnel in case of an emergency and determine what resources are available. One of your most important allies will be the local emergency medical services (EMS) system. An EMS system is a network of qualified emergency services personnel who use community resources and equipment to provide emergency care to victims of injury or sudden illness.

Posting Emergency Telephone Numbers. Although the telephone number for the local EMS system is 911 in many parts of the country, some areas may not have 911 service. Post the area's EMS system telephone number at every telephone and on the **crash cart** (the rolling cart of emergency supplies and equipment) or first-aid tray. Every office employee should know this number. If the community has no EMS system, post the telephone number of the local ambulance or rescue squad. You should also post the telephone numbers of the nearest fire company, police station, poison control center, women's shelter, rape hot line, and drug and alcohol center.

When you call the EMS system for medical assistance and transport, speak clearly and calmly to the dispatcher. Be prepared to provide the following information:

- Your name, telephone number, and location
- Nature of the emergency
- Number of people in need of help
- Condition of the injured or ill patient(s)
- Summary of the first aid that has been given
- Directions on how to reach the location of the emergency

Do not hang up until the dispatcher gives you permission to do so.

Common Emergency and First-Aid Supplies. The crash cart or tray contains basic drugs, supplies, and equipment for medical emergencies. Most crash carts also contain a first-aid kit with supplies for managing minor injuries and ailments. Figure 31-1 lists the usual items in a first-aid kit.

Contents of a First-Aid Kit

- Absorbent cotton (sterile)
- Adhesive dressings in various sizes
- Adhesive tape
- Airway or mouthpiece
- Analgesics, such as aspirin or acetaminophen
- Antiseptic solution
- Antiseptic wipes
- Calamine lotion
- Chemical hot and cold packs
- Disposable gloves
- Elastic bandages in various sizes
- First-aid book
- Ipecac syrup (two bottles)
- Personal protective equipment: gloves, mask and goggles or face shield, gown, shower cap, booties, pocket mask or mouth shield
- Scissors
- Splints in various sizes
- Sterile gauze pads in various sizes
- Sterile rolls of gauze
- Sugar packets
- Triangular bandage
- Tweezers
- Waterproof flashlight with extra batteries

Figure 31-1. These supplies are often included in a first-aid kit.

The actual contents of the crash cart or tray may vary slightly from practice to practice. Become familiar with these contents and know where they are located in the office. Procedure 31-1 describes how to check and restock the essential items on a crash cart.

Guidelines for Handling Emergencies

A medical emergency requires you to take certain steps. You are not responsible for diagnosing or providing medical care other than first aid. You are expected, however, to note the presence of serious conditions that threaten the patient's life. Then take appropriate action, but perform only those procedures that you have been trained to perform.

First, do a primary survey by assessing the patient's **a**irway, **b**reathing, and **c**irculation (ABCs). Then perform a secondary survey by examining the rest of the body for signs of illness or injury. Procedure 31-2 provides guidelines for performing an emergency assessment. After taking whatever emergency steps are appropriate to your findings, call the EMS system for medical help if the physician is not already by your side.

Sometimes a patient or a patient's family member calls the medical office with an emergency. If you are responsible for handling telephone calls, be prepared to triage the injuries by telephone. Triaging is the classification of injuries according to severity, urgency of treatment, and place for treatment.

To handle emergency calls, follow the practice's telephone triage protocols. For example, if a parent calls to say her daughter has broken her arm and the child's bone is visible, tell her to call the local EMS system for immediate care and transport to the hospital. If, however, a parent calls to say her son swallowed half a bottle of baby bath, tell her to remain calm and give her the telephone number of the poison control center. Depending on circumstances, you may offer to make the necessary telephone call yourself.

Adhere to the following general guidelines in any emergency situation.

- Stay calm.
- Reassure the patient.
- Act in a confident, organized manner.

Personal Protection. Whenever you administer first aid and emergency treatment, try to reduce or eliminate the risk of exposing yourself and others to infection. Follow Universal Precautions and assume that all blood and body fluids are infected with blood-borne pathogens. To protect yourself and others, take the following basic precautions. Include personal protective equipment (PPE) in your first-aid kit at work and at home. Standard PPE includes gloves, goggles and mask or face shield, gown, shower cap, and booties. A pocket mask or mouth shield provides personal protection when you perform rescue breathing. Plan to use specific PPE based on the condition of the patient. Table 31-1 provides examples of PPE

PROCEDURE 31-1

Stocking the Crash Cart

Objective: To ensure that the crash cart includes all appropriate drugs, supplies, and equipment needed for emergencies

OSHA Guidelines: This procedure does not involve exposure to blood, body fluids, or tissues.

Materials: Protocol for or list of crash cart items, crash cart

Method

1. Review the office protocol for or list of items that should be on the crash cart.
2. Check the drugs on the crash cart against the list. Restock those that were used, and replace those that have passed their expiration date. Crash cart drugs typically include the following:
   - Activated charcoal
   - Amobarbital sodium (Amytal Sodium)
   - Apomorphine hydrochloride
   - Atropine
   - Dextrose 50%
   - Diazepam (Valium)
   - Digoxin (Lanoxin)
   - Diphenhydramine hydrochloride (Benadryl)
   - Epinephrine, injectable
   - Furosemide (Lasix)
   - Glucagon
   - Glucose paste or tablets
   - Insulin (regular or a variety)
   - Intravenous dextrose in saline and intravenous dextrose in water
   - Ipecac syrup
   - Isoproterenol hydrochloride (Isuprel), aerosol inhaler and injectable
   - Lactated Ringer's solution
   - Lidocaine (Xylocaine), injectable
   - Metaraminol (Aramine)
   - Methylprednisolone tablets
   - Nitroglycerin tablets
   - Phenobarbital, injectable
   - Phenytoin (Dilantin)
   - Saline solution, isotonic (0.9%)
   - Sodium bicarbonate, injectable
   - Sterile water for injection
3. Check the supplies on the crash cart against the list. Restock items that were used, and make sure the packaging of supplies on the cart has not been opened. Crash cart supplies typically include the following:
   - Adhesive tape
   - Constricting band or tourniquet
   - Dressing supplies (alcohol wipes, rolls of gauze, bandage strips, bandage scissors)
   - Intravenous tubing, venipuncture devices, and butterfly needles
   - Padded tongue blades
   - Personal protective equipment
   - Syringes and needles in various sizes
4. Check the equipment on the crash cart against the list, and examine it to make sure that it is in working order. Restock equipment that is missing or broken. Crash cart equipment typically includes the following:
   - Airways in assorted sizes
   - Ambu-bag, a trademark for a breathing bag used to assist respiratory ventilation
   - Defibrillator (electrical device that shocks the heart to restore normal beating)
   - Endotracheal tubes in various sizes
   - Oxygen tank with oxygen mask and cannula
5. Check miscellaneous items on the crash cart against the list, and restock as needed. Miscellaneous crash cart items typically include the following:
   - Orange juice
   - Sugar packets

to use in various emergency situations. When in doubt, wear more PPE than you may think is called for.

Wear gloves if you expect hand contact with blood, mucous membranes, torn skin, or potentially contaminated articles or surfaces. In addition, if you have any cuts or lesions, wear PPE over the affected area.

Minimize splashing, splattering, or spraying of blood or other body fluids when performing first aid. If blood or other body fluids splash into your eyes, nose, or mouth, flush the area with water as soon as possible.

Wash your hands thoroughly with soap and water after removing the gloves. Also wash other skin surfaces that have come in contact with blood or other body fluids. Do not touch your mouth, nose, or eyes, and do not eat or drink after providing emergency care until you have washed your hands thoroughly. If you have been exposed to blood or other body fluids, be sure to tell the doctor. You may need postexposure treatment.

PROCEDURE 31-2

Performing an Emergency Assessment

Objective: To assess a medical emergency quickly and accurately

OSHA Guidelines

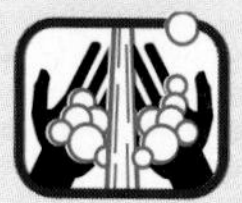 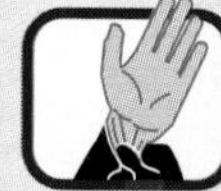 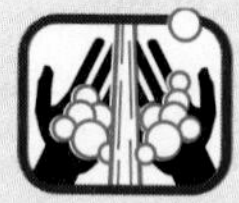

Materials: Penlight, patient's chart, pen

Method

1. Wash your hands and put on examination gloves if possible.
2. Talk to the patient to determine the level of consciousness.
3. If the patient can communicate clearly, ask what happened. If not, ask someone who observed the incident.
4. If you cannot determine the patient's medical history, check for a medical identification card or bracelet.
5. Assess the patient's ABCs (airway, breathing, and circulation), and begin rescue breathing or cardiopulmonary resuscitation (CPR) as needed (see Procedure 31-3).
6. Assess for injury, observing the body from head to toe. Palpate gently.
7. Observe the skin for pallor (paleness) or cyanosis (a bluish tint). If the patient is dark-skinned, observe for pallor or cyanosis on the inside of the lips and mouth.
8. Check the pulse for regularity and strength.
9. Check the eyes for pupil size. Using a penlight, assess pupil response to light.
10. Document your findings and report them to the doctor or emergency medical technician (EMT).
11. Assist the doctor or EMT as requested.
12. Remove the gloves and wash your hands.

Documentation. Document all office emergencies in the patient's chart. Be sure to include your assessment, treatment given, and the patient's response. If the patient was transported to another facility, record the location. Include the date and time with the documentation, as well as your signature and credentials.

Accidental Injuries

No matter where you encounter an emergency, your knowledge and certifications should enable you to provide first aid for the patient until a physician or EMT ar-

Table 31-1

Personal Protective Equipment for Emergencies

Equipment	Conditions for Use	Sample Emergencies Requiring Equipment
Gloves	Chance of contact with blood or other body secretions during emergency	Open wound, eye trauma
Goggles and mask or face shield and possibly shower cap	Chance of blood or other body secretions splattering	Bleeding, vomiting, most emergency care for small children (because of squirming)
Gown and possibly booties	Chance of contact with excessive bleeding	Childbirth, severe nosebleed
Pocket mask or mouth shield	Need for CPR or rescue breathing	Heart attack, respiratory arrest

rives. To help you become familiar with how to handle various emergency situations, the following sections present accidental injuries, common illnesses, and less common illnesses.

Accidental injuries that may call for emergency medical intervention include the following:

- Bites and stings
- Burns
- Choking
- Ear trauma
- Eye trauma
- Falls
- Fractures and dislocations
- Head injuries
- Hemorrhaging
- Multiple injuries
- Poisoning
- Sprains and strains
- Weather-related injuries
- Wounds

Bites and Stings

Dog and cat bites and bee, wasp, and hornet stings are fairly common. Less common are snakebites and spider bites, which you are more likely to encounter in certain parts of the country, such as Florida or the Southwest, than in other areas.

Animal Bites. An animal bite may bruise the skin, tear it, or leave a puncture wound. A wound that tears the skin should be seen by a doctor and may need to be reported to the police, animal control officer, and local health department. If the animal can be found, it should be checked for rabies. Then, depending on the animal's rabies vaccination status, the animal may need to be quarantined. If the animal is a probable carrier of rabies and cannot be found, the doctor may administer antirabies serum to the patient as a precaution.

Dogs, cats, skunks, squirrels, raccoons, bats, and foxes are more likely to carry rabies than other animals. Hamsters, gerbils, guinea pigs, and mice are rarely infected by the rabies virus.

Human bites can raise concerns about transmitting the human immunodeficiency virus (HIV) or hepatitis B virus. HIV can be transmitted only if the bite breaks the skin and if the biter has bleeding gums. Hepatitis B virus may be transmitted by a human bite that punctures the skin. In this case a series of three injections is required to immunize against hepatitis B.

Immediate care for bites calls for washing the area thoroughly with antiseptic soap and water. (If the bite caused a puncture wound, try to make it bleed to flush out bacteria. Then wash the area with soap and water.) Apply an antibiotic ointment and a dry, sterile dressing. The doctor will administer tetanus toxoid if the patient has not received it in the last 7 to 10 years.

Insect Stings. Insect stings are merely a nuisance to most patients. The site of the sting can become red, swollen, itchy, and painful. If the patient was stung by a honeybee, you must first remove the stinger, because it still has the ability to release venom. Remove the stinger by scraping the skin with a credit card or other flat, hard, sharp object. Be careful not to release more venom. Avoid using your fingers or tweezers, because squeezing the stinger may force more venom into the wound. (If you cannot remove the stinger, call the physician.) Wash the skin with soap and water. Apply ice to the site after the stinger is removed to reduce the pain and swelling. Later apply a paste of baking soda or a dressing soaked in aloe vera juice or vinegar to reduce discomfort and itching.

A sting can be deadly to a patient who is allergic to the insect venom, because anaphylaxis can develop. The symptoms of and treatment for anaphylaxis are described later in this chapter.

Snakebites. Poisonous snakes in the United States include rattlesnakes, water moccasins (or cottonmouths), copperheads, and coral snakes. Because snakes are cold-blooded, they often lie on rocks to warm themselves. Most bites occur when a person steps onto, sits down on, or reaches over or between rocks where a snake is sunning itself.

The bites of most poisonous snakes produce similar symptoms: one or two puncture marks, pain, and swelling at the site; rapid pulse; nausea; vomiting; and perhaps unconsciousness and seizures. If possible, get a description of the snake so the EMS team or the hospital can procure the proper antivenin (a substance that counteracts the snake poison) ahead of time. Snakebites are dangerous, but with proper intervention, they rarely lead to death.

If a patient has been bitten by a snake that may be poisonous, call a doctor or the EMS system. If the patient must walk, have him walk slowly to prevent dispersion of the poison through the circulation. To care for a poisonous snakebite while you await help, wash the area gently with soap and water. Then apply a clean or sterile dressing. If possible, immobilize the injured part, and position it below heart level. Do not apply ice or a tourniquet, and do not cut or suction the wound.

Spider Bites. Only two types of spiders in the United States are a serious threat to health: the black widow spider, which has a red hourglass mark on its abdomen, and the brown recluse spider, which has a violin-shaped mark on its back. The black widow bite causes swelling and pain at the site, as well as nausea, vomiting, rigid abdomen, fever, rash, and difficulty breathing or swallowing. The brown recluse bite causes severe swelling and tenderness and, eventually, ulceration along the nerve closest to the location of the bite.

You are not expected to classify spiders and their bites accurately. Therefore, any patient bitten by a spider must be seen by a physician. To care for a patient with a spider bite, wash the area thoroughly with soap and water.

Apply an ice pack to the area to reduce swelling and pain. If possible, keep the area below heart level to prevent the poison from spreading. Healing of the bite can sometimes take several months.

Burns

Burns involve tissue injury that occurs from heat, chemicals, electricity, or radiation. Be sure that you teach patients about emergency treatment for burns as well as any follow-up care prescribed by the physician.

Classifications of Burns. The severity of a burn is determined by the depth and extent of the burn area, the source of the burn, the age of the patient, body regions burned, and other patient illnesses and injuries. When classifying burns, use the categories minor, moderate, and major. These categories take into account all the factors that determine severity. For example, a burn might be considered minor although it damages all skin layers if it affects only a small area of one leg on an otherwise healthy person. A major burn includes any burn in children younger than age 2, electrical burns, burns complicated by fractures or serious trauma, and burns on the hands, face, feet, or perineum.

Burns classified according to the depth of skin damage are called first-degree, second-degree, and third-degree (see Figure 31-2). In a first-degree burn, the epidermis is damaged and the skin is reddened. Blisters result from a second-degree burn, in which part of the dermis is destroyed. A third-degree burn damages all the skin layers.

First-Degree, or Superficial, Burns. A first-degree burn causes pain and makes the surrounding skin turn red. It is equivalent to a sunburn. Treat first-degree burns by applying cold-water dressings or by immersing the affected area in cold water. Gently pat the area dry, and apply a dry, sterile dressing. Do not use greasy ointments, butter, or other substances because they prevent oxygen from reaching the wound and will have to be scrubbed off before any treatment can be administered. Scrubbing would be very painful.

Second-Degree, or Partial-Thickness, Burns. Second-degree burns extend deeper into the skin than first-degree burns. They cause blistering, along with pain and redness. Immerse second-degree burns in cold water until the pain subsides. Then gently pat the area dry, taking care not to break blisters, and apply a dry, sterile dressing. Do not apply antiseptic ointment unless the doctor orders it. If the arms or legs are affected, elevate them to reduce swelling.

Third-Degree, or Full-Thickness, Burns. Third-degree burns, such as those received in a fire, involve all layers of skin and demand immediate emergency medical assistance. While you wait for the EMS team, do not remove charred or adhered clothing from the patient. Cover the burns and

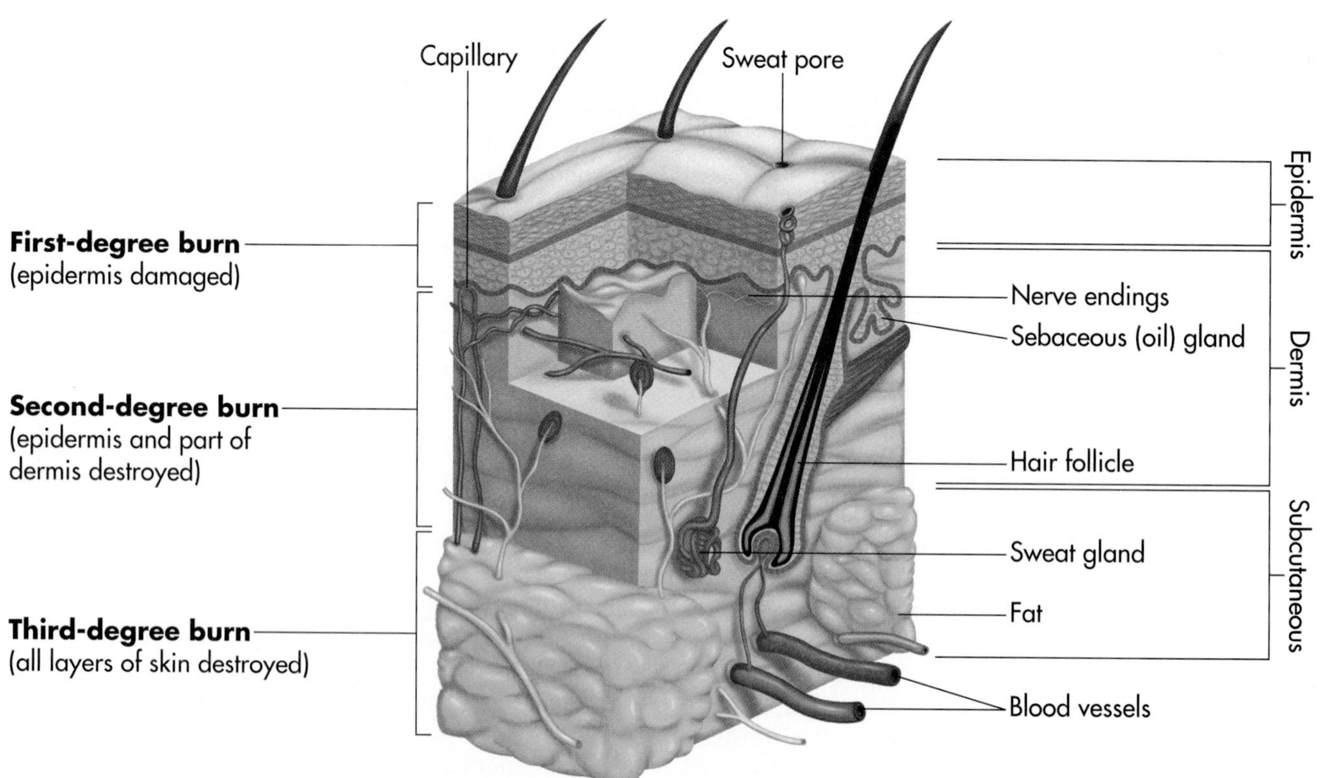

Figure 31-2. The depth of skin damage is one factor used to determine the severity of burns.

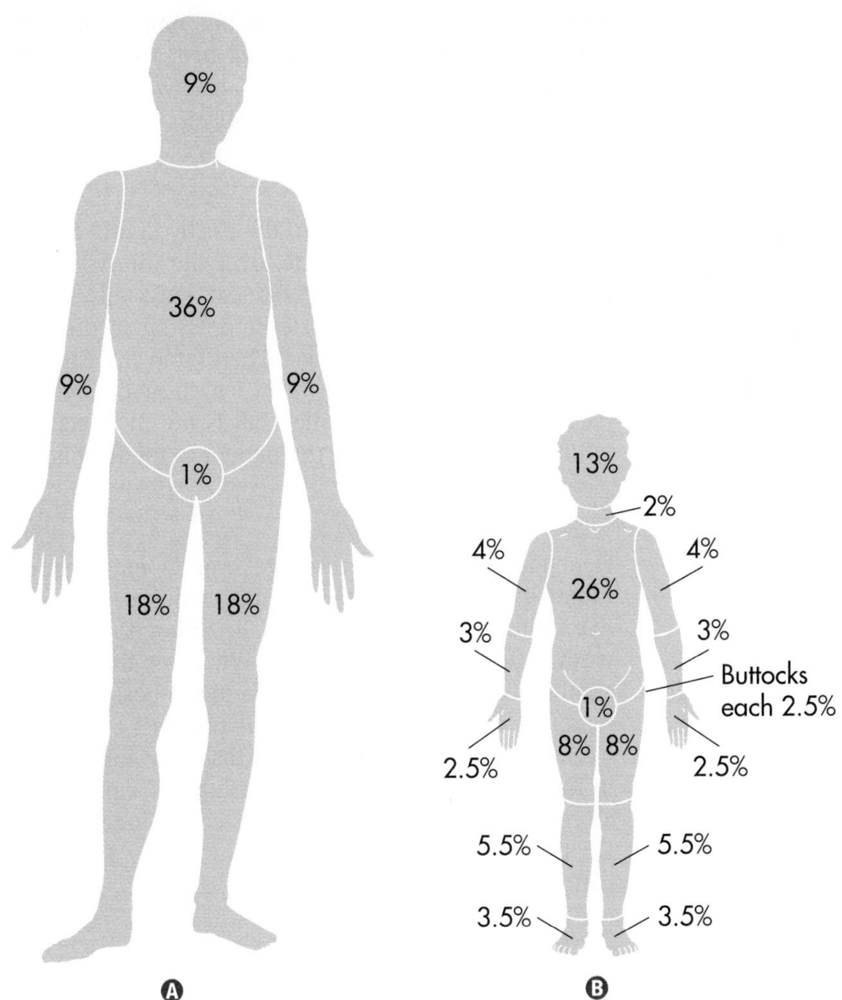

Figure 31-3. A. Use the rule of nines to calculate the percentage of body surface affected by burns in adults. Except for the genital region, percentage figures combine front and back surfaces. **B.** In children, use the percentages based on the Lund and Browder chart. These numbers take into account that children's body proportions differ from those of adults.

adhered clothing with thick, sterile dressings. If the hands, arms, or legs are burned, elevate them above the heart. Keep the patient warm and provide reassurance. Check to see whether the patient is suffering from smoke inhalation. Signs of smoke inhalation include difficulty breathing (often accompanied by coughing), smoky-smelling breath, or black residue in the patient's mouth and nose. If any of these signs are present, gently move the patient into a sitting position and monitor her breathing. Third-degree burns are usually not painful at first because of nerve damage.

Estimating the Extent of the Burn. Various methods are used to estimate the extent of the burn area (see Figure 31-3). To calculate the amount of skin surface burned on an adult, use the rule of nines. This rule assigns each of the following areas 9% of the body surface: the head and neck, each upper limb, the chest, the abdomen, the upper back, the lower back and buttocks, the front of each lower limb, and the back of each lower limb. These areas make up 99% of the body's surface. The genital region is the remaining 1%. The figures to use when making calculations in children are shown in Figure 31-3.

Particular Types of Burns. Some types of burns may require special treatment. They include chemical burns and thermal burns.

Chemical burns are more likely to affect workers at chemical or industrial facilities than people in the home. To treat this type of burn, flood the area with large amounts of water, then cover it with a dry dressing. Call the EMS team to transport the patient to the hospital.

Thermal burns may be caused by contact with hot liquids, steam, flames, radiation, excessive heat from fire, or hot objects. Call the EMS team immediately for victims of such burns. If you need to stop the burning process, use water to cool a burning substance, or use a wet cloth or blanket to put out a flame.

Choking

Choking occurs when food or a foreign object blocks a person's trachea, or windpipe. The main symptom of a choking emergency is the inability to speak. A choking person who cannot talk may give the universal sign of choking—a hand up to the throat and a fearful look. If you see someone giving this sign, be prepared to act promptly. First, approach the person and ask, "Are you choking?" If he can speak or cough, the airway is only partially obstructed. He should be able to dislodge the object on his own.

If the person cannot speak or cough, ask if you can help him. If he signals yes, then perform the Heimlich

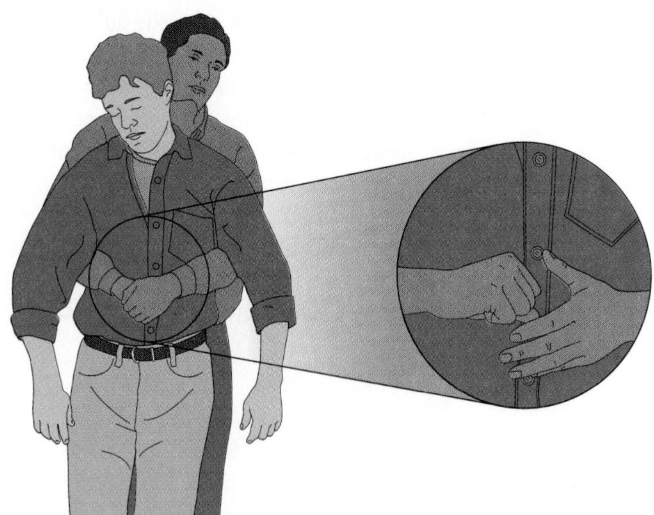

Figure 31-4. Perform abdominal thrusts on a conscious choking victim.

maneuver. Stand behind the person, and wrap your arms around his waist. Place the thumb side of your fist against his abdomen, slightly above the navel and below the **xiphoid process,** the lower extension of the breastbone. Grasp your fist with your other hand and press into the abdomen with quick upward thrusts. Continue until the object is ejected. The Heimlich maneuver is illustrated in Figure 31-4. Encourage all patients to learn the Heimlich maneuver, particularly those who care for children or the elderly.

If the victim loses consciousness, slowly lower him to the floor, and place him on his back. Straddle his thigh area. Open the person's mouth to check for a foreign body. If you see one, sweep it out with your fingers, as illustrated in Figure 31-5. Place the heel of one hand against the victim's abdomen, between the navel and the xiphoid process. Place the other hand on top of the first one. Press up toward the diaphragm with quick thrusts. Continue administering thrusts until the patient expels the foreign object, medical assistance arrives, or you no longer have the strength to continue. Stop periodically to check the person's mouth for a foreign body.

Attempt to ventilate the victim through rescue breathing. If this is not successful, continue with thrusts and sweeps and ventilation attempts until the airway is clear. If the person is still not breathing independently when the airway is clear, begin CPR. Procedure 31-3 describes how to perform CPR.

If an infant is choking, turn him upside down over your forearm and give five sharp blows to the back, between the shoulder blades. Next, quickly turn him over, protecting the head and neck between your forearms in a sandwich fashion, and give five quick chest thrusts with two fingers in the middle of the sternum between the nipples, as illustrated in Figure 31-12.

If a pregnant woman or an obese person is choking and you cannot encircle her abdomen with your arms, stand behind her and encircle her under the armpits. Place the thumb side of your fist over the center of the breastbone, and exert five quick backward thrusts. This procedure is illustrated in Figure 31-13.

Ear Trauma

Treat any cut or laceration to the ear by lightly applying a bandage, with even pressure, over the injury. It may be possible to reattach a severed ear surgically. Carefully wrap the severed ear in a sterile dressing secured with a self-adherent gauze bandage. Then wrap the ear in plastic, label it, and place it in an ice chest or over an ice pack so that it is kept chilled but is not in direct contact with the ice. Send it with the patient to the hospital.

Eye Trauma

Depending on its severity, eye trauma may require no more than an ice pack, or it may require hospital care. Eye trauma may result from a fall, a blow to the eye, or a wound from a pointed object. Whatever the cause, you should carefully examine the eye to the best of your ability and notify the physician of the patient's condition.

Eye injuries are commonly caused by foreign objects in the eye. Tiny specks cause tearing and can be painful. To remove them, use moistened sterile gauze or a tissue. Do not use a cotton ball, because it may leave behind cotton wisps that can irritate the eye.

Falls

If a patient falls from a chair or an examining table and cannot get up, call for help. Do not move him until the doctor or an EMT examines him. Move him only in a life-threatening situation, such as if the building is on fire. Arrange for transport to the hospital, and document the fall and injury in the patient's chart.

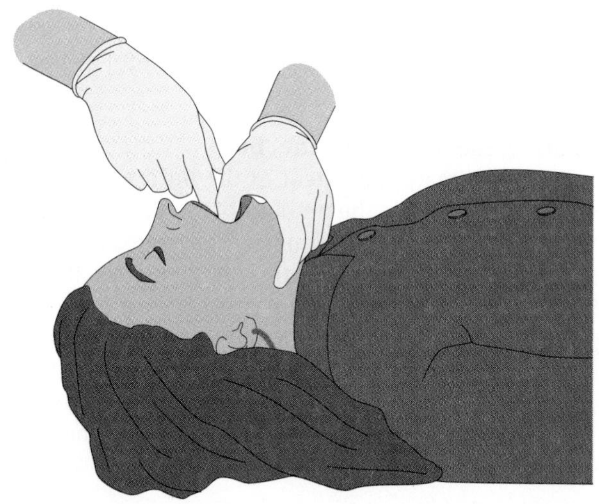

Figure 31-5. Use a finger sweep to remove a foreign object from the mouth.

PROCEDURE 31-3

Performing Cardiopulmonary Resuscitation (CPR)

Objective: To provide ventilation and blood circulation for a patient who shows none

OSHA Guidelines

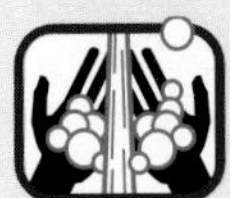
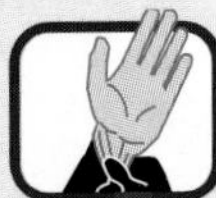
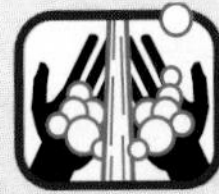

Materials: Mouth shield or, if you are not in the office, a piece of plastic with a hole for the mouth

Method

1. Shake the patient and ask, "Are you all right?" If there is no response, call the EMS system, or ask someone else to call.
2. Wash your hands and put on examination gloves if possible.
3. If the patient is not on her back, roll her whole body over.
4. Open the patient's airway by lifting her chin gently with one hand, while pushing back on her forehead with the other hand (see Figure 31-6).
5. If you suspect a neck injury, use the modified jaw thrust instead. To do this maneuver, put your fingers behind the jawbone just below the ear, and push the jaw forward (see Figure 31-7).
6. Place your ear close to the patient's mouth, and keep your eyes on her chest and stomach. Look for chest and abdominal movement. Listen for the sound of air moving. Feel for breath on your cheek. These signs indicate that the patient is breathing.
7. If you do not see, hear, or feel breathing, begin rescue breathing, as shown in Figure 31-8. Turn the hand you are resting on the patient's forehead so that you can also use it to pinch her nose.
8. Place a mouth shield over the patient's mouth, and take a deep breath. Place your mouth on the shield over the patient's mouth, making a seal. Then blow into her mouth. Pause and then blow into her mouth again. Watch to see that the patient's chest rises with the breaths.

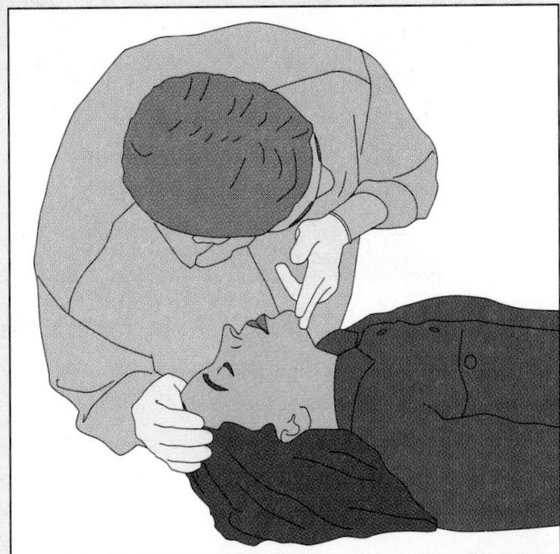

Figure 31-6. Use the head tilt-chin lift maneuver to open an airway.

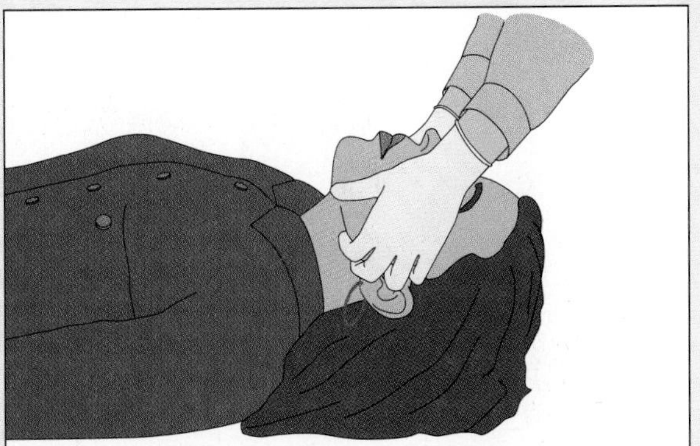

Figure 31-7. Use the jaw thrust maneuver for a patient with a neck injury.

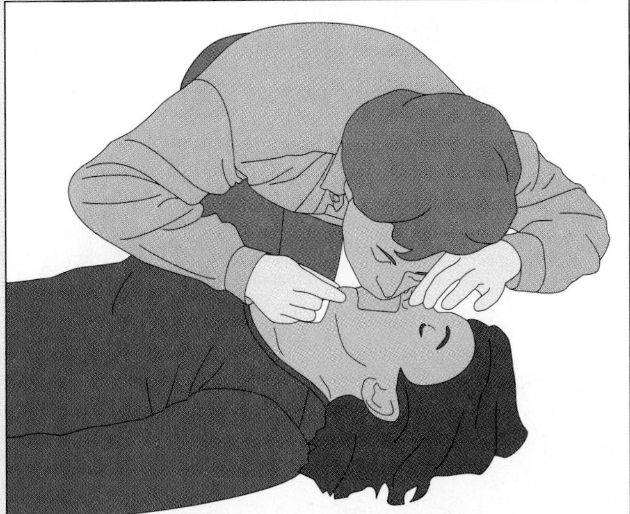

Figure 31-8. Perform mouth-to-mouth rescue breathing.

continued

PROCEDURE 31-3 continued

Performing Cardiopulmonary Resuscitation (CPR)

9. If you cannot make a good mouth-to-mouth seal, try mouth-to-nose breathing if needed (see Figure 31-9).
10. If the patient has a tracheostomy, breathe into the stoma after closing off the mouth and nose.
11. Next locate the carotid pulse to check for a heartbeat. To find the carotid artery, locate the larynx and slide the tips of your index and middle fingers into the groove beside the larynx. If you do not feel a pulse, start artificial circulation.
12. Locate the end of the sternum, which is called the xiphoid process. To do this quickly, run your index and middle fingers across the lower margin of the ribs to the notch where they meet. Place the two fingers flat on the chest at this spot. Place the heel of your other hand on the midline of the sternum, next to the index finger (see Figure 31-10).
13. With the heel of your hand in position, place your other hand on top of it and interlace your fingers. Straighten your arms and lock your elbows. Position your shoulders directly over your hands so that your thrust is downward (see Figure 31-11).
14. Depress the sternum 1½ to 2 inches for an adult. Release the compression completely, but keep your elbows locked and your hands on the chest.
15. Do four sets of 15 compressions and 2 breaths over a 1-minute period (5 compressions and 1 breath for a 1-minute period if it is a two-person rescue). Then check the pulse.
16. If the patient has a pulse but is not breathing, start rescue breathing. If the patient has no pulse and is not breathing, continue CPR until the patient regains consciousness or help arrives. Stop and take a pulse every few minutes.
17. Assist EMS personnel as requested.
18. Remove the gloves and wash your hands.

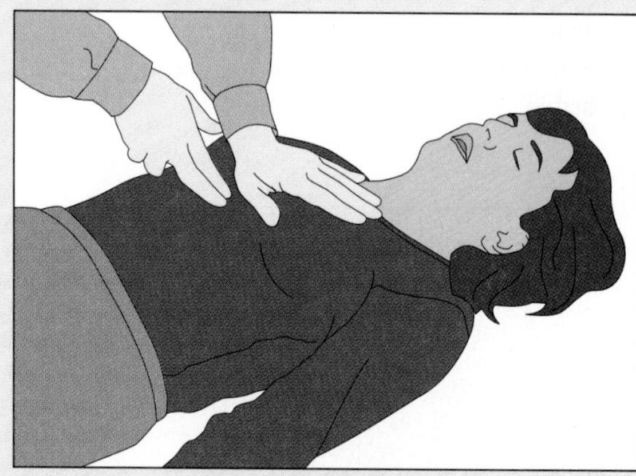

Figure 31-10. Place your hands at the xiphoid process.

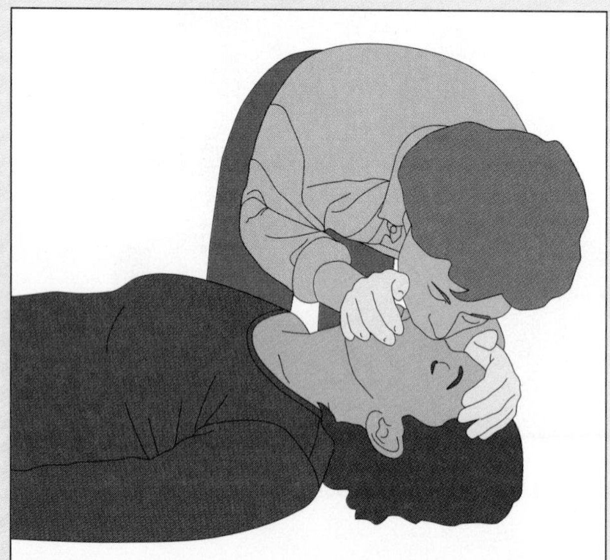

Figure 31-9. Use mouth-to-nose breathing if mouth-to-mouth breathing is not possible.

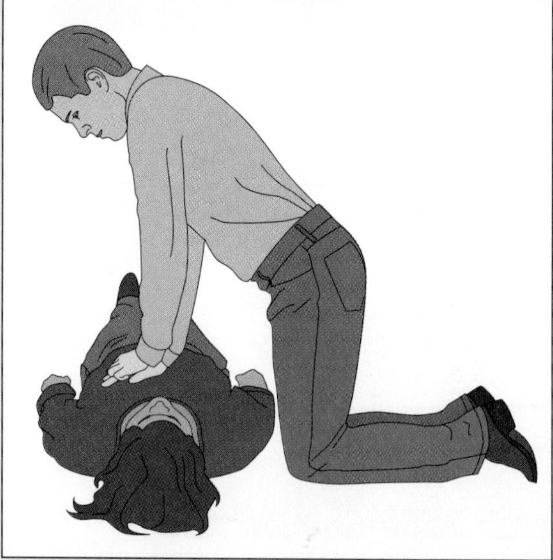

Figure 31-11. Align your shoulders directly over the victim's sternum, with your elbows locked.

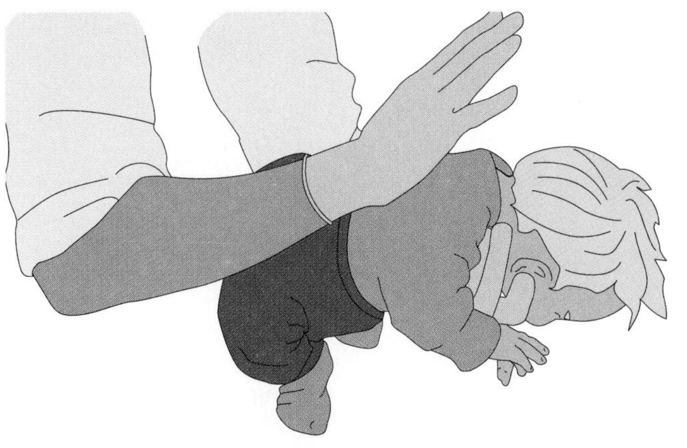

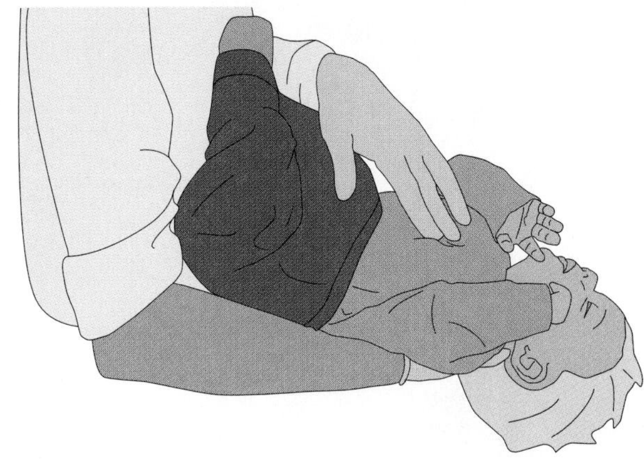

Figure 31-12. Use back blows and two-finger chest thrusts for a choking infant.

If the fall results in only a bump, apply ice and observe for bruises and swelling. Give the patient time to collect himself. Be sure to notify the doctor, who should examine the patient. Then document the fall, the injury, and the treatment in the patient's chart.

Falls are not limited to the physician's office, of course. Follow these procedures wherever you encounter someone who has fallen.

Fractures and Dislocations

A fracture is a break in a bone. Fractures are categorized in several ways (see Figure 31-14). Complete fractures go across the entire bone; incomplete fractures go through only part of the bone. Comminuted fractures are those in which the bone has broken into several fragments. In a greenstick fracture, the bone is bent, but only one side is fractured. Greenstick fractures occur most often in children because their bones are still soft and pliable. A fracture is simple, or closed, if it does not cause a break in the skin. In open, or compound, fractures, the bone breaks through the skin.

A **dislocation** is the displacement of a bone end from the joint. Both fractures and dislocations usually result from accidents or sports injuries. They can cause pain, loss of function, deformity, swelling, and discoloration. The injury is usually diagnosed by x-ray.

Treatment of fractures and dislocations depends on factors such as the nature of the injury and the patient's age and physical condition. The basic emergency steps are:

- Immobilization to reduce pain and continuing damage to soft tissue.
- Reduction, or moving the bone back into the proper position, for some fractures.

Immobilization is sometimes provided by the application of a splint or cast. The purpose of both splints and casts is to keep an injured body part in place and protect it as it heals. A **splint** is an appliance used for conditions that do not require rigid immobilization or, as a temporary measure, for those in which swelling is anticipated. A **cast** is a rigid, external dressing, usually made of plaster or fiberglass, that is molded to the contours of the body part to which it is applied. You may assist the physician with the application of a cast (see Figure 31-15). You may also educate the patient about these basic elements of cast care.

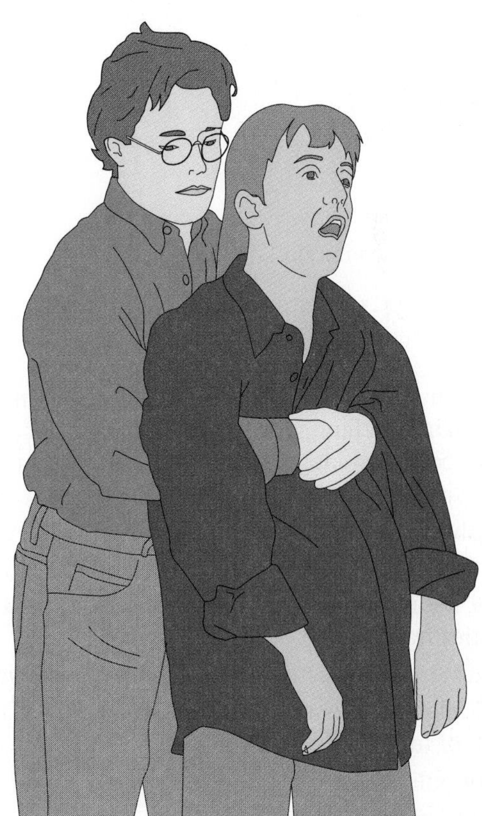

Figure 31-13. Use a chest thrust for a choking victim who is pregnant or obese.

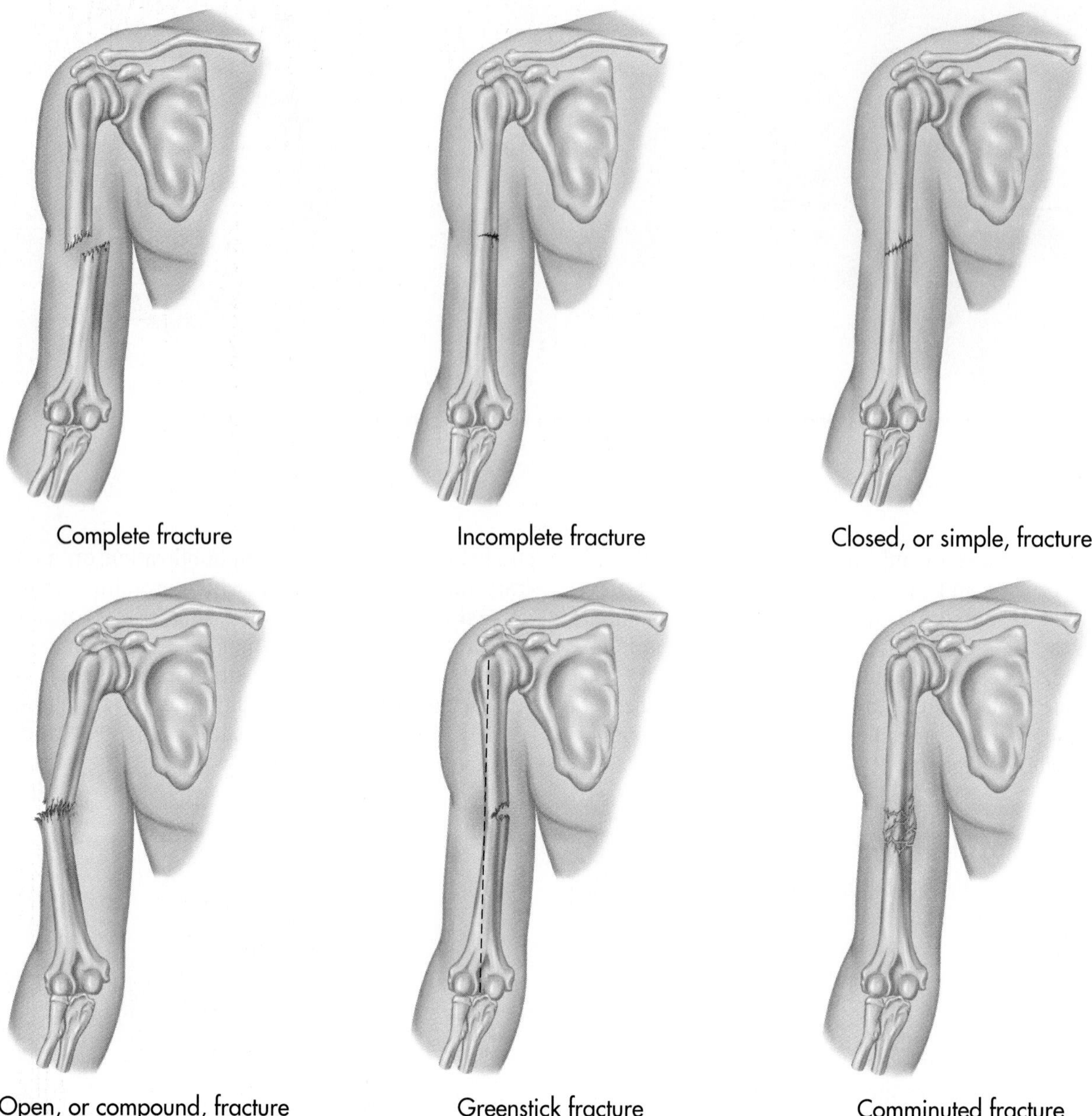

Figure 31-14. These illustrations show various types of fractures.

- Report any of the following to the physician immediately: pain, swelling, discoloration of exposed portions, lack of pulsation and warmth, or the inability to move exposed parts.
- Keep the casted extremity elevated for the first day.
- Avoid indenting the cast until it is completely dry.
- Check the movement and sensation of the visible extremities frequently.
- Restrict strenuous activities for the first few days.
- Avoid allowing the affected limb to hang down for any length of time.
- Do not put anything inside the cast.
- Keep the cast dry.
- Follow the physician's orders regarding restrictions of activities.

Head Injuries

Head injuries include concussions, contusions, fractures, intracranial bleeding, and scalp hematomas and lacerations. Some head injuries can be life-threatening and require immediate medical attention.

Concussion. A **concussion** is a jarring injury to the brain. It is the most common type of head injury. Someone who has a concussion may lose consciousness. Temporary loss of vision, pallor (paleness), listlessness, memory loss, or vomiting can also occur. Symptoms may disappear rapidly or last up to 24 hours. A concussion may produce slow intracranial bleeding. Teach the patient and the patient's family basic precautions after this type of injury. See "Educating the Patient" for more information on concussions.

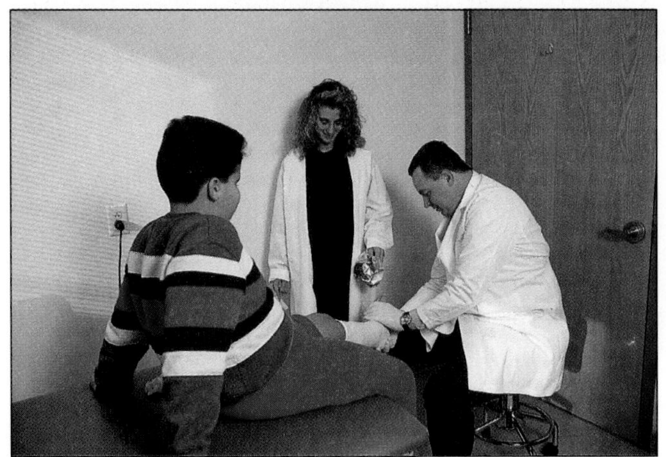

Figure 31-15. Patients should be instructed to keep the cast dry and to notify the physician if they have pain or unusual sensations.

Severe Head Injuries. Contusions, fractures, and intracranial bleeding cause symptoms similar to, but more profound than, symptoms of concussions. Symptoms to look for are leakage of clear or bloody fluid from the ears or nose, seizures, and respiratory arrest. A patient with a severe head injury requires immediate hospitalization. Your priority is to maintain the patient's airway and to begin rescue breathing or CPR if needed.

Scalp Hematomas and Lacerations. A **hematoma** is a swelling caused by blood under the skin. A scalp hematoma causes a bump on the head. This swelling can be reduced by applying ice immediately after the injury. Because blood vessels in the scalp are close to the skin, scalp lacerations often bleed profusely and look worse than they really are. Apply direct pressure to stop bleeding from a scalp laceration, wash the area with soap and water, and apply a dry, sterile dressing over the area.

Hemorrhaging

Hemorrhaging (heavy or uncontrollable bleeding) is generally the result of an injury. It may also be caused by an illness. The first-aid treatment remains the same in both cases. Bleeding can be internal or external. When administering first aid to a patient who may have internal bleeding, cover the patient with a blanket for warmth, keep the patient quiet and calm, and get medical help immediately.

Control external bleeding to prevent rapid blood loss and shock. Use direct pressure, apply additional dressings as needed, elevate the bleeding body part, and put pressure over a pressure point, as described in Procedure 31-4. Then transport the patient to an emergency care facility.

As a last resort, if medical help is more than an hour away, you may need to use a tourniquet (Figure 31-17) to save a person's life. You apply a tourniquet over the main pressure point just above the wound and tighten the tourniquet until the bleeding stops. Many people do not recommend applying a tourniquet in any situation because it may be difficult to judge when a person's life is at stake. Keep in mind that application of a tourniquet to a person's limb almost surely leads to loss of the limb.

Multiple Injuries

Sometimes a patient sustains more than one type of injury—for example, an arm fracture, head injury, lacerations, and internal bleeding. Multiple injuries often result from a car accident or a fall. If you need to assist a patient with multiple injuries, assess the ABCs and perform CPR if needed. Then call (or have someone else call) the EMS system or the physician. Once you have ensured an open airway, breathing, and circulation, perform first aid for the most life-threatening injuries first.

EDUCATING THE PATIENT

Concussion

Because a concussion can cause intracranial bleeding, handle gently a patient who is being treated for this type of injury. If bleeding is slow, it might take up to 24 hours to produce symptoms. Because intracranial bleeding may require brain surgery, use the following patient education guidelines to help ensure patient safety after a concussion.

- Inform the patient that the first 24 hours after the injury are the most critical.
- Tell the patient to refrain from strenuous activity, to rest, and to return to regular activity gradually.
- Instruct the patient to avoid using pain medicines other than acetaminophen, unless the drugs are approved by the physician.
- Advise the patient to eat lightly, especially if nausea and vomiting occur.
- Tell a family member to check on the patient every few hours. The family member should make sure the patient knows his own name, his location, and the name of the family member.
- Instruct the family member to call for medical assistance immediately if the patient shows signs of intracranial bleeding. Signs may include increasing confusion, sluggishness, or irritability; personality changes; seizures; persistent headache; blurred vision; abnormal eye movement; or staggering gait.

PROCEDURE 31-4

Stopping Bleeding

Objective: To stop bleeding and minimize blood loss

OSHA Guidelines

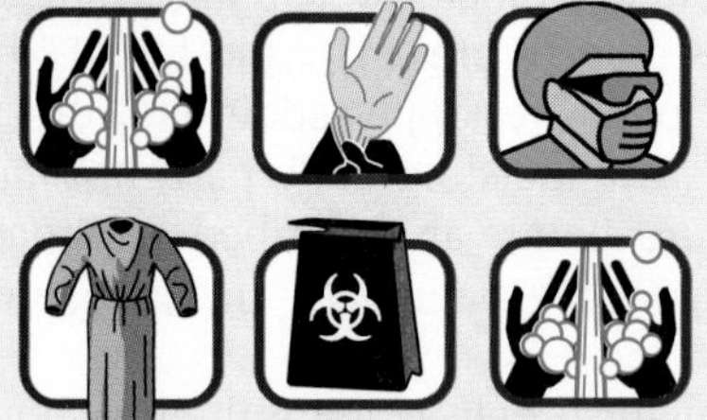

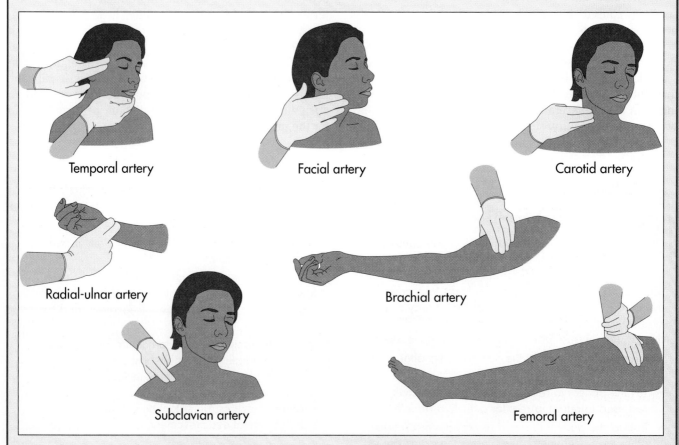

Materials: Clean or sterile dressings

Method

1. If you have time, wash your hands and put on examination gloves, face protection, and a gown to protect yourself from splatters, splashes, and sprays.
2. Using a clean or sterile dressing, apply direct pressure over the wound.
3. If blood soaks through the dressing, do not remove it. Apply an additional dressing over the original one.
4. Elevate the body part that is bleeding.
5. If direct pressure and elevation do not stop the bleeding, apply pressure over the nearest pressure point between the bleeding and the heart (see Figure 31-16). For example, if the wound is on the lower arm, apply pressure on the brachial artery. For a lower-leg wound, apply pressure on the femoral artery in the groin.
6. When the doctor or EMT arrives, assist as requested.
7. After the patient has been transferred to a hospital, properly dispose of contaminated materials.
8. Remove the gloves and wash your hands.

Temporal artery

Facial artery

Carotid artery

Radial-ulnar artery

Brachial artery

Subclavian artery

Femoral artery

Figure 31-16. Apply pressure on these pressure points to stop bleeding.

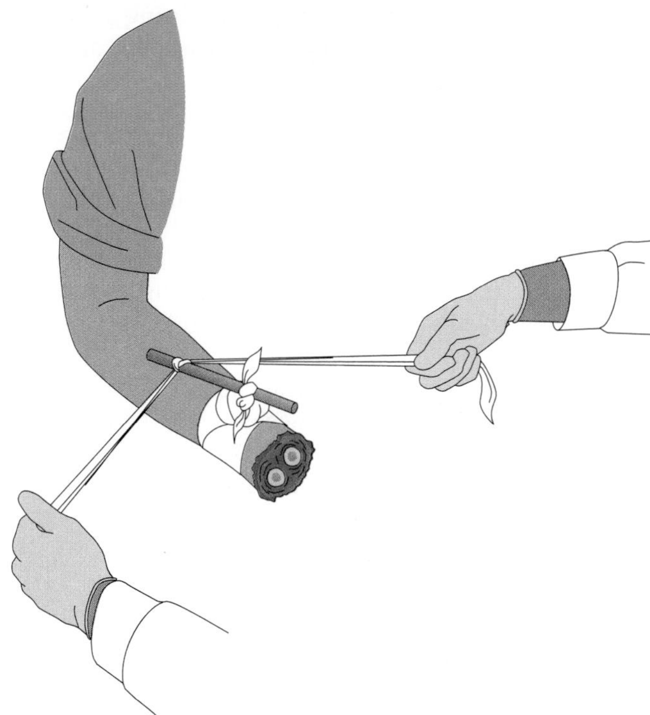

Figure 31-17. Apply a tourniquet only as a last resort, that is, if bleeding cannot be stopped and the patient is likely to die as a result.

Poisoning

A poison is a substance that produces harmful effects if it enters the body. Poisoning is serious and it can result in death or permanent injury if immediate medical care is not provided.

In addition to being able to handle a poisoning emergency, you need to educate patients in how to do the same. You should teach them about the symptoms of and treatment for the different types of poisoning. Provide them with pamphlets that describe the procedures to follow and stickers with the telephone number of the regional poison control center.

The majority of accidental poisonings happen to children under the age of 5. Young children are not necessarily put off by strong smells or burning sensations when they swallow something. Common causes of poisoning in children are household cleaning products, household plants, and medications. Poisons can also be caused by improperly prepared or contaminated food. These types of poisons are ingested, or swallowed.

Poisoning that results from coming in contact with plants, such as poison ivy, poison sumac, and poison oak, is common and generally fairly minor. This type of poisoning is referred to as absorbed poisoning. It can be serious, however, if the poisoning occurs over a large surface of the body.

Poisons can also be inhaled. This situation occurs when a person inhales a poisonous gas such as carbon monoxide or the fumes from burning poisonous plants.

Ingested Poisons. Poison that is swallowed remains in the stomach only a short time. Most of it is absorbed while in the small intestine. Symptoms of poisoning include abdominal pain and cramping; nausea; vomiting; diarrhea; odor, stains, or burns around or in the mouth; drowsiness; and unconsciousness. You should also suspect poisoning if packages containing poisonous substances are near a person who has one or more of these symptoms.

It is extremely important to call a poison control center (if available), hospital emergency room, doctor, or the EMS system for instructions if you think a patient has swallowed a poison. When you call, you will need to know the following:

- The patient's age
- The name of the poison
- The amount of poison swallowed
- When the poison was swallowed
- Whether or not the person has vomited
- How much time it will take to get the patient to a medical facility

Poisons vary in their toxicity. Some cause damage right away, whereas others cause damage several hours later. If the patient is alert and not having convulsions, follow these steps.

1. Call the regional poison control center.
2. Dilute the poison by directing the patient to drink one or two glasses of water or milk as quickly as possible. Assist as needed.
3. Induce vomiting with ipecac syrup if directed by the poison control center.
4. Seek immediate medical attention.

Do not induce vomiting unless directed by a medical authority. The patient may have ingested a strong acid, alkali, or petroleum product, such as chlorine bleach or gasoline. These products may cause further damage to the throat and esophagus during vomiting. If you do not know what the patient ingested, never induce vomiting.

Turn the patient on his left side. This position delays stomach emptying by several hours and prevents aspiration if the patient vomits. Take both poison container and vomited material to the hospital for inspection.

Food poisoning, another type of ingested poisoning, can occur when bacteria produce toxins in food. **Botulism,** for example, results from eating improperly canned or preserved foods that have been contaminated with the bacterium *Clostridium botulinum.* Symptoms appear within 12 to 36 hours after eating contaminated food. Initial symptoms include dry mouth, sore throat, weakness, vomiting, and diarrhea.

Food poisoning is often difficult to detect because the signs and symptoms vary greatly. A patient with food poisoning usually has abdominal pain, nausea, vomiting, gas, frequent bowel sounds, and diarrhea. Chills, joint pain, and excessive sweating may also occur. If you suspect that a patient has food poisoning, call the poison control center, and arrange for immediate transport to the hospital.

Absorbed Poisons. Most people have had the red, itchy rash that results from contact with poison ivy, poison sumac, or poison oak. In some people, however, the rash may be accompanied by a generalized swelling, burning eyes, headache, fever, and abnormal pulse or respirations.

To treat a patient who has come in contact with an absorbed poison, call the regional poison control center. Have the patient immediately remove all contaminated clothing. Then wash the affected skin thoroughly with soap and water, drench it with alcohol, and rinse well. To help relieve symptoms, apply wet compresses soaked with calamine lotion. Also suggest baths in colloidal oatmeal or applications of a paste made from 3 tsp baking soda and 1 tsp water to soothe the itching. If the rash is severe, the doctor may prescribe a corticosteroid ointment. Tell the patient to seek medical assistance if a fever or swelling develops.

Inhaled Poisons. A patient may inhale poisons by breathing air contaminated by chemicals in the workplace or by a malfunctioning stove or furnace in the home. The patient may not realize she has been exposed to a poisonous gas until symptoms arise. Even then, a patient may merely suspect the flu, because some symptoms of inhalation poisoning mimic those of influenza. Common symptoms include headache, tinnitus (ringing in the ears), angina (chest pain), shortness of breath, muscle weakness, nausea, vomiting, confusion, and dizziness, followed by blurred or double vision, difficulty breathing, unconsciousness, and cardiac arrest. Also, a patient who has facial burns may have sustained an inhalation injury.

To treat poisoning by inhalation, first get the patient into fresh air. If you are escorting a patient from a poisoned area, hold your breath to avoid inhaling the poison. Have someone call the EMS system or the regional poison control center. Loosen tight-fitting clothing and wrap the patient in a blanket to prevent shock. Check the ABCs and begin CPR if needed. Expect the EMS team to treat the patient with 100% oxygen.

Carbon monoxide is a major cause of inhalation poisoning in the home. It is a colorless and odorless natural gas produced by incomplete combustion of organic fuels, such as coal, wood, or gasoline. Carbon monoxide is especially dangerous in closed spaces because, when inhaled, it replaces oxygen in the blood. If you suspect carbon monoxide poisoning, look for clues in the environment such as a malfunctioning furnace or a car engine left running in a closed space such as a garage.

Mild carbon monoxide poisoning can cause headache and flulike symptoms without fever. Moderate poisoning may cause tinnitus, drowsiness, severe seizures, coma, and cardiopulmonary problems. Because the gas is odorless, people are often unaware they are being poisoned. They may fall asleep, lapse into unconsciousness, and die.

Sprains and Strains

Sprains and strains often result from sports injuries and accidents. A **sprain** is an injury characterized by partial tearing of a ligament that supports a joint, such as the ankle. A sprain may also involve injuries to tendons, muscles, and local blood vessels and contusions of the surrounding soft tissue. A **strain** is a muscle injury that results from overexertion. For example, back strain may occur when a person carries a heavy load.

Symptoms of a sprain include swelling, tenderness, pain during movement, and local discoloration. If you suspect a sprain, splint the joint, apply ice, and call the EMS system if needed. Inform the patient that an x-ray may be required to confirm that there is no fracture. A strain causes pain on motion. In most cases it should be examined by a physician, who may prescribe rest, application of heat, and a muscle relaxant.

Weather-Related Injuries

Exposure to extreme cold, extreme heat, and the sun's damaging rays can cause weather-related injuries. These injuries may require emergency medical attention.

Frostbite. When body tissues are exposed to below-freezing temperatures, frostbite can occur. Frostbite causes ice crystals to form between tissue cells, and these crystals enlarge as they extract water from the cells. Frostbite also causes obstruction to the blood supply in the form of blood clots. This aspect of frostbite prevents blood from flowing to the tissues and causes additional, severe damage to cells.

Symptoms of frostbite include white, waxy, or grayish yellow skin. The affected body part feels cold, tingling, and painful. The skin surface may feel crusty and the underlying tissue soft in comparison. If the frostbite is deep, the body part may feel cold and hard and not be sensitive to pain. Blisters may appear after rewarming.

Treat frostbite by wrapping warm clothing or blankets around the affected body part or placing it in contact with another body part that is warm. Do not rub or massage the affected area, or you may cause further damage to the frozen tissue. Call for medical assistance. If you are in a remote area, use the wet rapid rewarming method. This method involves placing the affected part in warm (100° to 104°F) water. Hot water should be added at regular intervals to keep the temperature of the bath stable. As an alternative method, you can heat the affected area with warm compresses. Because warming may cause pain, administer aspirin or acetaminophen. Continue rewarming for 20 to 40 minutes. After the affected area becomes soft, place dry, sterile gauze between skin surfaces, such as between the toes or the fingers or between the ear and the side of the head. Do not massage the skin or break blisters.

Heatstroke. Heatstroke results from prolonged exposure to high temperatures and humidity. This condition may lead to excessive loss of fluids (dehydration) and insufficient blood in the circulatory system (hypovolemic shock). High body temperature can damage tissues and organs throughout the body. If untreated, the patient will die. People most susceptible to heatstroke are children, the elderly, athletes, and patients who are obese, are diabetic, or have circulatory problems or other chronic illnesses.

Symptoms of heatstroke include hot, dry skin; high body temperature; altered mental state; rapid pulse; rapid breathing; dizziness; and weakness. If you suspect that a patient has heatstroke, check the patient's ABCs, and call the EMS system. Move the patient to a cool place, and remove outer clothing unless it is made of light cotton or other light fabric. Also, cool the patient with any means available, such as gentle spraying with a hose, movement to an air-conditioned place, vigorous fanning, or application of a wet sheet. If the humidity is above 75%, place ice packs on the patient's groin and armpits. Stop cooling when the patient's mental state improves. Keep the patient's head and shoulders slightly elevated.

Sunburn. Do not dismiss a sunburn as trivial. It is a burn that can cause redness, tenderness, pain, swelling, blisters, and peeling skin. It can lead to skin damage or cancer later in life.

Soak sunburned skin in cool water to help reduce the heat. Apply cold compresses, and later calamine lotion, to bring relief from the burning sensation. Have the patient elevate the legs and arms to prevent swelling. The patient should also drink plenty of water and take a pain reliever.

Educate the patient about the importance of using sunscreen and reapplying it every 2 to 3 hours when outdoors. Advise the patient to stay out of direct sunlight between 10:00 A.M. and 2:00 P.M., because the sun's rays are strongest during that period.

Wounds

A wound is an injury in which the skin or tissues under the skin are damaged. Wounds can be either open or closed. Figure 31-18 shows the various types of wounds.

Open Wounds. An open wound is a break in the skin or mucous membrane. Types of open wounds include incisions, lacerations, abrasions, and punctures.

Incisions and Lacerations. An incision is a clean and smooth cut, such as that from a kitchen knife. A laceration has jagged edges, as may result when a child steps on a piece of broken glass in the sand at the beach. Care of

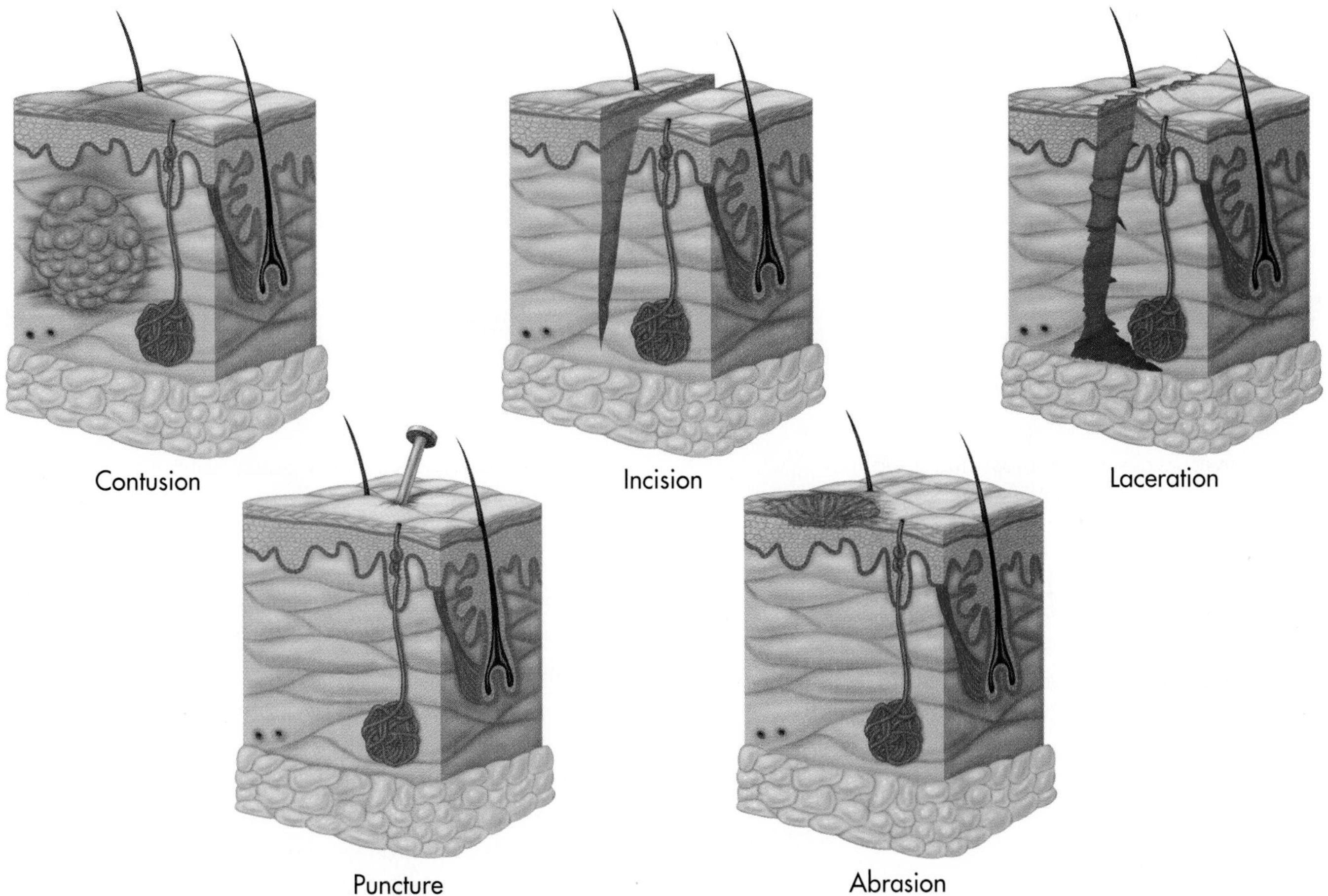

Figure 31-18. Different types of wounds produce different degrees of tissue damage.

minor incisions and lacerations involves controlling bleeding by covering the wound with a clean or sterile dressing and applying direct pressure. After the bleeding stops, clean and dress the wound. Procedure 31-5 explains how to clean minor wounds. Teach the patient the importance of keeping the wound clean and checking for signs of infection, such as heat, redness, pain, and swelling.

If the wound is deep and involves muscle, tendons, the face, the genitals, the mouth, or the tongue, control the bleeding with direct pressure to the wound (with a sterile dressing or clean cloth held against its surface), elevation, and use of pressure points. Contact the doctor and, if necessary, the EMS system.

Abrasions. An abrasion is a scraping of the skin, as when someone slides across gravel during a softball game. Abrasions require washing with soap and water. Be sure to remove all the dirt and debris to prevent tattooing (dark discoloration under the skin). Minor abrasions do not need a dressing or bandage, but large ones do. Various types of bandaging are shown in Figure 31-19. As with any wound, teach the patient to watch for signs of infection.

Punctures. A puncture wound is a small hole created by a piercing object, such as a bullet, knife, nail, or animal tooth. Puncture wounds are a potential breeding ground for tetanus bacteria, because the bacteria can live and thrive in the absence of oxygen. Allow the wound to bleed freely for a few minutes to help wash out bacteria. Then clean the wound with soap and water, and apply a dry, sterile dressing. If the patient has not had a tetanus toxoid immunization in the past 7 to 10 years, inform the physician so that one can be ordered.

Closed Wounds. A closed wound is an injury that occurs inside the body without breaking the skin. Closed wounds, which are usually called **contusions** (bruises), are caused by a blunt object striking the tissue. This action produces broken blood vessels and internal, localized bleeding (hematoma) below the area that has been struck. Treat such a wound with cold compresses to reduce swelling. The affected area will turn from black and blue to green to yellow as blood pigments oxidize. Inform the patient that these color changes are part of the normal healing process.

Common Illnesses

A variety of common illnesses frequently call for emergency medical intervention. As a patient educator, you can help ensure that patients recognize the symptoms of these illnesses and know when to call for medical assistance. Teaching patients the importance of following physician's orders for follow-up care is also your responsibility. Common illnesses include the following:

- Abdominal pain
- Asthma
- Dehydration
- Diarrhea
- Fainting
- Fever
- Hyperventilation
- Nosebleed
- Tachycardia
- Vomiting

Abdominal Pain

Acute abdominal pain that occurs suddenly and is accompanied by fever may indicate an emergency that requires surgery. The pain may involve spasmodic contrac-

PROCEDURE 31-5

Cleaning Minor Wounds

Objective: To clean and dress minor wounds

OSHA Guidelines

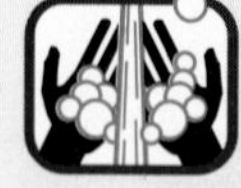
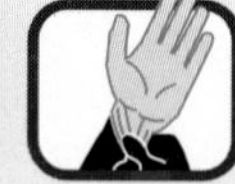

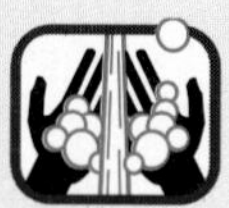

Materials: Sterile gauze squares, basin, antiseptic soap, warm water, sterile dressing

Method

1. Wash your hands and put on examination gloves.
2. Dip several gauze squares in a basin of warm, soapy water.
3. Wash the wound from the center outward to avoid bringing contaminants from the surrounding skin into the wound. Use a new gauze square for each cleansing motion.
4. As you wash, remove debris that could cause infection.
5. Rinse the area thoroughly, preferably by placing the wound under warm, running water.
6. Pat the wound dry with sterile gauze squares.
7. Cover the wound with a dry, sterile dressing. Bandage the dressing in place.
8. Properly dispose of contaminated materials.
9. Remove the gloves and wash your hands.
10. Instruct the patient on wound care.
11. Record the procedure in the patient's chart.

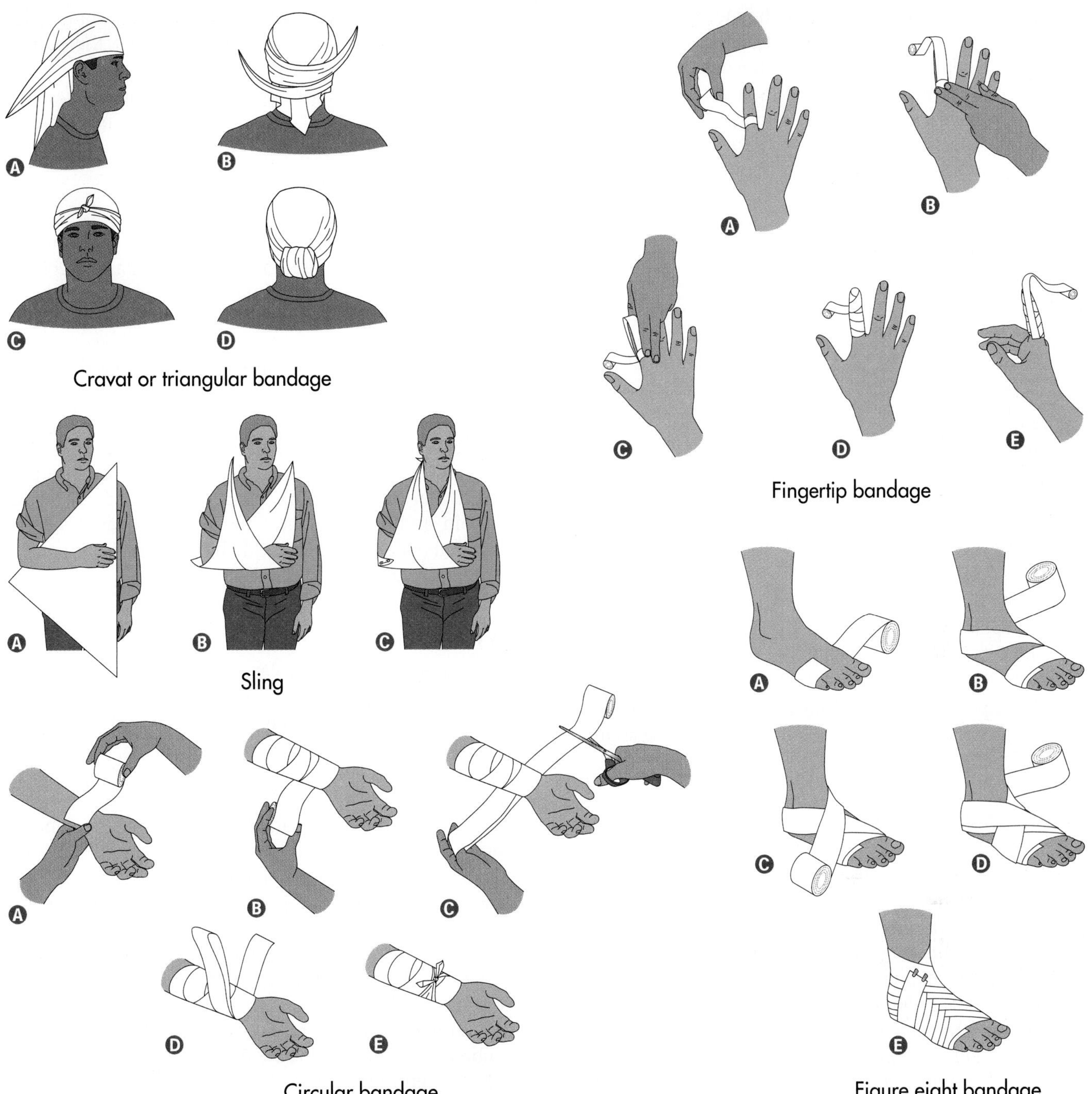

Figure 31-19. Apply a bandage, as needed, to a wound.

tions. It may feel knifelike or ache dully, and it may be localized or may radiate. The location of the pain gives clues to its cause. Acute pain in the right upper quadrant, for example, may signal a gallbladder attack. Pain in the right lower quadrant may indicate appendicitis.

Other causes include internal hemorrhage, intestinal perforation or obstruction, peptic ulcer, and hernia. In women, pelvic pain can indicate a gynecologic problem. Obviously, trauma to the area, such as wounds or blows, can produce acute abdominal pain.

While waiting for patient transport, have the patient lie on his back with his knees flexed (unless there is a wound or swelling in the abdomen). This position lets the abdominal muscles relax. Keep the patient quiet and warm, and act calm and concerned. Do not give anything by mouth, and keep an emesis basin handy in case the patient vomits. Do not apply heat to the abdomen because heat may exacerbate inflammation. Monitor the patient's pulse and consciousness, and check for signs of shock.

Asthma

Asthma is a common disorder caused by spasmodic narrowing of the bronchi. It is often an inherited tendency—that is, several members of one family may suffer from it. A patient who is having an acute attack wheezes, coughs, and is short of breath. She may become frightened and feel as if she cannot get enough air. If you spot an asthma attack, check the patient's ABCs, and notify the doctor at once. You may assist the patient in using a respiratory inhaler if she carries one with her. If directed, administer a mininebulizer treatment with a bronchodilator (drug that opens the bronchi), such as albuterol (Proventil) or epinephrine.

Dehydration

Dehydration results from a lack of adequate water in the body. The body's fluid intake is not sufficient to meet its fluid needs. Severe dehydration can result from vomiting, excessive heat and sweating, diarrhea, or lack of food or fluid intake. The following are symptoms of dehydration:

- Extreme thirst
- Tiredness
- Light-headedness
- Abdominal or muscle cramping
- Confusion (especially in elderly people)

Perform the following steps to administer first aid to a dehydrated person.

1. Move the victim into the shade or to a cool area.
2. To replace lost fluids, give the victim water, tea, fruit juice, a commercial electrolyte replacement fluid, or clear broth.
3. If symptoms persist or are accompanied by nausea, diarrhea, or convulsions, call for the EMS system or a physician.

Diarrhea (Acute)

Acute diarrhea can be caused by an intestinal infection, food poisoning, a bowel disorder, or the side effects of medication. Severe diarrhea causes dehydration and dangerous electrolyte imbalances that can lead to shock. Symptoms of shock include rapid pulse, low blood pressure, and pale, clammy skin.

Help the patient lie on his back and elevate his legs. Report the patient's condition to the doctor. As directed, prepare to assist in administering intravenous fluids to correct dehydration and restore electrolytes and to draw blood for testing.

Fainting (Syncope)

Fainting, or syncope, is a partial or complete loss of consciousness. It usually follows a decrease in the amount of blood flow to the brain. Before fainting, patients may feel weak, dizzy, cold, or nauseated. They may perspire or look pale and anxious.

If you are with a patient who feels as if she is going to faint, tell her to lower her head between her legs and to breathe deeply. Stay with her until the feeling passes. If the patient is having difficulty breathing or faints, lay her flat on her back with her feet slightly elevated. Loosen tight clothing and apply a cold cloth to her face. Observe the patient carefully, monitoring her breathing and level of consciousness. Observe for weakness in her arms and legs. Let her rest for at least 10 minutes after she regains full consciousness. Notify the physician that the patient fainted.

If your efforts do not revive a patient who has fainted, call the physician and the EMS system. The patient may be slipping into a coma.

Fever

Fever is a common clinical sign that often indicates infection. Mild or moderate fever can accompany a cold or an upset stomach. It can usually be managed with aspirin or acetaminophen. A fever of 106°F or higher (hyperthermia) is dangerous, however, because irreversible brain damage can occur if the fever is not lowered immediately.

If a patient's temperature is dangerously high, you must proceed at once to check the other vital signs and the level of consciousness. Notify the doctor and be prepared to start rapid cooling measures. Place ice packs on the groin and axilla, or give the patient a tepid sponge bath. If the patient is a child, be prepared to manage seizures (discussed later in this chapter).

Hyperventilation

Some patients who are under a great deal of stress lack the skills to deal with the stress effectively. They may seem anxious, frazzled, and more emotional than average patients. Patients under stress may begin to hyperventilate, or breathe too rapidly and too deeply. This breathing disturbs the normal balance of oxygen and carbon dioxide in the blood, and the carbon dioxide concentration falls below normal levels. Patients who are hyperventilating may also feel light-headed and as if they cannot get enough air. In addition, they may have chest pain and feel apprehensive.

Move a hyperventilating patient to a quiet area. Have the patient breathe into a paper bag, sealed tightly around the nose and mouth. Coach the patient to take slow, normal breaths. This procedure causes the patient to rebreathe exhaled carbon dioxide so that blood gas levels can return to normal.

Nosebleed

Nosebleed, or **epistaxis,** can occur for a variety of reasons. They include blowing the nose too hard, local irritation or dryness, frequent sneezing, fragile or superficial blood vessels, high blood pressure, a blow to the nose, and a foreign body in the nose. Nosebleeds are common in children, especially at night.

Treat a nosebleed by having the patient sit up with the head tilted forward to prevent blood from running down the back of the throat. Next, have the patient gently pinch the nostrils shut at the bottom for at least 5 minutes. If that does not stop the bleeding, apply an ice pack or cold compress to the nose and face, and continue to pinch the nostrils. If the bleeding cannot be controlled, arrange for transport to the office or to a hospital for cauterization or nasal packing.

Tachycardia

Tachycardia is a rapid heart rate, generally in excess of 100 beats per minute. A patient with tachycardia may report having **palpitations,** unusually rapid, strong, or irregular pulsations of the heart. He may feel as if his heart is pounding. Help the patient lie down, take his vital signs, and if instructed, obtain an electrocardiogram (ECG). (Electrocardiography is discussed in Chapter 39.) If tachycardia is accompanied by low blood pressure and light-headedness, notify the physician immediately. These symptoms indicate that the patient could faint or go into shock. Remain with the patient and keep him calm. If directed, obtain another ECG.

Vomiting

Vomiting is a symptom common to many disorders, ranging from food poisoning to various infections. When severe, it can lead to dehydration and dangerous changes in electrolyte levels, especially in patients who are very young, very old, or diabetic or who also have diarrhea. Because these problems can be severe, notify the doctor and provide appropriate care. Procedure 31-6 describes how to provide emergency care for a patient who is vomiting.

Less Common Illnesses

Even though some illnesses are less common than those previously discussed, you should still be familiar enough with them so that you can handle them effectively if a physician or EMT is not immediately available. Educate patients about symptoms they may encounter that require emergency medical intervention, as well as how important follow-up care is when they are recovering from such illnesses. Less common illnesses that may require emergency medical intervention include the following:

- Anaphylaxis
- Bacterial meningitis
- Diabetic emergencies
- Gallbladder attack
- Heart attack
- Hematemesis
- Obstetric emergencies
- Respiratory arrest
- Seizures
- Shock
- Stroke
- Toxic shock syndrome
- Viral encephalitis

PROCEDURE 31-6

Caring for a Patient Who Is Vomiting

Objective: To increase comfort and minimize complications, such as aspiration, for a patient who is vomiting

OSHA Guidelines

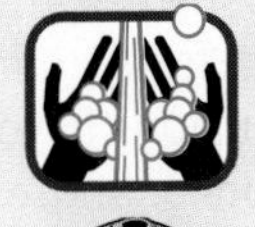
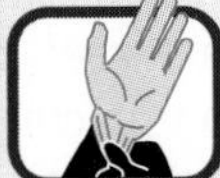

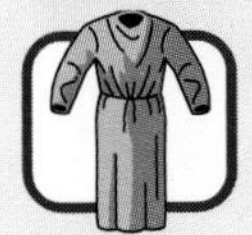
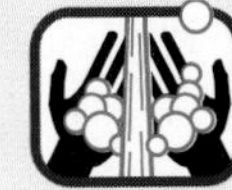

Materials: Emesis basin, cool compress, cup of cool water, paper tissues or a towel, and (if ordered) intravenous fluids and electrolytes and an antinausea drug

Method

1. Wash your hands and put on examination gloves and other PPE.
2. Ask the patient when and how the vomiting started and how frequently it occurs. Find out whether she is nauseated or in pain.
3. Give the patient an emesis basin to collect vomit. Observe and document its amount, color, odor, and consistency. Particularly note blood, bile, undigested food, or feces in the vomit.
4. Place a cool compress on the patient's forehead to make her more comfortable. Offer water and paper tissues or a towel to clean her mouth.
5. Monitor for signs of dehydration, such as confusion, irritability, and flushed, dry skin. Also monitor for signs of electrolyte imbalances, such as leg cramps or an irregular pulse.
6. If requested, assist by laying out supplies and equipment for the physician to use in administering intravenous fluids and electrolytes. Administer an antinausea drug if prescribed.
7. Prepare the patient for diagnostic tests if instructed.
8. Remove the gloves and wash your hands.

Anaphylaxis

Anaphylaxis, or anaphylactic shock, is a severe, often life-threatening allergic reaction. The reaction can be immediate or delayed up to 2 hours. It happens to people who have become sensitized to certain substances. For example, it can result from eating a type of food, being stung by an insect, or taking a particular type of medication, such as penicillin.

The first sign of anaphylaxis usually comes from the patient's skin. It becomes itchy, turns red, feels hot, and develops hives. The face may also become puffy. The throat may swell so that the patient has trouble breathing and swallowing and feels as if he has a "lump in the throat." Other symptoms include pallor, perspiration, and a weak, rapid, irregular pulse. If you detect these symptoms or if the patient becomes restless, has a headache, or says that his throat feels as if it is closing up, take the following steps immediately.

Check the ABCs and then notify the doctor. As directed, administer epinephrine, oral antihistamines, and oxygen, and help the patient sit up. After the patient receives epinephrine, monitor his vital signs every 2 to 3 minutes. Note skin color and monitor the airway. If he does not recover quickly, arrange for immediate transport to the hospital.

When severely allergic patients stabilize, the doctor prescribes an epinephrine autoinjector for patients to carry with them. You are responsible for teaching patients how to use this device. See "Educating the Patient" in Chapter 38 for directions.

Because of the possibility of anaphylaxis, a patient who has just received any type of injection should routinely be kept in the office for 20 to 30 minutes of observation. This procedure reduces the possibility that an allergic reaction to the medication will occur while the patient is unattended.

A less severe allergic reaction to drugs or certain foods may cause sneezing, itching, slight swelling of the skin, rash, or hives. This type of reaction can usually be controlled with diphenhydramine hydrochloride (Benadryl) or another antihistamine. The patient should be monitored closely, however, to make sure the condition does not progress to anaphylaxis.

Bacterial Meningitis

Bacterial meningitis is almost always a complication of another bacterial infection, such as otitis media (middle ear infection) or pneumonia. Therefore, first find out whether the patient currently has or recently has had a bacterial infection. The signs of bacterial meningitis are fever, chills, headache, and vomiting. If the patient has these signs and then develops a fever of 102°F, becomes less alert, has altered respirations, or experiences seizures, the infection has progressed to a dangerous state.

If these signs are present, assess the ABCs and notify the physician of the change in the patient's condition. Expect to arrange for transport to the hospital, where the patient will be treated with intravenous antibiotics.

Diabetic Emergencies

Diabetes is a fairly common disorder of carbohydrate metabolism (see Chapter 28). The body needs insulin, a hormone secreted by the pancreas, to use blood sugar to fuel body cells. Insulin secretion is impaired in patients with diabetes.

You can teach patients who have diabetes or who are at risk for diabetes how to recognize early signs of **hypoglycemia** (low blood sugar) and **hyperglycemia** (high blood sugar) before these conditions become medical emergencies. Symptoms of hypoglycemia include dizziness; headache; hunger; weakness; full, rapid pulse; and pallor. Symptoms of hyperglycemia include dry mouth, intense thirst, muscle weakness, and blurred vision. You should also be familiar with the signs and symptoms of the two most common diabetic emergencies you will encounter: insulin shock and diabetic coma.

Insulin Shock. Insulin shock is basically very severe hypoglycemia, in which a patient has too little sugar in the blood. Insulin shock occurs when insulin levels are so high that they move too much sugar from the blood into cells. Symptoms include rapid pulse; shallow respiration; hunger; profuse sweating; pale, cool, clammy skin; double vision; tremors; restlessness; confusion; and possibly fainting. Insulin shock can usually be corrected with administration of some form of sugar (candy, juice, or regular soda for a conscious patient or a sprinkle of table sugar on the tongue for an unconscious patient). If the cause of a diabetic emergency is unknown, give sugar. Patients will improve quickly if the cause is insulin shock and will not be harmed if the cause is diabetic coma, provided they are then transported to the hospital.

Diabetic Coma. Diabetic coma is the end result of severe hyperglycemia, in which a patient has too much sugar in the blood. It occurs when insulin levels are insufficient to move blood sugar into body cells. Its symptoms include rapid, deep gulping breaths; flushed, warm, dry skin; thirst; acetone breath (a sweet or fruity odor from the mouth); and disorientation or confusion. If you suspect diabetic coma, notify the doctor at once, and expect to arrange transport to the hospital.

Gallbladder Attack (Acute)

A classic acute gallbladder attack occurs after a person eats a high-fat meal rich in cholesterol. The patient may wake up in the night with acute abdominal pain (gallbladder colic) in the right upper quadrant. The pain is caused by inflammation of the gallbladder, usually related to gallstones obstructing the cystic duct, through which bile is secreted by the gallbladder. The pain may radiate to the back between the shoulder blades or be localized in the epigastric region (the upper central region of the abdomen) and the front chest area. The at-

MULTISKILL FOCUS

CPR Instructor

To gain medical assistant credentials, you must fulfill the requirements of either the American Association of Medical Assistants (for a Certified Medical Assistant) or the American Medical Technologists (for a Registered Medical Assistant). After obtaining your medical assistant certification or registration, you may wish to acquire additional skills in specialty areas through course work or on-the-job training. Although this course work or training may not lead to an additional certification or degree, it will enable you to expand your role in the medical office and advance your career as the demand for multiskilled health professionals increases.

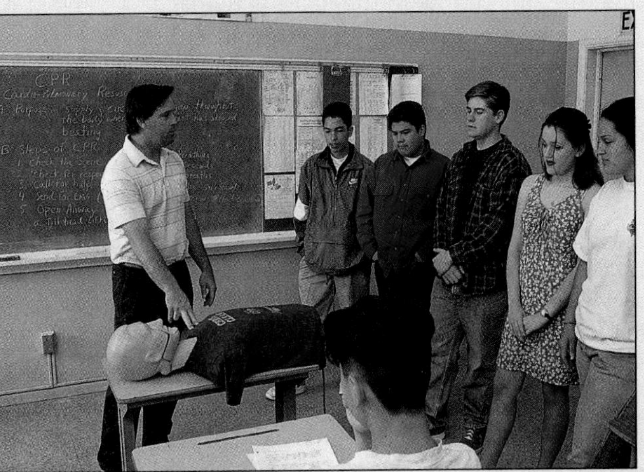

Skills and Duties

A CPR (cardiopulmonary resuscitation) instructor provides people with the knowledge and skills necessary to help save a person's life in an emergency. He teaches his students how to:

- Call for help.
- Help sustain life.
- Reduce pain.
- Minimize the consequences of injury or sudden illness until professional medical help arrives.

To teach a CPR class, an instructor must plan and coordinate the course in conjunction with a local American Red Cross unit or American Heart Association affiliate. He demonstrates the appropriate skills to his students and observes their technique. He then provides constructive feedback as they learn skills and make decisions regarding the appropriate action to take in an emergency.

The instructor is responsible for identifying participants who are having difficulty with the skills. He must develop effective strategies to help these students meet the course objectives. At the end of the course, the CPR instructor submits completed course records to the local American Red Cross chapter or American Heart Association affiliate.

Workplace Settings

CPR instructors teach classes in a variety of settings, including schools and universities, community rooms, camps, religious institutions, and medical clinics. Some employers, such as operators of swimming pools, camps, and day-care facilities, may require CPR instruction as a condition of employment.

Education

To be certified as a CPR instructor by the Red Cross, you must be at least 17 years old. In addition, you must complete two Red Cross courses. The first, the instructor candidate training course, provides instruction in teaching methods, evaluation, and reporting. After completing this course, you will be awarded an instructor candidate training certificate, which qualifies you to take the first aid and CPR instructor course. You must then pass a written test with a grade of 80% or better to gain certification. CPR instructors must teach one class every 2 years for recertification from the Red Cross.

The American Heart Association also provides training for CPR instructors. You must first pass the basic life support course for health-care providers, which teaches CPR skills. You then must take the instructor course, which covers teaching methods. After passing the instructor course, you must coteach a CPR class with an experienced instructor, who will monitor your performance. You will then become an approved instructor. CPR instructors affiliated with the American Heart Association are required to teach a minimum of two classes a year. The association has no minimum age to become an instructor.

CPR instructors may be paid or work as volunteers. There is no specific salary range for the job.

Where to Go for More Information

American Heart Association
National Center
7272 Greenville Avenue
Dallas, TX 75231-4596
(800) 242-8721, or call your local center

American Red Cross
17th and D Streets, NW
Washington, DC 20006
(202) 728-6400, or call your local chapter

tack may be accompanied by nausea and vomiting. The pain is usually so severe that the patient seeks medical attention; many patients think they are having a heart attack.

Gallbladder attacks caused by gallstones are more common among women who are over 40 and obese, and the frequency of attacks increases with age (especially after age 65). Diagnosis is usually made with the help of ultrasonography. The patient may require surgery to remove the gallstones.

Heart Attack

A heart attack, or **myocardial infarction** (MI), occurs when the blood flow to the heart is reduced as a result of blockage in the coronary arteries or their branches. Chest pain is the cardinal symptom of a heart attack. The patient may describe the pain as crushing, burning, heavy, aching, or like that of indigestion. The pain may radiate down the left arm or into the jaw, throat, or both shoulders. It may be accompanied by shortness of breath, sweating, nausea, and vomiting. The patient may be pale and have a feeling of doom. If you cannot easily detect pallor (paleness) because the patient has dark skin, check the patient's inner lip for paleness. Elderly patients may experience atypical symptoms of a heart attack, such as jaw pain, because responses to pain diminish during the aging process. The pain of a heart attack is not relieved by nitroglycerin.

If you think a patient is having a heart attack, notify the physician and EMS system immediately. Do not let the patient walk. Loosen tight clothing and have the patient sit up to aid breathing. The physician may order you to administer oxygen at 4 to 6 L per minute; make sure that no one in the area is smoking. Stay with the patient, observe the ABCs, and begin CPR if required. If directed, obtain an ECG. Take apical and radial pulses, as instructed by the physician. Be prepared to obtain medication from the crash cart.

Hematemesis

Hematemesis is the vomiting of blood. A patient who vomits bright red blood may have a gastrointestinal disorder, such as a bleeding ulcer. A patient who vomits blood that looks like coffee grounds may have slow bleeding into the stomach.

Quickly check the vital signs of a patient with hematemesis. If pulse and breathing are rapid and blood pressure is low, the patient may be going into shock. Notify the doctor immediately, and get the crash cart to help the doctor start an intravenous line to replace lost fluid. Then call the EMS system.

Obstetric Emergencies

If you work in an obstetric practice, you may see emergencies that are unique to this specialty. Although the physician handles most obstetric emergencies, you can assist by asking the patient specific questions about her problem so that the physician can decide what treatment is necessary.

Set up written protocols to handle these situations. For example, if the patient calls from home and reports gushing vaginal bleeding, your protocol may be to call the EMS system for her and tell her to lie down with her feet elevated. If the patient has a miscarriage, have her bring the expelled tissue with her to the office or hospital.

If you work in an obstetrician's office, you must also know how to assist a physician with an emergency childbirth. If there is no physician present when the emergency occurs, however, whether it is inside or outside the office, summon help and begin the procedure on your own. Never try to delay delivery when a birth is imminent. Procedure 31-7 describes how to assist with an emergency childbirth.

Respiratory Arrest

Respiratory arrest, or lack of breathing, is usually preceded by symptoms of respiratory distress. Symptoms include difficulty breathing, rapid breathing, palpitations, racing pulse, high or low blood pressure, sweating, pale or bluish skin, and decreasing level of consciousness. If a patient shows these symptoms, notify the doctor right away. If the patient develops respiratory arrest, have someone call the doctor and the EMS system while you perform CPR, as described in Procedure 31-3.

Seizures

A **seizure,** or convulsion, is a series of violent and involuntary contractions of the muscles. Seizures are usually related to brain malfunctions that can result from diseased or injured brain tissues. A seizure may be caused by high fever, epilepsy (a brain disorder that causes seizures with varying severity), meningitis, diabetic states, and many other medical problems.

Follow this emergency care for seizure patients.

1. Remove objects that may cause injury.
2. Place the patient on the floor or the ground. If possible, position him on his side with his head turned to the side to help keep the airway open and unobstructed by the tongue. This position is especially important if the patient vomits, to prevent aspiration of vomitus into the lungs.
3. Loosen restrictive clothing.
4. Protect the patient from injury, but do not try to hold him still during convulsions.
5. After convulsions end, keep the patient at rest, positioned for drainage from the mouth.
6. Make sure the patient is breathing. If he is not, begin rescue breathing.
7. Take vital signs and monitor respirations closely.
8. Move the patient to an examination room, or have him taken to a medical facility.

Shock

Generally speaking, shock is a life-threatening state associated with failure of the cardiovascular system. It can bring to a stop all normal metabolic functions. This condition prevents the vital organs from receiving blood.

Early symptoms of shock include restlessness; irritability; fear; rapid pulse; pale, cool skin; and increased respiratory rate. Treat a patient in shock by elevating the feet 8 to 12 inches. If you suspect a head injury, however, keep the patient flat or elevate the head and shoulders slightly. Monitor the ABCs and take steps to control

PROCEDURE 31-7

Assisting With Emergency Childbirth

Objective: To assist in performing an emergency childbirth

OSHA Guidelines

Materials: Clean cloths, sterile or clean sheets or towels, two sterile clamps or two pieces of string boiled in water for at least 10 minutes, sterile scissors, plastic bag, soft blankets or towels

Method

1. Ask the woman her name and age, how far apart her contractions are (about two per minute signals that the birth is near), if her water has broken, and if she feels straining or pressure as if the baby is coming.
2. Help remove the woman's lower clothing.
3. Explain that you are about to do a visual inspection to see if the baby's head is in position. Ask the woman to lie on her back with her thighs spread, her knees flexed, and her feet flat. Examine her to see if there is crowning (a bulging at the vaginal opening from the baby's head) (see Figure 31-20).
4. If the head is crowning, childbirth is imminent. Place clean cloths under the woman's buttocks, and use sterile sheets or towels (if they are available) to cover her legs and stomach.
5. Wash your hands thoroughly and put on examination gloves. If other PPE is available, put it on now.
6. At this point the physician would begin to take steps to deliver the baby, and you would position yourself at the woman's head to provide emotional support and help in case she vomited. If no physician is available, you may have to proceed on your own. In that case position yourself at the woman's side so that you have a constant view of the vaginal opening.
7. Talk to the woman and encourage her to relax between contractions while allowing the delivery to proceed naturally.
8. Position your gloved hands at the woman's vaginal opening when the baby's head starts to appear. Do not touch her skin.
9. Place one hand below the baby's head as it is delivered. Spread your fingers evenly around the baby's head to support it so that it does not touch the mother's anal area. Use your other hand to help cradle the baby's head (see Figure 31-21). Never pull on the baby.
10. If the umbilical cord is wrapped around the baby's neck, gently loosen the cord and slide it over the baby's head.
11. If the amniotic sac has not broken by the time the baby's head is delivered, use your finger to puncture the membrane. Then pull the membranes away from the baby's mouth and nose.

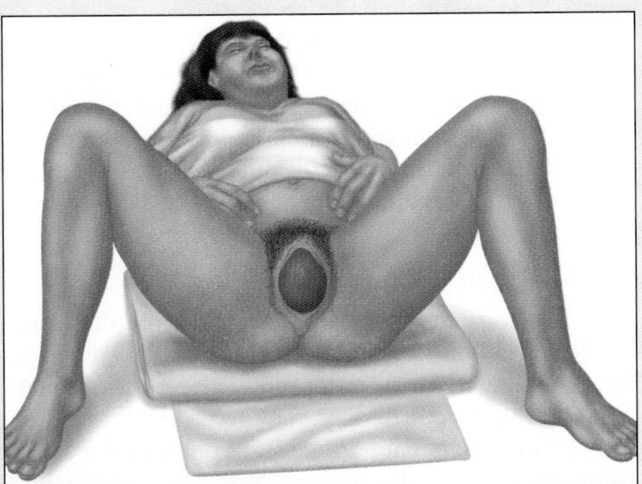

Figure 31-20. Crowning occurs when part of the baby's head becomes visible with each contraction.

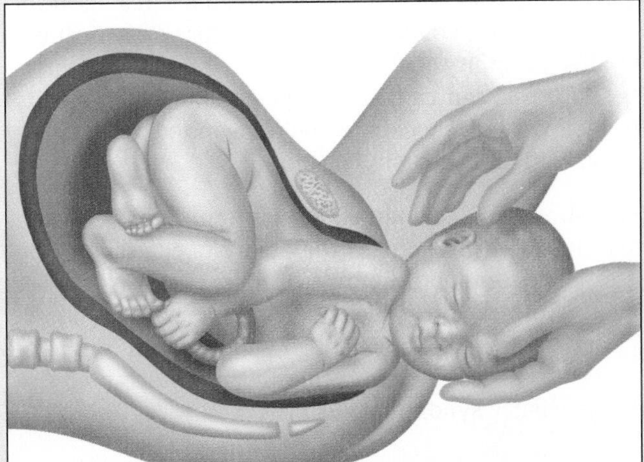

Figure 31-21. Support the baby's head with one hand while using the other hand to cradle the baby's head.

continued

PROCEDURE 31-7 continued

12. Wipe blood or mucus from the baby's mouth with a clean cloth.
13. Continue to support the baby's head as the shoulders emerge. The upper shoulder will deliver first, followed quickly by the lower shoulder.
14. After the feet are delivered, lay the baby on his side with the head slightly lower than the body. Keep the baby at the same level as the mother until you cut the umbilical cord.
15. If the baby is not breathing, lower the head, raise the lower part of the body, and tap the soles of the feet. If the baby is still not breathing, begin rescue breathing through the mouth and nose as directed in this chapter.
16. To cut the cord, wait several minutes, until pulsations stop. Use the clamps or pieces of string to tie the cord in two places: 6 inches from the baby and again about 12 inches from the baby (Figure 31-22).
17. Use sterilized scissors to cut the cord in between the placement of the two clamps or pieces of string.
18. Within 10 minutes of the baby's birth, the placenta will begin to expel. Save it in a plastic bag for further examination.
19. Keep the mother and baby warm by wrapping them in towels or blankets. Do not touch the baby any more than necessary.
20. Massage the mother's abdomen just below the navel every few minutes to control internal bleeding.
21. Arrange for transport of the mother and baby to the hospital.

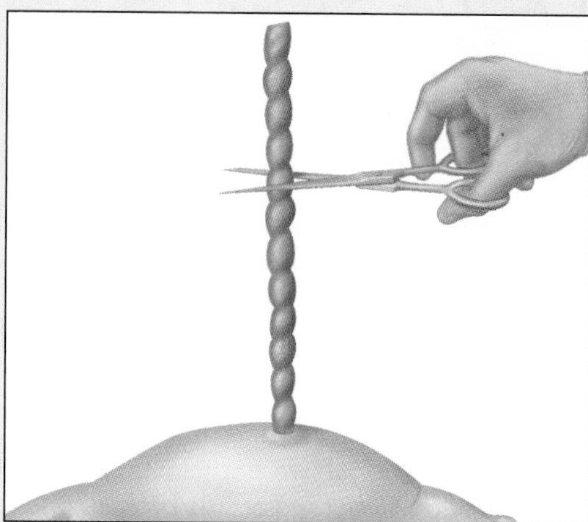

Figure 31-22. The infant must be breathing on his own before you clamp (or tie) and cut the umbilical cord.

bleeding. If the patient is chilly, wrap the patient in a blanket. Call the EMS system.

Several types of shock are possible. Anaphylactic shock, or anaphylaxis, is usually associated with an allergic reaction, as previously discussed. Hypovolemic shock and septic shock are two other types of shock.

Hypovolemic Shock. **Hypovolemic shock** results from insufficient blood volume in the circulatory system. It occurs after an injury that causes major fluid loss. Hemorrhage or burns can cause this type of fluid loss. Patients with hypovolemic shock must be transported to an emergency facility immediately.

Septic Shock. **Septic shock** results from massive, widespread infection that affects the ability of the blood vessels to circulate blood. Common causes are urinary tract infection (especially in older adults), postpartum infection, and a variety of infections in patients with immunosuppression (as caused by chemotherapy or acquired immunodeficiency syndrome [AIDS]).

Stroke

A stroke, or cerebrovascular accident (CVA), occurs when the blood supply to the brain is impaired. This impairment may cause temporary or permanent damage, depending on how long the brain cells are deprived of oxygen.

A minor stroke can cause headache, confusion, dizziness, tinnitus, minor speech difficulties, personality changes, weakness of the limbs, and memory loss. A major stroke typically produces loss of consciousness, paralysis on one side of the body, difficulty swallowing, loss of bladder and bowel control, slurred or garbled speech, and unequal pupil size.

If a patient has a stroke in the office, notify the physician at once, and call the EMS system. Maintain the patient's airway by turning the head toward the affected side to allow secretions to drain out rather than be aspirated. Loosen tight clothing. If directed by the physician, monitor vital signs and administer oxygen.

Toxic Shock Syndrome

Toxic shock syndrome (TSS) is an acute infection caused by the bacterium *Staphylococcus aureas.* The toxin produced by the bacterium can enter the body through a break in the skin or through the uterus. Although the infection is most common in menstruating women who are using tampons at the time of onset, the link between tampon use and TSS is unclear.

TSS symptoms include high fever, intense muscle aches, vomiting, diarrhea, headache, bouts of violent shivering, vaginal discharge, red eyes, and a decreased level of consciousness. A sign specific to TSS is a deep red rash on the palms of the hands and the soles of the feet. This skin then sloughs off. A menstruating patient with these symptoms should be instructed to remove the tampon immediately and replace it with a sanitary napkin.

TSS is treated in the medical office with intravenous antibiotics and fluids. The patient will require hospitalization, however.

Viral Encephalitis

Viral encephalitis is a severe inflammation of the brain caused directly by a virus or secondary to a complication resulting from a viral infection. Viral encephalitis may result from an epidemic, or it may arise sporadically. This condition requires accurate identification and prompt treatment. Symptoms develop suddenly, beginning with fever, headache, and vomiting. They quickly progress to stiff neck and back, decreased level of consciousness (from drowsiness to coma), and paralysis and seizures.

The level of consciousness must be monitored frequently in a patient with viral encephalitis. Prepare the patient for treatment with antiviral drugs, and arrange for transport to a hospital for a spinal tap and other diagnostic tests.

Common Psychosocial Emergencies

You will probably encounter psychosocial emergencies in the medical office at some point. These may result from drug or alcohol abuse, spousal abuse, child abuse, or elder abuse. Handle these situations as you were directed in Chapters 24 and 27. If you encounter patients who have overdosed on drugs, exhibit violent behavior, mention suicide, or have been raped, follow the specific clinical responsibilities described in this section.

You may also be responsible for referring patients with psychosocial emergencies to resources in the community. Some of these resources are listed in Table 31-2.

A patient who is overdosing on drugs can suffer serious medical problems and can even die. If a patient who has taken an overdose is brought to the medical office, call the EMS system immediately, and arrange for transport to the hospital.

Patients on drugs may become violent during withdrawal from the substance or while under the influence. If, at any time, a patient becomes aggressive or threatening,

Table 31-2

Resources for Patient Assistance

Resource	Contact Information
Al-Anon and Alateen	(800) 356-9996
Alcoholics Anonymous	(800) 356-9996 (public information) (800) 344-2666 (meeting information)
Child Abuse Hotline	(800) 422-4453
Mothers Against Drunk Driving (MADD)	(800) 438-6233
Narcotics Anonymous	P.O. Box 9999 Van Nuys, CA 91409
National Center on Child Abuse and Neglect	(800) 394-3366
National Clearinghouse for Alcohol and Drug Abuse Information	P.O. Box 2345 Rockville, MD 20847 (800) SAY-NO-TO
National Coalition Against Domestic Violence	(202) 638-6388
National Coalition Against Sexual Assault	(202) 483-7165
National Committee to Prevent Child Abuse	(312) 663-3520
National Council on Child Abuse and Family Violence	(800) 222-2000
National Domestic Violence Hotline	(800) 799-7233

continued

Table 31-2 continued

Resources for Patient Assistance

Resource	Contact Information
National Families in Action Drug Information Center	2296 Henderson Mill Road Suite 300 Atlanta, GA 30345 (770) 934-6364
National Institute on Drug Abuse Cocaine Hotline	(800) 662-HELP
National Organization for Victim Assistance (NOVA)	(800) TRY-NOVA
National Parents' Resource Institute for Drug Abuse (PRIDE) Drug Information Services	(800) 853-7867
Students Against Driving Drunk (SADD)	(508) 481-3568

follow office protocol for handling violent behavior. The protocol should state when to call the police, how to document the incident, and when to notify the insurance carrier.

During a psychosocial emergency, a patient may tell you he is so depressed that he has thought about killing himself. Allow the patient to talk freely. Listen carefully without interrupting. Whenever a patient mentions suicide or talks about life in ways that make you suspect suicidal tendencies, discuss your suspicions with the physician. Take comments on suicide seriously, no matter how casual they may seem.

Victims of rape may be of any age and either gender, but more than 90% are women. If a patient says she has been raped, provide privacy. Limit the number of people who ask her questions. She may feel traumatized, embarrassed, and fearful. Do not make her go through the office routine at this time.

If the physician asks you to speak to the patient, explain to her that you are legally required to contact the police so that they can file a report. The patient can decide later whether she wishes to press charges.

Contact the local rape hot line, and request that a rape counselor come to the office to stay with the patient during the examination and police report procedures. The physician should be familiar with state laws for collecting specimens and the protocol for caring for a rape victim.

Ensuring that a specimen is obtained from the victim and is correctly identified, is under the uninterrupted control of authorized personnel, and has not been altered or replaced is called establishing **chain of custody.** This procedure is required for medicolegal issues, such as evidence of rape, as well as for drug tests for illicit drug use. If the chain between the victim and the specimen cannot be proved to have remained unbroken, the specimen must be considered invalid.

The first link in the chain of custody is collecting the specimen. Semen specimens are commonly collected for typing in a rape examination. Other samples collected from the victim's body and clothing may include hair and skin that can help identify the offender.

Proper specimen identification is important. Without it, the chain of custody is broken at the beginning. If you are responsible for collecting the specimen, you must be sure the specimen is collected from the correct patient and that no one tampers with it. The chain of custody form (see Figure 31-23) must be completed correctly, and the patient may be required to sign or initial the form as well.

Multiple copies of the form are used as a safeguard system. One copy, usually the original, accompanies the specimen in a sealed envelope. Another copy is attached to the outside of the envelope so that each person who handles the specimen can initial the form. A third copy is usually retained in the patient's file.

These general procedures help maintain an intact chain of custody. Always refer to your office's procedures to make sure you are meeting all relevant requirements.

The Patient Under Stress

In emergency situations patients and family members are under a great deal of stress. You must realize that people react differently to emergency situations. You can learn how to detect signs of extreme stress by being alert for patients whose behavior varies from that previously observed or who cannot focus or follow directions.

Your role during many emergency situations may be to keep victims and their families and friends calm. You can promote calmness by listening carefully and giving your full attention. Your first priority, at all times, is the victim's well-being. If he is very distraught, for example, hold his hand while the doctor examines him. If one of

CHAIN OF CUSTODY FORM

SPECIMEN I.D. NO:

MADISON CLINICAL LABORATORY

195 North Parkway
Madison, WA 90869
(608) 555-3030

STEP 1—TO BE COMPLETED BY COLLECTOR OR EMPLOYER REPRESENTATIVE.

Employer Name, Address, and I.D. No.: OR Medical Review Officer Name and Address:

____

____

____

Donor Social Security No. or Employee I.D. No.: ______________

Donor I.D. verified: ❒ Photo I.D. ❒ Employer Representative ______________
Signature

Reason for test: (check one) ❒ Preemployment ❒ Random ❒ Postaccident
❒ Periodic ❒ Reasonable suspicion/cause
❒ Return to duty ❒ Other (specify)

Test(s) to be performed: ______________ Total tests ordered: ☐

Type of specimen obtained: ❒ Urine ❒ Blood ❒ Semen ❒ Other (specify)

Submit only one specimen with each requisition.

STEP 2—TO BE COMPLETED BY COLLECTOR.

For urine specimens, read temperature within 4 minutes of collection.
Check here if specimen temperature is within range. ❒ Yes, 90˚–100˚F/32˚–38˚C
Or record actual temperature here: ______________

STEP 3—TO BE COMPLETED BY COLLECTOR.

Collection site: ______________ Address ______________

City ______________ State ______ Zip ______________ Phone ______________

Collection date: ______________ Time: ______________ ❒ a.m. ❒ p.m.

I certify that the specimen identified on this form is the specimen presented to me by the donor identified in step 1 above, and that it was collected, labeled, and sealed in the donor's presence.

Collector's name: ______________ Signature of collector ______________

STEP 4—TO BE INITIATED BY DONOR AND COMPLETED AS NECESSARY THEREAFTER.

Purpose of change	Released by Signature	Received by Signature	Date
A. Provide specimen for testing			
B. Shipment to Laboratory			
C.			

Comments:

STEP 5—TO BE COMPLETED BY THE LABORATORY:

Specimen package seal(s) intact when received in lab? ❒ Yes ❒ No. If no, explain.

Laboratory receiver's initials ______________

Copy 1 - Original - Must accompany specimen to laboratory.

Figure 31-23. The chain of custody form provides documentation that specific specimen collection safeguards have been followed.

his relatives is crying and causing him to become emotional, suggest that the relative do something to help—for example, fill out paperwork in another room.

You may face special challenges when communicating with victims during emergencies. Victims may not speak your language, or they may have a visual or hearing impairment. In such instances, follow these guidelines.

- Use gestures throughout the process for non-English-speaking victims. Continue to speak, however, because they may be able to understand some English.
- Tell patients who have visual impairments what you are going to do before you do it, and maintain voice and touch contact while caring for them.
- Ask patients who have hearing impairments whether they can read lips. If they can, speak slowly to them and never turn away while you are speaking. If they cannot read lips, communicate by writing and using gestures. At all times try to remain face-to-face and keep direct physical contact.

Educating the Patient

During minor medical emergencies, after major emergencies have been resolved, and during routine office visits, you can educate patients about ways to prevent and handle various medical emergencies. For example, you might tell them how to contact the local American Red Cross office, post notices of upcoming classes the Red Cross offers, and encourage patients and family members to learn basic first aid. You might also develop a first-aid kit checklist and make it available to patients and families.

Make sure that all family members, including children, are familiar with the local EMS system and know how to contact it in an emergency. Suggest that families keep emergency numbers by the telephone. In addition, teach parents how to childproof their home for children of various ages. Remember that childproofing differs for different children—for example, for children who can crawl as opposed to children who can walk.

Provide brief, easy-to-read handouts to reinforce the information you present to patients. Prepare handouts in multiple languages if you provide care for non-English-speaking patients. Find and use patient education resources for the types of patients seen by the practice. For example, if you work in an obstetric office, obtain educational materials for pregnant and postpartum patients from companies that provide pregnancy-related products. Ask company representatives what materials are available. Many companies provide free videos and booklets.

Disasters

Your skills in dealing with emergencies, including first-aid and CPR training, will be an enormous help to your community in the event of a disaster. To be fully effective, you must also be familiar with standard protocols for responding to disasters. Table 31-3 shows ways that

Table 31-3

Assisting in Disasters

Type of Disaster	Action to Take
Weather disaster, such as flood or hurricane	Report to community command post. Have your credentials with you. Receive identifying tag or vest and assignment. Accept only assignment that is appropriate for your abilities. Expect to be part of team. Document medical care victim receives on person's disaster tag.
Office fire	Activate alarm system. Use fire extinguisher if fire is confined to small container, such as trash can. Turn off oxygen. Shut windows and doors. Seal doors with wet cloths to prevent smoke from entering. If evacuation is necessary, proceed quietly and calmly. Direct ambulatory patients and family members to appropriate exit route. Assist patients who need help leaving building.

you can help in certain types of disasters. You may even want to participate in fire or other disaster drills to familiarize yourself with emergency procedures.

Disasters can occur in any community. Two of the most common types of disasters are floods and hurricanes. One of the biggest floods in the United States occurred in the Midwest in the summer of 1993. Even before national disaster relief personnel could respond, local medical personnel were called to the scene to triage injured and displaced residents. In this type of disaster, many people suffer from emotional shock (which often results in physical problems), injuries, and illnesses. These people require skilled medical assistance.

In a disaster, you may be asked to perform triage. When you perform triage, you give each injured victim a tag that classifies the person as emergent (needing immediate care), urgent (needing care within several hours), nonurgent (needing care when time is not critical), or dead. The triage process is outlined in Procedure 31-8.

Summary

A medical emergency can occur anywhere—in a doctor's office, at home, in a restaurant, or on the street. The more you learn about handling each type of medical emergency, the more valuable your contributions to the situation become. You can make a substantial, positive difference in the health and lives of people who face medical emergencies to which you respond.

Always notify the doctor or the local EMS system when you encounter a medical emergency. Do not, at any time, perform procedures you have not been trained to do. Use common sense, assess the situation and the patient's condition, and provide first aid until a doctor or EMT arrives.

Patients having a medical emergency are often under extreme stress. Remember to stay calm and communicate clearly. Communicating with non-English-speaking patients and those with visual or hearing impairments requires special skills. You can develop these skills through educational and training programs you seek out or during routine office visits with these patients.

You may not be present when medical emergencies occur, so patients need to know how to respond to emergency circumstances. Take every opportunity to educate patients about preventing and responding to medical emergencies. Remember to draw on community resources when you provide information or support to patients and their families. There will always be opportunities to expand your knowledge, skills, and network for dealing with medical emergencies in your medical assisting work.

PROCEDURE 31-8

Performing Triage in a Disaster

Objective: To prioritize disaster victims

OSHA Guidelines

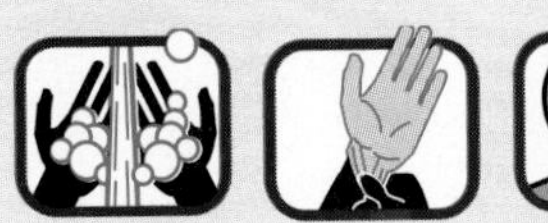
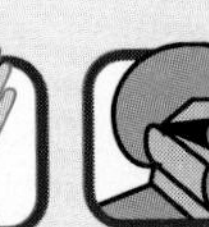
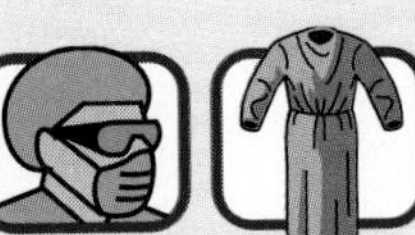

Materials: Disaster tag and pen

Method

1. Wash your hands and put on examination gloves and other PPE if available.
2. Quickly assess each victim.
3. Sort victims by type of injury and need for care, classifying them as emergent, urgent, nonurgent, or dead.
4. Label the emergent patients no. 1, and send them to appropriate treatment stations immediately. Emergent patients, such as those who are in shock or who are hemorrhaging, need immediate care.
5. Label the urgent patients no. 2, and send them to basic first-aid stations. Urgent patients need care within the next several hours. Such patients may have lacerations that can be dressed quickly to stop the bleeding but can wait for suturing.
6. Label nonurgent patients no. 3, and send them to volunteers who will be empathic and provide refreshments. Nonurgent patients are those for whom timing of treatment is not critical, such as patients who have no physical injuries but who are emotionally upset.
7. Label patients who are dead no. 4. Ensure that the bodies are moved to an area where they will be safe until they can be identified and proper action can be taken.

Chapter Review

Discussion Questions

1. What should you do to prepare the medical office for emergencies?
2. How would you assist a person who was bleeding from accidental injuries if you had no personal protective equipment with you?
3. Why should you be certified in first aid and CPR?

Critical Thinking Questions

1. Raoul Perez, age 27, is a patient with diabetes who comes to the office for treatment of an upper respiratory infection. While in the waiting room, he begins to sweat profusely and becomes restless and confused. What should you do and why?
2. Jennifer Myers, one of the office secretaries, confesses to you that she has become addicted to painkillers. She asks for your help, but she does not want you to tell anyone about her problem because she is afraid of losing her job. What should you do?
3. Elizabeth Sumner, age 39, has visited the office many times. Today, however, you notice that she is disheveled and anxious. After you greet her, she describes general, nonspecific complaints in a sad, tired tone of voice. What should you do?

Application Activities

1. Demonstrate first aid for choking, using mock abdominal thrusts on a classmate. Switch roles and have the classmate demonstrate the variations needed for a pregnant or obese patient. Critique each other's technique.
2. Demonstrate on a classmate how to stop bleeding from a large laceration on the lower arm. Switch roles and critique each other's technique.
3. As a class, divide into one large group and one small group. Students in the large group should role-play victims of a natural disaster such as an earthquake. Students in the small group should role-play medical assistants helping at the scene of the disaster. The victims should describe and role-play their conditions. On the basis of the descriptions and apparent conditions, the medical assistants should perform triage on the group of victims.

Further Readings

Advanced Cardiac Life Support. Dallas: American Heart Association, 1994.

American Red Cross. *Standard First Aid.* St. Louis, MO: Mosby–Year Book, 1992.

McAfee, Robert E. "Violence in America: Making a Difference One Patient at a Time." *The Professional Medical Assistant,* January/February 1996, 5–9.

National Safety Council. *Handbook of First Aid.* Boston: Jones and Bartlett, 1995.

Professional Guide to Signs and Symptoms. Springhouse, PA: Springhouse, 1993.

Psychosocial Crises, Clinical Skillbuilders Series. Springhouse, PA: Springhouse, 1992.

Standards and Guidelines for Cardiopulmonary Resuscitation and Emergency Care. Dallas: American Heart Association, 1992.

Wheeler, Sheila Quilter. *Telephone Triage: Theory, Practice, and Protocol Development.* Albany, NY: Delmar, 1993.

Section Four

Physician's Office Laboratory Procedures

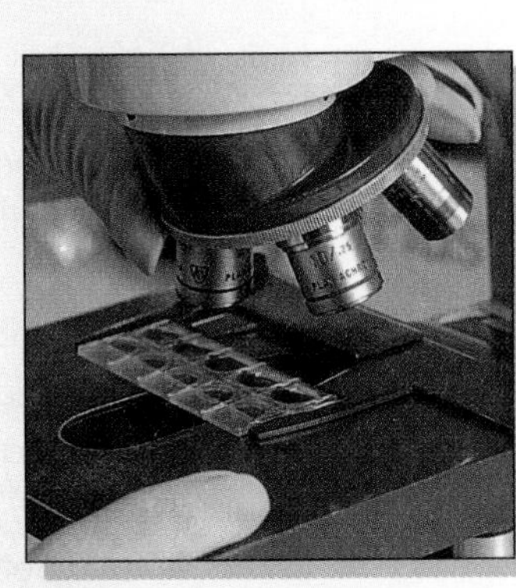

AREAS OF COMPETENCE

1997 ROLE DELINEATION STUDY

CLINICAL

- **Fundamental Principles**
- **Diagnostic Orders**
- **Patient Care**

GENERAL (Transdisciplinary)

- **Communication Skills**
- **Legal Concepts**

CHAPTER LIST

Laboratory Equipment and Safety

CHAPTER OUTLINE

- The Role of Laboratory Testing in Patient Care
- The Medical Assistant's Role
- Use of Laboratory Equipment
- Safety in the Laboratory
- Quality Assurance Programs
- Communicating With the Patient
- Record Keeping

OBJECTIVES

After completing Chapter 32, you will be able to:

- Describe the purpose of the physician's office laboratory.
- List the medical assistant's duties in the physician's office laboratory.
- Identify important pieces of laboratory equipment.
- Operate a microscope.
- Identify the regulatory controls governing procedures completed in the physician's office laboratory.
- Identify measures to prevent accidents.
- Describe correct waste disposal procedures.
- Describe the need for quality assurance and quality control programs.
- Maintain accurate documentation, including all logs related to quality control.
- List common reference materials to consult for information on procedures performed in the physician's office laboratory.
- Communicate with patients regarding test preparation and follow-up.
- Identify the medical assistant's record-keeping responsibilities.

AREAS OF COMPETENCE

1997 ROLE DELINEATION STUDY

CLINICAL

Fundamental Principles

- Apply principles of aseptic technique and infection control
- Comply with quality assurance practices
- Screen and follow up patient test results

Diagnostic Orders

- Collect and process specimens

continued

Key Terms

artifact
biohazard symbol
centrifuge
Certificate of Waiver tests
Clinical Laboratory Improvement Amendments of 1988 (CLIA '88)
compound microscope
control sample
electron microscope
hazard label
Material Safety Data Sheet (MSDS)
objective
ocular
oil-immersion objective
optical microscope
photometer
physician's office laboratory (POL)
proficiency testing program
qualitative test response
quality assurance program
quality control program
quantitative test result
reagent
reference laboratory
standard
10× lens

AREAS OF COMPETENCE continued

GENERAL (Transdisciplinary)

Legal Concepts

- Prepare and maintain medical records
- Follow federal, state, and local legal guidelines
- Maintain awareness of federal and state health care legislation and regulations
- Comply with established risk management and safety procedures
- Recognize professional credentialing criteria

The Role of Laboratory Testing in Patient Care

Laboratory analysis of blood, urine, or other body fluids and substances provides three kinds of information about a patient. First, regular monitoring through laboratory tests, such as those that are part of an annual examination, can help a physician identify possible diseases or other problems. Second, specific tests can help confirm or contradict a physician's initial diagnosis. Third, laboratory testing can help a physician determine and monitor the proper dosage of a patient's medication.

Kinds of Laboratories

Some physicians prefer to have all laboratory tests performed by a **reference laboratory,** a laboratory owned and operated by an organization outside the practice. Other physicians choose to have some tests completed by the reference laboratory and some completed in the office in the **physician's office laboratory (POL).**

There are advantages and disadvantages to each method of managing laboratory analyses. Reference laboratories often have technological resources beyond those available in the POL. Using a reference laboratory frees a physician's staff from testing duties and allows more time for patient care. Furthermore, some managed care companies have contracts with laboratory companies requiring their subscribers to use a specific reference laboratory. On the other hand, processing tests in the POL produces quicker turnaround and eliminates the need for the patient to travel to other test locations.

The Purpose of the Physician's Office Laboratory

Office policy determines which tests, if any, will be performed at your location and which tests will be performed by a reference laboratory. A POL, such as the one shown in Figure 32-1, is responsible for accurate and timely processing of routine tests, usually involving blood or urine, and for reporting test results to the physician. (A reference laboratory offers a complete range of tests in all specialties and subspecialties: cytology, toxicology, immunology, blood banking, urinalysis, histology, serology, chemistry, microbiology, and hematology. A POL generally limits tests to those involving chemistry, hematology, microbiology, and urinalysis.)

A POL usually processes chemical analyses, hematologic tests, microbiologic tests, and urinalyses. Chemical analyses are performed on blood and its components, urine, and other body fluids. Hematologic tests usually use samples of whole blood to identify problems with the count, size, or shape of blood cells that could indicate disease. Microbiologic tests examine blood, urine, sputum, reproductive fluids, and fluids from wounds to identify the presence of pathogenic organisms such as bacteria, viruses, fungi, protozoans, and parasites. Semen

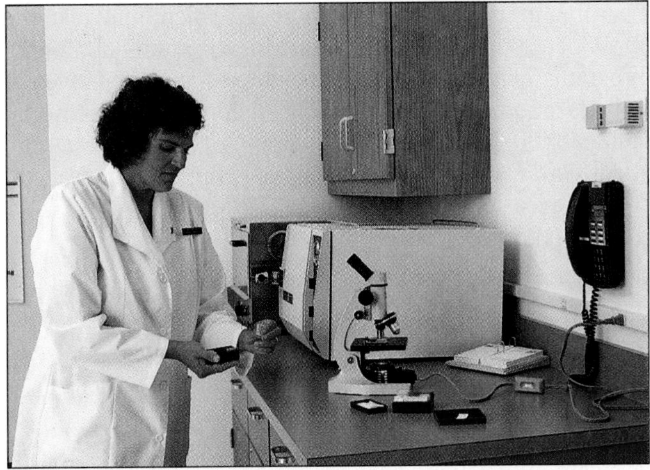

Figure 32-1. A physician's office laboratory (POL) may be simple or elaborate, depending on what tests the office performs.

may be examined microscopically to determine sperm levels, appearance, and motility. Urinalysis includes chemical analysis of the urine sample, analysis of its physical characteristics, and microscopic examination of the sample to detect disease states.

The Medical Assistant's Role

As a medical assistant, you may be responsible for processing tests done in the POL, including preparing the patient for the test, collecting the sample, completing the test, reporting the results to the physician, and communicating information about the test from the physician to the patient. Your role in the POL requires you to integrate a great deal of information to serve both the physician and the patient effectively. You will need to master the following subjects:

- Use of laboratory equipment
- Regulations governing laboratory practices and procedures
- Precautions for accident prevention
- Waste disposal requirements
- Housekeeping and maintenance routines
- Quality assurance and control procedures
- Technical aspects of specimen collection and test processing, including expected results
- Communication with patients
- Reporting of test results to the physician
- Record keeping of test specimens, procedures, and results
- Inventory and ordering of equipment and supplies
- Use of reference materials in the POL

Use of Laboratory Equipment

Learning to use a specific piece of equipment may take the form of on-the-job training, or you may attend training programs conducted by manufacturers' representatives at your location or at their training centers. You must be familiar with the operation of common laboratory equipment. You will routinely use the following equipment:

- Autoclave
- Centrifuge
- Microscope
- Electronic equipment
- Equipment used for measurement

Autoclave

A steam autoclave is used to sterilize, or eradicate all organisms on, the surfaces of instruments and equipment before they are used on a patient or in testing procedures. Use of the autoclave is discussed in Chapter 20.

Centrifuge

A **centrifuge** is a device for spinning a specimen at high speed until it separates into its component parts. The centrifuge in a POL is generally used to separate whole blood samples into blood components or to prepare urine samples for examination. Use of a centrifuge is described in greater detail in Chapter 34.

Microscope

The instrument used most often in a POL is the microscope. Common uses of the microscope are the examination of blood smears, blood cell counts, and identification of microorganisms in body fluid samples.

The usual microscope in a POL is an **optical microscope** (Figure 32-2). An optical microscope uses light, concentrated through a condenser and focused through the object being examined, to project an image. Most optical microscopes in POLs are **compound microscopes,** which use two lenses to magnify the image created by the condensed light.

You may see images that have been produced by an electron microscope in a research or reference laboratory. Instead of using a beam of light, the **electron microscope** uses a beam of electrons. Whereas the best optical microscopes can magnify an image several thousand times, an electron microscope can magnify an image several million times. Use of this highly specialized piece of equipment requires extensive training. An electron microscope is not usually found in the POL, because it is expensive and unnecessarily sophisticated for routine specimen examination.

You must be able to operate an optical microscope correctly. First you need to become familiar with the component parts.

Oculars. The **oculars** are the eyepieces through which you view the image. A microscope is either monocular, with a single eyepiece, or binocular, with two eyepieces. You can adjust the oculars on a binocular microscope to compensate for differences in visual acuity between your right and left eyes. You can also adjust the distance between oculars to match the distance between your eyes. The ocular contains a magnifying lens that usually magnifies an image ten times. Such a lens is called a **10× lens**.

Objectives. The ocular or oculars lead to the nosepiece, which contains the **objectives.** An objective contains another magnifying lens. Generally, microscopes used in the POL have a three-piece objective system. The three objectives are mounted on a swivel base, the nosepiece. An objective is moved into position directly under the ocular when needed.

Two of the objectives are dry objectives, which means there is air space between the specimen under examination and the objective. Condensed light passes through the specimen and the air space above the specimen as it travels toward the objective lens. These dry objectives

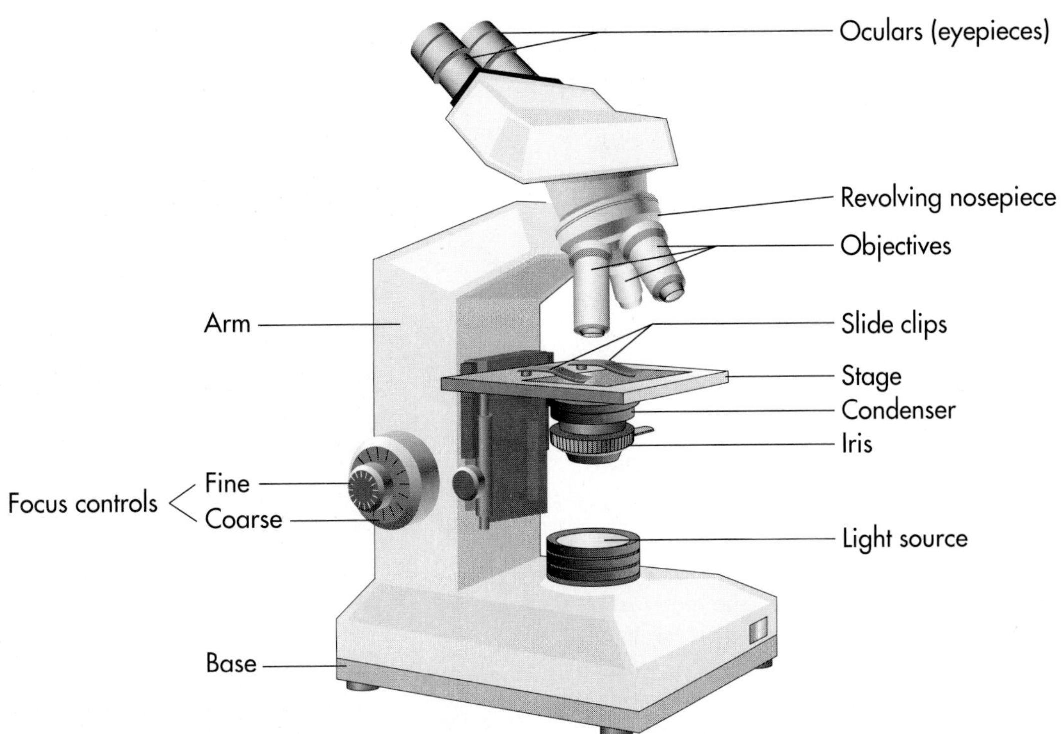

Figure 32-2. The microscope is the most heavily used piece of equipment in a POL.

are low- and high-power lenses, usually 10× and 40× respectively. When the low-power objective lens is combined with the ocular lenses, the total magnification factor is 100× (10× times 10×). The high-power lens and ocular lenses yield a magnification factor of 400×.

The third objective is an **oil-immersion objective.** It is designed to be lowered into a drop of immersion oil placed directly above the prepared specimen under examination. This design eliminates the air space between the microscope slide and the objective, where some of the light scatters beyond the objective. Placing the end of the objective in oil reduces the loss of light. A much sharper, brighter image results, allowing for greater magnification. An oil-immersion objective has a magnification factor of 100×. Combined with the ocular lenses, the total magnification factor is 1000×. The oil-immersion objective is used for specimens that need extreme magnification, such as blood smears.

Arm and Focus Controls. The ocular(s) and objectives, collectively referred to as the body tube, are attached to the base of the microscope by the arm. When moving a microscope, use one hand to grasp the arm and the other hand to support the base. (Never carry a microscope with one hand or by just the arm.) If the microscope has an electrical cord, make sure it is loosely coiled and secured with a wire tie or an elastic band.

The microscope arm is also the location of the focus controls. There are two focus controls: coarse and fine. These controls move the body tube up and down to bring into focus the object being examined.

Stage and Substage. The objectives and oculars are focused on a specimen placed on the stage of the microscope. The stage is the platform on which rests the specimen slide, held in place by metal clips. Under the stage is the substage containing the condenser, which concentrates the light being directed through the sample, and the iris. The iris is a diaphragm that opens and closes like the shutter of a camera to increase or decrease the amount of light illuminating the specimen. The stage is controlled by the stage mechanisms, which control left-right and forward-backward movements of the stage, allowing you to examine different areas of the specimen without reseating the slide.

Light Source. Under the stage and substage assemblies is the light source. Most POL microscopes use a built-in electric light source, and most of these are equipped with controls that allow you to adjust the light intensity. In place of a built-in light source, some microscopes use a mirror, which gathers and focuses light from a microscope lamp onto the specimen.

Specimen Slides and Coverslip. Although the specimen slide is not technically part of the microscope assembly, it is necessary for using the microscope. All specimens must be placed on slides. Many specimens also require a coverslip, or cover glass. The slide and coverslip support and position the specimen. They also prevent contamination of the microscope by the specimen. Specimens that are to be stained or immersed in oil, such as blood smears, do not require coverslips.

MULTISKILL FOCUS

Medical Laboratory Assistant

To gain medical assistant credentials, you must fulfill the requirements of either the American Association of Medical Assistants (for a Certified Medical Assistant) or the American Medical Technologists (for a Registered Medical Assistant). After obtaining your medical assistant certification or registration, you may wish to acquire additional skills in specialty areas through course work or on-the-job training. Although this course work or training may not lead to an additional certification or degree, it will enable you to expand your role in the medical office and advance your career as the demand for multiskilled health professionals increases.

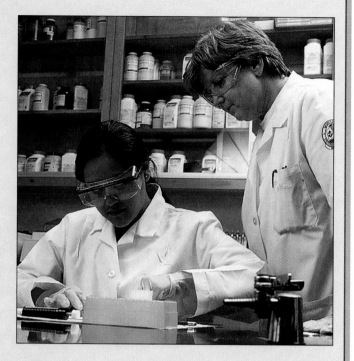

Skills and Duties

A medical laboratory assistant conducts laboratory tests on specimens of body fluids and tissue. She may test samples to diagnose disease, to develop new treatments to combat disease, or to evaluate the success of existing treatments. A medical laboratory assistant works under the supervision of a medical laboratory technician or physician.

The assistant uses sophisticated laboratory equipment to collect, process, and analyze samples of body fluids and tissue. She may prepare slides of the samples for viewing under the microscope or separate components within the samples for further testing. As part of the testing process, the assistant labels all samples and fills out reports of the analyses for the physician. She also sterilizes laboratory instruments and checks laboratory equipment to make sure it is fully functional.

The range of tests performed by a particular medical laboratory assistant will vary, depending on the type of laboratory in which she works. For example, an assistant who works in a small rural laboratory may perform a wide variety of tests, whereas an assistant working in a large reference laboratory may only perform tests of a single type. Some procedures require specialized knowledge and training. A medical laboratory assistant's education and experience will determine the complexity of the tests she may perform.

Workplace Settings

Medical laboratory assistants usually work in a hospital, clinic, or research center. An increasing number are also finding work at medical laboratories that run tests for hospitals and physicians. Medical laboratory assistants usually work a standard 40-hour week, although hospital laboratories sometimes require some evening and weekend shifts.

Education

A medical laboratory assistant must have a high school diploma or the equivalent. Some assistants acquire their additional training on the job, but most are trained in a certified program. The Commission on Accreditation of Allied Health Education Programs certifies more than 100 training programs, which range in length from 1 to 2 years, at vocational schools and community colleges. In some cases students may be able to combine courses in medical assisting with a liberal arts program to gain an associate's degree in medical laboratory technology.

Certification as a medical laboratory assistant is not required, but it is helpful in getting a job and advancing to other positions. In addition, some states require that medical laboratory assistants, along with all other laboratory staff, be licensed.

Where to Go for More Information

American Medical Technologists
710 Higgins Road
Park Ridge, IL 60068
(847) 823-5169

American Society of Clinical Pathologists
2100 West Harrison Street
Chicago, IL 60612
(312) 738-1336

National Accrediting Agency for Clinical Laboratory Services
8410 West Bryn Mawr Avenue, Suite 670
Chicago, IL 60631
(312) 714-8880

Using an Optical Microscope. To use an optical microscope, you must be able to focus it using each of the three objectives. Procedure 32-1 describes how to operate an optical microscope correctly.

You will also be responsible for the proper care and maintenance of the optical microscope in your office. Related concerns and techniques are described in "Caution: Handle With Care."

Electronic Equipment

Electronic equipment is used in the POL because it is more accurate, safer, and more efficient than manual methods; generally requires little maintenance; and does not require extensive training prior to its use. A wide variety of tasks, such as record keeping and retrieval, cell counting, and complex chemical analyses, are performed with electronic equipment. Manufacturers' instructions for operation and maintenance must be followed to ensure safety, efficiency, and reliable results.

A **photometer,** which measures light intensity, is a basic electronic component of many pieces of analytic laboratory equipment. A handheld glucometer (Figure 32-8), for example, contains a photometer that measures reflected light. A glucometer is used by patients with diabetes and by clinical personnel to monitor blood glucose levels.

Equipment Used for Measurement

Precise measurement is critical in the POL because it produces accurate test results. Much of the measurement required in the POL is built into the electronic equipment or premeasured kits you will use. You still must perform various measurements, however, when blood, semen, urine, and other body fluids are analyzed using manual tests. For example, in the sedimentation rate test that measures the rate at which red blood cells settle in a vertical column of blood, you measure the clear plasma at the top of the column after the settling period. Some reagents also require measuring.

Metric system units are commonly used in the POL. For information on metric system weight, height, and temperature measurements, see Chapter 24. To learn how to convert between measurement systems, see Chapter 38.

A variety of equipment is used to provide accurate measurements. You must take these measurements care-

PROCEDURE 32-1

Using a Microscope

Objective: To correctly focus the microscope using each of the three objectives for examination of a prepared specimen slide

OSHA Guidelines

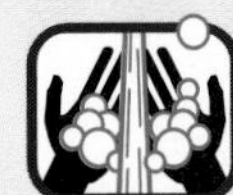 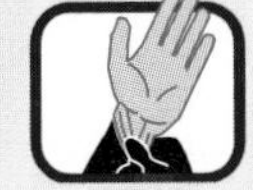   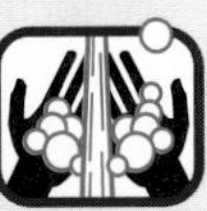 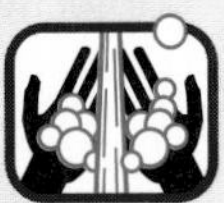

Materials: Microscope, lens paper, lens cleaner, prepared specimen slide, immersion oil, tissues

Method

1. Wash your hands and put on examination gloves.
2. Remove the protective cover from the microscope. Examine the microscope to make sure that it is clean and that all parts are intact.
3. Plug in the microscope and make sure the light is working. If you need to replace the bulb, refer to the manufacturer's guidelines. (Be sure to note bulb replacements in the maintenance log for the microscope.) Turn the light off before cleaning the lenses.
4. Clean the lenses and oculars with lens paper. Avoid touching the lenses with anything except lens paper. Pay careful attention to the oculars. They are easily dirtied by dust and eye makeup. If a lens is particularly dirty, use a small amount of lens cleaner. Oil-immersion lenses are prone to oil buildup if not cleaned properly. Too much lens cleaner, however, can loosen the cement that holds the lens in place.
5. Place the specimen slide on the stage. Slide the edges of the slide under the slide clips to secure the slide to the stage (Figure 32-3).

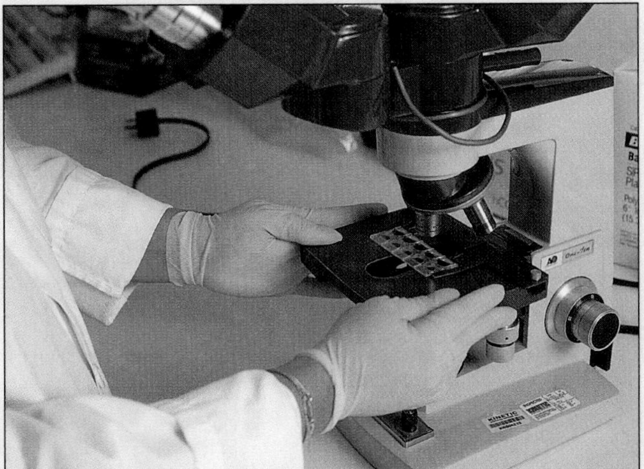

Figure 32-3. Carefully secure the specimen slide on the stage of the microscope.

continued

PROCEDURE 32-1 continued

Using a Microscope

6. Adjust the distance between the oculars to a position of comfort. You have correctly adjusted the oculars when the field you see through the eyepieces is a merged field, not separate left and right fields.
7. Adjust the objectives so that the low-power (10×) objective points directly at the specimen slide, as shown in Figure 32-4. Before swiveling the objective assembly, be sure you have sufficient space for the objective. Raise the body tube by using the coarse adjustment control, and lower the stage as needed. If the objective assembly is too close to the stage, you may hit the specimen slide and crack it. The specimen is then contaminated and cannot be used. The objective may also be damaged.
8. Turn on the light and, using the iris controls, adjust the amount of light illuminating the specimen so that the light fills the field but does not "wash out" the image. (At this point you are not examining the specimen image for focus but adjusting the overall light level.)

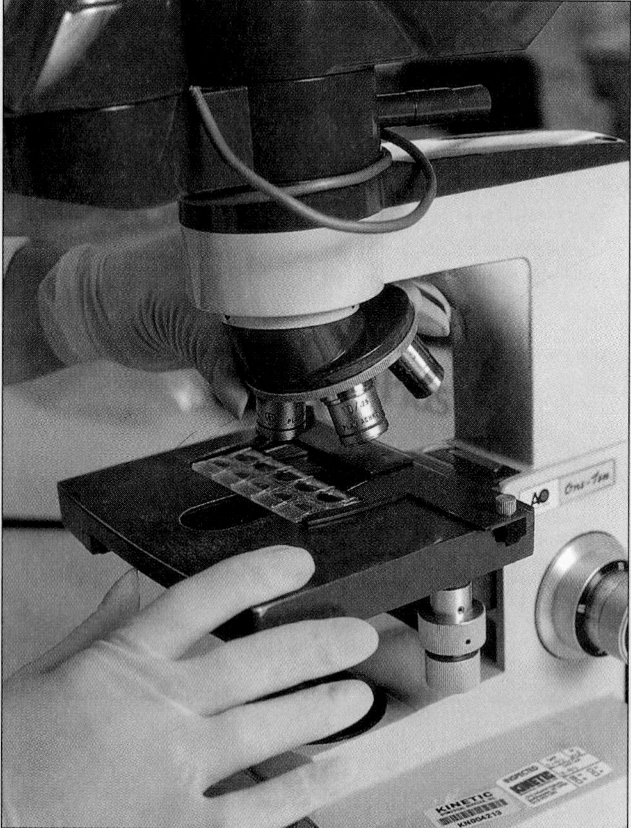

Figure 32-4. Move the low-power objective into position above the specimen slide.

9. Observe the microscope from one side, and slowly lower the body tube to move the objective closer to the stage and specimen slide. This adjustment is shown in Figure 32-5. If you used the stage controls to lower the stage away from the objectives, you may also need to adjust those controls. Again, take care not to strike the stage with the objective. The objective should almost meet the specimen slide but not touch it.
10. Look through the oculars and use the coarse focus control to slowly adjust the image. If necessary, adjust the amount of light coming through the iris.
11. Continue using the fine focus control to adjust the image. When the image is correctly adjusted, the specimen will be clearly visible, and the field illumination will be bright enough to show details but not so bright that it is uncomfortable to view.
12. Switch to the high-power (40×) objective. Most microscopes can be switched from the low-power objective to the high-power objective without your having to use the coarse focus adjustments again. Use the fine focus controls to view the specimen clearly.
13. Rotate the objective assembly so that no objective points directly at the stage and specimen slide. You will now have enough room to apply a small drop of immersion oil to the slide. (Only dry slides, without coverslips, are used with the oil-immersion objective.)

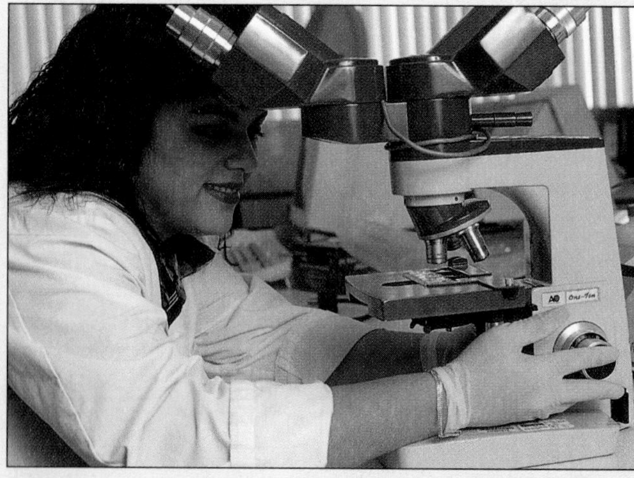

Figure 32-5. When lowering the objective toward the stage and specimen slide, observe the microscope from the side to be sure you do not hit the stage with the objective and crack the slide.

14. Apply a small drop of immersion oil to the specimen slide, as shown in Figure 32-6.
15. Swing the oil-immersion (100×) objective over the stage and specimen slide. Gently lower the objective so that it is surrounded by the immersion oil.
16. Examine the image and adjust the amount of light and focus as needed. To eliminate air bubbles in the immersion oil, gently move the stage left and right.
17. After you have examined the specimen as required by the testing procedure, lower the stage and raise the objectives.
18. Remove the slide. Dispose of it or store it as required by the testing procedure. If you must dispose of the slide, be sure to use the appropriate biohazardous waste container. If you must store the slide, remove the immersion oil with a tissue.
19. Clean the microscope stage, ocular lenses, and objectives (Figure 32-7). Be careful to remove all traces of immersion oil from the stage and oil-immersion objective.
20. Turn off the light. Unplug the microscope if that is your laboratory's standard operating procedure.
21. Rotate the objective assembly so that the low-power objective points toward the stage. Lower the objective so that it comes close to but does not rest on the stage.
22. Cover the microscope with its protective cover. Check the work area to be sure you have cleaned everything correctly and disposed of all waste material.
23. Remove the gloves and wash your hands.

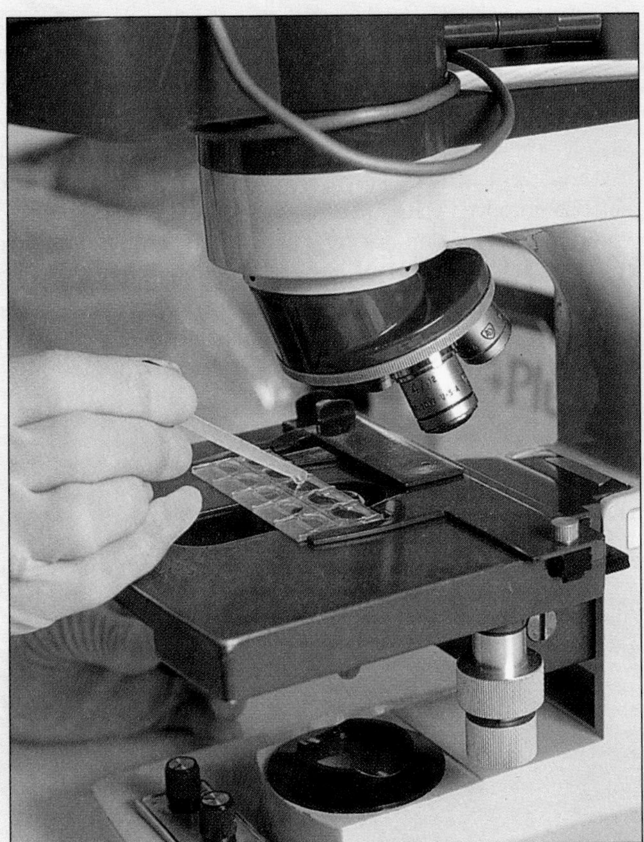

Figure 32-6. Place a small drop of immersion oil directly on the dry specimen.

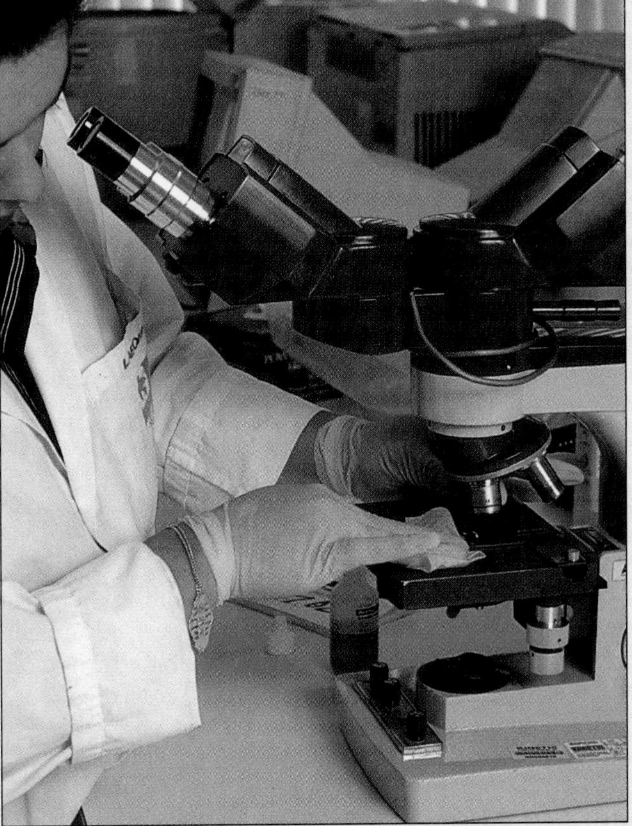

Figure 32-7. You need to remove all traces of immersion oil when you clean the microscope stage, ocular lenses, and objectives.

CAUTION HANDLE WITH CARE

Care and Maintenance of the Microscope

The microscope is the workhorse of the POL. For it to provide trouble-free service, however, it must be well cared for. Dust, oil, and other contaminants cause major problems with microscopes. Careless cleaning and haphazard storage will also eventually cause problems. These problems may include mechanical difficulties with the microscope or contamination of the specimen being examined. Foreign objects visible through a microscope, but unrelated to the specimen, are called **artifacts** and may be misinterpreted when the specimen is examined.

Clean the microscope after each use. Inspect the body tube, arm, and stage to make sure they are free from dust and other contaminants. Clean the ocular and objective lenses with lens paper, not tissue or other products. Tissue fibers are a common artifact. The eyepiece is an area in which skin oil, dust, and eye makeup may collect, posing a risk of disease transmission and making images difficult to see. Use lens-cleaning products according to the manufacturers' guidelines. Excess amounts of these products may dissolve the cement holding the lenses in place, rendering the microscope useless.

When not in use, the microscope should be stored under its plastic cover. If there is a power cord, wrap it loosely around the base, and secure it with a twist tie or elastic band. Lower the low-power objective close to the stage and center the stage.

If the microscope must be moved, hold it by the arm, and support it under the base. Carry the cord so that it does not dangle and pose a tripping hazard. Place the microscope on a sturdy table or bench, away from the edge.

fully for them to be of value in the final test results. You must calibrate blood-collecting equipment, such as syringes and capillary tubes, for exact measurement in certain tests. Other types of measuring equipment include:

- Pipettes, either mechanical or manual, which are used to measure small amounts of liquids.
- Volumetric or graduated flasks or beakers, which are used to measure the relatively large amounts of liquids necessary for reagents.
- A hemocytometer, which is a slide calibrated to the exact measurements needed to count blood cells and sperm under a microscope.
- Thermometers, generally in degrees centigrade, which are used to provide legal documentation that refrigerators, bacterial incubators, and other appliances maintain the precise temperature range required for accurate laboratory work.

Safety in the Laboratory

Safety is a primary concern in any laboratory environment. It is especially important in a physician's office laboratory because patients as well as laboratory workers may be at risk. For your own protection, as well as that of patients and coworkers, you must always be aware of and observe guidelines for laboratory safety.

Occupational Safety and Health Administration

The Occupational Safety and Health Administration (OSHA) was created within the Department of Labor as a result of legislation passed in 1970 (the Occupational Safety and Health Acts) to protect the safety of employees in the workplace. OSHA's duties include the creation and enforcement of both general safety standards and standards for specific industries and operations. In general, if a specific standard exists, its guidelines must be followed, but if no specific standard has been developed, the "general duty clause" takes effect. This clause requires an employer to maintain a workplace free from hazards that are recognized as likely to cause death or serious injury. OSHA also acts to enforce guidelines developed by the Centers for Disease Control and Prevention (CDC), in particular the guidelines for Universal Precautions. Copies of these guidelines can be obtained from many sources, including local OSHA offices, the

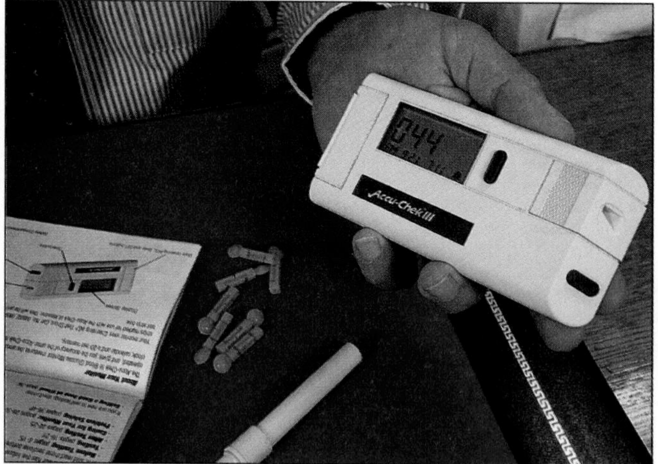

Figure 32-8. A handheld glucometer translates the amount of reflected light into the level of glucose in a blood sample.

CDC in Atlanta, Georgia, many industrial organizations throughout the country, and the Internet.

Important regulations or guidelines with which you should be familiar as you work as a medical assistant include the following:

- Universal Precautions
- Hazard Communication Standard
- OSHA Bloodborne Pathogens Standard
- Hazardous Waste Operations and Emergency Response Final Rule

Universal Precautions. As discussed in Chapter 19 and elsewhere, the general concept behind Universal Precautions is to assume that all blood, blood products, human tissue, and certain body fluids (including semen, vaginal secretions, saliva from dental procedures, cerebrospinal fluid, synovial fluid, pleural fluid, peritoneal fluid, pericardial fluid, and amniotic fluid) are contaminated with blood-borne pathogens. (Breast milk is not on the official list of transmission agents covered by Universal Precautions, but it is treated as such because it is believed that HIV has been transmitted from mother to child through breast milk.)

It has become common practice in the medical office to use Universal Precautions when handling all body fluids, excretions, and secretions. If you have any doubt about whether you need to take precautions, take them. Even though some substances do not present a risk of transmitting blood-borne pathogens, they may present a high risk of transmitting bacteria, viruses, or parasites. Follow these guidelines.

- Wear gloves when handling all body fluids, secretions, and excretions.
- Change gloves every time you move from patient to patient as you collect specimens for testing.
- Wash your hands immediately after removing used gloves.
- Wear other protective gear such as eye protection and face masks during procedures in which there is a risk that droplets or spray may come in contact with your eyes, nose, or mouth.
- Take special care to avoid injury from sharp or pointed instruments or equipment. Although gloves protect you from surface exposure to potentially infected substances, they offer little protection against exposure from needle sticks or cuts. Never use needles or other sharp instruments unnecessarily.
- Use only recommended instruments and equipment. A once common laboratory technique that has been discontinued is the use of a mouth pipette (a type of calibrated glass or plastic straw) to transfer specimens. Under no circumstances should you use a mouth pipette to transfer blood from one collection device to another.
- Take care when transporting specimens to the laboratory and when moving specimens in the laboratory to prevent spills and splashes.
- If a work surface becomes contaminated because of spilling or splashing, disinfect the area completely before beginning any other procedure.
- Dispose of waste products carefully and correctly.
- Be sure to remove protective gear before leaving the laboratory.

Hazard Communication Standard. The Hazard Communication Standard requires that employees receive training regarding workplace hazards, including how to interpret documentation about hazardous substances that pose an exposure threat. Hazardous materials must be correctly labeled, and employees must have access to information about the materials. The information must include the measures employees can take to protect themselves against harm from these substances.

Biohazard Labels. All containers used to store waste products, blood, blood products, or other specimens that may be contaminated with blood-borne pathogens are considered biohazardous. They must be clearly marked with the **biohazard symbol,** as shown in Figure 32-9. The biohazard symbol label must be bright orange-red and clearly lettered so that no one can mistake the meaning of the warning. Labels should be securely attached to containers.

In addition to using individual biohazard labels to identify particular containers, warning signs must be posted in the laboratory itself. These signs, such as the one shown in Figure 32-10, identify the presence of biohazardous material and list important safeguards to follow.

Material Safety Data Sheets. **Material Safety Data Sheets (MSDSs)** contain information about hazardous chemicals or other substances. A sample MSDS is shown in Figure 32-11. Each MSDS must contain the following information about the product it describes:

- Substance name, as it appears on the container label
- Chemical name(s) of each ingredient
- Common name(s) of each ingredient

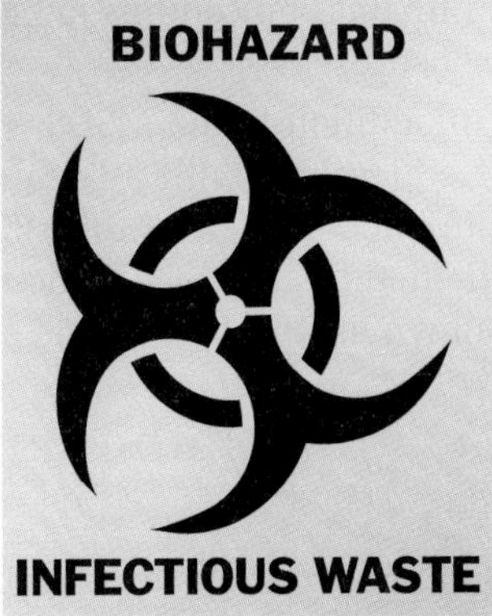

Figure 32-9. The biohazard symbol identifies material that has been exposed to potentially contaminated substances such as blood, blood products, or other body fluids.

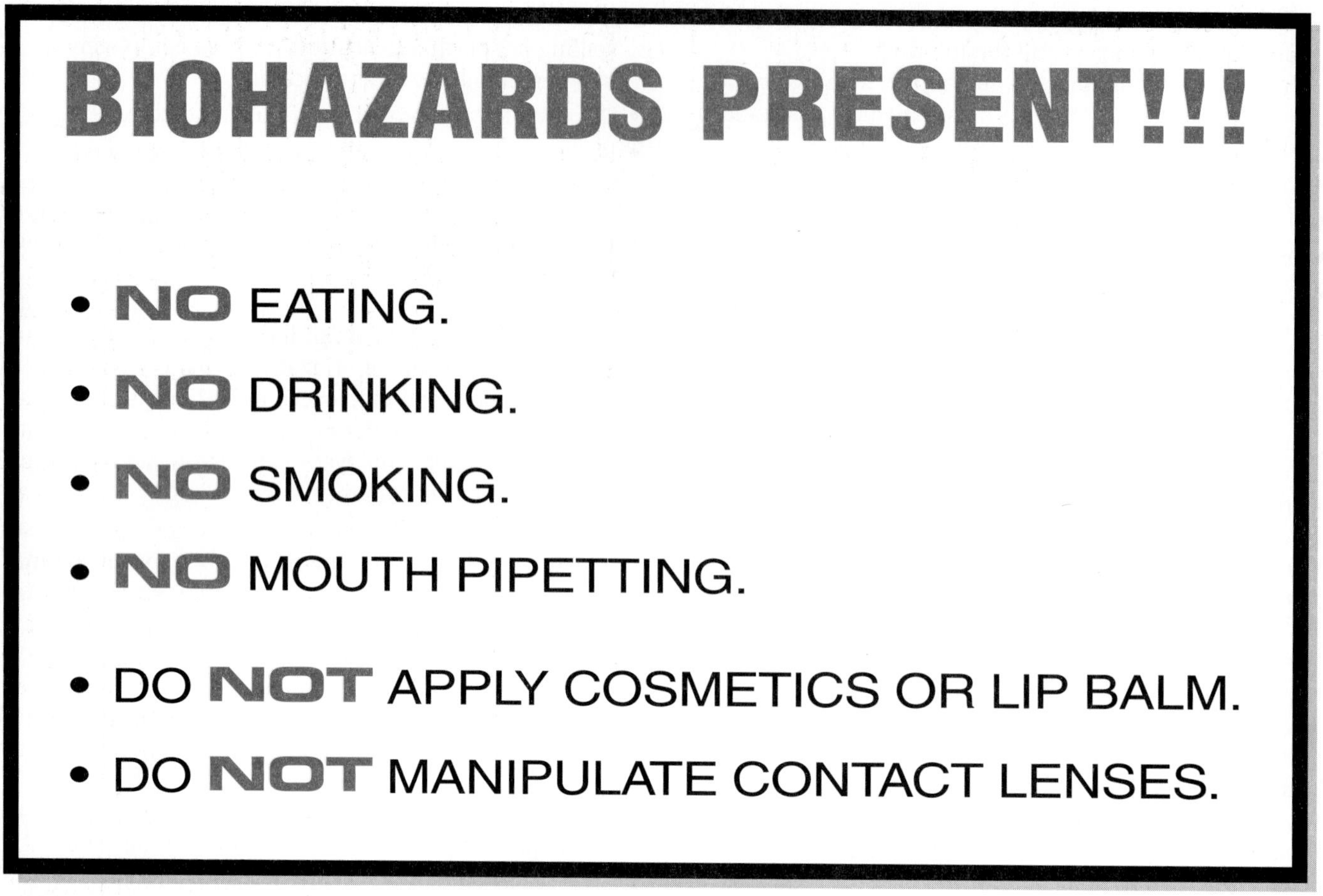

BIOHAZARDS PRESENT!!!

- NO EATING.
- NO DRINKING.
- NO SMOKING.
- NO MOUTH PIPETTING.
- DO NOT APPLY COSMETICS OR LIP BALM.
- DO NOT MANIPULATE CONTACT LENSES.

Figure 32-10. The biohazard warning sign alerts personnel to the presence of potentially contaminated substances and advises them about safety guidelines.

- Chemical characteristics of the product (boiling point, specific gravity, melting point, appearance, odor)
- Physical hazards posed by the product (fire, vapor pressure)
- Health hazards posed by the product (carcinogenicity [ability to cause cancer], routes and methods of entry, signs and symptoms of exposure)
- Guidelines for safe handling of the substance
- Emergency and first-aid procedures to be followed in the event of exposure

Hazard Labels. In addition to the MSDS, each hazardous substance must be identified with a hazard label. A **hazard label** is a shortened version of the MSDS that is permanently affixed to the substance container. A sample hazard label is shown in Figure 32-12.

OSHA Bloodborne Pathogens Standard

The OSHA Bloodborne Pathogens Standard identifies methods for reducing the risk of transmission of bloodborne pathogens, specifically the hepatitis B virus (HBV) and the human immunodeficiency virus (HIV). HIV is the virus that causes acquired immunodeficiency syndrome (AIDS). The standard identifies laboratory procedures that must be followed to prevent occupational exposure. It also describes the procedure that must be followed in the event of exposure to one of these viruses. To be in compliance with this standard, an employer must meet the following requirements.

- A written OSHA Exposure Control Plan must be created and updated annually or whenever procedures that require exposure to potentially contaminated material are added or changed. The plan must be available to all employees and to authorized OSHA authorities.
- Training must be provided to all employees describing the documentation mandated by the standard. This documentation includes the symptoms, methods of transmission, and epidemiology of infectious diseases caused by blood-borne pathogens. Employees must also be instructed in the use of personal protective equipment, Universal Precautions, and engineering controls designed to prevent exposure. Procedures to follow in the event of exposure or emergency situations must also be part of the training.
- The employer must make hepatitis B vaccine available to all employees who are at risk for occupational exposure. Employees must either receive the vaccination or decline it in writing. The employer must maintain

MATERIAL SAFETY DATA SHEET

WAVICIDE-01

Date Issued:

SECTION 1 **IDENTIFICATION**

Manufacturers Name and Address: Wave Energy Systems, Inc.
25 Mansard Court
Wayne, NJ 07470

Phone: 1-800-252-1125
Fax: (201) 633-1023

Hazardous Chemicals: *Glutaraldehyde*
Routes of entry: *Inhalation* ✓ *Skin/Eye* ✓ *Ingestion* ✓

Product Name: WAVICIDE-01 (2.5% aqueous glutaraldehyde solution)

Product Code: 0104 (case of 4 gallons) or 0112 (case of 12 quarts)

Product Type/General Information: Chemical Sterilant/Disinfectant

EPA Registration Number: 15136-1

Chemical Name: (active ingredient) 2.5% glutaraldehyde

PRECAUTIONARY LABELING
(HMIS Rating System)

Health	3
Flammability:	0
Reactivity:	0
Physical Hazard:	None

The New Jersey Poison Control Center has been provided information for use in medical emergencies involving this product. Call 1-800-962-1253.

SECTION 2 **HAZARDOUS INGREDIENTS/IDENTITY INFORMATION**

WAVICIDE-01 contains the following hazardous ingredients at concentrations greater than 1.0%:

CHEMICAL COMPONENTS	CAS%	% w/v	OSHA PEL	ACGIH TLV
Glutaraldehyde (active ingredient)	111-30-8	2.5	0.2 ppm[1]	0.2 ppm

WAVICIDE-01 contains no hazardous ingredients listed as carcinogens or potential carcinogens by the National Toxicology Program (NTP), International Agency on Cancer (IARC) or OSHA, and present at a concentration greater than 0.1%:

[1] The OSHA Permissible Exposure Level (PEL) for glutaraldehyde was invalidated in 1992 by court order. However, the PEL may remain valid in some OSHA approved state plans, and also can be enforced by federal OSHA under its General Duty Clause.

SECTION 3 **PHYSICAL/CHEMICAL CHARACTERISTICS**

Boiling Point:	100°C/212°F	**Evaporation Rate:**	0.81 (Butyl Acetate = 1)
Specific Gravity:	1.005 - 1.013	**Solubility (H_2O):**	Complete
Vapor Pressure:	16.9 mm Hg	**Appearance & Color:**	A clear, slightly yellow liquid with typical aldehyde odor and added lemon scent.
Melting point:	N/A	**pH:**	Approximately 6.30
Vapor Density:	1.1 (air = 1)	**Molecular Weight:**	100.11 (glutaraldehyde)
Freezing Point:	0°C/32°F (same as water)	**Odor Threshold:**	0.04 ppm, detectable (ACGIH)

SECTION 4 **FIRE AND EXPLOSION HAZARD DATA**

Flash Point (Test Method): None (Tag Closed Cup ASTM D 56)

Special Fire Fighting Procedures: Self-Contained Breathing Apparatus (SCBA) and protective clothing should be worn when fighting chemical fires.

Unusual Fire and Explosion Hazards: None known **Extinguishing Media:** Carbon dioxide, foam, dry chemical.

SECTION 5 **REACTIVITY DATA**

Stability: Unstable______ Stable ✓ **Hazardous Polymerization:** May Occur______ Will Not Occur ✓

Hazardous Decomposition Products: Thermal decomposition may produce carbon dioxide and or carbon monoxide.

Conditions and Materials to Avoid: Alkaline (pH > 10) and acidic (pH < 3) materials catalyze an aldol-type condensation (exothermic but not expected to be violent). Avoid High temperatures above 40°C/104°F and or evaporation of H_2O.

Figure 32-11. This two-page Material Safety Data Sheet (MSDS), as required by OSHA, contains important information about each hazardous substance used in the POL. (Courtesy of Wave Energy Systems, Inc., Wayne, NJ.)

Date Issued:

SECTION 6 — HEALTH HAZARD DATA

Routes of Entry: *Inhalation:* ✓ *Skin:* ✓ *Ingestion:* ✓ *Eyes:* ✓

Signs and Symptoms Associated With Overexposure (one-time or repeated):

Ingestion: May cause irritation and possibly chemical burns of the mouth, throat, stomach and esophagus. May produce discomfort in the mouth, throat, chest and abdomen, nausea, vomiting, diarrhea, dizziness, faintness, drowsiness, thirst and weakness.

Eyes: Solution contact may cause damage, including severe corneal injury, which could permanently impair vision if prompt first-aid and medical treatment are not obtained. Vapors may cause stinging sensation in the eye with excess tear production, blinking, and redness of the conjuntiva.

Skin: Direct solution contact may cause skin irritation or aggravation of an existing dermatitis. May also cause skin to turn a harmless yellow or brown color.

Inhalation: Vapor is irritating to the respiratory tract. May cause stinging sensations in the nose and throat, chest discomfort and tightening, difficulty with breathing and headache. May also aggravate pre-existing asthma and pulmonary disease.

Emergency and First Aid Procedure:

Ingestion: DO NOT INDUCE VOMITING. Drink large quantities of water and call a physician immediately
NOTE TO PHYSICIAN: Probable mucosal damage from oral exposure may contraindicate the use of gastric lavage.

Eyes: Immediately flush eyes with water and continue washing for at least 15 minutes. Obtain medical attention immediately, and follow up with an ophthalmologist.

Skin: Immediately remove contaminated clothing and flush skin with soap and water for a minimum of 15 minutes. If irritation persists, seek medical attention. Wash or discard contaminated clothing.

Inhalation: Remove to fresh air. Give artificial respiration if not breathing. If breathing is difficult, oxygen may be given by qualified personnel. If irritation persists, seek medical help.

Medical Conditions Generally Aggravated by Overexposure: See above.

SECTION 7 — PRECAUTIONS FOR SAFE HANDLING AND USE

Steps to be Taken if Material is Released or Spilled: Wear suitable protective equipment, including nitrile gloves, chemically resistant gown or apron, and protective eyewear (safety glasses or shield). A full face respirator , or half-face respirator with gas proof goggles, both worn with organic vapor cartridges, is recommended for small spills. A respirator is essential for large spills, or if you experience discomfort watery eyes, nasal or respiratory irritation) due to inadequate ventilation. For **small spills of 1 gallon or less**, gather up a bucket, household ammonia, and a sponge or mop. Don protective equipment and mix approximately 1 cup of ammonia with 1 cup of water in the bucket. Mop or sponge the ammonia mixture into the spill until thoroughly combined (about 2 minutes). Wipe or mop up resulting mixture and discard down the drain with a copious amount of water. Rinse bucket, mop or sponge with water, and give spill area a final wipe or mop with fresh water. Re-rinse all equipment, and allow spill area to dry. For **large spills of more than 1 gallon**, remove people from immediate spill area, and isolate until cleaned up. Don protective equipment including a respirator with organic vapor cartridges. Contain spill with absorbent material, ie. towels. Add approximately 228 grams of sodium bisulfite powder per gallon of WAVICIDE-01 spilled (aqueous sodium hydroxide and ammonium will also neutralize glutaraldehyde). With a sponge, mix neutralizing chemical into spill, and allow 5 minutes for deactivation to occur. Discard resulting mixture according to your facility's waste disposal guidelines. Mop spill area with fresh water. Rinse out all equipment (bucket, mop, towels) with large amounts of water. If paper towels were used, dispose of in a tightly closed trash bag. Let spill area dry, and if possible increase ventilation. Once glutaraldehyde odor is below allowable levels (TLV), the area may be released from isolation.

Waste Disposal Method: Dispose of WAVICIDE-01 after 30 days of re-use, or the MEC Indicator shows the solution is below it's minimum effective concentration (1.7% w/v), which ever is sooner. This may be accomplished by pouring solution down drain in accordance with state and local regulations. Flush with a large quantity of water. Do not reuse empty containers. Rinse thoroughly with water and dispose of in trash.

Precautions to be Taken in Handling and Storing: WAVICIDE-01 should be stored in it's original sealed container at controlled room temperature (15°C/50°F to 30°C/85°F).

Precautionary Labeling: Avoid contact with eyes, prolonged and repeated contact with skin, and contamination with food.

SECTION 8 — TRANSPORATATION DATA & ADDITIONAL INFORMATION

Proper Shipping Name: 2.5% Glutaraldehyde Solution **DOT (ground):** Not regulated **IATA (air):** Not Regulated **IMO (ocean):** Not Regulated

Hazard Class: None **Labels:** None needed **Packaging:** None **ID#:** None **Special Instructions:** None **Reportable Quantity:** None

SECTION 9 — CONTROL MEASURES

Eye Protection: Safety glasses, goggles or face shield recommended when working with WAVICIDE-01. An eye wash, and full face respirator with organic vapor cartridges or half face respirator with gas proof goggles and organic vapor cartridges should be available for emergency situations.

Ventilation: WAVICIDE-01 should be used in closed containers with tight fitting lids. The working area should be large enough with ventilation necessary to keep the level of atmospheric glutaraldehyde below the Threshold Limit Value (TLV). If the solution vapors are irritating to eyes and nose, the TLV is probably being exceeded, and additional ventilation may be necessary. A fume hood or self contained fume absorber may be appropriate for this purpose. Any ventilation should pull fumes away from worker and towards the floor.

Skin Protection: Nitrile gloves and a chemical resistant gown or apron should be worn when working with WAVICIDE-01. Rubber boots may be needed to contain large spills.

Respiratory Protection: None required if glutaraldehyde vapor levels are below the TLV. A full face respirator with organic vapor cartridges or SCBA should be available for emergencies.

SECTION 10 — SPECIAL REQUIREMENTS

None

Figure 32-11. Material Safety Data Sheet (continued)

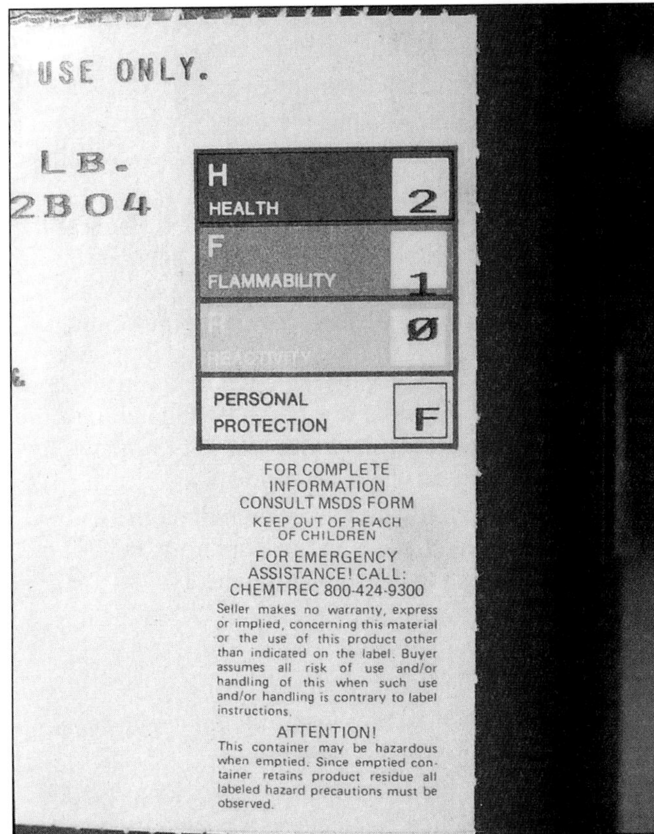

Figure 32-12. A hazard label is a condensed version of the MSDS and displays important information about a substance. It must be permanently affixed to the substance container.

documentation of vaccinations and refusals. Employees who initially decline the vaccine are free to reverse their decision at any point during their employment.

Hazardous Waste Operations and Emergency Response Final Rule. OSHA regulations also extend to the disposal of waste products generated during laboratory procedures. Hazardous waste products include the following:

- Blood
- Blood products
- Body fluids
- Body tissues
- Cultures
- Vaccines, killed or attenuated (live but weakened)
- Sharps
- Gloves
- Specula
- Inoculating loops
- Paper products contaminated with body fluids

Hazardous waste must be disposed of in properly constructed and labeled containers. Containers for sharps must be puncture-proof, leak-resistant, and rigid (Figure 32-13). Needles should be dropped into the sharps container without bending, breaking, or recapping them and with as little extra handling as possible. Other waste must be placed in plastic bags clearly labeled to identify the infectious contents. All biohazardous waste containers should be placed as close as possible to the area in which the waste is generated. This last procedure is followed to reduce the risk of spillage on the way to the disposal container.

Accident Prevention Guidelines

Work in the POL exposes you to hazards of four main types: physical, fire and electrical, chemical, and biologic. The following safeguards reduce the risk in one or more of these hazard categories. For example, by handling chemical containers carefully and correctly, you protect yourself from harmful chemical exposure as well as from physical injury from broken glass or other materials.

Physical Safety. There are many ways to ensure physical safety in the laboratory. You must understand and apply all the appropriate safeguards. Because accidents can happen, however, post emergency numbers in multiple locations throughout the laboratory. Once each quarter make sure the numbers are accurate and up to date.

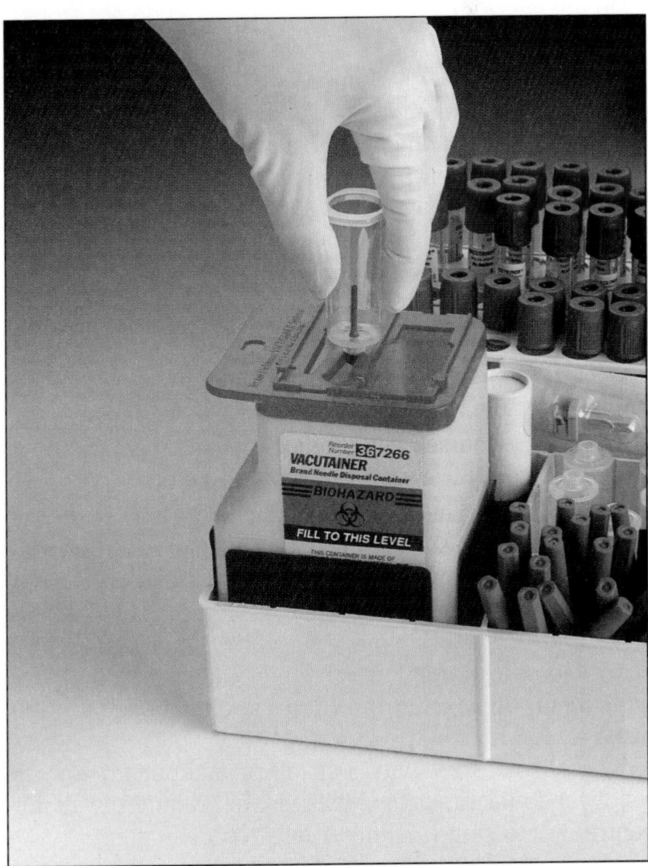

Figure 32-13. A sharps disposal container is a receptacle for used needles, lancets, specimen slides, and other disposable pointed or edged instruments, supplies, and equipment.

Some safeguards come under the heading of common sense. Their application requires no special knowledge.

- Walk, do not run, in the laboratory. Be careful when carrying objects through the laboratory, especially when approaching blind corners.
- Close all cabinet and closet doors and all desk and worktable drawers.
- Never use damaged equipment or supplies, such as cracked or chipped glassware.
- Do not overextend your reach when attempting to grasp supplies. Use only approved equipment, such as stepladders or stools, to reach high shelves. Do not climb onto chairs, desks, or tables to reach anything.
- When lifting an object, squat close to the object. Keep your back straight but not rigid. Lift the item by pushing up with your legs, not by pulling with your back. Hold the load firmly with both hands, close to your body. If necessary, put on a back-support belt before attempting to move heavy loads.

Being aware of the laboratory environment will help you protect your health and well-being. For example:

- Adjust your seat to the correct position to prevent back strain.
- If you are using a computer, take frequent breaks to reduce eyestrain and hand cramping.
- Do not eat or drink in the laboratory, and do not store food there. Never use laboratory supplies, such as beakers or flasks, for eating or drinking.
- Do not put anything in your mouth while working in the laboratory. (Some people have a habit of chewing on the end of their pencils, for example.)
- Do not apply makeup or insert contact lenses in the laboratory.
- Familiarize yourself with the location of the first-aid kit. If you are responsible for the kit in your area, check it weekly to make sure that it is adequately stocked with supplies and that expiration dates on medications have not passed.
- Familiarize yourself with the location and operation of the emergency eyewash and shower stations.

Wear appropriate protective gear and clothing in the laboratory. Use heat-resistant mitts or gloves to prevent burns. Wear sturdy, low-heeled, closed-toe shoes with rubber soles to prevent injury if you drop or spill something and to avoid slipping. Do not wear dangling jewelry or loose clothing that could get caught in laboratory equipment. Keep hair pulled back or covered for the same reason.

When you work with laboratory equipment, always follow manufacturers' guidelines. For example, wait for centrifuges to stop spinning before you open them.

Many laboratory materials and supplies require special handling and precautions.

- Store caustic chemicals and other hazardous substances below eye level to reduce the risk of upsetting the container and spilling the substance into your eyes.
- Do not attempt to grasp bottles, jars, or other containers if your hands or the containers are wet.
- Close containers immediately after use.
- Clean up spills immediately. If the floor is wet, either dry it or use appropriate warning devices to alert others to the hazard.
- Clean up broken glass with a broom. Do not handle the debris. If the material is biohazardous, use tongs or forceps to pick up the glass. Package the pieces in a sturdy container with a label identifying the contents.

Fire and Electrical Safety. The equipment and materials used in the POL make it especially vulnerable to fire and electrical hazards. It is critical for you to know how to respond to a fire or electrical accident.

- Familiarize yourself with the location of all fire extinguishers and fire blankets in the laboratory. Review the floor plan, noting the location of fire exits.
- Make sure you know how to operate the fire extinguishers.
- Participate in all office fire drills.
- Familiarize yourself with the location of circuit breakers and emergency power shutoffs.

It is, of course, never acceptable to smoke in the laboratory. Keep your area clear of clutter, such as boxes or empty storage containers. Such materials can feed, or even start, a fire. The following safeguards reduce electrical hazards.

- Avoid using extension cords. If they must be used, be sure the circuit is not overloaded. Tape extension cords to the floor to avoid tripping.
- Repair or replace equipment that has a broken or frayed cord.
- Dry your hands before working with electrical devices.
- Do not position electrical devices near sinks, faucets, or other sources of water. Be sure electrical cords do not run through water.

Work in the laboratory may sometimes require that you use a flame. Special precautions are essential in such circumstances.

- If you must use an open flame, extinguish it immediately after use.
- When using an open flame, be careful to keep your hair, clothing, and jewelry away from the flame source.
- If you must use a chemical in a procedure that requires an open flame, double-check the MSDS to identify the level of risk of fire for that chemical. If necessary, bring a fire extinguisher to the area in which you will be working.
- Never lean over an open flame.
- Never leave an open flame unattended.
- Turn off gas valves immediately after use. If you must use an open flame in the vicinity of a gas valve, always double-check to be sure the gas is off. Make sure there is adequate ventilation.

Chemical Safety. Familiarize yourself with the MSDS and hazard label of every chemical you will use during a procedure. If the MSDS indicates the need for special equipment or conditions to use a chemical safely, be sure you meet the requirements before beginning to work with the substance. General precautions as you prepare include the following.

- Wear protective gear to prevent harm to your skin or damage to your clothing. (Be sure to remove the protective gear before leaving the laboratory.)
- Always carry chemical containers with both hands as you gather supplies.
- Make sure you work in an area that is properly ventilated.

When you are ready to begin work, adhere to these guidelines.

- If you must smell the chemicals you are using, do not hold them directly under your nose. Instead, hold them a few inches away, and fan air across them and toward your nose.
- Work inside a fume hood if the chemical vapor is hazardous.
- Wear a personal ventilation device when working with certain chemicals, as specified by the MSDS.
- Never combine chemicals in ways not specifically required in test procedures.
- Mouth pipetting is prohibited at all times.
- If you are combining acids with other substances, always add the acid to the other substance. Adding substances to acid increases the risk of splashing.
- If you encounter a spill of an unknown chemical substance, do not pour any other chemicals on it. Clean it up, following strict hazardous waste control procedures. Never touch an unknown substance with your bare hands.

Biologic Safety. You will work with test specimens that may be contaminated with blood-borne or other pathogens. Treat every specimen as if it were contaminated.

- Follow Universal Precautions.
- If you have any cuts, lesions, or sores, do not expose yourself to potentially contaminated material. Consult your supervisor if you have any doubt about whether you can safely perform test procedures.
- Wash your hands before and after every procedure and whenever you come in contact with a potentially contaminated substance.
- Wear gloves at all times. Use other protective gear as appropriate to prevent exposing your eyes, nose, and mouth to potentially contaminated material.
- Mouth pipetting is prohibited at all times. Use specially made rubber suction bulbs to draw specimens mechanically.
- Work in a biologic safety cabinet (similar to a fume hood) when completing procedures that are likely to generate droplet sprays or splashes of potentially contaminated material.
- When transferring a blood specimen from a collection tube to another container, cover the tube stopper with an absorbent pad or a commercial stopper remover to prevent spray or splatter from the tube. Do not rock the stopper back and forth, because this could cause the tube to break. Always remove the stopper by opening it away from your face so that the vapor pressure flows away from you. Place the stopper on a sterile gauze pad while you work with the collection tube. Do not allow the stopper to come in contact with other work surfaces. Keep the collection tube stoppered unless you are actively using it.
- Establish clean and dirty areas in the laboratory. Place all used instruments and equipment in the dirty area for sanitization, disinfection, and sterilization.
- Disinfect your work area at least once a day with a 10% bleach solution or a germ-killing solution approved by the Environmental Protection Agency (EPA). If a spill occurs, immediately disinfect the work area.
- Dispose of waste products immediately.
- Dispose of needles in the appropriate sharps container. Do not bend, break, or recap a used needle, and never reuse a disposable needle.
- If an instrument or piece of equipment must be serviced, be sure it has been decontaminated first.
- If you use a bleach solution for disinfection, change it daily.

Accident Reporting. Despite all precautions, accidents still occur in the laboratory. Armed with an understanding of the materials with which you are working and basic first-aid procedures, you should be able to deal with most emergencies. Your office should also have written procedures to follow in the event of an accident. Familiarize yourself with the procedures beforehand so that you will know what to do if an accident occurs.

Your first responsibility is to ensure your safety and that of your colleagues and patients. If someone is injured as a result of an accident, administer first aid if required, and take steps to ensure that appropriate health-care personnel take charge of the injured person.

If exposure to spilled chemicals or other substances does not pose a threat, clean up the spill. Take precautions to prevent any of the spilled substances from coming in contact with your skin or clothes. Use appropriate cleaning products for spilled chemicals. Do not touch broken pieces of glass with your hands. Use tongs or a broom and dustpan to pick up the pieces.

Disinfect the surfaces on which the substance spilled. Soaking surfaces with a 10% bleach solution, made fresh each day, is usually sufficient to remove any contamination from blood, blood products, or body fluids.

Report the accident to your supervisor or other personnel as required by your office's policies. If the accident involves exposure to blood or blood products, OSHA regulations require that several steps be followed:

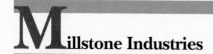

Central State Division
Incident Report

Name of Injured Employee ______________________

Department ______________________ Job Title ______________________

Supervisor ______________________

Date of Accident ______________________ Time ______________________

Nature of Injury ______________________

Was injured acting in a regular line of duty? ______________________

Was first aid given? __________ By whom? ______________________

Was designated emergency contact notified? ______________________

Did injured receive medical treatment? ______________________

Was injured tested for infection? ______________ If no, why not? ______________

Did injured go to ER? ______________ Other? ______________

Did injured leave work? ______________ Date ______________ Hour ______________ A.M. P.M.

Did injured return to work? ______________ Date ______________ Hour ______________ A.M. P.M.

Other Parties Involved ______________________

Names of Witnesses ______________________

Describe where and how accident occurred. ______________________

What, in your opinion, caused the accident? ______________________

Has anything been done to prevent a similar accident? ______________________

Has the hazard causing the injury been reported by telephone or in writing? ______________________

______________ Date ______________ Employee's Signature

______________ Date ______________ Supervisor's Signature

IF TREATMENT IS NEEDED, TAKE THE ORIGINAL AND DUPLICATE OF THIS FORM TO THE EMERGENCY ROOM.

This part for Employee Health Office use only

Was incident investigated? ______________________

Has injured had follow-up medical care? ______________________

Comments ______________________

Original copy to Employee Health Office *Duplicate copy to supervisor*

Figure 32-14. In the event of an accident or exposure incident in the POL, OSHA regulations require completion of an incident report form.

1. Immediate cleaning of the area, including disinfection of contaminated surfaces and sterilization of contaminated instruments and equipment
2. Notification of a designated emergency contact, as identified in your office's safety manual
3. Documentation of the incident on a form similar to that shown in Figure 32-14, including the names of all parties involved, the names of witnesses, a description of the incident, and a record of medical treatments given to those involved
4. Medical evaluation and follow-up examination of the employees involved
5. Written evaluation of the medical condition of the involved individuals, as well as testing for infection provided that such testing does not violate confidentiality regulations

Housekeeping

There is a high risk of serious contamination in the laboratory. Laboratory housekeeping duties are designed to reduce the risk of disease transmission. Great care must be taken to ensure that these duties are done correctly and regularly. Guidelines to ensure good operating procedures and to reduce the risk of infection are as follows.

- Refer to your office's written policies and procedures to ensure that you are performing housekeeping duties correctly and according to schedule.
- Immediately clean up spills or splashes of potentially contaminated material. Depending on the material, you may need to use special hazardous waste control products, such as those shown in Figure 32-15. Be sure to dry the area if appropriate, or clearly indicate that the area is still wet.
- Clean laboratory equipment immediately after use. Contaminants often become hard to remove if they are left on for a long time.
- Dispose of waste products carefully and correctly. Use extreme caution when handling and disposing of sharps. Procedure 32-2 describes how to dispose of biohazardous waste properly.

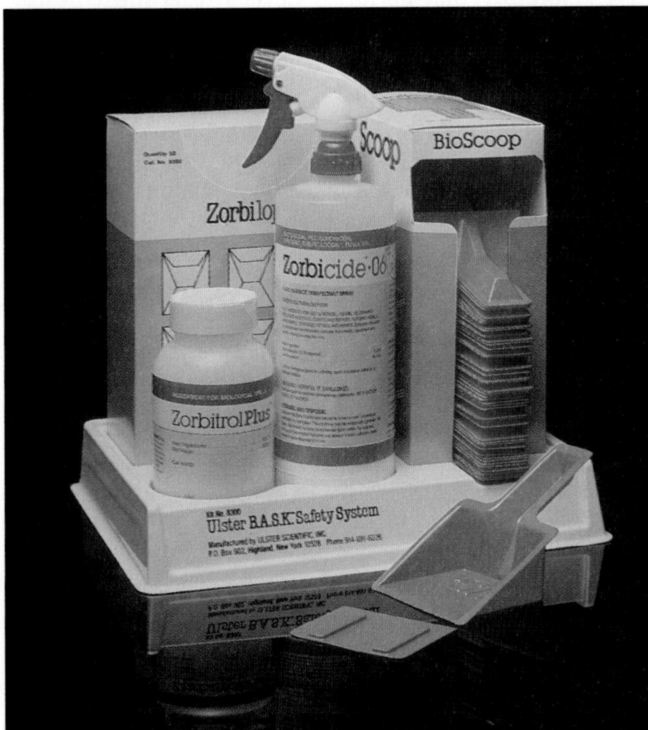

Figure 32-15. Certain substances require cleanup with specially formulated products such as these.

Quality Assurance Programs

The operation of a POL can have a significant impact on the health of the patients who depend on the medical practice for care. Accurate testing of specimens from patients is a primary concern. A **quality assurance program** is designed to monitor the quality of the patient care a medical laboratory provides.

Clinical Laboratory Improvement Amendments

In response to public concern over the accuracy of laboratory tests, Congress enacted the **Clinical Laboratory Improvement Amendments of 1988 (CLIA '88).** This law placed all laboratory facilities that conduct tests for diagnosing, preventing, or treating human disease or for assessing human health under federal regulations administered by the Health Care Financing Administration (HCFA) and the CDC. State governments have the ability to implement their own standards, which must be at least as stringent as federal standards. If your state has its own standards, your office will operate under those standards. The state health department provides information about which standards to follow in a given locale.

CLIA '88 has had a major impact on office laboratories. Because of the complexity of the regulations and the expense required to meet them, many doctors have closed their laboratories or sharply reduced the number of tests they perform. Several attempts have been made to change the federal legislation, including an effort to exempt POLs from the regulations. As the health-care debate continues, you may see changes in laboratory operations as a result of changes in CLIA '88 regulations.

As updated and implemented in 1992, CLIA '88 standards apply to four areas of laboratory operation: standards, fees, enforcement, and accreditation programs. Most of the regulations relate to laboratory standards. The specific standards that must be met depend on the test. Tests have been divided into three categories, based on complexity. They are Certificate of Waiver tests; Level I tests, of moderate complexity; and Level II tests, of high complexity.

Certificate of Waiver Tests. The **Certificate of Waiver tests,** as listed in Figure 32-16, are laboratory tests defined as follows.

PROCEDURE 32-2

Disposing of Biohazardous Waste

Objective: To correctly dispose of contaminated waste products, including sharps and contaminated cleaning and paper products

OSHA Guidelines

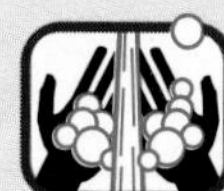 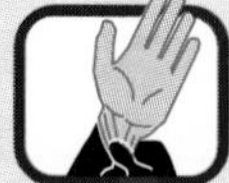 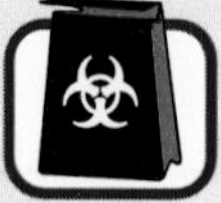 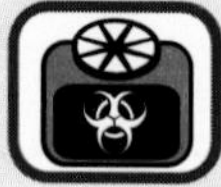 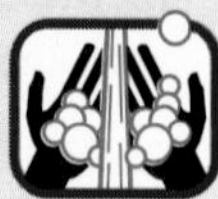

Materials: Biohazardous waste containers, gloves, waste materials

Method

To dispose of sharps or other materials that pose a danger of cutting, slicing, or puncturing the skin:

1. While wearing gloves, hold the article by the unpointed or blunt end.
2. Drop the object directly into an approved container. (If you are using an evacuation system, unscrew the needle and allow it to drop into the receptacle.) The container should be puncture-proof, with rigid sides and a tight-fitting lid.
3. If you are disposing of a needle, do not bend, break, or attempt to recap the needle before disposal. If the needle is equipped with a safety shield, slide the shield over the needle, and drop the entire assembly into the sharps container.
4. When the container is two-thirds full, replace it with an empty container. Depending on your office's procedures, the container and its contents may be sterilized before further disposal, or they may be collected by an authorized waste management agency.
5. Remove the gloves and wash your hands.

To dispose of contaminated paper waste:

1. While wearing gloves deposit the materials in a properly marked biohazardous waste container. A standard biohazardous waste container has an inner plastic liner, either red or orange and marked with the biohazard symbol, and a puncture-proof outer shell, also marked with the biohazard symbol.
2. If the container is full, secure the inner liner and place it in the appropriate area for biohazardous waste. (Biohazardous waste must be held in an area separate from regular waste and trash.)
3. Remove the gloves and wash your hands.

- The tests pose an insignificant risk to the patient if they are performed or interpreted incorrectly.
- The procedures involved are simple and accurate to such a degree that the risk of obtaining incorrect results is minimal.
- The tests have been approved by the Food and Drug Administration (FDA) for use by patients at home.

If laboratory management decides to perform these tests only, the office may apply for a Certificate of Waiver. When the certificate is granted, the laboratory is exempt from meeting various CLIA '88 standards that apply to the other two test categories. Such laboratories, however, are subject to the following: (1) random inspections to ensure that laboratories operating under a Certificate of Waiver are performing only those tests that qualify for the waiver and (2) investigation of the laboratory if there is any reason to believe the laboratory is not operating safely or if there have been complaints against the laboratory.

Level I Tests. Level I tests are moderately complex and make up approximately 75% of all tests performed in the laboratory. Among these tests are blood cell counts and cholesterol screening. Test procedures falling into the Level I category include studies involving bacteriology, mycobacteriology, mycology, parasitology, virology, immunology, chemistry, hematology, and immunohematology.

A laboratory that performs Level I tests must be run by a pathologist who has an MD or PhD degree. Technicians performing the tests must have training beyond the high school level as defined by CLIA '88 regulations. All personnel must participate in a quality assurance program for laboratory procedures, and the laboratory is subject to periodic unannounced inspections and proficiency testing.

Level II Tests. Level II tests are considered high-complexity procedures. They include more complicated tests in the specialties and subspecialties included in Level I; any test in clinical cytogenics, histopathology, histocompatibility, and cytology; and any test not yet categorized by the HCFA. Manufacturers' guidelines for testing products are often the best source for discovering the HCFA determination for a test. The HCFA publishes a directory of all Level I and Level II tests.

Like a laboratory that conducts Level I tests, a laboratory that conducts Level II tests is subject to inspection, proficiency testing, and participation in a quality assurance program, and it must be headed by a medical doctor or a scientist who has a PhD degree. Testing procedures can be performed only by qualified laboratory personnel, whose training exceeds that provided by high schools and is defined by CLIA '88 regulations.

Every quality assurance program must include the

Certificate of Waiver Tests

Urine tests

- Urinalysis by dipstick (reagent strip) or tablet reagent (nonautomated) for bilirubin, glucose, hemoglobin, ketone, leukocytes, nitrite, pH, protein, specific gravity, and urobilinogen
- Ovulation (visual color comparison tests)
- Pregnancy (visual color comparison tests)

Blood tests

- Erythrocyte sedimentation rate (ESR), nonautomated
- Hemoglobin by copper sulfate, nonautomated
- Spun microhematocrit
- Blood glucose (using devices approved by the FDA for home use)
- Fecal occult blood
- Hemoglobin by single analyte instruments, automated

Figure 32-16. A POL that performs only these tests is exempt from CLIA '88 standards once the POL has been granted a Certificate of Waiver.

following components, in a measurable and structured system, to satisfy CLIA '88 requirements:

- Quality control
- Instrument and equipment maintenance
- Proficiency testing
- Training and continuing education
- Standard operating procedures documentation

Quality Control and Maintenance

A **quality control program** is one component of a quality assurance program. The focus of the quality control program is to ensure accuracy in test results through careful monitoring of test procedures. To be in compliance with quality control standards, a laboratory must follow certain procedures.

Calibration. Testing equipment must be calibrated regularly, in accordance with manufacturers' guidelines. Calibration ensures that the equipment is operating correctly. Each calibration must be recorded in a quality control log, such as the one shown in Figure 32-17. Calibration routines are performed on a set of standards. A **standard** is a specimen, like the patient specimens you would normally process with the equipment except that the value for each standard is already known. The calibration procedure requires that the test equipment yield the correct results for the standards supplied. Calibration routines are run on the standards alone, never with patient samples. They are used exclusively to ensure that the equipment is performing according to manufacturers' specifications.

Control Samples. **Control samples** are similar to standards in that they are specimens like those taken from a patient and have known values. Unlike standards, however, control samples are used every time a patient sample is processed. Using a control sample serves as a check on the accuracy of the test. If the patient and control samples both yield irregular results, there may be an error in the test procedure.

The control samples for certain laboratory procedures show normal (negative) and abnormal (positive) results. Generally, positive and negative control samples are used with tests that yield a **qualitative test response** (the substance for which one is testing is either present or absent).

Quality Control Daily Log

Name of Unit	Glucose Control Solution	Strip Lot No./ Exp. Date	Low Control Value 35–65 mg/dL	High Control Value 175–235 mg/dL	Analyzed By	Date	Remedial Action Taken If Control Values Abnormal	Retest After Remedial Action Taken
XYZ Glucometer	Check-strip control solution	Lot 851 10/15/99	39 mg/dL	230 mg/dL	MSM	1/17/99		
Mitchell Drugs Glucometer	Check-strip control solution	Lot 851 10/15/99	50 mg/dL	267 mg/dL	MSM	1/17/99	Machine cleaned	220 mg/dL high value
XYZ Glucometer	Check-strip control solution	Lot 851 10/15/99	Unable to read	Unable to read	LMC	1/18/99	Battery changed	38 mg/dL low 198 mg/dL high
Mitchell Drugs Glucometer	Check-strip control solution	Lot 851 10/15/99	45 mg/dL	226 mg/dL	LMC	1/18/99		

Figure 32-17. The quality control log shows the completion of every quality control check conducted on a piece of equipment.

Urine Reagent Strip Control Log											Control Solution		Exp. Date ______	Lot # ______
Reagent Strip / Lot # & Exp. Date	Test	Specific Gravity	pH	Protein	Glucose	Ketone	Bilirubin	Blood	Nitrite	Urobi-linogen	Control Test Date	Remedial Action Taken If Reading Is Abnormal	Retest Date	Technician Initials
	Reagent Strip Expected Range													
	Test Results													
	Reagent Strip Expected Range													
	Test Results													

Figure 32-18. The reagent control log shows the quality testing performed on every batch or lot of reagent products.

Other control samples are formulated to show when results fall within a normal range. These samples are used for tests that yield **quantitative test results** (the concentration of a test substance in a specimen). At least two control samples containing different concentrations of the test substance should be run for quantitative tests.

Reagent Control. Control samples or standards are also run every time one opens a new supply of testing products, such as staining materials, culture media, and reagents. **Reagents** are chemicals or chemically treated substances used in test procedures. A reagent is formulated to react in specific ways when exposed under specific conditions. One example of a reagent is the chemically coated strip used in blood glucose monitoring. A visual change on the reagent strip (also called a dipstick) occurs in the presence of glucose in a blood sample. To ensure the quality of reagents, you should keep a reagent control log. If a defective reagent test is identified, it can be tracked to its source. A sample reagent control log is shown in Figure 32-18.

Maintenance. Testing instruments and equipment must be properly maintained, and all maintenance procedures must be documented. Follow manufacturers' guidelines for performing instrument and equipment maintenance. A maintenance log provides a complete record of all work performed on an instrument or a piece of equipment (Figure 32-19).

Documentation. A quality control program depends first on careful adherence to procedures designed to identify problems with equipment calibration, errors in testing procedures, and defective testing supplies. The second component of a quality control program is the careful documentation of all procedures. Besides maintaining the quality control log, the reagent control log, and the equip-

Acme Medical Supplies

Equipment Maintenance Record

Practice Russo and Russo Medical Associates

Name of Equipment Acme Microscope Model ABC-123

Location Lab **Purchase Date** 12/1/97

Date	Cleaning	Maintenance/Repair	Technician Initials
6/5	Microscope	Cleaned	CJC
6/11	Microscope high objective	Cleaned	DWM
6/14	Microscope	Changed bulb	CJC
6/16	Microscope eyepiece	Lens cover replaced	CJC
6/17	Microscope high objective	Cleaned	CJC

Figure 32-19. A maintenance log must be kept for every piece of laboratory equipment. All work done on the equipment must be recorded in the log.

ment maintenance log, you will also complete the following records as part of a quality control program:

- Reference laboratory log, which lists specimens sent to another laboratory for testing
- Daily workload log, which shows all procedures completed during the workday

Proficiency Testing

All laboratories that perform Level I and Level II tests as identified by CLIA '88 must participate in a proficiency testing program. **Proficiency testing programs** measure the accuracy of test results and adherence to standard operating procedures. Generally, proficiency tests include two parts: (1) a control sample from the proficiency testing organization engaged by your laboratory and (2) forms that must be completed to record the steps in the testing procedure. The control sample is processed normally, under the same conditions as any patient sample. The results, the forms, and sometimes the control samples are returned to the proficiency testing organization, which then informs your office of whether it has passed or failed the test. A passing mark means that your laboratory can continue to perform that particular test. A failing mark can mean that your laboratory must discontinue that test and possibly other tests as well.

Training, Continuing Education, and Documentation

One of your employer's responsibilities is to provide opportunities for employee training and continuing education. Another is to provide written reference materials and documentation for all procedures conducted in the POL. Your responsibility is to consult reference materials and take part in available training to keep your skills sharpened and up to date.

It may seem unnecessary to refer to written instructions for procedures you do many times a day. Changes can be made in a procedure for many reasons, however, and you must be aware of these changes. Here are some reference materials with which you should be familiar:

- Material Safety Data Sheets
- Standard operating procedures
- Safety manuals
- Equipment manufacturers' user or reference guides
- Clinical Laboratory Technical Procedure Manuals
- Regulatory documentation (OSHA standards, CLIA '88 requirements)
- Maintenance and housekeeping schedules

Communicating With the Patient

In your job as a medical assistant, you will be involved with patients before they submit samples for laboratory testing, during the specimen collection procedure, and after the physician has interpreted the test results. It is your responsibility to ensure that patients understand what is expected of them every step of the way.

Before the Test

Certain tests require patients to prepare by fasting or restricting fluid intake. It is your duty to explain test preparations. Use simple, nontechnical language and check with patients to be sure they understand the information. In some cases providing a written instruction sheet may be helpful.

Explaining the reason for the preparation can help ensure compliance or unearth potential problems. For example, if you explain to a patient that he is to refrain from drinking anything for a particular period, he might ask whether that includes the water he uses to take a certain medication. You can then make sure the patient receives the answers he will need for carrying out the physician's orders in light of his own circumstances.

If you are the person who collects specimens, you need to determine whether patients have correctly completed required test preparations. Test results are invalid in some cases if patients fail to follow test preparation guidelines. When preparations have not been completed correctly, discuss the situation with the physician or other appropriate staff member as required by your office to determine whether the specimen should still be collected. If the specimen is not collected, document the reason the test was not carried out as requested. Review the guidelines for specimen collection with the patient, and schedule another appointment if appropriate.

During Specimen Collection

The instructions you deliver to patients during specimen collection vary with the nature of the specimen. Always deliver instructions clearly and in language patients can understand. Do not assume that patients do not need to hear the instructions, even if they have had the test before. Explain what you must do and what patients must do before moving to each new step in the process.

Patients are understandably nervous during many collection procedures. In addition to communicating technical information, you should provide any helpful advice that may make the test easier. Also provide reassurance as appropriate. For example, if a patient asks whether the blood-drawing procedure is painful, explain that she may feel a sharp stick or stinging sensation when the needle is inserted but that she should feel no pain after that. Let the patient be your guide in determining how much information to provide. Some people want to know every detail, whereas others prefer to know as little as possible.

One important aspect of communicating with patients about testing procedures is your nonverbal communication skills. Even if you deliver accurate technical information and answer every question patients have, there can still be a breakdown in communication if your nonverbal signals do not support your verbal message. Follow these guidelines to ensure that your nonverbal actions are helping, not hindering, the communication process.

- Strike a balance between a strict, businesslike attitude and overly familiar friendliness. Your actions must impress on the patient that you are well informed about the procedure involved and that you care about the patient's understanding of it.
- Treat the patient with respect. Address the patient by name, using the appropriate courtesy title unless you have been invited to use the patient's first name or the patient is a child. Provide privacy during specimen collection. Privacy needs may be met by using a separate room or contained area for drawing blood, for example; a private bathroom is best for collecting urine specimens.
- Recognize that the patient may be under stress because of the test procedure or the pending results. Some patients may be familiar with the test procedures, but others may not know what to expect. You may need to repeat instructions or explain what you are doing more than one time. Remain calm and patient—never be abrupt or condescending.
- Direct your attention to the patient, particularly during a procedure that might be uncomfortable, such as drawing blood. Unless an emergency develops, pay attention to nothing else at that time.

After Specimen Collection

If the patient must follow particular guidelines after you collect the specimen, explain them. Commonly, posttest instructions deal with care of venipuncture sites, signs and symptoms of infection, additional or continuing dietary restrictions, and the schedule for further testing if it is necessary.

When the Test Results Return

When you receive the tests results, do not communicate them to the patient but to the doctor. Only the doctor is qualified to interpret test results for the patient. Your role in reporting results comes after the doctor examines the test information and prepares a report. Sometimes the doctor discusses the results with the patient. At other times you will be asked to convey the test results to the patient, along with instructions from the doctor. Answer only those patient questions that are within the range of your knowledge and experience. If the patient needs more information than you can provide, refer the patient to the doctor.

Record Keeping

The importance of accurate and complete record keeping can be summed up in one statement: If it is not written down, it was not done. This motto applies to all your duties as a medical assistant. Besides recording information about quality control and equipment maintenance, you will be called on to handle inventory control, record test results in patient records, and keep track of every specimen that passes through your hands. You may need to use standard abbreviations for measures when recording test results. Figure 32-20 provides a list of common abbreviations used in the laboratory.

Inventory Control

You will be responsible for taking inventory of equipment and supplies to ensure that the POL never runs out of them. To do so, you will keep a list of items that are used routinely and reordered systematically. Establish a regular schedule for counting items in the POL, perhaps every week or so. Then estimate when you will probably need to reorder an item—and put the date on your calendar.

Patient Records

When recording test results, it is your responsibility to identify unusual findings. Many offices require that out-of-range test results be circled or underlined in red. Follow the procedure established by your office. Test results are not communicated to the patient until the physician has had the opportunity to review the information. The physician usually initials or otherwise marks the records after examining them.

Specimen Identification

All specimens must be clearly identified with the patient's name, the patient's identification code if your office uses one, the date and time the specimen was collected, the initials of the person who collected the

Abbreviations for Common Laboratory Measures

cm = centimeter
cm^3 = cubic centimeter
dL = deciliter
fl oz = fluid ounce
g = gram
L = liter
lb = pound
m = meter
mg = milligram
mL = milliliter
mm = millimeter
mm Hg = millimeters of mercury
oz = ounce
pt = pint
QNS = quantity not sufficient
qt = quart
U = unit
wt = weight

Figure 32-20. You may encounter these common abbreviations when recording patients' test results.

specimen, the physician's name, and other information as required by the test procedure or your office. If you encounter an unidentified or incorrectly identified specimen, you must make an effort to track it to its source. The specimen will probably be discarded or destroyed, however, because there is no guarantee that it was identified correctly. Even if you do manage to identify it, it may have been compromised in some way.

Summary

The physician's office laboratory offers many opportunities for interesting and satisfying work in your role as a medical assistant. Those opportunities carry with them the responsibility to maintain and improve your technical skills; to stay abreast of technological, legislative, and regulatory developments; to take every precaution to prevent the transmission of disease and the occurrence of accidents or emergency situations; and to seek ways to improve the quality of patient care.

Keeping a level head and applying common sense will go a long way toward making your work in the laboratory efficient and accurate. Take time to do a procedure correctly the first time. Avoid shortcuts—they lead to mistakes and lost time.

The quantity of information you will need to learn, integrate, and convey to the patient through your actions and educational efforts may be daunting at first. As you gain understanding and confidence in your skills, however, much of it will become routine.

32 Chapter Review

Discussion Questions

1. Identify five common physical hazards in the laboratory and the steps you can take to eliminate them.
2. What responsibilities does an employer have under the OSHA Bloodborne Pathogens Standard?
3. Describe the three criteria used to determine a Certificate of Waiver test.

Critical Thinking Questions

1. You are about to examine a slide that you have clipped to the microscope stage. As you are adjusting the image, the microscope light goes out. What should you do?
2. While you are holding a vial of blood, it slips out of your hand and breaks. What should you do?
3. You have just completed an analysis of a control sample and a patient sample. Both samples yield abnormal results. What is the most likely cause, and what steps should you take next?

Application Activities

1. Examine a prepared slide under a microscope. With a partner, practice bringing the slide specimen into focus with each objective. Partners should check each other's work.
2. Obtain a Material Safety Data Sheet, and review the information on it. Explain to another student what hazards the substance poses, what measures can be taken to avoid injury from the substance, and what steps should be taken in the event of an accident.
3. With another student acting as your patient, explain the preparations necessary for a common blood test. Prepare a set of written instructions, but before giving them to the "patient," ask him to repeat the oral instructions you gave. Compare the patient's version to your written instructions to see how clearly you conveyed the preparation information.

Further Readings

Clinical Laboratory Technical Procedure Manuals. 2d ed. Villanova, PA: National Committee for Clinical Laboratory Standards, 1992.

Gianelli, Diane M. "Office Labs May Be CLIA-Free." *American Medical News,* 25 April 1995, 1.

Laboratory Medicine. Chicago: American Society of Clinical Pathologists, monthly.

Newsome, Rebecca. "OSHA Regulations for the Physician's Office." *The Professional Medical Assistant,* January/February 1991, 17–18.

Occupational Safety and Health Administration. *Personal Protective Equipment.* Washington, DC: U.S. Department of Labor, 1995.

Palko, Tom, and Hilda Palko. *Laboratory Procedures for the Medical Office.* Columbus, OH: Glencoe/McGraw-Hill, 1996.

Physician's Office Laboratory Guidelines, Procedure Manual. 2d ed. Villanova, PA: National Committee for Clinical Laboratory Standards, 1992.

Collecting, Processing, and Testing Urine Specimens

CHAPTER OUTLINE

- The Role of the Medical Assistant
- Anatomy and Physiology of the Urinary System
- Obtaining Specimens
- Urinalysis

OBJECTIVES

After completing Chapter 33, you will be able to:

- Describe the characteristics of urine, including its formation, physical composition, and chemical properties.
- Explain how to instruct patients in specimen collection.
- Identify guidelines to follow when collecting urine specimens.
- Describe proper procedures for collecting various urine specimens.
- Explain the process of urinary catheterization.
- List special considerations that may require you to alter guidelines when collecting urine specimens.
- Explain how to maintain the chain of custody when processing urine specimens.
- Explain how to preserve and store urine specimens.
- Describe the process of urinalysis and its purpose.
- Identify the physical characteristics present in normal urine specimens.
- Identify the chemicals that may be found in urine specimens.
- Identify the elements categorized and counted as a result of microscopic examination of urine specimens.

AREAS OF COMPETENCE

1997 ROLE DELINEATION STUDY

CLINICAL

Fundamental Principles

- Apply principles of aseptic technique and infection control

Diagnostic Orders

- Collect and process specimens
- Perform diagnostic tests

continued

Key Terms

anuria
bilirubin
bilirubinuria
cast
catheterization
clean-catch midstream urine specimen
crystal
drainage catheter
first morning urine specimen
glomerular filtration
glycosuria
hematuria
hemoglobinuria
myoglobinuria
nocturia
oliguria
phenylketonuria (PKU)
proteinuria
random urine specimen
refractometer
splinting catheter
supernatant
timed urine specimen
24-hour urine specimen
urinalysis
urinary catheter
urinary pH
urine specific gravity
urinometer
urobilinogen

AREAS OF COMPETENCE continued

GENERAL (Transdisciplinary)

Communication Skills

- Adapt communications to individual's ability to understand

The Role of the Medical Assistant

You will help collect, process, and test urine specimens. To perform your duties, you need to know about the anatomy and physiology of the kidneys, how urine is formed, and what its normal contents are. This information will help you collect various specimen types, process them, and perform urinalysis on them. Dealing with a variety of patient groups who require special care, including elderly patients and pediatric patients, will also be an important part of your job as a medical assistant.

Although you will not generally be dealing with blood-borne pathogens when obtaining and processing urine specimens, you will deal with potentially infectious body waste. For this reason you must take precautions to protect yourself, the patient, and others in the environment from transmitting disease-causing microorganisms. Most medical offices use Universal Precautions when dealing with urine. (See Chapters 19, 20, and 21 for detailed information on these precautions.) During all procedures you must be sure to wear adequate personal protective equipment (PPE), handle and dispose of specimens properly, dispose of used supplies and equipment properly, and sanitize, disinfect, and/or sterilize all reusable equipment.

Anatomy and Physiology of the Urinary System

The urinary system comprises two kidneys, two ureters, a bladder, and a urethra. The kidneys are located behind the peritoneum on either side of the lumbar spine. They remove excess water from the body and waste products from the blood in the form of urine. The urine then drains through the ureters and into the urinary bladder. The urinary bladder stores urine until it leaves the body through the urethra. The ureters, bladder, and urethra make up the urinary tract.

Formation of Urine in the Kidney

Urine formation is essentially a filtering process that occurs in the nephrons. Nephrons are the structural and functional units of the kidney (see Figure 33-1). Each kidney contains about a million nephrons, each of which is capable of forming urine.

Glomerular filtration occurs as blood moves through a tight ball of capillaries called the glomerulus. The glomerular capsule (Bowman's capsule) surrounds the glomerulus. Filtered fluid collects in this capsule, which is the functional beginning of the nephron. A capillary bed surrounds the winding tubule that makes up the rest of the nephron structure. Reabsorption of water, nutrients, and some electrolytes returns these substances to the blood as the filtered fluid passes through the long tubule. Other electrolytes and some additional substances are secreted from the blood into the tubule. Urine is the fluid that flows out of the nephron into the collecting tubule, passes through the funnel-shaped renal pelvis, leaves the kidney, and is carried down the ureter to the bladder.

The specific function of the nephron is to remove certain end products of metabolism from the blood plasma. Because the nephron allows for reabsorption of water and some electrolytes back into the blood, the nephron also plays a vital role in maintaining normal fluid balance in the body.

Physical Composition and Chemical Properties

Urine is made up of 95% water and 5% waste products and other dissolved chemicals. Components other than water include urea, uric acid, ammonia, calcium, creatinine, sodium, chloride, potassium, sulfates, phosphates, bicarbonates, hydrogen ions, urochrome, urobilinogen, a few red blood cells, and a few white blood cells. If a patient is taking any drugs that are excreted renally, the drugs may also show up in the urine. Urine in males may contain a few sperm cells.

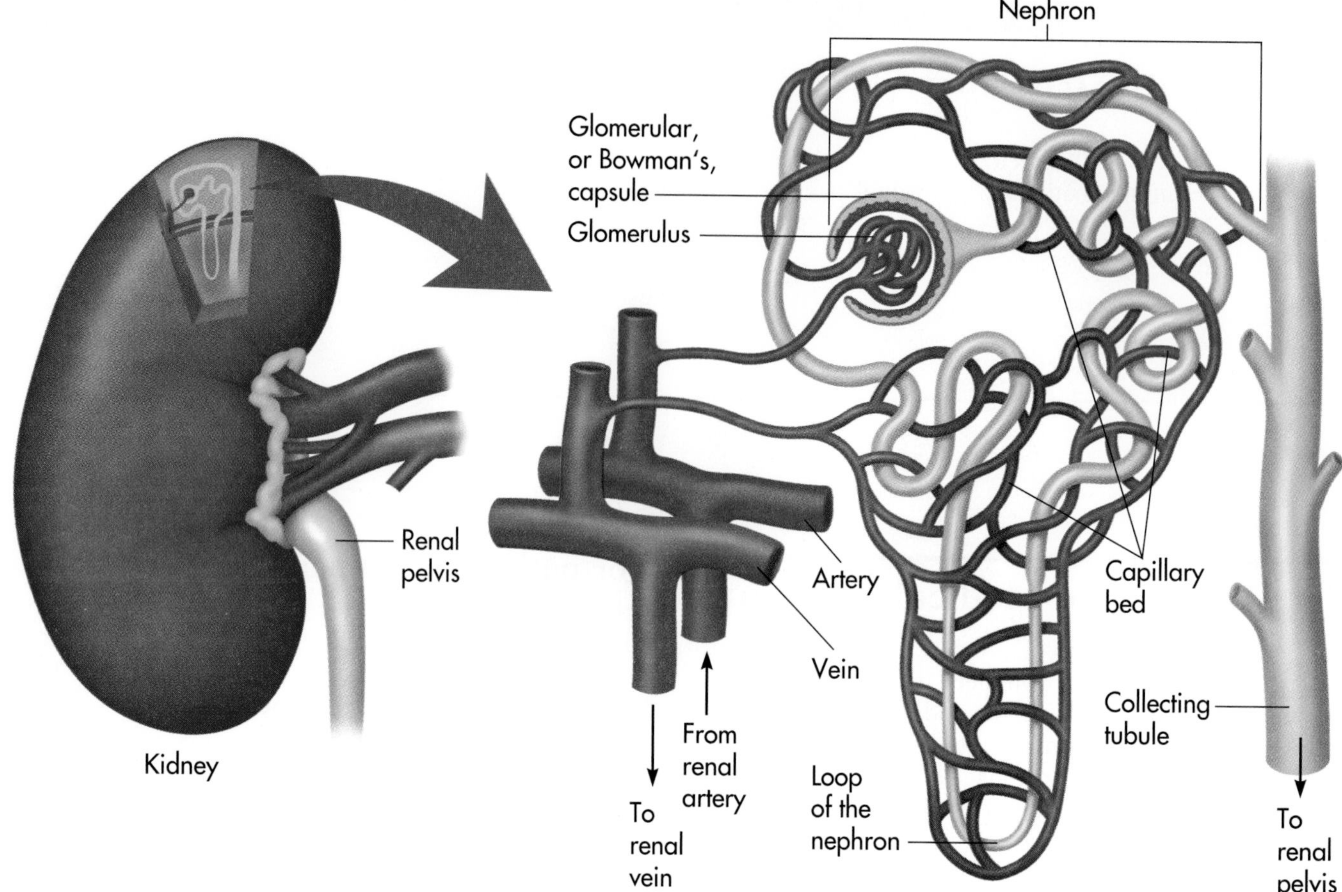

Figure 33-1. Urine is formed in the nephron, a long tubular structure, during a complex filtering process.

Obtaining Specimens

It is essential to collect, store, and preserve urine specimens in ways that do not alter their physical, chemical, or microscopic properties. You must follow guidelines each time you obtain specimens and instruct patients in the proper guidelines to follow.

General Collection Guidelines

When you collect urine specimens from patients, follow these guidelines.

- Make sure you are following the procedure that is specified for the urine test that will be performed.
- Use the type of specimen container indicated by the laboratory. If a patient must bring in a specimen, be sure that the container is provided by the physician's office or that the container is appropriate for the testing protocol.
- Label the specimen container before giving it to the patient or upon receipt of a container that the patient provides. Include the patient's name, the physician's name, the date and time of collection, and the initials of the person collecting the sample. Label the side of the specimen container, not the lid, because lids may be lost or switched.
- If the patient is having an invasive test, such as catheterization, always explain the procedure to the patient completely, using simple, clear language.
- If you are assisting in the collection process, wash your hands before and after the procedure, and wear gloves during the procedure.
- Complete all necessary paperwork, recording the collection in the patient's chart and making sure you use the correct request slip for the test that has been ordered.

Patients need to collect a urine specimen at home in many instances. It is your responsibility to give patients instructions for obtaining the specific type of specimen. In addition, provide them with the following general instructions.

- Urinate into the container indicated by the laboratory. In most instances urinate into a widemouthed, throwaway, spouted specimen container as instructed. Do not add anything to the container except the urine.
- If the collection container contains liquid or powdered preservative, do not pour it out.

- If any of the preservative spills on you, wash the area immediately and contact the physician's office.
- Always refrigerate the labeled collection container or keep it in a cooler or pail filled with ice.
- Be sure to keep the lid on the container.

Specimen Types

Many different tests are performed on urine. You may need to obtain different types of specimens for different tests. Specimens vary in two ways: in the method used to collect them and in the time frame in which they are collected.

Whenever you collect a specimen, you must follow the steps in the procedure exactly—or have the patient follow them exactly. Quality assurance is essential in the physician's office laboratory. As discussed in Chapter 32, control samples must be used every time you test patient specimens. These are the types of urine specimens:

- Random
- First morning
- Clean-catch midstream
- Timed
- 24-hour

Random Urine Specimen. The **random urine specimen** is the most common type of sample. It is a single urine specimen taken at any time of the day. A random urine specimen is collected in a clean, dry container. If the doctor is requesting that a culture be done on the specimen, provide the patient with a sterile container.

If the collection of a random urine specimen is to be done at the doctor's office, supply the patient with a urine specimen container. Show the patient to the bathroom, and ask the patient to void a few ounces of urine into the specimen cup and to leave the cup on the sink. Retrieve the specimen when the patient leaves the bathroom, pour it into a container, cover the container, and attach a properly completed label and requisition slip. Transport the specimen to the laboratory immediately. Urine specimens should be processed within 1 hour of collection. If this is not possible, refrigerate the specimens. Before processing refrigerated specimens, however, allow them to come to room temperature. If specimens will be shipped to an outside laboratory, chemical preservatives are added.

If patients are to collect a random urine specimen at home, have them use the container indicated by the laboratory. Either provide patients with a urine specimen container or instruct them to use a clean, widemouthed glass jar with a tight-fitting lid. Explain that a household dishwasher provides hot enough water to disinfect a jar adequately. Tell patients to refrigerate specimens until they bring them to the doctor's office and to keep them cool during transport.

First Morning Urine Specimen. The **first morning urine specimen** is collected after a night's sleep. This type of specimen contains greater concentrations of substances that collect over time than do specimens taken during the day. A urine specimen container or clean, dry jar is used to collect the urine as per the laboratory's request.

Clean-Catch Midstream Urine Specimen. The **clean-catch midstream urine specimen,** sometimes referred to as midvoid, may be collected and submitted for culturing to identify the number and the types of pathogens present. The presence of clinical symptoms or unexplained bacteria in a urinalysis specimen is an indication for urine culture. This method is not like other urine tests in which urine is simply voided into a specimen container. Instead, the clean-catch midstream method requires special cleansing of the external genitalia to avoid contamination by organisms residing near the urethral meatus (the external opening of the urethra). The only other way to obtain a specimen without this type of contamination is through catheterization, a procedure not routinely recommended because of the risk of infection. Procedure 33-1 describes how to perform this technique and how to instruct patients to collect a clean-catch midstream urine specimen.

Timed Urine Specimen. A physician may order a **timed urine specimen** to measure a patient's urinary output or to analyze substances (see the discussion of the 24-hour urine specimen also). First determine whether the required time period means that the patient must collect the specimen at home. If so, provide the patient with the proper collection container; written instructions on the process, including preservation of the specimen; and the following oral instructions.

- Discard the first specimen.
- Then collect *all* urine for the specified time (2 to 24 hours).
- Be sure the urine does not mix with stool or toilet paper.
- Keep the sample refrigerated until returning it to the physician's office or laboratory.

24-Hour Urine Specimen. A **24-hour urine specimen** is collected over a 24-hour period and is used to complete a quantitative and qualitative analysis of one or more substances, such as sodium, chloride, and calcium. You need to instruct the patient in the proper collection process. If an outside laboratory will be testing the specimen, you will receive protocols for collection, preservation, and transport. See "Educating the Patient" for specific information on the 24-hour collection process.

Catheterization

A **urinary catheter** is a sterile plastic tube inserted to provide urinary drainage. Such a catheter may be inserted into the kidney, the ureter, or the bladder. **Catheterization** is the procedure during which the catheter is inserted. Catheterization is performed for various reasons, including to:

- Relieve urinary retention.

PROCEDURE 33-1

Collecting a Clean-Catch Midstream Urine Specimen

Objective: To collect a urine specimen that is free from contamination

OSHA Guidelines

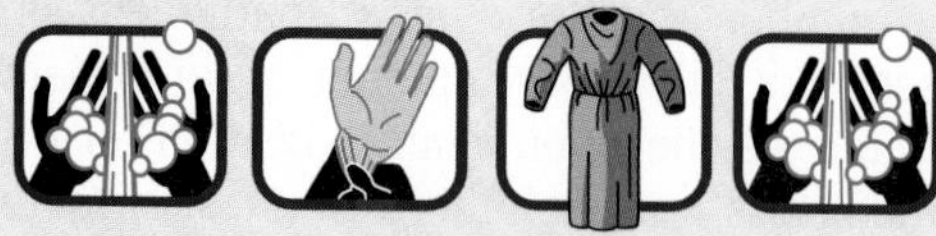

Materials: Dry, sterile urine container with lid; label; written instructions (if the patient is to perform procedure independently); antiseptic towelettes

Method

1. Confirm the patient's identity and be sure all forms are correctly completed.
2. Label the sterile urine specimen container with the patient's name, the physician's name, the date and time of collection, and the initials of the person collecting the specimen.

When the patient will be completing the procedure independently:

3. Explain the procedure in detail. Provide the patient with written instructions and the labeled sterile specimen container.
4. Confirm that the patient understands the instructions, especially not to touch the inside of the specimen container and to refrigerate the specimen until bringing it to the physician's office.

When you are assisting a patient:

3. Explain the procedure and how you will be assisting in the collection.
4. Wash your hands and put on examination gloves.

When you are assisting in the collection for female patients:

5. Remove the lid from the specimen container, and place the lid upside down on a flat surface.
6. Use three antiseptic towelettes to clean the perineal area by spreading the labia and wiping from front to back. Wipe with the first towelette on one side and discard it. Wipe with the second towelette on the other side and discard it. Wipe with the third towelette down the middle and discard it. To remove soap residue that could cause a higher pH and affect chemical test results, rinse the area once from front to back with water.
7. Keeping the patient's labia spread to avoid contamination, tell her to urinate into the toilet. After she has expressed a small amount of urine, instruct her to stop the flow.
8. Position the specimen container close to but not touching the patient.
9. Tell the patient to start urinating again. Collect the necessary amount of urine in the container. (If the patient cannot stop the urine flow, move the container into the urine flow and collect the specimen anyway.)
10. Allow the patient to finish urinating. Place the lid back on the collection container.
11. Remove the gloves and wash your hands.
12. Complete the test request slip, and record the collection in the patient's chart.

When you are assisting in the collection for male patients:

5. Remove the lid from the specimen container, and place the lid upside down on a flat surface.
6. If the patient is circumcised, use an antiseptic towelette to clean the head of the penis. Wipe with a second towelette directly across the urethral opening. If the patient is uncircumcised, retract the foreskin before cleaning the penis. To remove soap residue that could cause a higher pH and affect chemical test results, rinse the area once from front to back with water.
7. Keeping an uncircumcised patient's foreskin retracted, tell the patient to urinate into the toilet. After he has expressed a small amount of urine, instruct him to stop the flow.
8. Position the specimen container close to but not touching the patient.
9. Tell the patient to start urinating again. Collect the necessary amount of urine in the container. (If the patient cannot stop the urine flow, move the container into the urine flow and collect the specimen anyway.)
10. Allow the patient to finish urinating. Place the lid back on the collection container.
11. Remove the gloves and wash your hands.
12. Complete the test request slip, and record the collection in the patient's chart.

- Obtain a sterile urine specimen from a patient.
- Measure the amount of residual urine in the bladder to determine how much urine remains after normal voiding. (Patient voids and is then catheterized; more than 50 mL is considered abnormal.)
- Obtain a urine specimen if the patient cannot void naturally.
- Instill chemotherapy as a treatment for bladder cancer.
- Empty the bladder before and during surgery and before some diagnostic examinations.

EDUCATING THE PATIENT

How to Collect a 24-Hour Urine Specimen

When a patient needs to collect a 24-hour urine specimen, you must explain the procedure thoroughly and provide explicit written instructions. Be sure the patient understands that she must collect all her urine over the 24-hour period.

Provide the patient with a labeled sterile urine container with a lid. Tell her that at the start of the observation period (usually early in the morning), she should void and discard that specimen. Then every time she voids for the next 24 hours, she must collect the entire amount in the sterile container.

Tell the patient that the urine will be tested for substances that are released sporadically into the urine. Thus, it is extremely important to avoid using a bedpan, urinal, or toilet tissue, which could retain the substances for which the test is being done. Instead, the patient should urinate directly into a small collection container and then pour the urine into the large urine specimen container. Explain that the small container must be sanitized between uses with soap and warm water.

Explain that the large specimen container may have a preservative in it to prevent contamination and other alterations in the specimen. Instruct the patient to keep the specimen covered and in the refrigerator when not in use during the collection period. Emphasize the need to deliver the specimen to the doctor's office or laboratory as soon as possible after the 24-hour period is over, keeping the specimen cool during transport.

There are two primary types of urinary catheters:

- **Drainage catheters,** which are used to withdraw fluids and include an indwelling urethral (Foley) catheter placed in the bladder, a retention catheter in the renal pelvis, a ureteral catheter, a catheter for drainage through a wound that leads to the bladder (cystostomy tube), and a straight catheter to collect specimens or instill medications
- **Splinting catheters,** which are inserted after plastic repair of the ureter and must remain in place for at least a week after surgery

Catheterization is not routinely recommended because it can introduce infection. Some states do not permit medical assistants to perform catheterization, and in most health-care institutions, only a physician or nurse can insert or withdraw a catheter. Check the protocol in your state. If you cannot perform the procedure, you may be asked to assemble the necessary supplies and to assist the physician during it.

Catheterization performed in a physician's office is usually done for diagnostic purposes. Specially prepared catheterization kits that contain all necessary instruments and supplies are available. These kits include a sterile instrument pack that is used to create a sterile field for the procedure.

If a patient is incontinent, the physician may use a bladder-drainage catheter to help drain the bladder and keep the patient dry. Another type of drainage catheter, the ureteral, is inserted into the ureter to help drain urine.

The indwelling urethral (Foley) catheter is designed to stay in place within the bladder (Figure 33-2). It consists of two tubes, one inside the other. The inside tube is connected to a balloon, which is filled with water or air to keep the catheter from slipping out of the bladder. Urine travels through the bladder and drains from the outside tube into a soft plastic container. The physician may order a leg bag to attach to the patient's thigh. To prevent backflow into the patient's bladder, the container must always be lower than the bladder.

Special Considerations

When you obtain a urine specimen from a patient or take a history of a patient who may have a urinary problem, you need to consider the patient's sex, condition, and age. Some patients may require special care during collection procedures.

Special Considerations in Male and Female Patients. Depending on the test, you may need to alter guidelines for collecting urine specimens from a male or female patient. For example, Procedure 33-1 describes how to assist in collecting a clean-catch urine specimen from a female patient and from a male patient. In addition, when you take a medical history on a male or female patient, you will need to ask particular questions as part of your assessment. For example, if a female patient leaks urine when laughing or coughing, she may have bladder dysfunction, which would affect collecting a 24-hour urine specimen.

Special Considerations in Pregnant Patients. Pregnant women normally have increased urinary frequency. They may also be prone to urinary tract infections. At each prenatal visit pregnant women must have their urine checked for abnormal levels of glucose (a screening test for diabetes) and abnormal levels of protein (a screening test for preeclampsia or renal problems).

Ask a pregnant patient whether she has any pain during urination or in the kidney area. A positive response may indicate a urinary tract infection or kidney stones. Also ask about urine leakage and whether she has previously been pregnant. Leakage may occur in a woman who has had multiple births, because the pressure of the fetus on the bladder or delivery of the baby may have

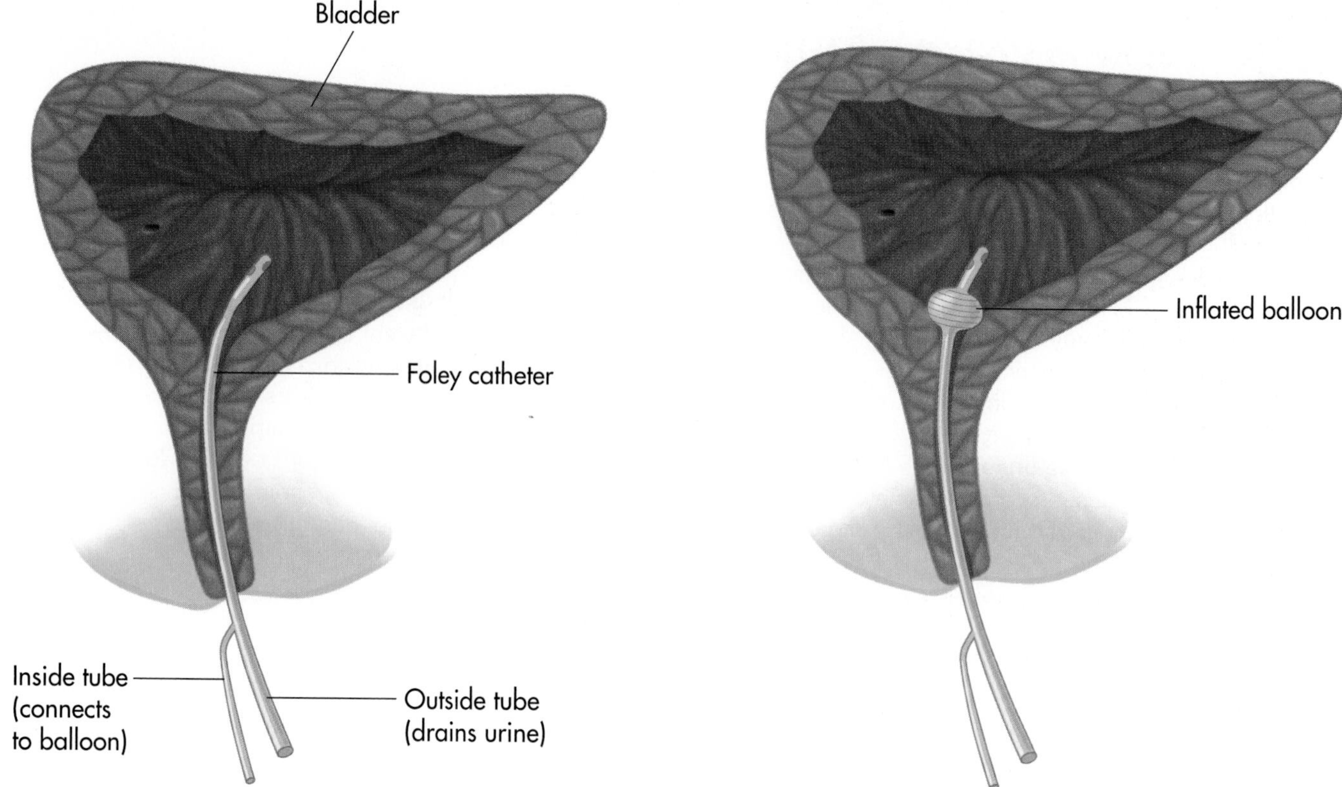

Figure 33-2. A Foley catheter stays in place within the bladder and has a collection container that is emptied periodically.

weakened the patient's bladder control. Additionally, ask whether any of the babies were delivered by forceps, which can injure urinary and genital structures.

Special Considerations in Elderly Patients. When you collect urine specimens from elderly patients, you must consider several points.

- Bladder muscles weaken with age, often leading to incomplete bladder emptying and chronic urine retention, which can cause urinary tract infection, **nocturia** (excessive nighttime urination), and incontinence. This condition can interfere with collecting a 24-hour urine specimen.
- Weakening of the supports of the uterus may cause it to prolapse (work its way down the vaginal canal). The uterus pulls with it the vaginal walls, bladder, and rectum. This weakening, which is often the result of several childbirths, may not occur until a woman is postmenopausal. Symptoms include pressure, incontinence, and urinary retention. Normal activities, such as walking up the stairs, can aggravate the problem. This condition can interfere with collecting a 24-hour specimen.
- Find out whether the patient ever loses bladder control. If so, ask whether it occurs suddenly or whether a feeling of intense pressure precedes it. These symptoms can be a sign of weakening of the bladder muscles, which can interfere with collecting a 24-hour specimen.
- Keep in mind that some elderly patients need assistance in providing a urine specimen. For example, you may have to accompany the patient to the bathroom and hold the specimen container. (Wash your hands before and after doing so, and wear gloves while providing this help.)
- If necessary, offer repeated explanations or reminders about the procedure or the specimens that need to be provided.

Special Considerations in Pediatric Patients. When you collect a urine specimen from a pediatric patient, involve the child (if age-appropriate) and the parents or guardians. Explain the procedure thoroughly and ask specific questions, including the following.

- If the child is in diapers, ask whether there is a problem of persistent diaper rash. (Rash may indicate a change in urine composition because of renal dysfunction.)
- Is the child excessively thirsty? (In this case the patient may not be taking in enough fluids for the amount of urine being excreted. Excessive thirst, combined with increased urinary frequency and volume, is symptomatic of diabetes.)

- Has the child experienced any difficulty urinating or a urine stream change? (These signs may suggest an obstruction in the urinary tract.)
- Does the child cry when urinating? (If so, the child may have pain or burning on urination, which can indicate a urinary tract infection.)
- If the child is in diapers, ask how many diapers are wet each day. Has the number changed recently? (Responses to these questions can rule out or confirm a urine volume change. For example, a child with a fever and increased perspiration might experience decreased urine volume.)
- Has the child experienced deterioration in bladder control, such as bed-wetting (enuresis)? (The child may be under stress or may have a small bladder capacity or a urinary tract infection.)
- If the child is having problems with toilet training and is more than 4 years old, ask whether the child learned to sit, stand, and talk at the age-appropriate times. (If so, the child may have a urinary system dysfunction.)

When you collect a urine specimen from a child who is toilet-trained, follow the same procedures as for an adult. If the child is an infant or not toilet-trained, however, follow the steps outlined in Procedure 33-2.

PROCEDURE 33-2

Collecting a Urine Specimen From a Pediatric Patient

Objective: To collect a urine specimen from an infant or a child who is not toilet-trained

OSHA Guidelines

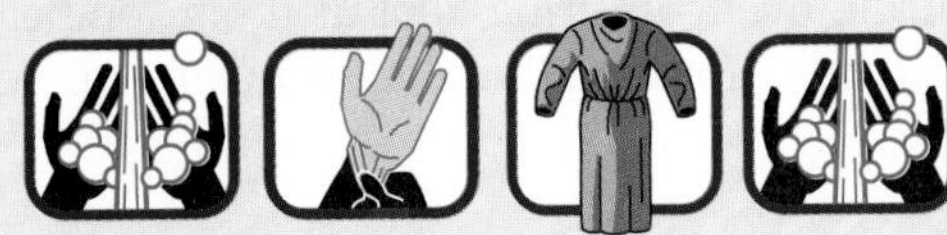

Materials: Urine specimen bottle or container, label, sterile cotton balls, soapy water, sterile water, plastic disposable urine collection bag

Method

1. Confirm the patient's identity and be sure all forms are correctly completed.
2. Label the urine specimen container with the patient's name, the physician's name, the date and time of collection, and your initials.
3. Explain the procedure to the child (if age-appropriate) and to the parents or guardians.
4. Wash your hands and put on examination gloves.
5. Have the parents pull the child's pants down and take off the diaper.
6. Position the child with the genitalia exposed.
7. Clean the genitalia. For a male patient, wipe the tip of the penis with a soapy cotton ball, and then rinse it with a cotton ball saturated with sterile water. Allow to air-dry. For a female patient, use soapy cotton balls to clean the labia majora from front to back, using one cotton ball for each wipe. Again, use cotton balls saturated in sterile water to rinse the area, and allow it to air-dry.
8. Remove the paper backing from the plastic urine collection bag, and apply the sticky, adhesive surface over the penis and scrotum (in a male patient) or vulva (in a female patient), as shown in Figure 33-3. Seal tightly to avoid leaks. Do not include the child's rectum within the collection bag or cover it with the adhesive surface.
9. Diaper the child.
10. Remove the gloves and wash your hands.
11. Check the collection bag every half-hour for urine. You must open the diaper to check; do not just feel the diaper.
12. If the child has voided, wash your hands and put on examination gloves.
13. Remove the diaper, take off the urine collection bag very carefully so that you do not irritate the child's skin, wash off the adhesive residue, rinse, and pat dry.
14. Diaper the child.
15. Place the specimen in the specimen container and cover it.
16. Remove the gloves and wash your hands.
17. Complete the test request slip, and record the collection in the patient's chart.

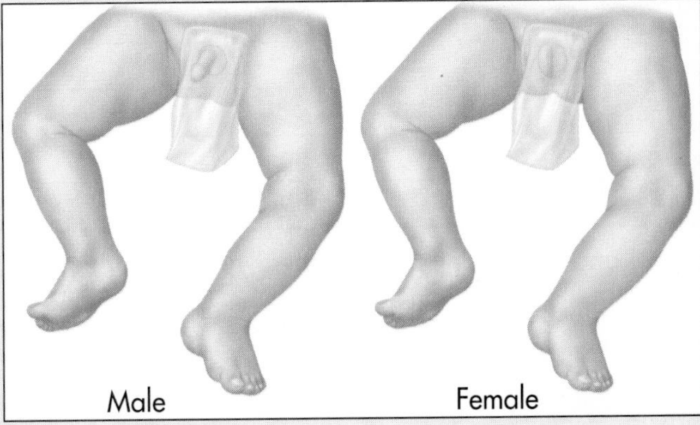

Figure 33-3. When you apply a pediatric urine bag, make sure there are no leaks.

Establishing Chain of Custody

Occasionally you may need to obtain urine specimens for drug and alcohol analysis. When you do so, you must establish a proper chain of custody.

The general approach to establishing chain of custody is described in Chapter 31. Because supplying a specimen for drug and alcohol testing could be self-incriminating, other requirements also apply. Begin by thoroughly explaining the procedure to the patient and having the patient sign a consent form. Figure 33-4 shows a typical consent form used when testing a urine specimen for drugs. This form states the purpose of the test and gives you permission to collect the specimen, prepare it for transport to the laboratory for analysis, and release the results to the agency requesting the test (such as a prospective or current employer). Distribute copies of this form to the medical review officer, laboratory, patient, collector, and employer or other requesting party.

Inform the patient that medications (both prescription and nonprescription), drugs, and alcohol will show up in the test results. Encourage the patient to list on the consent form all substances consumed in the last 30 days, including what was taken and how much.

The chain of custody form, described in Chapter 31, indicates the source of the urine sample. This form verifies that the patient whose name is on the laboratory request and consent forms is the same person who provided the sealed specimen sent to the laboratory. You will take the steps that follow to confirm that the specimen is from the correct patient.

Give the patient a special collection bottle. Tell him that you must read the temperature of the specimen within 4 minutes of collection and note the temperature on the chain of custody form. (A just-voided specimen will be close to body temperature.)

Explain that no water may be running in the bathroom while the patient provides the sample. While the patient is inside the bathroom, stand outside the door and listen to make sure the patient actually urinates into the collection container. Take the specimen bottle from the patient as he leaves the bathroom.

Preservation and Storage

Proper preservation and storage of specimens are essential. Changes that affect the chemical and microscopic properties of urine occur in urine kept at room temperature for more than 1 hour. Such changes invalidate cer-

Crossroads Medical Center
Newfield, New Jersey 07655-3213
201-555-4000

Drug Screen Consent Form

A urine drug test is required by____________________ as part of your pre-employment screening. Please provide us with a list of all medications that you are presently taking.

____

____

____

____

____

I understand that my prospective or continued employment is contingent on a successful screening.

Date: __________ Signature:____________________

Witness:______________________________

Figure 33-4. A consent form is a legal requirement when urine is collected for drug testing.

tain test results. If you leave a specimen unpreserved by any means for more than 1 hour, changes occur in the urine that affect the results of all urine testing—physical, chemical, and microscopic.

Refrigeration is the most common method for storing and preserving urine. It prevents bacterial growth in a specimen for at least 24 hours. Refrigeration can cause other changes in the urine, however, that may affect the physical characteristics of sediment and specific gravity. Bringing the specimen back to room temperature before testing will correct these problems. You can use chemical preservatives to preserve specimens, especially 24-hour specimens or those that must be sent a long distance to a laboratory.

Urinalysis

Urinalysis is the evaluation of urine by various types of testing methods to obtain information about body health and disease. Urinalysis consists of three types of testing:

- Physical
- Chemical
- Microscopic

There are normal values for all tests done on urine. The normal value for a specific substance may be negative or none, or it may be a range in concentration. Urine test results within normal ranges indicate health and normality.

Table 33-1

Standard Urine Values

Test	Value
Acetoacetate	None
Acetone	None
Albumin, qualitative	Negative
Albumin, quantitative	10–140 mg/L (24 hours)
Ammonia	140–1500 mg/24 hours
Bacteria (culture)	<10,000 colonies/mL
Bilirubin	Negative
Blood, occult	Negative
Calcium, quantitative	100–300 mg/24 hours
Casts	Rare/high-power field
Catecholamines, total	<100 μg/24 hours
Chloride	110–120 mEq/24 hours
Chorionic gonadotropin	Negative
Color	Pale yellow to dark amber
Creatine, nonpregnant women/men	<100 mg/24 hours (or <6% of creatinine)
Creatine, pregnant women	≤12% of creatinine
Creatinine, men	1.0–1.9 g/24 hours
Creatinine, women	0.8–1.7 g/24 hours
Crystals	Negative
Cystine and cysteine	<38.1 mg/24 hours
Estrogens, men	4–25 μg/g creatinine/24 hours
Estrogens, women	
Follicular	7–65 μg/g creatinine/24 hours
Midcycle	32–104 μg/g creatinine/24 hours
Luteal	8–135 μg/g creatinine/24 hours
Glucose, qualitative	Negative
Glucose, quantitative	50–500 mg/24 hours
Ketones	Negative
Lead	0.021–0.038 mg/L
Odor	Distinctly aromatic
pH	4.5–8.0
Phenylpyruvic acid	Negative
Phosphorus	0.4–1.3 g/24 hours
Potassium	40–80 mEq/24 hours
Protein (Bence Jones protein/free light chains)	Negative
Red blood cells	0–3/high-power field
Sodium	80–180 mEq/24 hours
Specific gravity, single specimen	1.005–1.030
Specific gravity, 24-hour specimen	1.015–1.025
Turbidity	Clear
Urea nitrogen	12–20 g/24 hours
Uric acid	0.25–0.75 g/24 hours
Urobilinogen, quantitative	1.0–4.0 mg/24 hours
Urobilinogen, semiquantitative	≤1 E. U./2 hours
Volume, adult females	600–1600 mL/24 hours
Volume, adult males	800–1800 mL/24 hours
Volume, children	3–4 times adult rate/kg
White blood cells	0–8/high-power field

Table 33-1 identifies normal values for a variety of urine tests. Because a urine test is a screening test, all abnormal values must be followed up with a confirmatory test.

Urinalysis is done as part of a general physical examination to screen for certain substances or to diagnose various medical conditions (see Table 33-2). For example, daily urine output provides a picture of renal function. With adequate fluid intake, the average adult daily urine output is 1250 mL per 24 hours. When total intake and output measurements are not approximately equal, urinary tract dysfunction may be the cause.

The urinary system works with other body systems to help the body function normally. Therefore, a disorder in another body system can affect urinary function. For ex-

Table 33-2

Common Urine Tests According to Clinical Condition

Clinical Condition or Suspected Disease	Types of Urine Testing
Acidosis	Reagent strip* for pH Specific gravity
Alkalosis (metabolic, respiratory)	Reagent strip* for pH Specific gravity
Diabetes mellitus	Odor (fruity) Microscopic examination for fatty, waxy casts Reagent strip* for ketonuria, glycosuria Specific gravity
Drug abuse	Gas chromatography–mass spectrometry**
Genitourinary infections (prostatitis, urethritis, vaginitis)	Cultures for bacteria, yeasts, parasites Microscopic examination for bacteria, RBCs
Human immunodeficiency virus (HIV)	Culture for virus (antibiotic added to kill bacteria) Other tests as indicated by specific symptoms
Hypercalcemia	Microscopic examination for calcium oxalate crystals Specific gravity
Hypertension	Microscopic examination for casts (hyaline, RBC) Specific gravity
Infectious diseases (bacterial) or other inflammatory diseases	Color and odor Cultures for bacteria, yeasts, viruses Microscopic examination for bacteria, WBCs, RBC casts (in severe cases) Reagent strip* for bacteria Turbidity
Metabolic disorders (except diabetes mellitus)	Color Microscopic examination for cystine crystals Reagent strip* for ketonuria, fructosuria, galactosuria, pentosuria, pH
Nephron disorders (nephrotic syndrome, glomerulonephritis, nephrosis, nephrolithiasis, pyelonephritis)	Color Microscopic examination for casts (epithelial, fatty, waxy, RBC), RBCs Reagent strip* for proteinuria Specific gravity Turbidity
Phenylketonuria	Color Reagent strip* for pH

continued

Table 33-2 continued

Clinical Condition or Suspected Disease	Types of Urine Testing
Poisoning (arsenic, cadmium, lead, mercury)	Color Mass spectrometry**
Polycystic kidney disease	Proteinuria Urinary volume
Pregnancy	Reagent strip* for human chorionic gonadotropin (HCG)
Renal infections (acute glomerulonephritis, nephrotic syndrome, pyelonephritis, pyogenic infection)	Color Microscopic examination for epithelial cells (especially with tubular degeneration), numerous casts (granular, hyaline, WBC), RBCs, WBCs Radioimmunoassay (RIA)** Reagent strip* for bacteria, albumin Specific gravity Turbidity Urinary volume
Renal disease, renal failure, severe renal damage, acute renal failure, renal tubular degeneration	Microscopic examination for epithelial cells (especially with tubular degeneration), numerous casts (hyaline, fatty, waxy, RBC) Reagent strip* for proteinuria (albumin), pH Specific gravity Turbidity Urinary volume
Sickle cell anemia	RBC casts
Starvation, dietary imbalance, extreme change in diet, dehydration	Color Odor (fruity) Reagent strip* for ketonuria Specific gravity
Urinary tract infection or mild inflammation (cystitis, pyelonephritis)	Color and odor Cultures for bacteria, yeasts, viruses Microscopic examination for bacteria, WBC casts, RBCs, WBCs Reagent strip* for bacteria, albumin, pH Specific gravity Turbidity
Urinary obstruction (tumor, trauma, inflammation)	Color Microscopic examination for RBCs Specific gravity Urinary volume

*Federal listings of waived tests refer to these as dipstick tests.

**Drug screening and some other common urine tests must be performed by a forensic laboratory or other laboratory capable of performing gas chromatography, mass spectrometry, and radioimmunoassay.

ample, the kidneys interact with the nervous system to help regulate blood pressure and control urination. Thus, a nervous system disorder can affect the circulatory and urinary systems. The cardiovascular system delivers blood to the kidneys for filtration, and the kidneys regulate fluid balance, which helps maintain circulation of blood and myocardial function. A cardiovascular system disorder can allow blood to be delivered to the kidneys at a pressure inadequate for filtration, which would affect urinary system function.

Physical Examination and Testing of Urine Specimens

The first step in urinalysis is the visual examination of physical characteristics. Prior to starting the physical examination, it is essential to check the specimen for proper labeling. As part of quality assurance, examine it to make sure there is no visible contamination and that no more than 1 hour has passed since collection (or since the sample was refrigerated and brought back to room temperature). These physical characteristics are examined:

- Color and turbidity
- Volume
- Odor
- Specific gravity

Color and Turbidity. Normal urine ranges from pale yellow (straw-colored) to dark amber. The color, which comes from a yellow pigment called urochrome, depends

Table 33-3

Urine Color and Turbidity: Possible Causes

Color and Turbidity	Pathologic Causes	Other Causes
Colorless or pale straw color (dilute)	Diabetes, anxiety, chronic renal disease	Diuretic therapy, excessive fluid intake (water, beer, coffee)
Cloudy	Infection, inflammation, glomerular nephritis	Vegetarian diet
Milky white	Fats, pus	Amorphous phosphates, spermatozoa
Dark yellow, dark amber (concentrated)	Acute febrile disease, vomiting or diarrhea (fluid loss or dehydration)	Low fluid intake, excessive sweating
Yellow-brown	Excessive RBC destruction, bile duct obstruction, diminished liver-cell function, bilirubin	
Orange-yellow, orange-red, orange-brown	Excessive RBC destruction, diminished liver-cell function, bile, hepatitis, urobilinuria, obstructive jaundice, hematuria	Drugs (such as pyridium, rifampin), dyes
Salmon pink		Amorphous urates
Cloudy red	RBCs, excessive destruction of skeletal or cardiac muscle	
Bright yellow or red	RBCs (hemorrhage, myoglobin, hemoglobin), excessive destruction of skeletal or cardiac muscle, porphyria	Beets, drugs (such as phenazopyridine hydrochloride), dyes (such as food coloring and contrast media)
Dark red, red-brown	Porphyria, RBCs (menstrual contamination, hemorrhage, hemoglobin), blood from previous hemorrhage	
Green, blue-green	Biliverdin, *Pseudomonas* organisms, oxidation of bilirubin	Vitamin B, methylene blue, asparagus (for green)
Green-brown	Bile duct obstruction	
Brownish black	Methemoglobin, melanin	Drugs (levodopa)
Dark brown or black	Acute glomerulonephritis	Drugs (nitrofurantoin, chlorpromazine, iron preparations)

on food or fluid intake, medications (including vitamin supplements), and waste products present in the urine. In general, a pale color indicates dilute urine, and a dark color indicates concentrated urine.

You will assess urine for turbidity, or cloudiness, by noting whether the urine is clear, slightly cloudy, cloudy, or very cloudy. Typically, urine is clear, although cloudy urine does not always indicate an abnormal condition.

The color of urine and any turbidity that is present can reveal medical conditions that require treatment. Table 33-3 provides more information on variations in urine color and turbidity and the possible causes or sources of these variations. Both pathologic (resulting from disease) and nonpathologic causes are noted.

Volume. Normal urine volume, or output, varies according to the patient's age. Normal adult urine volume is 600 to 1800 mL per 24 hours (average of 1250 mL per 24 hours). Infants and children have smaller total urine volumes, although they produce more urine per unit of body weight. Urine volume is typically measured on a timed specimen (such as a 24-hour urine specimen) rather than a random specimen.

Oliguria, insufficient production (or volume) of urine, occurs in such conditions as dehydration, decreased fluid intake, shock, and renal disease. The absence of urine production is called **anuria.** Renal or urethral obstruction and renal failure can cause anuria.

Odor. Although the odor of urine is not typically recorded or considered a significant indicator of disease, it can provide clues about the body's condition. The odor of normal, freshly voided urine is distinct but not unpleasant and is sometimes characterized as aromatic. After urine has been standing for a while, bacteria in the specimen decompose the urea, which causes an odor similar to ammonia.

Diseases, the presence of bacteria, and particular foods (such as asparagus and garlic) can cause changes in urine odor. For example, in the presence of urinary tract infections, urine is foul-smelling, and in patients with uncontrolled diabetes, the smell is characterized as fruity (because of the presence of ketones). Phenylketonuria, a congenital metabolic disease, produces a strange, "mousy" odor in an infant's wet diaper.

Specific Gravity. Urine specific gravity is a measure of the concentration or amount of substances dissolved in urine. Because the kidneys remove metabolic wastes and other substances from the blood, the specific gravity of the urine they produce is an indicator of kidney function. The physician's office laboratory uses any of three methods to determine specific gravity:

- Urinometer
- Refractometer
- Reagent strip (dipstick)

Specific gravity is a relative measure that is always compared to a standard. The standard for liquids is distilled water, which contains no dissolved substances.

$$\text{Specific gravity} = \frac{\text{weight of sample}}{\text{weight of distilled water}}$$

The specific gravity of distilled water is 1.000. You use special equipment to test for specific gravity (Figure 33-5).

The normal range of urine specific gravity is 1.005 to 1.030. Specific gravity fluctuates throughout the day in response to fluid intake. A first morning urine specimen normally has a higher specific gravity than a specimen provided later in the day. An increase in urine specific gravity indicates that the kidneys cannot properly dilute the urine. The urine then becomes more concentrated, causing it to darken. Increased specific gravity may indicate such conditions as a urinary tract infection, dehydration (for example, from fever, vomiting, or diarrhea), adrenal insufficiency, hepatic disease, or congestive heart failure. A decrease in the specific gravity of urine causes a lighter than normal urine color, may indicate that the kidneys cannot properly concentrate the urine, and may suggest such conditions as overhydration (excess fluid in the body), diabetes insipidus, chronic renal disease, or systemic lupus erythematosus.

Urinometer Measurement. A **urinometer** is a sealed glass float with a calibrated scale on the stem. The level at which a urinometer floats in a urine specimen is proportional to the urine's specific gravity. You must calibrate a

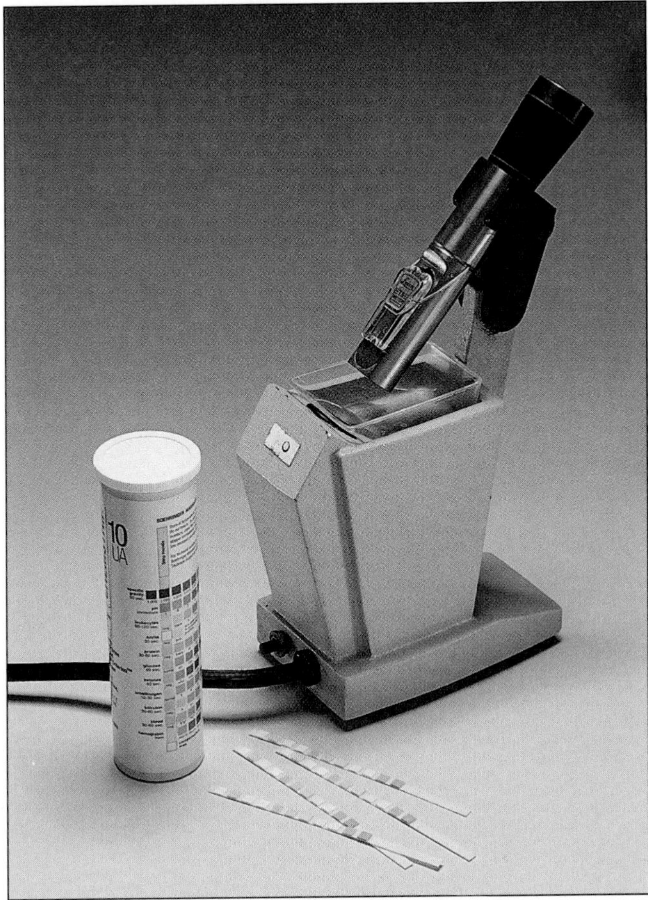

Figure 33-5. Specific gravity is commonly determined using a refractometer or reagent strips.

PROCEDURE 33-3

Measuring Specific Gravity With a Urinometer

Objective: To measure the specific gravity of a urine specimen with a urinometer

OSHA Guidelines

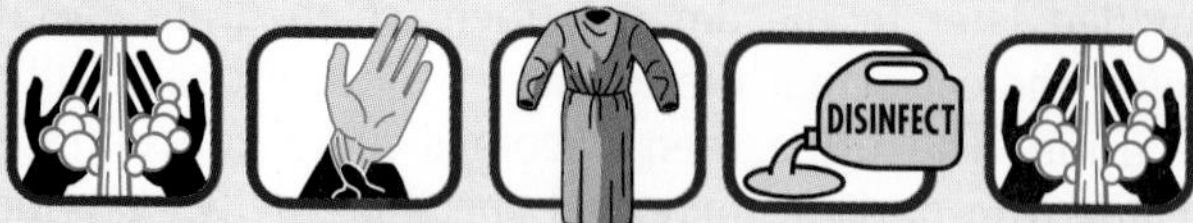

Materials: Urine specimen, laboratory report form, distilled water, urinometer, glass cylinder

Method

1. Wash your hands and put on examination gloves.
2. Check the specimen for proper labeling, and examine it to make sure that there is no visible contamination and that no more than 1 hour has passed since collection (or since the specimen has been removed from the refrigerator and brought back to room temperature).
3. If the urine specimen is refrigerated, allow it to warm to room temperature to avoid erroneous results.
4. Swirl the specimen to mix it thoroughly.
5. Confirm that the urinometer has been calibrated that day. If not, follow steps 6 through 9, using distilled water (at room temperature) in place of urine. If the specific gravity value is not 1.000, a new urinometer may be needed.
6. Using the specimen, fill the glass cylinder two-thirds to three-fourths full. (If you do not have enough liquid to make the urinometer float freely, you cannot use this method to determine specific gravity. Write QNS [quantity not sufficient] on the laboratory report form.)
7. Place the cylinder on a level surface; carefully introduce the urinometer into the specimen in the cylinder, and use the stem of the urinometer to gently spin the float (Figure 33-6).
8. Watch the bottom of the meniscus (the curve in the air-to-liquid surface of the specimen in the cylinder) at eye level.
9. As soon as the urinometer stops spinning, read the value on the scale where the bottom of the meniscus touches the stem of the urinometer (Figure 33-7).
10. Repeat the process of floating the urinometer and reading the results to obtain duplicate readings and ensure quality control. (Remove the stem and dry it completely before performing repeat tests.)
11. Record each result on the laboratory report form.
12. Sanitize and disinfect the urinometer and glass cylinder. (Do not use heat to disinfect the urinometer, because it could damage the instrument.) Put the urinometer and cylinder away when they are dry.
13. Clean and disinfect the work area.
14. Remove the gloves and wash your hands.
15. Record each result in the patient's chart.

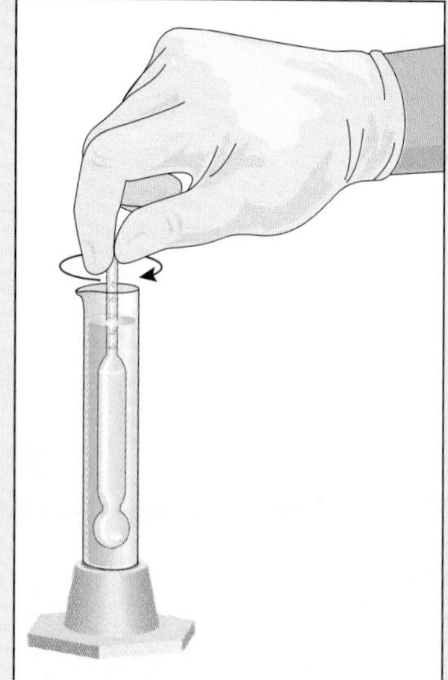

Figure 33-6. Gently spin the stem to ensure that the urinometer is floating freely.

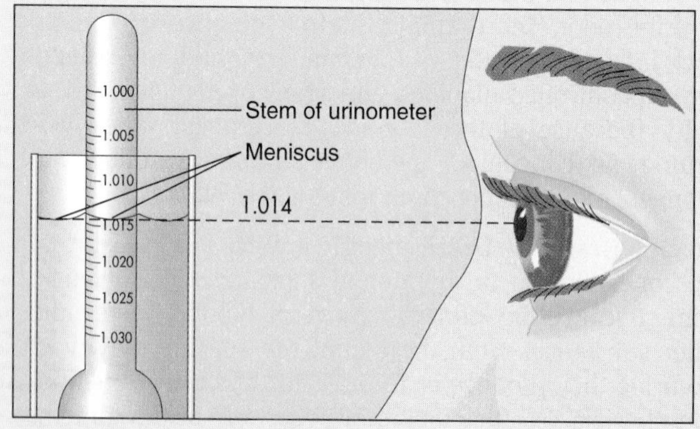

Figure 33-7. When the urinometer stops spinning, read the value on the scale.

urinometer each day with distilled water to ensure accuracy. When the float is placed in the cylinder containing distilled water, it should stabilize at the 1.000 level. You must have at least 15 mL of urine to accurately determine specific gravity with a urinometer, and the urine must be at room temperature. Procedure 33-3 describes how to measure specific gravity with a urinometer.

Refractometer Measurement. A **refractometer** is an optical instrument that measures the refraction, or bending, of light as it passes through a liquid. The degree of refraction, or refractive index, is proportional to the amount of dissolved material in the liquid. You must calibrate a refractometer each day with distilled water by setting the instrument at 1.000 with the set screw. Two standard solutions (solutions of known specific gravity) are also used to ensure accuracy. Advantages of using a refractometer to measure urine specific gravity are that the process takes little time and requires little urine. Only a drop of urine is used for this determination, so a volume of urine too small for urinometer testing may be measured by a refractometer. Procedure 33-4 describes how to measure specific gravity with a refractometer.

Reagent Strip Measurement. You may use special reagent strips, or dipsticks, to test for specific gravity. Test pads along these plastic strips contain chemicals that react with substances in the urine and change color in precise

PROCEDURE 33-4

Measuring Specific Gravity With a Refractometer

Objective: To measure the specific gravity of a urine specimen with a refractometer

OSHA Guidelines

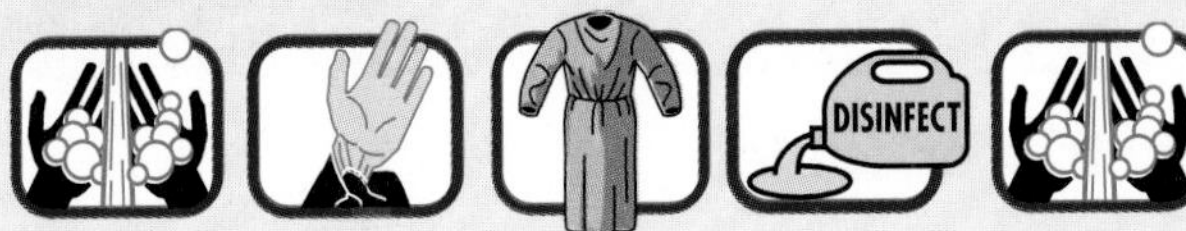

Materials: Urine specimen, refractometer, dropper, laboratory report form

Method

1. Wash your hands and put on examination gloves.
2. Check the specimen for proper labeling, and examine it to make sure that there is no visible contamination and that no more than 1 hour has passed since collection (or since the specimen has been removed from the refrigerator and brought back to room temperature).
3. Swirl the specimen to mix it thoroughly.
4. Confirm that the refractometer has been calibrated that day. If not, you must calibrate it with distilled water. You must also use two standard solutions as controls to check the accuracy of the refractometer. Follow steps 6 through 11, using each of the three samples in place of the specimen. Clean the refractometer and the dropper after each use, and record the calibration values in the quality control log.
5. Open the hinged lid of the refractometer.
6. Draw up a small amount of the specimen into the dropper.
7. Place one drop of the specimen under the cover.
8. Close the lid.
9. Turn on the light, and look into the eyepiece of the refractometer. As the light passes through the specimen, the refractometer measures the refraction of the light and displays the refractive index on a scale on the right with corresponding specific gravity values on the left (see Figure 33-8).
10. Read the specific gravity value at the line where light and dark meet.
11. Record the value on the laboratory report form.
12. Sanitize and disinfect the refractometer and the dropper. Put them away when they are dry.
13. Clean and disinfect the work area.
14. Remove the gloves and wash your hands.
15. Record the value in the patient's chart.

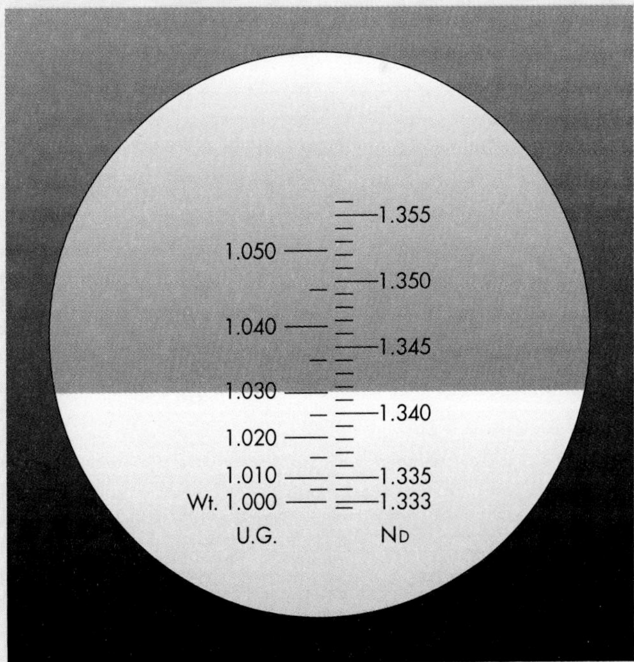

Figure 33-8. A refractometer uses light refraction to measure specific gravity.

ways. The reagent strip container includes a color chart for interpreting color changes on the test pads. When you evaluate urine specific gravity in this way, keep in mind that this type of test depends on precisely timed intervals identified by the manufacturer. Follow all directions exactly. The general steps for using reagent strips are as follows.

1. Wash your hands and put on examination gloves.
2. Identify the specimen.
3. After checking the expiration date on the reagent strip container (never use expired strips), remove a reagent strip from the container, holding the strip in your hand or placing it on a clean paper towel. Immediately replace the cap on the container.
4. Swirl the specimen to mix it thoroughly.
5. Note the time and simultaneously dip the strip into the urine and quickly remove it.
6. Draw the reagent strip across the specimen container's lip to remove excess urine.
7. Hold the strip horizontally and, after waiting for the specified time interval, compare the strip to the color chart on the container.
8. Read the value that corresponds to the matching color (for specific gravity in this case), and record the value on the laboratory report form.
9. Remove the gloves and wash your hands.
10. Place the laboratory report form in the patient's chart.

Chemical Testing of Urine Specimens

As a medical assistant, you may be asked to perform chemical tests on urine. Prior to performing chemical tests, always check for proper identification on the urine specimen to be tested. Chemical testing is usually done with reagent strips or tablets. It can also be performed with certain automated machines that use photometry.

The doctor orders chemical testing of urine to determine the status of body processes such as carbohydrate metabolism, liver or kidney function, or acid-base balance. Other reasons for chemical testing include deter-

Table 33-4

Some Common Chemical Analyses by Reagent Strip or Tablet

Substance Test Indicates	Manufacturer of Test Strip or Tablet	Name of Test Strip or Tablet
Albumin (a protein)	Bayer	Albustix
		Multistix
	Boehringer Mannheim	Chemstrip
Bacteria (screen)	Bayer	Multistix
	Boehringer Mannheim	Chemstrip
Bilirubin	Bayer	Ictotest*
		Bili-Labstix
		Multistix
	Boehringer Mannheim	Chemstrip
Blood		
Red blood cells (as hemoglobin)	Bayer	Multistix
		Labstix
		Hema-Combistix
		Hemastix
	Boehringer Mannheim	Chemstrip
White blood cells (as leukocytes)	Bayer	Leucostix
		Multistix
	Boehringer Mannheim	Chemstrip

continued

mining the presence of drugs, toxic environmental substances, or infections.

Testing With Reagent Strips or Tablets. As already described in the discussion of specific gravity, reagents (on plastic strips or in tablets) are chemicals that react with a particular substance in urine and change color in precise ways. These changes indicate the presence of that substance and the amount or concentration of the substance in the urine specimen. For example, when a reagent strip is used to test for ketones, the reacted color on the strip will correspond either to a specific concentration of ketone bodies, such as acetoacetic acid, or to no ketones present.

Reagent strips are used to test urine for a number of substances. In addition to ketones, these substances include nitrite, pH, blood, bilirubin, glucose, protein, and leukocytes. The tests and the usual reagent strips used in the tests are listed in Table 33-4.

There are numerous trade names for urine reagent strips, or dipsticks, and tablets (for example, Multistix, Chemstrip, and Acetest). Not all reagents are reactive for the same chemicals. You must choose the appropriate strip or tablet according to the chemical test requested. All reagent strips and tablets are used once and discarded.

Follow the exact directions that come with the reagent strips or tablets to ensure accurate results. For quality assurance, take these basic precautions: Keep strips and tablets in tightly closed containers in a cool, dry area. Never remove them from the container until immediately before testing. Examine strips for discoloration before use; discard discolored strips. Check the expiration date on the bottle; do not use strips or tablets that have expired. Use strips within 6 months of opening the container. Every time you open a new supply of reagents, run control samples to check for proper operation.

Although the process is essentially the same for all reagent strip tests, there are variations in time intervals before reading results. Some reagent strips are designed to test for several substances at once. The basic procedure for using reagent strips for chemical tests is

Table 33-4 continued

Substance Test Indicates	Manufacturer of Test Strip or Tablet	Name of Test Strip or Tablet
Glucose	Bayer	Clinistix
		Clinitest*
	Lilly	TesTape
Ketone bodies		
Acetoacetate	Bayer	Acetest*
		Ketostix
		Labstix
		Multistix
	Boehringer Mannheim	Chemstrip
Acetone	Bayer	Acetest*
	Boehringer Mannheim	Chemstrip
pH	Bayer	Hema-Combistix
		Combistix
		Multistix
		Bili-Labstix
		Labstix
	Boehringer Mannheim	Chemstrip

*These reagent tablet tests are often used to confirm questionable results seen on reagent strip tests.

the same as that described in the discussion of specific gravity.

Tests based on reagent tablets are confirmatory for various substances in urine. These tests take longer to perform and may be used when reagent strip tests are inconclusive. Reagent tablet tests generally involve putting a drop of urine on the tablet, putting a drop of urine on a special mat (Ictotest), or putting a tablet in a few drops of urine or diluted urine. Procedure 33-5 describes how to perform the Acetest (a typical reagent tablet test) to confirm the presence of ketones in the urine.

Ketone Bodies. Ketone bodies (or ketones) are intermediary products of fat and protein metabolism in the body. They include acetone, acetoacetic acid, and β-hydroxybutyric acid. Only the first two substances can be determined by reagent strip or tablet test. Normally, there are no ketones in urine. The presence of ketones in the urine may indicate that a patient is following a low-carbohydrate diet, or it may indicate that the patient has a condition such as starvation, excessive vomiting, or diabetes mellitus. Because ketones evaporate at room temperature, be sure to test urine immediately or cover the specimen tightly and refrigerate it until testing can be done.

pH. **Urinary pH** is a measure of the degree of acidity or alkalinity of the urine. Determination of pH can provide information about a patient's metabolic status, diet, medications being taken, and several conditions. The normal pH of freshly voided urine ranges from 4.5 to 8.0. The average urine pH is 6.0, which is slightly acidic. A pH of 7.0 is neutral, a lower pH is acidic, and a higher one is alkaline. Patients with alkaline urine may have such conditions as urinary tract infection or metabolic or respiratory alkalosis. Those with acidic urine may have such conditions as phenylketonuria or acidosis. Reagent strip, or dipstick, tests on both urine and blood are used to measure pH in the body. (See Chapter 34 for information on blood tests for pH.)

Blood. A patient who has blood in the urine may be menstruating, have a urinary tract infection, or have trauma or bleeding in the kidneys. To test for blood in urine, use a reagent strip that reacts with hemoglobin. There are two indicators on the strip. One is for nonhemolyzed blood, the other for hemolyzed blood.

Colors on the strip range from orange through green to dark blue and may indicate **hematuria** (the presence of blood in the urine) caused by cystitis; kidney stones; menstruation; or ureteral, bladder, or urethral irritation.

PROCEDURE 33-5

Performing a Reagent Tablet Test

Objective: To perform the Acetest on a urine specimen to confirm the presence of ketones

OSHA Guidelines

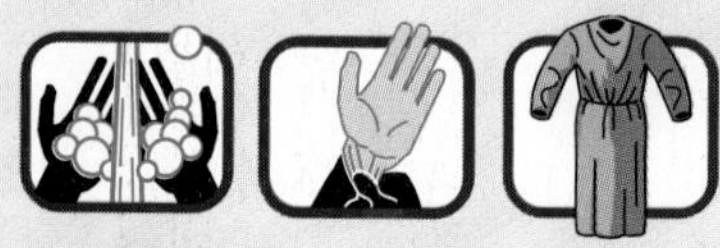

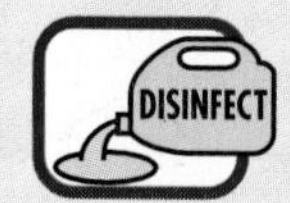

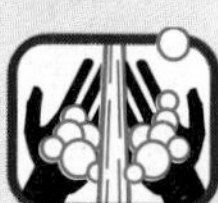

Materials: Urine specimen, laboratory report form, color chart, medicine dropper or disposable plastic pipette, Acetest reagent tablets, paper cup of water for rinsing dropper, white paper

Method

1. Wash your hands and put on examination gloves.
2. Check the specimen for proper labeling, and examine it to make sure that there is no visible contamination and that no more than 1 hour has passed since collection (or the specimen has been removed from the refrigerator and brought back to room temperature).
3. Swirl the specimen to mix it thoroughly.
4. Place a piece of white paper on the working surface.
5. Tap one Acetest tablet into the lid of its container, without touching the tablet. Then tap the tablet from the lid onto the white paper.
6. Draw up a small amount of urine from the specimen into the medicine dropper or pipette.
7. Put one drop of urine on the tablet.
8. Wait 30 seconds; a color should appear if the test is positive.
9. Compare the tablet color with the color on the chart and match.
10. Read the result from the chart indicating the amount of ketones (acetone and acetoacetic acid only) in the urine specimen.
11. Record the amount on the laboratory report form.
12. Discard used disposable supplies; rinse the dropper with clean water.
13. Clean and disinfect the work area.
14. Remove the gloves and wash your hands.
15. Record the result in the patient's chart.

The presence of free hemoglobin in the urine is known as **hemoglobinuria,** a rare condition caused by transfusion reactions, malaria, drug reactions, snakebites, or severe burns. Injured or damaged muscle tissue—such as occurs in crushing injuries, myocardial infarction, muscular dystrophy, or injuries during contact sports—can cause **myoglobinuria** (the presence of myoglobin in the urine). Reagent strip testing does not distinguish between these two conditions.

Bilirubin and Urobilinogen. When hemoglobin breaks down, it converts into conjugated bilirubin in the liver and then to urobilinogen in the intestines. Presence of the bile pigment **bilirubin** in the urine (**bilirubinuria**) is one of the first signs of liver disease or conditions that involve the liver. When bilirubin is present, urine turns yellow-brown to greenish orange. You usually use a reagent strip to test for bilirubin.

Although **urobilinogen** is present in the urine in small amounts, elevated levels of this colorless compound formed in the intestines may indicate increased red blood cell destruction or liver disease. Lack of urobilinogen in the urine may suggest total bile duct obstruction, as a result of which urobilinogen is not formed in the intestines or reabsorbed in the circulation. To test for urobilinogen, you use reagent strips.

Testing for either bilirubin or urobilinogen must be performed on a fresh urine specimen. Bilirubin decomposes rapidly in bright light to form biliverdin, which is not detected by the reagent strip test for bilirubin. Urobilinogen breaks down to urobilin on standing.

Glucose. Glucose is present in patients with normal urine, but only in small quantities not detectable by the reagent strip test for glucose. **Glycosuria** (the presence of significant glucose in the urine) is common in patients with diabetes. Blood is more commonly tested for glucose than urine is, because reagent strip or tablet tests may show false-negative results when used for testing urine.

Protein. Although a small amount of protein is excreted in the urine every day, an excess of protein in the urine (**proteinuria**) usually indicates renal disease. Proteinuria is also common in pregnant patients or after heavy exercise.

Nitrite. The presence of nitrite in the urine suggests a bacterial infection of the urinary tract. The test is not definitive, however, because some bacteria cannot convert nitrate to nitrite. Also, if an insufficient number of bacteria are present in the urine or if the urine has not incubated long enough in the bladder for a reaction to take place, a negative nitrite test can occur. The best urine specimen to test for nitrites is the first morning specimen.

When testing for urinary nitrite, you must test the urine immediately or refrigerate the specimen. Bacteria can multiply in a specimen that is allowed to sit at room temperature, thus causing a false-positive test result. Bacteria can also further metabolize the nitrite already produced, thus causing a false-negative result.

Leukocytes. Leukocytes appear in the urine in urinary tract or renal infections. Use strip tests for leukocyte esterase, a chemical seen when leukocytes are present, to test for leukocytes.

Phenylketones. The presence of phenylketones in a patient's urine indicates **phenylketonuria (PKU),** a genetically inherited disorder in which the body cannot properly metabolize the nutrient phenylalanine. This disorder causes phenylketones to accumulate in the bloodstream, resulting in mental retardation. PKU can be treated successfully by limiting dietary intake of phenylalanine, which makes up 5% of all natural protein, from early infancy. Although urine can be tested for the presence of phenylketones, blood testing is routine for newborns before discharge, at least 24 hours after birth.

Other Types of Chemical Testing. There are other types of chemical tests that may be performed on urine specimens. They generally involve testing for electrolytes and osmolality. Because these tests are performed in an outside laboratory rather than in a physician's office laboratory, you do not need to know the steps in each procedure.

Microscopic Examination of Urine Specimens

You may perform a microscopic examination of urine to view formed elements found in urine sediment that you would not be able to see without the aid of a microscope. You will use a centrifuge to obtain sediment for analysis. A centrifuge spins test tubes containing fluid at speeds that cause heavier substances in the fluid to settle to the bottom of the tubes.

During microscopic examination, elements that are categorized and counted include the cells, casts, crystals, yeast, bacteria, and parasites that form sediment (precipitate) after urine is centrifuged. You may use the KOVA System, manufactured by Hycor Biomedical, Irvine, California, to prepare urine sediment for microscopic examination. When you use the KOVA System, the sediment is evenly distributed to four calibrated chambers before the microscopic elements are counted. Procedure 33-6 describes how to process a urine specimen for microscopic examination of sediment.

Cells. High-power magnification is used to classify and count cells. Three types of cells are found in urine (Figure 33-13, p. 682):

- Epithelial cells
- White blood cells
- Red blood cells

Epithelial Cells. Epithelial cells are classified as round, transitional, or squamous. Round epithelial cells can be round to oval and have a large, oval, and sometimes

PROCEDURE 33-6

Processing a Urine Specimen for Microscopic Examination of Sediment

Objective: To prepare a slide for microscopic examination of urine sediment

OSHA Guidelines

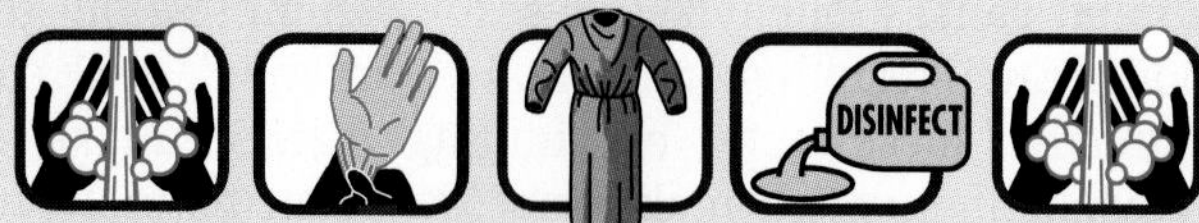

Materials: Fresh urine specimen, two glass or plastic test tubes, water, centrifuge, tapered pipette, glass slide with coverslip, microscope with light source, laboratory report form

Method

1. Wash your hands and put on examination gloves.
2. Check the specimen for proper labeling, and examine it to make sure that there is no visible contamination and that no more than 1 hour has passed since collection (or since the specimen has been removed from the refrigerator and brought back to room temperature).
3. Swirl the urine specimen to mix it thoroughly.
4. Pour approximately 10 mL of urine into one test tube and 10 mL of plain water into the other (Figure 33-9).
5. Balance the centrifuge by placing the test tubes on either side (Figure 33-10).
6. Make sure the lid is secure, and set the centrifuge timer (Figure 33-11) for 3 to 5 minutes.
7. Set the speed as prescribed by your office's protocol (usually 1500 to 2000 revolutions per minute) and start the centrifuge.
8. After the centrifuge stops, lift out the tube containing the urine, and carefully pour most of the liquid portion—called the **supernatant**—down the drain in the sink (Figure 33-12).

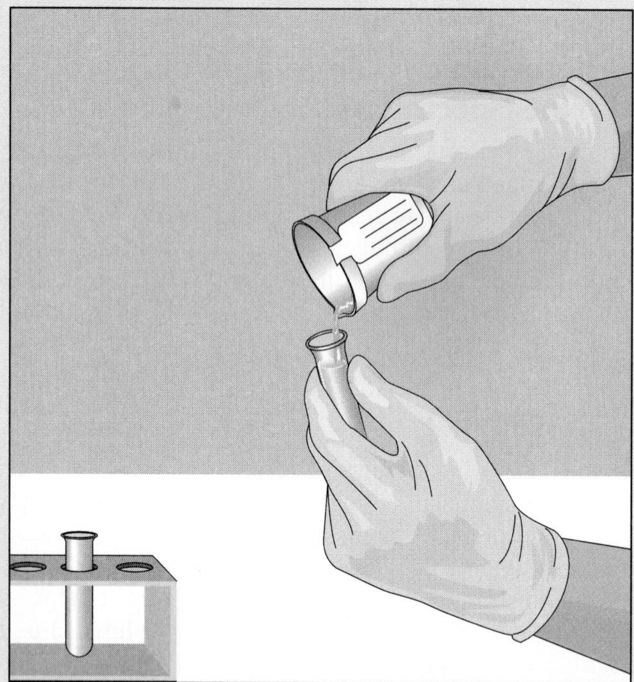

Figure 33-9. Fill one test tube with approximately 10 mL of urine and the other with 10 mL of water.

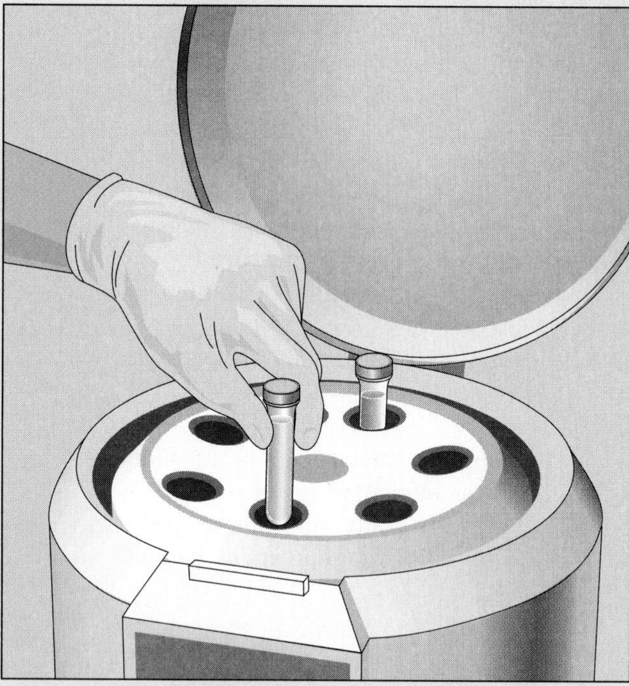

Figure 33-10. The centrifuge must be balanced by placing one test tube on each side.

eccentric nucleus. Although a few of these cells appear normally in urine, several may indicate tubular damage in the kidneys.

Transitional epithelial cells line the urinary tract from the renal pelvis (the beginning of the ureter) to the upper portion of the urethra. They can be round to oval and may have a tail and, occasionally, two nuclei. Like the round epithelial cell, a few appear normally in urine, but several may indicate tubular damage.

Squamous epithelial cells line the lower portion of the genitourinary tract. They are large, flat, irregular cells with a small, round, centrally located nucleus. They

9. A few drops of urine should remain in the bottom of the test tube with any sediment. Mix the urine and sediment together by gently tapping the bottom of the tube on the palm of your hand.
10. Use the tapered pipette to obtain a drop or two of urine sediment. Place the drops in the center of a clean glass slide.
11. Place the coverslip over the specimen, allow it to settle, and place it on the stage of the microscope.
12. Correctly focus the microscope as directed in Procedure 32-1.

Note: Most medical assistants are trained to perform this procedure only up to this point. After this, the physician usually examines the specimen. You may, however, be asked to clean the items after the examination is completed. The remaining steps are provided for your information.

13. Use a dim light and view the slide under the low-power objective.
14. Switch to the high-power objective. View any casts, cells, and crystals. Adjust the slide position so that you can view it from at least ten different fields. Turn off the light after the examination is completed.
15. Record the observations on the laboratory report form.
16. Properly dispose of used disposable materials.
17. Sanitize and disinfect nondisposable items; put them away when they are dry.
18. Clean and disinfect the work area.
19. Remove the gloves and wash your hands.
20. Record the observations in the patient's chart.

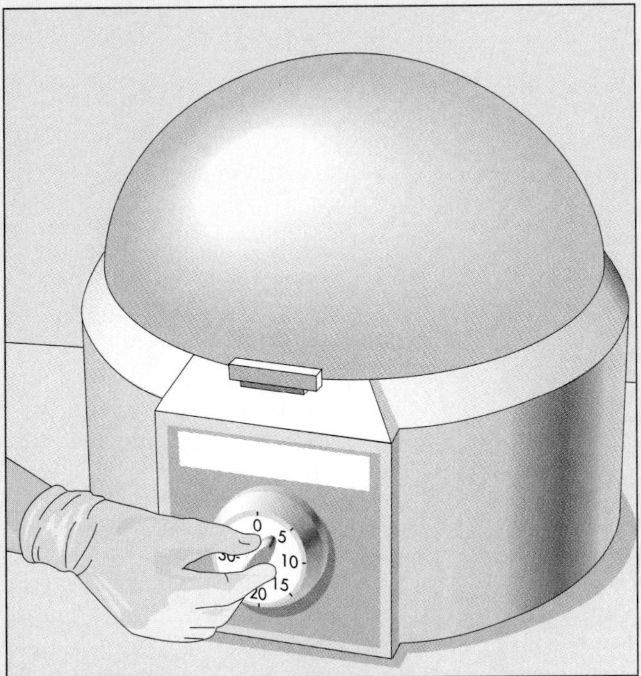

Figure 33-11. Set the centrifuge timer for 3 to 5 minutes.

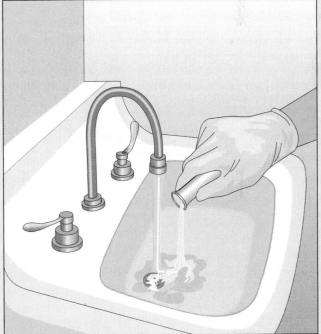

Figure 33-12. Make sure you do not lose any sediment when you pour off the urine.

often occur in sheets or clumps and can be easily recognized under low-power magnification.

White Blood Cells. White blood cells are larger than red blood cells, have a granular appearance, and usually contain a multilobed nucleus. They are typically found in large numbers (greater than the normal zero to eight per high-power field) in the urine if inflammation is present or if the specimen was contaminated during collection.

Red Blood Cells. Red blood cells can be pale, round, nongranular, and flat or biconcave. They have no nucleus and enter the urinary tract during inflammation or injury. From zero to three red blood cells per high-power field in

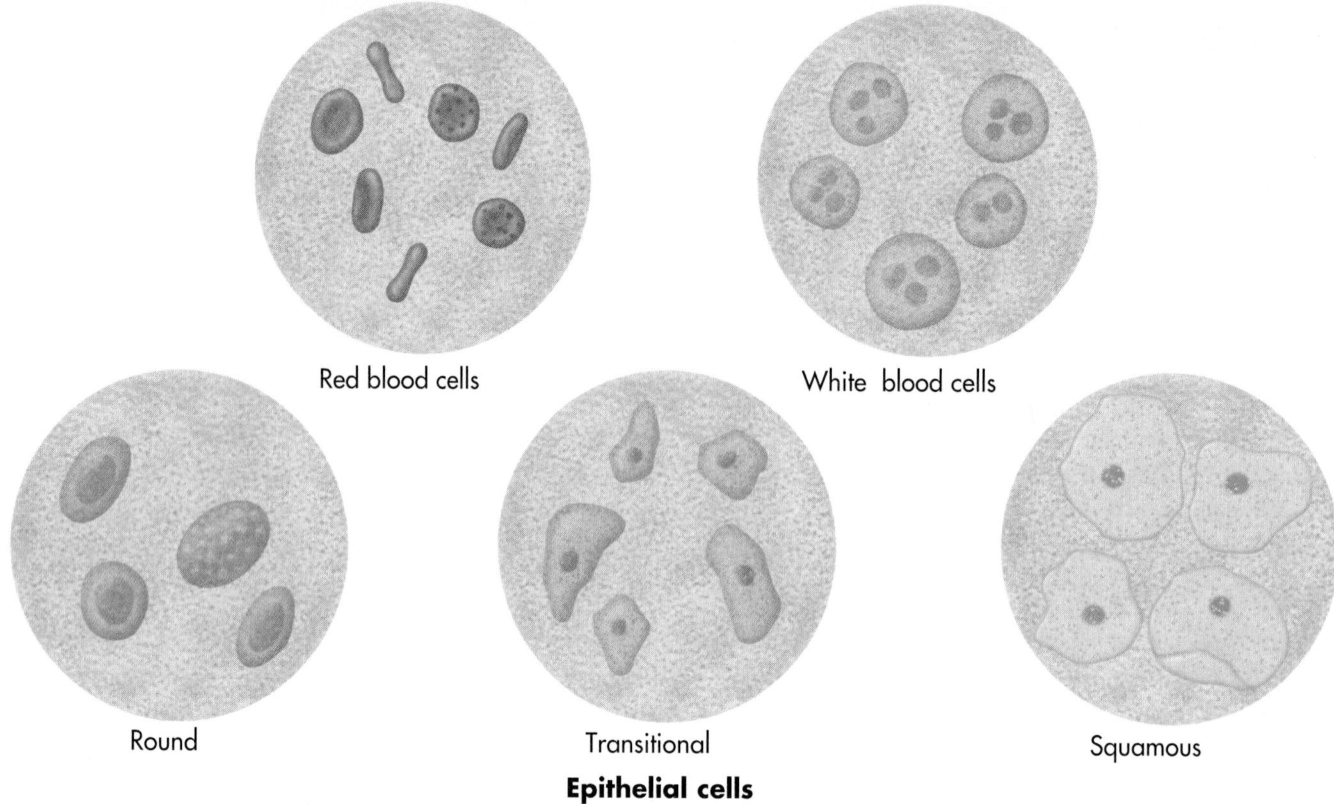

Figure 33-13. The number and types of cells found in urine constitute important diagnostic information about a patient's condition.

urine is normal. Numerous red blood cells may indicate a variety of problems, however, including urinary infection, obstruction, inflammation, trauma, or tumor.

Casts. **Casts,** which are cylinder-shaped elements with flat or rounded ends, form when protein from the breakdown of cells accumulates and precipitates in the kidney tubules and is washed into the urine. The protein then assumes the size and shape of the tubules. Casts differ in composition and size (Figure 33-14). Classified according to their appearance and composition, casts can indicate renal pathologic conditions or can be caused by strenuous exercise. Types of casts include the following:

- Hyaline casts, which are pale, transparent, and shaped like cylinders, with rounded ends and parallel sides. Composed of protein, they form because of diminished urine flow through individual nephrons. They are present in patients with kidney disease or in people who have exercised strenuously.
- Granular casts, which resemble hyaline casts and can also result from kidney disease or strenuous exercise. The granules are believed to come from degeneration of cellular inclusions.
- Red blood cell casts, which always indicate an abnormality and are hyaline casts with embedded red cells. Because of the red blood cells, these casts sometimes appear brown.
- White blood cell casts, which are hyaline casts with leukocytes. These casts typically have a multilobed nucleus and may indicate pyelonephritis, which is an inflammation of the kidney and renal pelvis.
- Epithelial cell casts, which contain embedded renal tubular epithelial cells and indicate excessive kidney damage. Causes include shock, renal ischemia, heavy-metal poisoning, certain allergic reactions, and nephrotoxic drugs. These casts are often confused with white blood cell casts.
- Waxy casts, which are rare, yellow, glassy, brittle, smooth, and homogeneous structures with cracks or fissures and squared or broken ends. These casts occur with severe renal disease.

Crystals. **Crystals,** naturally produced solids of definite form, are commonly seen in urine specimens, especially those permitted to cool. They usually do not indicate a significant disorder, except when found in large numbers in patients with kidney stones and in a few pathologic conditions (such as hypercalcemia and some inborn errors of metabolism). Figure 33-15 shows common crystals found in urine specimens. Because different substances tend to crystallize in urine that is acidic and in urine that is alkaline, or basic, it is important to determine the pH of a patient's urine before you try to identify any crystals that are present.

Yeast Cells. Yeast cells, which are usually oval and may show budding, may be confused with red blood cells. Yeast cells in urine sediment are associated with genitourinary tract infection, external genitalia contamination,

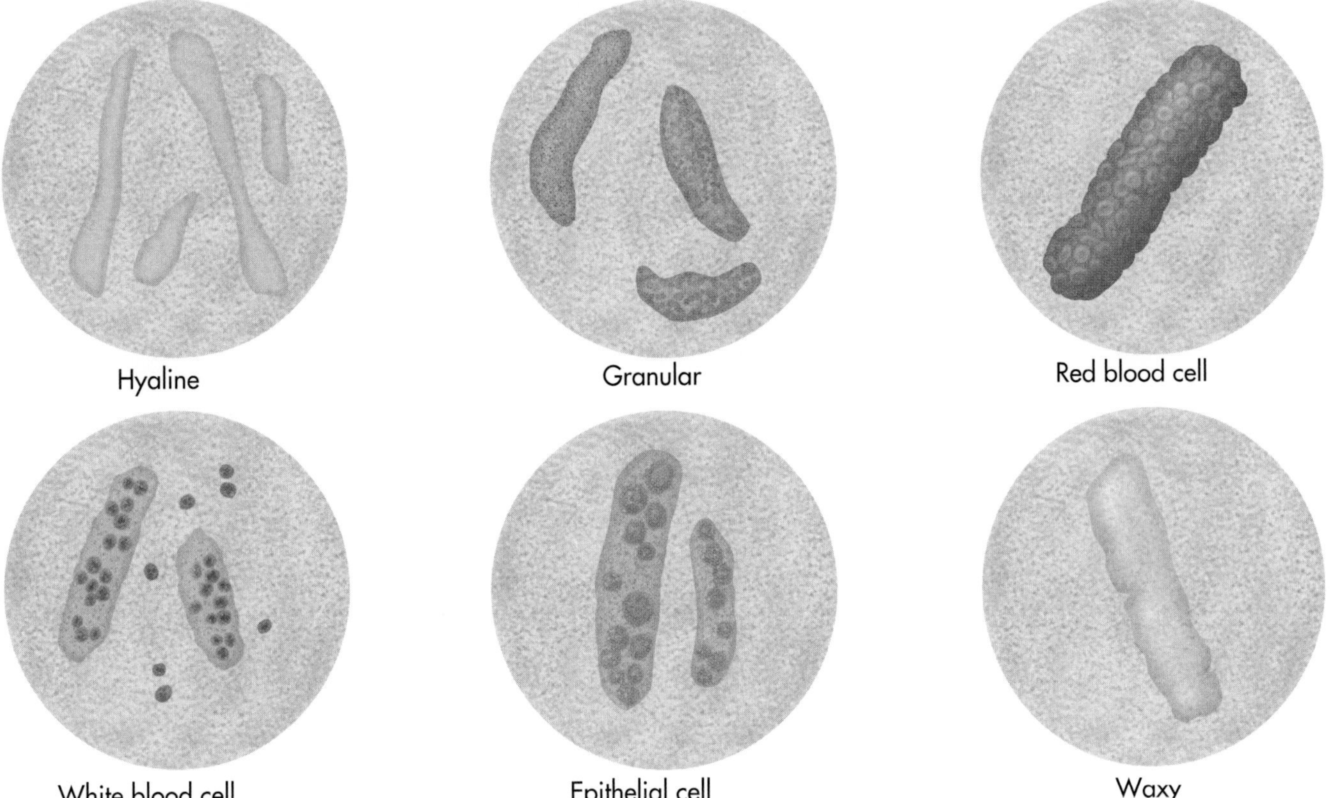

Figure 33-14. Casts, which are shaped like cylinders with flat or rounded ends, are formed when protein accumulates in the kidney tubules and is washed into the urine.

vaginitis, urethritis, and prostatitis. These cells are also commonly seen in the urine of patients with diabetes.

Bacteria. Although a few bacteria are normally found in urine, urinary tract infection may be indicated if the urine has bacteria along with a putrid odor and numerous white blood cells. Bacteria under high-power magnification appear rod- or cocci-shaped.

Parasites. The presence of parasites in sediment may signal genitourinary tract infection or external genitalia contamination. The most common urinary parasite, *Trichomonas vaginalis* (a pear-shaped protozoan with four flagella), is typically found in vaginal disorders but may also appear in males. When a urine specimen is cooled, *Trichomonas* organisms die.

Summary

The volume and physical, chemical, and microscopic characteristics of urine provide a great deal of information about a patient's health. Although invasive collection methods are sometimes necessary, routine urine specimens can be obtained by noninvasive, painless means. Urinalysis is the most common diagnostic test performed in doctors' offices.

You will have a substantial role in collecting, processing, and testing urine specimens. You will need to understand the urinary tract system and the basic characteristics of urine, including how it is formed, its physical composition, its chemical properties, and its microscopic characteristics.

Assisting patients and instructing them in the procedures required to collect different types of specimens are important aspects of your job. You must understand the purposes and procedures for collecting random specimens, first morning specimens, clean-catch midstream specimens, timed specimens, and 24-hour specimens. Throughout all collecting and processing procedures, you must practice quality assurance and employ precautions to avoid spreading disease-causing microorganisms.

When obtaining and processing specimens, you need to follow general guidelines as well as take into account special considerations for specific groups of patients. You are responsible for ensuring that specimens are preserved and stored so that they are not contaminated or otherwise altered.

You may perform some tests on urine and prepare urine specimens for evaluation by the doctor. In either case you must be able to distinguish between normal and abnormal findings concerning the physical, chemical, and microscopic characteristics of urine.

Urinalysis provides important information to the doctor. You play a significant role in seeing that the specimen has been properly collected, processed, and tested, so that the information obtained from the analysis is useful and accurate.

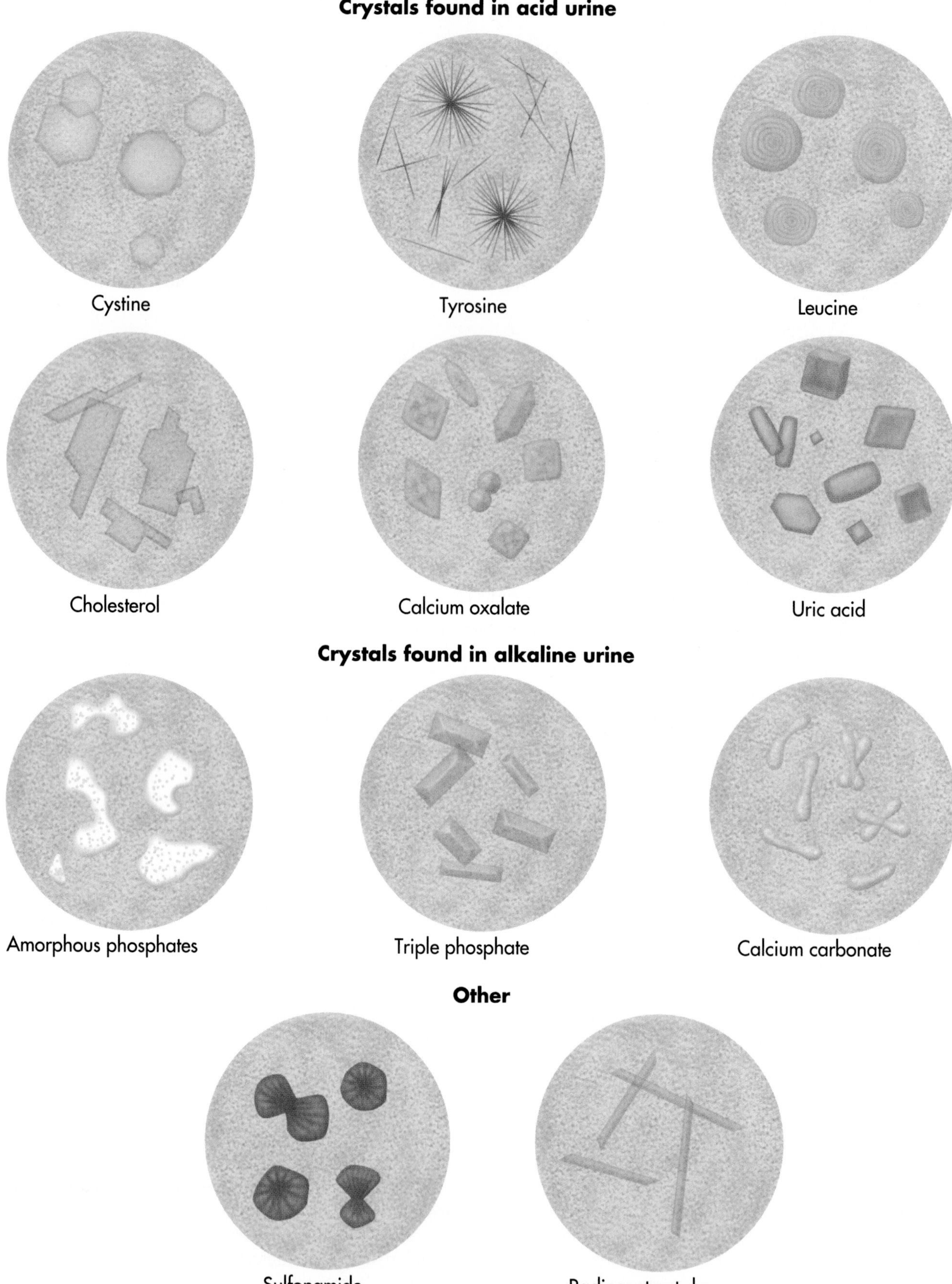

Figure 33-15. You should be able to identify common crystals in urine and what they mean.

33 Chapter Review

Discussion Questions

1. When is it worth putting the patient at risk for infection to insert a catheter?
2. List the physical characteristics of a urine sample that should be observed during routine urinalysis. What would you look for in each characteristic?
3. List guidelines that, when followed, help ensure that a patient successfully obtains a clean-catch midstream specimen at home.

Critical Thinking Questions

1. While performing a routine examination of a urine specimen, you find that it is colorless and that the odor is fruity. What pathologic condition could cause this reaction, and which reagent strip tests could you perform to confirm the cause?
2. Compare and contrast quality assurance for physical and chemical testing of urine specimens.
3. After collecting a clean-catch midstream urine specimen, a patient gives it to you. You notice that the container lid is not on the container and the patient is holding the container by its side, with his thumb inside the container. What should you do about this sample? Why?

Application Activities

1. Using a doll, demonstrate the correct method for applying a urine collection bag to a female infant.
2. Demonstrate the correct method for preparing a slide for microscopic examination of sediment.
3. Working with another student acting in the role of patient, explain the recommended procedure for collecting a 24-hour urine specimen. Ask appropriate questions to ensure that the "patient" understands the procedure. Then switch roles so that each student has the opportunity to play each role.

Further Readings

Barnett, Beatrice. *Urine-Therapy—It May Save Your Life.* Margate, FL: Lifestyle Institute, 1992.

Bridgen, Malcom L., and Ann Leadbeater. "Stick 'Em Up: Optimizing Results With Urinalysis Dipsticks." *Medical Laboratory Observer* 26, no. 6 (June 1994): 32–36.

"Clinical Validation Study of Cancer Diagnostic Test Announced." *Cancer Biotechnology Weekly,* 26 February 1996, 7.

Kunin, Calvin M. *Urinary Tract Infections: Detection, Prevention and Management.* 5th ed. Baltimore: Williams & Wilkins, 1996.

Scarre, Shelly S. *Urinalysis: Methods, Diagnostics, Influence of Sexually Transmitted Diseases and Abuse-Injury Implications.* Washington, DC: ABBE Publications, 1995.

Tietz, Norbert W., ed. *Clinical Guide to Laboratory Tests.* 3d ed. Philadelphia: W. B. Saunders, 1995.

"Urine Test Detects HIV-Positive Subjects in Study." *AIDS Weekly,* 5 September 1994, 15.

Urine Testing for Drugs of Abuse. New York: Gordon, 1991.

USP DI-Volume II Advice for the Patient: Drug Information in Lay Language. Rockville, MD: United States Pharmacopeial Convention, 1995.

Collecting, Processing, and Testing Blood Specimens

CHAPTER OUTLINE

- The Role of the Medical Assistant
- The Functions and Composition of Blood
- Collecting Blood Specimens
- Responding to Patient Needs
- Performing Common Blood Tests

OBJECTIVES

After completing Chapter 34, you will be able to:

- Discuss the composition and function of blood.
- Describe the process for collecting a blood specimen.
- Explain the importance of confirming patients' identities and correctly identifying blood samples.
- Describe how to perform venipuncture and capillary puncture procedures.
- Identify the equipment and supplies required for blood-drawing procedures.
- Discuss the correct procedures for disposing of waste generated during blood-drawing procedures.
- Discuss common fears and concerns of patients and how to ease these fears.
- Develop techniques for helping patients with special needs, including children, the elderly, patients at risk for uncontrolled bleeding, and difficult patients.
- Identify common blood tests and explain their purposes.
- Perform certain blood tests.

AREAS OF COMPETENCE

1997 ROLE DELINEATION STUDY

CLINICAL

Fundamental Principles

- Apply principles of aseptic technique and infection control

Diagnostic Orders

- Collect and process specimens
- Perform diagnostic tests

GENERAL (Transdisciplinary)

Communication Skills

- Adapt communications to individual's ability to understand

Key Terms

basophil
B lymphocyte
buffy coat
capillary puncture
coagulation
eosinophil
erythrocyte
erythrocyte sedimentation rate (ESR)
formed elements
granular leukocyte
hematocrit
hematology
hemocytometer
hemoglobin
hemolysis
lancet
leukocyte
micropipette
monocyte
morphology
neutrophil
nongranular leukocyte
packed red blood cells
phagocytosis
phlebotomy
plasma
platelet
pyrogen
serum
thrombocyte
T lymphocyte
venipuncture
whole blood

The Role of the Medical Assistant

The examination of blood can provide extensive information about a patient's condition. You may be asked to collect and process blood specimens for examination in your work as a medical assistant. A basic understanding of the anatomy and physiology of the circulatory system, as discussed in Chapter 23, will help you properly perform these tasks. You will also need a working knowledge of the functions of blood and the kinds of cells that make up blood tissue.

You will use several techniques to obtain blood specimens. **Phlebotomy** is the insertion of a needle or cannula (small tube) into a vein for the purpose of withdrawing blood. Phlebotomists receive special training in phlebotomy; drawing blood is the main, if not exclusive, task in their work. Smaller blood samples may be obtained by using a small, disposable instrument to pierce surface capillaries. You must be able to perform such procedures accurately so that the sample is appropriate for the ordered tests. You must also be skilled in putting the patient at ease during this procedure. Your reassuring manner, ability to handle technical problems, and careful preparation for answering many kinds of questions will be important to your success in this area.

You must understand how to process blood specimens and conduct various blood tests, particularly if you work in a laboratory. Finally, to make sure the test results are handled efficiently and accurately, you must be able to complete the necessary paperwork. All these skills are essential, regardless of whether you collect blood specimens in a physician's office laboratory (POL), hospital, or laboratory drawing station.

The Functions and Composition of Blood

The circulatory system transports blood throughout the body. The heart of the average adult pumps 8 to 12 pints of blood through more than 70,000 miles of veins, arteries, and capillaries each day. Blood is a complex and dynamic tissue that is essential to life and health.

Hematology is the study of blood, and hematologists study its functions and composition. Blood has many functions, all of which are important to the overall health of the body. Blood does all of the following:

- Distributes oxygen, nutrients, and hormones to body cells
- Eliminates waste products from body cells
- Attacks infecting organisms or pathogens
- Maintains acid-base balance
- Regulates body temperature

Blood is composed of four parts: **plasma** (the liquid in which other components are suspended), red blood cells, white blood cells, and platelets (thrombocytes). The plasma, or fluid part of blood, forms 55% of blood volume. The red blood cells, white blood cells, and platelets comprise the other 45% of blood volume, which is known as the **formed elements** (see Figure 34-1). **Whole blood** is the total volume of plasma and formed elements.

Red Blood Cells

Red blood cells (RBCs), or **erythrocytes,** play a vital role in internal respiration (the exchange of gases between blood and body cells). Blood transports oxygen to body cells in two forms. About 98% of the oxygen is bound to **hemoglobin,** the main component of erythrocytes. The other 2% to 3% of the oxygen is dissolved in plasma. In addition, erythrocytes transport carbon dioxide from body cells to the lungs, although most carbon dioxide is carried in plasma. Healthy RBCs are disk-shaped and have concave sides (biconcave). Hemoglobin, a protein that contains iron, gives RBCs their rusty red color. A mature erythrocyte contains no nucleus.

White Blood Cells

White blood cells (WBCs), or **leukocytes,** protect the body against infection. (The function of WBCs as part of the body's defense against disease is discussed in Chapter 19.) Leukocytes are divided into two primary groups: **granular leukocytes** (also known as polymorphonuclear leukocytes) and **nongranular leukocytes** (also known as agranular or mononuclear leukocytes). The division is based on the type of nucleus and cytoplasm in the cell. Each type of leukocyte performs a specific defense function, and the shape of each is suited to its role.

Granular Leukocytes. Granular, or polymorphonuclear, leukocytes have segmented nuclei and granulated cytoplasm. The three types of granular leukocytes are basophils, eosinophils, and neutrophils. **Basophils** produce the chemical histamine, which aids the body in controlling allergic reactions and other exaggerated immunologic responses. **Eosinophils** capture invading bacteria and antigen-antibody complexes through **phagocytosis,** or the engulfing of the invader. The number of eosinophils increases during allergic reactions and in response to parasitic infections. **Neutrophils** aid in phagocytosis by attacking bacterial invaders. They are also responsible for the release of **pyrogens,** which cause fever.

Nongranular Leukocytes. Nongranular leukocytes have solid nuclei and clear cytoplasm. The two types of nongranular leukocytes are lymphocytes and monocytes. Lymphocytes are divided into two groups: B lymphocytes and T lymphocytes. **B lymphocytes** produce antibodies

MULTISKILL FOCUS

Phlebotomist

To gain medical assistant credentials, you must fulfill the requirements of either the American Association of Medical Assistants (for a Certified Medical Assistant) or the American Medical Technologists (for a Registered Medical Assistant). After obtaining your medical assistant certification or registration, you may wish to acquire additional skills in specialty areas through course work or on-the-job training. Although this course work or training may not lead to an additional certification or degree, it will enable you to expand your role in the medical office and advance your career as the demand for multiskilled health professionals increases.

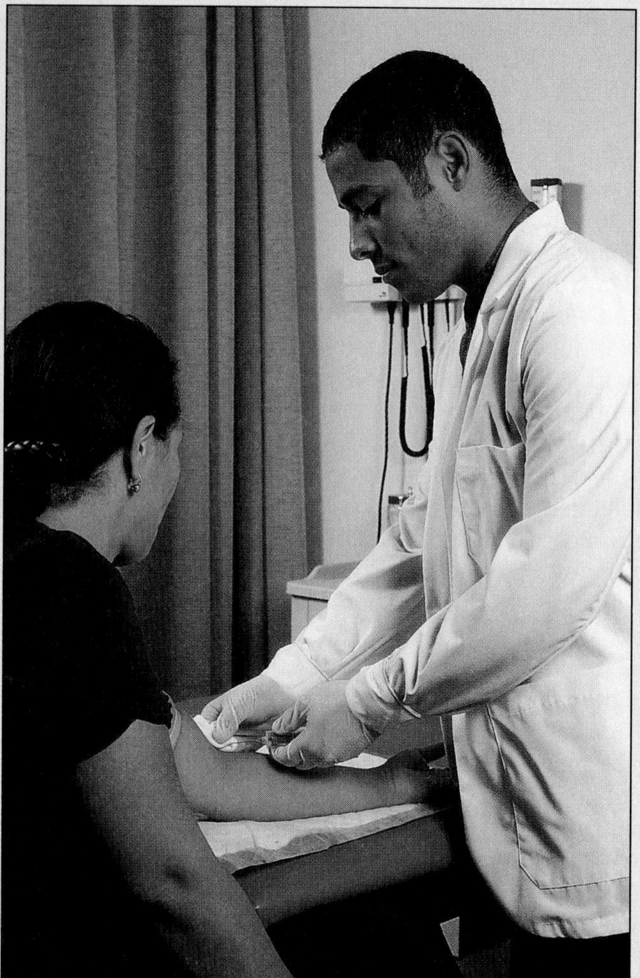

Skills and Duties

Traditionally, a phlebotomist's job has been to draw blood from patients for analysis. Today, however, phlebotomists perform many additional duties. Many phlebotomists now perform simple tests on blood samples at the patient's hospital bedside or in close proximity to the patient. This "point of care" testing speeds physician diagnoses, often reducing the length of a patient's stay in the hospital.

Other phlebotomists are trained to perform patient care functions, which differ from hospital to hospital. For example, they may run electrocardiogram equipment, change beds, deliver trays, or transport patients. While phlebotomists in the past worked primarily in the hospital laboratory, today's phlebotomists work closely with the nursing department and have more direct contact with patients.

Blood collection remains the mainstay of a phlebotomist's job. As part of this process, a phlebotomist performs administrative duties such as documenting the collected blood samples and labeling specimens. A phlebotomist may also administer a health-related questionnaire to the patient if one is required by the physician or an insurance company.

Workplace Settings

Most phlebotomists work in a hospital setting. Others are employed in laboratories, physicians' offices, and health departments. Some phlebotomists work with homebound individuals in nursing homes or private residences.

The job market for phlebotomists is good, provided that they are cross-trained in other specialties. Most institutions prefer phlebotomists who have additional training in areas such as performing blood tests.

Education

Most states require phlebotomists to be certified. The American Society of Phlebotomy Technicians (ASPT) is one of the bodies that provides certification.

To take the ASPT's national phlebotomy examination, you must either have 6 months of full-time work experience (or 1 year of part-time work experience), or graduate from an accredited phlebotomy training program. A high school diploma or general equivalency diploma (GED) is needed to enroll in such a program. To receive full certification, candidates must have at least 100 successful, documented vein punctures and 25 successful, documented skin punctures.

Where to Go for More Information

American Society of Clinical Pathologists
2100 West Harrison
Chicago, IL 60612
(312) 738-1336

American Society of Phlebotomy Technicians
P.O. Box 1831
Hickory, NC 28603
(704) 322-1334

National Phlebotomy Association
5615 Landover Road
Hyattsville, MD 20784
(301) 386-4200

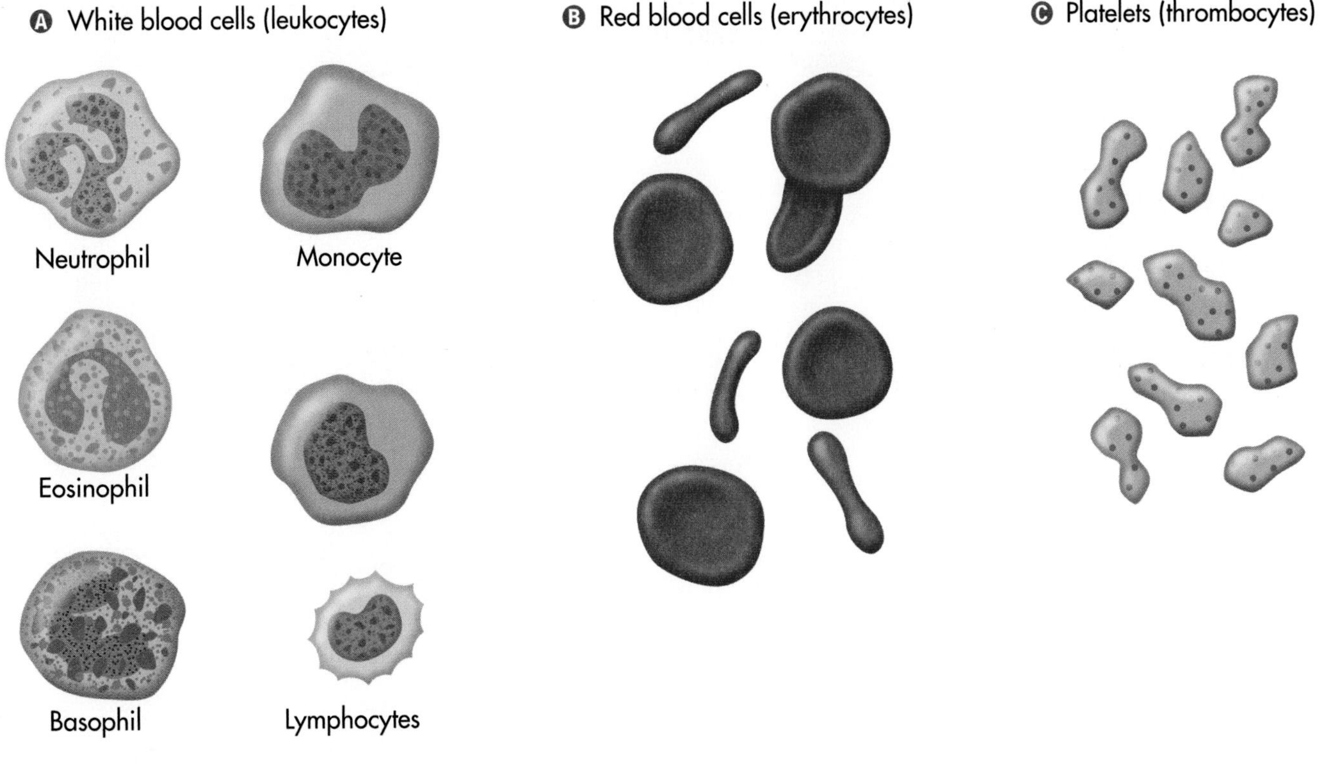

Figure 34-1. The formed elements of the blood are (a) white blood cells, (b) red blood cells, and (c) platelets.

to combat specific pathogens. **T lymphocytes** regulate immunologic response. T lymphocytes are further classified as helper T cells and suppressor T cells. T cells are the cells attacked by human immunodeficiency virus (HIV), the virus that causes acquired immunodeficiency syndrome (AIDS). **Monocytes** are large white blood cells with oval or horseshoe-shaped nuclei. They also defend the body by phagocytosis, recognizing and destroying foreign organisms and particles.

Platelets

Platelets, or **thrombocytes,** are fragments of cytoplasm (the part of the cell that surrounds the nucleus) that are smaller than either RBCs or WBCs. Platelets are irregular in shape and have no nucleus. These cell fragments are crucial to clot formation.

Plasma and Serum

Plasma is a clear, yellow liquid in which the formed elements of blood are suspended. Plasma is nearly 90% water; it also contains about 9% protein and 1% other substances in suspension (see Figure 34-2). These other substances include carbohydrates, fats, gases, mineral salts, protective substances, and waste products.

Serum is the clear, yellow liquid that remains after a blood clot forms. It differs from plasma in that it does not contain fibrinogen, a protein involved in clotting. The fibrinogen converts into fibrin (a sticky protein) and traps formed elements of the blood in a clot. The process of clotting is called **coagulation.**

Blood Types or Groups

An individual's RBCs may carry one or both of two major antigens on their surface. These antigens are known as A and B. The presence or absence of these antigens determines the blood type or group to which that person's blood belongs. Blood that contains neither A nor B antigen is designated O.

In addition to antigens, an individual's blood may contain certain antibodies. Blood that carries only the A antigen contains anti-B antibodies, and blood that carries only the B antigen contains anti-A antibodies. Blood that carries neither antigen contains both anti-A and anti-B antibodies, whereas blood that carries both antigens contains neither anti-A nor anti-B antibodies.

Blood is carefully matched before a blood transfusion. If a patient is given incompatible blood, the antibodies in the patient's blood will combine with the antigens in the transfused blood. This reaction leads to clumping of the RBCs and possible **hemolysis** (the rupturing of red blood cells, which releases hemoglobin). The released hemoglobin can block the renal tubules and cause kidney failure and death.

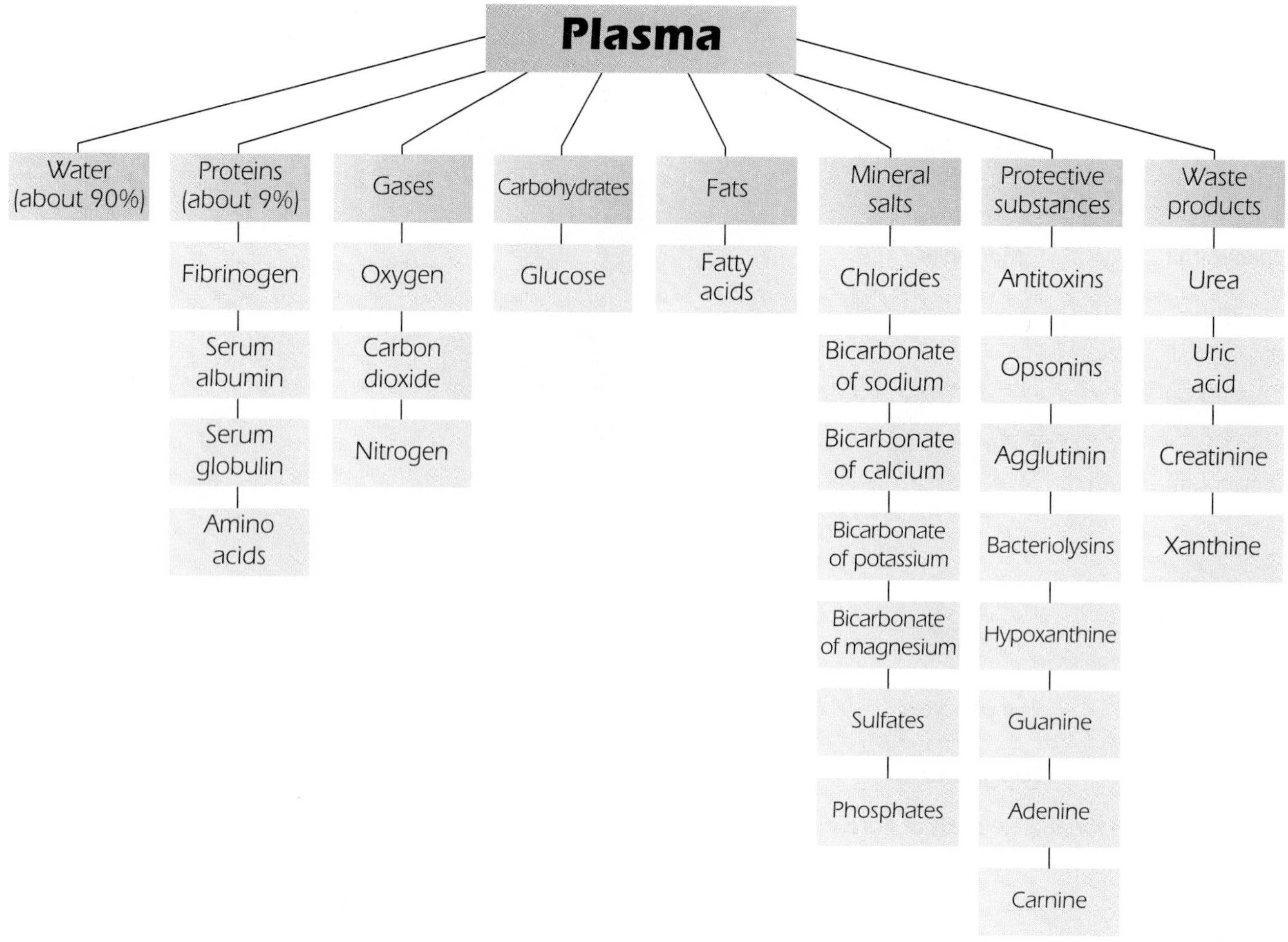

Figure 34-2. A wide variety of substances account for about 10% of plasma by volume. The remainder is water.

Hematologists can determine blood type by mixing a blood specimen with serum containing different antibodies and noting the clumping reactions that occur. The most common system for identifying blood types is the ABO system. The ABO system designates the two major antigens A and B and consists of four groups:

- A: only the A antigen (and anti-B antibodies) present
- B: only the B antigen (and anti-A antibodies) present
- AB: both A and B antigens (and neither antibodies) present
- O: neither A nor B antigen (but both antibodies) present

In addition to the ABO classification, another important blood identifier is the Rh factor. The Rh factor, so named because it was discovered through research on the rhesus monkey, is another antigen found on the surface of the RBC. Approximately 85% of people have the Rh factor in their blood, and their blood type is considered to be Rh positive (Rh+). The other 15% are Rh negative (Rh-). Like the antigens that identify the main group to which a sample belongs, the Rh antigen is also capable of generating a similar, potentially fatal, antigen-antibody reaction.

In these two classification systems, blood is identified by type and Rh factor. The following list identifies eight combinations and the approximate percentage of the population with each type, according to the American Red Cross:

- Type A+: 34%
- Type A-: 6%
- Type B+: 8%
- Type B-: 2%
- Type AB+: 3%
- Type AB-: 1%
- Type O+: 39%
- Type O-: 7%

In addition to these main classifications, several rare blood types appear in specific populations.

Type O negative (O-) is considered the universal donor because it lacks the A, B, and Rh antigens. Type AB positive (AB+) is considered the universal recipient because it will not react with donated blood from any blood group. Note that recipient and donor must be compatible with regard to A and B antigens as well as the Rh factor for transfusion to be safe.

Collecting Blood Specimens

There is a standard process for drawing blood specimens. Following these steps will enable you to perform the procedure smoothly, accurately, and safely and ensure that documentation is completed properly.

Reading and Interpreting the Test Order

The first steps in preparing to draw blood for testing are to review the written testing request and to assemble the equipment and supplies. The patient should arrive with a laboratory request form if you are working in a physician's office laboratory or a laboratory drawing station. You will probably receive a test order from your supervisor if you are working in a hospital.

Reviewing the Test Order. It is essential to first review the patient's blood-collection order to determine what tests will be run. Many tests require expedited or special handling to ensure accurate results.

Your office will have specific collection procedures for each type of test. If you have any questions about these procedures, ask your supervisor. If you will be sending the blood specimen to a reference laboratory for testing, make sure you know its requirements. The cost of reprocessing a test far surpasses the extra time needed to be sure of the process requirements.

When reviewing the test order, you will need to know the meaning of certain abbreviations. Many abbreviations used in laboratory work and their meanings are presented in Figure 34-3. If you are ever in doubt or if the resources in your office or laboratory do not provide the answers you need, ask the doctor or your supervisor.

Assembling the Equipment and Supplies. Specific blood-drawing equipment and collection devices vary with the type of test. Make sure you have the appropriate equipment to collect all necessary samples if more than one test is ordered. All specimen-collection tubes, slides, and other containers should be labeled immediately after collection with the patient's name, the date and time of collection, the initials of the person collecting the specimen, and other information as required by the test procedure or your office. Some offices use an identification code for each patient.

Common Abbreviations Used in Blood Tests

Abbreviation	Meaning	Abbreviation	Meaning
Ab	antibody	AST	aspartate aminotransferase
ABO	classification system for four blood groups	AT-III	antithrombin III
AcAc	acetoacetate	B	blood (whole blood)
ACE	angiotensin-converting enzyme	Baso	basophil
ACT	activated coagulation time	BCA	breast cancer antigen
ACTH	adrenocorticotropic hormone	BJP	Bence Jones protein
ADH	antidiuretic hormone	BT	bleeding time
AFB	acid-fast bacillus	BUN	blood urea nitrogen
AFP	alpha-fetoprotein	Ca; Ca^{++}	calcium
Ag	antigen	CA	cancer antigen
AG	anion gap	CBC	complete blood (cell) count
A/G R	albumin-globulin ratio	CEA	carcinoembryonic antigen
AHF	antihemolytic factor	CHE	cholinesterase
Alb	albumin	CK	creatine kinase
Alc	alcohol	CMV	cytomegalovirus
ALG	antilymphocyte globulin	CN-	cyanide anion
ALP; alk phos	alkaline phosphatase	CO	carbon monoxide
ALT	alanine aminotransferase	CO_2	carbon dioxide
ANA	antinuclear antibody	COHb	carboxyhemoglobin
APAP	acetaminophen	Cr	creatinine
APTT	activated partial thromboplastin time	CrCl	creatinine clearance
ASA	acetylsalicylic acid (aspirin)	CT	calcitonin

continued

Figure 34-3. These abbreviations are routinely used in blood tests.

Common Abbreviations Used in Blood Tests continued

Abbreviation	Meaning
DAF	decay accelerating factor
DHEA	dehydroepiandrosterone, unconjugated
Diff	differential (blood cell count)
EBNA	Epstein-Barr virus nuclear antigen
EBV	Epstein-Barr virus
EDTA	ethylenediaminetetraacetic acid
Eos	eosinophil
EP	electrophoresis
Eq	equivalent
ERP	estrogen receptor protein
ESR	erythrocyte sedimentation rate
FBS	fasting blood sugar
FFA	free fatty acids
FSH	follicle-stimulating hormone (follitropin)
FT_4	free thyroxine
FT_4I	free thyroxine index
GFR	glomerular filtration rate
GH	growth hormone
GHRH	growth hormone–releasing hormone
GnRH	gonadotropin-releasing hormone
GTT	glucose tolerance test
HA	hemagglutination
HAI	hemagglutination inhibition test
HAV	hepatitis A virus
Hb; Hgb	hemoglobin
HbCO	carboxyhemoglobin
HBV	hepatitis B virus
HCG; hCG	human chorionic gonadotropin
Hct	hematocrit
HCV	hepatitis C virus
HDL	high-density lipoprotein
HDV	hepatitis delta virus
HGH; hGH	human growth hormone
HIV	human immunodeficiency virus
HLA	human leukocyte antigen
HPV	human papilloma virus
HSV	herpes simplex virus
HTLV	human T-cell lymphotrophic virus
Ig	immunoglobulin
IgE	immunoglobulin E
INH	inhibitor
IV	intravenous
L	liver
LD; LDH	lactate dehydrogenase
LDL	low-density lipoprotein
LH	luteinizing hormone
LMWH	low-molecular-weight heparin
Lytes	electrolytes
MCV	mean cell volume
MetHb	methemoglobin
MLC	mixed lymphocyte culture
MONO	monocyte
MPV	mean platelet volume
MSAFP	maternal serum alpha-fetoprotein
NE	norepinephrine
NPN	nonprotein nitrogen
OGTT	oral glucose tolerance test
P	plasma
PAP	prostatic acid phosphatase
PB	protein binding
PBG	porphobilinogen
PCT	prothrombin consumption time
PCV	packed cell volume (hematocrit)
P_i	inorganic phosphate
PKU	phenylketonuria
PLT	platelet
PMN	polymorphonuclear (leukocyte; neutrophil)
PRL	prolactin
PSA	prostate-specific antigen
PT	prothrombin time
PTH	parathyroid hormone
PTT	partial thromboplastin time
PV	plasma volume
PZP	pregnancy zone protein
RAIU	thyroid uptake of radioactive iodine
RBC	red blood cell; red blood (cell) count
RBP	retinol-binding protein
RCM	red cell mass
RCV	red cell volume
RDW	red cell distribution of width
Retic	reticulocyte
RF	rheumatoid factor; relative fluorescence unit
Rh	rhesus factor
RIA	radioimmunoassay
rT_3	reverse triiodothyronine
S	serum
Segs	segmented polymorphonuclear leukocyte
SPE	serum protein electrophoresis
T_3	triiodothyronine
T_4	thyroxine
TBG	thyroxine-binding globulin
TBV	total blood volume
TG	triglyceride
TRH	thyrotropin-releasing hormone
TSH	thyroid-stimulating hormone
VDRL	Venereal Disease Research Laboratory (test for syphilis)
VLDL	very-low-density lipoprotein
WB	Western blot
WBC	white blood cell; white blood (cell) count

Source: Adapted from Norbert W. Tietz, ed., *Clinical Guide to Laboratory Tests*, 3d ed. (Philadelphia: W. B. Saunders, 1995).

Alcohol and cotton balls or alcohol wipes, sterile gauze, and adhesive bandages are standard supplies for procedures during which blood is drawn from a vein or capillaries. Alcohol causes inaccurate results for certain tests, however, so for these tests, povidone iodine or benzalkonium chloride is used. You will need a tourniquet (a flat, broad length of vinyl or rubber or a piece of fabric with a Velcro closure) for **venipuncture,** the puncture of a vein—usually performed with a needle for the purpose of drawing blood.

Preparing Patients

After you review the test order and assemble the necessary equipment and supplies, take a moment to relax, gather your thoughts, and consider your purpose. This may strike you as odd advice, but your calm and positive demeanor helps establish the best possible relationship with a patient who may be uneasy about having blood drawn. The moment you use to relax and focus may save you time and save patients unnecessary discomfort by contributing to a quick, efficient procedure.

Greeting and Identifying Patients. Greet patients pleasantly, introduce yourself, and explain that you will be drawing some blood. It is essential to identify patients correctly before you begin the procedure. Ask patients to state their full name, and be sure you hear both the first and last names correctly. Verify that the name the patient gives is the name on the order. (In some facilities, the phlebotomist may ask for a Social Security number or a patient ID or chart number to further identify the patient.)

Confirming Pretest Preparation. The presence and level of certain substances in blood are affected by food and fluid intake or by other activities in daily life. Some tests require that the patient follow certain pretest restrictions. The purpose behind these restrictions is either to minimize the influence of the restricted food on the blood or to stress the body to see how it responds, as indicated by the blood.

One test that requires patients to follow pretest instructions closely is the glucose tolerance test, which measures a patient's ability to metabolize carbohydrates. This test is used to detect hypoglycemia and diabetes mellitus. You instruct the patient to eat a diet high in carbohydrates for the 3 days before the test and to fast for the 8 to 12 hours before the appointment. After initial blood and urine samples are taken, the patient ingests a measured dose of glucose solution. Blood and urine samples are then taken at prescribed intervals as ordered by the physician. The glucose levels in the samples are often graphed for the physician's review.

Before you draw blood for any test, determine whether the patient has complied with pretest instructions. If the patient has not followed pretest instructions, explain that the test cannot be performed. Make a note on the order, and report the information to the physician or your supervisor.

Explaining the Procedure and Safety Precautions. Explain to the patient the procedure you will use to obtain the blood specimen for testing. Be clear and brief when you describe what you will do; too much detail leaves some patients queasy. You must follow Universal Precautions during all phlebotomy procedures, as described in "Caution: Handle With Care." These precautions may be second nature to you, but they may raise concerns in the patient. Explain the need for each of the preventive measures you are taking in language the patient can understand. Assure the patient that these measures protect against exposure to infection.

Establishing a Chain of Custody. You will need to follow specific guidelines to establish a chain of custody for blood samples drawn for drug and alcohol analysis. (Chapter 31 explains general chain of custody procedures.) Because donating a specimen for drug and alcohol testing is potentially self-incriminating, the patient must sign a consent form for the testing. (This form is discussed in Chapter 33.) Although the clerical procedures for blood tests for drug and alcohol analysis are similar to those for urine tests, blood tests differ because you can confirm by direct observation that a blood specimen has been taken from the patient in question.

Handling an Exposure Incident. When you adhere to Universal Precautions, the risk of exposure to bloodborne pathogens is very small. Accidents can occur, however. If you suffer a needle stick or other injury that results in exposure to blood or blood products from another person, you must report the incident to the appropriate staff members immediately. Wash the injured area carefully and apply a sterile bandage. Record the time and date of the incident, the names of the people involved, and the nature of the exposure. Depending on the situation, you may receive medications. You and the other person involved will be asked to undergo blood testing and be involved in follow-up studies. The Occupational Safety and Health Administration (OSHA) requires every employer to have an established procedure for handling exposure incidents.

Drawing Blood

Some, but not all, states permit medical assistants to obtain blood samples. Your office will clarify which duties, if any, you may perform related to phlebotomy procedures. If your duties include collecting blood samples, you will obtain them either through venipuncture or capillary puncture. You must understand when these techniques are used and know how to perform them.

Venipuncture. Venipuncture requires puncturing a vein with a needle and collecting blood into either a tube or a syringe. The most common sites for venipuncture are the median cubital and cephalic veins of the forearm, although other sites may be used if the primary site is unacceptable. Figure 34-4 shows the veins in the antecubital fossa (the small depression inside the bend of the elbow) and the forearm that are used for venipuncture.

CAUTION HANDLE WITH CARE

Phlebotomy and Personal Protective Equipment

The Centers for Disease Control and Prevention (CDC) has classified all phlebotomy procedures as a risk for exposure to contaminated blood or blood products. You must use appropriate protective equipment during all phlebotomy procedures. Remember, it is up to you to protect yourself and the patient.

Gloves
Gloves are the first line of defense during a phlebotomy procedure. They protect against spills and splashing of contaminated blood. Wash your hands and put on clean examination gloves that fit snugly before you work with each patient. Remove the gloves, dispose of them in a biohazardous waste container, and wash your hands after working with each patient.

Garments
Garments such as laboratory coats and aprons can protect your clothing from spills and splashes and provide a measure of protection from contaminated materials. Some garments are designed to resist penetration by blood or blood products. You may find it necessary to wear such garments when drawing blood or performing blood tests.

Masks and Protective Eyewear
Mucous membranes are especially vulnerable to invasion by infectious agents. Use masks and protective eyewear to help safeguard mucous membranes in your mouth, nose, and eyes from infection.

Masks help protect your mouth and nose from splashes or sprays of blood or blood products. You cannot predict when exposure to blood may occur. Accidental puncture of an artery during a phlebotomy procedure could result in a spray of blood. Blood may also spray or splash accidentally during some testing protocols. Most medical assistants do not routinely wear masks for phlebotomy procedures, however, once they have achieved proficiency in performing them.

Goggles can protect your eyes from splashing and spraying during blood drawing or testing. Health-care workers in dental offices often wear goggles because patient treatments can easily expose workers to contaminated blood or bloody saliva.

Clear plastic face shields combine the protection of masks and goggles. They are often used during major surgical procedures. You may use a face shield if you do extensive testing on blood specimens. Face shields are not usually worn when drawing blood.

Personal protective equipment works two ways: it protects you from a patient's contaminated blood, and it also protects the patient from infectious agents you may be carrying. By using PPE correctly, you will make your workplace a safer place for you and the patients.

Various instruments are used to perform venipuncture. Practice using the devices so that your technique is smooth, steady, and competent.

Evacuation Systems. Evacuation systems, the most common of which is the VACUTAINER system (manufactured by Becton Dickinson VACUTAINER Systems, Franklin Lakes, New Jersey), use a special double-pointed needle, a plastic needle holder/adapter, and collection tubes (see Figure 34-5). The collection tubes are sealed to create a slight vacuum. You insert the covered inner point of the needle into one end of the holder/adapter and the first collection tube into the other end. Remove the plastic cap from the outer needle of the assembled system. Hold the needle at a 15° angle to the patient's arm, and puncture the patient's vein with the needle. Then press the collection tube fully onto the covered needle tip, piercing the stopper and allowing the vacuum to help draw blood into the collection tube. Procedure 34-1 explains how to use an evacuation system to draw a blood sample.

An evacuation system has several advantages over other methods of blood collection. It is easy to collect several samples from one venipuncture site using the interchangeable vacuum collection tubes. Tubes are calibrated by evacuation to collect the exact amount of blood required. Some collection tubes are prepared with additives needed to correctly process the blood sample for testing, such as anticoagulants. Finally, because there is no need to transfer blood from a collection syringe to a sample tube, the potential for exposure to contaminated blood is reduced.

Needle and Syringe Systems. An evacuation system is not the best choice for drawing blood in every case. For example, if the patient has small or fragile veins, the vacuum created when the collection tube is pressed over the needle point can cause the veins to collapse. You may collect blood using a sterile needle and syringe assembly when an evacuation system is not suitable, such as when the patient is elderly or difficult to stick. You can use a smaller needle and control the vacuum in the syringe by pulling the plunger back slowly. Other aspects of the procedure are essentially the same, except that the blood sample is collected in the syringe and must immediately be transferred to a collection tube.

Butterfly Systems. You may also use a butterfly system, or winged infusion set, when you work with patients who have small or fragile veins. Flexible wings attached to the needle simplify needle insertion. A length of flexible tubing (either 5 or 12 inches, approximately) connects the needle to the collection device. The inserted

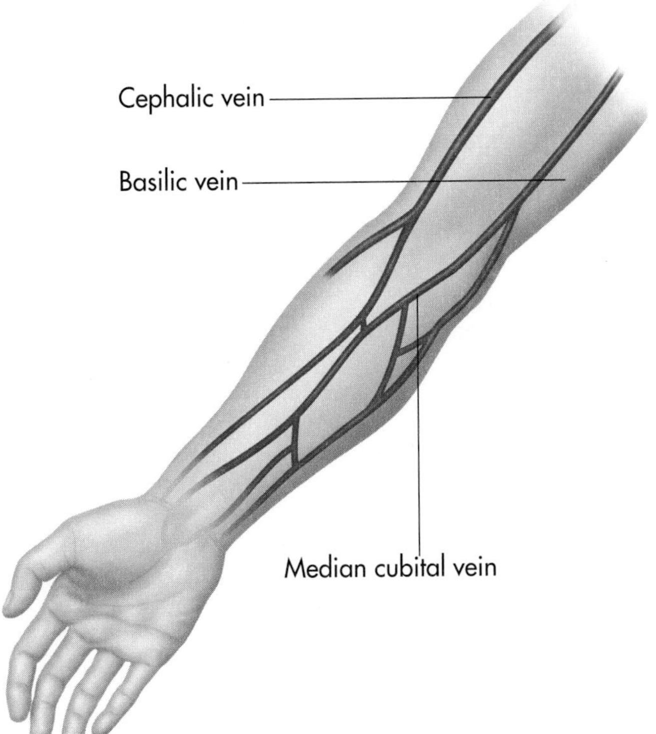

Figure 34-4. Veins commonly used for venipuncture include the cephalic vein, the basilic vein, and the median cubital vein.

needle remains completely undisturbed while the collection device is manipulated. Because it is motionless, the needle causes less trauma to the vein and surrounding tissue than do other systems for venipuncture. A butterfly system generally uses a smaller needle (23 gauge) than other venipuncture techniques do. A butterfly system can be used with an evacuated collection tube or a syringe (see Figure 34-11, p. 698).

Collection Tubes. No matter which method is used to collect blood, the samples must immediately be mixed with the appropriate additives in the correct collection tubes before they are transported to the laboratory for testing. The stoppers of the tubes are different colors, each color identifying the type of additives (if any) they contain (see Figure 34-12, p. 698). These additives must be compatible with the laboratory process the sample will undergo. Each laboratory may choose which tubes to use for a particular test.

Additives include anticoagulants and other materials that help preserve or process a sample for particular types of testing. When you collect a blood sample, double-check that you are using the appropriate collection tubes for the tests ordered. You must also fill the tubes in a specific order to preserve the integrity of the blood sample. Each laboratory requires a specific order of draw for collection tubes. The National Committee for Clinical Laboratory Standards also publishes its recommended order of draw. Table 34-1, p. 699, identifies collection tube stopper colors, additives present in the tubes, and types of tests, in a typical order of draw.

Needle Shields. Although gloves provide good protection against blood spills and splashes, they provide little protection against needle sticks or slices. To address this problem, manufacturers of medical equipment have developed adaptable needle shields. These devices fit over existing blood-drawing systems to protect medical personnel from needle injuries. One such device is the Saf-T Clik shielded blood needle adapter manufactured by Winfield Medical, San Diego, California (see Figure 34-13, p. 699).

Capillary Puncture. **Capillary puncture** requires a superficial puncture of the skin with a sharp point. Compared with venipuncture, capillary puncture releases a smaller amount of blood. The blood may be collected in small, calibrated glass tubes. It may also be collected on glass microscope slides or applied to reagent strips (or dipsticks), which are specially treated paper or plastic strips used in specific diagnostic tests.

Capillary puncture in adults and children is usually performed on the great (middle) finger or the ring finger. (Use the patient's nondominant hand for this procedure if possible.) The puncture should be made slightly off

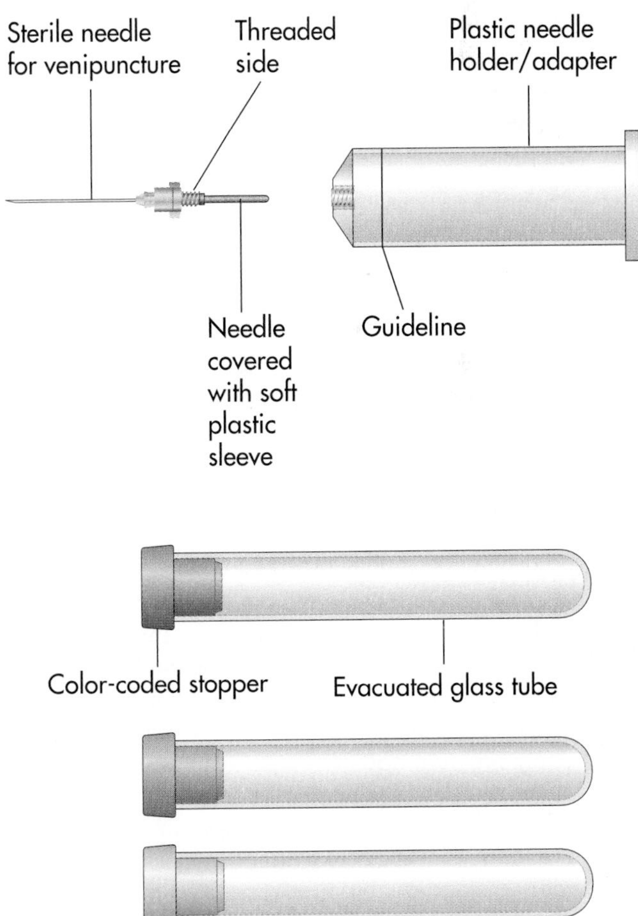

Figure 34-5. The VACUTAINER system uses interchangeable collection tubes that allow you to draw several blood specimens from the same venipuncture site.

PROCEDURE 34-1

Performing Venipuncture Using an Evacuation System

Objective: To collect a venous blood sample using an evacuation system

OSHA Guidelines

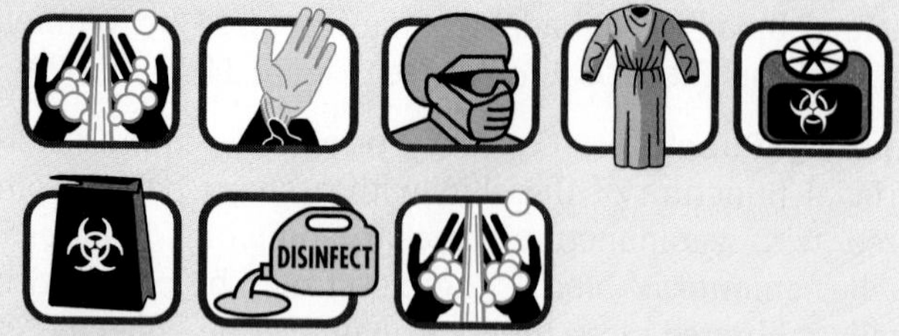

Materials: VACUTAINER components (needle, needle holder/adapter, collection tubes), antiseptic and cotton balls or antiseptic wipes, tourniquet, sterile gauze squares, sterile adhesive bandages

Method

1. Review the laboratory request form, and make sure you have the necessary supplies.
2. Greet the patient, confirm the patient's identity, and introduce yourself.
3. Explain the purpose of the procedure, and confirm that the patient has followed the physician's special instructions.
4. Make sure the patient is sitting in a venipuncture chair or is lying down.
5. Wash your hands. Put on examination gloves.
6. Prepare the needle holder/adapter assembly by inserting the threaded side of the needle into the adapter and twisting the adapter in a clockwise direction. Push the first collection tube into the other end of the needle holder/adapter until the outer edge of the collection tube stopper meets the guideline.
7. Ask the patient whether one arm is better than the other for the venipuncture. The chosen arm should be positioned slightly downward (see Figure 34-6).
8. Apply the tourniquet to the patient's upper arm midway between the elbow and the shoulder. Wrap the tourniquet around the patient's arm and cross the ends. Holding one end of the tourniquet against the patient's arm, stretch the other end to apply pressure against the patient's skin. Pull a loop of the stretched end under the end held tightly against the patient's skin, as shown in Figure 34-7. The tourniquet should be tight enough to cause the veins to stand out but should not stop the flow of blood. You should still be able to feel the patient's radial pulse. Ask the patient to make a fist and release it several times to make the veins in the forearm stand out more prominently.

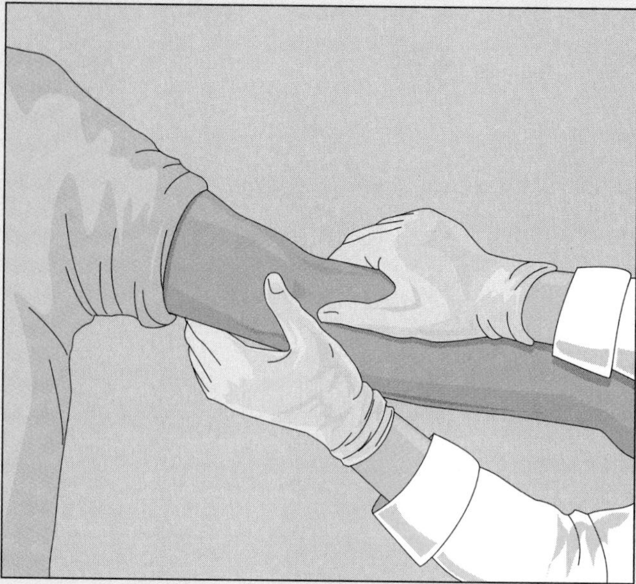

Figure 34-6. The patient's arm should be positioned slightly downward for a venipuncture.

9. Palpate the proposed site, and use your index finger to locate the vein, as shown in Figure 34-8. The vein will feel like a small tube with some elasticity. If you feel a pulsing beat, you have located an artery. If you cannot locate the vein within 1 minute, release the tourniquet and allow blood to flow freely for 1 to 2 minutes. Then reapply the tourniquet and try again to locate the vein.
10. After locating the vein, clean the area with a cotton ball moistened with antiseptic or an antiseptic wipe. Use a circular motion to clean the area, starting at the center and working outward. Allow the site to air-dry, or use the same circular motion to wipe the area dry with a sterile gauze square.

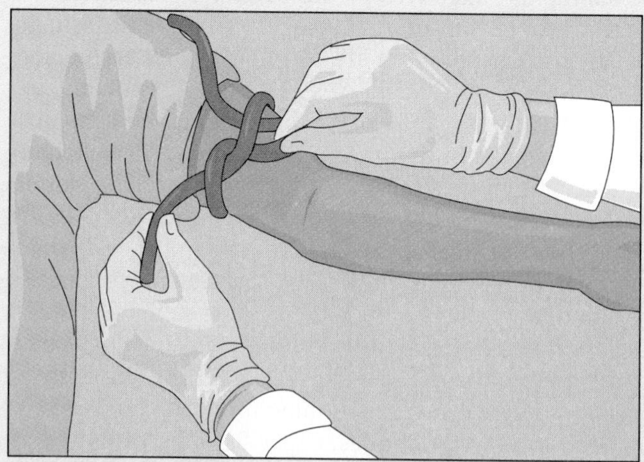

Figure 34-7. Applying a tourniquet makes it easier to find a patient's vein when you are drawing blood.

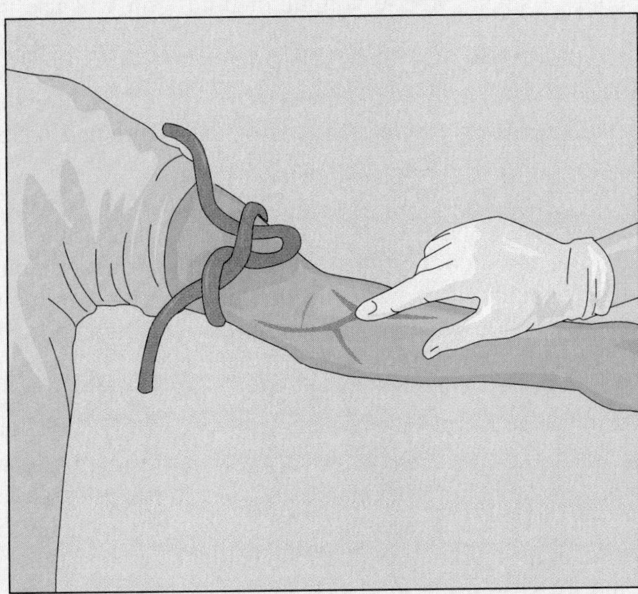

Figure 34-8. Use your index finger to locate the vein.

11. Remove the plastic cap from the outer point of the needle cover, and ask the patient to tighten the fist. Hold the patient's skin taut above and below the insertion site. With a steady and quick motion, insert the needle—held at a 15° angle, bevel side up, and aligned parallel to the vein—into the vein (see Figure 34-9). You will feel a slight resistance as the needle tip penetrates the vein wall. Penetrate to a depth of ¼ to ½ inch. Grasp the holder/adapter between your index and great (middle) fingers. Using your thumb, seat the collection tube firmly into place over the needle point, puncturing the rubber stopper. Blood will begin to flow into the collection tube.
12. Fill each tube until the blood stops running to ensure the correct proportion of blood to additives. Switch tubes as needed by pulling one tube out of the adapter and inserting the next in a smooth and steady motion. (The soft plastic cover on the inner point of the needle retracts as each tube is inserted and recovers the needle point as each tube is removed.)
13. Once blood is flowing steadily, ask the patient to release the fist, and untie the tourniquet by pulling the end of the tucked-in loop. The tourniquet should, in general, be left on no longer than 1 minute. (Longer periods may cause hemoconcentration, an increase in the blood-cell-to-plasma ratio, and invalidate test results.) You must remove the tourniquet before you withdraw the needle from the vein. (Removing the tourniquet releases pressure on the vein.)
14. As you withdraw the needle in a smooth and steady motion, place a sterile gauze square over the insertion site (Figure 34-10). Dispose of the needle immediately. Instruct the patient to hold the gauze pad in place with slight pressure. The patient should keep the arm straight and slightly elevated for several minutes.
15. If the collection tubes contain additives, you will need to invert them slowly several times to mix the chemical agent and the blood sample.
16. Label specimens and complete the paperwork.
17. Check the patient's condition and the puncture site for bleeding. Replace the sterile gauze square with a sterile adhesive bandage.
18. Properly dispose of used supplies and disposable instruments, and disinfect the work area.
19. Remove the gloves and wash your hands.
20. Instruct the patient about care of the puncture site.
21. Document the procedure in the patient's chart.

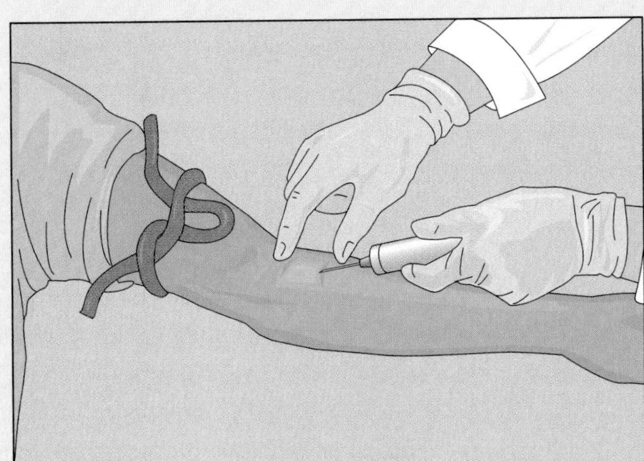

Figure 34-9. When performing venipuncture, hold the needle at a 15° angle.

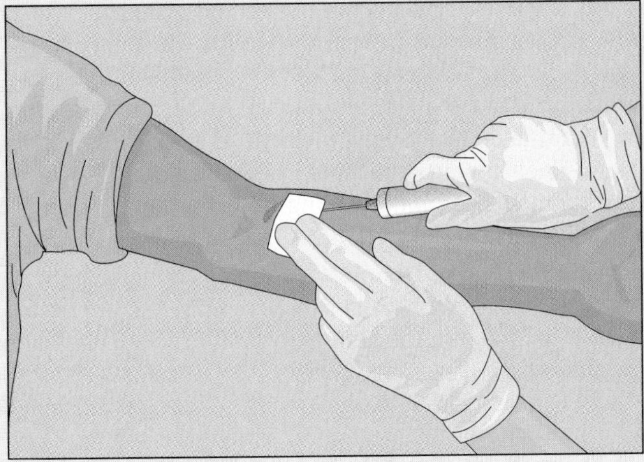

Figure 34-10. Place a sterile gauze square over the insertion site as you withdraw the needle.

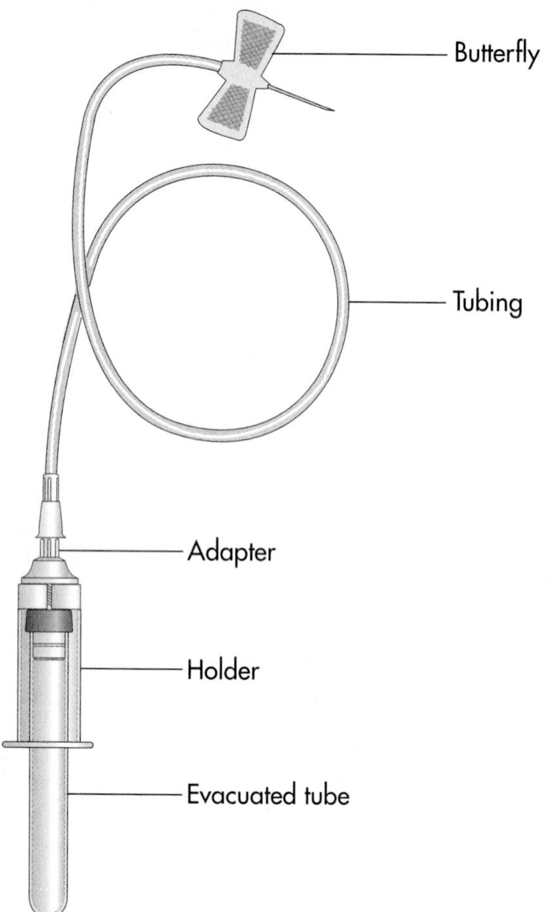

Figure 34-11. Once inserted, the needle of a butterfly system remains undisturbed during specimen collection.

center on the pad of the fingertip. Capillary puncture in infants is usually performed on one of the outer edges of the underside of the heel. An alternate site for both children and adults is the lower part of the earlobe, unless the patient's ear is pierced.

Lancets. Lancets are used in the capillary puncture technique. This technique is employed when the amount of blood required for a specific procedure is not very large or when technical difficulties prevent use of the venipuncture technique. A **lancet** is a small, disposable instrument with a sharp point used to puncture the skin and make a shallow incision (between 2.0 and 3.0 mm deep for an adult and no deeper than 2.4 mm for an infant). The blood welling up from the incision is then collected.

Automatic Puncturing Devices. Automatic puncturing devices are loaded with a lancet. Because the depth to which they puncture the skin is mechanically controlled, they are more accurate than the traditional lancet method. These spring-loaded devices have disposable platforms that rest on the finger. Different platforms are used, depending on the desired depth of the puncture. Both the lancet and the platform should be discarded after use. Some companies also manufacture completely disposable devices, which come individually wrapped and are used only once.

Micropipettes. A pipette is a calibrated glass tube for measuring fluids. A **micropipette** is a small pipette that holds a small, precise volume of fluid. You will use micropipettes to collect capillary blood for some tests. Capillary tubes, with a single calibration mark, are also used to collect capillary blood for certain tests. Procedure 34-2 explains how to perform a capillary puncture and collect a sample of capillary blood.

UNOPETTES. The UNOPETTE (manufactured by Becton Dickinson VACUTAINER Systems) is a disposable micropipette blood-diluting system used to perform manual blood counts. It allows collection of a specific volume of capillary blood and subsequent mixing of the blood with a specific volume of diluting fluid. Several types of UNOPETTES are available for performing various blood counts. Procedure 34-3 explains how to fill a UNOPETTE.

MICROTAINER Tubes. MICROTAINER tubes (manufactured by Becton Dickinson VACUTAINER Systems) are small plastic tubes that have a widemouthed collector, similar to a funnel, which allows blood to flow quickly and freely into the tube. Like collection tubes in an evacuation system, MICROTAINER tubes have different colored tops indicating which, if any, additives they contain.

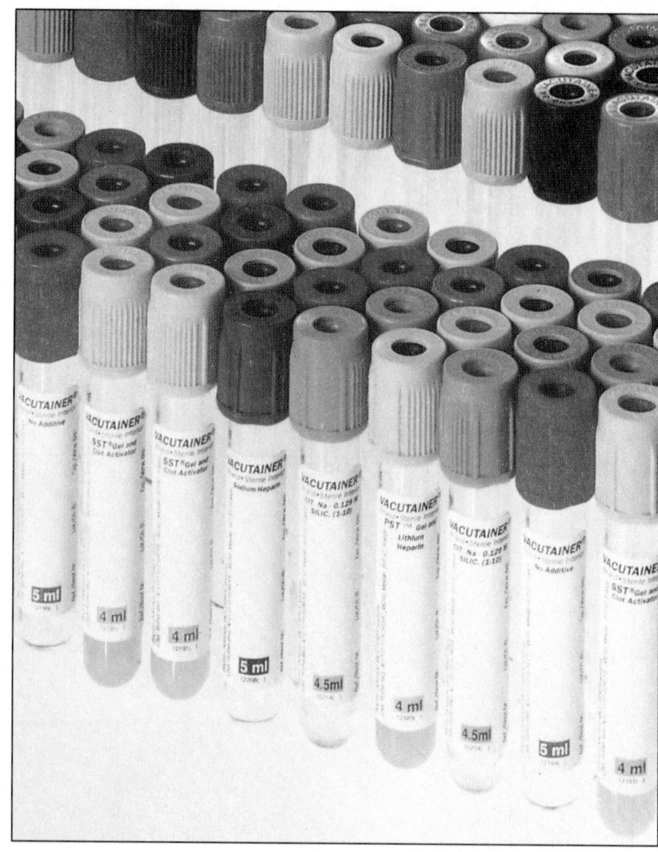

Figure 34-12. Special color-coded stoppers on collection tubes indicate which additives are present and, therefore, which types of laboratory tests may be performed on each blood specimen.

Table 34-1

Blood-Collection Tubes

Stopper Color	Additive	Test Types
Yellow	Sodium polyanetholesulfonate	Plasma cultures
Red	None	Blood chemistries, AIDS antibody, viral studies, serologic tests, blood grouping and typing
Red/black (tiger stripes)	Silicone serum separator	Tests requiring blood serum
Blue	Sodium citrate (anticoagulant)	Coagulation studies
Green	Sodium heparin (anticoagulant)	Electrolyte studies, arterial blood gases
Lavender	Ethylenediaminetetraacetic acid (EDTA) (anticoagulant)	Hematology studies
Gray	Potassium oxalate or sodium fluoride (anticoagulant)	Blood glucose

Reagent Products. Several common tests do not require processing of fluid blood samples. For these tests, you may apply droplets of freshly collected blood to chemically treated paper or plastic reagent strips (dipsticks) or add freshly collected blood droplets to small containers holding chemicals that react in the presence of specific substances or microorganisms. Some of the blood tests performed in this way are those for determining blood glucose levels, sickle cell anemia, infectious mononucleosis, and rheumatoid arthritis.

Smear Slides. You may need to apply a drop of freshly collected blood to a prepared microscope slide for some tests. More commonly, a smear slide is prepared in the laboratory from a blood sample containing an anticoagulant, for examination under a microscope.

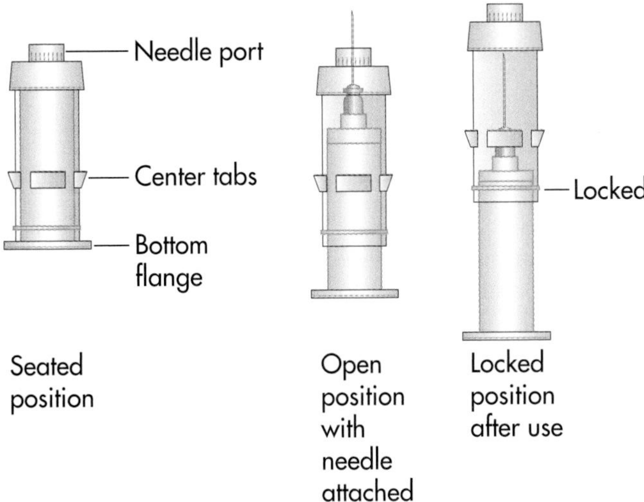

Figure 34-13. Devices such as the Saf-T Clik needle shield help prevent needle injuries.

Responding to Patient Needs

Many patients are anxious when they have a blood test, and some patients have special needs or present special problems that make drawing blood challenging. Anxiety about blood tests may stem from a variety of concerns. Special needs may be related to a patient's age group or a medical condition. Some problems involve difficulty obtaining a blood sample or the patient's physiological or emotional response to a procedure. Being aware of possible sources of patient anxiety and understanding a wide range of special concerns can help you respond to patient needs with sensitivity and competence.

Patient Fears and Concerns

Some patients express their fears or concerns directly. Other patients ask questions that highlight their fears. Providing more information or a complete understanding is reassuring to many patients. For others, the information serves only to confuse, overwhelm, or create more fear. You must decide how much information to give each patient and be prepared to answer questions.

Patients sometimes ask questions that are not appropriate for you to answer. A patient may ask you about his prognosis, medical condition, blood type, or other medical information. It is not appropriate for you to discuss these topics with the patient. Tell the patient that only the physician can answer such questions. There are some commonly expressed fears and concerns to which you should respond, however.

PROCEDURE 34-2

Performing Capillary Puncture

Objective: To collect a capillary blood sample using the finger puncture method

OSHA Guidelines

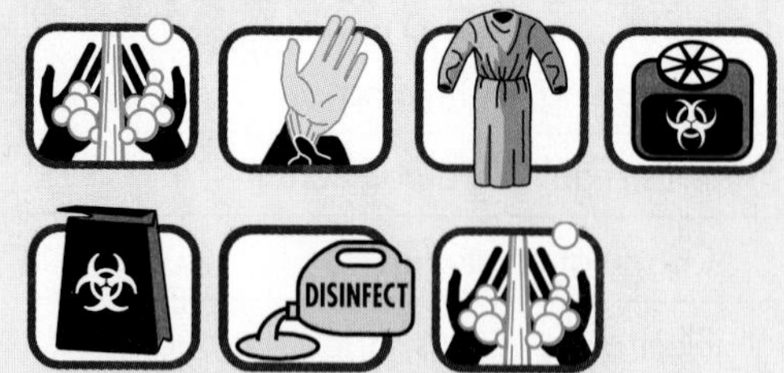

Materials: Capillary puncture device (lancet or automatic puncture device such as Autolet or Glucolet), antiseptic and cotton balls or antiseptic wipes, sterile gauze squares, sterile adhesive bandages, reagent strips, micropipettes, smear slides

Method

1. Review the laboratory request form, and make sure you have the necessary supplies.
2. Greet the patient, confirm the patient's identity, and introduce yourself.
3. Explain the purpose of the procedure, and confirm that the patient has followed the doctor's special instructions.
4. Make sure the patient is sitting in the venipuncture chair or is lying down.
5. Wash your hands. Put on examination gloves.
6. Examine the patient's hands to determine which finger to use for the procedure. Avoid fingers that are swollen, bruised, scarred, or calloused. Generally, the ring and great (middle) fingers are the best choices. If you notice that the patient's hands are cold, you may want to warm them between your own, have the patient put them in a warm basin of water or under warm running water, or wrap them in a warm cloth. Warming the patient's hands improves circulation.
7. Prepare the patient's finger with a gentle "milking" or rubbing motion toward the fingertip. Keep the patient's hand below heart level so that gravity helps the blood flow.
8. Clean the area with a cotton ball moistened with antiseptic or an antiseptic wipe. Allow the site to air-dry, or wipe the area dry with a sterile gauze square.
9. Hold the patient's finger between your thumb and forefinger. Hold the lancet or automatic puncture device at a right angle to the patient's fingerprint, as shown in Figure 34-14. Puncture the skin on the pad of the fingertip with a quick, sharp motion. The depth to which you puncture the skin is generally determined by the length of the lancet point. Most automatic puncturing devices are designed to penetrate to the correct depth.
10. Allow a drop of blood to form at the end of the patient's finger. If the blood droplet is slow in forming, apply steady pressure (Figure 34-15).

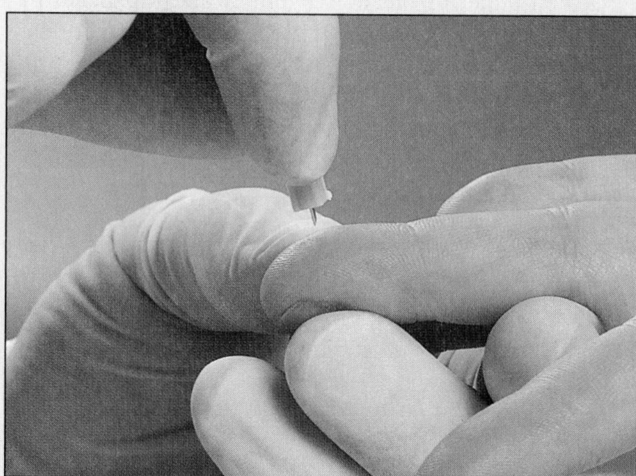

Figure 34-14. Hold the lancet or automatic puncture device at a right angle to the patient's fingerprint.

Pain. The question that medical assistants performing phlebotomy probably hear most often is, Will this hurt? Never lie to a patient who asks this question. Inform the patient that he will feel a stick just as the lancet or point of the needle is inserted but that this pain goes away almost immediately. Tell a patient who seems particularly nervous to take a deep breath and let it out slowly. Also suggest that the patient focus on something else in the room or close his eyes and relax during the procedure.

A patient may express concern and report a previous unpleasant experience with blood testing. Listen to the patient's concerns. Describe what you will do to reduce discomfort and what the patient can do to be more at ease. Let the patient know that you will help him sit comfortably or lie down while the blood sample is being obtained. Tell the patient to let you know if he begins to feel light-headed. You might also ask the patient whether one arm is better to use than the other. Many patients have had blood drawn before and can tell you which sites were successful. Consulting the patient helps the patient feel more in control and provides you with important information.

Avoid milking the patient's finger, because it dilutes the blood sample with tissue fluid and causes hemolysis.

11. Wipe away the first droplet of blood. (This droplet is usually contaminated with tissue fluids released when the skin is punctured.) Then fill the collection devices, as described.

    Micropipettes: Hold the tip of the tube just to the edge of the blood droplet. The tube will fill through capillary action. If you are preparing microhematocrit tubes, you need to seal one end of each tube with clay sealant. (See Procedure 34-7 for this process.)

    Reagent strips: With some reagent strips (dipsticks), you must touch the strip to the blood drop but not smear it; with other strips, you must smear it. Follow the manufacturer's guidelines.

    Smear slides: Gently touch the blood droplet to the smear slide and process the slide as described in Procedure 34-6.

12. After you have collected the required samples, dispose of the lancet immediately. Then wipe the patient's finger with a sterile gauze square (Figure 34-16). Instruct the patient to apply pressure to stop the bleeding.
13. Label specimens and complete the paperwork. Some tests, such as glucose monitoring, must be completed immediately.
14. Check the puncture site for bleeding. If necessary, replace the sterile gauze square with a sterile adhesive bandage.
15. Properly dispose of used supplies and disposable instruments, and disinfect the work area.
16. Remove the gloves and wash your hands.
17. Instruct the patient about care of the puncture site.
18. Document the procedure in the patient's chart. (If the test has been completed, include the results.)

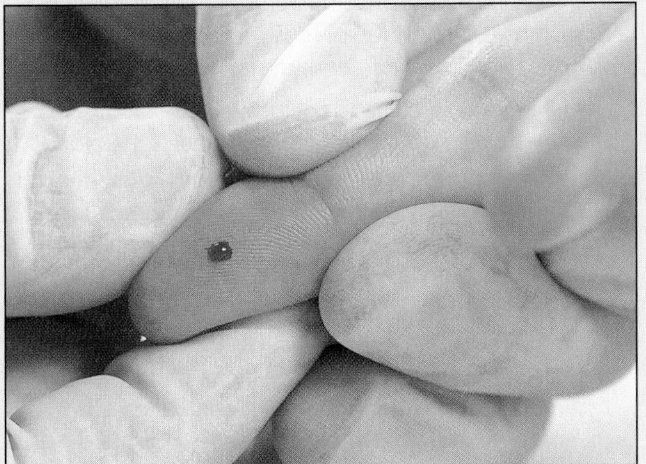

Figure 34-15. Apply steady pressure to the patient's finger, but do not milk it.

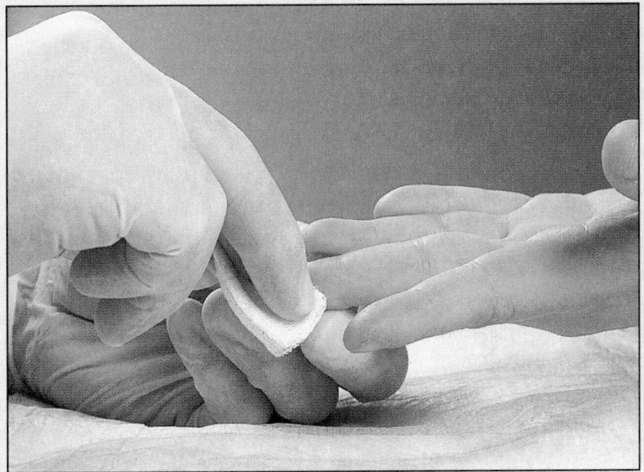

Figure 34-16. Use a sterile gauze square to wipe remaining blood from the patient's finger.

Bruises or Scars. Some patients may express fear of getting a bruise or scar from a blood test. Explain that some bruising is possible but that it will fade within a few days. Most bruising is caused by a hematoma, which occurs when blood leaks out of the vein and collects under the skin. Hematomas can be prevented by releasing the tourniquet before withdrawing the needle and applying proper pressure over the puncture site after the needle has been withdrawn. Bruising is common with fair-skinned patients. Scars, on the other hand, are unlikely.

Serious Diagnosis. Patient fears are not always rational. One fear patients express is that the more tubes of blood you require, the more serious their condition must be. Patients may also fear that a blood test is being done to help the doctor diagnose an extremely serious disease.

You can help relieve a patient's fears by explaining that a blood test is one of the best ways to obtain an overall picture of health (emphasize health, not disease). Note that blood tests show what is normal about the blood, as well as any abnormalities. You might also explain that several samples are being taken because the blood used

PROCEDURE 34-3

Filling a UNOPETTE

Objective: To fill a UNOPETTE for use in blood chemistry testing

OSHA Guidelines

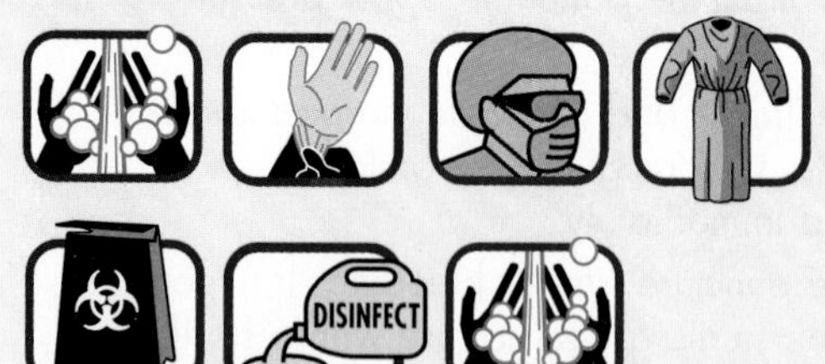

Materials: Blood specimen (either from a capillary puncture or a specimen tube containing anticoagulated blood), UNOPETTE (self-filling diluting micropipette), wooden applicator sticks, gauze squares

Method

1. Wash your hands and put on examination gloves.
2. Prepare the UNOPETTE by using the protective shield on the micropipette to puncture the seal on the reservoir. Set the reservoir aside. Figure 34-17 shows the components of the pipette system.
3. If you will be using blood from a capillary puncture, follow the instructions in Procedure 34-2 to express a drop of blood from the patient's finger or heel. If you will be using a venous blood sample, check the specimen for proper labeling, uncap the specimen tube and, using wooden applicator sticks, remove any coagulated blood from the inside rim of the tube.
4. Remove the shield from the micropipette of the UNOPETTE. Touch the tip of the tube to the blood sample (Figure 34-18). The tube will take up the correct amount through capillary action.
5. Pull the micropipette away from the sample, holding it carefully to prevent spillage. Wipe the outside of the tube with clean gauze to remove excess blood. Do not let the gauze come in contact with the blood in the tube, as the gauze will absorb some of the blood.
6. Hold the micropipette in one hand, and grasp the reservoir between the thumb and forefinger of the other hand. Squeeze the reservoir sides slightly to create a vacuum inside the reservoir.
7. Cap the overflow end of the micropipette with the index finger of the hand in which you are holding the tube. While still holding the sides of the reservoir, insert the end of the tube into the reservoir. Release the sides of the reservoir, and remove your finger from the overflow end of the micropipette, allowing the vacuum to draw the

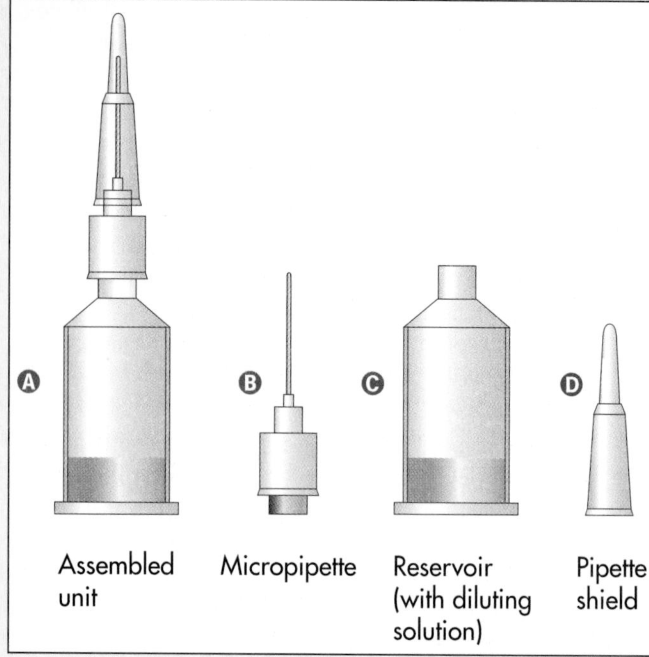

Figure 34-17. A disposable micropipette blood-diluting system such as (a) the UNOPETTE is composed of (b) a micropipette, (c) a reservoir, and (d) a pipette shield.

in blood tests is processed in different ways; the blood collected for one test cannot be used in another.

Blood testing may also be done to determine how well and at what levels medications are acting in the blood. Explain that the doctor may want to see how much medication is in the blood to better manage the prescribed dosage. When a patient needs repeated tests for drug levels, explain that the tests show how the body is using the medication.

Contracting a Disease From the Procedure. Probably the greatest fear of patients undergoing blood tests is contracting HIV, AIDS, or hepatitis B virus (HBV). Although many people are now well informed about how AIDS and other serious diseases are contracted, it is understandable for a patient to worry about blood-borne pathogens. Do not dismiss the patient's concerns, and do not downplay the importance of following Universal Precautions.

Explain the precautions you will take to prevent the spread of infection. Allow the patient to see you wash your hands and put on new gloves before you begin to take the blood sample. Stress that the needle is sterile. Explain that you have not touched the needle and that it

sample out of the tube, through the overflow chamber, and into the reservoir.

8. Squeeze the reservoir several times to force the sample through the tube and into the overflow chamber to "rinse" the overflow chamber and tube, as shown in Figure 34-19. (Be careful not to squeeze so hard that blood comes out of the overflow chamber.)
9. Cap the overflow chamber with your finger again, and gently invert the reservoir and micropipette assembly to ensure complete mixing of the sample with the diluting fluid (see Figure 34-20). Replace the pipette shield to prevent evaporation.
10. If required by the test procedure, allow the sample to settle for the prescribed amount of time.
11. Properly dispose of used supplies, and disinfect the work area.
12. Remove the gloves and wash your hands.

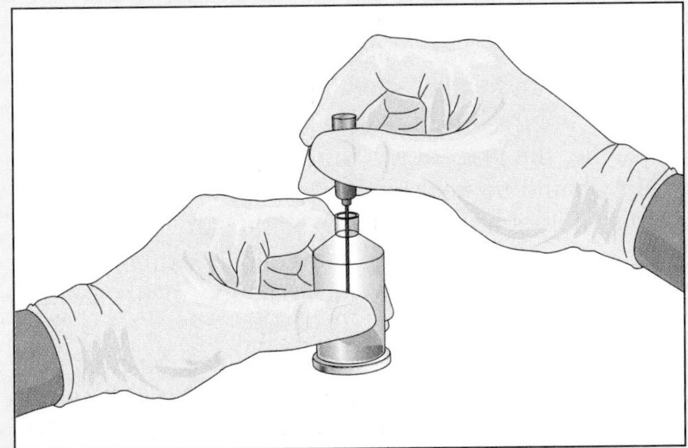

Figure 34-19. Squeeze the reservoir several times to force blood through the tube into the overflow chamber.

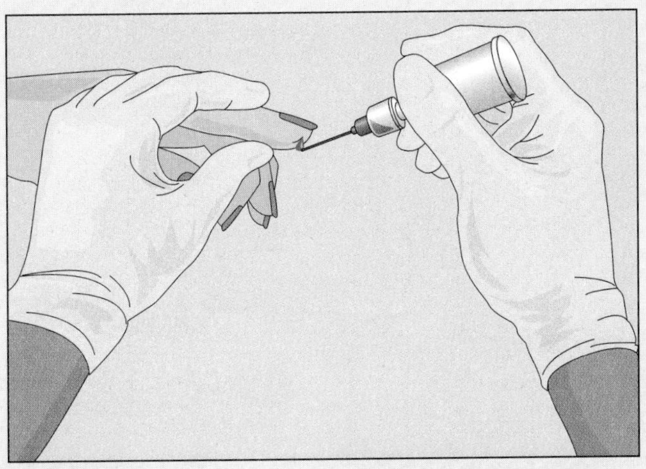

Figure 34-18. Remove the shield from the micropipette, and touch the tip of the pipette to the blood specimen.

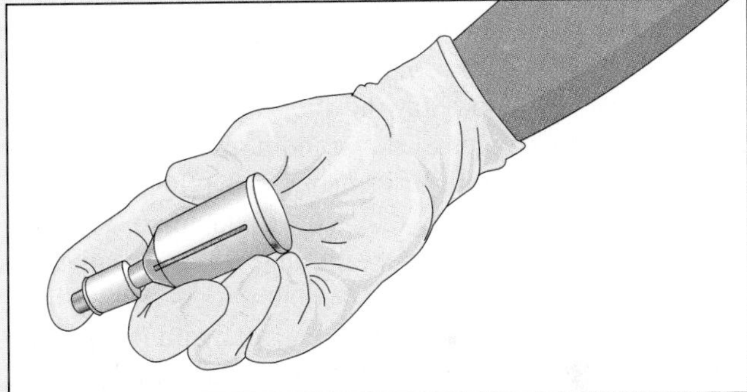

Figure 34-20. Invert the reservoir and micropipette assembly to ensure complete mixing of the blood with diluting fluid.

will be discarded when you finish. Let the patient see you put the needle in the sharps container.

Use this opportunity to educate the patient about the transmission of AIDS. Emphasize that AIDS, and other infections transmitted by blood, can be transmitted only when there is direct contact with contaminated blood or other body fluids. Explain that your gloves protect both you and the patient by providing a barrier to infection transmission from one person to another. Explain that your other protective equipment, such as goggles or a mask, also helps prevent the spread of infection.

Special Considerations

You will encounter a variety of patients, some of whom have special needs, as you collect blood specimens. You will find yourself in many different kinds of situations, some of them problematic. Some special needs and problematic situations are fairly common, and you must be prepared to deal with them.

Children. It is a challenge to explain blood-drawing procedures to children. Many children become visibly upset by the situation. If possible, it is best to talk with the parents or caregivers before working with the child.

The adults can provide the best insight into how their child handles stressful situations.

Your primary concern when working with infants is to complete tests correctly. Because an infant's veins are often too small for adequate blood collection, the best site for drawing blood is usually the heel.

When working with children, address them directly. Speak clearly in a calm, soothing voice, and explain the procedure briefly in terms they can understand. If they ask whether the process will hurt, be honest. Very young children should be held by their parent or guardian or a coworker during a venipuncture or capillary puncture to prevent them from moving. If a child is extremely distressed, it may be best to go on to another patient while the child calms down.

After you have begun the procedure, give the child status reports such as, We're almost finished! You've been very brave. This information helps calm nervous parents or caregivers as well.

When the procedure is complete, offer a compliment on some aspect of the child's behavior. Gather your supplies and samples as quickly as possible to avoid alarming the child with the sight of blood-collection tubes. If parents or caregivers have questions, encourage them to discuss the tests with the child's physician.

Elderly Patients. The challenges presented by elderly patients may test your technical skills as well as your interpersonal skills. Physically, some older adults are frail and may not withstand blood-drawing procedures as easily as younger patients. Changes in skin condition often make elderly patients more prone to bruising and other injuries. Decreased circulation may make it difficult to collect enough blood for an adequate sampling. Elderly patients with impaired hearing may have trouble understanding instructions and answering questions. Patients with dementia may also be unable to understand what you are saying.

When you communicate with an elderly patient, speak in clear, low-pitched tones. High-pitched voices are more difficult for people with hearing impairments to understand. When asking questions, give the patient time to answer, and confirm the response to prevent misunderstandings. Avoid both overly simple yes or no questions that the patient might answer without thinking and overly complex questions that might confuse the patient. Take your time with the procedure, and explain it in language the patient can understand.

Patients at Risk for Uncontrolled Bleeding. Patients who have hemophilia or are taking blood-thinning medications are at risk for uncontrolled bleeding at the collection site. (Hemophilia is a disorder in which the blood does not coagulate at a wound or puncture site.) Be especially careful and alert as you follow the standard procedures for collecting a blood specimen. In addition, hold a cotton ball over the puncture site for at least 5 minutes to make sure bleeding has stopped completely. If uncontrolled bleeding does occur, call the physician immediately.

Difficult Patients. You may encounter a particular challenge in working with a patient either because of technical problems or because of personality issues. Being prepared for these situations is the best method for coping with them.

The Difficult Venipuncture. There will be times when you simply cannot get a good blood sample. If your first attempt at drawing blood fails, try again at another site. Give the patient (and yourself) a short break, and make an attempt on the other arm, for instance. Sometimes the veins in one arm are easier to work with than the veins in the other arm. If you cannot get a good sample on the second try, stop. Ask for assistance from your supervisor or the doctor.

Fainting Patients. It is impossible to predict which patients will have a reaction to a blood-drawing procedure. Generally, however, an ill patient is more likely to experience a reaction than a well patient. The best way to deal with this potential problem is to position every patient so that, if fainting does occur, no injury will result.

Have patients sit in a special venipuncture chair (see Figure 34-21). These chairs are designed to help prevent

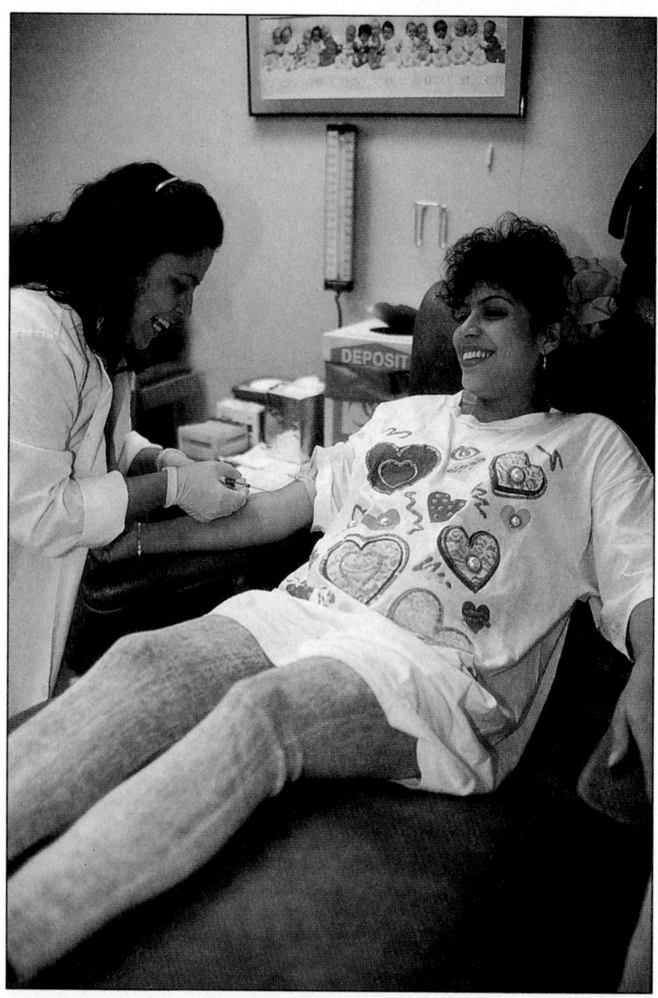

Figure 34-21. Venipuncture chairs are designed to make blood drawing easier and to prevent patients from falling if they should faint.

patients from sliding to the floor in the event of fainting. If your office is not equipped with a venipuncture chair, have patients lie down on an examination table. A patient who has a history of fainting or feels ill should lie down with feet elevated or knees drawn up while you complete the procedure.

If a patient does faint and the needle is still in the vein, release the tourniquet and withdraw the needle quickly and steadily. Apply pressure to the site. Most people revive promptly, and no other action is required. Do not leave the patient alone. Notify the doctor that the patient fainted, and ask the doctor whether you should continue with the procedure.

If there is a more severe reaction, notify the appropriate staff member and remain with the patient. If the patient is in a chair and begins to slide out, raise the safety arm and gently lower the patient to the floor. Protect the patient's head at all times, and make sure she is breathing easily. The doctor should examine the patient before you move her. Follow the doctor's instructions.

When the patient begins to recover, assist her into a sitting position and then to a chair or couch. The patient should rest until she feels strong enough to walk—usually about 15 minutes. When the patient feels steady, she should be led to another area of the office, such as the patient reception area. At this point another staff member usually becomes responsible for the patient's care and determines when she can leave.

Angry or Violent Patients. Some patients are extremely resistant to having blood drawn. Although their objections may seem illogical, remember that people often do not think as clearly in moments of high emotion as they normally do.

Encourage a patient who is mildly upset and wants to argue about the need for the blood test to let you take the sample and then discuss the situation with the doctor. If you convince the patient to submit to the test, complete the procedure quickly and accurately. Avoid arguing with the patient.

Do not force the issue with a patient who becomes violent or refuses outright to submit to the procedure. A patient does have the right to refuse testing or treatment. Under no circumstances should you attempt to physically force a patient to give a blood sample. Never endanger yourself, other patients, or your colleagues by refusing to back down from an angry or violent patient. Report the problem to the appropriate staff, make a note on the order, and follow other established procedures.

Performing Common Blood Tests

Many blood tests are routinely ordered as part of a complete general examination to determine a patient's overall health. The results of individual tests can provide information that aids in the diagnosis of specific conditions, diseases, and disorders, as noted in Table 34-2.

Table 34-2

Common Blood Tests and the Conditions They Help Identify

Substance Identified or Quantified	Part of Blood Tested	Indication, Disease, or Disorder
Acetone	Serum or plasma	Diabetic or fasting metabolic ketoacidosis
Alanine aminotransferase (ALT)	Serum	Liver disorders
Alpha-fetoprotein (AFP)	Fetal serum	Fetal liver and gastrointestinal tract status, hepatitis
Amylase	Serum	Drug toxicity, parotid or pancreas disorders
Angiotensin-converting enzyme (ACE)	Serum	Lung cancer, sarcoidosis, acute or chronic bronchitis
Antidiuretic hormone (ADH)	Plasma	Syndrome of inappropriate ADH, Guillain-Barré syndrome, brain tumor
Aspartate aminotransferase (AST)	Serum	Liver disease (including viral hepatitis), infectious mononucleosis, damaged heart or skeletal muscle
Bilirubin	Serum	Liver disease, fructose intolerance, hypothyroidism
Blood urea nitrogen (BUN)	Serum or plasma	Kidney disorders

continued

Table 34-2 continued

Substance Identified or Quantified	Part of Blood Tested	Indication, Disease, or Disorder
Cancer antigens (numbers 125, 15-3, 549, 72-4), tumor-associated glycoprotein (TAG)	Serum	Specific cancers identified, depending on antigen tested
Calcium, total (fasting)	Serum	Hyperparathyroidism, malignant disease with bone involvement
Carbon dioxide, total	Venous serum or plasma	Acidosis or alkalosis (acid-base balance)
Cholesterol, total	Serum or plasma	Hyperlipoproteinemia, coronary artery disease, atherosclerosis
Creatine kinase (CK)	Serum	Muscular dystrophies, Reye's syndrome, heart disease, shock, some neoplasms
Erythrocyte count (RBC)	Whole blood	Anemia
Erythrocyte sedimentation rate (ESR)	Whole blood	Infectious diseases, malignant neoplasms, sickle cell anemia
Glucose (fasting)	Whole blood	Pancreatic function, ability of intravenous insulin to offset diet in diabetes mellitus
Glucose (fasting—tolerance test)	Serum	Diabetes mellitus, hypoglycemia
Lactate dehydrogenase (LD)	Serum	Anemia, viral hepatitis, shock, hypoxia, hyperthermia
Leukocyte count (WBC)	Whole blood	Leukemia, infection, leukocytosis
Phenylalanine	Plasma	Hyperphenylalaninemia, obesity, phenylketonuria
Potassium (K^+) and sodium (Na^+)	Serum	Fluid-electrolyte balance
Prostatic acid phosphatase (PAP)	Serum	Prostatic cancer
Sickle cells	Whole blood	Sickle cell anemia
Thyroid-stimulating hormone (TSH), triiodothyronine (T_3), thyroxine (T_4)	Serum	Thyroid function
Uric acid	Serum	Gout, leukemia

The number of blood tests routinely performed in POLs has declined since the implementation of Clinical Laboratory Improvement Amendments of 1988 (CLIA '88) regulations. Many POLs now perform only waivered tests. Each POL is different, however, and regulations do change. Check with your employer about what tests your office performs regularly. You should be familiar with a wide range of tests and the steps involved with each even if you do not anticipate performing them.

You may encounter several chemical substances while performing your responsibilities in the laboratory. Chemicals you might encounter in laboratory work include the following:

- Anticoagulants, which cause the blood to remain in a liquid, uncoagulated state
- Serum separators, which form a gel-like barrier between serum and the clot in a coagulated blood sample
- Stains, which color particular cells, making microscopic studies easier to complete

Anticoagulants or serum separators are always present in blood-collection tubes and do not need to be added to the sample.

You must be absolutely clear about which chemicals are used for which tests and the precise amounts involved. It is also important to understand the purpose of blood tests so you can educate patients. You must, in addition, know the range of normal test values so you can be aware of potential problems and note them for the doctor's attention. Table 34-3 shows the normal ranges for a variety of blood tests.

Hematologic Tests

Hematologic tests are commonly performed in routine blood testing. These tests can be performed on venous or capillary whole blood samples. Hematologic tests include blood cell counts, morphologic studies, coagulation tests, and the nonautomated erythrocyte sedimentation rate test.

Blood Counts. Whole blood, as described earlier, contains the formed elements (red blood cells, white blood cells, platelets) and the fluid portion (plasma). The total number of blood cells and the percentage of the whole sample that each type represents can tell the physician a

Table 34-3

Normal Ranges for Blood Tests

Blood Test	Blood Component Tested	Normal Range
Blood counts		
Red blood cells (erythrocytes)		
Men	Whole blood	4.3–5.7 × 10^6 cells/µL
Women	Whole blood	3.8–5.1 × 10^6 cells/µL
White blood cells (leukocytes)	Whole blood	4.5–11.0 × 10^3 cells/µL
Platelets	Whole blood	150–400 × 10^3 cells/µL
Differential		
Neutrophils	Whole blood	60%–70%
Eosinophils	Whole blood	1%–4%
Basophils	Whole blood	0%–0.5%
Lymphocytes	Whole blood	20%–30%
Monocytes	Whole blood	2%–6%
Hematocrit (Hct)	Whole blood	
Men		39%–49%
Women		35%–45%
Hemoglobin (Hb, Hgb)	Whole blood	
Men		13.2–17.3 g/dL
Women		11.7–16.0 g/dL
Erythrocyte sedimentation rate (ESR)		
Wintrobe	Whole blood	
Men		0–5 mm/hour
Women		0–15 mm/hour
Westergren	Whole blood	
Men		0–15 mm/hour
Women		0–20 mm/hour

continued

Table 34-3 continued

Blood Test	Blood Component Tested	Normal Range
Coagulation tests		
Prothrombin time (PT)	Plasma	11–15 seconds
Bleeding time	Whole blood	2–7 minutes
Blood gases (collected anaerobically)		
Partial pressure of carbon dioxide ($PaCO_2$)	Arterial blood	
Men		35–48 mm Hg
Women		32–45 mm Hg
Partial pressure of oxygen (PaO_2)	Arterial blood	83–108 mm Hg
Total carbon dioxide (CO_2)	Venous serum or plasma	23–29 mEq/L
Electrolytes		
Bicarbonate (HCO_3^-)	Arterial plasma	21–28 mEq/L
	Venous plasma	27–29 mEq/L
Calcium (Ca^{++})	Serum	8.6–10.0 mg/dL
Chloride (Cl^-)	Serum, plasma	98–108 mEq/L
Potassium (K^+)	Serum	3.5–5.1 mEq/L
Sodium (Na^+)	Serum	136–145 mEq/L
Chemical and serologic tests		
Alpha-fetoprotein (AFP)	Serum	
Fetal, first trimester		20–400 mg/dL
Adult		<15 ng/mL
Alanine aminotransferase (ALT)	Serum	
Men		10–40 U/L
Women		7–35 U/L
Aspartate aminotransferase (AST, formerly SGOT)	Serum	
Men		11–26 U/L
Women		10–20 U/L
Bilirubin, total direct	Serum	0.3–1.2 mg/dL
Blood urea nitrogen (BUN)	Serum, plasma	6–20 mg/dL
Carcinoembryonic antigen (CEA)	Serum	<5.0 ng/mL
Cholesterol, total	Serum, plasma	
Men		158–277 mg/dL
Women		162–285 mg/dL

continued

Table 34-3 continued

Blood Test	Blood Component Tested	Normal Range
Chemical and serologic tests (continued)		
Cholesterol, total (continued)		
High-density lipoproteins (HDLs)	Serum, plasma	
Men		28–63 mg/dL
Women		37–92 mg/dL
Low-density lipoproteins (LDLs)	Serum, plasma	
Men		89–197 mg/dL
Women		88–201 mg/dL
Creatine kinase (CK)	Serum, plasma	
Men		38–174 U/L
Women		26–140 U/L
Creatinine	Serum, plasma	
Men		0.9–1.3 mg/dL
Women		0.6–1.2 mg/dL
Cytomegalovirus (CMV)	Serum	None
Epstein-Barr virus (EBV)	Whole blood	None
Glucose (fasting blood sugar, FBS)	Serum	74–120 mg/dL
Group A β-hemolytic streptococci	Serum	None
Human immunodeficiency virus (HIV) antibodies	Serum, plasma	None
Insulin	Serum	<17 μU/mL
Iron, total	Serum	
Men		65–175 μg/dL
Women		50–170 μg/dL
Ketone bodies (as acetoacetate)	Serum, plasma	None
Lactate dehydrogenase (LD)	Serum, plasma	140–280 U/L
pH	Arterial blood	7.35–7.45
	Venous blood	7.32–7.43
Proteins	Serum	
Total		6.2–8.0 g/dL
Albumin		3.4–4.8 g/dL
Fibrinogen		200–400 mg/dL
Uric acid	Serum	
Men		4.4–7.6 mg/dL
Women		2.3–6.6 mg/dL

great deal about a patient's condition. A physician can order an individual test or a complete blood (cell) count (CBC), which includes the following tests:

- Red blood (cell) count (RBC), which is the total number of red blood cells in a sample
- White blood (cell) count (WBC), which is the total number of white blood cells in a sample
- Differential white blood cell count, which is the number of each type of white blood cell (basophils, eosinophils, neutrophils, lymphocytes, and monocytes) in the first 100 leukocytes of a sample
- Platelet count (automated), which is the number of platelets in a sample, or a platelet estimate, which indicates whether the amount of platelets is adequate
- **Hematocrit** determination, which identifies how much of the volume of a sample is made up of red blood cells after the sample has been spun in a centrifuge; expressed as a percentage
- Hemoglobin determination, which measures the amount of hemoglobin in the sample

Most POLs use automated equipment for performing blood counts, but you need to know how to perform blood counts manually. This competency provides a backup for the automated instrumentation and puts you in a better position to recognize unusual findings among automated results. All manual counts are estimates. The types of blood cell counts differ in sample preparation and in the equipment and methods used.

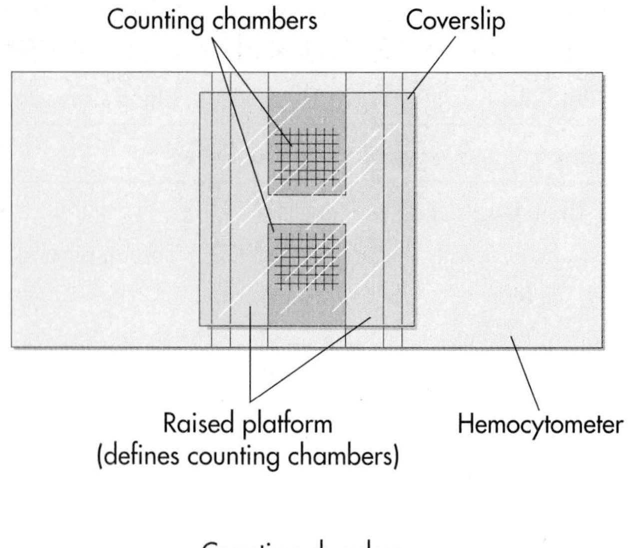

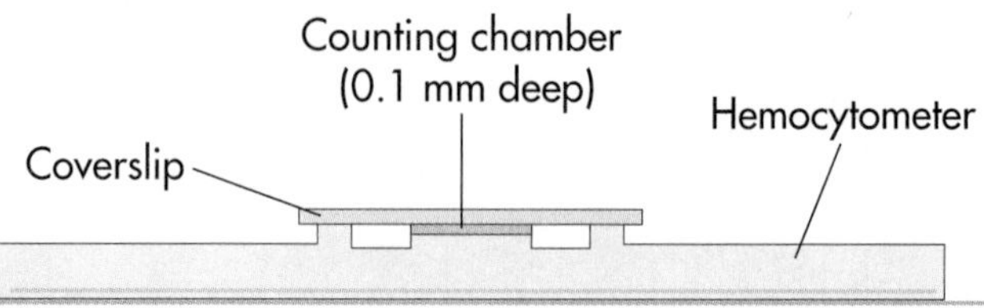

Figure 34-22. You can count the number of blood cells in a blood specimen by using a hemocytometer.

Overall Cell Counts. You will use a diluted sample and a hemocytometer when you count RBCs or WBCs. A **hemocytometer** is a special microscope slide that allows you to count blood cells by examining a diluted blood sample under the microscope. The hemocytometer is thicker than the average microscope slide, with a raised platform shaped like a capital H (see Figure 34-22). The top and bottom slots of the H are the counting chambers. Etched into the slide under each chamber is a grid of fine lines, which helps you count individual cells. A hemocytometer coverslip is placed on top of the chamber, spreading the sample to a uniform depth of 0.1 mm. Procedure 34-4 explains how to charge, or fill, a hemocytometer.

Cells in a fluid blood specimen are too numerous to count accurately, so samples are diluted before counting for both manual and automated counts. The dilution factor and diluting substance for RBCs differ from those for WBCs. For this reason RBC and WBC counts are performed on separately prepared samples on separate slides. Procedure 34-5 describes how to perform a blood cell count using a hemocytometer.

Differential Cell Counts. You will prepare a blood smear slide and stain the smear for a differential cell count. Procedure 34-6 details preparation of a blood smear slide. When you carry out this process correctly, there will be a region of the slide where blood cells are dense but lie in a single plane (not stacked or bunched together.) This is the region where you will count the cells.

A polychromatic (multicolored) stain such as Wright's stain simplifies a differential cell count. The blue and red-orange dyes (methylene blue and eosin, respectively) stain cell structures in ways that identify each of the five types of white blood cells. When stained, neutrophils have a dark purple nucleus and pale pink cytoplasm containing fine pink or lavender granules. Basophils have a purple nucleus and light purple cytoplasm that contains large, blue-black granules. Eosinophils can be identified by the purple nucleus and the bright orange granules in pink cytoplasm. Lymphocytes appear as a large, dark purple nucleus surrounded by a small amount of blue cytoplasm. The fifth type of leukocytes, monocytes, are the largest and have gray-blue cytoplasm.

Figure 34-29 shows the zigzag pattern for counting leukocytes visible in the field when using the microscope's oil-immersion objective. Follow this pattern and count the first 100 leukocytes, recording the count by leukocyte type on a differential cell counter. Each cell type is expressed as a percentage of the 100 leukocytes counted. You may estimate the platelet count by averaging the count in 10 to 15 fields.

Hematocrit. You measure a patient's hematocrit percentage by collecting a small sample of the patient's blood in

PROCEDURE 34-4

Charging (Filling) a Hemocytometer

Objective: To prepare a hemocytometer slide for viewing

OSHA Guidelines

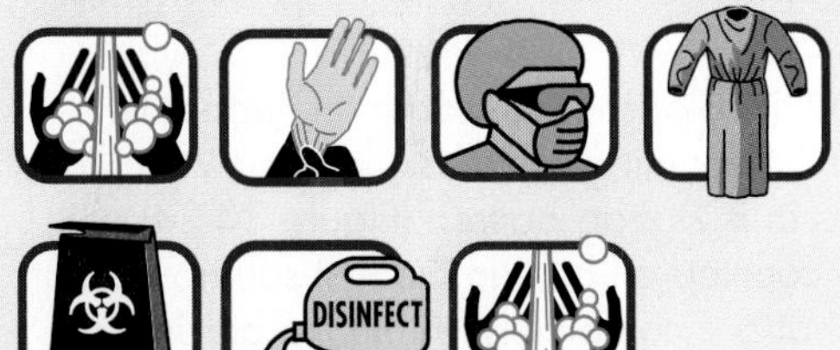

Materials: UNOPETTE (self-filling diluting micropipette) containing a blood specimen, hemocytometer slide, hemocytometer coverslip, 70% alcohol, lens paper, sterile gauze squares, petri dish with dampened filter paper

Method

1. Wash your hands and put on examination gloves.
2. Clean the hemocytometer slide and hemocytometer coverslip with 70% alcohol and lens paper. Double-check the slide and coverslip to make sure neither is scratched nor cracked.
3. Position the coverslip over the counting chamber of the hemocytometer.
4. Convert the UNOPETTE to a dropper by removing the capillary tube assembly from the reservoir and reversing it so that the capillary tube becomes a dropper tube.
5. Invert the reservoir and squeeze the sides gently to release three or four drops of diluted blood onto a sterile gauze square. Discard the gauze square.
6. Maintaining slight pressure on the sides of the reservoir, touch the tip of the dropper tube to the underside edge of the coverslip in the loading area of the hemocytometer. The sample will flow onto the slide through capillary action. The dropper tip must touch the edge of the coverslip for capillary action to occur. Fill both sides of the counting chamber.
7. Allow the chamber to sit undisturbed for 1 or 2 minutes in a petri dish lined with moist filter paper. Do not allow the slide to dry out. (The waiting period allows the cells to settle into a single plane, making them easier to count. Evaporation damages the sample, however, and renders it useless.)
8. Properly dispose of used supplies, and disinfect the work area.
9. Remove the gloves and wash your hands.

a microhematocrit tube, sealing the tube, and spinning it in a centrifuge. This process is described in Procedure 34-7, p. 716. During this process heavier red blood cells move to one end of the tube, whereas lighter plasma moves to the other end. Between the RBCs, also called the **packed red blood cells,** and the plasma is the buffy coat (see Figure 34-34, p. 718). The **buffy coat** contains the white blood cells and platelets.

Always run two samples of the patient's blood specimen. After removing each sample from the centrifuge, compare the column of packed RBCs with a standard hematocrit gauge. Read on the gauge the percentage of total blood volume represented by the RBCs. Average the readings of the two patient samples. (The samples should be within 2% of each other.)

Hemoglobin. Hemoglobin resides within the red blood cells. You will determine the concentration of hemoglobin in the blood by lysing (rupturing) the red blood cells (hemolysis) and evaluating the color of the sample. This procedure may be done with a hemoglobinometer—a handheld device that makes color evaluation less subjective than older methods of visual matching with color samples. Blood specimens mixed with a reagent, such as Drabkin's reagent, undergo a color reaction that can be quantified by reading color intensity in a photoelectric colorimeter.

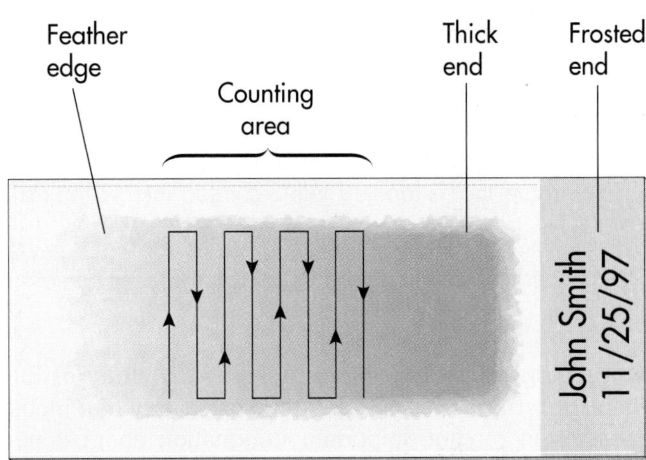

Figure 34-29. Follow this pattern when counting leukocytes visible in the field under the oil-immersion objective of the microscope.

PROCEDURE 34-5

Completing a Blood Cell Count Using a Hemocytometer

Objective: To count white blood cells (WBCs) and red blood cells (RBCs) in separately prepared portions of a blood specimen

OSHA Guidelines

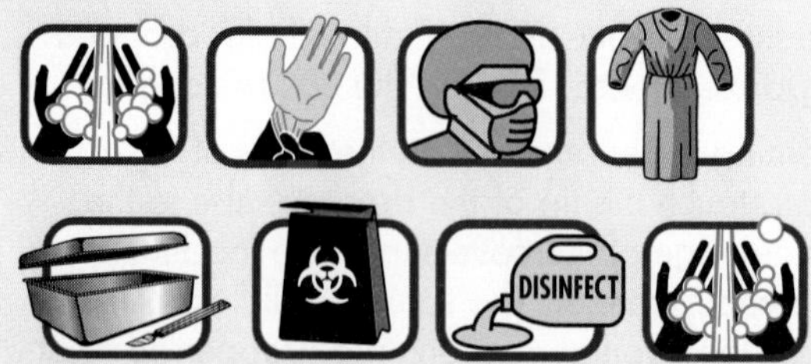

Materials: Two prepared hemocytometer slides with hemocytometer coverslips (one for WBCs, one for RBCs), microscope, tally counter

Method

1. Wash your hands and put on examination gloves.
2. Move the prepared WBC hemocytometer slide to the microscope stage, being careful to keep the slide level. Note that the microscope stage must be in the lowered position to allow you to place the hemocytometer on it without damage to the slide.
3. Adjust the microscope so that a counting chamber (the top or bottom slot of the H-shaped, raised platform) is positioned over the light source. Adjust the microscope so that the counting chamber is illuminated with the lowest light setting.
4. Look at the microscope from the side as you slowly raise the stage to position the slide close to the 10× objective. (Watching from the side allows you to see how far you can adjust the microscope without touching the slide. If you touch the objective to the coverslip, you must prepare a new slide.)
5. Focus the microscope until you can see the counting lines on the slide, as shown in Figure 34-23. Note that the grid consists of nine squares, with each square that is labeled WBC divided into 16 boxes. These squares are used to count white blood cells. The center square is divided into 25 boxes, with each box further divided into 16 tiny blocks. This square is used to count red blood cells.
6. To count white blood cells, start in the upper left square of the counting chamber, labeled WBC, and count cells in a zigzag pattern (Figure 34-24) until you have counted all cells in the first square. Count the cells that are completely within the borders of each box in the square and the cells that touch the top and left outer edges of the square. Do not count cells that touch the right or bottom outer edges of the square. Click the hand counter once for each

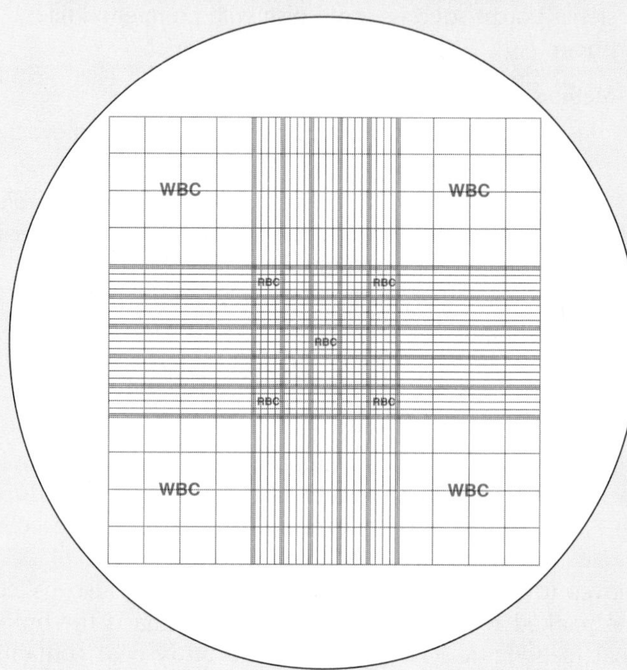

Figure 34-23. Different areas of the hemocytometer grid are used for counting white blood cells (WBCs) and red blood cells (RBCs). Red blood cells are counted under higher magnification than are white blood cells.

Morphologic Studies. **Morphology** is the study of the shape or form of objects. A morphologic study of a blood sample can provide important information about a patient's condition. During a morphologic study on blood, a blood smear is examined, and the appearance and shape of cells in the sample are recorded. Special note is made of abnormal cell size, shape, or content and abnormal organization of cells. A morphologic study is often performed just after the differential count and platelet estimate on the same blood smear slide. Morphologic studies require special training and are not routinely done by medical assistants.

Coagulation Tests. A physician may order coagulation tests to identify potential bleeding problems before surgical procedures. A regular schedule of coagulation tests

cell in the square. When you finish with the upper left square, record the number that appears on the hand counter, reset the counter to zero, and move to the upper right, lower right, and lower left squares labeled WBC. Repeat the counting process and record each square's total. Move to the other counting chamber and count all four squares.

Review the totals. The eight square totals should vary by no more than 10 cells. Total the four squares of each side, and multiply the result by 50. The two chamber totals should vary by no more than 1000 cells. If your totals show a larger variance, the hemocytometer has been filled unevenly, and the procedure must be repeated. Calculate the average result by adding the two chamber totals and dividing that number by 2. Round off the result to the nearest 100 cells.

7. To count red blood cells, repeat steps 1 through 5 with the RBC slide, using the 40× objective and bringing the center square into focus. Start in the upper left box of the square labeled RBC, and count cells in a zigzag pattern until all cells in the first box have been counted. Count the cells completely within the borders of each block in the box and cells touching the top and left outer edges of the box. Do not count cells touching the right or bottom edges of the box. Click the hand counter once for each cell in the box. When you finish with the upper left box, record the number on the hand counter, reset the counter to zero, and move to the upper right, lower right, lower left, and center boxes labeled RBC. Repeat the counting process and record each box's total. Move to the other counting chamber, and count all five boxes.

   Review the totals. The ten box totals should vary by no more than 20 cells. Total the five boxes of each side, and multiply the result by 10,000. The two chamber totals should vary by no more than 300,000 cells. If your totals show a larger variance, the hemocytometer has been filled unevenly, and the procedure must be repeated. Calculate the average result by adding the two chamber totals and dividing that number by 2. Round off the result to the nearest 100 cells.

8. Remove the hemocytometer from the microscope. Sanitize and disinfect both the hemocytometer slides and coverslips. Disinfect the work area.
9. Remove the gloves and wash your hands.
10. Record each result in the patient's chart. Be sure to identify abnormal results.

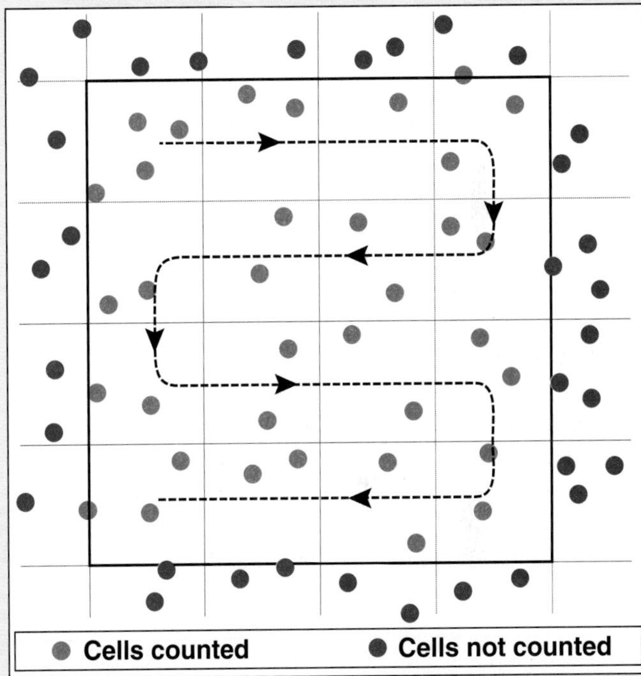

Figure 34-24. Use the same zigzag pattern to count either red blood cells or white blood cells.

may be ordered to monitor therapeutic drug levels when a patient is receiving medications such as heparin or warfarin (Coumadin). Coagulation studies include the prothrombin time (PT) and partial thromboplastin time (PTT) tests. These tests are usually performed using automated devices such as the Coaguchek Plus, manufactured by Boehringer Mannheim Diagnostics, Indianapolis, Indiana. These systems monitor the changing pattern of light transmission through the sample as coagulation occurs. Medical assistants sometimes perform such coagulation studies.

Erythrocyte Sedimentation Rate. The nonautomated **erythrocyte sedimentation rate (ESR)** test measures the rate at which red blood cells, the heaviest blood component, settle to the bottom of a blood sample. You will

PROCEDURE 34-6

Preparing a Blood Smear Slide

Objective: To prepare a blood specimen to be used in a morphologic or other study

OSHA Guidelines

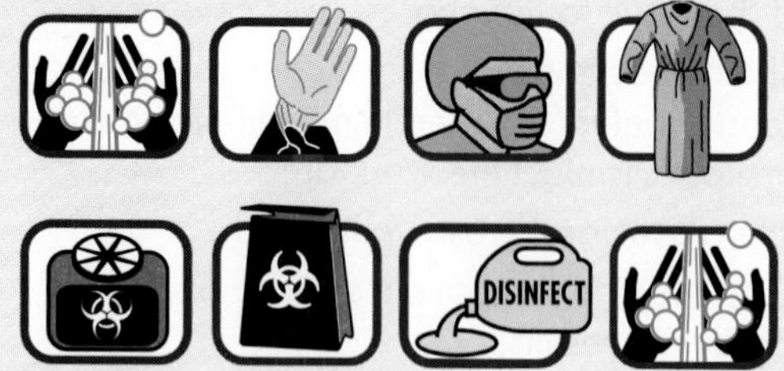

Materials: Blood specimen (either from a capillary puncture or a specimen tube containing anticoagulated blood), capillary tubes, sterile gauze squares, slide with frosted end, wooden applicator sticks

Method

1. Wash your hands and put on examination gloves.
2. If you will be using blood from a capillary puncture, follow the steps in Procedure 34-2 to express a drop of blood from the patient's finger. If you will be using a venous sample, check the specimen for proper labeling, uncap the specimen tube, and use wooden applicator sticks to remove any coagulated blood from the inside rim of the tube.
3. Touch the tip of the capillary tube to the blood specimen. The tube will take up the correct amount through capillary action.
4. Pull the capillary tube away from the sample, holding it carefully to prevent spillage. Wipe the outside of the capillary tube with a sterile gauze square to remove excess blood.
5. With the slide on the work surface, hold the capillary tube in one hand and the frosted end of the slide against the work surface with the other.
6. Apply a drop of blood to the slide, about ¾ inch from the frosted end, as shown in Figure 34-25. Place the capillary tube in a safe location to prevent spillage.
7. Pick up the spreader slide with your dominant hand. Hold the slide at approximately a 30° to 35° angle. Place the edge of the spreader slide on the smear slide close to the unfrosted end. Pull the spreader slide toward the frosted end until the spreader slide touches the blood drop (see Figure 34-26). Capillary action will spread the droplet along the edge of the spreader slide.
8. As soon as the drop spreads out to cover most of the spreader slide edge, push the spreader slide back toward the unfrosted end of the smear slide,

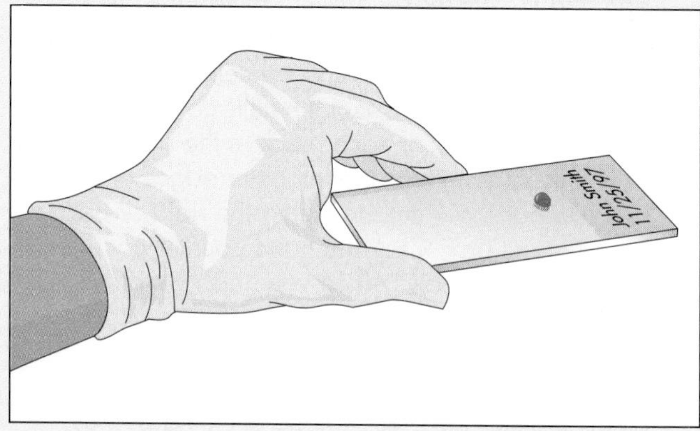

Figure 34-25. Apply a drop of blood to the slide about ¾ inch from the frosted end.

transfer freshly collected, anticoagulated blood to a calibrated tube and place the tube in a sedimentation rack to run this test (see Figure 34-35, p. 718). You examine the tube an hour later to determine how far the red blood cells have fallen. Test results are recorded as millimeters per hour (mm/hr). Several standard testing systems are used, including the Westergren and Wintrobe systems. You must adhere closely to each manufacturer's instructions when using these systems, because ESR test results are sensitive to factors such as the temperature and freshness of the samples, precise position of the sample tube, and vibrations affecting the tube or the rack.

Chemical Tests

Blood chemistry analysis examines several dozen chemicals found in human blood. Tables 34-2 and 34-3 include many chemical tests on blood. Highly detailed studies are rarely performed in the POL because they require expensive, sophisticated equipment and techniques. Complex testing is also subject to strict CLIA '88 regulations that increase the administrative work and the need for more highly trained personnel. These types of tests, therefore, are commonly performed at an independent test laboratory. Automated equipment for analyzing blood chem-

pulling the sample across the slide behind it, as shown in Figure 34-27. Maintain the 30° to 35° angle.

9. As you near the unfrosted end of the smear slide, gently lift the spreader slide away from it, still maintaining the angle, as shown in Figure 34-28. The resulting smear should be approximately 1½ inches long, preferably with a margin of empty slide on all sides. The smear should be thicker on the frosted end of the slide.
10. Properly label the slide, allow it to dry, and follow the manufacturer's directions for staining it for the required tests.
11. Properly dispose of used supplies, and disinfect the work area.
12. Remove the gloves and wash your hands.

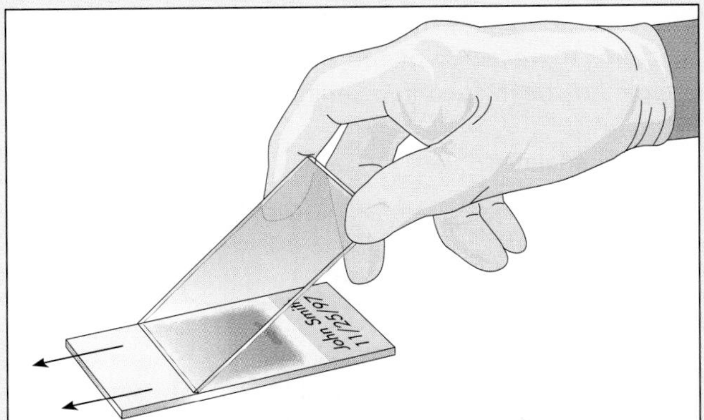

Figure 34-27. When the drop covers most of the spreader slide edge, push the spreader slide back toward the unfrosted end of the smear slide.

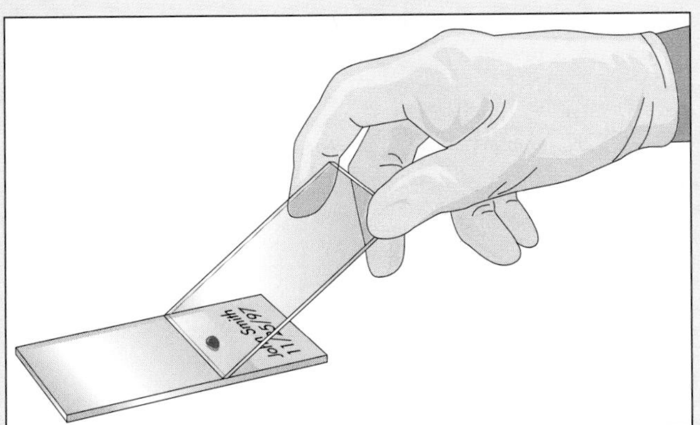

Figure 34-26. Hold the spreader slide at a 30° to 35° angle. Pull the spreader slide toward the frosted end until it touches the drop of blood.

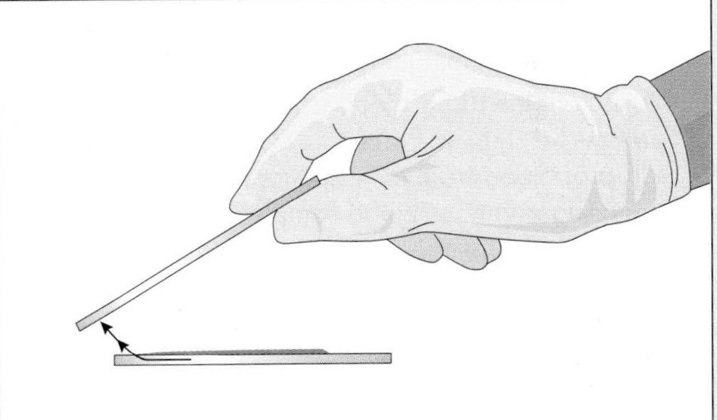

Figure 34-28. Lift the spreader slide away from the smear slide, maintaining a 30° to 35° angle. The smear should be thicker on the frosted end of the slide.

istry, however, is becoming more available, less expensive, and simpler to operate than it was in the past. This trend makes it more likely that you may use automated equipment to perform some types of blood chemistry tests. Keeping abreast of new developments will help prepare you for possible changes in your laboratory duties.

Some tests of blood chemistry are routinely performed in the POL. Blood glucose monitoring, for example, is often performed by a medical assistant or by a patient. Glucose monitoring systems require the use of sterile lancets to perform a capillary puncture. You will collect the blood on reagent strips that change color in accordance with glucose levels present in the blood. The level is determined either by comparing the color on the strip with color standards provided with the reagent strips or by feeding the strip into a handheld reading device. You will also teach patients to perform this kind of test at home. Be sure to stress the importance of following the manufacturer's guidelines for correct operation of a testing device.

Serologic Tests

Serologic tests detect the presence of specific substances in a blood sample. The terms *serologic test* and *immunoassay* refer to the introduction of an antigen or antibody into the

PROCEDURE 34-7

Measuring Hematocrit Percentage After Centrifuge

Objective: To identify the percentage of a blood specimen represented by red blood cells after the sample has been spun in a centrifuge

OSHA Guidelines

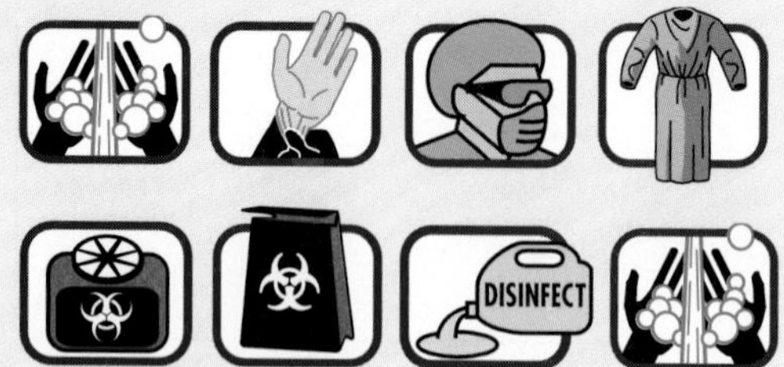

Materials: Blood specimen (either from a capillary puncture or a specimen tube containing anticoagulated blood), microhematocrit tube, sealant tray containing sealing clay, centrifuge, hematocrit gauge, wooden applicator sticks, gauze squares

Method

1. Wash your hands and put on examination gloves.
2. If you will be using blood from a capillary puncture, follow the steps in Procedure 34-2 to express a drop of blood from the patient's finger. If you will be using a venous blood sample, check the specimen for proper labeling, uncap the specimen tube, and use wooden applicator sticks to remove any coagulated blood from the inside rim of the tube.
3. Touch the tip of one of the microhematocrit tubes to the blood sample, as shown in Figure 34-30. The tube will take up the correct amount through capillary action.
4. Pull the microhematocrit tube away from the sample, holding it carefully to prevent spillage. Wipe the outside of the microhematocrit tube with a gauze square to remove excess blood.
5. Hold the microhematocrit tube in one hand, with a gloved finger over one end to prevent leakage, and press the other end of the tube gently into the clay in the sealant tray (Figure 34-31). The clay plug must completely seal the end of the tube.
6. Repeat the process to fill another microhematocrit tube. Tubes must be processed in pairs to maintain a balance in the centrifuge.
7. Place the tubes in the centrifuge, with the sealed ends pointing outward (see Figure 34-32). If you are processing more than one sample, record the position identification number in the patient's chart to track the sample.

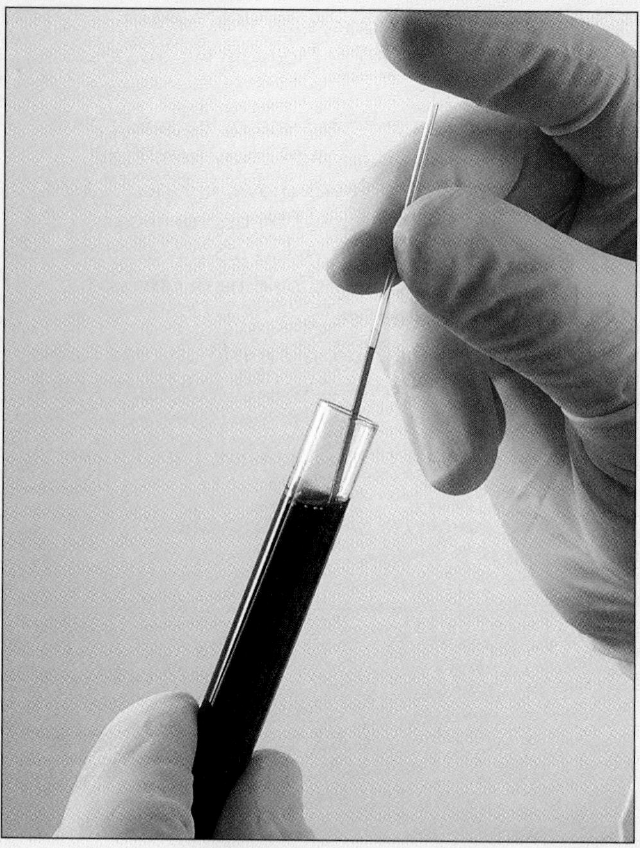

Figure 34-30. Touch the tip of one of the microhematocrit tubes to the blood specimen.

8. Seal the centrifuge chamber.
9. Run the centrifuge for the required time, usually between 3 and 5 minutes. Allow the centrifuge to come to a complete stop before unsealing it.
10. Determine the hematocrit percentage by comparing the column of packed red blood cells in the microhematocrit tubes with the hematocrit gauge, as shown in Figure 34-33. Position each tube so that the boundary between sealing clay and red blood cells is at zero on the gauge. Some centrifuges are equipped with gauges, but others require separate handheld gauges.
11. Record the percentage value on the gauge that corresponds to the top of the column of red blood cells for each tube. Compare the two results. They should not vary by more than 2%. If you record a greater variance, at least one of the tubes was filled incorrectly, and you must repeat the test.
12. Calculate the average result by adding the two tube figures and dividing that number by 2.

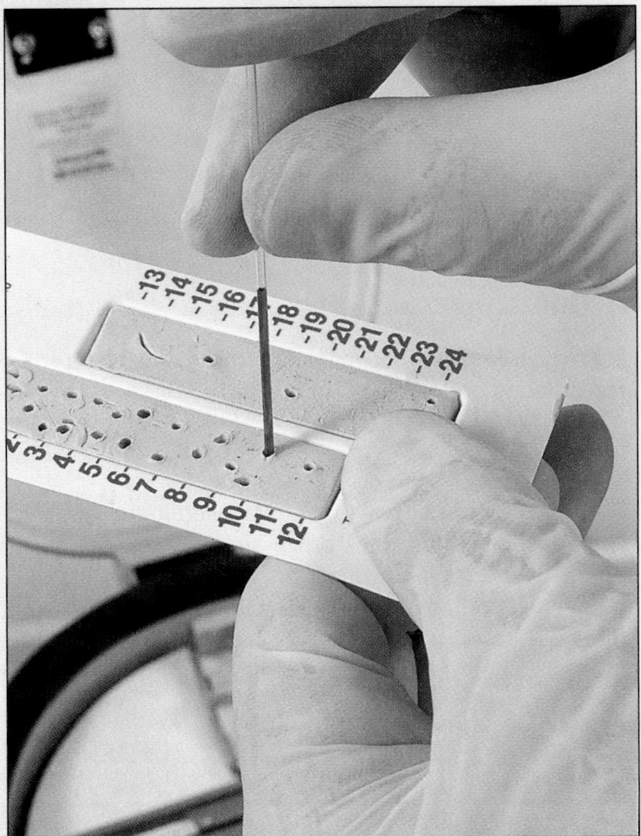

Figure 34-31. Press the end of the tube into the clay in the sealant tray.

13. Properly dispose of used supplies, and clean and disinfect the equipment and the area.
14. Remove the gloves and wash your hands.
15. Record the test result in the patient's chart. Be sure to identify abnormal results.

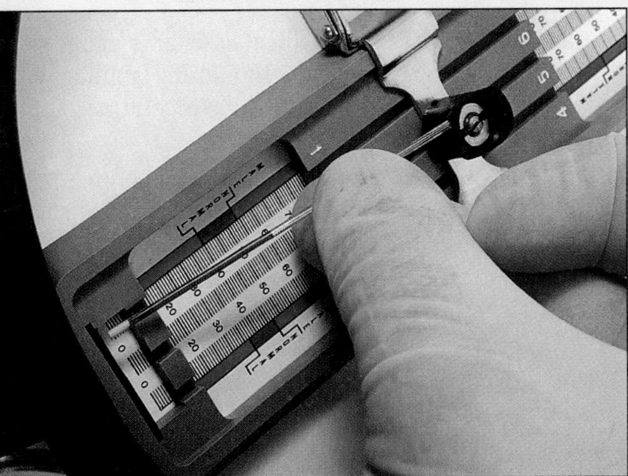

Figure 34-32. Be sure to place the tubes in the centrifuge so that the sealed ends are pointing outward.

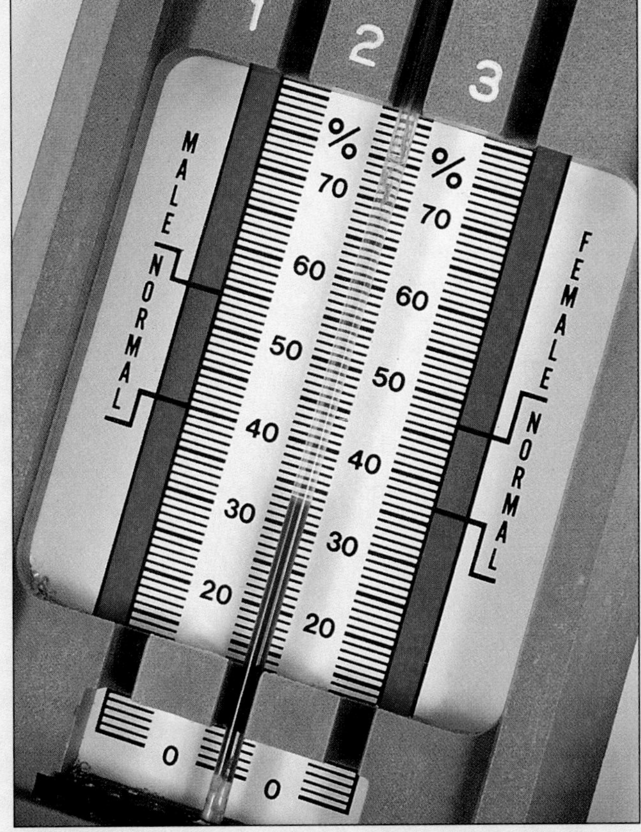

Figure 34-33. Compare the column of packed red blood cells in the microhematocrit tube with the hematocrit gauge to determine the hematocrit percentage.

specimen and the detection of a specific reaction to the antigen or antibody. Serologic testing methods can be used to detect disease antibodies, drugs, hormones, and vitamins in the blood and to determine blood types. They are also used to test urine and other body fluids.

Immunoassays. Although medical assistants usually do not perform immunoassays, you should be familiar with several immunoassay methods that have common applications. These methods include:

- Western blot, in which antigens are blotted onto special filter paper for examination. Western blot tests are generally used to confirm HIV infection diagnosis.
- Radioimmunoassay (RIA), in which radioisotopes are used to "tag" antibodies. RIA tests are extremely sensitive and generally performed in a reference laboratory.
- Enzyme-linked immunosorbent assay (ELISA), in which enzyme-labeled antigens and substances that can absorb antigens generate reactions to specific antibodies. These reactions are identified through visual or photoelectric color detection. HIV infection is diagnosed using an ELISA test.
- Immunofluorescent antibody (IFA) test, in which dye, visible when the sample is examined under a fluorescent microscope, colors specific antibodies.

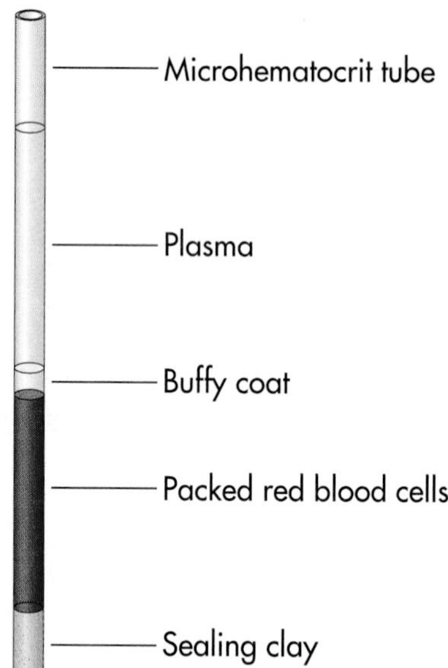

Figure 34-34. Blood in a centrifuged microhematocrit tube separates into packed red blood cells, the buffy coat, and plasma.

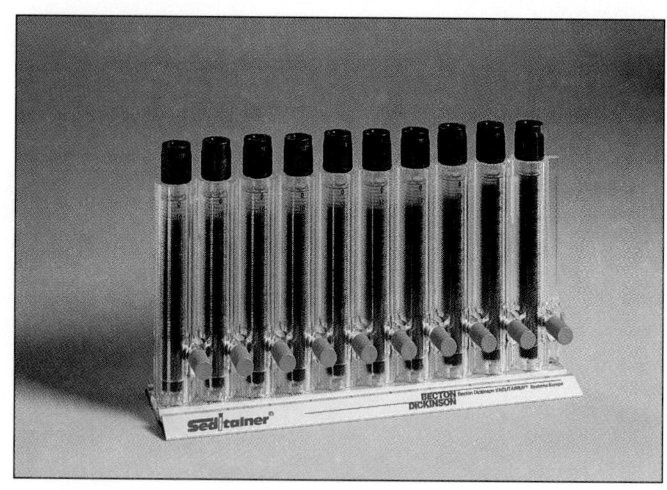

Figure 34-35. The sedimentation rack holds blood specimens steady and level for the ESR test.

Rapid Screening Tests. Several serologic tests have been developed for quick processing. Some, such as early pregnancy tests performed on urine, are available for home use. When you use tests of this type or explain their use to a patient, keep in mind that the manufacturer's guidelines must be carefully followed to ensure accurate results.

Summary

Successful phlebotomy procedures require not only superior technical skills but also excellent interpersonal communication skills. When you are confident in your ability to perform venipuncture and capillary puncture techniques and in your understanding of common blood tests, you impart confidence to the patient. You should know what pretest instructions the patient should follow and what the patient can expect during the test.

As a medical assistant, you may be called on to complete certain testing procedures or to explain the purpose of tests to the patient. Therefore, it is important to understand the basics of blood composition and the common blood tests a patient might undergo. You can make the difference between a successfully drawn, accurately evaluated blood specimen and one that must be drawn again from a confused, unhappy patient.

34 Chapter Review

Discussion Questions

1. Identify the major components of whole blood.
2. Explain the differences between venipuncture and capillary puncture techniques.
3. Identify four types of blood tests you might perform on a patient.

Critical Thinking Questions

1. You encounter an abbreviation on the laboratory order that you have never seen before. It could be read one of several ways, or it might be a mistake. What should you do?
2. Upon opening a centrifuge to complete a hematocrit percentage determination, you discover that one of the capillary tubes appears to be empty. What is the likely explanation, and what should be done now?
3. Consider a situation in which you need to take a blood sample from a mildly angry patient. Describe how you would deal with this patient.

Application Activities

1. With a partner, practice each step of the capillary puncture process on each other until you can smoothly execute each step. Critique each other's work.
2. Practice creating a smoothly drawn smear slide. Have a classmate critique your work.
3. With a classmate, role-play a situation in which a medical assistant must calm a child who is fearful about having a blood test. Then switch roles and offer suggestions for improving each other's communication skills.

Further Readings

"Cholesterol Testing Under Fire." *Science News,* 2 March 1996, 37.

Elinskas, Amy. "B-G-T-E-S-T: A Basic Review." *RN* 56 (June 1993): 49.

Kader, A. G. "How Safe Is Our Blood Supply?" *American Health* 15 (June 1996): 78–79.

Lieser, Carol S. "Easing Children's Procedural Pain." *American Journal of Nursing* 95, no. 11 (November 1995): 17.

Pendergraph, Garland. *Handbook of Phlebotomy.* 3d ed. Baltimore: Williams & Wilkins, 1992.

Tietz, Norbert W., ed. *Clinical Guide to Laboratory Tests.* 3d ed. Philadelphia: W. B. Saunders, 1995.

Travis, J. "AIDS Update '96." *Science News,* 23 March 1996, 184–186.

Westfall, Jo. "When Drawing Blood Draws Questions." *Medical Laboratory Observer* 26 (December 1994): 32.

Introduction to Microbiology

CHAPTER OUTLINE

- Microbiology and the Role of the Medical Assistant
- How Microorganisms Cause Disease
- Classification and Naming of Microorganisms
- Viruses
- Bacteria
- Protozoans
- Fungi
- Multicellular Parasites
- How Infections Are Diagnosed
- Specimen Collection
- Transporting Specimens to an Outside Laboratory
- Direct Examination of Specimens
- Preparation and Examination of Stained Specimens
- Culturing Specimens in the Medical Office
- Determining Antimicrobial Sensitivity
- Quality Control in the Medical Office

OBJECTIVES

After completing Chapter 35, you will be able to:

- Define microbiology.
- Describe how microorganisms cause disease.
- Describe how microorganisms are classified and named.
- Explain how viruses, bacteria, protozoans, fungi, and parasites differ and give examples of each.
- Describe the process involved in diagnosing an infection.
- List general guidelines for obtaining specimens.
- Describe how throat culture, urine, sputum, wound, and stool specimens are obtained.
- Explain how to transport specimens to outside laboratories.
- Describe two techniques used in the direct examination of culture specimens.
- Explain how to prepare and examine stained specimens.
- Describe how to culture specimens in the medical office.
- Explain how cultures are interpreted.
- Describe how to perform an antimicrobial sensitivity determination.
- Explain how to implement quality control measures in the microbiology laboratory.

Key Terms

acid-fast stain
aerobe
agar
anaerobe
antimicrobial
bacillus
coccus
colony
culture
culture and sensitivity (C & S)
culture medium
etiologic agent
facultative
fungus
gram-negative
gram-positive
Gram's stain
keratin
KOH mount
microbiology
mold
mordant
O and P specimen
parasite
protozoan
qualitative analysis
quality control (QC)
quantitative analysis
smear
spirillum
stain
vibrio
virus
wet mount
yeast

AREAS OF COMPETENCE
1997 ROLE DELINEATION STUDY

CLINICAL

Fundamental Principles

- Apply principles of aseptic technique and infection control
- Comply with quality assurance practices

Diagnostic Orders

- Collect and process specimens
- Perform diagnostic tests

Patient Care

- Obtain patient history and vital signs

GENERAL (Transdisciplinary)

Legal Concepts

- Document accurately

Microbiology and the Role of the Medical Assistant

Microbiology is the study of microorganisms—simple forms of life that are microscopic (visible only through a microscope) and are commonly made up of a single cell. Microorganisms are found everywhere. Some microorganisms are normally found on the skin and within the human body; they are called normal flora. They do not typically cause disease. Instead, they perform a number of important functions. For example, microorganisms in the intestines produce vitamins and help digest food. They also help protect the body from infection.

Many microorganisms cause infections. These microorganisms are referred to as pathogenic, or disease-causing. Infections can be mild, as in the case of the common cold. Infections can, however, sometimes lead to serious conditions. The proper diagnosis and treatment of infections are essential to restoring good health.

You may assist the physician in performing a number of microbiologic procedures that aid in diagnosing and treating infectious diseases. The types of microbiologic procedures you may be required to perform in the medical office include obtaining specimens or assisting the physician in doing so, preparing specimens for direct examination by the physician, and preparing specimens for transportation to a microbiology laboratory for identification.

Some physicians' offices have their own laboratories and are equipped to perform certain microbiology procedures. If this is the case in your office, you may be required to perform additional microbiologic procedures.

How Microorganisms Cause Disease

Anton van Leeuwenhoek first observed single-celled organisms through a microscope more than 300 years ago. It was not until much later, however, that microorganisms were identified as the cause of disease, through the works of scientists such as Louis Pasteur and Robert Koch.

Microorganisms can cause disease in a variety of ways. They may use up nutrients or other materials needed by the cells and tissues they invade. Microorganisms may damage body cells directly by reproducing themselves within cells, or the presence of microorganisms may make body cells the targets of the body's own defenses. Some microorganisms produce toxins, or poisons, that damage cells and tissues. Infecting microorganisms, or toxins they produce, may remain localized or may travel throughout the body, damaging or killing cells and tissues. The resulting symptoms include local swelling, pain, warmth, and redness, along with generalized symptoms of fever, tiredness, aches, and weakness. Infection by certain organisms may also cause skin reactions, gastrointestinal upset, or other symptoms.

Pathogenic organisms can be transmitted from one person to another in one of two ways:

- Through direct person-to-person contact, such as touching
- Through indirect contact, as with vectors, contaminated objects, droplets expelled in the air, or contaminated food or drink

The microorganisms that make up our normal flora, in addition to intact skin and mucous membranes, act as a barrier against infection by certain pathogens. Even these protective microorganisms, however, can cause infection if they invade other areas of the body.

Classification and Naming of Microorganisms

There are many different types of microorganisms, several of which can cause disease. Scientists classify microorganisms on the basis of their structure. Common classifications of microorganisms include the following:

- Subcellular, which consist of hereditary material, either deoxyribonucleic acid (DNA) or ribonucleic acid (RNA), surrounded by a protein coat
- Prokaryotic, which have a simple cell structure with no nucleus and no organelles in the cytoplasm
- Eukaryotic, which have a complex cell structure containing a nucleus and specialized organelles in the cytoplasm

Table 35-1 lists the characteristics that distinguish these classifications, as well as the types of microorganisms found in the classifications. Types of microorganisms include the following:

- Viruses
- Bacteria
- Protozoans
- Fungi
- Multicellular parasites

These types may be further divided into special groups that share certain characteristics. For example, within the bacteria are the special groups mycobacteria and rickettsiae, within each of which the members share distinct characteristics.

Specific microorganisms are named in a standard way, using two words. The first word refers to the genus (a category of biologic classification between the family and the species) to which the microorganism belongs. The second word refers to the particular species of the organism. Each species represents a distinct kind of microorganism. For

Table 35-1

Classifications of Microorganisms

Classification	Characteristics	Examples
Subcellular	Noncellular Nucleic acid surrounded by protein coat	Viruses
Prokaryotic cells	Simple structure Single chromosome No organelles	Bacteria
Eukaryotic cells	Highly structured Nucleus and cytoplasm Organelles	Protozoans, fungi, parasites

example, within the bacteria is the *Staphylococcus* genus. Then within that genus are various species such as *Staphylococcus aureus* and *Staphylococcus epidermidis*. Although the two bacteria belong to the same genus, they differ greatly in their ability to cause disease.

Viruses

Viruses are among the smallest known infectious agents. They cannot be seen with a regular microscope. Viruses are a simpler life form than the cell, consisting only of nucleic acid surrounded by a protein coat, as shown in Figure 35-1. Because of this fact, viruses can live and grow only within the living cells of other organisms.

Many viruses cause disease in people. Viruses are the cause of many of the common illnesses and conditions seen frequently in the medical office, including the common cold, influenza, chickenpox, croup, hepatitis, mononucleosis, and warts. Other illnesses caused by viruses are acquired immunodeficiency syndrome (AIDS), mumps, rubella, measles, encephalitis, and herpes. Vaccines are available to protect people from many of these viruses.

Bacteria

Bacteria are single-celled prokaryotic organisms that reproduce very quickly and are one of the major causes of disease. Under the right conditions—the right temperature, the right nutrients, and moisture—bacterial cells can double in number in 15 to 30 minutes. This rapid reproduction is one reason why untreated infections can be dangerous.

Classification and Identification

There are many different kinds of bacteria and many ways to identify them. Bacteria can be classified according to their shape, their ability to retain certain dyes, their ability to grow with or without air, and certain biochemical reac-

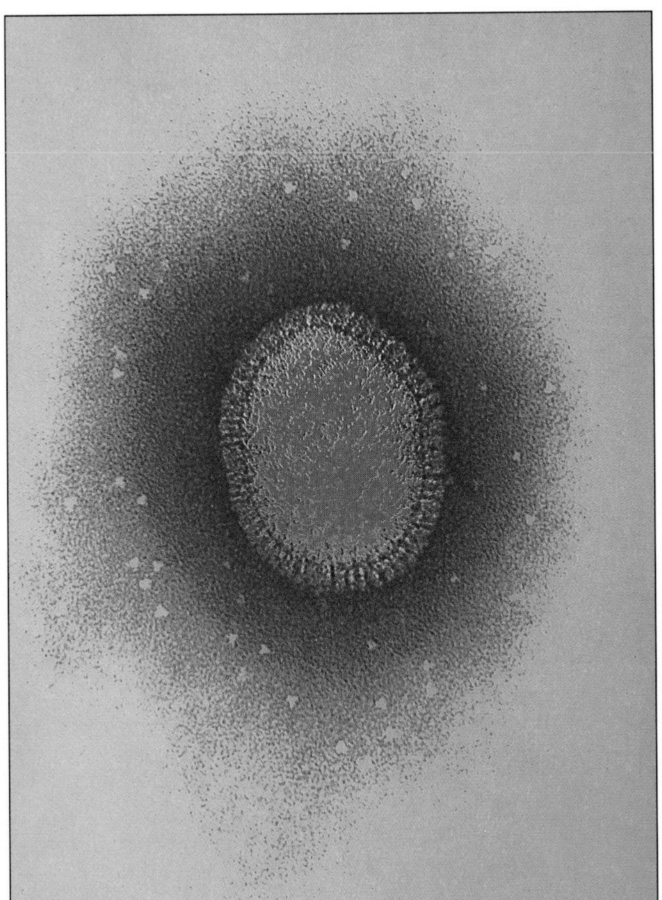

A

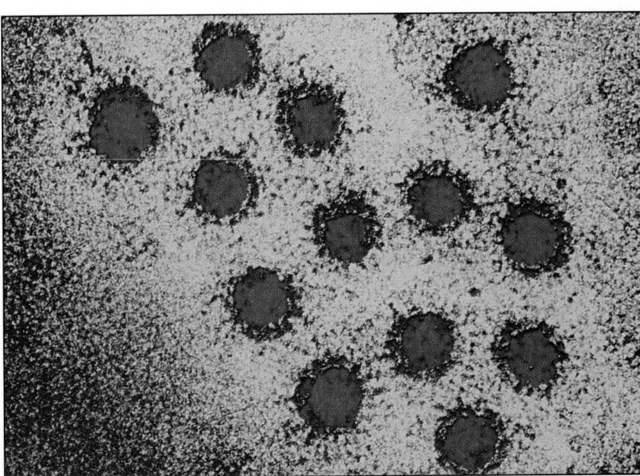

B

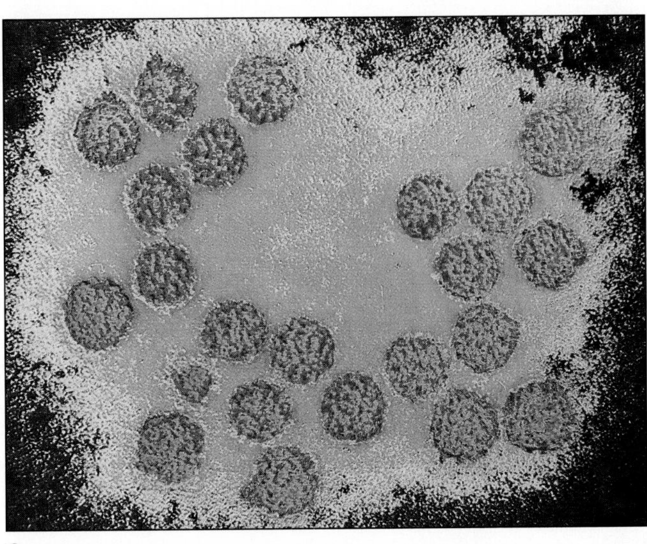

C

Figure 35-1. Three types of viral diseases often seen in medical offices are (a) influenza, (b) hepatitis, and (c) warts.

tions. Table 35-2 lists some of the major groups of bacteria, with distinguishing characteristics and a few examples.

Shape. The most common way to classify bacteria is according to their shape. A **coccus** (plural, cocci) is spherical, round, or ovoid; a **bacillus** (plural, bacilli) is rod-shaped; a **spirillum** (plural, spirilla) is spiral-shaped; and a **vibrio** (plural, vibrios) is comma-shaped. Figure 35-2 illustrates the four shapes.

- Cocci can be further divided into three types. Staphylococci are grapelike clusters of cocci commonly found on the skin. One species of this microorganism causes a variety of infections, including boils, acne, abscesses, food poisoning, and a type of pneumonia. Diplococci are pairs of cocci. The causative agents for gonorrhea and some forms of meningitis are diplococci. Streptococci are cocci that grow in chains. These microorganisms are responsible for infections such as strep throat, certain types of pneumonia, and rheumatic fever.
- Bacilli, or rod-shaped bacteria, are responsible for a wide variety of infections, including gastroenteritis, tuberculosis, pneumonia, whooping cough, urinary tract infections, botulism, and tetanus.
- Spirilla, or spiral-shaped bacteria, are responsible for infections such as syphilis and Lyme disease.

Table 35-2

Some Major Groups of Bacteria

Gram-Positive Bacteria

Shape	Characteristic	Genus	Species
Spherical, round, or ovoid	Grow in clusters	*Staphylococcus*	*aureus epidermidis*
	Grow in chains	*Streptococcus*	*pyogenes pneumoniae*
Straight rod	Aerobic	*Bacillus*	*subtilis*
	Anaerobic	*Clostridium*	*botulinum tetani*

Gram-Negative Bacteria

Shape	Characteristic	Genus	Species
Spherical, round, or ovoid	Aerobic	*Neisseria*	*meningitidis gonorrhoeae*
Straight rod	Aerobic	*Pseudomonas* *Haemophilus*	*aeruginosa* *influenzae*
	Facultative	*Escherichia* *Salmonella* *Shigella*	*coli* *typhi* *dysenteriae*
Comma	Facultative	*Vibrio*	*cholerae*
Spiral	Move by undulating	*Treponema*	*pallidum*

Other Groups

Shape	Characteristic	Genus	Species
Straight, curved, or branched rod	Acid-fast	*Mycobacterium*	*tuberculosis*
Variable	No rigid cell wall Intracellular parasite	*Mycoplasma* *Rickettsia*	*pneumoniae* *rickettsii*
Spherical, round, or ovoid	Intracellular parasite	*Chlamydia*	*trachomatis*

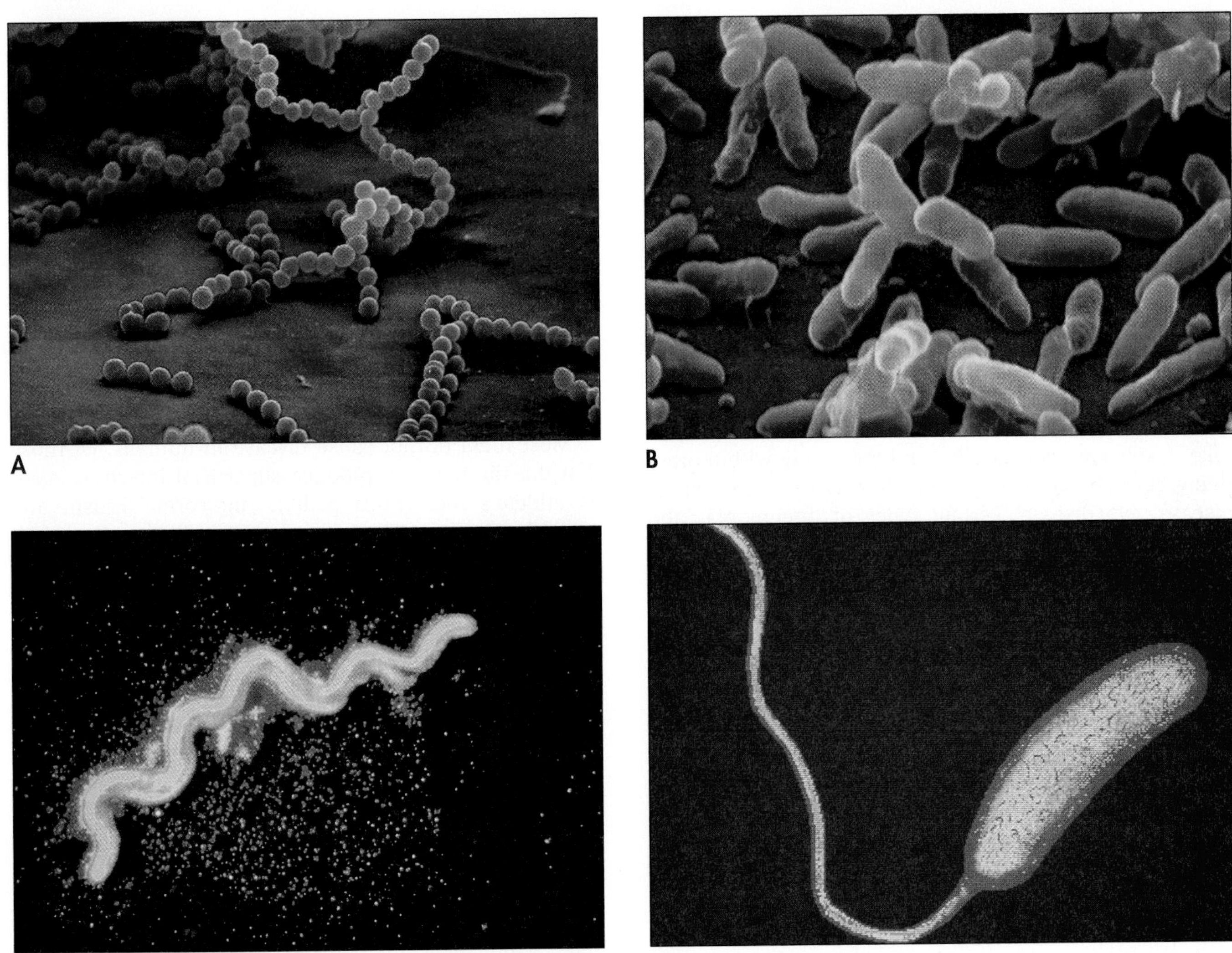

Figure 35-2. The four bacterial classifications by shape are (a) coccus, (b) bacillus, (c) spirillum, and (d) vibrio.

- Vibrios, or comma-shaped bacteria, are responsible for diseases such as cholera and some cases of food poisoning.

Ability to Retain Certain Dyes. In addition to their shape, bacteria are commonly classified by how they react to certain stains. A **stain** is a solution of a dye or group of dyes that imparts a color to microorganisms. The most common staining procedure in use today is the **Gram's stain,** a method of staining that differentiates bacteria according to the chemical composition of their cell walls. This procedure is often performed in the medical office. Another important stain is the **acid-fast stain,** a staining procedure for identifying bacteria with a waxy cell wall. The bacteria that cause tuberculosis can be stained with this procedure.

Ability to Grow in the Presence or Absence of Air. Bacteria that grow best in the presence of oxygen are referred to as **aerobes.** Those that grow best in the absence of oxygen are referred to as **anaerobes.** Organisms that can grow in either environment are referred to as being **facultative.** Although most common bacteria are aerobes, many of the bacteria that make up the normal flora of the body are anaerobes. Not surprisingly, anaerobes are often responsible for infections within the body.

Biochemical Reactions. Many closely related bacteria can be differentiated from one another only by certain biochemical reactions that occur within the bacterial cell. One way to identify a particular bacterial strain is to look at what type of sugars the bacteria can use as food.

Special Groups of Bacteria

Several groups of bacteria have certain characteristics that set them apart from most other bacteria. These include the mycobacteria, rickettsiae, chlamydiae, and mycoplasmas.

Mycobacteria. Mycobacteria are rod-shaped bacilli with a distinct cell wall that differs from that of most bacteria. Certain types of mycobacteria cause disease in humans. For example, *Mycobacterium tuberculosis* causes the respiratory disease tuberculosis, and *Mycobacterium leprae* causes leprosy.

Rickettsiae. Rickettsiae are very small bacteria that can live and grow only within other living cells. Rickettsiae are commonly found in insects such as ticks and mites but may be transmitted to humans through bites. Rickettsiae are responsible for diseases such as Rocky Mountain spotted fever and typhus.

Chlamydiae. Chlamydiae are organisms that differ from other bacteria in the structure of their cell walls. Like rickettsiae, they can live and grow only within other living cells. In humans, chlamydiae can cause venereal disease, eye disease, certain types of pneumonia, and certain types of heart disease.

Mycoplasmas. Mycoplasmas are small bacteria that completely lack the rigid cell wall of other bacteria. These bacteria cause a variety of human diseases, including venereal disease and a form of pneumonia.

Protozoans

Protozoans are single-celled eukaryotic organisms that are generally much larger than bacteria. Protozoans are found in soil and water, and most do not cause disease in people. Certain protozoans are pathogenic, however, and cause diseases such as malaria (see Figure 35-3), amebic dysentery (a type of diarrhea), and trichomoniasis vaginitis (a type of venereal disease). Protozoal diseases are a leading cause of death in developing countries because the lack of proper sanitation in some areas promotes their spread. These diseases are also common in patients with depressed immune systems.

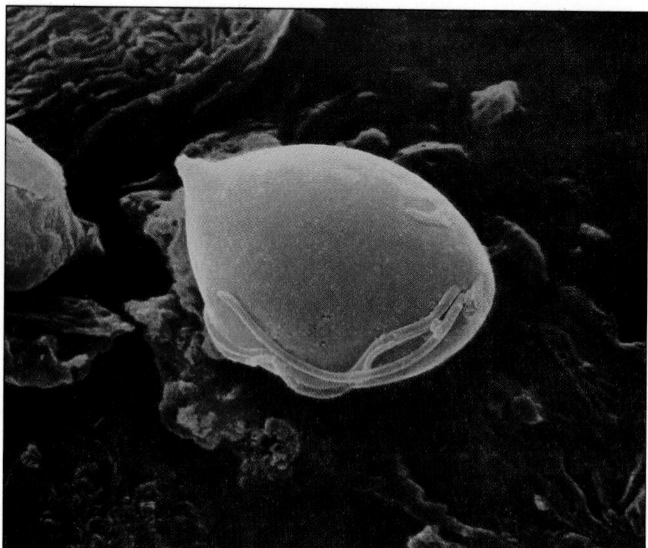

Figure 35-3. The protozoan *Trichomonus vaginalis* causes a venereal disease in humans.

Fungi

A **fungus** (plural, fungi) is a eukaryotic organism that has a rigid cell wall at some stage in the life cycle. Fungi that grow mainly as single-celled organisms that reproduce by budding are referred to as **yeasts,** whereas fungi that grow into large, fuzzy, multicelled organisms that produce spores are called **molds.** Figure 35-4 shows the differences between these two types of fungi.

Most fungi do not cause disease in humans. Of those that do, the majority produce superficial infections such as athlete's foot (tinea pedis), ringworm, thrush, and vaginal yeast infections. Fungi can produce serious, life-threatening illness, however, when they infect the body's internal tissues. This kind of infection can occur when patients have a depressed immune system, as in patients who are undergoing treatment for cancer and patients with AIDS.

Multicellular Parasites

A **parasite** is an organism that lives on or in another organism and uses that other organism for its own nourishment, or for some other advantage, to the detriment of the host organism. Viruses, rickettsiae, chlamydiae, and some protozoans are parasitic. Multicellular organisms can also be parasitic, and some of these organisms are microscopic during all or part of their lives. An infection caused by a parasite is called an infestation. Multicellular parasites that cause human disease include certain worms and insects, as illustrated in Figure 35-5.

Parasitic Worms

People can be infected with a parasitic worm by ingesting its eggs or an immature form of the worm or by having the parasite penetrate the skin. As with the protozoans, infestation by these parasites is more common in developing nations that have poor sanitation.

Worms that infect people include roundworms, flatworms, and tapeworms. Roundworms can occur in the intestines, as in the case of pinworms, a common infection in children. Other roundworms, such as *Trichinella,* are found in muscle tissue. *Trichinella spiralis,* which causes the infection trichinosis, enters the human body in infected meat eaten raw or insufficiently cooked. People may also get flatworms and tapeworms by eating undercooked meats. A trained medical professional must inspect a patient's stool for the presence of the parasite or its eggs to diagnose an intestinal infection with a parasitic worm.

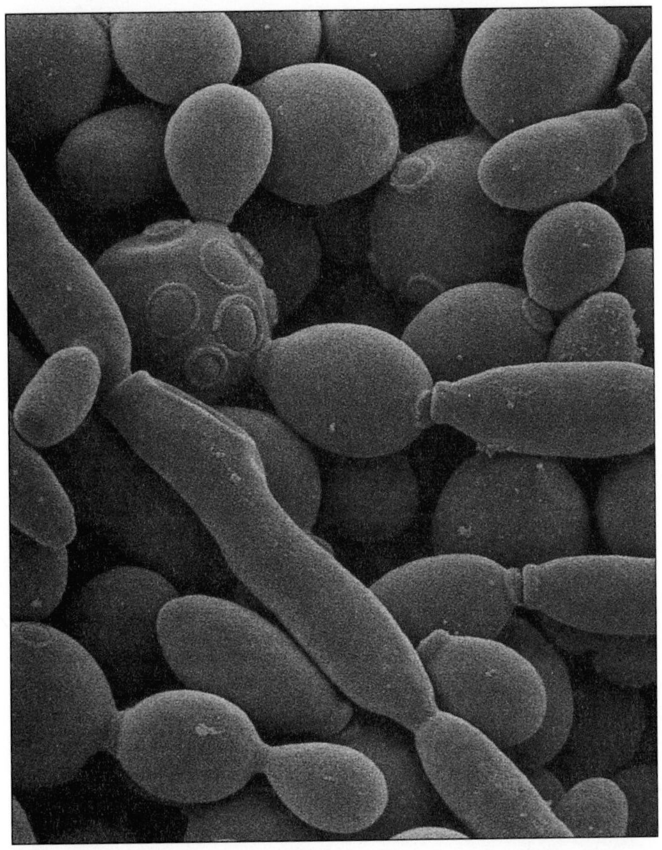

A

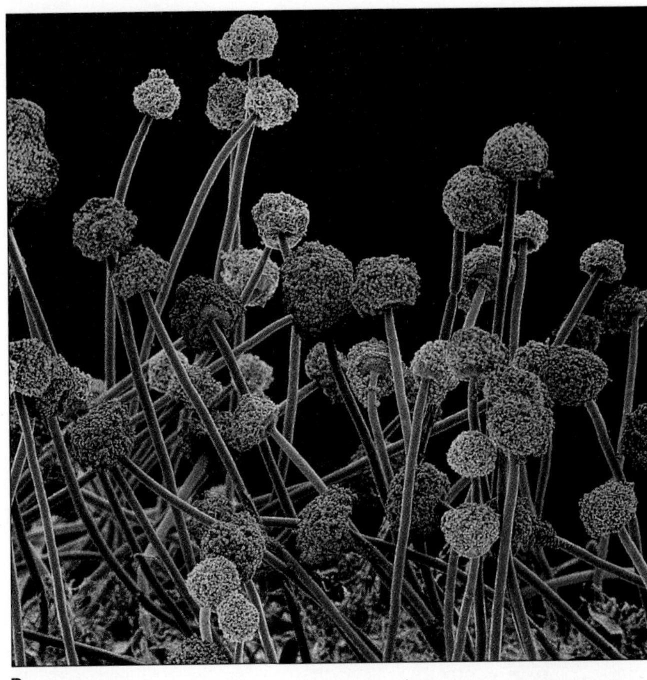

B

Figure 35-4. Because fungi lack the ability to make their own food, they depend on other life forms. **A.** Single-celled fungi are called yeasts. **B.** Multicelled fungi are called molds.

Parasitic Insects

Insects that can bite or burrow under the skin include mosquitoes, ticks, lice, and mites. These insects spread many viral, bacterial (including rickettsial), and protozoal diseases. The causative organisms can live in the insects' bodies and enter people's bodies when they are bitten by the insects. Such diseases include Lyme disease, malaria, Rocky Mountain spotted fever, and encephalitis. Infestations such as scabies that are caused by some lice and mites are considered parasitic diseases.

How Infections Are Diagnosed

To assist with the diagnosis and treatment of an infection, you must work closely with other members of the medical team. The basic steps in diagnosis and treatment are summarized in Figure 35-6.

Step 1. Examine the Patient

When a patient comes into the office with signs or symptoms that suggest an infection, begin by taking the patient's vital signs and noting the patient's complaints. On the basis of these findings and examination of the patient, the doctor can make a presumptive, or tentative, clinical diagnosis.

In many cases signs and symptoms of a particular infection are so characteristic of the disease that the doctor need not perform additional tests to reach a diagnosis. An example might be a case of chickenpox or mumps. At other times, however, the doctor needs to gather additional information to confirm a diagnosis and determine the cause.

Step 2. Obtain One or More Specimens

To determine the cause of an infection, you may need to obtain material from one or more areas of the patient's body. Label each specimen properly and include with it the physician's presumptive diagnosis. If the sample is to be transported to an outside laboratory, ensure that it is transported in such a way that any pathogenic organisms remain alive (and safely contained) during transit.

Step 3. Examine the Specimen Directly

You must sometimes obtain more than one specimen from each site. The doctor or specially trained laboratory or microbiology personnel will then directly examine one

A

B

C

D

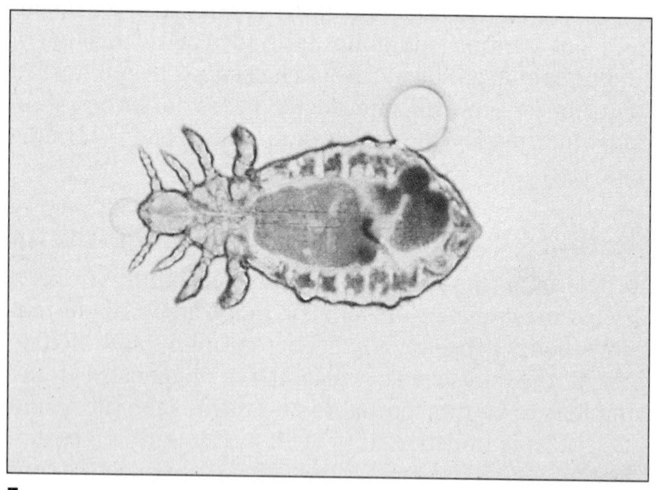

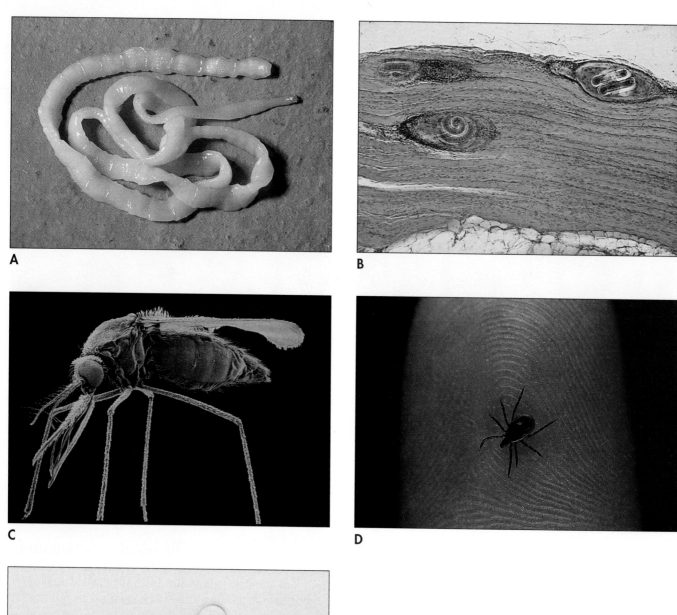

E

Figure 35-5. Parasitic worms, such as (a) tapeworms and (b) *Trichinella,* cause disease in humans when they are ingested. Parasitic insects, such as (c) mosquitoes, (d) deer ticks, and (e) mites, cause disease by biting or burrowing into the skin.

specimen under the microscope. The specimen may be viewed in one of two ways:

- As a **wet mount,** a preparation of a specimen in a liquid that allows the organisms to remain alive and mobile while they are being identified
- As a **smear,** in which a specimen is spread thinly and unevenly across a slide

If you make a smear, allow it to dry and stain or treat it as ordered before it is examined microscopically. In some cases direct examination allows the doctor to make a presumptive diagnosis of the offending microorganism.

Step 4. Culture the Specimen

If the physician still needs a more definitive identification of the microorganism, you may perform a **culture,** in which a sample of the specimen is placed in or on a substance that allows microorganisms to grow. A **culture medium** is a substance that contains all the nutrients a particular type of microorganism needs. Most media come in the form of a semisolid gel. The particular medium is chosen according to the site from which the specimen was obtained and the suspected cause of infection. After you inoculate (place a sample of the specimen in or on) the medium, place it in an incubator (a chamber that can be set to a specific temperature and humidity) to allow the microorganism to grow.

The culture is examined visually and microscopically after a specified time, and a preliminary identification is made. The physician sets up additional tests to confirm the identification of the microorganism that has been

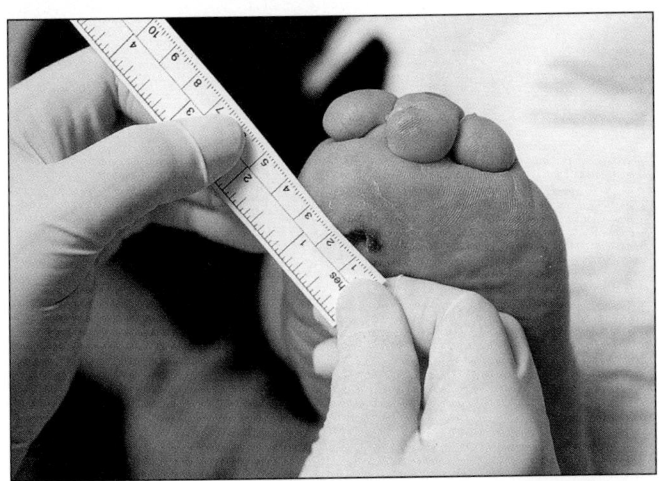

A

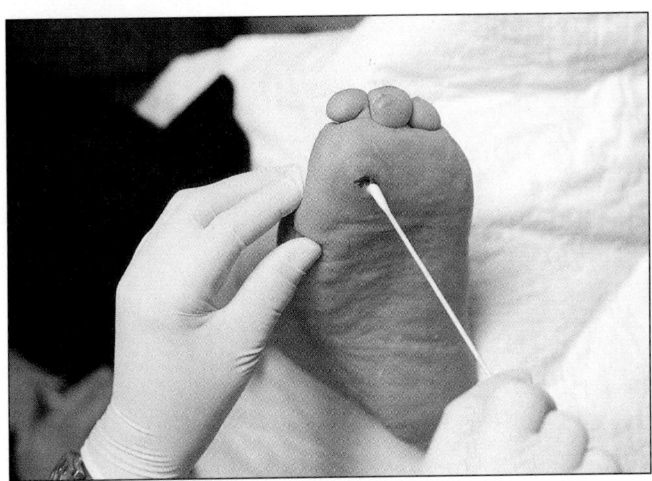

B

C

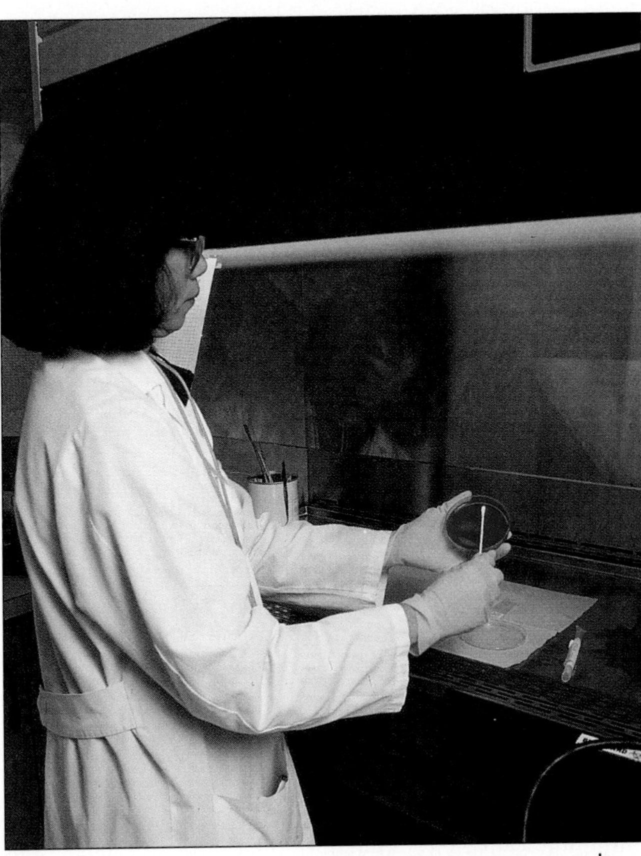

D

Figure 35-6. The steps in diagnosis and treatment of an infection: **A.** Examine the patient. **B.** Obtain one or more specimens. **C.** Examine the specimen directly, by wet mount or smear. **D.** Culture the specimen.

continued

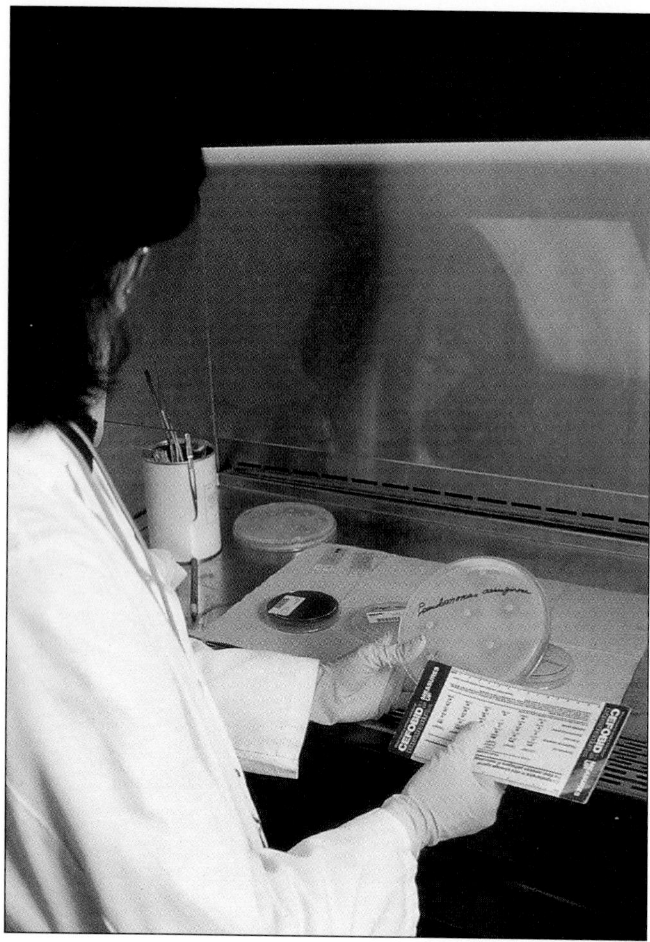

E

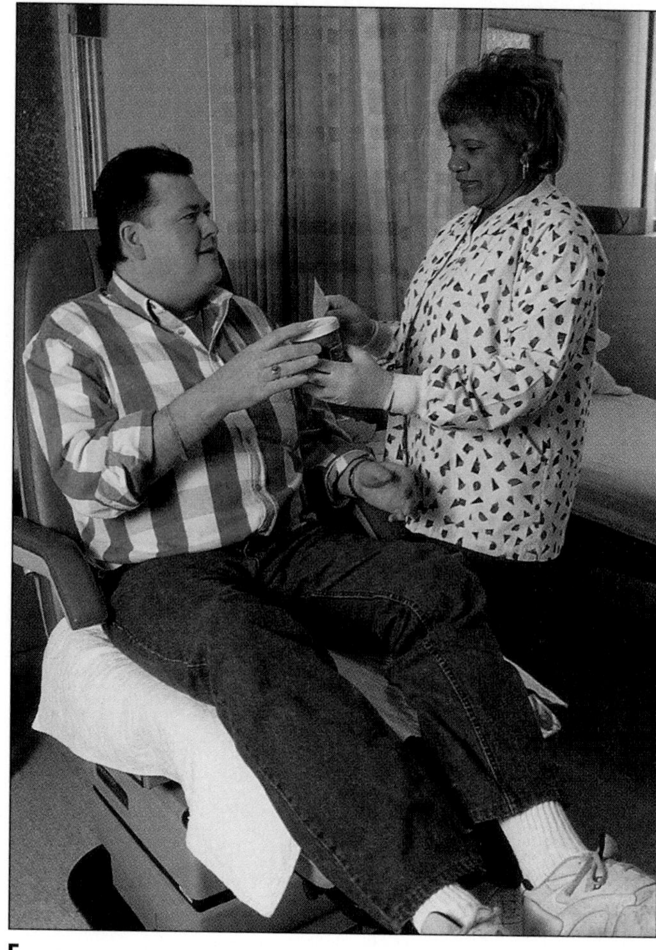

F

Figure 35-6. (continued)
E. Determine the culture's antibiotic sensitivity. **F.** Treat the patient as ordered by the physician.

isolated from the specimen. Most microbiology laboratories and some physicians' office laboratories are equipped to grow routine bacterial cultures and some fungal cultures. Physicians' office laboratories, in particular, may have to send out other types of cultures, such as virus cultures, to a specialized laboratory for identification.

Step 5. Determine the Culture's Antibiotic Sensitivity

In many cases of bacterial infection, a **culture and sensitivity (C & S)** is performed. This procedure involves culturing a specimen and then testing the isolated bacterium's susceptibility (sensitivity) to certain antibiotics. The results help the doctor determine which antibiotics might be most effective in treating the infection.

Step 6. Treat the Patient as Ordered by the Physician

On the basis of identification of the microorganism and antibiotic sensitivity, if determined, the physician can prescribe an **antimicrobial.** This agent, which kills microorganisms or suppresses their growth, should help clear up the patient's infection.

Specimen Collection

Perhaps the most important step in isolating and identifying a microorganism as the cause of an infection is collecting the specimen. If you do not collect the specimen properly, the organism may not grow in culture so that it can be identified. The result may be an untreated infection. Furthermore, if the specimen becomes contaminated during collection and the contaminant is mistakenly identified as the cause of the infection, the patient may receive incorrect or even harmful therapy.

In addition to vaginal specimens (discussed in detail in Chapter 27), the most common types of culture specimens involve the following:

- Throat
- Urine
- Sputum
- Wound
- Stool

Tissue samples removed during minor surgical procedures may be sent for microbiologic analysis, but it is more common to send these types of samples to a pathology laboratory for examination. Rather than checking for infectious disease, the pathology laboratory checks the sample for other types of diseases or abnormalities. There are important differences between preparing a specimen for pathologic study and preparing one for microbiologic analysis. For information on the former, read "Caution: Handle With Care."

Specimen-Collection Devices

To help ensure optimal recovery of microorganisms, you must use the appropriate collection device or specimen container. This container is usually provided by the laboratory where the specimen is going to be analyzed. Special collection devices are available for the collection of sputum, urine, and stool specimens, as shown in Figure 35-7. These containers are designed with large openings to allow collection of the specimen with minimal chance of contamination. They also have tight-fitting caps to prevent leakage and contamination.

Sterile Swabs. The most common device for obtaining cultures is the sterile swab. They vary in the absorbent material at the tip and in the composition of the shaft (Figure 35-8).

Although cotton is absorbent, it is no longer used for culture swabs, because natural chemicals in cotton inhibit the growth of certain microorganisms. Polyester, rayon, or calcium alginate fibers are preferred. Most swabs used to collect routine specimens have a wooden or plastic shaft for rigidity. There are also swabs with a small tip and a flexible wire shaft made especially for culturing hard-to-reach areas and obtaining pediatric specimens. Some collection containers contain two swabs—one for a culture and one for a smear.

Collection and Transport Systems. Sterile, self-contained systems for obtaining and transporting specimens are commercially available from many suppliers. The CULTURETTE Collection and Transport System, manufactured by Becton Dickinson Microbiology Systems of Sparks, Maryland, is a well-known example. The unit, shown in Figure 35-9, contains a polyester swab and a small, thin-walled glass vial of transport medium in a plastic sleeve. If a specimen will not be tested within 30 minutes after it is obtained, the swab is replaced in the sleeve, and the glass vial is crushed between the thumb and the index finger. The moisture and nutrients provided

CAUTION
HANDLE WITH CARE

Preparing and Transporting Specimens for Pathologic Study

Tissue samples are often sent to an outside laboratory for pathologic evaluation to determine whether disease or abnormalities are present. In the laboratory the structure of the tissue is examined both macroscopically (by the naked eye) and microscopically. (This microscopic observation of tissue is known as histology.) Pathology specimens must be handled differently from those prepared for microbiologic analysis.

Collection of the Specimen

Most tissue samples to be sent to a pathology laboratory are collected in a sterile specimen cup. Some specimens (such as a Pap smear), however, are collected with a swab or a scraper and smeared on a slide. In either case a preservative or fixative must be used to preserve the appearance of the tissue and cells so that an accurate assessment can be made. The most common preservative for solid tissue samples is formalin. A fixative such as polyvinyl alcohol (PVA) is often used for slides.

Occasionally a single tissue specimen is sent for both microbiologic and pathologic evaluation. It may be necessary to divide the sample between two specimen containers because the two samples must be handled differently. The specimen for pathologic testing is simply placed in formalin. A specimen for microbiologic culturing, on the other hand, must be handled in as sterile a manner as possible. In addition, a culture specimen must *not* be exposed to formalin, because formalin will kill microorganisms present in the sample.

If a slide needs to be prepared for pathologic examination, the sample is smeared onto the labeled slide, a fixative is sprayed or applied, and the slide is allowed to dry. The specimen must not be allowed to dry out before the fixative is applied, or the slide will be difficult to interpret.

Transportation to the Laboratory

A pathology specimen container should be securely closed and placed in a zipper-type plastic bag, with the requisition form attached to the outside. Special cardboard slide holders are used to transport slides. The requisition form should be wrapped around the slide holder and secured with a rubber band.

Pathology specimens are transported to the laboratory in the same way as microbiologic specimens. (Refer to Procedure 35-2 for the correct method for transporting microbiologic specimens to outside laboratories.) Specimens that will not be picked up right away should be refrigerated.

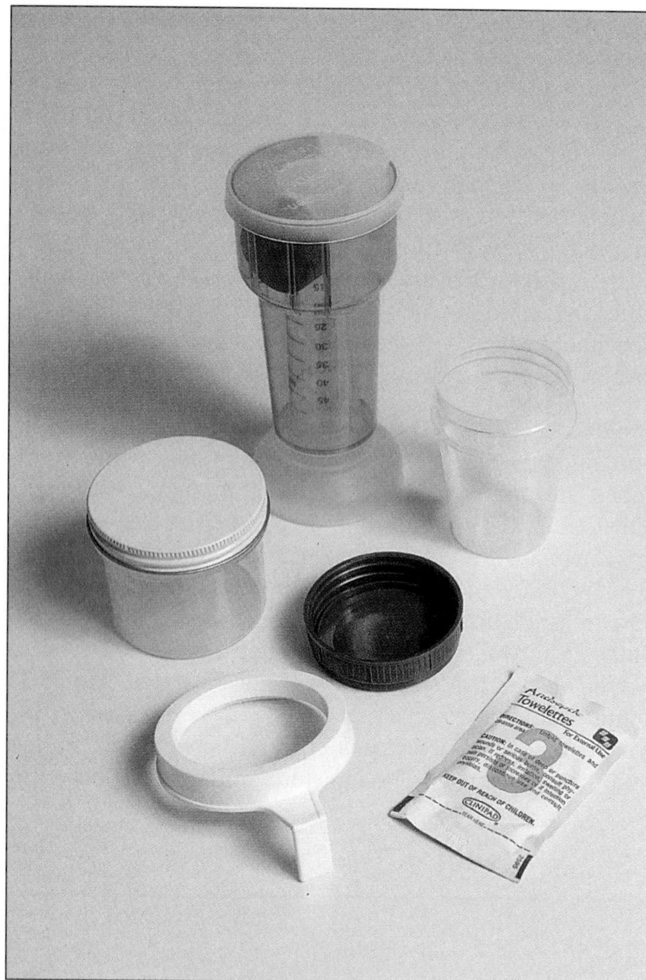

Figure 35-7. You may use specially designed collection containers to collect sputum, urine, and stool specimens.

by the transport medium help keep the bacteria alive during transport to the laboratory.

Several collection systems are also available for culturing anaerobic organisms. These systems provide a means of generating an oxygen-free environment so that the anaerobic organisms remain viable (alive and able to reproduce) during transport.

Specimen-Collection Guidelines

To collect specimens properly, you should follow a number of general guidelines.

- Obtain the specimen with great care to avoid causing the patient harm, discomfort, or undue embarrassment. If patients are to collect specimens on their own, give them clear, detailed instructions along with the proper container.
- Collect the material from a site where the organism is most likely to be found and where contamination is least likely to occur. For example, the best location to obtain a specimen for diagnosing strep throat is at the back of the throat in the area of the tonsils. A properly collected sputum specimen should contain mucus that is coughed up from the respiratory tract, but it should not contain saliva, which is a contaminant.
- Obtain the specimen at a time that allows optimal chance of recovery of the microorganism. Knowledge of the infectious disease process allows the doctor to determine the best time to collect a specimen. For example, certain viruses are more readily isolated during the early, symptomatic stage of an illness.
- Use appropriate collection devices, specimen containers, transport systems, and culture media to ensure optimal recovery of microorganisms. The purpose of such equipment and materials is to preserve the viability of any microorganisms so that they will grow in culture. Special collection devices are available for certain body areas or suspected pathogens.
- Obtain a sufficient quantity of the specimen for performing the requested procedures. If, for example, both a culture and a direct examination of a swabbed specimen will be done, you must collect two specimens. Each procedure requires its own sample.
- Obtain the specimen before antimicrobial therapy begins. If the patient is already taking an antibiotic, note this fact on the laboratory request form, or ask the doctor whether you should obtain the specimen.

After correctly collecting the specimen, you must label the container and include the appropriate requisition form. The label should contain the following information:

- Patient's name and identification number (if appropriate)
- Source (collection site) of the specimen
- Date and time of collection
- Doctor's name
- Your initials (if you obtained the specimen)

The requisition form should include the following information:

- Patient's name, address, and identification number
- Patient's age and gender

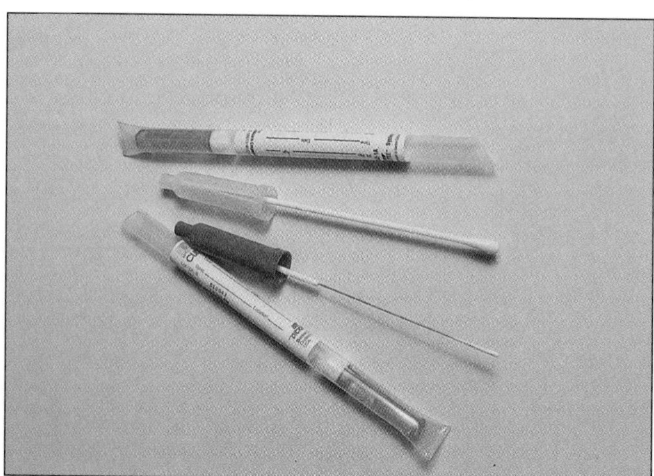

Figure 35-8. Sterile swabs vary in size and in material.

- Patient's insurance billing information
- Type and source of the microbiologic specimen (for example, discharge from wound, big toe)
- Date and time of microbiologic specimen collection
- Test requested
- Medications the patient is currently receiving
- Doctor's presumptive diagnosis
- Doctor's name, address, and phone number
- Special instructions or orders

Throat Culture Specimens

A microbiologic procedure frequently performed in a medical office is obtaining a throat culture. The doctor may request a culture on patients with signs or symptoms of an upper respiratory, throat, or sinus infection. Identification of the microorganism responsible for the infection allows the doctor to treat the patient as effectively as possible.

In most cases the doctor wants to determine whether the patient has strep throat, an infection caused by the bacterium *Streptococcus pyogenes*. It is particularly important to diagnose and treat this infection because, left untreated, strep throat can lead to complications such as rheumatic fever. Rheumatic fever is an inflammation of the heart tissue that occurs more frequently in school-age children than in any other population.

When you obtain a throat culture specimen, you must avoid touching any structures inside the mouth, because this will contaminate the specimen. The correct technique for obtaining a throat culture specimen is outlined in Procedure 35-1.

Many doctors order rapid strep tests done if strep is suspected. Antigen-antibody test kits for strep are available in a variety of brands. They provide immediate indications of the presence of the strep antigen on a throat swab, sparing the patient the expense and waiting period associated with having a culture done. (A test kit for mononucleosis provides similar information, but the specimen used is blood instead of a throat swab.)

If your office does not culture microbiologic specimens, you need to use a sterile collection system to obtain the specimen. If your office has the equipment to perform its own cultures, use a sterile swab and inoculate a culture plate directly with the swab. Specimens to be evaluated in the office should be cultured immediately after collection.

Urine Specimens

To minimize contaminants in urine specimens, it is important to obtain a clean-catch midstream specimen. You must process urine specimens within an hour of collection or refrigerate them to prevent continued bacterial growth. (Collection of urine specimens for culturing is discussed in detail in Chapter 33.)

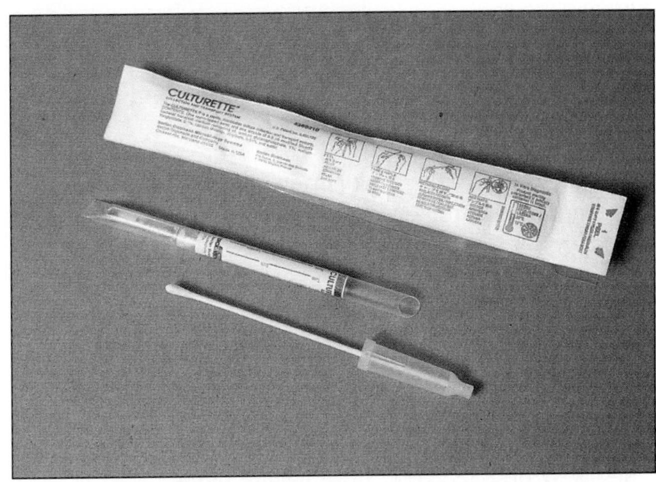

Figure 35-9. The CULTURETTE is used to obtain and transport microbiologic specimens to outside laboratories. (Courtesy of Becton Dickinson Microbiology Systems)

Sputum Specimens

To obtain sputum specimens, have the patient expectorate (cough up) mucus from the lungs into a wide-mouthed specimen container. Beforehand instruct the patient to avoid contaminating the specimen with saliva. If sputum specimens are not cultured right away, they should be refrigerated.

Observe Universal Precautions whenever you handle sputum samples. Wear a face shield or mask and goggles when collecting such a specimen, especially if the patient is coughing. Even when tuberculosis is not suspected, the potential for transmission of this type of bacteria always exists.

Wound Specimens

You usually obtain specimens from infected wounds and lesions by swabbing. The procedure is similar to that of a throat culture. Be sure you obtain representative material from a deep area and a surface area of the wound without contaminating the swab by touching areas outside the site.

Stool Specimens

If the physician suspects that the patient has certain diseases, such as cancer or colitis, or bacterial, protozoal, or parasitic infections, you may need to obtain stool specimens. The collection technique varies with the suspected microorganism. Although both you and the patient may be embarrassed to discuss instructions for collecting stool specimens, do not let this interfere with proper specimen collection.

Patients must collect stool specimens properly so they are not contaminated with urine or water from the toilet, both of which can lead to inaccurate results. Patients can collect stool specimens on a clean paper plate, in a clean waxed-paper carton, or in a container or on collection

PROCEDURE 35-1

Obtaining a Throat Culture Specimen

Objective: To isolate a pathogenic microorganism from the throat or to rule out strep throat

OSHA Guidelines

Materials: Tongue depressor, sterile collection system or sterile swab plus blood agar culture plate

Method

1. Identify the patient, introduce yourself, and explain the procedure.
2. Assemble the necessary supplies; label the culture plate if used.
3. Wash your hands and put on examination gloves and goggles and a mask or a face shield. (The patient may cough while you swab the throat.)
4. Have the patient assume a sitting position. (Having a small child lie down rather than sit may make the process easier. If the child refuses to open the mouth, gently squeeze the nostrils shut. The child will eventually open the mouth to breathe. Enlist the help of the parent to restrain the child's hands if necessary.)
5. Open the collection system or sterile swab package by peeling the wrapper halfway down; remove the swab with your dominant hand.

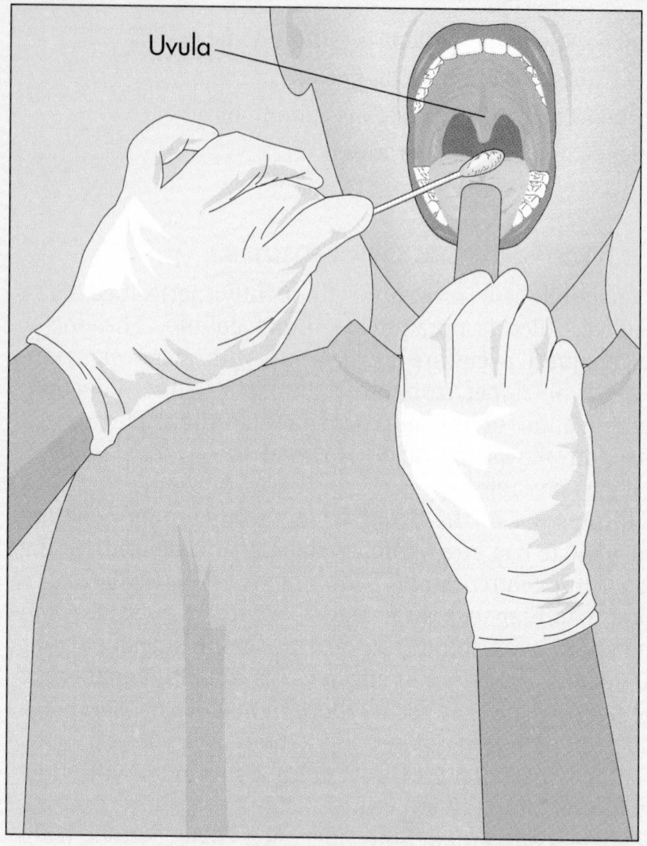

Figure 35-10. When obtaining a throat culture specimen, swab the back of the throat in the area of the tonsils on each side, taking care to avoid touching the uvula.

tissue that you provide. Another way to collect a stool specimen is to place plastic wrap loosely over the toilet seat with enough material to form a collection pocket in the middle. Patients then use a tongue depressor to place a portion of the sample in a specimen container with a tight-fitting lid.

Suspected Bacterial Infection. Bacterial infections caused by species of the *Shigella* or *Salmonella* genus can cause loose, bloody, or mucus-tinged stools. A doctor who suspects that a patient has one of these types of infections may request that a stool specimen be obtained for culture.

Successful recovery of these pathogenic bacteria from a stool specimen depends on timely inoculation of special culture media. The doctor may request obtaining a sample in the office whenever possible to avoid delay in processing the specimen. Several types of culture media promote the growth of intestinal pathogens while suppressing the growth of other microorganisms.

Suspected Protozoal or Parasitic Infection. In cases of a suspected protozoal or parasitic infection, the physician may request what is known as an **O and P specimen,** short for an ova and parasites specimen. This type of stool sample is examined for the presence of certain forms of protozoans or parasites, including their eggs (ova).

When a physician requests an O and P test, obtain both a fresh and a preserved stool specimen. A fresh specimen is examined both macroscopically and microscopically for the presence of microorganisms. A preserved specimen is also necessary because certain forms of these organisms are destroyed within a short time after leaving the body and may not be detected in the fresh specimen. You must always obtain a preserved specimen when stool samples are sent to an outside laboratory.

Special stool collection kits are available. They contain a specimen container for a fresh sample, along

6. Ask the patient to tilt back the head and open the mouth as wide as possible.
7. With your other hand, depress the patient's tongue with the tongue depressor.
8. Ask the patient to say Ah.
9. Insert the swab and quickly swab the back of the throat in the area of the tonsils (Figure 35-10), twirling the swab over representative areas on both sides of the throat. (Avoid touching the uvula, the soft tissue hanging from the roof of the mouth, because touching it will make the patient gag and will contaminate the specimen.)
10. Remove the swab and then the tongue depressor from the patient's mouth.
11. Discard the tongue depressor in a biohazardous waste container.

To transport the specimen to a reference laboratory:

12. Immediately insert the swab back into the plastic sleeve, being careful not to touch the outside of the sleeve with the swab.
13. Crush the vial of transport medium to moisten the tip of the swab (Figure 35-11).
14. Label the collection system and arrange for transport to the laboratory.

To prepare the specimen for evaluation in the physician's office laboratory:

12. Immediately inoculate the culture plate with the swab, using a back-and-forth motion.

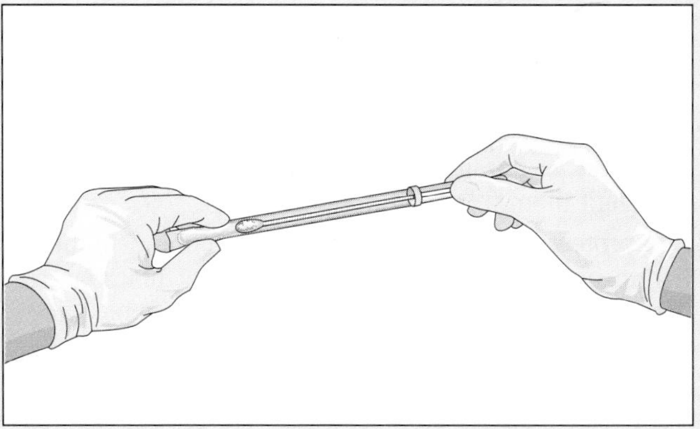

Figure 35-11. The transport medium released from the crushed capsule keeps microorganisms alive while in transit to the laboratory for culturing.

13. Discard the swab in a biohazardous waste container.
14. Place the culture plate in the incubator.

When finished with all specimens:

15. Remove the gloves and wash your hands.
16. Document the procedure in the patient's chart.

with vials of two types of preservatives, formalin (a dilute solution of formaldehyde) and polyvinyl alcohol (PVA). Instruct the patient to place the stool sample in the specimen container and to mix portions of the specimen in each of the preservative vials. The laboratory will examine all specimens for the presence of microorganisms.

When a physician suspects that a patient has a protozoal or parasitic infection, he will request that a series of at least three stool specimens be examined. Three specimens are required because different diagnostic forms of the microorganism may be present in the stool at different times. The presence of the microorganism could be missed with only one sample. Because certain medications can interfere with detection of these microorganisms, the patient may be asked to refrain from using medications such as antidiarrheal compounds, antacids, and mineral oil laxatives for at least a week before samples are obtained.

Transporting Specimens to an Outside Laboratory

Some physicians' offices do not perform microbiologic testing. They choose to send their culture specimens to an outside laboratory. In addition, many specialized microbiologic procedures cannot be performed routinely in the office laboratory and must be sent out. One example of a specialized procedure is a virus culture. Culturing and identifying viruses require special techniques and equipment that are almost never found in a physician's office laboratory. Culturing a specimen for bacteria such as chlamydia is also a procedure that requires special techniques.

Your Main Objectives

When you collect and transport a microbiologic specimen to an outside laboratory, you have three main objectives:

1. To be sure you follow the proper collection procedures and use the proper collection device. Most laboratories have specific directions for sample collection and packaging that you must follow. A laboratory may even provide specific containers in which to collect and transport samples. If you collect or package any specimens improperly, the laboratory may not accept them for testing.
2. To maintain the samples in a state as close to their original as possible. You must take specific steps to prevent them from deteriorating.
3. To protect anyone who handles a specimen container from exposure to potentially infectious material. To do so, ensure that the specimen container has a tight-fitting lid. As extra protection against leakage, place the specimen container in a secondary container or zipper-type plastic bag. The laboratory usually provides such a bag.

Methods of Transportation

Specimens that are to be tested by an outside laboratory may be transported there in one of three ways:

- During regularly scheduled daily pickups by the laboratory
- During an as-needed pickup by the laboratory
- Through the mail

Pickup by the laboratory is the most reliable and timely method of transporting microbiologic specimens. Although each laboratory has its own procedure, the general steps for preparing specimens for transport to a laboratory are outlined in Procedure 35-2.

Sending Specimens by Mail

There may be times when you must send a specimen through the mail to a special reference laboratory for a test that is not normally done by a local laboratory. The U.S. Postal Service accepts a package containing microbiologic specimens as long as the total volume of specimen material is less than 50 mL and it is packaged under strict regulations specified by the U.S. Public Health Service.

When sending specimens through the mail, pack them securely with adequate cushioning material to prevent breakage and leakage. Leakage can not only contaminate the specimen but also put mail handlers at risk of contamination with infectious materials. The proper technique for packaging and labeling microbiologic specimens is outlined by the Centers for Disease Control and Prevention (CDC) and shown in Figure 35-12.

Securely close the primary culture container, and surround it with enough absorbent packing material to absorb the entire fluid contents if the container were to

PROCEDURE 35-2

Preparing Microbiologic Specimens for Transport to an Outside Laboratory

Objective: To properly prepare a microbiologic specimen for transport to an outside laboratory

OSHA Guidelines

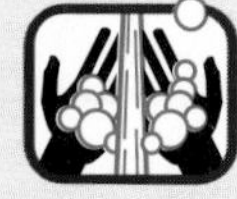
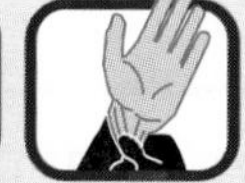

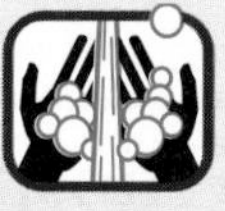

Materials: Specimen-collection device, requisition form, secondary container or zipper-type plastic bag

Method

1. Wash your hands and put on examination gloves (and goggles and a mask or a face shield if you are collecting a microbiologic throat culture specimen).
2. Obtain the microbiologic culture specimen.
    a. Use the collection system specified by the outside laboratory for the test requested.
    b. Label the microbiologic specimen-collection device at the time of collection.
    c. Collect the microbiologic specimen according to the guidelines provided by the laboratory and office procedure.
3. Remove the gloves and wash your hands.
4. Complete the test requisition form.
5. Place the microbiologic specimen container in a secondary container or zipper-type plastic bag.
6. Attach the test requisition form to the outside of the secondary container or bag, per laboratory policy.
7. Log the microbiologic specimen in the list of outgoing specimens.
8. Store the microbiologic specimen according to guidelines provided by the laboratory for that type of specimen (for example, refrigerated, frozen, or 37°C).
9. Call the laboratory for pickup of the microbiologic specimen, or hold it until the next scheduled pickup.
10. At the time of pickup ensure that the carrier takes all microbiologic specimens that are logged and scheduled to be picked up.
11. If you are ever unsure about collection or transportation details, call the laboratory.

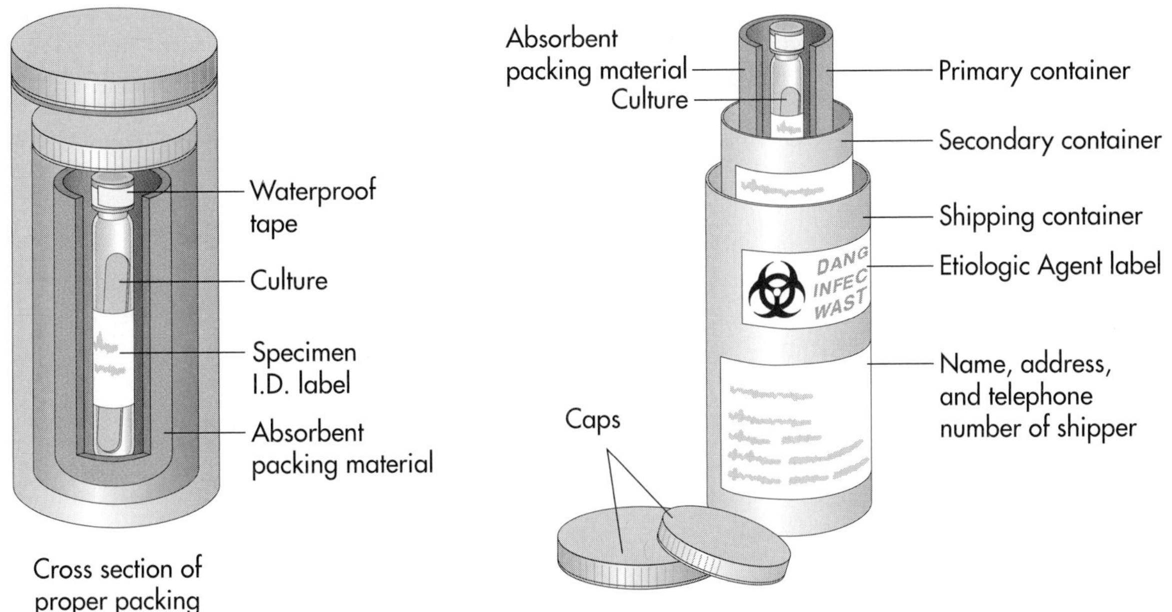

Figure 35-12. When packaging and labeling a specimen for mail delivery, you must follow the procedures set by the CDC, based on U.S. Public Health Service regulations.

leak. Place these items together in a secondary container, commonly a metal container with a screw-top or snap-on lid. Then place the secondary container in an outer shipping carton made of cardboard or Styrofoam.

If you must keep a specimen cold or frozen, place dry ice outside the secondary container. Use an outer shipping carton that is constructed to permit release of carbon dioxide gas as the dry ice sublimates (turns into vapor). Use enough cushioning material with the dry ice to prevent the secondary container from moving around as the dry ice sublimates. Then label the package to indicate that it contains dry ice (considered a hazardous material.)

In addition to the address label, microbiologic specimens sent through the mail must have an Etiologic Agent label affixed to the package, as shown in Figure 35-12. This label uses the biohazard symbol to serve as notice to the carrier of the nature of the contents. The term **etiologic agent** refers to a living microorganism or its toxin that may cause human disease.

Direct Examination of Specimens

At times, the physician may directly examine the specimen under a microscope to detect the presence of microorganisms or to identify them. The physician may perform this procedure in the office to get the information needed to initiate treatment immediately.

Two types of procedures that allow direct examination of microbiologic specimens are preparing wet mounts and preparing potassium hydroxide (KOH) mounts. You may be required to perform these procedures as part of your duties.

Wet Mounts

A wet mount permits quick identification of many microorganisms. Wet mounts are easy to prepare.

1. Wearing examination gloves, mix a small amount of the specimen with a drop of normal saline (0.9% sodium chloride [NaCl] solution) on a glass slide.
2. Apply a coverslip over the mixture.
3. Provide the doctor with the slide for direct examination under the microscope.

If you obtain a specimen from a body site that is normally sterile, detection of microorganisms on a wet mount immediately tells the doctor whether there is infection. Wet mounts are also useful in determining whether a microorganism is motile, or able to move, which helps in identifying the microorganisms.

Potassium Hydroxide (KOH) Mounts

A **KOH mount** is a type of mount used when a physician suspects that a patient has a fungal infection of the skin, nails, or hair. It is difficult to visualize a fungus directly in these types of specimens because the body produces a tough, hard protein called **keratin,** which often masks any fungus present. The chemical potassium hydroxide (KOH) is added to the specimen to dissolve the keratin and allow visualization of any fungus.

To prepare a KOH mount, follow these steps.

1. Wearing examination gloves, suspend the specimen of skin, hair, or nails in a drop of 10% KOH on a glass slide.
2. Apply a coverslip.
3. Allow the specimen to sit at room temperature for 30 minutes to dissolve the keratin. To speed up this process, gently heat (do not boil) the slide in the flame of a Bunsen burner.
4. Provide the physician with the slide to examine for microscopic evidence of fungal structures.

Preparation and Examination of Stained Specimens

Although wet mounts are a useful tool for detecting microorganisms, microorganisms and their structures can be seen more clearly when you stain them with a dye or group of dyes. As with wet mounts and KOH mounts, the doctor can make a quick, tentative diagnosis with stained specimens. A stained specimen also enables the doctor to differentiate between types of infections, such as bacterial and yeast infections, or between bacterial infections of one type and another. Stains also help doctors identify microorganisms that have grown on culture plates.

Preparation of Smears

The first step in staining a microbiologic specimen is to prepare a smear. To do so, simply apply a small amount of the specimen to a glass slide. Allow the sample to dry, and briefly heat the slide to "fix" the sample to the slide so that it does not wash off during the staining process. The steps in preparing a specimen smear are described in detail in Procedure 35-3.

Gram's Stain

The stain that is most frequently used for microscopic examination of bacteriologic specimens is the Gram's stain. A Gram's stain is a simple procedure that you can easily

PROCEDURE 35-3

Preparing a Microbiologic Specimen Smear

Objective: To prepare a smear of a microbiologic specimen for staining

OSHA Guidelines

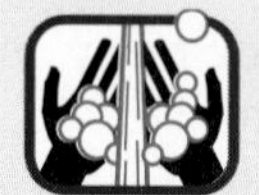
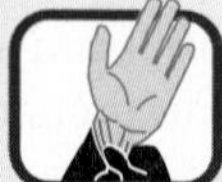
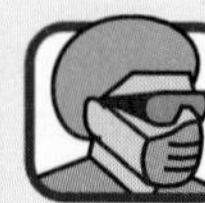

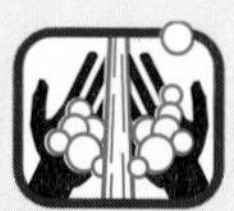

Materials: Glass slide with frosted end, pencil, specimen swab, Bunsen burner, forceps

Method

1. Wash your hands and put on examination gloves.
2. Assemble all the necessary items.
3. Use a pencil to label the frosted end of the slide with the patient's name.
4. Roll the specimen swab evenly over the smooth part of the slide, making sure that all areas of the swab touch the slide (Figure 35-13).
5. Discard the swab in a biohazardous waste container. (Retain the microbiologic specimen for culture as necessary or according to office policy.)
6. Allow the smear to air-dry. Do not wave the slide to dry it, because this may spread pathogens or contaminate the slide.
7. Heat-fix the slide by holding the frosted end with forceps and passing the clear part of the slide, with the smear side up, through the flame of a Bunsen burner three or four times. (Your office may use an alternate procedure for fixing the slide, such as flooding the smear with alcohol, allowing it to sit for a few minutes, and either pouring off the remaining liquid or allowing the smear to air-dry. Pap smear slides must be fixed with a chemical spray within 10 seconds. Chlamydia slides come with their own fixative.)
8. Allow the slide to cool before staining the smear.
9. Return the materials to their proper location.
10. Remove the gloves and wash your hands.

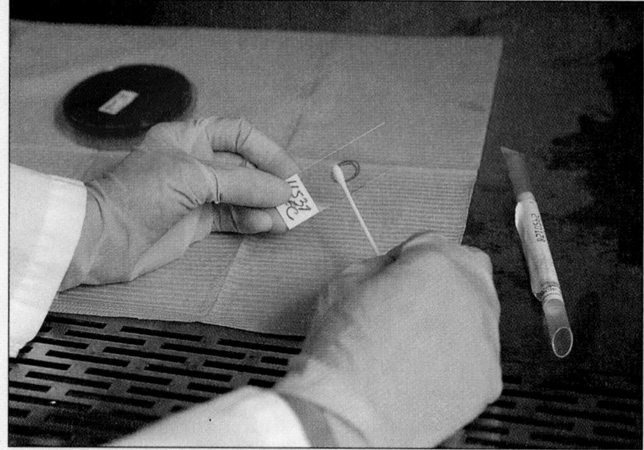

Figure 35-13. Rolling the swab ensures that representative microorganisms collected on it are deposited on the slide.

perform in the medical office. The steps for performing a Gram's stain are outlined in Procedure 35-4.

A Gram's stain involves performing a series of staining and washing steps on the heat-fixed smear. First, apply a purple stain called crystal violet (also known as gentian violet) to the smear. After washing the slide in water, apply iodine. The iodine acts as a **mordant,** a substance that can intensify or deepen the response of a specimen to a stain. Iodine helps bind the dye to the bacterial cell wall. After washing the slide again in water, apply a decolorizing solution (alcohol or acetone-alcohol). Certain bacterial species retain the purple dye even after the decolorizer is added. These bacteria appear blue or violet and are referred to as being **gram-positive.**

Other bacteria lose their purple color when the decolorizer is added. To allow the physician to visualize these bacteria, apply a red counterstain (safranin) to the smear. Bacteria that lose the purple color and pick up the red color of the safranin are referred to as being **gram-negative.** Figure 35-15 illustrates gram-positive and gram-negative bacteria.

On the bases of a bacterium's staining characteristics and the shape and arrangement of cells, the physician can make a presumptive identification of an organism. For example, clusters of cocci that appear gram-positive typically suggest an infection with staphylococci.

Besides bacteria, other types of microorganisms, such as protozoans and parasites, can often be visualized with the Gram's stain. Since the Gram's stain is typically not the best type of stain for these microorganisms, however, the physician may order another type of stain.

PROCEDURE 35-4

Performing a Gram's Stain

Objective: To make bacteria present in a specimen smear visible for microscopic identification

OSHA Guidelines

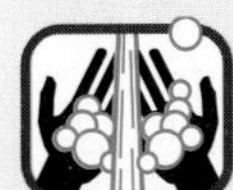
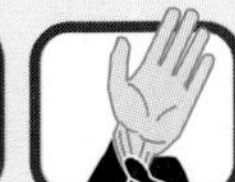
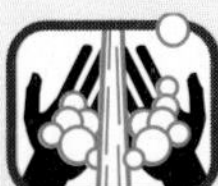

Materials: Heat-fixed smear, slide staining rack and tray, crystal violet dye, iodine solution, alcohol or acetone-alcohol decolorizer, safranin dye, wash bottle filled with water, forceps, blotting paper or paper towels (optional)

Method

1. Assemble all the necessary supplies.
2. Wash your hands and put on examination gloves.
3. Place the heat-fixed smear on a level staining rack and tray, with the smear side up.
4. Completely cover the specimen area of the slide with the crystal violet stain (Figure 35-14a). (Many commercially available Gram's stain solutions have flip-up bottle caps that allow you to dispense stain by the drop. If the stain bottle you are using does not have an attached dropper cap, use an eyedropper.)
5. Allow the stain to sit for 1 minute; wash the slide thoroughly with water from the wash bottle (Figure 35-14b).
6. Use the forceps to hold the slide at the frosted end, tilting the slide to remove excess water.
7. Place the slide flat on the rack again, and completely cover the specimen area with iodine solution (Figure 35-14c).
8. Allow the iodine to remain for 1 minute; wash the slide thoroughly with water (Figure 35-14d).
9. Use the forceps to hold and tilt the slide to remove excess water.
10. While still tilting the slide, apply the alcohol or decolorizer drop by drop until no more purple color washes off (Figure 35-14e). (This step usually takes no more than 10 seconds.)
11. Wash the slide thoroughly with water (Figure 35-14f); use the forceps to hold and tip the slide to remove excess water.
12. Completely cover the specimen with safranin dye (Figure 35-14g).
13. Allow the safranin to remain for 1 minute; wash the slide thoroughly with water (Figure 35-14h).
14. Use the forceps to hold the stained smear by the frosted end, and carefully wipe the back of the slide to remove excess stain.
15. Place the smear in a vertical position and allow it to air-dry. (The smear may be blotted lightly between blotting paper or paper towels to hasten drying [Figure 35-14i]. Take care not to rub the slide, or the specimen may be damaged.)
16. Sanitize and disinfect the work area.
17. Remove the gloves and wash your hands.

continued

A Apply crystal violet. Wait 1 minute.

B Wash slide with water.

C Apply iodine solution. Wait 1 minute.

D Wash slide with water.

E Apply decolorizing solution.

F Wash slide with water.

G Apply safranin dye to slide. Wait 1 minute.

H Wash slide with water.

I Blot and allow slide to air-dry.

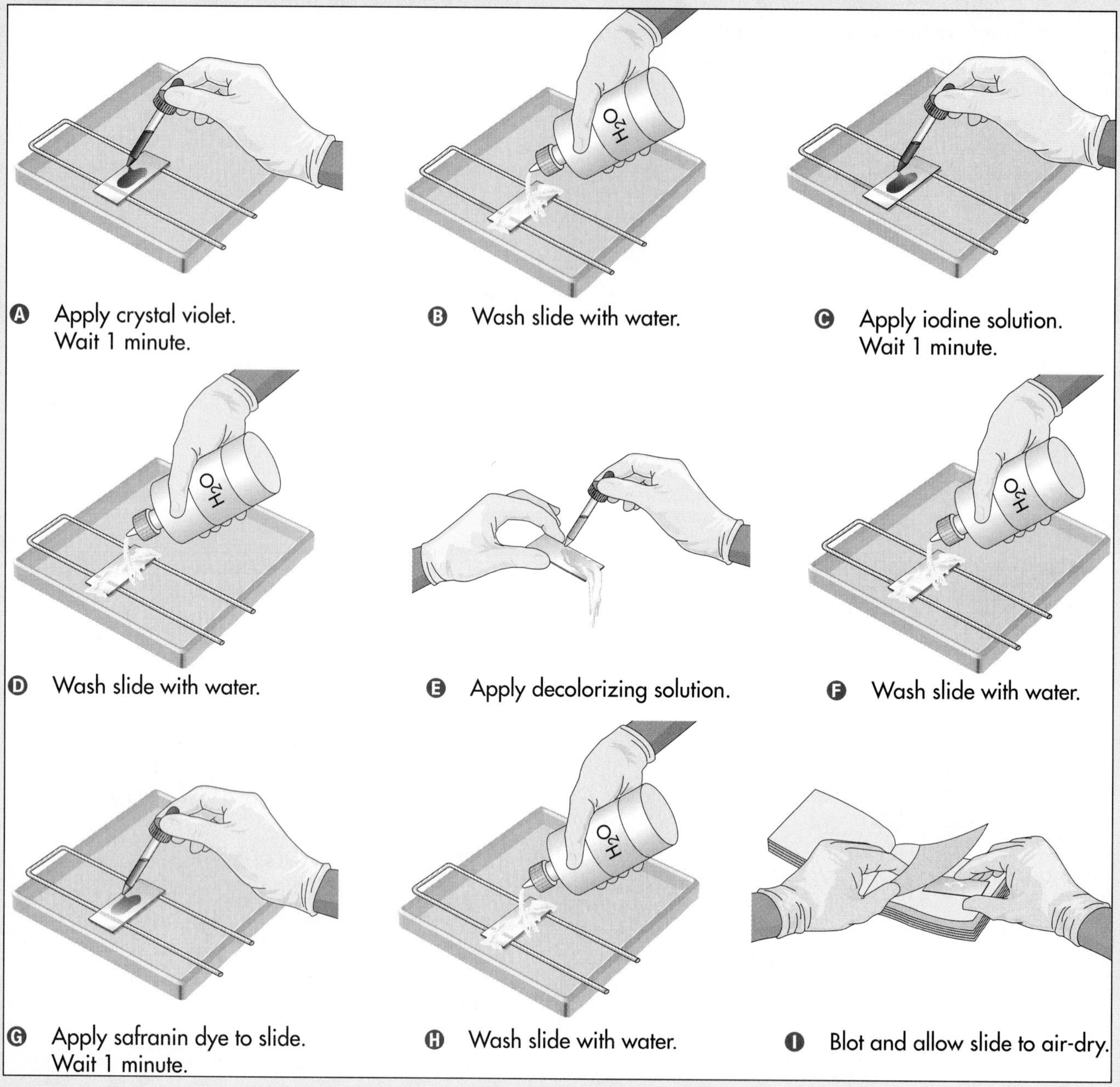

Figure 35-14. The procedure for performing a Gram's stain on a microbiologic specimen involves covering the specimen with a series of stains, water washes, and alcohol in a specific order, for precise periods of time.

Culturing Specimens in the Medical Office

If your medical office is equipped with a laboratory and if you have the necessary on-the-job training or additional courses, you may be required to culture certain specimens. It is, however, becoming more common for doctors' offices to send specimens to outside laboratories because of Clinical Laboratory Improvement Amendments of 1988 (CLIA '88) guidelines and the additional requirements concerning personnel and administrative work.

Culturing involves placing a sample of the specimen on or in a specialized culture medium. This medium contains nutrients that enable microorganisms such as bacteria and fungi to grow. The medium is placed in an incubator set at 37°C (body temperature), the optimal temperature

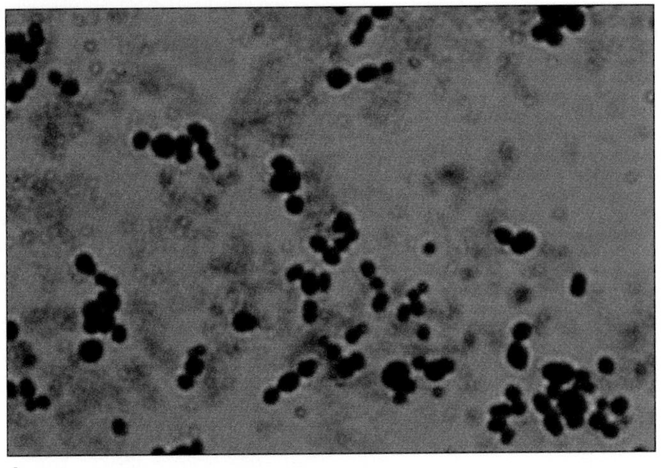

A

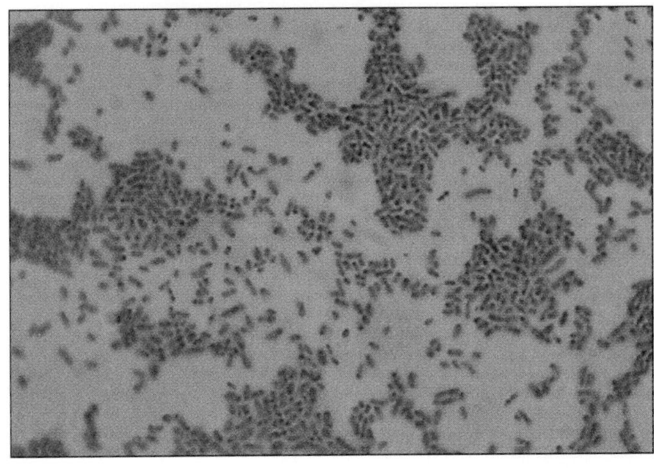

B

Figure 35-15. **A.** Gram-positive organisms appear blue or violet after staining. **B.** Gram-negative organisms appear red.

for growth. As the microorganism multiplies, a **colony**—a distinct group of the organisms—can be seen on the surface of the culture medium. The microorganism is identified according to the colony appearance, its staining characteristics, and certain biochemical reactions.

Culture Media

Culture media come in liquid, semisolid, and solid forms. In the medical office you will most likely work with a semisolid. The medium contains **agar,** a gelatinlike substance derived from seaweed that gives the medium its consistency. This form of medium comes commercially prepared in culture plates—round, covered glass or plastic dishes also called petri dishes.

When using petri dishes, handle them only on the outside, so that they do not become contaminated. You can avoid introducing contaminants by storing the petri dishes with the agar side up. Use the palm of your hand to pick up the agar-containing part of the dish when you are ready to inoculate it with a specimen.

Types of Media. Many different types of semisolid media are commercially available. The type of medium used for culturing depends on the type of suspected organism and the site from which the specimen is obtained. Some types allow the growth of only certain kinds of bacteria while inhibiting the growth of others. These types are referred to as selective media. Selective media are commonly used for specimens that normally contain bacteria, such as stool or vaginal samples.

Other types of media support the growth of most organisms and are referred to as nonselective media. The most common type of culture medium used in the laboratory is blood agar, a nonselective medium. Blood agar gets its red color from sheep's blood. Comparing the growth of a specimen on selective and nonselective media often provides important information about the microorganisms present.

You will typically use a blood agar plate when you culture a throat swab specimen. The organism that causes strep throat (*Streptococcus pyogenes*) can be identified when it grows on blood agar because it destroys the blood cells in the agar, leaving a clear zone surrounding each colony. This process of red blood cell destruction is referred to as hemolysis.

Special Culture Units. Small physicians' office laboratories often use commercial culture units with specific culturing purposes. Units for performing rapid urine culture, such as Uricult (manufactured by Orion Diagnostica, Somerset, New Jersey), are typical. Uricult consists of a small vial that has a double-sided paddle attached to a screw-on top (Figure 35-16). Each side of the paddle

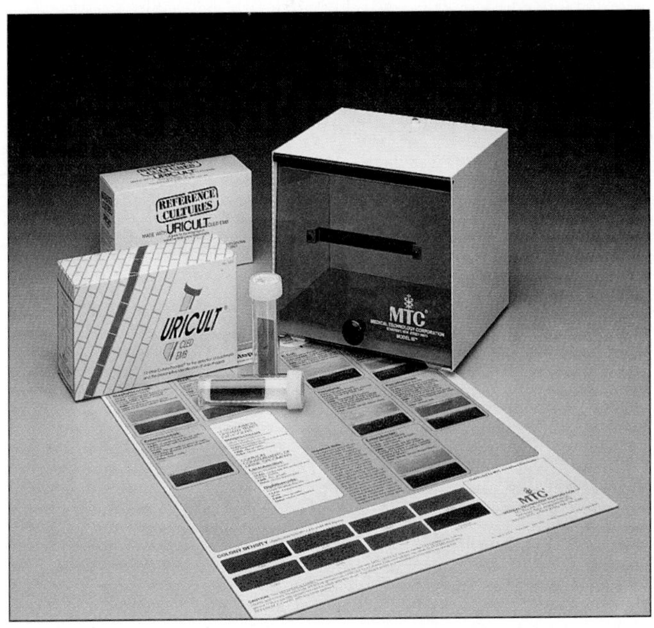

Figure 35-16. One common urine culture device consists of a lid and attached double-sided paddle that screws into a vial.

contains a different type of medium on its surface. To culture a urine specimen, simply dip the media paddle into the clean-catch midstream urine specimen or catheterized specimen, coating both sides of the paddle. Then remove the paddle from the specimen, screw it into the vial, and place it upright in the incubator for 18 to 24 hours. If bacteria are present, they will grow on the surfaces of the media. Other units for culturing urine, throat specimens, vaginal specimens, and blood are also simple to use. These units usually enable you to obtain an estimate of the number of bacteria in the sample in addition to identifying the bacteria.

Inoculating a Culture Plate

Inoculating a culture plate involves transferring some or all of the specimen onto the plate. Before inoculating a plate, label it on the bottom (agar side) rather than the lid, because the lid can be lost or switched. Label the plate with the patient's name, doctor's name, source of the sample, date and time of inoculation, and your initials. You can apply a label or write the information with a grease pencil or permanent marker.

In the case of a specimen swab, inoculate the plate by streaking the swab across the plate. Bacterial colonies can be identified by their appearance. This determination of the type of pathogen is referred to as a **qualitative analysis** of the specimen.

To perform a qualitative analysis of a specimen such as urine, introduce only a small portion of the specimen onto the plate. A wire inoculating loop is used for this purpose. A loop is a small circle of wire attached to a long handle. When this loop is dipped into the specimen, a small amount of liquid can be transferred to the plate.

In addition, you may need to perform a separate determination of the number of bacteria present in specimens such as urine. This determination is referred to as a **quantitative analysis.** A quantitative analysis is important with a specimen such as urine because a few bacteria may contaminate a urine sample during collection. A true infection is confirmed by the presence of a certain number of bacteria; any number beneath this level is typically considered contamination.

Inoculating for Qualitative Analysis. To inoculate an agar plate for qualitative analysis, perform the first pass with a culture swab (as with a throat culture) or an inoculating loop (as with a urine culture). If you use a culture swab, roll and streak it back and forth across an area covering roughly one-third of the culture plate to deposit the microorganisms. When using an inoculating loop, spread the material by streaking the loop across one-third of the plate in the same back-and-forth pattern. Figure 35-17 shows the correct pattern for inoculating a plate.

Because there may be a great many microorganisms in the specimen, you need to streak the inoculated (first-pass) area with a sterile loop to separate out individual colonies that can be identified on the remaining areas of the culture plate. Unless you use a sterile disposable loop, first sterilize the loop by heating it in a bacterial loop incinerator (Palko and Palko, 1996, fig. 26.4) until it glows red. Allow the loop to cool, and pass it once across the inoculated area of the plate to pick up a small number of microorganisms. Then streak it in a back-and-forth pattern over the second one-third of the plate. Next pass it once across the second inoculated area of the plate, and streak it back and forth over the last one-third of the

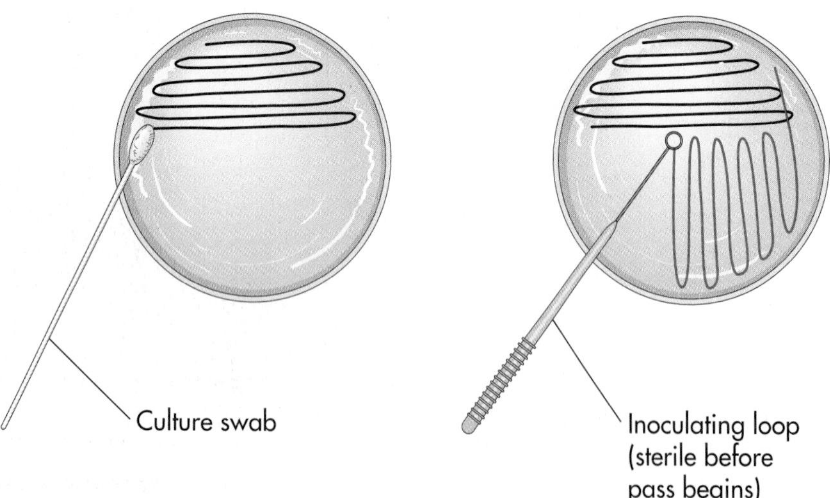
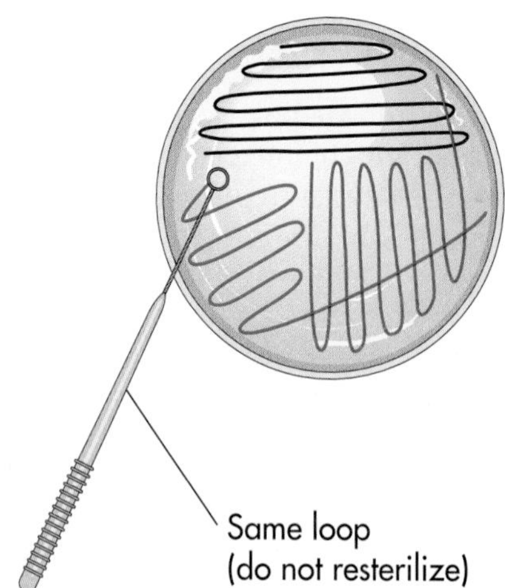

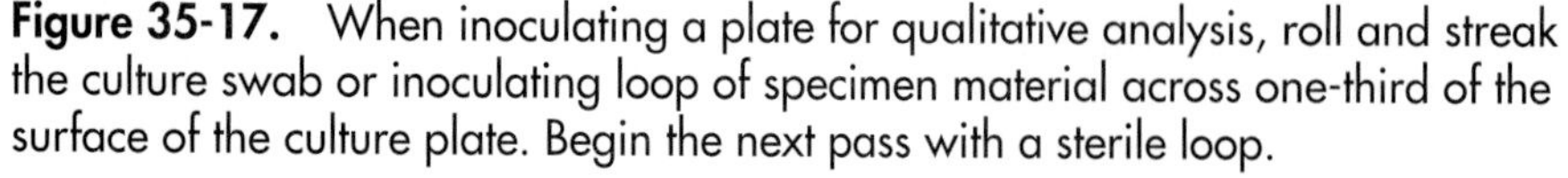

Figure 35-17. When inoculating a plate for qualitative analysis, roll and streak the culture swab or inoculating loop of specimen material across one-third of the surface of the culture plate. Begin the next pass with a sterile loop.

plate. Each successive pass serves to reduce the concentration of the microorganisms. This procedure allows isolated colonies, or colony-forming units, to be observed in the area of the last pass of the loop, as Figure 35-18 shows.

In the case of throat cultures, the physician may simply want you to screen the sample to see whether streptococcal organisms are present. You may not need to use a loop to spread the microorganisms; the swab will be sufficient, as described in Procedure 35-1, when preparing the specimen for screening.

Inoculating for Quantitative Analysis. To perform a quantitative analysis of a urine specimen, use a calibrated loop to withdraw a portion of urine from the sample. The wire circle on a calibrated loop is a precise size that picks up an exact volume of liquid when it is dipped into the specimen. For example, calibrated loops may allow you to pick up either 0.01 or 0.001 mL of liquid.

When you perform a quantitative analysis, be sure the urine specimen is well mixed before taking the sample. Mixing is required because the microorganisms may settle to the bottom of the specimen cup. Sterilize, cool, and dip the calibrated loop into the sample. Transfer the entire volume to the surface of an agar plate by making a single streak down the center of the plate. Next spread the specimen evenly across the plate at a right angle to the initial streak, using the same loop (without sterilizing it). Turn the plate and spread the material again, at a right angle to the last streak, over the entire surface. Figure 35-19 illustrates this technique.

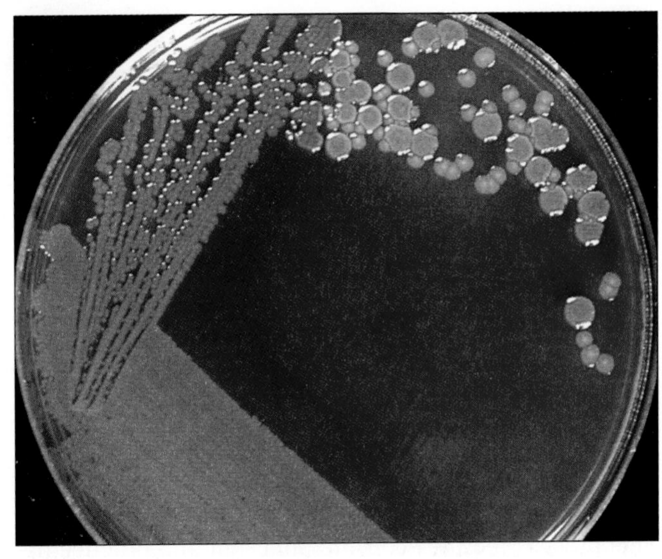

Figure 35-18. You can see individual colony-forming units in the last third of an inoculated culture plate.

After the microorganisms are allowed to grow for 24 hours, estimate the number of microorganisms by counting the number of colonies that appear on the surface of the plate. For example, if you use a 0.001-mL loop to streak the plate and 50 colonies grow, multiply the 50 colonies by 1000 to obtain the number of colonies per milliliter. In this case you would estimate that there are 50,000 colony-forming units per milliliter of urine. You must be especially careful that your counts and calculations are correct so that the doctor has accurate information on which to base a diagnosis.

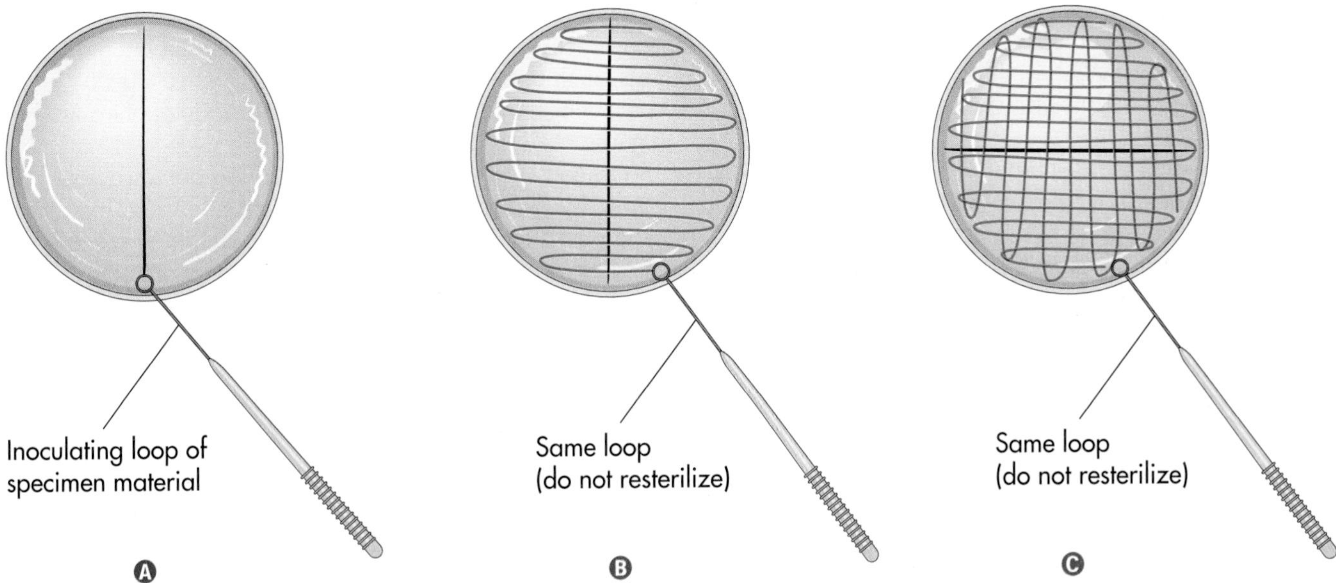

Figure 35-19. When inoculating a plate for quantitative analysis, (a) streak the loop down the center of the plate. Next (b) streak the loop at right angles to the first inoculation. Then (c) turn the plate 90°, and streak the entire surface once more.

Incubating Culture Plates

After inoculating a plate, place it in an incubator set at 35° to 37°C (human body temperature) to allow the bacteria to grow. Plates are always incubated with the agar side up, so that any moisture that collects in the plate will fall on the inside of the lid and not on the growing surface of the agar. How long plates are allowed to grow varies with the type of culture. Most bacteria grow sufficiently within 24 hours, but some require 48 hours. Fungi typically take longer to grow than bacteria and may grow at a slightly lower temperature (35° to 36°C).

Interpreting Cultures

After incubation, cultures are assessed for growth and interpreted. Pathogens may be identified at this time. This process requires considerable skill and practice because pathogens must often be differentiated from normal flora. This step may be performed by the physician, a microbiologist, or a medical assistant who has been properly trained to do so through on-the-job training or additional course work. "Tips for the Office" discusses the types of qualifications and training you need to interpret cultures.

The process of interpreting a culture typically involves several determinations. The characteristics of the colonies growing on the agar are noted, along with their relative numbers. In addition, any changes in the media surrounding the colonies are noted, because these changes may reflect certain characteristics of the microorganism.

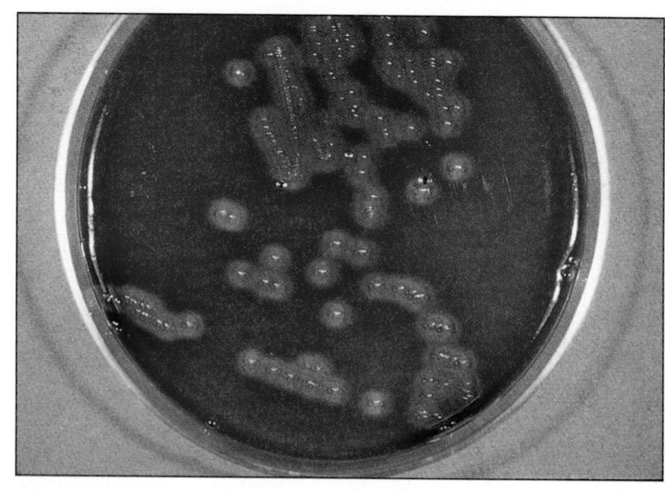

Figure 35-20. A positive strep throat culture contains distinctive colonies surrounded by areas of hemolysis.

The physician decides at this point whether additional procedures are required. In the case of a throat culture, the presence of colonies of a characteristic shape, size, and color, surrounded by areas of hemolysis, suggests strep throat, as shown in Figure 35-20. A Gram's stain

Tips FOR THE OFFICE

Obtaining Additional Training in Microbiology

Identifying microorganisms in culture specimens requires considerable skill and practice. In a microbiology laboratory, these tests may be performed by medical technologists (MTs), medical laboratory technicians (MLTs), or other health professionals, including medical assistants who have received special training.

These classifications differ in the amount of education and training required. Medical technologists, also called clinical laboratory scientists, must earn a bachelor's degree and undergo 1 year of clinical training. Medical laboratory technicians must have completed a 2-year program at an accredited college (or the equivalent amount of course work), be a graduate of an accredited professional school or armed forces school, or hold certification in another related field while completing specific on-the-job training. Certification for both MTs and MLTs requires successful completion of a national certifying examination. In addition to certification, some states require MTs and MLTs to obtain a state license to work in a laboratory.

As part of their training, MTs and MLTs routinely receive instruction in microbiology. They also learn the clinical laboratory skills involved in identifying microorganisms. As part of your current medical assistant curriculum, you are learning the basic principles of microbiology and some of the techniques of specimen collection and processing. To be able to perform microbiologic tests, such as sensitivity tests, and interpret cultures of specimens, however, you would need additional training.

You can learn these types of skills and advance your career by taking part in the continuing education programs your office has to offer. Local colleges or schools of allied health may also offer clinical microbiology courses. Such a course will enable you to become proficient in performing microbiologic identification. All laboratories, including those in the doctor's office, require employees to participate in a proficiency testing program, according to guidelines set forth by the Clinical Laboratory Improvement Amendments of 1988 (CLIA '88).

Developing clinical skills in the area of microbiology can be challenging and satisfying. These skills will contribute to your office's efficiency and ability to provide high-quality patient care. Additional training in microbiology will also enhance your career by making you more valuable to any medical practice or facility.

and determination of bacterial shape may be all of the steps that are necessary for a confirmed diagnosis. Many cultures, however, require additional biochemical and, in some cases, serologic tests for definitive identification of the pathogen.

Determining Antimicrobial Sensitivity

After a particular bacterial (or sometimes fungal) pathogen is identified, the organism's sensitivity (also called susceptibility) to several different antimicrobial agents must be determined. This information enables the doctor to choose an agent for treating the infection that is likely to be effective in curing it. If your office does not perform antimicrobial sensitivity tests but, instead, receives reports on them from reference laboratories, the results are reported as sensitive (no growth), intermediate (little growth), or resistant (overgrown).

Performing an antimicrobial sensitivity test involves taking a sample of the isolated pathogen, suspending it in a small amount of liquid medium, and streaking it evenly on the surface of a culture plate. Small disks of filter paper containing various antimicrobial agents are placed on top of the inoculated agar plate. Although this step can be done manually using sterile forceps, a special dispenser that is often used places all the disks down at once (Figure 35-21).

The plate is then incubated at 37°C, and the results are evaluated the following day. If a particular antimicrobial agent is effective against the microorganism, there will be a clear zone around the disk, indicating that the growth was inhibited in the area of the agent, as seen in Figure 35-22. If there is growth right up to the disk, it means that the agent is not effective against the organism. Each zone is measured in millimeters and compared to a standard chart to determine the degree of effectiveness of the antimicrobial agent. The doctor uses these results to choose an effective antimicrobial agent to treat the patient.

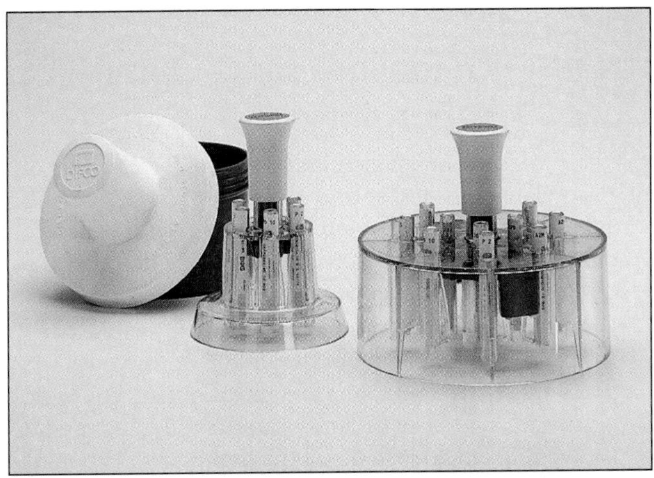

Figure 35-21. Antimicrobial disk dispensers simplify placement of antimicrobial disks, help ensure that each disk contains a single antimicrobial agent, and reduce the probability of contaminating the culture.

Quality Control in the Medical Office

Medical offices are required to have a **quality control (QC)** system in place, which is an ongoing system to evaluate the quality of medical care being provided. Although quality is sometimes difficult to define, most people would agree that high-quality care involves achieving the best possible medical outcome for each patient while attending to both the patient's and the family's needs. Quality control in the medical office provides an objective means of defining, monitoring, and correcting potential problems that affect the quality of care.

Part of quality control in the medical office includes risk management, strategies for helping to minimize the chances of accidents or the risk of infection. These strategies include following general safety rules and regulations and Universal Precautions. Keep in mind that, in practice, medical offices use Universal Precautions when obtaining and handling all types of specimens, not only those capable of transmitting bloodborne pathogens.

Quality control involves an ongoing assessment of the reliability and quality of the work performed. As with all laboratory procedures, quality control in the microbiology laboratory of a medical office is particularly important in achieving quality assurance.

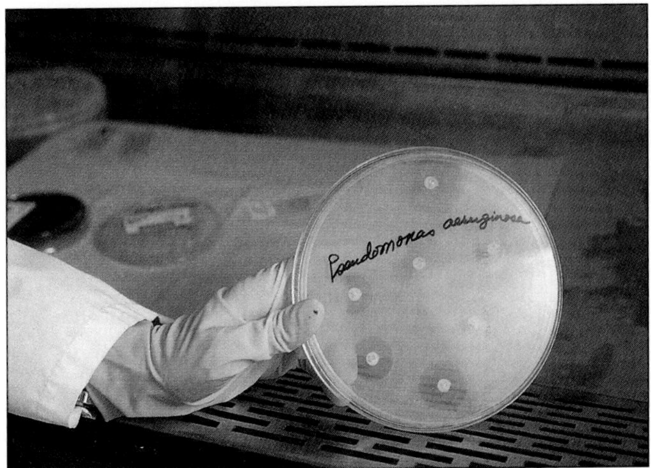

Figure 35-22. The effectiveness of different antimicrobial agents against an organism is apparent when an antimicrobial sensitivity test is performed.

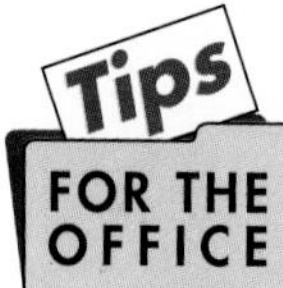

Guidelines for a Quality Control Program in a Microbiology Laboratory

To maintain the highest possible standards of patient care and safety, all facets of a medical laboratory must be checked and monitored. The essential components of a quality control program in a microbiology laboratory include the following:

- Developing an up-to-date procedures manual. This manual is one of the most important documents in the laboratory. The procedures manual directs day-to-day activities and ensures that proper procedures are followed. It should include all general policies, regulations, and procedures, including those involving quality control and the transport of specimens to outside laboratories. The manual should be placed in a binder and kept in a location where all employees can refer to it. At least once a year, the laboratory director or supervisor should update and revise the manual.
- Monitoring laboratory equipment. A quality control program should include a preventive maintenance program for all laboratory equipment to ensure proper functioning. All equipment should be checked and cleaned at regular intervals. Temperatures of refrigerators, freezers, heating blocks, water baths, and incubators should be checked daily with an accurate standardized thermometer. Autoclaves should be tested each week with a spore strip to check sterility, and pH meters must be tested for accuracy using pH-calibrating solutions. A tachometer should be used to check the revolutions per minute of serology rotators and centrifuges. (All centrifuges must have lids.) Safety hoods should be checked two to four times per year to make certain that they permit adequate air flow. The results of all quality control tests should be documented each time a test is performed.
- Monitoring media, supplies, and reagents. Media should be periodically checked for sterility and the ability to grow certain strains of stock organisms. Stains and reagents should also be checked with control organisms to ensure accurate results. Each culture tube, plate of medium, and reagent should be labeled as to its content and its preparation and expiration dates.
- Ensuring qualified personnel. Only qualified personnel should be hired, and employees should be offered an effective continuing education program. All personnel should be given the opportunity to learn new skills. This procedure benefits the laboratory and can also help advance employees' careers. Proficiency testing of blind samples may be used as teaching exercises and should be made available to all interested personnel.
- Ensuring adequate space. One issue of quality control and safety in the laboratory that is often overlooked is the allocation of sufficient work space for personnel. A minimum of 100 sq ft of work space for each full-time equivalent employee is recommended. Safety and high-quality performance are enhanced when there is sufficient space to perform each task.

Quality Control in the Microbiology Laboratory

Quality control is necessary in several areas in a microbiology laboratory. All media, staining solutions, and reagents (chemicals and chemically treated substances used in test procedures) should be evaluated frequently for effectiveness. Media must also be evaluated for sterility. Equipment such as refrigerators, freezers, and incubators should be properly maintained, cleaned, and checked for accuracy of temperature. The essential components of a quality control program as established by the College of American Pathologists are outlined in "Tips for the Office."

The Impact of CLIA '88

In addition to an internal quality control program, all laboratories must incorporate the appropriate policies and procedures to comply with CLIA '88. (See Chapter 32 for a full discussion of CLIA '88.) A substantial part of these requirements involves proper documentation of laboratory policies and procedures, materials, and personnel qualifications and training. If a laboratory has a good quality control program in place, it is likely that the required guidelines are already being followed.

In addition, any laboratory that performs certain procedures must enroll and participate in an approved proficiency testing program. A proficiency testing program monitors the quality of a laboratory's test results. The procedures in a microbiology laboratory that require proficiency testing include those classified as moderately complex or highly complex. An example of a moderately complex procedure is performing a culture and sensitivity test.

Proficiency testing involves culturing, identifying, and determining the sensitivity of blind specimen samples, that is, samples that are unknown to laboratory personnel. The results are then checked for accuracy. If you perform these types of procedures in the medical office, you may be asked to participate in the proficiency testing program.

Summary

A variety of microorganisms can cause infection. They are a major cause of disease in humans. As a medical assistant, you play an important role in the diagnosis and treatment of infection.

Collecting a microbiologic specimen is the most important step in diagnosing an infection. To ensure accurate results, you must use the correct collection device and technique. Then you must process the specimen or transport it to the laboratory in a timely manner to enable recovery of microorganisms.

The process of identification often begins when the doctor examines the fresh or stained specimen. Most specimens are cultured and incubated, and the resultant growth is evaluated. The antibiotic sensitivity of an isolated pathogen can then be determined to aid the doctor in making treatment decisions.

Quality control in the microbiology laboratory is an important factor in ensuring high-quality medical care. The focus and attention you bring to this part of your work will pay handsome dividends in terms of patient care, laboratory safety, and personal satisfaction. Developing your clinical skills will be an asset to the office and will allow you to advance in your career.

35 Chapter Review

Discussion Questions

1. Name five types of microorganisms, and give an example of a disease caused by each.
2. Explain the difference between a qualitative and a quantitative analysis of a microbiologic specimen.
3. Define quality control in a medical office. What are the most important parts of quality control? Why?

Critical Thinking Questions

1. You need to do a throat culture on an ordinarily active 4-year-old boy. How would you explain the procedure to the child, and what might you say to gain his cooperation?
2. The laboratory pickup service has arrived to pick up specimens. You find that a sputum specimen has been left out at room temperature all day. What should you do?
3. You have just explained to a patient how to collect a stool specimen at home, but the patient seems disgusted with the prospect. How can you make the collection process seem easier and less distasteful?

Application Activities

1. With your instructor's approval, practice performing a throat culture on a partner.
2. Use one of your throat culture specimens to inoculate a blood agar plate. Incubate the culture and observe the appearance of normal throat flora.
3. Fill out a laboratory request form for a microbiology test being sent to a reference laboratory.

Further Readings

Acceptance of Hazardous, Restricted, or Perishable Matter. Publication 52. Washington, DC: U.S. Postal Service, April 1990.

Burton, Gwendolyn R. W., and Paul G. Engelkirk. *Microbiology for the Health Sciences.* 5th ed. Philadelphia: Lippincott-Raven, 1996.

Fabian, Denise. "Handling Laboratory Specimens in a Medical Office." *The Professional Medical Assistant,* January/February 1991, 6–7.

Koneman, Elmer W., et al. *Color Atlas and Textbook of Diagnostic Microbiology.* 4th ed. Philadelphia: J. B. Lippincott, 1992.

Levinson, Warren E., and Ernest Jawetz. *Medical Microbiology & Immunology. Examination & Board Review.* 3d ed. Norwalk, CT: Appleton & Lange, 1994.

Palko, Tom, and Hilda Palko. *Laboratory Procedures for the Medical Office.* Columbus, OH: Glencoe/McGraw-Hill, 1996.

Woods, Gail L., and John A. Washington. "The Clinician and the Microbiology Laboratory." In *Mandell, Douglas, and Bennett's Principles and Practice of Infectious Diseases,* 4th ed., edited by Gerald L. Mandell, John E. Bennett, and Raphael Dolin. New York: Churchill Livingstone, 1995, 169–199.

Section Five

Nutrition, Pharmacology, and Diagnostic Equipment

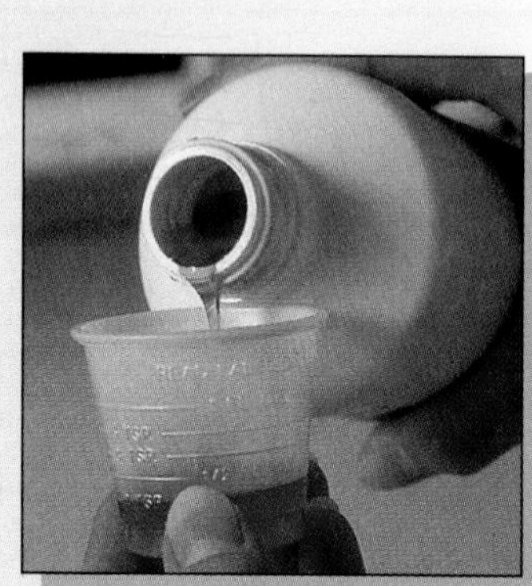

AREAS OF COMPETENCE

1997 ROLE DELINEATION STUDY

CLINICAL

- **Fundamental Principles**
- **Diagnostic Orders**
- **Patient Care**

GENERAL (Transdisciplinary)

- **Legal Concepts**
- **Instruction**

CHAPTER LIST

Nutrition and Special Diets

CHAPTER OUTLINE

- The Role of Diet in Health
- Daily Energy Requirements
- Nutrients
- Dietary Guidelines
- Assessing Nutritional Levels
- Modifying Diets
- Eating Disorders
- Patient Education

OBJECTIVES

After completing Chapter 36, you will be able to:

- Explain why a medical assistant needs to understand the role of diet in health.
- Describe how the body uses food.
- Explain the role of calories in the diet.
- Identify the seven basic food components and explain the major functions of each.
- List the Dietary Guidelines for Americans.
- Explain how the Food Guide Pyramid can be used to plan a nutritious, well-balanced diet.
- Describe the test used to assess body fat.
- Identify types of patients who require special diets and the modifications required for each group.
- Identify specific modified diets that may be ordered to treat or prevent certain conditions.
- Describe the warning signs, symptoms, and treatment for eating disorders.
- Describe techniques the medical assistant can use to effectively educate different types of patients about nutritional requirements.

AREAS OF COMPETENCE

1997 ROLE DELINEATION STUDY

GENERAL (Transdisciplinary)

Instruction

- Explain office policies and procedures
- Teach methods of health promotion and disease prevention
- Locate community resources and disseminate information

Key Terms

amino acid
anabolism
anorexia nervosa
antioxidant
behavior modification
bulimia
calorie
catabolism
cholesterol
complete protein
complex carbohydrate
fiber
food exchange
incomplete protein
lipoprotein
mineral
parenteral nutrition
saturated fat
skinfold test
triglyceride
unsaturated fat
vitamin

The Role of Diet in Health

You need to know what effect food has on health so that you can help patients meet their dietary requirements. Food is the body's source of nutrients, or substances the body needs to function properly. As you study nutrition, you will learn how the body uses nutrients as well as how and why people eat. People need specific types of foods to stay healthy or to regain their health after illness or surgery. People with specific conditions may also need to follow special diets.

You will work closely with the rest of the medical team to ensure that patients understand the role of diet in health and that they adhere to any diet prescribed by their physician or dietitian. A registered dietitian (RD) is a professional who uses the science of nutrition to design ways for people to obtain their optimal nourishment. Dietetics plays an important role in the health field. Dietitians work with physicians and the rest of the medical team to plan diets that are both therapeutic and realistic for patients.

Daily Energy Requirements

The human body requires the nutrients in food for three major purposes:

- To provide energy
- To build, repair, and maintain body tissues
- To regulate body processes

A person's daily energy requirements depend on many factors. To understand the relationship of food to good health, you need to understand how the body uses food.

Metabolism

Food must be broken down before the body can use it. This process is an integral part of metabolism. Metabolism is the sum of all the cellular processes that build, maintain, and supply energy to living tissue. During metabolism body tissue is built up and broken down, and heat and energy are produced.

Metabolism takes place in two phases. In **anabolism,** substances such as nutrients are changed into more complex substances and used to build body tissues. In **catabolism,** complex substances, including nutrients and body tissues, are broken down into simpler substances and converted into energy. The body uses this energy to maintain and repair itself. Of the energy people get from the food they eat, about 25% is directly used for bodily functions, and the rest becomes heat.

Each person's body requires a minimal amount of nutrients to carry on a basic level of metabolism to live. Each person's daily nutritional requirements vary with age, weight, percentage of body fat, activity level, state of health, and other variables. The body's metabolic rate, or speed of metabolism, can also be affected by many factors, such as pregnancy, malnutrition, and disease.

Calories

The amount of energy a food produces in the body is measured in kilocalories. A kilocalorie, commonly called a **calorie,** is the amount of energy needed to raise the temperature of 1 kg of water by 1°C. Foods differ in the number of calories they contain. The more calories in a food, the more available energy it has. Calories are also used to measure the energy the body uses during all activities and metabolic processes.

As mentioned, people's daily nutritional needs differ, depending on variables of age, weight, percentage of body fat, activity level, and state of health. If people eat an excess of calories—more than the body can use—the excess is stored as fat in the body. Conversely, lowering caloric intake causes the body to burn off stored fat for energy.

Depending on the food's weight (in grams) or volume, each food has a value in calories. Therefore, you can count the number of calories a person consumes by monitoring food intake and adding up the calories in each food serving. You can use a food calorie counter, such as those often found in cookbooks and in nutrition books, to look up caloric values. A calorie counter tells you, for instance, that 1 c of cooked carrots contains 50 calories or that 1 c of cooked corn kernels contains 130 calories. Calories are also listed on the labels of food packages.

You can estimate the number of calories a person burns during certain activities by consulting a chart similar to Table 36-1. You can see how many more calories a 190-lb person burns than a 120-lb person does during the same activity.

Nutrients

The body needs a variety of nutrients for energy, growth, repair, and basic processes. Seven basic food components provide these nutrients and work together to help keep the body healthy:

- Proteins
- Carbohydrates
- Fiber
- Lipids
- Vitamins
- Minerals
- Water

As the body digests foods that contain these components, it breaks them down so that it can use them. Of the seven components, only proteins, carbohydrates, and fats contain calories and provide the body with energy. The rest perform a variety of other essential functions.

Table 36-1

Calories Burned per Hour in Selected Activities

Activity	120-lb Person	190-lb Person
Bicycling	360	570
Football (touch)	288	456
Calisthenics	324	516
Handball	456	720
Hiking	300	480
Running (10 mph)	720	1140
Skiing		
(downhill)	426	672
(cross-country)	564	888
Soccer	456	720
Swimming	228	366
Tennis	330	522
Volleyball	258	408
Walking (2 mph)	156	252

Adapted from Marvin R. Levy et al., *Life & Health: Targeting Wellness* (New York: McGraw-Hill, 1992).

Proteins

Protein is the most essential nutrient for building and repairing cells and tissue. Therefore, it is especially important for people to get enough protein during illness and healing. Other major functions of protein are to:

- Help maintain the body's water balance.
- Assist with antibody production and disease resistance.
- Help maintain body heat.

The body makes protein out of **amino acids,** which are natural organic compounds found in plant and animal foods. Besides being used to build and maintain tissue, protein can be broken down to produce energy, especially if other energy sources are low. Each gram of protein contains 4 calories. Excess protein is broken down by the body and contributes to fat stores.

The optimal level of protein in a healthy person's diet is 10% to 20% of total caloric intake. More protein may be required during illnesses and recovery from injury. A deficiency in protein leads to weight loss and fatigue, malnutrition, extremely dry skin, lowered resistance to infection, and interference with normal growth processes.

Complete Proteins. There are 20 amino acids that are absolutely necessary to the body. The body can make 11 of them itself, but the remaining 9—called the essential amino acids—must be obtained through diet. Proteins that contain all 9 essential amino acids are called **complete proteins.** Complete proteins are found in animal food sources such as meat, fish, poultry, eggs (both the yolk and the white), and milk.

Adults who eat meat products are advised to eat lean meats to avoid ingesting too much fat, which can be harmful. For instance, poultry, especially if it is eaten without the skin and prepared by a low-fat cooking method such as grilling, is a good lean-meat choice. Low-fat or skim milk can be substituted for whole milk (except for children under the age of 2, who need more fat in their diet than do older children and adults).

Incomplete Proteins. Individual plant sources of food do not provide complete proteins. They provide **incomplete proteins**—proteins that lack one or more of the essential amino acids. Various plant sources such as nuts, dry beans, grains, and vegetables can be combined, however, to provide all nine essential amino

Natalie Miranda

acids. Figure 36-1 shows examples of foods containing incomplete proteins and complete proteins.

Planning for adequate protein intake and learning to combine protein foods to obtain all the essential amino acids are especially important for vegetarians (people who do not eat meat). Types of vegetarians include lacto-ovo-vegetarians, who eat no animal products except eggs and dairy products, and vegans, who eat no animal or dairy products at all. Although vegetarians may have to eat a larger quantity of foods than nonvegetarians to meet their daily nutritional needs, their diet offers advantages that include greater fiber intake and less fat. Figure 36-2 shows types of incomplete protein foods, such as rice and beans, that can be used in combination to provide complete proteins.

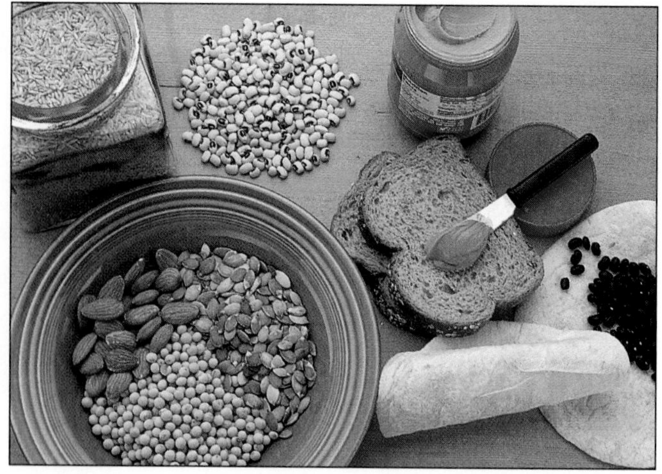

Figure 36-2. These foods, which contain incomplete protein, can be combined to make complete proteins.

Carbohydrates

Carbohydrates in food provide about two-thirds of a person's daily energy needs. Carbohydrates also provide heat, help metabolize fat, and help reserve protein for uses other than supplying energy. Each gram of carbohydrate contains 4 calories. The daily requirement for carbohydrates is 50% to 60% of total caloric intake. Carbohydrate deficiency leads to weight loss, protein loss, and fatigue.

There are two basic types of carbohydrates:

- Simple sugars, found in fruits, some vegetables, milk, and table sugar
- Complex carbohydrates, found in grain foods, such as breads, pastas, cereals, and rice; in some fruits and vegetables, such as potatoes, corn, broccoli, apples, and pears; and in legumes, such as peas, peanuts, and beans

Simple sugars are small molecules that consist of 1 or 2 sugar (saccharide) units. **Complex carbohydrates,** or polysaccharides, are long chains of sugar units. Starch is a type of complex carbohydrate that is a major source of energy from foods of plant origin. Fiber, another type of complex carbohydrate, is discussed below.

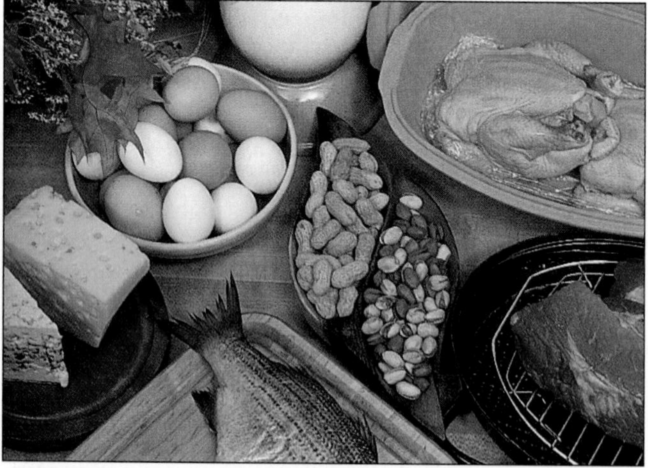

Figure 36-1. Foods such as meat, fish, poultry, eggs, and milk are complete proteins because they contain all the essential amino acids. Plant sources usually provide incomplete protein.

Carbohydrates used for immediate fuel are converted to glucose, a simple sugar that cells use for energy. An excess of carbohydrates is either stored in the liver and muscle cells as glycogen (long chains of glucose units—the animal equivalent of starch) or converted into and stored as fat. After the body's carbohydrate reserves are depleted, it starts burning fat.

Healthful, nutritive sources of carbohydrates include fruits and vegetables, pasta, cereal, and potatoes (see Figure 36-3). The American Dietetic Association suggests natural sources of carbohydrates with an emphasis on complex carbohydrates, such as vegetables, legumes, and whole grain breads and cereals. Sugary foods, such as sweet desserts, candy, and soft drinks, also contain carbohydrates, but they are high in calories and low in nutritional value.

Fiber

Fiber is in a separate category, although it is a type of complex carbohydrate. Fiber does not supply energy or heat to the body. It is the tough, stringy part of vegetables and grains. Fiber is not absorbed by the body, but it serves these important digestive functions:

- Increasing and softening the bulk of the stool, thus promoting normal defecation
- Absorbing organic wastes and toxins in the body so that they can be expelled
- Decreasing the rate of carbohydrate breakdown and absorption

Therapeutically, fiber can help treat and prevent constipation, hemorrhoids, diverticular disease, and irritable bowel syndrome. It is linked to reduced blood cholesterol levels, reduction of gallstone formation, control of diabetes, and reduction in the risk of certain types of cancer and other diseases. Too little fiber can result in an increased risk of colon cancer, hypercholesterolemia (high blood cholesterol), and increased blood glucose levels after eating. Too much fiber can cause constipation, diarrhea, and other gastrointestinal disorders and can impair mineral absorption.

The recommended amount of fiber for adults is 20 to 35 g a day. Because fiber works in conjunction with other substances and nutrients, it is advisable to get dietary fiber from a variety of food sources (see Figure 36-4). Adequate water intake is especially important for fiber to work properly.

Fiber can be classified as soluble or insoluble. Soluble fiber, found in foods such as oats, dry beans, barley, and some fruits and vegetables, is the type that tends to absorb fluid and swell when eaten. It slows the absorption of food from the digestive tract, helps control the blood sugar level of diabetics, lowers blood cholesterol levels, and softens and increases the bulk of stools. Insoluble fiber, found in the bran in whole wheat bread and brown rice, for example, promotes regular bowel movements by contributing to stool bulk.

Lipids

Lipids in the diet include dietary fats and fat-related substances. Fats are a concentrated source of energy that the body can store in large amounts. Each gram of fat contains 9 calories (more than twice the calorie content of proteins and carbohydrates). About 95% of the lipids from plant and animal sources of food are fats. These simple lipids, or **triglycerides,** consist of glycerol (an alcohol) and three fatty acids. Chemical qualities of the fatty acids in a triglyceride determine the fat's characteristic flavor and texture. About 5% of dietary lipids are compound lipids such as cholesterol. Compound lipids are fat-related substances that are important components of cell membranes, nervous tissue, and some hormones. Compound lipids are vital to the transport of all fatlike substances within the body.

Lipids assist with important body functions and are essential to growth and metabolism. Among this nutrient's jobs are the following:

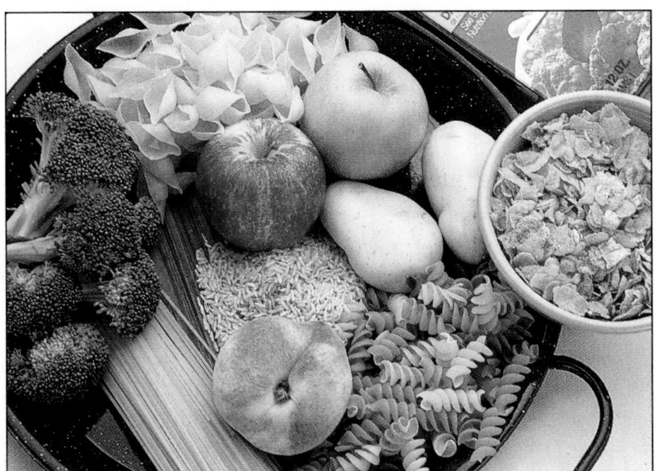

Figure 36-3. Healthful sources of carbohydrates are plentiful.

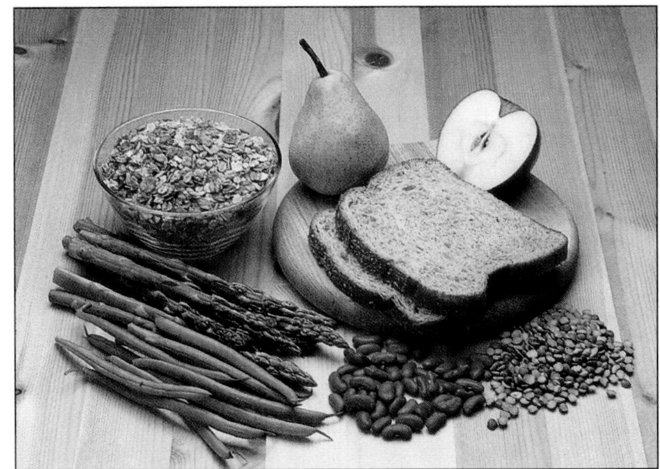

Figure 36-4. Dietary fiber serves many functions in the human body and is considered a basic food component.

- Providing a concentrated source of heat and energy
- Transporting fat-soluble vitamins
- Storing energy in the form of body fat, which insulates and protects the organs
- Providing a feeling of satiety, or fullness, because it is digested more slowly than other nutrients

A lipid deficiency can interfere with the body's absorption and utilization of vitamins and can cause fatigue and dry skin. An excess of lipids, particularly some dietary fats, however, can lead to increased levels of triglycerides and cholesterol in the blood and an increased risk of heart and artery disease and other diseases. It is recommended that adults obtain no more than 30% of their daily calories from fat sources. Cholesterol intake should be limited to 300 mg per day. People with heart disease and certain other diseases or risks may benefit from even lower levels of lipid intake.

Saturated and Unsaturated Fats. The fats in food can be classified as either saturated fats or unsaturated fats (see Figure 36-5). **Saturated fats** are derived primarily from animal sources and are usually solid at room temperature. They are found in meats and animal products such as butter, egg yolks, and whole milk. Coconut oil and palm oil are also saturated fats. Consumption of saturated fats should be restricted because these fats tend to raise blood cholesterol levels.

Unsaturated fats are usually liquid at room temperature. They include most vegetable oils. Unsaturated fats can be divided into two classes:

- Polyunsaturated fats, such as corn, soya, safflower, and sunflower oils
- Monounsaturated fats, such as peanut, canola, and olive oils

Unsaturated fats can also be hydrogenated (have hydrogen added to their structures) so that they become solid at room temperature, as with margarine. Unsaturated fats tend to lower blood cholesterol.

Natalie

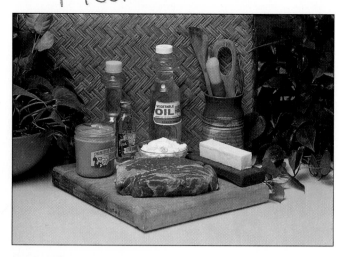

Figure 36-5. Foods that contain saturated fats include meat and butter. Most vegetable oils contain unsaturated fats.

The body needs essential fatty acids (primarily linoleic acid) for building and maintaining tissues. Because the body cannot produce these fatty acids, they must be supplied by food. Saturated fats in butter, egg yolks, and milk and unsaturated fats in corn, canola, sunflower, and safflower oils are good sources of essential fatty acids.

Cholesterol. **Cholesterol** is a fat-related substance produced by the liver that can also be obtained through dietary sources. Only animal-based foods contain cholesterol. It is essential to health because it:

- Serves as an integral part of cell membranes.
- Provides the structural basis for all steroid hormones and vitamin D.
- Serves as a constituent of bile, which aids in digestion.

Lipid Levels in the Blood. Lipids, like other nutrients, are carried throughout the body in the bloodstream. When blood lipid levels become excessive, however, they pose certain risks. Doctors often order blood tests to determine the level of triglycerides and cholesterol in their patients' blood as a measure of overall health. High levels of cholesterol, especially if accompanied by high levels of triglycerides, may indicate an increased risk of heart disease, stroke, and peripheral vascular disease.

Lipids are not soluble in water; fats (or oil) and water do not mix. Because the fluid portion of blood is 90% water, lipids are encased in large molecules that are fat-soluble on the inside and water-soluble on the outside. These large molecules, called **lipoproteins,** carry lipids such as cholesterol and triglycerides through the bloodstream. Low-density lipoproteins (LDLs) and high-density lipoproteins (HDLs) are the two main types of lipoproteins. Cholesterol in blood is identified as HDL or LDL, depending on which type of lipoprotein carries it. High levels of LDL cholesterol in blood are a primary risk factor for heart attacks. High levels of LDL cholesterol most commonly occur in people whose diets are high in saturated fats. HDL cholesterol, commonly referred to as good cholesterol, carries excess cholesterol away from arteries and back to the liver for breakdown and elimination.

Patients can often reduce elevated cholesterol levels by increasing exercise and intake of soluble fiber and decreasing the dietary intake of saturated fats. (Table 36-2 lists the saturated fat and cholesterol contents of various foods.) These measures tend to elevate the level of HDL cholesterol in the bloodstream and reduce the level of LDL cholesterol.

Vitamins

Vitamins are organic substances that are essential for normal body growth and maintenance and resistance to infection. Vitamins also help the body use other nutrients and assist in various body processes.

Most vitamins are absorbed directly through the digestive tract. They can be either water-soluble or fat-soluble. Water-soluble vitamins, such as vitamin C and the B vitamins, are not stored by the body and therefore must be replaced every day. Fat-soluble vitamins, such as vitamins A, D, E, and K, are stored for longer periods.

The amounts of vitamins the body needs are relatively small; however, a vitamin deficiency through lack of ingestion or absorption can lead to disease. Some vitamins can also cause health problems if taken in excess. Toxic levels of vitamin A, for example, can produce effects ranging from headache to liver damage. Because the level of vitamin intake is so essential to health, the Food and Nutrition Board of the National Research Council has established Recommended Dietary Allowances (RDAs) for vitamins. For detailed information on specific vitamins, see Table 36-3.

Eating a well-balanced, nutritious diet minimizes the likelihood of vitamin deficiency. Many manufactured foods are also vitamin-fortified. Even so, some people choose to augment their diets with vitamin supplements (see Figure 36-6). A physician or other member of the medical team may, in some instances, prescribe vitamin supplements for patients.

Minerals

Minerals are natural, inorganic substances the body needs to help build and maintain body tissues and carry on life functions. Depending on the relative amounts the body requires, minerals fall into two categories:

- Major minerals the body needs in fairly large quantities, including calcium, magnesium, and phosphorus
- Trace minerals the body needs in tiny amounts, including iron, iodine, zinc, selenium, copper, fluoride, chromium, manganese, and molybdenum

Minerals essential to good health include calcium, iron, iodine, zinc, copper, magnesium, phosphorus, fluoride, manganese, chromium, molybdenum, and selenium. Calcium, iron, and iodine are the minerals in which people are most often deficient. Most minerals are absorbed in the intestines, and any excess is eliminated.

Natasha Marie Valenzuela 28

Table 36-2

Saturated Fat and Cholesterol Contents of Various Foods

Food	Saturated Fat (g)	Cholesterol (mg)
Cheddar cheese (1 oz)	6.0	30
Mozzarella, part skim (1 oz)	3.1	15
Whole milk (1 c)	5.1	33
Skim milk (1 c)	0.3	4
Butter (1 tbsp)	7.1	31
Mayonnaise (1 tbsp)	1.7	8
Tuna in oil (3 oz)	1.4	55
Tuna in water (3 oz)	0.3	48
Lean ground beef, broiled (3 oz)	6.2	74
Leg of lamb, roasted (3 oz)	5.6	78
Bacon (3 slices)	3.3	16
Chicken breast, roasted (3 oz)	0.9	73

Source: U.S. Department of Agriculture

Minerals With Recommended Dietary Allowances. There are several minerals for which RDAs have been established. These minerals are calcium, iron, iodine, zinc, magnesium, phosphorus, and selenium.

Calcium. Calcium builds healthy bones and teeth, aids in blood clotting, and helps nerves and muscles function properly. It is found in dairy products, green leafy vegetables, broccoli, legumes, and the soft bones of sardines and salmon (Figure 36-7).

Calcium deficiency can cause poor bone growth and tooth development in children, osteoporosis in adults, and poor blood clotting. The normal requirement is 800 to 1200 mg per day.

Iron. Iron, one of the most important nutrients, is essential for the production of red blood cells, which transport oxygen throughout the body. It is also a component of enzymes needed for energy production. Although iron is found in a wide variety of foods, it is the most frequently deficient nutrient in people's diets. Liver, meat, poultry, fish, egg yolks, fortified breads and cereals, dark green vegetables, and dried fruits are good dietary sources of iron (Figure 36-8), although less than 20% of it is usually absorbed.

Iron deficiency can cause anemia, a blood disorder that results in fatigue, weakness, and impaired mental abilities. At toxic levels iron may increase the risk of coronary heart disease. The daily requirement is 10 to 15 mg.

Iodine. Iodine plays a vital role in the activities of the thyroid hormones, which are involved in reproduction, growth, nerve and muscle function, and the production of new blood cells. Deficiency can cause an enlarged thyroid gland, known as goiter. Iodine can be obtained in seafood, iodized salt, and seaweed products. The daily requirement is 150 µg.

Zinc. Zinc promotes normal growth and wound healing and participates in many cell activities that involve proteins, enzymes, and hormones. It is found in liver, lamb, beef, eggs, oysters, and whole grain breads and cereals, although it is not always easily absorbed. Deficiency can result in growth retardation, impaired taste and smell, and reduced immune function. The daily requirement is 12 to 15 mg.

Magnesium. Magnesium activates cell enzymes, helps metabolize proteins and carbohydrates, maintains the structural integrity of the heart and other muscles, and aids in muscle contraction. Good sources include green leafy vegetables, nuts, legumes, bananas, and whole grain products. A deficiency may result from persistent vomiting or diarrhea, kidney disease, general

Natasha Marie Valenzuela

Table 36-3

Vitamins

Vitamin	Functions	Adult RDA*	Food Sources	Deficiencies and/ or Toxicities
Vitamin A (retinol, provitamin, carotene)	Aids in night vision; cell growth and maintenance; normal reproductive function; health of skin, mucous membranes, and internal tracts	Males: 1000 µg retinol equivalents Females: 800 µg retinol equivalents	Milk fat; butter; egg yolks; meat; fish liver oil; liver; green, yellow, and orange leafy vegetables; yellow and orange fruits	Deficiency: night blindness; dry, rough skin; risk of internal infection Toxicity: headache, vomiting, joint pain, hair loss, jaundice, liver damage
Vitamin B_1 (thiamine)	Aids enzymes in breaking down and using carbohydrates; helps the nerves, muscles, and heart function efficiently	Males: 1.5 mg Females: 1.1 mg	Whole grains, brewer's yeast, organ meats, lean pork, beef, liver, legumes, seeds, nuts	Deficiency: beriberi with appetite loss, digestive problems, muscle weakness and deterioration, nervous disorders, heart failure
Vitamin B_2 (riboflavin)	Aids enzymes in metabolism of fats and proteins	Males: 1.2–1.5 mg Females: 1.0–1.1 mg	Dairy products, organ meats, green leafy vegetables, enriched and fortified grain products	Deficiency: cracks at lip corners, irritations at nasal angles, inflammation of the tongue, seborrheic dermatitis, anemia
Vitamin B_3 (niacin)	Aids enzymes in metabolism of carbohydrates and fats	Males: 15–19 mg Females: 13–15 mg	Meat, fish, poultry, enriched and fortified grain products	Deficiency: pellagra with dermatitis, diarrhea, inflammation of mucous membranes, dementia Toxicity: dilation of blood vessels; if sustained, abnormal liver function
Vitamin B_6 (pyridoxine)	Aids enzymes in synthesis of amino acids	Males: 2.0 mg Females: 1.6 mg	Chicken, fish, pork, liver, kidney, some vegetables, grains, nuts, legumes	Deficiency: convulsions, dermatitis, anemia Toxicity: loss of muscle coordination, severe sensory neuropathy
Folate (compounds)	Works with cobalamins in nucleic acid synthesis and metabolism of amino acids; maintains red blood cells	Males: 200 µg Females: 180 µg	Liver, yeast, legumes, green leafy vegetables, some fruits	Deficiency: glossitis, diarrhea, anemia, lethargy

continued

malnutrition, alcoholism, and the use of certain medications. The daily requirement is 280 mg for women and 350 mg for men.

Phosphorus. Phosphorus is involved in bone and tooth formation, chemical reactions in the body, and energy production. It is found in dairy foods, animal foods, fish, cereals, nuts, and legumes. A deficiency of phosphorus can cause gastrointestinal, blood cell, and other disorders. Toxicity is harmful as well. The daily requirement is 800 mg for adults 25 and over.

Natasha Marie Valenzuela

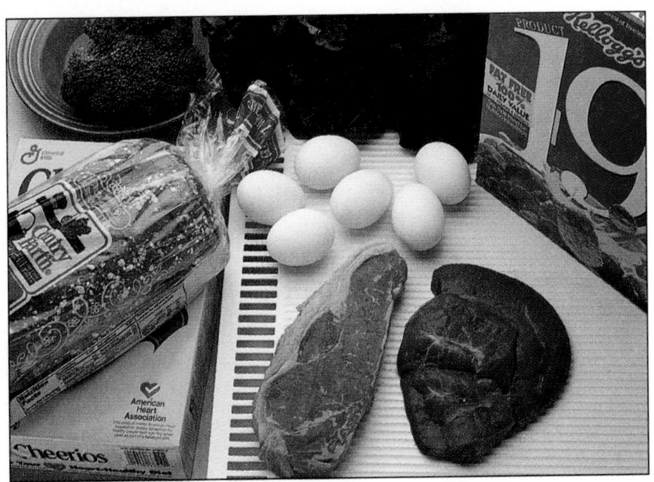

Figure 36-8. Iron, a mineral that is needed in small amounts, is found in a wide variety of foods.

to eight glasses of water a day to maintain a healthy water balance. The daily need for water varies with size and age, the temperatures to which someone is exposed, the degree of physical exertion, and the water content of the foods one eats. Someone who is eating mostly foods with a high water content, such as fruits and vegetables, can drink a little less water than someone who is eating mostly foods with a low water content.

If people get too little water or lose too much water through vomiting, diarrhea, burns, or perspiration, they become dehydrated. Signs and symptoms of dehydration include dry lips and mucous membranes, weakness, lethargy, decreased urine output, and increased thirst. Severe dehydration can lead to hypovolemia, a reduction in the volume of blood in the body. Severe hypovolemia can result in inadequate blood pressure that affects the functioning of the heart, central nervous system, and various organs—a condition known as hypovolemic shock. If dehydration progresses so that water is lost from body cells, death usually occurs within a few days.

Procedure 36-1 explains how to educate patients to drink the right amount of water each day to prevent dehydration. Make sure patients know whether they are to drink extra fluids to replace fluids lost in an illness or to help rid the body of waste.

Principal Electrolytes and Other Nutrients of Special Interest

The principal electrolytes are essential to normal body functioning. Other nutrients, such as antioxidants, also merit special mention.

Principal Electrolytes. Although the principal electrolytes in the body—sodium, potassium, and chloride—are often excluded from lists of nutrients, they are essential dietary components. Electrolytes play an important role in maintaining body functions, such as normal heart rhythm.

PROCEDURE 36-1

Educating Adult Patients About Daily Water Requirements

Objective: To teach patients how much water their bodies need to maintain health

OSHA Guidelines: This procedure does not involve exposure to blood, body fluids, or tissues.

Materials: Patient education literature, patient's chart, pen

Method

1. Explain to patients how important water is to the body. Point out the water content of the body and the many functions of water in the body: maintaining the body's fluid balance, lubricating the body's moving parts, transporting nutrients and secretions.
2. Add any comments applicable to an individual patient's health status—for example, issues related to medication use, physical activity, pregnancy, and so on. Be aware that some elderly patients purposely limit their fluid intake because of incontinence or physical limitations that make getting to a bathroom difficult.
3. Explain that people obtain water by drinking water and other fluids and by eating water-containing foods. On average, a person should drink six to eight glasses of water a day to maintain a healthy water balance in which intake equals excretion. People's daily need for water varies with size and age, the temperatures to which they are exposed, degree of physical exertion, and the water content of foods eaten. Make sure you reinforce the physician's or dietitian's recommendations for a particular patient's water needs.
4. Caution patients that soft drinks, coffee, and tea are not good substitutes for water and that it would be wise to filter out any harmful chemicals contained in the local tap water or to drink bottled water, if possible.
5. Provide patients with tips about reminders to drink the requisite amount of water. Some patients may benefit from using a water bottle of a particular size, so they know they have to drink, say, three full bottles of water each day (Figure 36-9). Another

continued

PROCEDURE 36-1 continued

Educating Adult Patients About Daily Water Requirements

helpful tip is to make a habit of drinking a glass of water at certain points in the daily routine, such as first thing in the morning and before lunch.

6. Remind patients that you and the physician are available to discuss any problems or questions.
7. Document any formal patient education sessions or significant exchanges with a patient in the patient's chart, noting whether the patient understood the information presented. Then initial the entry (Figure 36-10).

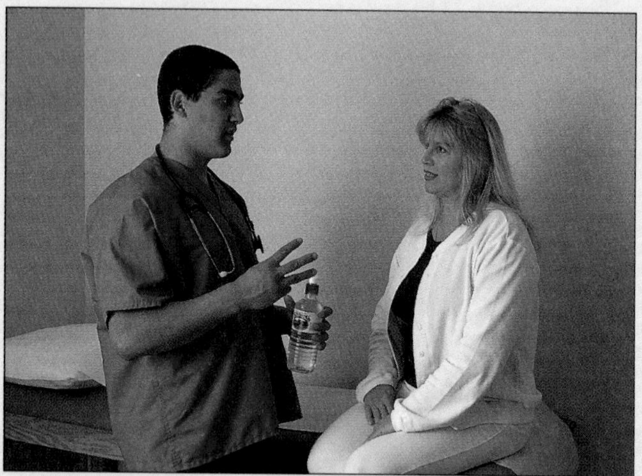

Figure 36-9. Using a personal water bottle that holds 16 oz, the patient can make a point of drinking three to four full bottles daily.

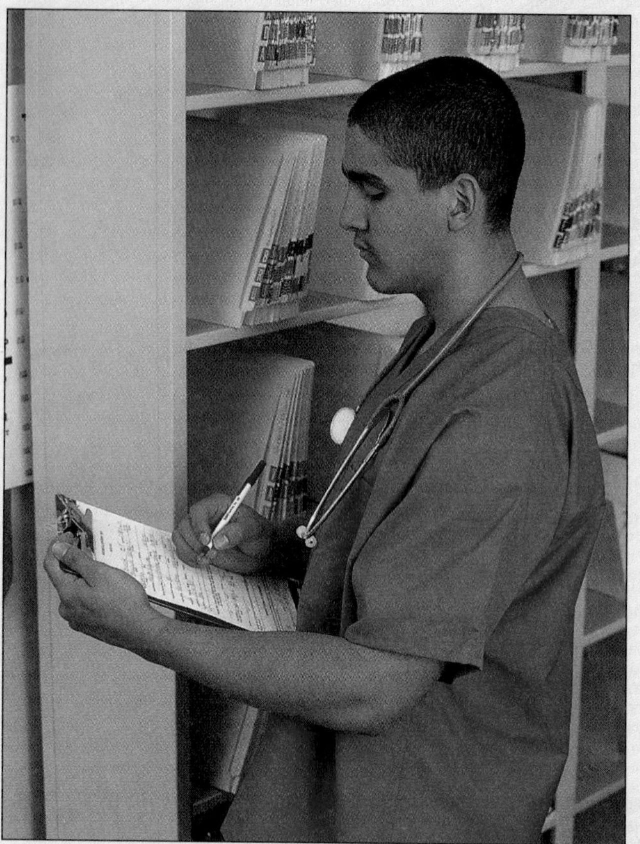

Figure 36-10. Always document patient education sessions in the patient's chart.

Sodium (Na) maintains fluid and acid-base balances, assists in the transport of glucose, and maintains normal conditions inside and outside cells. Salt is the main dietary source of sodium, and high salt intakes are normally associated with a diet high in processed foods. Too much sodium can be associated with high blood pressure in salt-sensitive individuals. Although many Americans consume far more, it is recommended that daily sodium intake be limited to 2.4 g or less.

Potassium (K) is a crucial element in the maintenance of muscle contraction and fluid and electrolyte balance. It contributes to acid-base balance and the transmission of nerve impulses. Its role in fluid balance helps regulate blood pressure. Potassium occurs in unprocessed foods, particularly in fruits such as bananas, raisins, and oranges; many vegetables; and fresh meats (Figure 36-11). The minimum requirement is 1600 to 2000 mg per day.

Chloride (Cl) is essential in maintaining fluid and electrolyte balance, and it is a necessary component of hydrochloric acid, secreted into the stomach during digestion of food. Because dietary chloride comes almost entirely from sodium chloride, sources are essentially the same as those of sodium.

Antioxidants. **Antioxidants** are chemical agents that fight certain cell-destroying chemical substances called free radicals. In fact, antioxidants may help ward off cancer and heart disease by neutralizing free radicals, byproducts of normal metabolism that may also form as a result of exposure to various damaging factors, such as cigarette smoke, alcohol, or x-rays. Antioxidants may be added to foods and cosmetics as preservatives. The nutrients beta-carotene, vitamin C, vitamin E, and selenium (Figure 36-12) are natural antioxidants.

Dietary Guidelines

A variety of dietary guidelines exist to help people get proper nutrition, reduce the occurrence of disease, and control their weight. These recommendations, which are

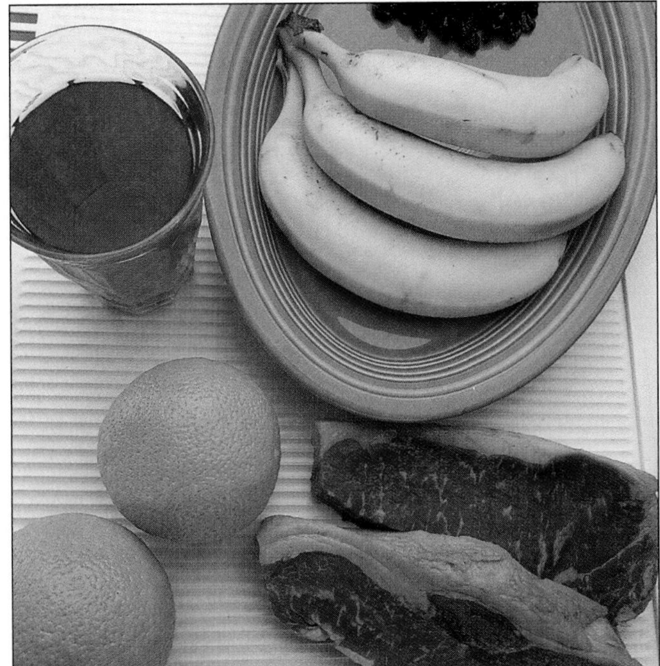

Figure 36-11. These foods are good sources of potassium.

issued by governmental agencies or private associations, are designed to encourage healthy eating habits.

Dietary guidelines suggest the types and quantities of food that people should eat each day. They may also contain recommendations about which types of foods to limit and which types of foods to increase.

Dietary Guidelines for Americans

The U.S. Department of Agriculture and the U.S. Department of Health and Human Services issued updated Dietary Guidelines for Americans in 1995. These guidelines encourage people to eat a balanced diet and to limit consumption of less nutritious foods. Here are their recommendations.

1. Eat a variety of foods to get the energy, protein, vitamins, minerals, and fiber you need for good health.
2. Balance the food you eat with physical activity—maintain or improve your weight to help reduce your chances of high blood pressure, heart disease, stroke, some types of cancer, and diabetes.
3. Choose a diet with plenty of grain products, vegetables, and fruits, which provide needed vitamins, minerals, fiber, and complex carbohydrates and can help you lower your intake of fat.
4. Choose a diet low in fat, saturated fat, and cholesterol to reduce your risk of heart attack and certain types of cancer.
5. Choose a diet moderate in sugars—a diet with lots of sugars has too many calories and too few nutrients and can contribute to tooth decay.
6. Choose a diet moderate in salt and sodium to help reduce your risk of high blood pressure.
7. If you drink alcoholic beverages, do so in moderation—alcoholic beverages supply calories, but little or no nutrients.

Food Guide Pyramid

In 1992 the U.S. Department of Agriculture introduced a new food pyramid, which serves as a nutritional guideline to replace previous pyramids, food wheels, and food groups. The pyramid is divided into six parts to show the quantities of food people should consume daily from each of five basic food groups (Figure 36-13). The sixth, and smallest, part of the pyramid represents fats, oils, and sweets, which should be eaten sparingly. The Food Guide Pyramid shows how the proportions of each basic food group contribute to a balanced diet.

Two symbols, a circle and a triangle, are used on the pyramid. The circle indicates fat that occurs naturally or is added, and the triangle indicates sugar that is added. These symbols show how fat and sugar—although they come mainly from fats, oils, and sweets—can occur naturally or be added to foods in the five basic food groups.

You can use the Food Guide Pyramid to explain nutritional guidelines to patients. If you post a colorful copy of it in your office—perhaps near the scale or on the wall of the examination room—you can use it as a visual aid when helping patients plan a balanced diet.

To help patients plan a balanced diet, you will need to know how much of a food equals a serving. For example, one serving of fruit equals one medium apple or orange, ½ c canned fruit, or ¾ c (6 oz) fruit juice. You should refer to a chart similar to Table 36-4, which lists serving sizes for foods in each of the basic food groups. Serving sizes for young children are smaller; for example,

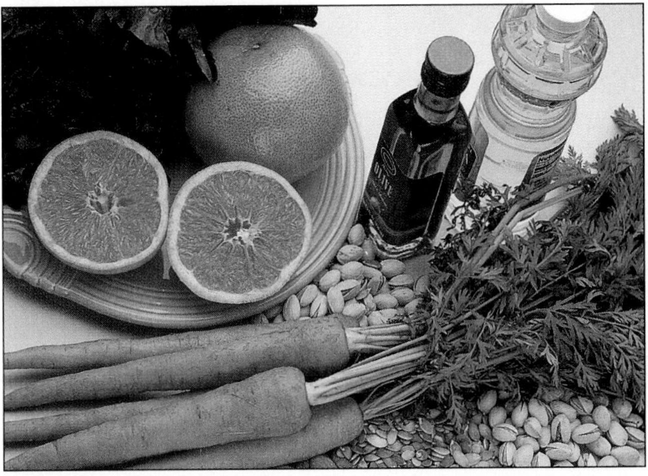

Figure 36-12. Antioxidants are substances in food that may offer protection against certain chronic diseases. Foods rich in beta-carotene, vitamin C, vitamin E, and selenium contain antioxidants.

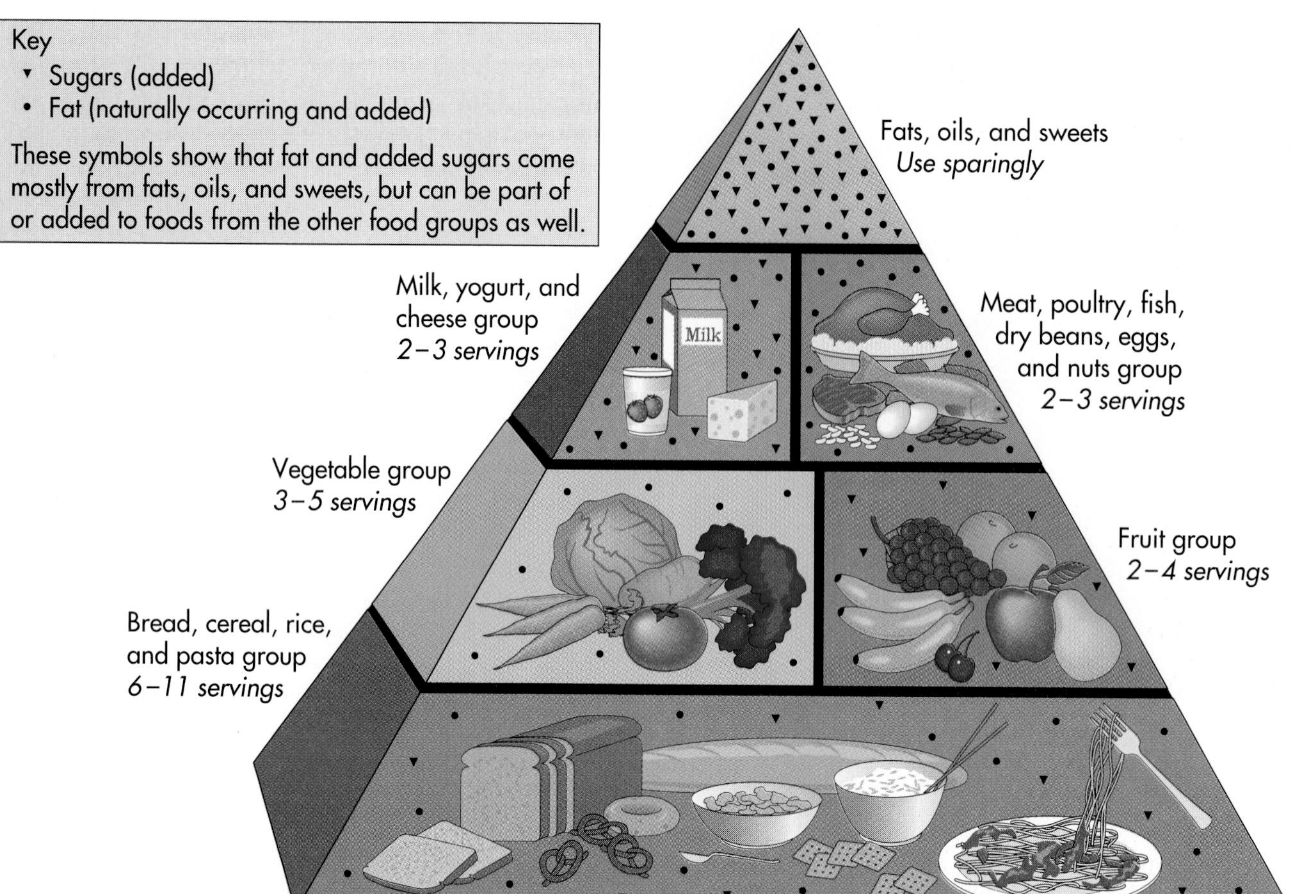

Figure 36-13. The U.S. Department of Agriculture's Food Guide Pyramid can be used to plan a nutritious, well-balanced diet.

serving sizes for toddlers and preschoolers are about half the sizes listed in the table.

The Food Guide Pyramid is a general guideline. It does not provide exact information about what to eat. Nutritional needs vary from person to person, depending on age, gender, and activity level (see Table 36-5). That is why the pyramid lists ranges of servings.

American Cancer Society Guidelines

The American Cancer Society has set forth the following guidelines to aid in the prevention of cancer.

1. Eat more high-fiber foods such as fruits, vegetables, and whole grain cereals.
2. Eat plenty of dark green and deep yellow fruits and vegetables rich in vitamins A and C.
3. Eat plenty of broccoli, cabbage, brussels sprouts, kohlrabi, and cauliflower.
4. Be moderate in consumption of salt-cured, smoked, and nitrite-cured foods, such as bacon and smoked sausage.
5. Cut down on total fat intake from animal sources and fats and oils.
6. Avoid obesity.
7. Be moderate in consumption of alcoholic beverages.

The American Cancer Society also advises that

> *high-fat diets may contribute to the development of cancers of the breast, colon, and prostate. High-fiber foods might help reduce risk of colon cancer. A varied diet containing plenty of vegetables and fruits rich in vitamins A and C may reduce risk for a wide range of cancers. Salt-cured, smoked, and nitrite-cured foods have been linked to esophagus and stomach cancer. (American Cancer Society, 1992)*

Assessing Nutritional Levels

Doctors assess a patient's nutritional status by analyzing age, health status, height, weight, type of body frame, body circumference, percentage of body fat, nutritional and exercise patterns, and energy needs. They accomplish this through direct measurement as well as through questionnaires and interviews. During the analysis, doctors take into account individual factors such as culture, beliefs, lifestyle, and education.

To measure fat as a percentage of body weight, doctors may perform a **skinfold test,** measuring the

Table 36-4

What Counts as a Serving?

Food Group	Food and Quantity
Bread, cereal, rice, and pasta	1 slice bread 1 oz ready-to-eat cereal ½ c cooked cereal, rice, or pasta
Vegetable	1 c raw leafy vegetables ½ c other vegetables—cooked or raw ¾ c vegetable juice
Fruit	1 medium apple, banana, or orange ½ c chopped, cooked, or canned fruit ¾ c fruit juice
Milk, yogurt, and cheese	1 c milk or yogurt 1½ oz natural cheese 2 oz process cheese
Meat, poultry, fish, dry beans, eggs, and nuts	2–3 oz cooked lean meat, poultry, or fish ½ c cooked dry beans or 1 egg counts as 1 oz lean meat 2 tbsp peanut butter or ⅓ c nuts counts as 1 oz meat

Source: Nutrition and Your Health: Dietary Guidelines for Americans, 4th ed. (Washington, DC: U.S. Department of Agriculture and U.S. Department of Health and Human Services, 1995).

Table 36-5

Number of Servings Required for Different Calorie Levels

Colorie Level (Common Individuals in Group)	About 1600 Many women, older adults	About 2200 Children, teen girls, most men, active women	About 2800 Teen boys, active men
Grain Products Group Servings	6	9	11
Vegetable Group Servings	3	4	5
Fruit Group Servings	2	3	4
Milk Group Servings	2–3*	2–3*	2–3*
Meat and Beans Group Servings	2 (5 oz total)	2 (6 oz total)	3 (7 oz total)
Total Fat (g)	53	73	93

Source: Nutrition and Your Health: Dietary Guidelines for Americans, 4th ed. (Washington, DC: U.S. Department of Agriculture and U.S. Department of Health and Human Services, 1995).

*Women who are pregnant or breast-feeding, teenagers, and young adults to age 24 need 3 servings.

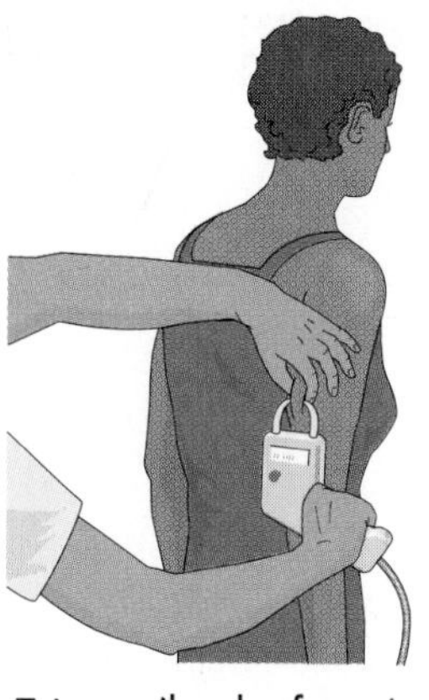

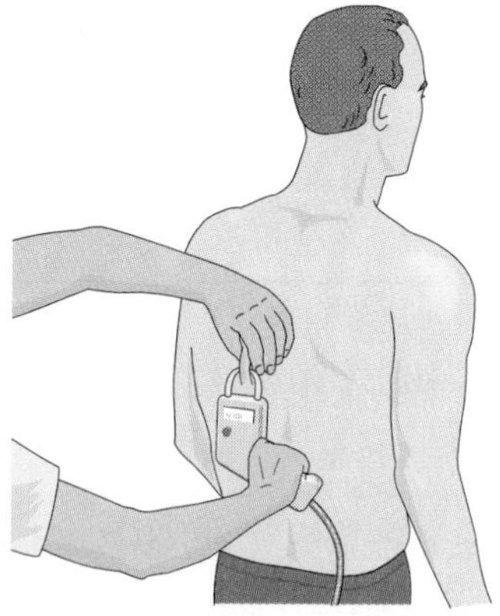

Triceps (back of arm)

Subscapular (below shoulder blade)

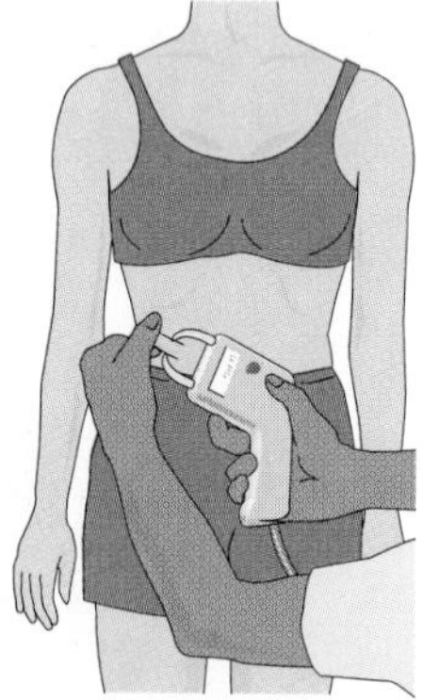

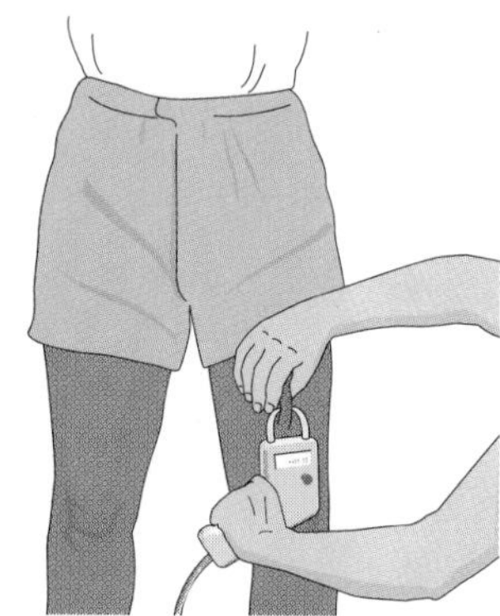

Suprailiac (above hipbone)

Thigh (front)

Figure 36-14. To estimate an individual's body fat percentage, a professional uses a tool called a caliper to measure the thickness of a fold of skin at one or more points on the body.

thickness of a fold of skin with a caliper (Figure 36-14). This measurement is often made on the triceps, midway between the shoulder and elbow. The test indicates the total percentage of fat, because about 50% of body fat is just below the skin and the volume of fat below the skin is related to the volume of inner fat. A trained individual must perform this test, which must be precise to be reliable.

The optimal percentage of body fat differs between men and women. For males younger than age 50, it is 10% to 14%; older than 50, 12% to 19%. In females younger than age 50, it is 14% to 23%; older than 50, 16% to 25%. Aging usually changes the ratio a bit because some muscle tissue is replaced by fat, even if weight remains constant.

Modifying Diets

A person's diet has a significant effect on health, appearance, and recovery from disease. After a physician or dietitian has established a patient's nutritional status, any necessary or beneficial dietary adjustments can be instituted. Dietary modification may be used alone or in combination with other therapies to prevent or treat illness. Factors affecting people's specific dietary needs may include pregnancy, injury, disease, vegetarianism, aging, genetic disorders, and substance abuse.

Adjustments in diet may involve any of the following:

- Restricting certain foods
- Emphasizing particular foods
- Changing daily caloric intake
- Changing the amount of a specific nutrient
- Changing textures of foods
- Altering the number of daily meals
- Changing variables such as bulk or spiciness

Physicians work with dietitians to determine the best diet therapy to initiate for individual patients. Diet therapy is based on many factors, including particular foods and nutrients associated with different diseases or body states.

Patients With Specific Nutritional Needs

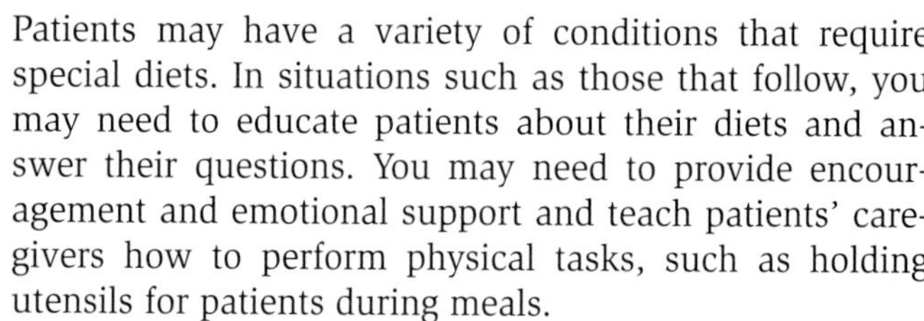

Patients may have a variety of conditions that require special diets. In situations such as those that follow, you may need to educate patients about their diets and answer their questions. You may need to provide encouragement and emotional support and teach patients' caregivers how to perform physical tasks, such as holding utensils for patients during meals.

Patients With Allergies. Some patients have food allergies. Allergic reactions to food can range from sneezing or a rash to the potentially fatal state of anaphylaxis, described in Chapter 31. The scratch test described in Chapter 28 is used to determine which foods cause an allergic reaction.

Usually specific foods must be eliminated from or restricted in an allergic patient's diet. Procedure 36-2 provides information on discussing with the patient potential dangers of common foods and reactions to those foods.

Some of the most common food allergens are wheat, milk, eggs, and chocolate. The doctor may confirm an allergy by eliminating and then reintroducing the patient's suspect foods one by one. The patient's allergy may decrease over time through systematic desensitization by means of allergy shots and other regimens.

If a food that is being eliminated or restricted was a primary source of nutrients for the patient, then the doctor must adjust the diet to include another source of those nutrients. For example, if a baby is allergic to milk, the doctor recommends a milk-substitute formula.

Patients With Anemia. Iron deficiency anemia, the most common type of anemia, is usually caused by chronic blood loss, a lack of iron in the diet, impaired intestinal absorption of iron, or an increased need for iron, as in pregnancy. A patient may need to take iron supple-

PROCEDURE 36-2

Alerting Patients With Food Allergies to the Dangers of Common Foods

Objective: To explain how patients can eliminate allergy-causing foods from their diets

OSHA Guidelines: This procedure does not involve exposure to blood, body fluids, or tissues.

Materials: Results of the patient's allergy tests, patient's chart, pen, patient education materials

Method

1. Identify the patient and introduce yourself.
2. Discuss the results of the patient's allergy tests (if available), reinforcing the physician's instructions. List the foods the patient has been found to be allergic to. Provide the patient with a checklist of those foods.
3. Discuss with the patient the possible allergic reactions those foods can cause.
4. Talk about how the patient can avoid or eliminate those foods from the diet. Point out that the patient needs to be alert to avoid the allergy-causing foods not only in their basic forms but also as ingredients in prepared dishes and packaged foods. (Patients allergic to peanuts, for example, should avoid products containing peanut oil as well as peanuts.) Tell the patient to read labels carefully and to inquire at restaurants about the use of those ingredients in dishes listed on the menu.
5. With the physician's or dietitian's consent, talk with the patient about the possibility of finding adequate substitutes for the foods if they are among the patient's favorites. Also discuss, if necessary, how the patient can obtain the nutrients in those foods from other sources (for example, the need for extra calcium sources if the patient is allergic to dairy products). Provide these explanations to the patient in writing, if appropriate, along with supplementary materials such as recipe pamphlets, a list of resources for obtaining food substitutes, and so on.
6. Discuss with the patient the procedures to follow if the allergy-causing foods are accidentally ingested.
7. Answer the patient's questions and remind the patient that you and the rest of the medical team are available if any questions or problems arise later on.
8. Document the patient education session or interchange in the patient's chart, indicate the patient's understanding, and initial the entry.

ments and ingest more dietary iron as part of the treatment for this disorder. Foods high in iron include liver, egg yolks, dark green vegetables, beans, some dried fruits, and fortified breads and cereals.

Patients With Cancer. Most patients being treated for cancer undergo weight loss resulting both from the cancer and from treatments involving radiation or chemotherapy. To help their bodies fight off the cancer, these patients must increase their caloric intake. It is especially important that they get enough protein, because protein is needed to regenerate cells to replace the cells destroyed by the cancer and cancer treatments. These patients may also need to increase their intake of B vitamins and vitamins A, C, D, and E to support tissue growth and repair and promote efficient metabolism and use of all nutrients in the diet.

Encourage patients with cancer to follow the diet the physician sets for them. Patients may find this difficult, because cancer often produces loss of appetite. They may also experience nausea and vomiting. Educate patients about ways to make food more appealing and easier to digest. Consuming small meals at frequent intervals may help. Patients may also follow a liquid diet. Bringing food to room temperature or chilling it slightly may reduce food odors that can trigger nausea.

Patients With Diabetes. A special diet is one of the foundations of treatment for diabetes. Dietary guidelines for patients with diabetes must not only provide them with adequate nutrition but also keep their blood sugar level under control and interact appropriately with medication. Patient education is especially important, because patients with diabetes must comfortably maintain the dietary modifications over a lifetime.

The diet a physician or dietitian prescribes for someone with diabetes includes a specific number of calories, meals per day, amount of carbohydrates, and amounts of other nutrients. As a way to simplify the diet, a system of **food exchanges** is used. All food exchanges in a particular food category provide the same amounts of protein, fat, and carbohydrates. Food exchange lists can be obtained from a registered dietitian or the American Diabetes Association.

The list of exchanges is divided into six categories—vegetables, fruits, breads, meats, fats, and milk—and indicates how large a portion of each food in a category is equal to one "exchange" of food in that category. This information tells patients what portions of specific foods are interchangeable and whether they are eating the correct amounts of those foods. The list includes a variety of foods from which patients make their selections. It is important that patients with diabetes not skip a meal, because skipping meals disturbs the balance of blood sugar and metabolism.

Patients with diabetes who are dependent on insulin should eat regular meals at consistent times. Skipping or delaying meals can result in hypoglycemia or an insulin reaction. Patients should work with a registered dietitian and their physician to create a meal plan that keeps blood glucose levels as close to normal as possible. The medical team specifies the proportion of carbohydrates and calories in meals, depending on the type of insulin patients use and the timing of injections.

Fiber is also important for patients who have diabetes. Fiber can sometimes prevent a sharp rise in blood glucose after a meal and may reduce the amount of insulin needed. It is therefore recommended that people with diabetes gradually increase their fiber intake until it is at about 45 g per day.

Patients Who Are Elderly. Universal nutritional guidelines for aging patients have not been developed. It is known, however, that energy and metabolic requirements usually decline with age, which calls for some dietary modification. The Food and Nutrition Board of the National Academy of Science recommends a 10% decrease in caloric intake for people over age 50 compared with that of young adults. Men and women above age 75 should decrease their intake another 10% to 15%. The exact adjustment, however, depends on the individual patient's condition and needs.

Because protein requirements do not change, elderly patients should select foods that provide ample protein in a smaller quantity of food. To achieve daily nutritional goals, patients may require supplements for iron, calcium, and other minerals, such as phosphorus and magnesium.

Because aging is often accompanied by decreased gastrointestinal muscle tone, elderly patients should increase their intake of high-fiber foods and drink plenty of water. Although all people need a certain amount of fat in their diet to help the body absorb vitamins, too much may lead to atherosclerosis. Elderly individuals should therefore keep fat intake to 20% of their total calories.

Certain factors can impair or impede eating in this age group and may even lead to malnutrition. If you recognize any of these factors, discuss them with the patient's doctor:

- Physical factors, such as chewing difficulty caused by tooth loss or poorly fitting dentures, swallowing difficulty, and lack of appetite caused by altered taste, smell, or sight
- Medications, which may adversely affect food intake or nutrient use
- Social factors, including apathy toward food caused by depression, grief, or loneliness
- Economic factors, including homelessness or lack of money for food or transportation

Patients With Heart Disease. Coronary heart disease is caused by atherosclerosis, which usually results from hyperlipidemia, or an excess of lipids in the bloodstream. Left untreated, this condition can lead to angina, heart attack, or stroke.

Patients can significantly lower their risk by reducing their blood cholesterol levels and losing weight if they are overweight. Patients who have coronary heart disease usually must reduce their consumption of fats to a level that provides less than 30% of their total caloric intake. Saturated fats should provide less than 10% of caloric intake. Patients who have had a heart attack or are at increased risk for a heart attack are also encouraged to increase their consumption of soluble fiber.

As a medical assistant, your role with these patients is to encourage them to follow the nutritional regimen prescribed by the doctor. Do not recommend other dietary changes. Instead, educate patients about ways to reduce the amount of fat in their diets, such as by substituting skim milk for whole milk.

Patients With Hypertension. Hypertension (high blood pressure) is a condition that affects more than 20% of American adults. Nutritional therapy for patients with hypertension involves the following:

- Restricting sodium intake to 2 to 3 g per day, especially in salt-sensitive individuals
- Increasing potassium intake through consumption of fresh fruits and vegetables
- Ensuring adequate calcium intake to meet an RDA of 800 mg
- Eliminating or reducing alcohol use
- Decreasing total fat intake and obtaining no more than 10% of calories from saturated fats

Patients With Lactose Sensitivity. Lactose is the sugar contained in human and animal milk. It must be broken down in the body by the enzyme lactase to enable the body to digest dairy products. In people from some parts of the world, lactase is present in the body until age 3 or 4, after which it all but disappears. As a result, after early childhood many people have trouble digesting foods that contain lactose and eliminate these foods from their diets. People who are especially sensitive to dietary lactose are often referred to as being lactose intolerant.

Chemical preparations can help a person digest lactose. Those preparations may be added to certain foods, such as ice cream, for lactose-sensitive people. If people with a lactose sensitivity choose to avoid dairy products, they need to be sure to obtain protein and calcium from other sources.

Patients Who Are Overweight. Overweight is a common problem: more than one-third of American adults are overweight. Overweight patients weigh 10% to 20% more than is recommended for their height and gender.

Patients who are more than 20% overweight are considered obese. Obesity can lead to medical complications such as elevated blood cholesterol levels, hypertension, diabetes, joint problems, respiratory problems, and heart disease.

Approaches to Weight Loss. Overweight may be approached with dietary modification alone, but an exercise program is usually included. Behavior modification is also a common element of weight-loss programs. In a weight-loss program, foods should be proportioned in accordance with the Food Guide Pyramid, and the diet should be appealing and enjoyable. The goal is to have the patient decrease daily caloric intake and increase physical activity at an appropriate rate while remaining comfortable and healthy.

Weight loss will not occur unless patients expend more energy than they consume. A physician or dietitian can calculate each person's daily caloric needs and determine how many calories must be cut from the diet and how much activity must be increased to result in weight loss. Foods that are high in nutrients but low in calories are desirable.

The **behavior modification** facet of weight loss includes such methods as keeping a food diary to pinpoint overeating patterns, controlling the stimuli associated with overeating, and providing rewards for successful behavior. You can help overweight patients in their weight-loss efforts by teaching them to:

- Eat slowly, because the message that the stomach is full takes 20 minutes to register with the brain.
- Eat five or six small meals daily.
- Be patient—reliable weight loss occurs over time, not immediately.

Motivation and Education. Because patients who are trying to lose weight may have trouble with motivation, they need as much support as possible. You can provide encouragement and education. You may be able to introduce the patient to low-calorie or low-fat recipes, for instance, and positively reinforce the patient's efforts by complimenting small, gradual successes.

You will no doubt need to explain that fad diets and diet drugs are seldom successful. Fad weight-loss methods can lead to vitamin, mineral, and protein deficiency; serious medical disorders; and even death. Tell patients to use the following criteria to identify fad diets. These diets:

- Promise ease and comfort in weight loss.
- Promise extremely quick weight loss.
- Include only a few foods, such as grapefruit or low-protein foods.
- Require the purchase of some secret ingredient or pill.
- Are often published in a book or magazine.

Truly effective weight-loss regimens usually involve the following.

- They include a variety of foods that contain adequate nutrients.
- They include an activity component.
- They may be safely followed over a long period of time.

An effective program should be one in which the patient is able to lose weight (including fat) gradually and constantly, with some plateaus, and then maintain the loss indefinitely afterward. You can help patients with the challenge of maintaining their weight loss by recommending a reputable weight-loss group or a support group that will help them make the necessary lifestyle changes and remain motivated.

Pediatric Patients. During the first year of life, an infant experiences the most rapid period of growth and development that occurs during the life span. Breast milk and commercially prepared formula contain the balance of nutrients that infants' bodies need during that period. Cow's milk does not meet these standards.

The pace of growth is steadier and slower during childhood, with growth spurts throughout. Nutritional needs change to reflect growth, maturation, and increasing activity levels. Vitamin D and calcium are critical to tooth and bone formation, and fluoride strengthens teeth. Hunger regulates food intake in young children, but forcing children to eat can promote eating habits that lead to obesity.

Patients Who Are Pregnant or Lactating. Nutrition is especially important during pregnancy, when it provides for normal growth and health of the baby as well as the health of the pregnant woman. Doctors recommend that pregnant women gain a certain amount of weight during each trimester of pregnancy, with a total weight gain of about 25 to 35 lb. The rate of weight gain should be 2 to 5 lb in the first trimester and about 1 lb per week after that. Gaining too little or too much weight during pregnancy can result in serious complications.

Among the nutritional guidelines for pregnant women are the following:

- An additional 10 to 15 g of protein a day in the form of meat, poultry, fish, eggs, and dairy products
- 1200 mg of calcium a day, preferably in the form of low-fat dairy products, such as skim milk
- 30 mg of iron a day through meat, liver, egg yolks, grains, leafy vegetables, nuts, dried fruits, legumes, and supplements (it is difficult to meet the daily need with food alone)
- Folic acid intake of 400 µg a day through leafy vegetables, yeast, and liver, as well as supplements
- Adequate fiber intake to prevent the constipation that often accompanies pregnancy
- Recommendations consistent with the Food Guide Pyramid and normal sodium and water intake

Breast-feeding has specific nutritional and dietary requirements as well, because breast milk is nutrient-rich and the body requires considerable energy and nutrients to produce it. The infant depends on this milk for the extensive growth that takes place during the first months of life. Lactating women need to consume an additional 500 calories and an additional 12 to 19 g of protein per day, as well as 260 to 280 μg of folic acid and 1200 mg of calcium.

Specific Modified Diets

Physicians may modify a patient's diet to treat or prevent certain conditions. Specific types of modified diets include changes in texture, nutrient level, frequency and timing of meals, and exclusions.

Texture. A patient may need changes in food consistency as a result of swallowing, chewing, or other gastrointestinal problems or to fulfill short-term needs that result from such events as laboratory tests or surgical procedures. The following special diets are based on texture.

- A clear-liquid diet consists solely of foods such as tea, broth, noncitrus juices, carbonated beverages, popsicles, and gelatin. A full-liquid diet is less restrictive and includes strained cooked cereals, plain ice cream, sherbet, pudding, and strained soups.
- A soft diet includes foods that are easy to chew, swallow, and digest. Foods patients cannot tolerate and those high in fiber are eliminated from this diet.
- All foods in a pureed diet are put through a strainer so that they are in the form of a semisolid. Pureed foods are easy to chew and swallow.
- A high-fiber diet contains large amounts of fiber (greater than 40 g) from sources such as fresh fruits, vegetables, and bran cereal. Physicians may prescribe this diet for patients with conditions such as diverticulosis and constipation. The diet increases the bulk of fecal matter and stimulates peristalsis (waves of alternating contraction and relaxation of the intestine that move contents through the intestine).

Nutrient Level. Doctors may make nutrient-level modifications in patients' diets before or after surgical or medical procedures or for patients who have specific conditions. The following are some special diets based on nutrient levels.

- Doctors may prescribe low-sodium diets for patients who suffer from disease conditions affecting the cardiovascular system, liver, pancreas, and gallbladder, including edema and hypertension. The typical American diet contains 2 to 5 g of sodium daily. For mild sodium restriction, daily intake is limited to 2 to 3 g; the patient reduces salt in cooking, adds no salt at the table, and avoids processed foods. Moderate sodium restriction allows 1 g per day; the patient adds no salt in cooking or at the table and limits high-sodium vegetables, meat, and milk. Severe restriction allows 500 mg per day and greatly limits high-sodium vegetables, meat, milk, and eggs.
- Doctors recommend low-cholesterol diets for patients with high blood cholesterol levels. Such diets involve replacing saturated fats with unsaturated fats, using low-fat or nonfat cooking methods, and restricting fatty foods.
- Doctors may prescribe reduced-calorie diets to promote weight loss in patients who are overweight.
- Doctors may recommend low-tyramine diets for patients who have migraine headaches and patients who are taking certain antidepressant drugs. The compound tyramine is found in aged cheeses, red wine, beer, cream, chocolate, and yeast.
- Doctors may order high-calorie, high-protein diets for patients who have infections, are recovering from burns or surgery, or have had weight loss caused by a severe illness. Food intake is increased to provide 3000 to 5000 calories per day. Protein usually accounts for the greatest caloric increase in these diets.
- Doctors may prescribe high-carbohydrate diets for patients with kidney diseases and some cardiac conditions.

You can help patients who need to make nutrient-level modifications by teaching them how to read food labels. All packaged foods carry a Nutrition Facts label that contains information on the ingredients, major nutrients, and recommended amounts of key nutrients in daily diets. Procedure 36-3 explains how to educate patients about reading food labels.

You can also teach patients how to interpret the terms on food labels (see Table 36-6). Understanding marketing terms simplifies the process of buying the right foods to meet special dietary needs.

Frequency and Timing of Meals. A patient's diet may also be modified by adjusting the standard three-meal pattern. The goal may be to eat six small meals rather than three large meals to minimize stress on organs affected by disease conditions—as in patients with ulcers or hiatal hernia. In other cases meals may simply be timed to follow tests or therapeutic procedures.

Exclusion of Certain Foods. Physicians may order that specific foods be omitted from patients' diets for health reasons.

- In a bland diet specific foods that cause irritation are eliminated, along with caffeine, alcohol, nicotine, aspirin, and some spices. A typical bland diet includes easily digested foods, such as mashed potatoes and gelatins. Raw fruits and vegetables, whole grain foods, and very hot or cold items are among foods to avoid. A physician may prescribe this type of diet for a patient with a peptic ulcer, for example.
- Exclusion diets are also prescribed for patients who have food intolerances. These diets must eliminate foods that contain the offending substances but still provide the nutrients needed for good health. Intolerance to lactose, the sugar in milk, is fairly common. Intolerance to the amino acid phenylalanine—a condition present at birth—is fairly rare but very serious. Infants born in hospitals in the United States are tested for this

intolerance because if these infants were to receive a standard diet, they would develop severe mental retardation. People with this condition, known as phenylketonuria (PKU), must be vigilant about checking labels on prepared foods as well as knowledgeable about the phenylalanine content of fresh foods.

Using Supplements and Parenteral Nutrition

When a patient has a loss or lack of appetite or cannot tolerate a normal meal, the doctor may prescribe a specially formulated food supplement that provides protein, carbohydrates, fat, vitamins, and minerals. A patient who is chronically ill, underweight, or anemic or who has just undergone surgery may take supplements orally or through a tube to the stomach or small intestine. If the supplement is being taken orally, encourage the patient to follow the prescribed directions.

When patients cannot tolerate receiving supplements enterally (by way of the digestive tract), they may be fed parenterally. **Parenteral nutrition** is provided to patients as specially prepared nutrients injected directly into their veins rather than given by mouth. Because a parenteral feeding bypasses the digestive system, the nutrients it contains must already be in a form the body can use as they enter the blood.

Patients Undergoing Drug Therapy

Drugs may change a patient's nutritional status and needs. Long-term drug therapy and multiple prescriptions make close nutritional monitoring a high priority.

Drug therapy can cause a change in food intake, a change in the body's absorption of a nutrient, or both.

PROCEDURE 36-3

Teaching Patients How to Read Food Labels

Objective: To explain how patients can use food labels to plan or follow a diet

OSHA Guidelines: This procedure does not involve exposure to blood, body fluids, or tissues.

Materials: Food labels from products

Method

1. Identify the patient and introduce yourself.
2. Explain that food labels can be used as a valuable source of information when planning or implementing a prescribed diet.
3. Using a label from a food package, such as the ice-cream label shown in Figure 36-15, point out the Nutrition Facts section.
4. Describe the various elements on the label—in this case the ice-cream label.
   - Serving size is the basis for the nutrition information provided. One serving of the ice cream is ½ c. There are 16 servings in the package of ice cream.
   - Calories and calories from fat show the proportion of fat calories in the product. One serving of the ice cream contains 170 calories; more than 45% of the calories come from fat.
   - The % Daily Value section shows how many grams (g) or milligrams (mg) of a variety of nutrients are contained in one serving. Then the percentage (%) of the recommended daily intake of each given nutrient (assuming a diet of 2000 calories a day) is shown. The ice cream contains 24% of a person's recommended daily saturated fat intake but only 3% of dietary fiber.

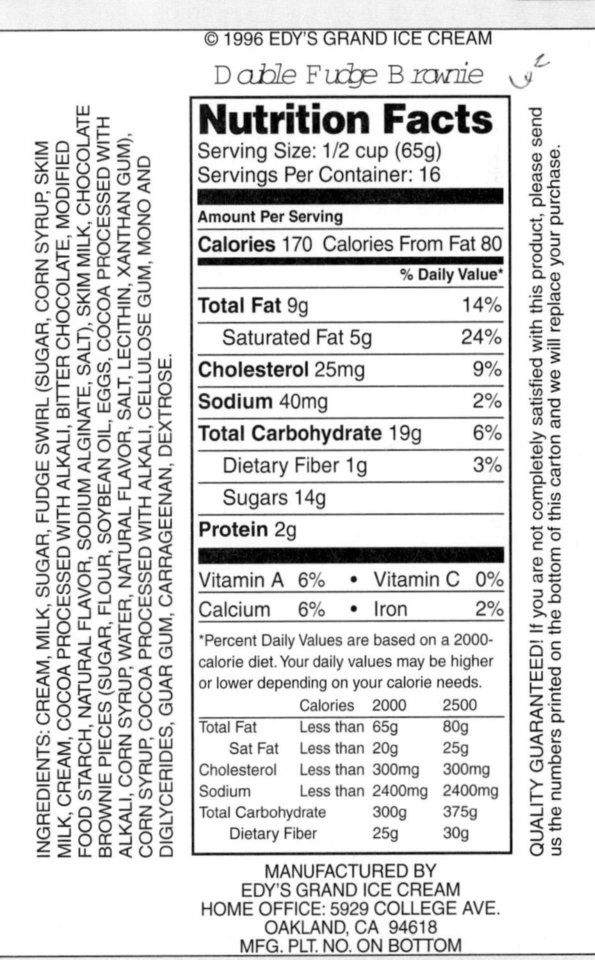

Figure 36-15. Food labels are a source of nutrition information. This label provides facts on the nutrients and ingredients contained in this product.

continued

PROCEDURE 36-3 continued

Teaching Patients How to Read Food Labels

- Recommendations for total amounts of various nutrients for both a 2000-calorie and a 2500-calorie diet are shown in chart form near the bottom of the label. These numbers provide the basis for the daily value percentages.
- Ingredients are listed in order from largest quantity to smallest quantity. In this half-gallon of ice cream, cream, milk, and sugar are the most abundant ingredients.

5. Inform the patient that a variety of similar products with significantly different nutritional values are often available. Explain that patients can use nutrition labels, such as those shown in Figures 36-15 and 36-16, to evaluate and compare such similar products. Patients must consider what a product contributes to their diets, not simply what it lacks. To do this, patients must read the entire label. Compared with the regular ice cream, the "no sugar added" ice cream contains less fat, fewer carbohydrates, and an extra gram of protein, but it contributes an additional 15 mg of sodium and lacks fiber. It also uses an artificial sweetener that contains phenylalanine.
6. Ask the patient to compare two other similar products and determine which would fit in better as part of a healthy, nutritious diet that meets that patient's individual needs.
7. Document the patient education session in the patient's chart, indicate the patient's understanding, and initial the entry.

© 1996 EDY'S GRAND ICE CREAM

No Sugar Added Butter Pecan

INGREDIENTS: MILK, SKIM MILK, SORBITOL, POLYDEXTROSE, MALTODEXTRIN, CREAM, ROASTED PECANS (PECANS, COCONUT OIL, BUTTER, SALT), WATER, BUTTER, NATURAL FLAVOR, CARAMEL COLOR, MONO AND DIGLYCERIDES, CELLULOSE GUM, XANTHAN GUM, CELLULOSE GEL, TURMERIC AND ANNATTO COLOR, SUNETT® ACESULFAME POTASSIUM, CARRAGEENAN, ASPARTAME.

SUNETT® IS A REGISTERED TRADEMARK OF HOECHST AG. PHENYLKETONURICS: CONTAINS PHENYLALANINE.

Nutrition Facts

Serving Size: 1/2 cup (62g)
Servings Per Container: 16

Amount Per Serving	
Calories 110 Calories From Fat 45	
	% Daily Value*
Total Fat 5.0g	7%
Saturated Fat 2.0g	9%
Cholesterol 10mg	3%
Sodium 55mg	9%
Total Carbohydrate 12g	4%
Dietary Fiber 0g	0%
Sugars 3g	
Sugar Alcohols 4g	
Protein 3g	

Vitamin A	4%	Vitamin C	0%
Calcium	8%	Iron	0%

*Percent Daily Values are based on a 2000-calorie diet. Your daily values may be higher or lower depending on your calorie needs.

	Calories	2,000	2,500
Total Fat	Less than	65g	80g
Sat Fat	Less than	20g	24g
Cholesterol	Less than	300mg	300mg
Sodium	Less than	2400mg	2400mg
Total Carbohydrate		300g	375g
Dietary Fiber		25g	30g

QUALITY GUARANTEED! If you are not completely satisfied with this product, please send us the numbers printed on the bottom of this carton and we will replace your purchase.

MANUFACTURED BY
EDY'S GRAND ICE CREAM
HOME OFFICE: 5929 COLLEGE AVE.
OAKLAND, CA 94618
MFG. PLT. NO. ON BOTTOM

Figure 36-16. By reading this label, a patient would learn that this ice cream contains less fat and fewer calories than regular ice cream.

Likewise, foods can interfere with the metabolism and action of a drug. For example, laxatives and certain other types of drugs may suppress the appetite. Antihistamines, alcohol, insulin, thyroid hormones, and some other drugs can stimulate appetite. Anesthetics can interfere with taste. Calcium in milk can diminish the absorption of some antibiotics. Be sure to discuss any possible interactions with the physician or dietitian before discussing diet and drug regimens with a patient.

Eating Disorders

Eating disorders, characterized by extremely harmful eating behavior, can lead to health problems. These disorders can damage the body and even cause death. They are most common in adolescent girls and young women, although 10% to 15% of patients with eating disorders are male. Figure 36-17 lists signs and symptoms of common types of eating disorders.

Anorexia Nervosa

Anorexia nervosa is an eating disorder in which people starve themselves. They fear that if they lose control of eating, they will become grossly overweight. They lose an excessive amount of weight and become malnourished, and women often stop menstruating. The typical patient with anorexia nervosa is a high-achieving, white female in her teens or early 20s. The numbers of children and middle-aged women who suffer from the disorder, however, have been increasing.

The cause of anorexia remains unknown, but risk factors include the following:

Table 36-6

Food Label Terms and Definitions

Term	Definition
Low calorie	Less than or equal to 40 calories per serving
Reduced calorie	At least 25% fewer calories per serving than the food it replaces
Cholesterol free	Less than or equal to 2 mg cholesterol per serving
Low cholesterol	Less than or equal to 20 mg cholesterol per serving
Reduced cholesterol	At least 25% less cholesterol per serving than the food it replaces
Low fat	Less than or equal to 3 g fat per serving
Reduced fat	At least 25% less fat per serving than the food it replaces
Sodium free	Less than or equal to 5 mg sodium per serving
Very low sodium	Less than or equal to 35 mg sodium per serving
Low sodium	Less than or equal to 140 mg sodium per serving
Reduced sodium	At least 25% less sodium per serving than the food it replaces

Source: U.S. Department of Health and Human Services, Food and Drug Administration

- Coming from a family that has problems with alcoholism
- Suffering a childhood trauma, such as sexual abuse (20% to 50% of patients were sexually abused)
- Having a high stress level
- Suffering from depression
- Suffering from shame and low self-esteem
- Having an extreme need to be in control

It has also been noted that anorexia tends to run in families. The victim of anorexia often uses food as a way to deal with the psychological effects of trauma by numbing the emotions or as a means of getting some measure of control in life. Anorexia can be precipitated by any major life change.

This disorder can be fatal. The first stage of treatment is to restore normal nutrition. Patients may need to be hospitalized and fed intravenously or by nasogastric tube, which enters through the nose and delivers food into the stomach. Hospitalization may be necessary, because patients with excessive weight loss may develop cardiac and other medical disorders. These patients may also be at risk for suicide. The hospital stay may eventually provide patients with the structure and support they need to establish healthy eating patterns.

Psychotherapy is a cornerstone of treatment protocol. Therapy usually involves a combination of one-on-one and group therapy. Therapy groups that are single-sex rather than coed are preferable because of the different gender and peer group issues men and women face. Doctors may prescribe medication for depression and anxiety. The later stages of treatment include teaching patients and their families about nutrition concepts.

Bulimia

Bulimia is an eating disorder in which people eat a large quantity of food in a short time (bingeing) and then attempt to counter the effects of bingeing by self-induced vomiting, use of laxatives or diuretics, and/or excessive exercise. People with bulimia may use such behavior to try to gain control of their lives and weight.

Bulimia can be triggered when a slightly overweight person diets but fails to achieve the goal. Episodes are usually frequent, rapid, and uncontrollable. The behavior may occur only during periods of stress.

People with bulimia often diet when not bingeing. Psychologically, they believe their worth depends on being thin. Behind their cheerful exterior, they usually feel depressed, lonely, ashamed, and empty.

Signs and Symptoms of Common Eating Disorders

Anorexia Nervosa

- Unexplained weight loss of at least 15%
- Self-starvation
- Excessive fear of gaining weight
- Malnourishment
- Cessation of menstruation in women
- Drastic reduction in food consumption
- Denial of feeling hungry
- Ritualistic eating habits
- Overexercising
- Unrealistic self-image as being obese
- Extremely controlled behavior

Bulimia

- Eating large quantities of food in a short period, followed by purging
- Pretexts for going to the bathroom after meals
- Using laxatives or diuretics to control weight
- Buying and consuming large quantities of food
- Feeling out of control while eating
- Maintaining a constant weight while eating a large amount of fattening foods
- Mood swings
- Awareness of having a disorder, but fear of not being able to stop
- Depression, self-deprecation, and guilt following the episodes

Binge Eating

- Bingeing on food, not followed by purging
- Weight gain

Figure 36-17. Be alert for these signs and symptoms of eating disorders when you work with patients.

Most bulimics who seek help are in their early 20s and report that they have been bulimic for 4 to 6 years. Because they are more likely to want and seek help, they are slightly easier to treat than anorexics.

Bulimia is usually not life-threatening, but it can cause the following serious health problems:

- Erosion of tooth enamel
- Enlarged salivary glands
- Lesions in the esophagus
- Stomach spasms
- Chemical and hormonal imbalances

As with anorexia, treatment involves a combination of psychotherapy and medication. Dental work, medication for depression and anxiety, nutritional counseling, and support groups may be used. The goal is to establish a healthy weight and good eating patterns as well as to resolve the psychosocial triggers.

Getting Help

Studies show an unsatisfactory rate of recovery from eating disorders; only about half of anorexic patients fully recover. The disorders can become chronic, with periods of remission and relapse. Chronic anorexia can be fatal, and many people who do recover from eating disorders remain preoccupied with food.

If you suspect that a patient has an eating disorder, be alert for the following eating or activity patterns that the patient might mention in conversation:

- Skipping two or more meals a day or limiting caloric intake to 500 or fewer calories a day
- Eating a very large amount of food in an uncontrollable manner over the course of 2 hours
- Eating large quantities of food without being hungry
- Using laxatives, excessive exercise, vomiting, diuretics, or other purges for weight control
- Avoiding social situations because they may interfere with a diet or exercise
- Feeling disgust, depression, and guilt after a binge
- Feeling that food controls life

Patient Education

Whenever you teach patients about nutrition and diet, you help them take steps to improve their health. In most instances a physician or dietitian gives the patient instructions, which you then reinforce. Patients may feel more comfortable asking you questions about their diet than asking other members of the medical team. They may think their concerns are too trivial or simple for the physician or dietitian.

Because of your frequent contact with patients, you can play a major role in education. You can teach patients about the role of nutrition in helping to prevent specific medical conditions. You can also teach patients how to be wise consumers when they shop by reading food package labels. You will be better equipped to educate patients and answer their questions if you have a solid knowledge of diet and nutrition and if you stay current with recent research findings. See "Educating the Patient" for information on the relevance of such research. Before discussing a diet with any patient, be sure you understand the regimen the physician or dietitian is recommending, as well as how to implement it.

If you are unsure of answers to any patient's questions, always ask the physician. Refer patients who have questions about meal patterns and food selections to the registered dietitian, if one is available.

EDUCATING THE PATIENT

Changes in Nutritional Recommendations

In the field of nutrition—as in other scientific fields—research continues to provide people with additional information. How that information is used and the speed with which it is communicated often depend on public service agencies and federal agencies responsible for nutritional guidance.

You can help answer patients' questions about the potential usefulness of new information by understanding the difference between initial research findings and those evaluated and endorsed by the government. In many cases information is not officially released or endorsed until the government has studied the facts and determined that they are accurate and concrete enough for public consideration. For example, initial findings have suggested the following information.

- Beta-carotene supplements may provide no benefit and may even be harmful.
- Certain fruit-derived flavenoids—pigmented antioxidants—may help halt the growth of cancer cells.
- Vitamin E may be effective in slowing the accumulation of artery-clogging plaque.
- Dark beer may reduce the risk of coronary artery disease.

Patients may read about research studies and ask whether they should make whatever dietary changes the findings suggest. You need to explain that such findings are preliminary and not formally approved by a government agency. Although the approval process is lengthy—requiring a significant amount of data and test results—it provides a system for protecting consumers from false nutritional claims.

Tell patients that once the government determines that a nutritional recommendation is warranted, it often acts on it. One example is the case of folate. Since the 1960s a number of studies have been conducted on the importance of folate in the diet. Over the years, those studies have yielded the following results.

- Folate offers protection from neural tube defects in unborn babies.
- Folate can reverse certain anemias.
- Folate may reduce the risk of cervical dysplasia.
- Folate appears to lower the likelihood of heart attacks.

As a result of these studies, the Department of Health and Human Services' Food and Drug Administration considered folate to be so important to all people that it approved the addition of folate to flour. Several nutrients have long been added to certain products to improve the products' nutritional value and to increase people's intake of important nutrients lacking in the general diet:

- Vitamin A and vitamin D, added to dairy products
- Iodine, added to salt
- Niacin, added to milled grain products
- Various vitamins and minerals, added to processed cereals

Explain to patients that nutritional recommendations change as scientists learn more about the ways various foods affect the human body and the exact amount of nutrients the body requires. Keep up to date on nutrition research so you can provide patients with the latest information and help them steer clear of unsubstantiated claims.

Your Role in Patient Education

When discussing dietary requirements with a patient, keep in mind that the patient is always the focus of nutritional care. Specific factors to take into account include the following:

- Any psychological or lifestyle factors that affect food choices and behaviors. Learn about the patient's dietary likes and dislikes, as well as religious or cultural restrictions, before you suggest the use of specific foods in meeting dietary requirements.
- The patient's age and family circumstances. For example, parents need to know the specifics about an infant's or a child's diet. An elderly person's diet needs to be physically and economically manageable as well as nutritious.
- Diseases and disorders. For example, if the patient has chewing or breathing problems or is nauseous, the doctor will have to prescribe treatments or medications to address those problems.
- The patient's psychological condition. You can learn a great deal about psychological status through discussion and nonverbal cues. For instance, you might look for signs that the patient is frustrated with the dietary changes or is in denial about a problem. The greater the rapport you develop with a patient, the more you will be able to help.

Remind patients that eating healthfully will help them feel and look better and help their bodies work better. When the doctor prescribes therapeutic diets, be sure patients are fully aware of the reasons they must follow the diets. Help patients set realistic goals, and praise them for even the smallest accomplishments. Offer positive reinforcement for current and new good food habits.

As with all patient education, teaching methods such as role playing, repetition of concepts, and the use of literature and other media reinforce your discussion. Use printed and audiovisual materials such as those shown in Figure 36-18 (available from health agencies and other sources) to illustrate your points.

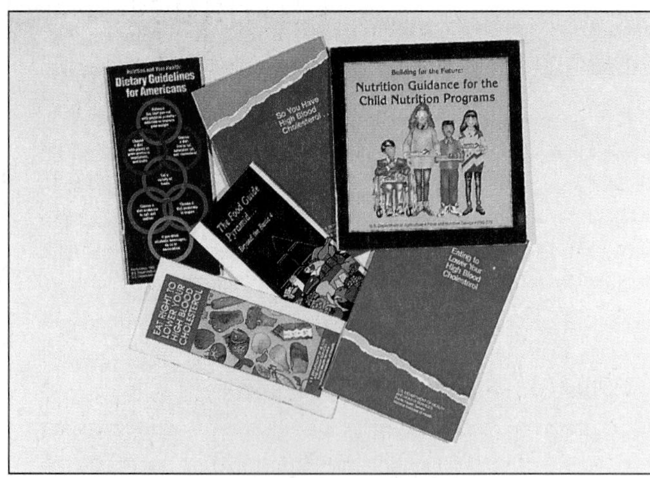

Figure 36-18. A variety of materials are available to help you teach patients about diet and nutrition.

Patient education sessions can be formal or informal and can take place at any appropriate time and place, such as in the office, over the telephone, or during a treatment or procedure. If possible, let patients decide which arrangements they prefer, or let them know the schedule in advance.

Patients need your support and empathy in working toward diet and nutrition goals, whether preventive or therapeutic. Follow these guidelines for best results when discussing diets with patients.

- Treat each patient as an individual with unique eating habits, knowledge of nutrition, and ability to learn.
- Teach a small amount of material at a time; 15- to 30-minute sessions are better than hour-long ones.
- Keep explanations at the level of the patient's understanding and vocabulary.
- Emphasize the patient's good eating behavior to reinforce it.
- Let the patient play an active role in the learning process—for example, by helping to plan the diet.
- Give the patient a written diet plan to take home, as well as any other helpful materials you have to offer.
- Suggest that the patient contact local support groups for people who are trying to maintain the same kind of diet.

Keep in mind that patient education has become increasingly important for patients receiving managed care. Managed care providers want to see documentation of preventive care in patients' charts. Failure to provide documentation can jeopardize a patient's insurance coverage.

Cultural Considerations

Eating is a personal and social activity, and cultural issues play an especially important part in diet and nutrition. A person's cultural heritage, religious background, family traditions, socioeconomic status, and personal beliefs help determine eating habits and preferences. Culture and lifestyle also help shape food purchasing and serving habits, likes and dislikes, meal timing and frequency, attitude toward food supplements, and tendency to snack.

Dietitians and nutritionists who design diets and recipes for patients know that to design successful diets, they must take into account cultural and lifestyle factors.

Table 36-7

Sources of Information About Specific Diet and Nutrition Issues

Organization	Address/Telephone Number
American Cancer Society	1599 Clifton Road NE Atlanta, GA 30329 (404) 320-3333
American Diabetes Association	National Center P.O. Box 25757 1660 Duke Street Alexandria, VA 22314 (703) 549-1500
American Dietetic Association	Suite 800 216 West Jackson Boulevard Chicago, IL 60606 (800) 366-1655 (Nutrition Hotline) (312) 899-0040 (Customer Service Ext. 5000)

continued

Table 36-7 continued

Sources of Information About Specific Diet and Nutrition Issues

Organization	Address/Telephone Number
American Heart Association	7320 Greenville Avenue Dallas, TX 75231 (214) 373-6300
Anorexia Nervosa and Related Eating Disorders, Inc.	P.O. Box 5102 Eugene, OR 97405 (541) 344-1144
National Association of Anorexia Nervosa and Associated Disorders	Box 7 Highland Park, IL 60035 (847) 831-3438
National Eating Disorders Organization	6655 South Yale Avenue Tulsa, OK 71436 (918) 481-4044
Overeaters Anonymous (OA)	P.O. Box 44020 Rio Rancho, NM 87174 (505) 891-2664

You can increase the effectiveness of your patient education if you become familiar with the food habits and beliefs common to your patients' cultural backgrounds. Learn to recognize the eating patterns belonging to different cultures, and make a special effort to familiarize yourself with the food preferences of the ethnic groups most commonly represented among the patients in the practice where you work.

Outside Resources for Patient Education

Many community health agencies and organizations offer patient education materials and information about specific diet and nutrition issues. Some of them are listed in Table 36-7. Investigate your own community to find others, and keep the information on file.

Summary

Nutrition is a complex, highly technical topic that touches people's daily lives. It is part of your job to make good nutrition understandable and achievable for patients. You will play a major role in educating patients about special diets and in helping them implement dietary changes as instructed by physicians and dietitians. Your knowledge of basic nutritional principles and current nutritional findings will help you perform these tasks with confidence and competence.

You will need a basic understanding of metabolism and the role of calories in the diet. You must also be familiar with the body's daily requirements for protein, carbohydrates, fiber, fat, vitamins, minerals, and water and which foods can fulfill these requirements. The more you learn about foods and their nutritional value, the better able you will be to educate patients about meeting their particular nutritional needs.

Whenever you work with patients, be alert for body weights significantly above or below the ideal. It is also important to recognize indications of eating patterns that may lead to health problems such as obesity, anorexia nervosa, and bulimia.

Your knowledge about nutrition will help you teach patients a major means of supporting and improving their overall health. In some cases your work in this area will help patients avoid or recover from life-threatening medical conditions.

36 Chapter Review

Discussion Questions

1. Compare and contrast the dietary guidelines described in the chapter. Name any additions you think should be made.
2. What signs might indicate that a person has an eating disorder? What should you do if a patient exhibits any of these signs?
3. What are some methods you can use to tailor your patient education about diet and nutrition to each patient's personal circumstances?

Critical Thinking Questions

1. A patient calls you, upset and concerned that her teenage daughter has decided to become a vegetarian and may not get proper nutrition. What could you say to her?
2. Keep track of all the foods you eat for 1 day. Using the Food Guide Pyramid and recommended serving sizes, place each food in a group and add up the number of servings you ate in each group. How would you rate your diet? How could you improve your diet?
3. A hypertensive patient needs to limit salt in her diet. Because of her busy and active lifestyle, however, she rarely has time to prepare fresh foods. Instead, she purchases prepackaged, processed foods. What suggestions could you offer for helping her keep her salt intake to a minimum?

Application Activities

1. Plan a well-balanced, health-promoting diet for 1 day for a 45-year-old man recently diagnosed with cardiovascular disease; do the same for a pregnant patient who is a lacto-ovo-vegetarian.
2. Have each member of the class report on the typical diet of a particular culture—Mexican, Asian, Mediterranean, Saudi, and so on. How does the diet satisfy nutritional requirements? In what areas is it outstanding or inadequate? How does the diet differ from a typical American diet?
3. Investigate and report on nutrient supplements that are not yet mainstream or are relatively new, such as garlic pills, shark cartilage, bee pollen, and ginseng. What is the nutritional composition of each? What are people trying to use them for? Why? Do most physicians agree that these supplements are beneficial or harmless? Do you agree with these physicians' assessments? Why or why not?

Further Readings

Barer-Stein, T. *You Eat What You Are: A Study of Ethnic Food Traditions.* Toronto: Culture Concepts, 1991.

Cancer Facts & Figures. Atlanta: American Cancer Society, 1992.

Eating and Exercise Disorders. Eugene, OR: Anorexia Nervosa and Related Eating Disorders, Inc., 1996.

Food Guide Pyramid Table Tents. Chicago: American Dietetic Association, 1996.

Lean Toward Health. Chicago: American Dietetic Association, 1995.

National Research Council. *Recommended Dietary Allowances.* 10th ed. Washington, DC: National Academy Press, 1989.

Nutrition and Your Health: Dietary Guidelines for Americans. 4th ed. Home and Garden Bulletin Number 232. Washington, DC: U.S. Department of Agriculture and U.S. Department of Health and Human Services, 1995.

Nutrition Fact Sheets. Chicago: American Dietetic Association, 1996.

Public Health Service. *Healthy People 2000: National Health Promotion and Disease Prevention Objectives.* DHHS Publication Number (PHS) 91-50213. Washington, DC: U.S. Department of Health and Human Services, 1991.

Toufexis, Anastasia. "The New Scoop on Vitamins." *Time,* 6 April 1992, 54–59.

Principles of Pharmacology

CHAPTER OUTLINE

- The Medical Assistant's Role in Pharmacology
- Drugs and Pharmacology
- Sources of Drugs
- The Food and Drug Administration (FDA)
- Pharmacodynamics
- Pharmacokinetics
- Pharmacotherapeutics
- Toxicology
- Sources of Drug Information
- Regulatory Function of the FDA
- Vaccines
- Patient Education About Drugs

OBJECTIVES

After completing Chapter 37, you will be able to:

- Describe the five categories of pharmacology.
- Differentiate between chemical, generic, and trade names for drugs.
- Describe the major drug categories.
- List the main sources of drug information.
- Contrast over-the-counter and prescription drugs.
- Compare the five schedules of controlled substances.
- Describe how to register a physician with the Drug Enforcement Administration (DEA) for permission to administer, dispense, and prescribe controlled drugs.
- Describe how vaccines work in the immune system.
- Identify patient education topics related to the use of nonprescription and prescription drugs.

AREAS OF COMPETENCE

1997 ROLE DELINEATION STUDY

CLINICAL

Patient Care

- Maintain medication and immunization records

GENERAL (Transdisciplinary)

Legal Concepts

- Document accurately

continued

Key Terms

absorption
administer
controlled substance
dispense
distribution
dosage
dose
efficacy
excretion
generic name
indication
labeling
narcotic
opioid
pharmaceutical
pharmacodynamics
pharmacognosy
pharmacokinetics
pharmacology
pharmacotherapeutics
prescribe
prescription
prescription drug
toxicology
trade name
vaccine

AREAS OF COMPETENCE continued

- Follow federal, state, and local legal guidelines
- Maintain awareness of federal and state health care legislation and regulations
- Maintain and dispose of regulated substances in compliance with government guidelines

Instruction

- Explain office policies and procedures

The Medical Assistant's Role in Pharmacology

You will be expected to have a basic knowledge of medications. There are increasing numbers of over-the-counter (OTC) drugs that were formerly available only with a **prescription,** a physician's written order to authorize the dispensing (and sometimes, administering) of drugs to a patient. The newly approved OTC drugs have been added to an array of drugs, many of which are available at supermarkets, that people purchase to treat themselves for ailments ranging from arthritis to colds to stomach ulcers.

As a medical assistant, you will need to be attentive to ensure that the physician is aware of all medications, both prescription and OTC, that a patient is taking. You also need to ask each patient about use of alcohol and recreational drugs (both past and present) as well as herbal remedies. You will need to educate the patient about the purpose of a drug and how to take the drug for maximum effectiveness and minimum adverse effects. As your state permits, you may also be asked to give drugs to a patient. Safe and effective drug therapy requires more of you than simply giving a drug or a prescription to a patient, however. Advanced skills that you will want to attain are described in "Tips for the Office."

To handle these important functions, you must understand pharmacologic principles, be able to translate prescriptions, and be prepared to answer basic patient questions (Figure 37-2). You must also adhere to legal requirements and keep accurate records.

Drugs and Pharmacology

A drug is a chemical compound used to prevent, diagnose, or treat a disease or other abnormal condition. The study of drugs is called **pharmacology.** A specialist in pharmacology is called a pharmacologist. Included in pharmacology are **pharmacognosy** (the study of characteristics of natural drugs and their sources), **pharmacodynamics** (the study of what drugs do to the body), **pharmacokinetics** (what the body does to drugs), **pharmacotherapeutics** (the study of how drugs are used to treat disease), and **toxicology** (the study of poisons or poisonous effects of drugs).

According to the Department of Justice's Drug Enforcement Administration (DEA) guidelines, a doctor **prescribes** a drug when he gives a patient a prescription to be filled by a pharmacy. To **administer** a drug is to give it directly by injection, by mouth, or by any other route that introduces the drug into a patient's body. A healthcare professional **dispenses** a drug by distributing it, in a properly labeled container, to a patient who is to use it.

Sources of Drugs

Many drugs originate as natural products. Many other drugs originate in the chemical laboratory, as chemists seek to improve existing drugs.

Natural Products

Most often, drugs originate as substances from natural products, such as plants, animals, minerals, bacteria, or fungi. Figure 37-3 shows examples of natural sources of drugs. A pharmacognosist is a pharmacologist who specializes in the study of the characteristics of these drugs and their sources.

Plants. Perhaps the oldest source of drugs is plants. For hundreds of years, drugs have been made from seeds, bulbs, roots, stems, buds, leaves, or other parts of plants. Two examples of plant-derived drugs are digitoxin, which comes from the foxglove plant, and quinine, which comes from cinchona tree bark. There are countless others, and new drugs are developed from plants almost daily.

Animals. Animals are also used as a source of drugs. Certain animal substances have been shown to be com-

Tips FOR THE OFFICE

Expanding Your Knowledge of Medications

In the area of patient care, the 1997 AAMA Role Delineation Chart lists drug preparation and administration as a basic skill for medical assistants. Before you can administer medications safely, you must have a full knowledge of pharmacologic principles. You must also be able to read and understand all

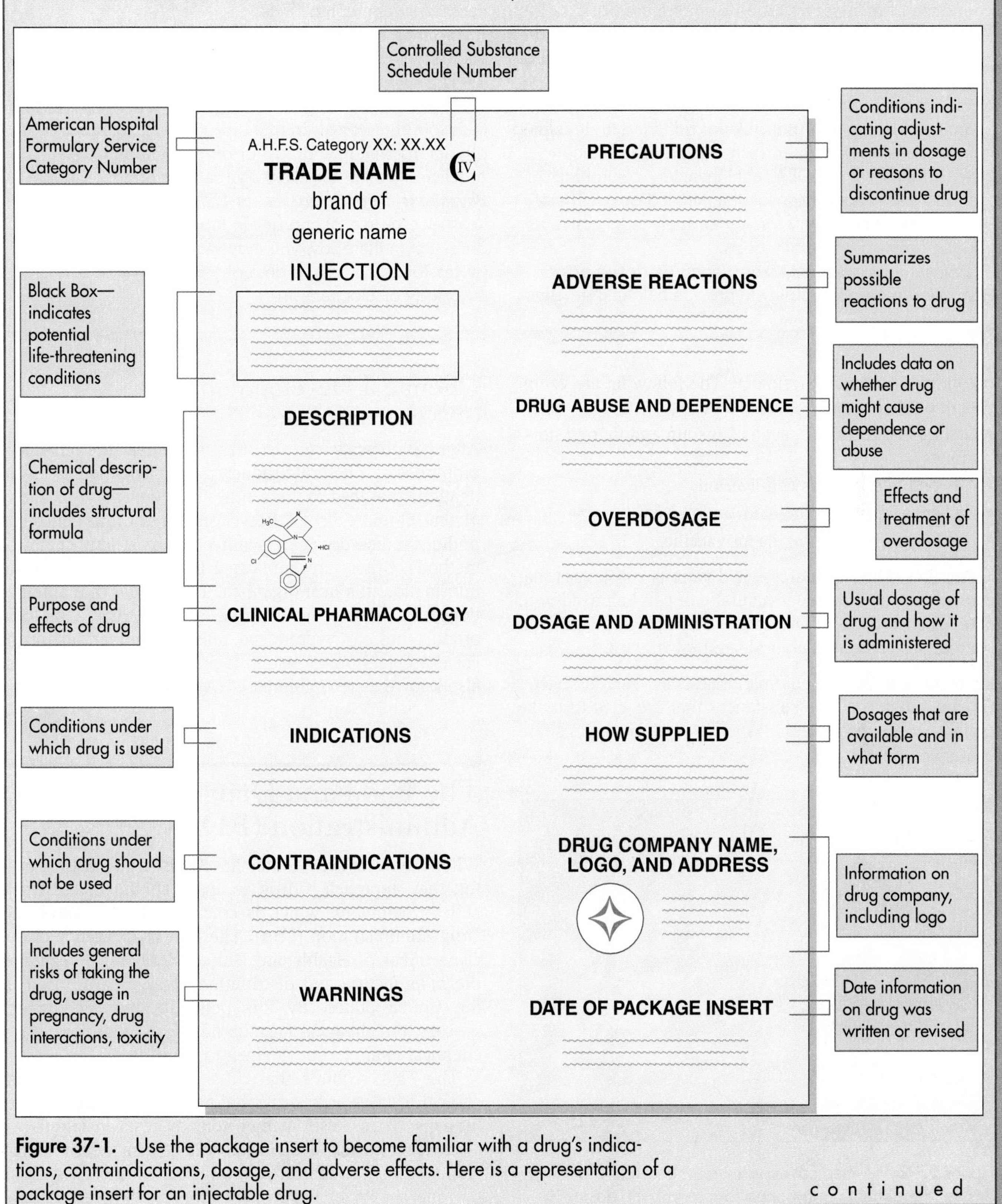

Figure 37-1. Use the package insert to become familiar with a drug's indications, contraindications, dosage, and adverse effects. Here is a representation of a package insert for an injectable drug.

continued

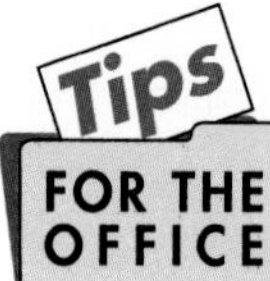

Expanding Your Knowledge of Medications continued

medical terms and abbreviations that appear on a prescription.

The Role Delineation Chart also includes the maintenance of medication records among the basic skills. You will need to use this skill whenever you record a patient's immunizations or transcribe prescription information.

Because controlled drugs are subject to many laws, you will be legally responsible for adhering to all related regulations. Laws require such activities as physician registration with the DEA, tight inventory control for drugs, and proper disposal of controlled drugs. These laws make it necessary for you to apply legal concepts to the practice on a daily basis.

Whenever a patient takes a nonprescription or prescription drug, your ability to provide helpful instructions will be vital. By educating the patient about how to use a drug properly, you will not only help the patient improve medically but also increase the probability of patient safety and compliance.

The most efficient way to prepare for all these responsibilities is to read the package inserts (see Figure 37-1) and drug labels that accompany all medications, whether they are drugs from drug company representatives (the samples given to the practice to acquaint physicians with new drugs) or drugs ordered by the practice. Another excellent source of information is the *Physicians' Desk Reference*, or *PDR*, which most practices receive free of charge. To learn more about how drugs act in the body, you may want to read articles in professional journals or do further course work in pharmacology or biochemistry.

patible with human physiology. The following are examples of animal substances used as drugs:

- Glandular substances, such as insulin and thyroid hormones
- Fats and oils, such as cod-liver oil
- Enzymes, such as pancreatin and pepsin
- Antiserums and antitoxins for vaccines

Minerals. Mineral sources yield various substances that can be used as they occur naturally or can be mixed with other substances. Two drugs derived from mineral sources are potassium chloride and mineral oil.

Bacteria and Fungi. Simple organisms, such as bacteria and fungi, produce substances that are used to make certain antibiotics. Cephalosporins and penicillins are examples.

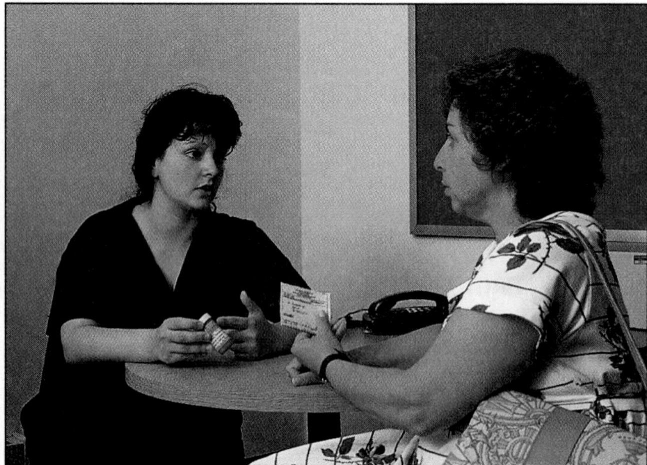

Figure 37-2. A medical assistant must be prepared to answer the patient's questions about a drug the doctor is prescribing.

Chemical Development of Natural Products

After a pharmacognosist has identified the chemical properties of a natural product, a chemist conducts investigations that lead to the synthesis (chemical duplication) of one or more drugs, based on the pharmacognosist's findings. Some drugs are synthesized by strictly chemical methods. Others are duplicated by manipulating genetic information in a host organism. These types of manipulations can cause a host organism to produce a biologic product ordinarily produced only in another organism. For example, human insulin is produced by these means, also known as recombinant DNA techniques.

The Food and Drug Administration (FDA)

When chemists believe they have a drug that will be useful, they approach a drug company for further research and development, which is controlled by the Food and Drug Administration (FDA). The FDA is an agency of the Department of Health and Human Services. It regulates the manufacture and distribution of every drug used in the United States. By this point in the development process, the chemical formula has been identified, and a chemical name has been given to the drug.

The FDA requires that drug manufacturers perform clinical tests on new drugs before the drugs are used by humans. These tests include toxicity tests in laboratory animals, followed by clinical studies (frequently called clinical trials) in controlled groups of volunteers, such as the one shown in Figure 37-4. Some volunteers are patients; others are healthy subjects.

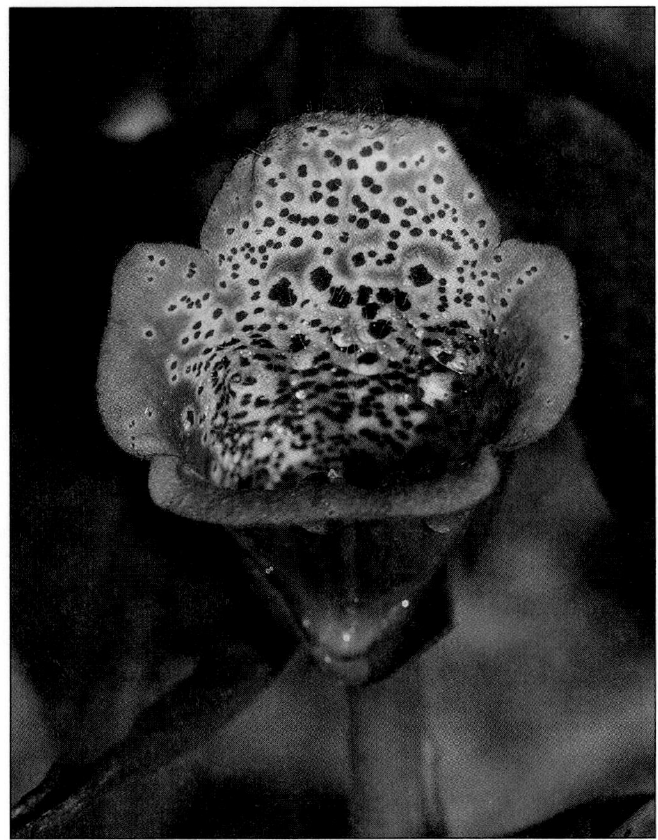

A

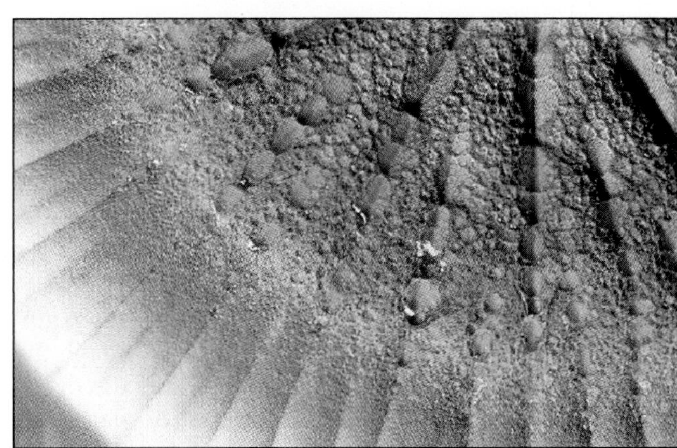

B

Figure 37-3. Many drugs originate as natural products. **A.** The foxglove plant is the source of digitoxin. **B.** Bacteria and yeasts are sources of many antibiotics.

Clinical tests are designed to consider the ratio of benefits to the risk of adverse side effects. If the clinical tests prove the drug is safe and effective, the FDA approves it for marketing. The manufacturer must continue to demonstrate the drug's safety and **efficacy** (therapeutic value) and must submit reports whenever it discovers unexpected adverse reactions. The FDA can withdraw a drug from the market at any time if evidence suggests that it is no longer safe or effective.

During the clinical trials the **pharmaceutical** (drug) company studies all aspects of the pharmacology of the new drug. When the company seeks approval from the FDA, it must document the pharmacodynamics, pharmacokinetics, safety (how many and what kind of adverse effects), and efficacy of the drug. In addition, it must present data regarding the **dose,** the amount of drug given at one time.

Pharmacodynamics

Pharmacodynamics is the study of what a drug does to the body, that is, the mechanism of action or how the drug works to produce a therapeutic effect. Pharmacodynamics includes the interaction between the drug and target cells or tissues and the body's response to that interaction.

For example, when a patient with diabetes takes insulin, the drug acts by allowing the movement of glucose across cell membranes. This movement makes the glucose available to cells to use as an energy source. The end effect is a decrease in the blood glucose level.

Pharmacokinetics

Pharmacokinetics is what the body does to a drug, that is, how the body absorbs, metabolizes, distributes, and excretes the drug. It is important to understand these processes so that you will be able to explain to patients

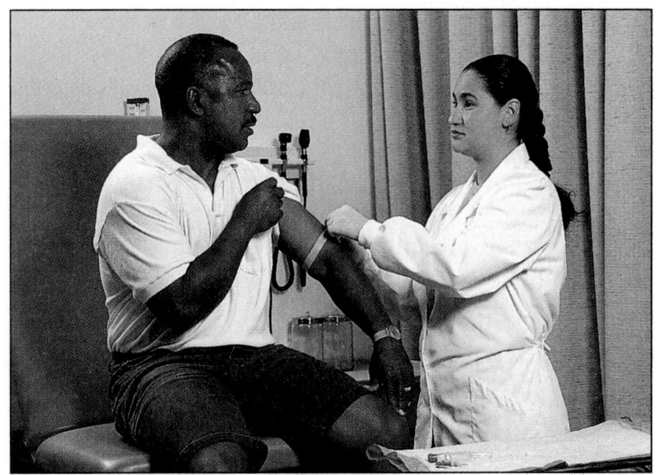

Figure 37-4. Tests such as blood tests provide baseline data on volunteers at the start of clinical trials.

the reasons for taking a particular drug with food or for drinking plenty of water while taking a drug.

Absorption

Absorption is the process of converting a drug from its dose form, such as a tablet or capsule, into a form the body can use. For example, tablets or capsules are absorbed through the stomach or intestines into the bloodstream. Water, food, or a particular food may either hinder or assist the absorption of a specific drug through the stomach or intestines. Some drugs may irritate the digestive organs if they are taken without food or water. Because of such possible reactions, patients must precisely follow instructions for taking a drug with plenty of water, with food, or without food.

Injected drugs are absorbed through the skin (intradermally), through the tissue just beneath the skin (subcutaneously), or through muscle (intramuscularly), depending on the type of injection. Absorption allows the drug to enter the bloodstream and pass into tissues. Drugs that are administered intravenously are directly available to target cells from the bloodstream.

The extent and rate of drug absorption depend on several factors. One factor is the route of administration (see Chapter 38). When the drug is administered by mouth, for example, coatings on tablets or capsules and the amount and type of food consumed with the drug may affect absorption. Other factors involve the characteristics of the drug itself. For example, insulin products vary in rate of absorption, depending on their mode of preparation.

Metabolism

Drug metabolism is the process by which drug molecules are transformed into simpler products called metabolites. This transformation usually occurs in the liver, where enzymes break down the drug. Some drugs, however, are metabolized in the kidneys. Metabolism can be affected by disease, a patient's age or genetic makeup, characteristics of the drug, or other factors.

When drugs metabolized in the liver are prescribed for either children or the elderly, the dose is likely to be lower than that prescribed for young adults. Metabolism in children and the elderly is different from metabolism in other patients; the drugs may remain in the body longer and possibly reach harmful levels. The same concern holds true for any patient with impaired liver or kidney function if prescribed drugs are metabolized in the affected organ.

Distribution

Distribution is the process of transporting a drug from its administration site, such as the muscle of an injection site, to its site of action. Distribution also pertains to the length of time a drug takes to achieve maximum or peak plasma levels, that is, the length of time between dosing and availability in the bloodstream.

Excretion

Excretion describes the manner in which a drug is eliminated from the body. Most drugs are eliminated in urine. Drugs may also be excreted in feces, perspiration, saliva, bile, exhaled air, and breast milk.

Pharmacotherapeutics

Pharmacotherapeutics is the study of how drugs are used to treat disease. This area of pharmacology is sometimes called clinical pharmacology.

Drug Names

One drug may have several different names, including the drug's official name (also known as the **generic name**), international nonproprietary name, chemical name, and **trade name** (brand or proprietary name). To demonstrate, the trade-name antibacterial drug prescribed by physicians as Keflex or Biocef is also identified by the following names:

- Cephalexin (generic name)
- Cefalexin (international nonproprietary name)
- 7-(D-α-amino-α-phenylacetomido)-3-methyl-3-cephem-4-carboxylic acid, monohydrate (chemical name)

As a medical assistant, you will probably need to use only generic or trade names. In general, think of the generic name of a drug as a simple form of its chemical name. For each new drug marketed by a drug manufacturer, the United States Adopted Names (USAN) Council selects a generic name. This name is nonproprietary; that is, it does not belong to any one manufacturer. A generic name is also considered a drug's official name, which is listed in the *United States Pharmacopeia/National Formulary.* The 50 drugs most commonly dispensed in 1996 are listed in Table 37-1 by generic name, trade name, and category of pharmacologic activity. Notice that a drug may appear in the table more than once if its dispensing record was high for multiple trade names or for generic and trade names.

A drug's trade name is selected by its manufacturer. It is protected by copyright and is the property of the manufacturer. When a new drug enters the market, its manufacturer has a patent on that drug, which means that no other manufacturer can make or sell the drug for 17 years. When the patent runs out, any manufacturer can sell the drug under the generic name or a different trade name. The original manufacturer, however, is the only one allowed to use the drug's original trade name. For example, the antibiotic cephalexin has two trade names, Keflex and Biocef. These names are owned by different manufacturers.

A physician may prescribe a drug by its generic or trade name. Because generic drugs are usually less expensive, most physicians try to prescribe them if

Table 37-1

The 50 Drugs Most Commonly Dispensed in U.S. Community Pharmacies in 1996

Generic Name	Trade Name*	Category of Pharmacologic Activity
Amoxicillin	Trimox	Antibiotic
Conjugated estrogens	Premarin Tabs	Conjugated estrogens
Levothyroxine sodium	Synthroid	Thyroid hormone
Hydrocodone bitartrate with acetaminophen	Generic (Watson)	Antitussive, analgesic, antipyretic
Ranitidine HCl	Zantac	Histamine H_2 (gastric) receptor antagonist
Fluoxetine	Prozac	Antidepressant
Enalapril maleate	Vasotec	Antihypertensive
Digoxin	Lanoxin	Cardiotonic
Nifedipine (extended release)	Procardia XL	Vasodilator
Sertraline HCl	Zoloft	Antidepressant
Warfarin sodium	Coumadin Tabs	Anticoagulant
Omeprazole	Prilosec	Gastric acid secretory depressant
Diltiazem	Cardizem CD	Vasodilator (coronary)
Amoxicillin	Amoxil	Antibiotic
Amlodipine besylate	Norvasc	Antianginal, antihypertensive
Loratadine	Claritin	Antihistamine
Furosemide	Generic (Mylan)	Diuretic
Lisinopril	Zestril	Antihypertensive
Triamterene with hydrochlorothiazide	Generic (CibaGeneva)	Diuretic
Amoxicillin with clavulanate potassium	Augmentin	Antibiotic
Clarithromycin	Biaxin	Antibiotic
Acetaminophen with codeine	Generic (Lemmon)	Analgesic
Amoxicillin	Generic (Biocraft)	Antibiotic
Azithromycin	Zithromax	Antibiotic
Simvastatin	Zocor	Antihyperlipidemic
Penicillin V potassium	Veetids	Antibiotic

continued

Table 37-1 continued

The 50 Drugs Most Commonly Dispensed in U.S. Community Pharmacies in 1996

Generic Name	Trade Name*	Category of Pharmacologic Activity
Ciprofloxacin HCl	Cipro	Antibiotic
Paroxetine HCl	Paxil	Antidepressant
Propoxyphene napsylate with acetaminophen	Generic (Mylan)	Analgesic, antipyretic
Albuterol (inhaler)	Proventil Aerosol	Bronchodilator
Tramadol HCl (tablets)	Ultram	Analgesic
Cephalexin	Generic (Biocraft)	Antibiotic
Norethindrone and ethinyl estradiol	Ortho-Novum 7/7/7	Progestin and estrogen (contraceptive)
Terazosin HCl	Hytrin	Alpha reductase inhibitor (for benign prostatic hypertrophy), antihypertensive
Lovastatin	Mevacor	Antihyperlipidemic, HMG-CoA reductase inhibitor
Albuterol (inhaler)	Generic (Warrick)	Bronchodilator
Insulin (human)	Humulin N	Antidiabetic
Phenytoin	Dilantin Kapseals	Anticonvulsant
Alprazolam	Generic (CibaGeneva)	Sedative-hypnotic
Metformin HCl	Glucophage	Antihyperglycemic
Ethinyl estradiol and levonorgestrel	Triphasil	Progestin (contraceptive)
Nabumetone	Relafen	NSAID
Potassium chloride	K-Dur 20	Replenisher (electrolyte)
Famotidine	Pepcid	Histamine H_2 (gastric) receptor antagonist
Zolpidem tartrate	Ambien	Hypnotic
Pravastatin sodium	Pravachol	Antihyperlipidemic
Fenfluramine	Pondimin	Anorexiant
Clonazepam	Klonopin	Anticonvulsant
Acetaminophen with codeine	Generic (Purepac)	Analgesic
Trimethoprim and sulfamethoxazole	Generic (Lemmon)	Antibiotic

Adapted from "The Top 200 Drugs," *American Druggist*, February 1997, 30–37.

*Many of the most commonly prescribed drugs are currently prescribed by generic name. The name of the manufacturer of a generic drug dispensed is listed in parentheses.

possible. Many states allow pharmacists to substitute a generic drug for a trade-name drug unless the physician specifies otherwise. In fact, most health insurance prescription plans now require the substitution of generic drugs for trade-name drugs (unless otherwise specified by a physician). Frequently, they also require the pharmacy to charge a higher copay amount for trade-name drugs than for generic drugs. Some prescription plans now offer a mail-in pharmacy through which a patient can obtain generic drugs with a reduced copayment or without any copayment.

Drug Categories

Drugs are categorized by their action on the body, general therapeutic effect, or the body system affected. Table 37-2 lists a variety of drug categories.

Table 37-2

Selected Drug Categories

Drug Category	Examples Generic Name (Trade Name)	Action of Drug
Analgesic	Acetaminophen (Tylenol) Acetylsalicylic acid, or aspirin Hydromorphone HCl (Dilaudid) Morphine sulfate (MS Contin) Oxycodone HCl (Percocet)	Relieves mild to severe pain
Anesthetic	Lidocaine HCl (Xylocaine) Tetracaine HCl (Pontocaine) Thiopental sodium (Pentothal Sodium)	Prevents sensation of pain (generally, locally, or topically)
Antacid	Aluminum hydroxide (Basaljel) Calcium carbonate (Tums) Magaldrate (Riopan)	Neutralizes stomach acid
Anthelmintic	Mebendazole (Vermox) Pyrantel pamoate (Combantrin, Antiminth)	Kills, paralyzes, or inhibits the growth of parasitic worms
Antiarrhythmic	Amiodarone HCl (Cordarone) Disopyramide phosphate (Norpace) Propranolol HCl (Inderal)	Normalizes heartbeat in cases of certain cardiac arrhythmias
Antibiotic	Cefaclor (Ceclor) Erythromycin (E-Mycin) Penicillin V potassium (Pen Vee K) Tetracycline HCl (Tetracap) Vancomycin HCl (Vancocin)	Kills microorganisms or inhibits or prevents their growth
Anticholinergic	Atropine sulfate (Isopto Atropine) Diclomine HCl (Bentyl) Scopolamine (Transderm-Scōp)	Blocks parasympathetic nerve impulses
Anticoagulant	Enoxaparin sodium (Lovenox) Heparin sodium (Hep-Lock) Warfarin sodium (Coumadin)	Prevents blood from clotting

continued

Table 37-2 continued

Selected Drug Categories

Drug Category	Examples Generic Name (Trade Name)	Action of Drug
Anticonvulsant	Clonazepam (Klonopin) Phenobarbital sodium (Luminol Sodium) Phenytoin (Dilantin) Primidone (Mysoline)	Relieves or controls seizures (convulsions)
Antidepressant (three types)		Relieves depression
Tricyclic	Amitriptyline HCl (Elavil) Doxepin HCl (Sinequan)	
Monoamine oxidase (MAO) inhibitors	Phenelzine sulfate (Nardil) Tranylcypromine sulfate (Parnate)	
Selective serotonin reuptake inhibitors (SSRIs)	Fluoxetine HCl (Prozac) Sertraline HCl (Zoloft)	
Antidiarrheal	Kaolin and pectin mixtures (Kaopectate) Loperamide HCl (Imodium) Tincture of opium (Paregoric)	Relieves diarrhea
Antidote	Acetylcysteine (Mucosil) for acetaminophen (Tylenol) Flumazenil (Romazicon) for benzodiazepines, such as diazepam (Valium) or alprazolam (Xanax) Naloxone HCl (Narcan) for narcotics, such as morphine	Counteracts action of specific drug class
Antiemetic	Dimenhydrinate (Dramamine) Prochlorperazine (Compazine) Trimethobenzamide HCl (Tigan)	Prevents or relieves nausea and vomiting
Antifungal	Amphotericin B (Fungizone) Griseofulvin (Grisactin) Nystatin (Mycostatin)	Kills or inhibits growth of fungi
Antihistamine	Cetirizine HCl (Zyrtec) Chlorpheniramine maleate (Chlor-Trimeton) Diphenhydramine HCl (Benadryl) Loratadine (Claritin) Terfenadine (Seldane)	Counteracts effects of histamine and relieves allergic symptoms
Antihypertensive	Atenolol (Tenormin) Doxazosin mesylate (Cardura) Methyldopa (Aldomet)	Reduces blood pressure

continued

Table 37-2 continued

Selected Drug Categories

Drug Category	Examples Generic Name (Trade Name)	Action of Drug
Anti-inflammatory (two types)		Reduces inflammation
Nonsteroidal (NSAIDs)	Ibuprofen (Advil) Ketoprofen (Orudis) Naproxen (Naprosyn)	
Steroids	Dexamethasone (Decadron) Methylprednisolone (Medrol) Prednisone (Deltasone)	
Antineoplastic	Dactinomycin (Cosmegen) Bleomycin sulfate (Blenoxane) Paclitaxel (Taxol) Tamoxifen citrate (Nolvadex)	Poisons cancerous cells
Antipsychotic	Chlorpromazine HCl (Thorazine) Clozapine (Clozaril) Haloperidol (Haldol) Risperidone (Risperdal) Thioridazine HCl (Mellaril)	Controls psychotic symptoms
Antipyretic	Acetaminophen (Tylenol) Acetylsalicylic acid, or aspirin	Reduces fever
Antiseptic	Isopropyl alcohol, 70% Povidone-iodine (Betadine)	Inhibits growth of microorganisms
Antitussive	Codeine Dextromethorphan hydrobromide (component of Robitussin DM)	Inhibits cough reflex
Bronchodilator	Albuterol (Proventil) Epinephrine (Epinephrine Mist) Isoproterenol HCl (Isuprel)	Dilates bronchi (airways in the lungs)
Cathartic (laxative)	Bisacodyl (Dulcolax) Magnesium hydroxide (Milk of Magnesia) Casanthranol (Peri-Colace)	Induces defecation, alleviates constipation
Contraceptive	Ethinyl estradiol and norgestimate (Ortho Cyclen) Norethindrone and ethinyl estradiol (Ortho-Novum) Norgestrel (Ovrette)	Reduces risk of pregnancy

continued

Table 37-2 continued

Selected Drug Categories

Drug Category	Examples Generic Name (Trade Name)	Action of Drug
Decongestant	Oxymetazoline HCl (Afrin) Phenylephrine HCl (Neo-Synephrine) Pseudoephedrine HCl (Sudafed)	Relieves nasal swelling and congestion
Diuretic	Hydrochlorothiazide (Hydrodiuril) Furosemide (Lasix) Mannitol	Increases urine output, reduces blood pressure and cardiac output
Emetic	Syrup of ipecac (Ipecac Syrup)	Induces vomiting
Expectorant	Guaifenesin (component of Robitussin) Terpin hydrate	Liquefies mucus in bronchi; allows expectoration of sputum, mucus, and phlegm
Hemostatic	Thrombin (Thrombogen) Phytonadione or vitamin K_1 (Mephyton)	Controls or stops bleeding by promoting coagulation
Hormone replacement	Insulin (Humulin) for pancreatic deficiency Hydrocortisone (Hydrocortone Acetate) for adrenocortical deficiency Levothyroxine sodium (Synthroid) for thyroid deficiency	Replaces or resolves hormone deficiency
Hypnotic (sleep-inducing) or sedative	Chloral hydrate (Noctec) Ethchlorvynol (Placidyl) Secobarbital sodium (Seconal Sodium)	Induces sleep or relaxation (depending on drug potency and dosage)
Muscle relaxant	Carisoprodol (Rela or Soma) Cyclobenzaprine HCl (Flexeril)	Relaxes skeletal muscles
Mydriatic	Atropine sulfate (Allergan) for ophthalmic use Phenylephrine HCl (Alcon Efrin) for ophthalmic use or (Neo-Synephrine HCl) for nasal use	Constricts vessels of eye or nasal passage, raises blood pressure, dilates pupil of eye in ophthalmic preparations
Stimulant	Amphetamine sulfate (Benzadrine) for central nervous system Caffeine (No-Doz) for central nervous system; also component of many analgesic formulations and coffee	Increases activity of brain and other organs, decreases appetite

continued

Table 37-2 continued

Selected Drug Categories

Drug Category	Examples Generic Name (Trade Name)	Action of Drug
Vasoconstrictor	Dopamine HCl (Intropin) Norepinephrine bitartrate (Levophed)	Constricts blood vessels, increases blood pressure
Vasodilator	Isosorbide mononitrate (Monoket) Nitroglycerin (Nitrostat) Reserpine (Serpasil); also component of other drugs	Dilates blood vessels, decreases blood pressure

Sources: Physicians' Desk Reference; U.S. Pharmacopeia Dictionary.
Note: Some drugs have a secondary category. When in doubt, check the *Physicians' Desk Reference* or *U.S. Pharmacopeia Dictionary.*

Indications and Labeling

An **indication** is the purpose or reason for using a drug. FDA-approved indications are part of a drug's **labeling.** Labeling also includes the form of the drug, such as tablet or liquid.

Regardless of category, some drugs may be used to treat several different conditions. Multiple uses are possible if the drug affects several body systems at once or if the drug's primary effect produces significant secondary effects in other body systems.

When a drug is used for multiple indications, one or more indications may not be in its labeling. Out-of-label prescribing is legal. Doctors who do it usually know from continuing education (seminars or journal articles) that such uses are generally accepted. For example, Benadryl (diphenhydramine) is an antihistamine used to treat allergic symptoms in both children and adults. Because it tends to make a patient sleepy but is safe for children, a pediatrician may use a low dose of Benadryl as a temporary sedative for a young child. Its use as a sedative, however, is not part of the labeling for Benadryl.

Another example of a drug with multiple uses is minoxidil. As a trade-name tablet, it is known as the antihypertensive Loniten; as a trade-name topical solution, it is known as the hair-growth stimulant Rogaine. In the case of minoxidil, both indications are approved, but the tablet labeling is for hypertension and the topical solution labeling is for hair growth.

It is important to be aware of these labeling considerations when dealing with questions from patients. Never assume that a drug is appropriate for only one use or that it is administered in only one form. Always consult the doctor or other sources of drug information before answering a patient's question.

Safety

The safety of a drug is determined by how many and what kinds of adverse effects are associated with it. An adverse effect may require immediate attention. It is not uncommon for a patient to call the physician's office with complaints of new symptoms soon after beginning therapy with a drug. Be alert for such complaints, because they could be signs of an adverse reaction to the drug or an interaction with another medication. These calls should be brought to the physician's attention. Some adverse effects are common whereas others are rare.

Efficacy

A patient may complain that a newly prescribed drug is not doing what the doctor said it would. There are a variety of explanations for such a complaint, including the following.

- The drug is working adequately, but the patient does not understand how it works.
- The **dosage** (size, frequency, and number of doses) needs to be adjusted.
- The drug has not yet reached a therapeutic level in the bloodstream.
- The wrong drug was prescribed, or the wrong drug was dispensed by the pharmacy (this is rare, but possible).
- Some drugs work better in some patients than in others; not every drug is for everyone (this is particularly true of antihistamines).
- Some forms of a drug work better than others, such as tablets versus injection.
- The generic drug does not work, but the trade-name drug does.

Kinds of Therapy

There are several descriptive terms for drug therapy. Depending on a patient's condition, the physician may use drugs for any of the following kinds of therapy:

- Acute: Drug is prescribed to improve a life-threatening or serious condition, such as epinephrine for severe allergic reaction.
- Empiric: Drug is prescribed according to experience or observation until blood or other tests prove another therapy to be appropriate, such as penicillin for suspected strep throat.
- Maintenance: Drug is prescribed to maintain a condition of health, especially in chronic disease, such as insulin for diabetes mellitus.
- Palliative: Drug is prescribed to reduce the severity of a condition or its accompanying pain, such as morphine for cancer.
- Prophylactic: Drug is prescribed to prevent a disease or condition, such as immunizations or birth control drugs.
- Replacement: Drug is prescribed to provide chemicals otherwise missing in a patient, such as hormone replacement therapy for a woman in menopause.
- Supportive: Drug is prescribed for a condition other than the primary disease until that disease resolves, such as a corticosteroid for severe allergic reactions.
- Supplemental: Drug or nutrients are prescribed to avoid deficiency, such as iron for a woman who is pregnant.

Toxicology

Toxicology is the study of the poisonous effects, or toxicity, of drugs, including adverse effects and drug interactions. Because you are likely to see evidence of only immediate toxic effects when administering a drug, this topic will be discussed in more detail in Chapter 38. You must be aware, however, of some possible toxic effects that may not be apparent right away:

- An adverse effect on a fetus when the drug crosses the placenta
- An adverse effect on infants when the drug passes easily into breast milk
- Adverse reactions reported in clinical trials, such as headache, drowsiness, gastric upset, or other effects
- An adverse effect in immunocompromised patients who are unable to metabolize a drug normally
- An adverse effect in pediatric or elderly patients or in patients with hypertension, diabetes mellitus, or other serious chronic conditions
- An adverse drug interaction when the drug is taken with another drug that is incompatible
- A carcinogenic (cancer-causing) effect in some patients

Nearly always, an adverse effect has been encountered in the clinical trials of a drug, and there will be mention of the adverse effect under that heading in the package insert or in accepted drug reference works. In the reports of clinical trials, however, the drug company must report *all* adverse effects noted during testing. As a result, effects that, at least theoretically, could not be caused by the drug are included. In dealing with patients who are about to begin drug therapy, it is best to avoid mentioning specific adverse effects associated with drugs. To do so could cause undue alarm, prompt patients to imagine they have the effects, or discourage patients from taking the needed medication. Always ask patients if they have any questions, and have the doctor answer patients' questions if they are drug-related. Because patients will receive lists of adverse effects from the pharmacist, encourage them to discuss concerns with the pharmacist or to call the doctor's office. Also encourage patients to inform the doctor of adverse effects they experience after beginning drug therapy.

Sources of Drug Information

It is important to keep several up-to-date sources of drug information in the office for when you or the doctor need detailed information about a specific drug. Sources to refer to include the *Physicians' Desk Reference* (Figure 37-5), *Drug Evaluations, United States Pharmacopeia/National Formulary,* and *American Hospital Formulary Service.*

Physicians' Desk Reference (PDR)

Medical Economics, Inc., of Oradell, New Jersey, publishes the *Physicians' Desk Reference,* or *PDR,* annually, along with supplements twice a year. It sends the book free to doctors' offices and sells it through bookstores. The company also publishes separate editions for generic, nonprescription, and ophthalmologic drugs, as well as a guide to drug interactions, adverse effects, and indications.

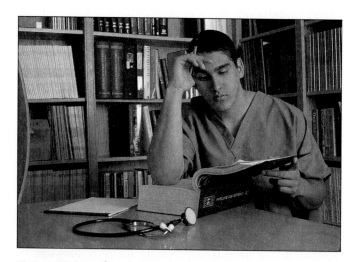

Figure 37-5. The *Physicians' Desk Reference* is one of several publications in which you can find current information on specific drugs.

The *PDR* presents information provided by pharmaceutical companies about more than 2500 prescription drugs. The *PDR* has color-coded directories of drug categories, generic names, and trade names. It also lists the names, addresses, emergency telephone numbers, and products available from each of the pharmaceutical companies.

The drug information section is divided according to manufacturer, and the drugs are then grouped alphabetically within each manufacturer's subsection. The information closely resembles that on drug package inserts, which are illustrated in "Tips for the Office." The package insert for each drug describes the drug, its purpose and effects (clinical pharmacology), indications, contraindications (conditions under which the drug should not be administered), warnings, precautions, adverse reactions, drug abuse and dependence, overdosage, dosage and administration, and how the drug is supplied (for example, tablets in different doses, liquid). Also included in this section are diagnostic compounds made by the drug companies.

A separate section is devoted to color photographs of common drugs in various forms, also grouped by manufacturer. Other sections on Poison Control Centers, controlled substances, and the system for reporting adverse reactions to vaccines could be important resources for you.

Drug Evaluations

Drug Evaluations is published once a year by the American Medical Association. It contains detailed information on more than 1000 drugs, including their names, efficacy, adverse reactions, and precautions.

United States Pharmacopeia/ National Formulary

The *United States Pharmacopeia/National Formulary,* or *USP/NF,* is the official source of drug standards in the United States and is published about every 5 years. By law, every drug sold under a name listed in the *USP/NF* must meet the strict standards of the *USP/NF.*

The *USP/NF* describes each drug approved by the federal government and lists its standards for purity, composition, and strength, as well as its uses, dosages, and storage. The *NF* portion of the book provides the chemical formulas of the drugs.

American Hospital Formulary Service (AHFS)

The American Society of Hospital Pharmacists in Bethesda, Maryland, publishes the *American Hospital Formulary Service,* or *AHFS.* It sells the two-volume set by subscription and provides four to six supplements each year. The *AHFS* lists generic names and is divided into sections based on drug actions.

Regulatory Function of the FDA

After the FDA approves a drug, it continues its regulatory function to protect patients and consumers. The FDA reviews new-indication proposals (applications from companies for new indications for a drug), OTC proposals (applications for OTC status of a prescription drug), and further clinical trial results. If an adverse effect appears many times, for example, the FDA may withdraw the causative drug from the market.

Drug Manufacturing

The FDA also regulates drug manufacturing. It ensures that drugs shipped between states have the proper identity, strength, purity, and quality. Each manufacturer must consistently identify each drug by a particular color, form, shape, size, and label. It must produce every dose at the same tested strength, using the exact formula approved by the FDA. The manufacturer must also use high-quality, contaminant-free ingredients.

Nonprescription, or Over-the-Counter, Drugs

A nonprescription, or over-the-counter (OTC), drug is one that the FDA has approved for use without the supervision of a licensed health-care practitioner. The consumer must follow the manufacturer's directions to use the drug safely. Some OTC drugs, such as aspirin and vitamin supplements, have been OTC drugs for many years. The number of prescription drugs that have been granted OTC status is increasing. Although OTC drugs are safe when used as directed on the package, patient education contributes significantly to their safe use.

Prescription Drugs

A **prescription drug** is one that can be used only by order of a physician and must be dispensed by a licensed health-care professional, such as a pharmacist, physician, podiatrist, or licensed midwife. Some prescription drugs are dispensed as over-the-counter medications at much lower dosages.

Controlled Substances

A **controlled substance** is a drug or drug product that is categorized as potentially dangerous and addictive. The greater the potential, the more severe the limitations on prescribing it. Use of these controlled drugs is strictly regulated by federal laws. States, municipalities, and institutions must adhere to these laws but may also impose their own regulations.

Comprehensive Drug Abuse Prevention and Control Act. The Comprehensive Drug Abuse Prevention and Control Act, also known as the Controlled Substances Act (CSA) of 1970, is the federal law that created the Drug Enforcement Administration (DEA) and strengthened drug enforcement authority. The CSA designates five schedules, according to degree of potential for a substance to be abused or used for a nontherapeutic effect. The five schedules and examples of substances in each are outlined in Table 37-3.

Drugs that are Schedule I substances have a high abuse potential or pose unacceptable dangers. In the United States these drugs are legal only for research. Doctors are not allowed to prescribe these drugs, which include heroin, LSD, marijuana, and peyote.

Drugs that are Schedule II substances have a high potential for abuse and may cause physical or psychological dependence. They do have therapeutic uses, however, for which they require written prescriptions. Prescriptions for these drugs may not be renewed. Examples of these drugs include dextroamphetamines (Dexedrine), secobarbital (Seconal), and opioids. **Opioids** are natural or synthetic drugs that produce opiumlike effects, such as codeine, morphine, and meperidine (Demerol). Government agencies use the popular term **narcotics** for opioids.

Drugs that are Schedule III substances have a lower abuse potential than drugs that are Schedule I or II substances and may cause moderate-to-low physical or psychological dependence. Prescriptions for these drugs may be given orally or in writing. Prescriptions may include refills, but refills are limited to five refills within 6 months of the original prescription. Benzphetamine (Didrex), butabarbital (Butisol), and methyltestosterone (Virilon) are examples of Schedule III drugs. Some drugs can belong to both Schedules II and III, depending on strength per tablet or capsule.

Drugs that are Schedule IV substances have a lower abuse potential than drugs that are Schedule III substances and have various therapeutic uses. Prescriptions may include refills, but refills are limited to five refills within 6 months of the original prescription. These drugs include pentazocine (Talwin), fenfluramine, and diazepam (Valium).

Drugs that are Schedule V substances have a lower abuse potential than drugs that are Schedule IV substances and have varied therapeutic uses. Most Schedule V drugs are dispensed like other nonopioid prescription drugs, but some may be dispensed without a prescription, depending on state regulations. Most of these drugs are antidiarrheals or antitussives that contain small amounts of opioids, such as codeine, dihydrocodeine, or diphenoxylate.

Sometimes the DEA reclassifies drugs. For example, a Schedule III drug may eventually be found to be less addictive than originally determined and therefore reclassified as a Schedule IV drug.

Controlled Substance Labeling. The Controlled Substances Act also set up a labeling system to identify controlled substances. An example of this label is shown in Figure 37-6. The large C means that the drug is a controlled substance, and the Roman numeral inside the C corresponds to the DEA schedule to which the drug belongs.

Doctor Registration. Under the CSA, doctors who administer, dispense, or prescribe any controlled substance must register with the DEA and must have a current state license to practice medicine and, if required, a state controlled substance license. They must also comply with all aspects of the CSA, as outlined in Procedure 37-1.

To register the doctor with the DEA, submit DEA Form-224 (Figure 37-7), called the Application for Regis-

Table 37-3

Schedules of Controlled Substances

Schedule	Abuse Potential	Examples
I	High	Heroin, LSD, methaqualone
II	High	Amphetamines, codeine, meperidine, morphine, secobarbital
III	Lower than Schedule II	Benzphetamine, butabarbital, methyltestosterone, talbutal
IV	Lower than Schedule III	Some benzodiazepines, chloral hydrate, fenfluramine, pentazocine
V	Lower than Schedule IV	Antitussives or antidiarrheals that combine small amounts of opioids (narcotics), such as codeine, dihydrocodeine, or diphenoxylate, with other drugs

Source: U.S. Department of Justice, *Physician's Manual,* March 1990.

tration Under Controlled Substances Act of 1970. Send the form and the appropriate fee to the Drug Enforcement Administration, Registration Unit, Central Station, P.O. Box 28083, Washington, DC 20038-8083, or the nearest regional office. This registration must be renewed every 3 years, with DEA Form-224a. The renewal steps are outlined in Procedure 37-2. The DEA should automatically send this form to the doctor's office at least 45 days before the renewal is due.

Doctors who administer or dispense drugs at more than one office must register at each location. Each registration is assigned a unique number, which identifies to suppliers and pharmacies that the doctor is properly authorized.

Ordering Drugs That Are Controlled Substances. A doctor who needs Schedule II drugs for the practice must order them by using the U.S. Official Order Forms–Schedules I & II (DEA Form-222), which you can obtain from the DEA (Figure 37-8). (DEA Form-222 is also used by research facilities such as pharmaceutical laboratories to order Schedule I drugs for research purposes; medicinal uses are not approved for Schedule I drugs.) One copy of the form goes to the DEA for overall surveillance of drug distribution. In most states this form can be used to obtain Schedule II drugs from the normal drug supplier.

When Schedule II drugs are ordered from an out-of-state company, some states require the doctor to send a copy of the purchase agreement (not the DEA Form-222) to the state attorney general's office within 24 hours of placing the order.

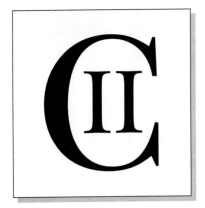

Figure 37-6. This symbol indicates that the drug is a Schedule II controlled substance.

Schedules III through V drugs require less complicated ordering. They require only the doctor's DEA registration number.

Drug Security. Always store drugs that are controlled substances in a locked cabinet or safe. If required by state law, use double locks for opioids. The doctor should keep the key(s) at all times, except when asking you to add to or take from the stock (if this is a task medical assistants are permitted to perform in your state). If controlled drugs are stolen from the doctor's

PROCEDURE 37-1

Helping the Physician Comply With the Controlled Substances Act of 1970

Objective: To comply with the Controlled Substances Act of 1970

OSHA Guidelines: This procedure does not involve exposure to blood, body fluids, or tissues.

Materials: DEA Form-224, DEA Form-222, DEA Form-41, pen

Method

1. Use DEA Form-224 (shown in Figure 37-7) to register the physician with the Drug Enforcement Administration. Be sure to register each office location where the physician administers or dispenses drugs in Schedules II through V. Renew all registrations every 3 years using DEA Form-224a.
2. Order Schedule II drugs using DEA Form-222, shown in Figure 37-8, as instructed by the physician. (Stocks of these drugs should be kept to a minimum.)
3. Include the physician's DEA registration number on every prescription for a drug in Schedules II through V.
4. Complete an inventory of all drugs in Schedules II through V every 2 years (as permitted in your state; this task may be reserved to other health-care professionals).
5. Store all drugs in Schedules II through V in a secure, locked safe or cabinet (as permitted in your state).
6. Keep accurate dispensing and inventory records for at least 2 years.
7. Dispose of expired or unused drugs according to the DEA regulations. Always complete DEA Form-41 (shown in Figure 37-9) when disposing of controlled drugs.

continued

DEA Form -224 (Aug 1994) OMB No. 1117-0014

APPLICATION FOR REGISTRATION
UNDER
CONTROLLED SUBSTANCES ACT OF 1970

Please **PRINT** or **TYPE** all entries.

No registration may be issued unless a completed application form has been received (21 CFR 1301.32).

Name (Last, First, Middle)

Proposed Business Address

City State Zip Code

DRUG ENFORCEMENT ADMINISTRATION
CENTRAL STATION
P.O. BOX 28083
WASHINGTON, D.C. 20038 – 8083
For **INFORMATION,** Call: **(202) 307 – 7255**

See "Privacy Act" information on reverse.

THIS BLOCK FOR DEA USE ONLY

REGISTRATION CLASSIFICATION: Submit Check or Money Order Payable to the **Drug Enforcement Administration** in amount indicated on enclosed fee schedule (3 year registration period).

• FEE MUST ACCOMPANY APPLICATION

1. BUSINESS ACTIVITY: (Check one box only)
   A ☐ Retail Pharmacy B ☐ Hospital/Clinic C ☐ Practitioner ________ *(Specify Medical Degree, e.g., DDS, DO, DVM, MD, NP, PA, etc.)* D ☐ Teaching Institution (Instructional purposes only)

2. SCHEDULES: (Check all applicable schedules in which you intend to handle controlled substances. See Schedules on Reverse of Instruction Sheet.)
   Schedule II ☐ Narcotic Schedule II ☐ Nonnarcotic Schedule III ☐ Narcotic Schedule III ☐ Nonnarcotic Schedule IV ☐ Schedule V ☐

3. ☐ CHECK HERE IF YOU REQUIRE ORDER FORMS.

4. **ALL APPLICANTS MUST ANSWER THE FOLLOWING:**
   (a) Are you currently authorized to prescribe, distribute, dispense, conduct research, or otherwise handle the controlled substances in the schedules for which you are applying, under the laws of the State or jurisdiction in which you are operating or propose to operate?
   ☐ YES – State License No. ________ ☐ NOT APPLICABLE ☐ PENDING
   ☐ YES – State Controlled Substance No. ________ ☐ NOT APPLICABLE ☐ PENDING
   (b) Has the applicant ever been convicted of a crime in connection with controlled substances under State or Federal law?
   ☐ YES ☐ NO
   (c) Has the applicant ever surrendered or had a Federal controlled substance registration revoked, suspended, restricted, or denied?
   ☐ YES ☐ NO
   (d) Has the applicant ever had a State professional license or controlled substance registration revoked, suspended, denied, restricted, or placed on probation?
   ☐ YES ☐ NO
   (e) If the applicant is a corporation (other than a corporation whose stock is owned and traded by the public), association, partnership, or pharmacy, has any officer, partner, stockholder or proprietor been convicted of a crime in connection with controlled substances under State or Federal law, or ever surrendered or had a Federal controlled substance registration revoked, suspended, restricted or denied, or ever had a State professional license or controlled substance registration revoked, suspended, denied, restricted, or placed on probation?
   ☐ YES ☐ NO ☐ NOT APPLICABLE

IF THE ANSWER TO QUESTION(S) (b), (c), (d), or (e) is YES, include a statement using the space provided on the REVERSE of this part.

Print or Type Name Here – Sign Below ________ Applicant's Business Phone No. ________

SIGN HERE ➤ Signature of applicant or authorized individual ________ Date ________

Title (If the applicant is a corporation, institution, or other entity, enter the TITLE of the person signing on behalf of the applicant (e.g., President, Dean, Procurement Officer, etc....))

5. CERTIFICATION FOR FEE EXEMPTION

☐ CHECK THIS BLOCK IF APPLICANT HEREON IS A FEDERAL, STATE, OR LOCAL GOVERNMENT OPERATED HOSPITAL OR INSTITUTION.

Practitioners cannot be exempted from payment of the fee. The undersigned hereby certifies that the applicant named hereon is a Federal, state, or local government operated hospital or institution, and is exempt from the payment of the application fee.

Signature of Certifying Official ________ Date ________

Print or Type Name ________

Print or Type Title ________

WARNING: **Section 843(a)(4) of Title 21, United States Code, states that any person who knowingly or intentionally furnishes false or fraudulent information in this application is subject to imprisonment for not more than four years, a fine of not more than $30,000.00 or both.**

Mail the Original and 1 copy with FEE to the above address. Retain 3rd copy for your records. **FEES ARE NOT REFUNDABLE.**

VOID

Figure 37-7. DEA Form-224 must be completed to register the physician with the Drug Enforcement Administration.

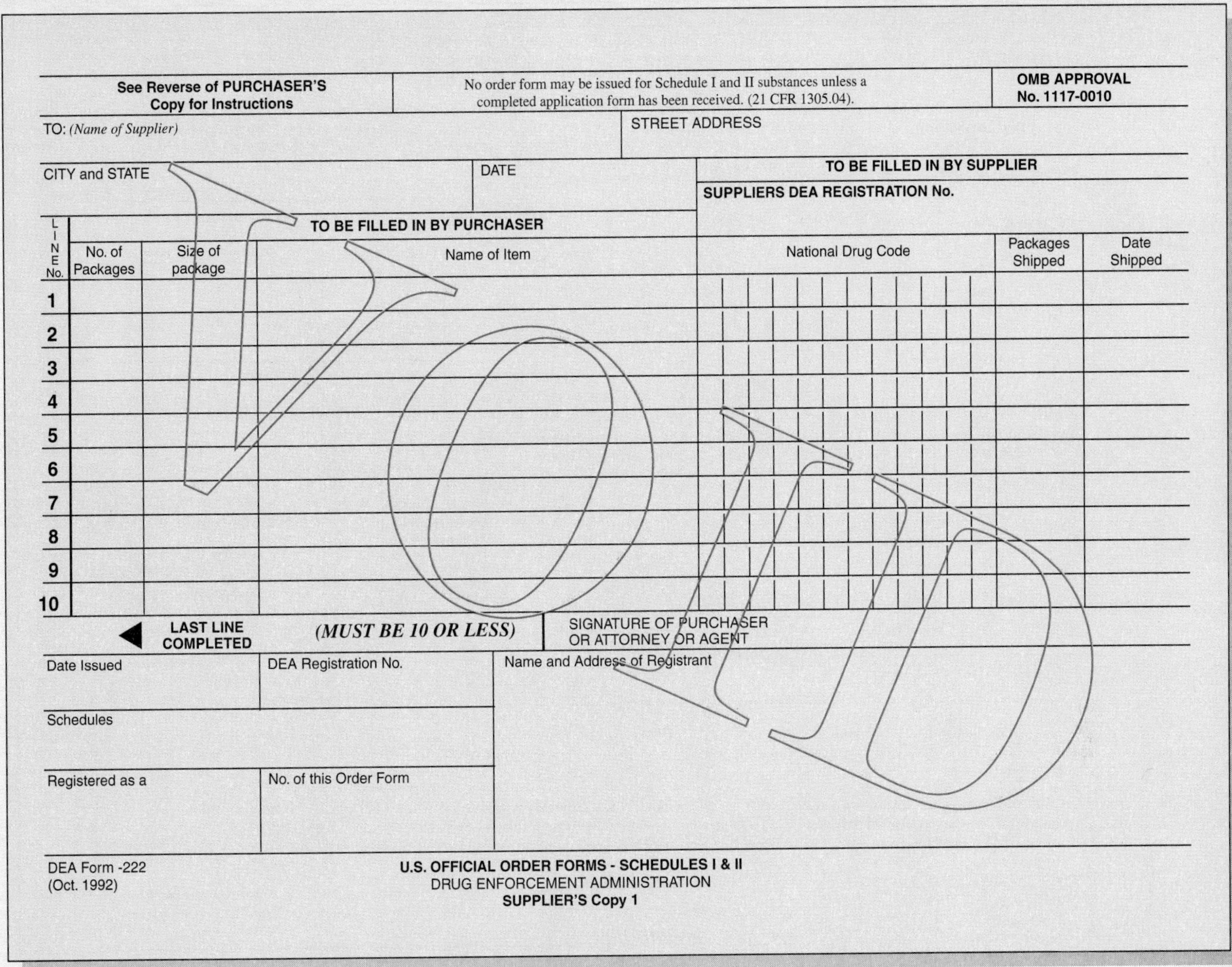

See Reverse of PURCHASER'S Copy for Instructions

No order form may be issued for Schedule I and II substances unless a completed application form has been received. (21 CFR 1305.04).

OMB APPROVAL No. 1117-0010

TO: *(Name of Supplier)*

STREET ADDRESS

CITY and STATE

DATE

TO BE FILLED IN BY SUPPLIER

SUPPLIERS DEA REGISTRATION No.

TO BE FILLED IN BY PURCHASER

LINE No.	No. of Packages	Size of package	Name of Item	National Drug Code	Packages Shipped	Date Shipped
1						
2						
3						
4						
5						
6						
7						
8						
9						
10						

◀ **LAST LINE COMPLETED** ***(MUST BE 10 OR LESS)***

SIGNATURE OF PURCHASER OR ATTORNEY OR AGENT

Date Issued

DEA Registration No.

Name and Address of Registrant

Schedules

Registered as a

No. of this Order Form

DEA Form -222 (Oct. 1992)

U.S. OFFICIAL ORDER FORMS - SCHEDULES I & II
DRUG ENFORCEMENT ADMINISTRATION
SUPPLIER'S Copy 1

VOID

Figure 37-8. Use DEA Form-222 to order Schedule II drugs.

continued

OMB Approval No. 1117-0007	DEPARTMENT OF JUSTICE/DRUG ENFORCEMENT ADMINISTRATION REGISTRANTS INVENTORY OF DRUGS SURRENDERED	PACKAGE No.

The following schedule is an inventory of controlled substances which is hereby surrendered to you for proper disposition.

FROM: *(Include Name, Street, City, State and ZIP Code in space provided below).*

Signature of applicant or authorized agent

Registrant's DEA Number

Registrant's Telephone Number

NOTE: CERTIFIED MAIL (Return Receipt Requested) IS REQUIRED FOR SHIPMENTS OF DRUGS VIA U.S. POSTAL SERVICE: See instructions on reverse of form.

NAME OF DRUG OF PREPARATION **Registrants will fill in Columns 1, 2, 3, and 4 Only.**	Number of Containers	CONTENTS *(Number of grams, tablets, ounces or other units per container)*	Controlled Substance Content *(Each Unit)*	**FOR DEA USE ONLY**		
				DISPOSITION	QUANTITY	
					GMS.	MGS.
1	*2*	*3*	*4*	*5*	*6*	*7*
1						
2						

The controlled substances surrendered in accordance with Title 21 of the Code of Federal Regulations, Section 1307.21, have been received in _______packages purporting to contain the drugs listed on this inventory and have been: **(1) Forwarded tape-sealed without opening; (2) Destroyed as indicated and the remainder forwarded tape-sealed after verifying contents; (3) Forwarded tape-sealed after verifying

DATE: _______________ **19** _____ **DESTROYED BY:** ______________________

••*Strike out lines not applicable* **WITNESSED BY:** ______________________

INSTRUCTIONS

1. List the name of the drug in column 1, the number of containers in column 2, the size of each container in column 3, and in column 4 the controlled substance content of each unit described in column 3; e.g., morphine sulfate tabs., 3 pkgs., 100 tabs., 1/4 gr. (16 mg.) or morphine sulfate tabs., 1 pkg., 83 tabs., 1/2 gr. (32 mg.), etc.
2. All packages included on a single line should be identical in name, content and controlled substance strength.
3. Prepare this form in quadruplicate. Mail two (2) copies of this form to the Special Agent in Charge, under separate cover. Enclose one additional copy in the shipment with the drugs. Retain one copy for your records. One copy will be returned to you as a receipt. No further receipt will be furnished to you unless specifically requested. Any further inquiries concerning these drugs should be addressed to the DEA District Office which serves your area.
4. There is no provision for payment for drugs surrendered. This is merely a service rendered to registrants enabling them to clear their stocks and records of unwanted items.
5. Drugs should be shipped tape-sealed via prepaid express or certified mail (return reciept requested) to Special Agent in Charge, Drug Enforcement Administration, of the DEA District Office which serves your area.

PRIVACY ACT INFORMATION

AUTHORITY: Section 307 of the Controlled Substances Act of 1970 (P.L. 91-513).
PURPOSE: To document the surrender of controlled substances which have been forwarded by registrants to DEA for disposal.
ROUTINE USES: This form is required by Federal Regulations for the surrender of unwanted Controlled Substances. Disclosures of information from this system are made to the following categories of users for the purposes stated.
A. Other Federal law enforcement and regulatory agencies for law enforcement and regulatory purposes.
B. State and local law enforcement and regulatory agencies for law enforcement and regulatory purposes.
EFFECT: Failure to document the surrender of unwanted Controlled Substances may result in prosecution for violation of the Controlled Substances Act.

Public reporting burden for this collection of information is estimated to average 30 minutes per response, including the time for reviewing instructions, searching existing data sources, gathering and maintaining the data needed, and completing and reviewing the collection of information. Send comments regarding this burden estimate or any other aspect of this collection of information, including suggestions for reducing this burden, to the Drug Enforcement Administration, Records Management Section, Washington, D.C. 20537; and to the Office of Management and Budget, Paperwork Reduction Project No. 1117-0007, Washington, D.C. 20503.

DEA Form – 41
(Jun. 1986)

Figure 37-9. Use DEA Form-41 to report disposal of controlled drugs.

PROCEDURE 37-2

Renewing the Physician's DEA Registration

Objective: To accurately complete DEA Form-224a to renew the physician's DEA registration on time

OSHA Guidelines: This procedure does not involve exposure to blood, body fluids, or tissues.

Materials: Calendar, tickler file (optional), DEA Form-224a, pen

Method

1. Calculate a period of 3 years from the date of the original registration or the most recent renewal. Note that date as the expiration date of the physician's DEA registration.
2. Subtract 45 days from the expiration date, and mark this date on the calendar as a reminder to submit renewal forms. You might also put a reminder to submit renewal forms in the physician's tickler file for that date.
3. If you receive registration renewal paperwork (DEA Form-224a) from the DEA well before the submission date, put it in a safe place until you can complete it and have the physician sign it.
4. If you do not receive renewal paperwork by the submission date, call your regional DEA office to request DEA Form-224a or send written notice that no form was received and a request for the renewal form to:

   Drug Enforcement Administration
   Registration Unit
   Central Station
   P.O. Box 28083
   Washington, DC 20038-8083
5. Before the expiration deadline, complete DEA Form-224a as instructed on the form, and have the physician sign it.
6. Submit the original and one copy of the completed form with the appropriate fee to the DEA so that it will arrive before the deadline. Keep one copy for the office records.

office, call the regional DEA office at once. Also notify the state bureau of narcotic enforcement and the local police. File all reports required by the DEA and other agencies as a follow-up.

Record Keeping. A doctor who administers or dispenses (as opposed to prescribes) controlled drugs to patients must maintain two types of records: dispensing records and inventory records. Note that these requirements do not apply to doctors who prescribe but neither administer nor dispense controlled drugs.

Dispensing Records. The dispensing record for Schedule II drugs must be kept separate from the patient's regular medical record. Each time a drug is administered or dispensed, the doctor must note the date, the patient's name and address, the drug, and the quantity dispensed.

The dispensing record for Schedules III through V drugs must include the same information. The record for these drugs may be kept in the patient's medical record unless the doctor charges for the drugs dispensed. All dispensing records must be kept for 2 years and are subject to inspection by the DEA.

Inventory Records. A doctor who regularly dispenses controlled drugs must also keep inventory records of all stock on hand. This regulation applies to all scheduled drugs. To take an inventory, count the amount of each drug on hand. Compare this amount with the amount of the drug ordered and the amount dispensed to patients.

The controlled drug inventory must be repeated every 2 years. You must include copies of invoices from drug suppliers in the inventory record. All inventories and records of Schedule II drugs must be kept separate from other records. Inventories and records of other controlled drugs must be separate or easily retrievable from ordinary business and professional records. All records on controlled drugs must be retained for 2 years and made available for inspection and copying by DEA officials if requested.

Disposing of Drugs. If the doctor asks you to dispose of any outdated, noncontrolled drugs, you may flush them down the toilet or put them in the trash, depending on state law. Incineration may be required for large amounts of injectable and topical drugs. In some instances the doctor may hire an outside company to incinerate the drugs. If not, you may ask the local hospital to incinerate them for you if this is permitted by state law.

If the doctor needs to dispose of controlled drugs, such as expired samples, obtain DEA Form-41 (Figure 37-9), called Registrants Inventory of Drugs Surrendered, which is available from the nearest DEA office. Complete the form, have the doctor sign it, and call the DEA to obtain instructions for disposal of the drugs. If you must ship them, use registered mail. After the drugs have been destroyed, the DEA will issue the doctor a receipt, which you should keep in a safe place.

If doctors terminate their medical practice, they must return their DEA registration certificate and any unused copies of DEA Form-222 to the nearest DEA office. To prevent unauthorized use, write the word *VOID* across the front of these forms. Regional DEA offices will tell doctors how to dispose of any remaining controlled drugs.

Writing Prescriptions

Any drug that is not available over the counter requires a prescription. According to the Controlled Substances Act, doctors may issue prescriptions for controlled drugs only in the schedules for which they are registered with the DEA.

You must be familiar with the terms and abbreviations used in prescriptions (Figure 37-10), and you must become familiar with the doctor's style of writing. With this knowledge, you will be able to administer the prescribed drugs accurately (if allowed in your state) and to discuss the prescription accurately with a patient or pharmacist.

Common Abbreviations Used in Prescriptions

Abbreviation	Meaning
ṫ	one
ṫṫ	two
ṫṫṫ	three
a̲	before
AA, āā	of each
a.c., ac	before meals
ad lib	as desired
amt	amount
aq.	aqueous
b.i.d., BID, bid	twice a day
c̄	with
cap, caps	capsules
cc	cubic centimeter
d	day
D/C, d/c	discontinue
Dil, dil	dilute
dr	dram
Dr	doctor
D/W	dextrose in water
Dx, dx	diagnosis
Fl, fl, fld	fluid
gal	gallon
gm, Gm, g	gram
gr	grain
gt, gtt	drop(s)
H, hr, h	hour
HS, h.s., hs	hour of sleep or at bedtime
IM	intramuscular
IU	international unit
IV	intravenous
kg	kilogram
L, l	liter
liq	liquid
m, min	minim
mcg, μg	microgram
mEq	milliequivalent
mEq/L	milliequivalents per liter
mg	milligram
mL, ml	milliliter
mm	millimeter
noc, noct	night
npo, NPO	nothing by mouth
NS	normal saline
o.d.	once a day
O.D., OD	right eye
oint	ointment
O.S., OS	left eye
O.U., OU	both eyes
oz	ounce
p̄	after, past
p.c., pc	after meals
per	by or with
po, per os	by mouth
PRN, p.r.n., prn	whenever necessary
pt	pint
Pt	patient
pulv	powder
q.	every
q.a.m., qam	every morning
q.d., qd	every day
q.h., qh	every hour
q2h, q2	every 2 hours
qhs	every night
q.i.d., qid	four times a day
qns, QNS	quantity not sufficient
qod	every other day
qs	quantity sufficient
℞, Rx	prescription, take
s̄	without
SC, s.c., SQ, subq, SubQ	subcutaneous
Sig	directions
sol	solution
ss	one-half
stat, STAT	immediately
subling, SL	sublingual
S/W	saline in water
tab	tablet
Tbsp, tbsp	tablespoon
t.i.d., tid	three times a day
tinc, tr, tinct	tincture
top	topically
tsp	teaspoon
ung, ungt	ointment
U	unit
wt	weight

Figure 37-10. Physicians use many abbreviations when they write prescriptions.

Every prescription has four basic parts: the superscription, inscription, subscription, and signature.

1. The superscription includes the date, the patient's full name and address, and the symbol ℞, which means "take thou" in Latin.
2. The inscription is the name of the drug (either generic or trade name) and the amount. It usually specifies the amount of drug in each dose of capsules, tablets, or suppositories in milligrams, such as Banthine 50 mg. The inscription for oral liquid drugs typically uses milligrams per milliliter, such as codeine sulfate 15 mg/5 mL. The inscription usually gives the amount for creams, ointments, and topical liquids as a percentage, such as Spectazole 1% cream.
3. The subscription contains the directions to the pharmacist. It includes the size of each dose, the total number or amount of the drug to be dispensed for this prescription, and the form of the drug, such as tablets.
4. The signature, or transcription, refers to patient instructions. These are nearly always written using the abbreviations shown in Figure 37-10. Instructions generally follow the abbreviation Sig, which means "mark" in Latin. Many of these instructions appear in Latin, which the pharmacist must translate. The pharmacist includes the translated patient instructions on the prescription drug label.

A prescription also includes these items:

- Doctor's name, office address and telephone number, and DEA registration number
- Doctor's signature
- Number of times the prescription can be refilled
- Indication of whether the pharmacist may substitute a generic version of a trade-name drug at the patient's request

Prescriptions may be typed or handwritten in ink or indelible pencil on a prescription blank. Prescriptions for multiple medications may be written on a different form from that used for a single medication (Figure 37-11). In some states a prescription for Schedule II drugs must be prepared in triplicate on an official Department of Justice prescription form. When this form is required, the doctor keeps one copy, and the pharmacist keeps the original and sends the endorsed second copy to the Department of Justice.

The doctor may have you prepare prescriptions for signing. Because the doctor is responsible for the accuracy of prescriptions, you must be sure to write them clearly and correctly.

Prescription Blanks. Prescription blanks make prescription writing convenient and efficient. They are usually preprinted with the doctor's name, address, telephone number, state license number, and DEA registration number. Most blanks also provide space for writing the patient's name and address, the date, and other information. Some blanks are printed on colored paper or have a background design to minimize the risk of alteration, counterfeiting, or loss. To prevent unauthorized use of prescription blanks, never leave them unattended. For tips on secure handling of prescription blanks, read "Caution: Handle With Care."

If something about a prescription arouses suspicion, the pharmacist who receives it may call the doctor's office to verify it. You should be able to check the patient's records and tell the pharmacist whether the doctor wrote a prescription for that patient. If the prescription is a forgery, notify the doctor and, if she gives you authorization, notify the DEA.

The doctor should not use a prescription to obtain drugs for office stock. When the office needs drugs (other than Schedule II drugs), they should be obtained from a

THOMAS A. McNEIL, MD
General Practice
50 East Elm Street, Sacramento, CA 94106
Telephone: (916) 555-5550

For *Scott J. Smith* Date *January 15, 1998*
Address *11123 Main Street, Sacramento, CA 94107*

Rx *Levothyroid 0.1mg*
Disp: #60
Sig: † tab 1 po q.d. 2

CAL. LIC. #G099111
DEA #AK08880002

Substitution permissible ____ yes ✔ ____ no *VOID*
Refill *2* Times
Thomas A. McNeil, MD

THOMAS A. McNEIL, MD
General Practice
CAL. LIC. #G099111 *50 East Elm Street, Sacramento, CA 94106*
DEA #AK08880002 Telephone: (916) 555-5550

For *Marjorie Smith* Date *January 7, 1998*
Address *11123 Main Street, Sacramento, CA 94107*

SIG:	LABEL MEDICATION	MG/CC	QUANTITY	REFILLS
Rx 1.	*Cyclobenzaprine*	*† tab 10mg po t.i.d.*	*90*	*∅*
Rx 2.	*Voltaren*	*† tab 50mg po b.i.d.*	*100*	*2*
Rx 3.	*Hydrocodone c̄ APAP*	*† tab 5/500mg po q4h prn pain*	*30*	*∅*
Rx 4.				
Rx 5.				

Substitution Permissible ____ yes ✔ ____ no *VOID*
Thomas A. McNeil, MD

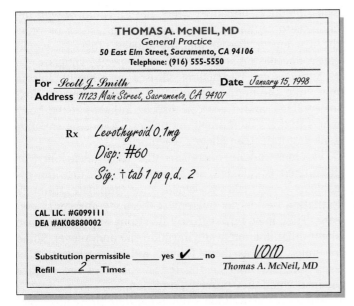

Figure 37-11. The physician may order drugs on a prescription blank (left) for a single medication or (right) for multiple medications.

CAUTION HANDLE WITH CARE

Secure Handling of Prescription Pads

Because prescription pads are small, substance abusers can easily steal a single prescription sheet or an entire pad and use it to obtain controlled substances. To keep prescription pads secure, handle them with caution and follow these tips.

Storage and Use

- Keep all prescription pads, except the pad the physician is currently using, in a locked cabinet or a locked drawer in the physician's desk.
- Remind the physician to carry the current pad at all times or to keep it out of sight but easily accessible for writing prescriptions.
- Never ask the physician to sign prescription blanks in advance.
- Never use prescription blanks as notepaper.
- Suggest that the physician write prescribed amounts of medication in numerals and words—for example, 25 (twenty-five) capsules.

Printing and Preparation

- Order printing in colored ink that is not reproducible.
- Order prescription blanks with attached no-carbon-required duplicates to provide a permanent record of all prescriptions written. Keep the duplicate in the patient's record.
- Order tinted prescription blanks to allow easy detection of erasures or correction fluid.
- See to it that the phrase "℞ not valid for narcotics, barbiturates, or amphetamines" or "Not valid for Schedule II or III drugs" is preprinted in the center of each prescription blank. Use higher security and separate prescription blanks for these drugs.
- Do *not* allow the physician's DEA registration number to be preprinted on separate prescription blanks for Schedule II or III drugs.
- Have a sequencing number preprinted on all prescription blanks so that a missing blank will be noticed quickly.

pharmacy with an order form. When the drugs are delivered, you should receive an invoice from the pharmacist.

Telephone Prescriptions. If requested by the doctor, you may telephone a new or renewal prescription to the patient's pharmacy. To do this, provide the pharmacist with the same information that would appear in a written prescription. You may not, however, telephone a prescription for a Schedule II drug. In an emergency situation, when a patient needs a drug immediately and no alternative is available, the doctor may telephone a prescription for a Schedule II drug. The amount must be limited to the period of emergency, and a written prescription must be sent to the pharmacist within 72 hours. The pharmacist must notify the DEA if a written prescription does not arrive within the specified time.

Vaccines

A **vaccine** is a special preparation made from microorganisms and administered to a person to produce reduced sensitivity to, or increased immunity to, an infectious disease. Vaccines are stored with the office supply of drugs and require similar handling. If you work in a pediatrician's office, you will handle the vaccines for childhood diseases. In an adult practice you can expect to see influenza vaccines and vaccines for diseases to which patients might be exposed in foreign travel.

It is important to know how vaccines work in the immune system. Immunity is discussed in detail in Chapter 19. Immunizations, particularly those for children, are discussed in Chapter 20. Adverse reactions to medications and vaccines are discussed in Chapter 38.

Through the action of the immune system, a patient can be protected from—or made not susceptible to—a disease. This immunity results from the formation of antibodies that destroy or alter disease-causing agents.

Antibody Formation

The human body creates antibodies in response to an invasion by an antigen (foreign substance). When an antigen enters the body, specialized white blood cells (lymphocytes) produce antibodies, which in turn combine with the antigens to neutralize them. This action arrests or prevents the reaction or disease that the antigen otherwise would cause. Specific antibodies always fight specific antigens.

Antigens can be bacteria, viruses, or other organisms that enter the body in spite of its natural defenses. Toxins, pollens, and drugs can also be antigens if the body reacts to them by forming antibodies. (Allergens are antigens that induce an allergic reaction.)

Vaccines contain organisms that have been killed or attenuated (weakened) in a laboratory. Because the organisms have been weakened, they stimulate antibody formation but do not overpower the body and cause disease. They may, however, still be strong enough to cause slight inflammation at the injection site and a fever. Some vaccines, such as those for the influenza viruses, may even produce some of the lesser effects of the disease against which they provide protection.

Immunizations made from organisms are called vaccines. Those made from the toxins of organisms are called toxoids. Some immunizations, such as polio vaccine, last a lifetime. Others, such as tetanus toxoid, do not. In the latter case booster immunizations must be used to stimulate the lymphocytes to produce antibodies again.

Timing of Immunizations

The Advisory Committee on Immunization Practices, the American Academy of Pediatrics, and the American Academy of Family Physicians jointly publish a schedule for immunizations (discussed in Chapter 20). This schedule covers children from infancy through 16 years of age. Just as children receive immunizations before exposure to disease, adults may receive immunizations for influenza or other diseases, including those to which an adult could be exposed during travel.

Patients are sometimes immunized after exposure. For example, if patients have been exposed to a serious disease and there is too little time for them to produce antibodies, they may receive an antiserum that contains antibodies to the disease-carrying organism. These immunizations are made from human or animal serum. If bacterial toxins (rather than bacteria) cause the disease, the patient may receive an antitoxin.

Antiserums and antitoxins must be used cautiously. They are usually reserved for life-threatening infectious diseases. Because patients can be allergic to substances in animal antiserums and antitoxins, human serums are usually preferred.

An example of a postexposure immunization is one given to a patient who has been exposed to hepatitis B virus (HBV). This patient should be given the antiserum hepatitis B immune globulin (HBV-Ig) within 7 days after exposure and again 28 to 30 days later. Because HBV-Ig is made from human serum, it causes relatively few adverse reactions. Another example involves a patient who may have been exposed to tetanus (lockjaw) organisms as the result of an injury such as a puncture wound. This patient may receive tetanus immune globulin (T-Ig, a human product) or tetanus antitoxin. Because tetanus antitoxin is made from horse serum, it may cause serious reactions in patients who are allergic to horses or horsehair.

For every vaccine in your medical office, you must be familiar with the indications, contraindications, dosages, administration routes, potential adverse effects, and methods of storage and handling. You must carefully read the package insert provided with each vaccine and, when necessary, consult drug reference books for further information.

Patient Education About Drugs

Your role as teacher cannot be underestimated with regard to drugs. In addition to providing specific instructions about different categories of drugs, you need to give your attention to all the drugs a patient is taking, whether prescription or over-the-counter.

Over-the-Counter Drugs

Even though patients can obtain OTC drugs without a prescription, they need to know several important facts to use them safely. That is why you should plan an education session with any patient whose medical history reveals use of OTC drugs or for whom a doctor has suggested an OTC drug.

In your patient education sessions, caution patients not to treat themselves with OTC drugs as a way to avoid medical care. For example, OTC drugs are available to treat recurrent yeast infections. Nonetheless, a patient should consult a doctor the first time she develops an infection.

Also inform patients that OTC drugs, which provide safe dosages for self-care only when used as directed, may not produce enough therapeutic benefit in some cases. In other cases they may mask symptoms or aggravate the problem.

Inform patients that many OTC drugs contain more than one active ingredient. These extra ingredients, such as aspirin or caffeine, can cause allergic or other undesirable effects.

It is important to advise patients that interactions can occur when a person takes more than one OTC drug at a time or takes an OTC and a prescription drug together. These interactions can lead to adverse reactions. For example, a patient who takes the prescription blood thinner warfarin (Coumadin) to prevent blood clots must avoid taking aspirin for pain relief. Taking these drugs together increases the risk of uncontrolled bleeding.

Prescription Drugs

Before patients begin drug therapy, you must inform them of certain considerations (such as when to take the drug) and drug safety precautions. As part of your patient education, provide instructions orally and, if possible, in writing. For commonly prescribed drugs, you may use preprinted information sheets published by the American Medical Association. Some pharmacies now routinely provide an information sheet with each dispensed drug. Figure 37-12 shows a sample of a drug information sheet.

Encouraging the Complete Medication List. Advise patients to inform the doctor of all drugs—prescription and OTC—they use regularly or periodically. Also advise patients to include past and present use of alcohol and recreational drugs as well as herbal remedies. When patients have more than one doctor, tell them to inform each doctor about all medications they are taking. Encourage them to keep up-to-date medication lists with dosages (some patients keep this information on their home computers). This information can help patients and health-care professionals prevent and monitor for drug interactions.

Encouraging the Complete Adverse Reaction List. Tell patients to inform each of their doctors of any adverse reactions (including allergic reactions) they have had to

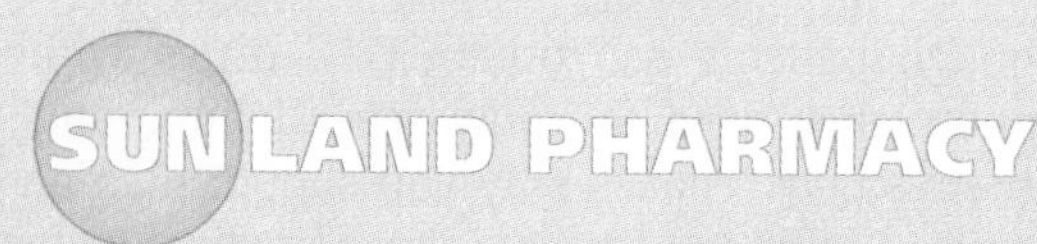

Patient Name: Jean Cranston
RX#: 711428172
Drug: Albuterol Inhalation Aerosol

COMMON USES:
To treat asthma, bronchitis, and other lung diseases.

HOW SHOULD I USE IT?
Follow your doctor's and/or the package instructions. Shake well before each use. Rinse mouth after each inhalation to avoid dryness. If breathing has not improved in 20 minutes, call doctor.

ARE THERE ANY SIDE EFFECTS?
Very unlikely, but report: Flushing, trembling, headache, nausea, vomiting, rapid heartbeat, chest pain, weakness, dizziness.

HOW DO I STORE THIS?
Store at room temperature away from moisture and sunlight. Do not puncture. Do not store in the bathroom. Rinse and clean inhaler regularly as described in package instructions.

Figure 37-12. Many pharmacies provide consumers with drug information sheets that accompany their prescriptions.

drugs. Previous adverse reactions may prompt a doctor to adjust a dosage or select a different drug. A history of drug allergies may contraindicate the use of a particular drug.

Educating for Patient Compliance. To help ensure that patients comply with instructions, confirm that they completely understand the name, dosage, and purpose of each drug prescribed for them. If patients must take more than one drug at a time, be sure they know the correct and relevant information for each one. Also teach patients to inform other health-care providers whenever there is a change in their medication regimen. In addition, cover each of the following points when educating patients about drugs.

- Explain how and when to take each drug to ensure its safety and effectiveness. Some drugs should be taken with food to minimize gastrointestinal irritation. Others should be taken on an empty stomach for proper absorption and metabolism. Some drugs must be taken once a day in the morning; others should be taken three or four times a day. If patients' medication schedules are complex, suggest that they create a chart, calendar, or diary to remind them of what drug to take and when, or create a schedule for them.
- Tell patients how long to take each drug. In the case of antibiotics, advise them to take all of the drug as scheduled, even if they feel better before finishing it. In the case of medicines prescribed for chronic disease, advise patients that they will need to continue taking the medication unless the doctor tells them to stop. Be aware that some drugs, such as prednisone, must be tapered off slowly to prevent adverse reactions.
- Explain how to identify possible adverse effects of each drug and safety measures related to adverse effects. For example, instruct patients to avoid certain activities, such as driving or operating machinery, while taking a drug that causes drowsiness. Also tell them to call the doctor if they experience adverse effects or any unusual reactions. If appropriate, inform patients that misuse of the drug may lead to dependence, and mention the dangers of drug dependence.
- Tell patients not to save old medications or share them with anyone else. Old medications and those taken by people other than the patient for whom they were prescribed can cause severe, unexpected adverse effects. Advise patients to check the expiration date on all drugs and to flush expired ones down the toilet.
- Suggest that patients avoid alcohol when taking a drug unless the doctor or pharmacist indicates otherwise. Alcohol interacts with some drugs, causing adverse effects, such as lethargy, confusion, or coma.
- Tell patients to ask their pharmacists where to store each medication. Some drugs must be refrigerated. Others should be kept in a dry, cool area. Drugs should not usually be kept in a hot, damp place, such as a bathroom. They must always be kept out of the reach of children.
- Tell patients to take their drugs in a well-lit area so they can read each drug label carefully before taking each dose. They should never assume that they are taking the right medication without reading the label on the container. If patients have poor vision, print the name of the drug and the dosage schedule clearly on a separate piece of paper or card to attach to the medication container.
- Instruct patients to call the doctor if they have any questions about their drug therapy.

Summary

Pharmacology is the study of drugs, or pharmaceuticals. The pharmacologist studies pharmacognosy, pharmacokinetics, pharmacodynamics, pharmacotherapeutics, and toxicology. Pharmacognosy is the study of the characteristics of natural drugs and their sources. Pharmacokinetics pertains to how the body absorbs, metabolizes, distributes, and excretes a drug. Pharmacodynamics relates to a drug's mechanism of action, or how it affects the body. Pharmacotherapeutics addresses the use of drugs to prevent or treat disease. Toxicology is the study of poisons and the toxic effects of drugs, including adverse effects or drug interactions.

Every drug has several names, including chemical, generic, and trade names. Based on its action, a drug can belong to one of many classifications. These data can be found in the *Physicians' Desk Reference* and other sources of drug information.

Patients can obtain nonprescription (over-the-counter) drugs without a physician's order. For prescription drugs, patients must have a physician's written (or oral) order. For drugs that have been classified as controlled substances because they are potentially dangerous and addictive, extensive regulations apply. The physician must be registered with the Drug Enforcement Administration and follow the legal requirements of the Controlled Substances Act of 1970 to administer, dispense, and prescribe these drugs.

Immunizations usually contain killed or weakened organisms. They are used to provide immunity against specific diseases. Childhood immunizations should follow a recommended schedule. Other immunizations should be given as the need arises.

No matter what type of drug a patient must take, your role as an educator is an important one. You need to teach patients about specific drugs and required safety precautions. When you educate a patient carefully and thoroughly about a drug, you enhance the likelihood of patient compliance and safety.

37 Chapter Review

Discussion Questions

1. Briefly describe the importance of knowing about pharmacodynamics and pharmacokinetics in your role as a medical assistant.
2. Distinguish between the chemical, generic, and trade names of a drug.
3. Give an example of a drug from each schedule of controlled substances stipulated by the CSA of 1970.

Critical Thinking Questions

1. Why do federal, state, and local governments prohibit or control the use of some drugs, such as heroin and steroids?
2. Why should children be immunized against diseases such as diphtheria and hepatitis B?
3. Why is patient education especially important for a patient who is receiving drug therapy?

Application Activities

1. Using the abbreviations in Figure 37-10, translate the following prescriptions:
   - triamterene 100 mg po b.i.d. p.c.
   - Benadryl 25–50 mg po hs prn insomnia
   - Rocephin 250 mg IM STAT
2. Using the *Physicians' Desk Reference,* find the information on indications, contraindications, warnings, drug abuse and dependence, and overdosage for each of the following drugs: Clinoril, fenfluramine hydrochloride, Lescol, Lopid, mirtazapine, quazepam, Sedapap, and Ventolin.
3. With your instructor, examine the required forms and discuss the prescribing requirements for controlled drugs in your state.

Further Readings

Edmunds, Marilyn W. *Introduction to Clinical Pharmacology.* 2d ed. St. Louis: Mosby–Year Book, 1995.

Gerlach, Mary Jo. *Nursing Pharmacology: Concepts and Activities.* Springhouse, PA: Springhouse, 1994.

Harvey, R., et al., eds. *Lippincott's Illustrated Reviews: Pharmacology.* Philadelphia: J. B. Lippincott, 1992.

Hill, John K. "Recognizing the Signs of Addiction." *The Professional Medical Assistant,* January/February 1994, 8–10.

Hitner, Henry, and Barbara T. Nagle. *Basic Pharmacology for Health Occupations.* 3d ed. Columbus, OH: Glencoe, 1993.

PDR Family Guide to Prescription Drugs. Oradell, NJ: Medical Economics, 1993.

"The Top 200 Drugs." *American Druggist,* February 1997, 30–37.

Williams, Bradley R., and Charold L. Bear. *Essentials of Clinical Pharmacology in Nursing.* 2d ed. Springhouse, PA: Springhouse, 1994.

Drug Administration

CHAPTER OUTLINE

- The Medical Assistant's Role in Drug Administration
- Scope of Practice
- Dosage Calculations
- Preparing to Administer a Drug
- Techniques of Administering Drugs
- Educating the Patient About Drug Administration
- Special Considerations
- Nonpharmacologic Pain Management

Key Terms

buccal
diluent
douche
infusion
intradermal (ID)
intramuscular (IM)
intravenous (IV)
ointment
route
solution
subcutaneous (SC)
sublingual
topical
transdermal
volume
Z-track method

OBJECTIVES

After completing Chapter 38, you will be able to:

- Discuss your responsibilities regarding drug administration.
- Perform dosage calculations accurately.
- Describe how to assess the patient before administering any drug.
- Identify the "seven rights" of drug administration.
- Describe the various techniques of drug administration you may be asked to perform.
- Compare different types of needles and syringes.
- Explain how to administer an intradermal, subcutaneous, or intramuscular injection.
- Explain what information you need to teach the patient about drug use, interactions, and adverse effects.
- Describe special considerations related to drug administration.
- Describe nonpharmacologic ways to manage pain.

AREAS OF COMPETENCE

1997 ROLE DELINEATION STUDY

CLINICAL

Fundamental Principles

- Apply principles of aseptic technique and infection control

Patient Care

- Prepare and administer medications and immunizations
- Maintain medication and immunization records

continued

AREAS OF COMPETENCE continued

GENERAL (Transdisciplinary)

Legal Concepts

- Document accurately

Instruction

- Explain office policies and procedures

The Medical Assistant's Role in Drug Administration

Drug administration is one of a medical assistant's most important—and most dangerous—duties. By following the procedures for proper drug administration, you can help restore patients to health. If you calculate dosages inaccurately, measure drugs incorrectly, or administer drugs improperly, however, patients' medications may have no therapeutic effect, may worsen their disease or abnormal condition, or may cause them to die.

To administer drugs safely and effectively to all patient groups, including pediatric, pregnant, and elderly patients, you must know and understand the principles of pharmacology presented in Chapter 37. In addition, you must be comfortable with basic mathematics so you can calculate both a dose (the amount of drug given at one time) and a dosage (the amount of drug given over time and its frequency), know the "seven rights" of drug administration, and be skilled in administering drugs in different ways. Furthermore, you must be comfortable with all aspects of drug administration to be able to assume your role as an educator, so that you can instruct patients about the drugs prescribed for them.

Because drug administration is a common and vital part of your job, you must familiarize yourself with the uses, contraindications, interactions, and adverse effects of common drugs. In particular, you should be familiar with the medications frequently prescribed in your practice. If you want to expand your knowledge, you can take further courses in pharmacology or biochemistry.

Remember that you share the responsibility for knowing a drug's usual dosage, **route** (the way a drug is introduced into the body), adverse effects, and special considerations. If you are unsure about any of these factors, check the *Physicians' Desk Reference* (*PDR*) or another source of drug information, as described in Chapter 37.

Scope of Practice

Many states have medical practice acts that define medical assistants' exact duties in drug administration. For example, an act may specify which drugs you are allowed to administer and by which routes. Because state laws vary, you need to research the scope of practice for medical assistants in the state where you will work.

Dosage Calculations

Before you can administer a drug, you may need to calculate the dose the physician has prescribed. To do so, you must understand various systems of measurement and ways to convert from one system to another.

Measurement Systems

In the United States three systems of measurement are used in pharmacology and drug administration. You must be able to use all three of these systems:

- Metric
- Apothecaries'
- Household

Although most drug manufacturers and doctors use the metric system, some doctors still use the older apothecaries' system. You must also be familiar with the household system, because most patients use household measures when taking medicines at home.

To understand drug measurement, focus primarily on remembering the basic unit of volume and weight for each system, as shown in Table 38-1. **Volume** refers to the amount of space a drug occupies. Weight refers to its heaviness.

Metric System. The basic units of volume and weight in the decimal-based metric system are liters (L) to measure volume and grams (g) to measure weight. Prefixes are added to these basic units of measurement to indicate multiples—such as dekaliter or kilogram—or fractions—such as milliliter or microgram. Common metric equivalents are presented in Table 38-2. Note that a cubic centimeter (cc) is the amount of space occupied by 1 mL. Therefore, cc and mL are used interchangeably in prescriptions.

Apothecaries' System. The apothecaries' system uses minims, fluidrams, fluidounces, pints, quarts, and gallons to measure volume. It measures weight by grains,

Table 38-1

Comparing Selected Metric and Apothecaries' Measures (Approximate Values)

Measures of Volume	Measures of Weight
Metric vs Apothecaries'	Metric vs Apothecaries'
1 milliliter (mL) = 15–16 minims (min, ♏)	0.06 gram (g) or 60 milligrams (mg) = 1 grain (gr)
4 mL = 1 fluidram (fl dr, f℈)	0.5 g or 500 mg = 7¾ gr
30 mL = 1 fluidounce (fl oz, f℥)	1 g or 1000 mg = 15 gr
500 mL = 1 pint (pt)	4 g = 1 dram (dr, ʒ)
1000 mL or 1 liter (L) = 1 quart (qt)	30 g = 1 ounce (oz, ℥)

scruples, drams, ounces, and pounds. Common apothecaries' equivalents are outlined in Table 38-3. The apothecaries' system also uses Roman numerals to indicate the amount of the drug. For example, ASA gr X means "10 grains of acetylsalicylic acid (aspirin)." Note that in the metric system, the amount precedes the unit, whereas in the apothecaries' system, the amount follows the unit. Although this system is less popular than it once was, some doctors still use it.

Household System. The only household units of measurement that are used to measure drugs are units of volume. These include drops, teaspoons, tablespoons, ounces, cups, pints, quarts, and gallons. Common household equivalents are shown in Table 38-4.

Conversions Between Measurement Systems

At times you may need to convert from one measurement system to another. Because of the difference in basic units of measure, you must remember that conversions between systems are only approximate equivalents. If you use a conversion chart, read it carefully before administering a drug. Check it several times, and place a ruler under the line you are reading to be absolutely sure you are reading the chart properly. When you must calculate conversions instead of using a conversion chart, use either the ratio or the fraction method.

Table 38-2

Common Metric Equivalents

Measures of Volume	Measures of Weight
0.001 liter (L) = 1 milliliter (mL) or 1 cubic centimeter (cc)	0.001 gram (g) or 1000 micrograms (μg) = 1 milligram (mg)
0.01 L = 1 centiliter (cL)	0.01 g = 1 centigram (cg)
0.1 L = 1 deciliter (dL)	0.1 g = 1 decigram (dg)
1 L = 1000 mL	1 g = 1000 mg or 0.001 kilogram (kg)
10 L = 1 dekaliter (daL)	10 g = 1 dekagram (dag)
100 L = 1 hectoliter (hL)	100 g = 1 hectogram (hg)
1000 L = 1 kiloliter (kL)	1000 g = 1 kg

Table 38-3

Common Apothecaries' Equivalents

Measures of Volume	Measures of Weight
60 minims (min, ♏) = 1 fluidram (fl dr, f℥)	20 grains (gr) = 1 scruple (scr, ℈)
8 fl dr = 1 fluidounce (fl oz, f℥)	60 gr or 3 scr = 1 dram (dr, ʒ)
16 fl oz = 1 pint (pt)	8 dr = 1 ounce (oz, ℥)
2 pt = 1 quart (qt)	12 oz = 1 pound (℔)
4 qt = 1 gallon (gal)	

Ratio Method. Suppose the doctor orders ASA gr X. Although this translates to 10 grains of aspirin in the apothecaries' system, the available tablets come in milligrams, a metric measurement. To convert from apothecaries' to metric measure, you must set up a ratio to solve for *x*, the unknown dose in milligrams. Follow these steps to convert the measurement.

1. Set up the first ratio:
$$x : 10 \text{ gr}$$
2. Next set up the second ratio with the standard equivalent between the available and ordered measurements:
$$60 \text{ mg} : 1 \text{ gr}$$
3. Then use both ratios in a proportional equation that reads, *x* is to 10 gr as 60 mg is to 1 gr. Mathematically, this is written:
$$x : 10 \text{ gr} :: 60 \text{ mg} : 1 \text{ gr}$$
4. To solve for *x*, multiply the outer and then the inner parts of the proportion:
$$x \times 1 \text{ gr} = 10 \text{ gr} \times 60 \text{ mg}$$
5. To solve for *x*, divide both sides of the equation by 1 gr, then do the arithmetic, canceling out like terms in each numerator (top of the fraction) and denominator (bottom of the fraction):
$$\frac{x \times \cancel{1 \text{ gr}}}{\cancel{1 \text{ gr}}} = \frac{10 \cancel{\text{gr}} \times 60 \text{ mg}}{1 \cancel{\text{gr}}}$$
$$x = \frac{10 \times 60 \text{ mg}}{1}$$
$$x = \frac{600 \text{ mg}}{1}$$
$$x = 600 \text{ mg}$$

Fraction Method. Suppose the physician orders 300 mg of aspirin in the metric system. The tablets, however, are labeled in grains, an apothecaries' measure. To make this conversion, follow these steps.

1. Set up a fraction with the ordered dose on the top and the unknown amount on the bottom:
$$\frac{300 \text{ mg}}{x}$$
2. Next set up a fraction with the standard equivalent. Make sure that for this fraction you use units of measure on the top and the bottom that match the units of measure on the top and the bottom of the first fraction:
$$\frac{60 \text{ mg}}{1 \text{ gr}}$$
3. Then set up a proportion with both fractions:
$$\frac{300 \text{ mg}}{x} = \frac{60 \text{ mg}}{1 \text{ gr}}$$
4. Now cross multiply. Multiply the bottom left number by the top right number, and multiply the top left number by the bottom right number:
$$x \times 60 \text{ mg} = 300 \text{ mg} \times 1 \text{ gr}$$

Table 38-4

Common Household Measurements

Measures of Volume
60 drops (gtt) = 1 teaspoon (tsp)
3 tsp = 1 tablespoon (tbsp)
6 tsp = 1 ounce (oz) or 2 tbsp
8 oz = 1 cup (c)
2 c = 1 pint (pt)
4 c = 1 quart (qt) or 2 pt

5. To solve for x, divide both sides of the equation by 60, then do the arithmetic, canceling out like terms in the top and bottom of each fraction:

$$\frac{x \times \cancel{60\text{ mg}}}{\cancel{60\text{ mg}}} = \frac{300\cancel{\text{ mg}} = 1\text{ gr}}{60\cancel{\text{ mg}}}$$

$$x = \frac{300 \times 1\text{ gr}}{60}$$

$$x = \frac{300\text{ gr}}{60}$$

$$x = 5\text{ gr}$$

Calculations and Drug Doses

You may occasionally need to do some calculations to provide a prescribed drug dose. You can use the ratio method or the fraction method to calculate the dose. Because a patient's health or life can depend on your calculations, take the time to check and recheck your arithmetic. If you need extra practice in calculations, consider buying and using a dosage calculation workbook.

Ratio Method. Suppose the doctor orders 500 mg of ampicillin, but each tablet contains only 250 mg. To calculate how to provide this dose, follow these steps.

1. Set up a ratio with the unknown number of tablets and the amount of the drug ordered:

$$x : 500\text{ mg}$$

2. Next set up a ratio with a single tablet and the amount of drug in a single tablet:

$$1\text{ tab} : 250\text{ mg}$$

3. Now put both of these ratios in a proportion:

$$x : 500\text{ mg} :: 1\text{ tab} : 250\text{ mg}$$

4. To solve for x, multiply the outer and then the inner parts of the proportion:

$$x \times 250\text{ mg} = 500\text{ mg} \times 1\text{ tab}$$

5. To solve for x, divide both sides of the equation by 250 mg, then do the arithmetic, canceling out like terms in the top and bottom of each fraction:

$$\frac{x \times \cancel{250\text{ mg}}}{\cancel{250\text{ mg}}} = \frac{500\cancel{\text{ mg}} \times 1\text{ tab}}{250\cancel{\text{ mg}}}$$

$$x = \frac{500\text{ tabs}}{250}$$

$$x = 2\text{ tabs}$$

As another example, the doctor orders 30 mg of Adalat, but each capsule contains only 10 mg. To calculate the prescribed drug dose using the ratio method, you would set up these equations:

$$x : 30\text{ mg}$$

$$1\text{ cap} : 10\text{ mg}$$

$$x : 30\text{ mg} :: 1\text{ cap} : 10\text{ mg}$$

$$x \times 10\text{ mg} = 30\text{ mg} \times 1\text{ cap}$$

$$\frac{x \times \cancel{10\text{ mg}}}{\cancel{10\text{ mg}}} = \frac{30\cancel{\text{ mg}} \times 1\text{ cap}}{10\cancel{\text{ mg}}}$$

$$x = \frac{30\text{ caps}}{10}$$

$$x = 3\text{ caps}$$

Fraction Method. For the same problem, you could use the fraction method to calculate how to provide the prescribed dose. Follow these steps for the fraction method.

1. Set up the first fraction with the dose ordered and the unknown number of capsules:

$$\frac{30\text{ mg}}{x}$$

2. Set up the second fraction with the amount of drug in a capsule and a single capsule:

$$\frac{10\text{ mg}}{1\text{ cap}}$$

3. Then use both fractions in a proportion:

$$\frac{30\text{ mg}}{x} = \frac{10\text{ mg}}{1\text{ cap}}$$

4. To solve for x, cross multiply. Remember to multiply the bottom left number by the top right number and multiply the top left number by the bottom right number:

$$x \times 10\text{ mg} = 30\text{ mg} \times 1\text{ cap}$$

5. To solve for x, divide both sides of the equation by 10 mg, then do the arithmetic, canceling out like terms in the top and bottom of each fraction:

$$\frac{x \times \cancel{10\text{ mg}}}{\cancel{10\text{ mg}}} = \frac{30\cancel{\text{ mg}} \times 1\text{ cap}}{10\cancel{\text{ mg}}}$$

$$x = \frac{30\text{ caps}}{10}$$

$$x = 3\text{ caps}$$

As another example, the doctor orders 120 mg of Armour thyroid but each tablet contains only 30 mg. To calculate the prescribed drug dose using the fraction method, you would set up these equations:

$$\frac{120\text{ mg}}{x}$$

$$\frac{30\text{ mg}}{1\text{ tab}}$$

$$\frac{120\text{ mg}}{x} = \frac{30\text{ mg}}{1\text{ tab}}$$

$$x \times 30\text{ mg} = 120\text{ mg} \times 1\text{ tab}$$

$$\frac{x \times \cancel{30\text{ mg}}}{\cancel{30\text{ mg}}} = \frac{120\cancel{\text{ mg}} \times 1\text{ tab}}{30\cancel{\text{ mg}}}$$

$$x = \frac{120\text{ tabs}}{30}$$

$$x = 4\text{ tabs}$$

Preparing to Administer a Drug

Drugs may be administered for either local or systemic effects. Generally, drugs that have local effects are applied directly to the skin, tissues, or mucous membranes. Drugs that produce systemic effects are administered by routes that allow the drug to be absorbed and distributed in the bloodstream throughout the body. The importance of extreme care with drug dose and route is described in "Caution: Handle With Care."

Before prescribing the route of administration for a drug, the doctor considers the drug's mechanism of action (described in the section on pharmacodynamics in Chapter 37); the drug's characteristics, cost, and availability; and the patient's physical and emotional state. The different routes of administration are described in Table 38-5 and discussed later in this chapter.

Assessment

Although the doctor gives the order to administer a drug, much of the responsibility is yours. Because you will often interview the patient, you must be alert to—and inform the doctor of—any change in the patient's condition that could affect drug therapy.

CAUTION HANDLE WITH CARE

Dose and Route in Drug Administration

In the 1997 AAMA Role Delineation Chart, drug preparation and administration are included among the basic clinical skills for patient care. They require close attention to detail, strong patient assessment skills, and expert technique.

You must give close attention to both dose and route of administration, especially when one depends on the other. Not only must you give extreme care to dose and route, but frequently you must also check and recheck the ordered form of the drug (for example, tablet or extended release capsule). In the following examples, this crucial relationship is illustrated.

1. Prochlorperazine (Compazine) is an antiemetic drug for acute nausea and vomiting. It is given to both children and adults. When the vomiting is so severe that a tablet or capsule cannot be swallowed, the drug is administered in injectable or suppository form. This drug is available in the following forms:
   - 10 mL multidose vials with 5 mg of drug per mL, written as 5 mg/mL
   - 2 mL single-dose vials 5 mg/mL
   - 4 fl oz bottles of syrup 5 mg/5 mL (5 mg/1 tsp)
   - 5 mg tablets
   - 10 mg tablets
   - 2 mL prefilled disposable syringes 5 mg/mL
   - 2½ mg suppositories
   - 5 mg suppositories
   - 25 mg suppositories
   - 10 mg extended release capsules
   - 15 mg extended release capsules

   Because so many forms of this drug are available, there is a high risk of error in choosing the correct form. In addition, the route of administration can determine how much drug is delivered in one dose. For example, note that suppositories are available in 2½-mg, 5-mg, and 25-mg forms. If the 2½-mg dose were written as 2.5 mg, there might be confusion with the 25-mg dose suppository. Thus the 2½-mg suppository is always written this way, even in the *PDR*. This clarification helps prevent a child's receiving the adult dose of 25 mg, which could result in serious complications to the central nervous system. This possible confusion is a good example of how much difference a decimal point can make.

   Note also that in the syrup there is a 5-mg dose of drug per 5 mL (1 tsp), whereas in the other liquid forms (vials and prefilled syringes), there is a 5-mg dose of drug per 1 mL. The injectable form is five times more concentrated than the syrup. Therefore, if you were to administer the same amount of injectable liquid as syrup to a patient, you would give the patient five times more drug than in the syrup. Just as a child could be endangered with the 25-mg suppository, an adult could be endangered with the wrong form of liquid. Because elderly patients often receive syrup forms of medication, this instruction could be particularly confusing.
2. Allergy shots must be administered subcutaneously rather than intramuscularly to allow slower absorption of the serum. Within 30 minutes, a wheal and redness will appear if the patient has an allergic reaction. In such a case the patient requires further close monitoring. If the serum were injected intramuscularly, this reaction would not only be hidden (because of the deeper administration), it would also occur more rapidly (because of the faster rate of absorption). In fact, the patient could go into anaphylaxis, or anaphylactic shock, without any warning.

Check and recheck every order and drug label to prevent confusion and incorrect administration. This procedure is always worth the time it takes.

Before administering a drug, ensure that the ordered dose is appropriate for the patient's age and weight. Check that the patient has no swelling or injury at the administration site. Also make sure there are no contraindications (allergy, other medical condition, or use of another drug that prevents the safe use of the ordered drug or route).

General Rules for Drug Administration

No matter what drug or administration route is ordered, follow these general rules when administering drugs.

- Give only the drugs the physician has ordered. Written orders are preferable, but oral orders are appropriate for emergencies. If you are unfamiliar with any aspect of a drug the physician orders, consult a drug reference work.
- Wash your hands before handling the drug. Prepare the drug in a well-lit area, away from distractions. Focus only on the task at hand.
- Calculate the dose if necessary. If you are unsure of your computation, ask another medical assistant, a nurse, or the physician to check it.
- Avoid leaving a prepared drug unattended, and never administer a drug that someone else has prepared.

Table 38-5

Routes and Methods of Drug Administration

Route and Drug Forms	Method
Buccal route Tablets	Place drug between patient's gum and cheek. To ensure absorption, tell patient to leave tablet there until it dissolves and not to chew or swallow it. No eating, drinking, or smoking until tablet is completely dissolved.
Intradermal route Solutions Powders for reconstitution	Administer drug by injection into upper layers of patient's skin.
Intramuscular route Solutions Powders for reconstitution	Administer drug by injection into muscle.
Intravenous route Solutions (often in bags of 250, 500, or 1000 mL) Powders for reconstitution Blood and blood products	Administer drug by injection or infusion into vein.
Inhalation therapy (nasal or oral) Aerosols Sprays Mists or steam	Administer drug by inhalation to reach respiratory tract.
Oral route Tablets Capsules Liquids Lozenges	Give drug to patient to swallow.
Ophthalmic (eye) or otic (ear) route Solutions Ointments	Apply drug, usually as drops, in patient's eye or ear.

continued

Table 38-5 continued

Routes and Methods of Drug Administration

Route and Drug Forms	Method
Rectal route Suppositories Solutions	Insert suppository into rectum. Administer solution as enema, using tube and nozzle.
Subcutaneous route Solutions Powders for reconstitution	Administer drug by injection into subcutaneous layer of skin.
Sublingual route Tablets Sprays	Place drug under patient's tongue. To ensure absorption, tell patient to leave tablet there until it dissolves and not to chew or swallow it. No eating, drinking, or smoking until tablet is completely dissolved.
Topical route Ointments Lotions Creams Tinctures Powders Sprays Solutions	Apply drug to patient's skin or rub into skin.
Transdermal route Patches	Apply drug to clean, dry, nonhairy area of skin.
Urethral route Solutions	Administer drug by instilling in bladder, using catheter.
Vaginal route Solutions Suppositories Ointments Foams Creams	Administer solution as douche, using tube and nozzle. Administer any other form by inserting into vagina with applicator.

- Ask the patient to state his name to ensure correct identification. Also ask the patient to tell you about any possible drug allergies. Do not rely on documentation in his chart; he may have developed a new allergy that has not yet been added to the record. Then verify any drug allergies in the chart.
- Be sure the physician is in the office when you administer a drug or vaccine. If the patient develops an anaphylactic reaction (sudden, severe allergic reaction) to the drug or vaccine, the physician must administer epinephrine. Some patients need to know how to administer this drug themselves. For information about epinephrine, see "Educating the Patient."
- After administering the drug, observe the patient for unexpected effects. Give the patient specific instructions about the effects of the drug as well as general information about drug use.
- If the patient refuses to take the drug, flush it down the toilet. Do *not* return it to the original container. Be sure to document the refusal in the patient's record and tell the physician.

EDUCATING THE PATIENT

Using an Epinephrine Autoinjector

If you are working in a medical office that treats people with allergies, you must be familiar with epinephrine so that you can teach patients how to self-administer the drug. Epinephrine is a drug used to treat allergies so severe that exposure to the allergen may be life-threatening. The following reactions indicate the possibility of anaphylaxis, or anaphylactic shock, a severe allergic reaction:

- Flushing
- Sharp drop in blood pressure
- Hives
- Difficulty breathing
- Difficulty swallowing
- Convulsions
- Vomiting
- Diarrhea and abdominal cramps

If a patient with a severe allergy experiences any or all of these symptoms, the reaction can be fatal unless emergency treatment is given immediately. Therefore, patients who cannot always control their exposure to an allergen—for example, bee or wasp venom—must have access to an epinephrine autoinjector for emergency intramuscular use.

These injectors, which are prepackaged (Figure 38-1), deliver either 0.3 mg of epinephrine—a single dose for an adult—or 0.15 mg of epinephrine—a single dose for a child. A patient who is exposed to the allergen should use the injector if the allergy is confirmed or if the allergy is suspected and signs of anaphylaxis appear.

Teach the patient to follow these steps when using an autoinjector.

1. Remove the autoinjector from the packaging (box and/or plastic tube).
2. Pull back the gray cap.
3. Place the black tip of the injector on the outside of the upper thigh. (The injector can go through clothing.)
4. Press firmly into the thigh and hold for 10 seconds.
5. Remove the autoinjector and massage the injection site for a few minutes.
6. Call your physician or go to the emergency room of a nearby hospital. An autoinjector is designed as emergency supportive therapy only. It is not a replacement or substitute for immediate medical or hospital care.

Make sure the patient is thoroughly familiar with the parts of the autoinjector, how to activate it, how to use it, and what to do next. Ask the patient to explain the use of the autoinjector to you, as if you had never seen one. This approach not only reinforces the patient's understanding of the process but also improves the patient's self-confidence and points out any possible misconceptions. If the patient is very young or otherwise unable to use the autoinjector reliably, teach a family member or companion how to perform the process.

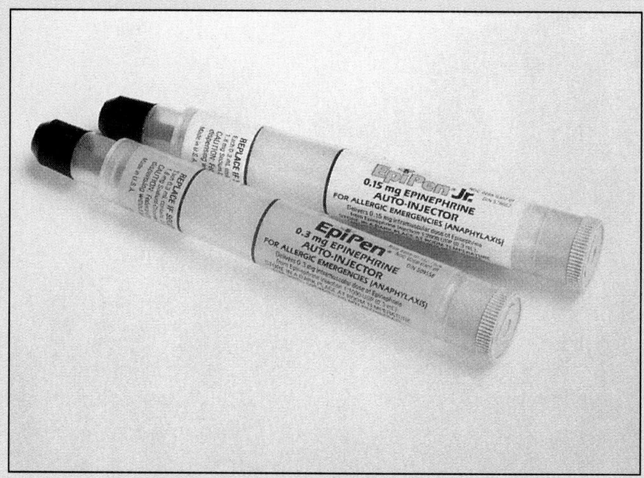

Figure 38-1. Epinephrine autoinjectors come prepackaged, containing the correct amount of the drug for an adult or a child (the junior unit).

- If you make an error in drug administration, tell the physician immediately.
- Document immediately the drug and dose administered; never document administration before giving medicine.

To master your administration techniques, practice with classmates. When on the job, ask a coworker, perhaps a nurse or a more experienced medical assistant, to critique your technique.

"Seven Rights" of Drug Administration

When administering any drug, whether medication or vaccine, observe the "seven rights" of drug administration. *Never* deviate from these seven steps. Adhering to these "rights" helps ensure that you administer the drug correctly. The seven rights refer to the following:

- Right patient
- Right drug

- Right dose
- Right time
- Right route
- Right technique
- Right documentation

Right Patient. Always check the name on the order for a drug or vaccine in the patient's chart; then ask the patient to tell you her name. Be especially careful with a forgetful or confused patient, because she might answer to any name. Have a confused patient state her name, or check her name with an attending family member.

Right Drug. Carefully compare the name of the prescribed drug or vaccine in the patient's chart with the label on the drug container. As you check the drug name on the label, look at the expiration date. Never use a drug that has passed this date.

If you are unfamiliar with the drug, look it up in the *PDR* or other drug reference. Also, never prepare a drug from a container with a damaged or handwritten label. To ensure accuracy, read the label three times:

1. When you obtain the drug container from the cabinet
2. When you pour or prepare the drug from the container
3. When you put the container back in the cabinet (before leaving the medication room)

Right Dose. Compare the dose on the order in the patient's chart with the dose you prepare. To obtain the right dose, read the label closely. Do not confuse the dose contained in one tablet with the number of tablets in the container.

Right Time. Be sure to give the drug at the right time. If it must be given after meals, make sure the patient has eaten recently. For certain drugs, you must ensure that it is the correct time of day and the correct time in a series of doses. Timing is crucial with allergy shots because of possible reactions.

Right Route. Double-check to make sure the administration route you are preparing to use matches the route the doctor ordered. Check that the patient can receive the drug by this route and that the route seems appropriate. For example, if the patient has an injury at the specified injection site, consult the doctor for a possible alternative site or a different route.

Right Technique. Always use the proper administration technique. If you have not given a drug or vaccine by the ordered route recently, review the technique before administering the drug.

Right Documentation. Document the procedure immediately after administering the drug or vaccine to the patient. Do not wait until later, and do not document before administration. Be sure to include the date, time, drug or vaccine name, dose, administration route, patient reaction, patient education about the drug, and your initials. If the drug is a controlled substance, also document it on the controlled substance inventory record. Remember that correct documentation demands neat handwriting that others who care for the patient can read easily.

Techniques of Administering Drugs

The doctor may ask you to administer drugs by one of the routes outlined in Table 38-5. Because most patients take a prescription to a pharmacy to be filled and then take oral drugs at home, you rarely need to administer these drugs in the office. You are likely, however, to be asked to do the following.

- Place drugs in the patient's mouth between the cheek and gum or under the tongue.
- Administer a drug by any means other than by mouth (if permitted in your state).
- Demonstrate how to use an inhaler.
- Apply topical drugs (those applied to the skin).
- Administer or assist in administering drugs into the urethra, vagina, or rectum.
- Administer medications to the eye or ear.

These duties require you to master a variety of techniques to give drugs safely by any route.

Oral Administration

Drugs for oral administration include tablets, capsules, lozenges, and liquids. These drugs are absorbed relatively slowly as they travel along the gastrointestinal (GI) tract.

Oral administration is contraindicated in patients who have severe nausea, are comatose, or cannot swallow. Certain drugs are ineffective when administered orally, because the digestive process changes them chemically to an ineffective form or does not deliver them to the bloodstream quickly enough.

Many drugs, however, are most effective when given orally. These include antibiotics, vitamins, throat lozenges, and cough syrups. Although these drugs are familiar to most people, as a medical assistant, you must follow certain steps to ensure that the patient understands the drug and that the drug is administered safely and effectively. The steps for oral administration are outlined in Procedure 38-1.

Buccal and Sublingual Administration

Although buccal and sublingual drugs are placed in the mouth, they do not continue along the GI tract. Instead, they dissolve and are absorbed in the **buccal** area (between the cheek and gum) or the **sublingual** area (under the tongue), where they are placed. The medication is absorbed through tissue that is rich in capillaries, and the drug enters the bloodstream directly. Because the drug does not pass into the stomach or intestines before absorption, it produces a therapeutic effect more quickly than do oral drugs.

PROCEDURE 38-1

Administering Oral Drugs

Objective: To safely administer an oral drug to a patient

OSHA Guidelines: This procedure does not involve exposure to blood, body fluids, or tissues.

Materials: Drug order (in patient chart), container of oral drug, small paper cup (for tablets, capsules, or caplets) or plastic calibrated medicine cup (for liquids), glass of water or juice, straw (optional), package insert or drug information sheet

Method

1. Wash your hands.
2. Select the ordered drug (tablet, capsule, or liquid).
3. Check the "seven rights," comparing information against the drug order.
4. If you are unfamiliar with the drug, check the *PDR* or other drug reference, read the package insert, or speak with the physician. Determine whether the drug may be taken with or followed by water or juice.
5. Ask the patient about any drug or food allergies. If the patient is not allergic to the ordered drug or other ingredients used to prepare it, proceed.
6. Perform any calculations needed to provide the prescribed dose. If you are unsure of your calculations, check them with a coworker or the physician.

If You Must Give Tablets or Capsules

7. Open the container and tap the correct number into the cap (Figure 38-2). Do not touch the inside of the cap because it is sterile. If you pour out too many tablets or capsules and you have not touched them, tap the excess back into the container.
8. Tap the tablets or capsules from the cap into the paper cup.
9. Re-cap the container.
10. Give the patient the cup along with a glass of water or juice. If the patient finds it easier to drink with a straw, unwrap the straw and place it in the fluid. If patients have difficulty swallowing pills, have them drink some water or juice before putting the pills in the mouth. This additional fluid makes the pills float and allows patients to swallow quickly.

If You Must Give a Liquid Drug

7. If the liquid is a suspension, shake it well.
8. Locate the mark on the medicine cup for the prescribed dose. Keeping your thumbnail on the mark, hold the cup at eye level and pour the correct amount of the drug. To prevent liquid drips from obscuring the label, keep the label side of the bottle on top as you pour (Figure 38-3), or put your palm over it.

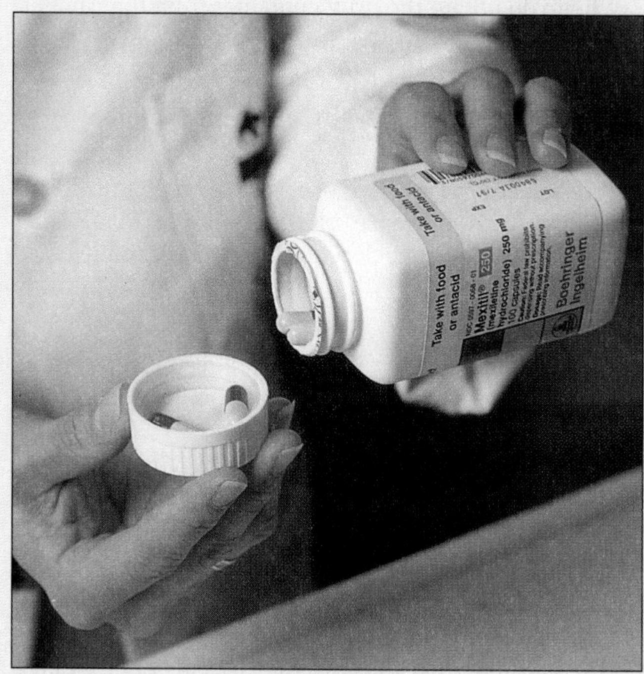

Figure 38-2. Tap tablets gently into the cap.

Specially formulated tablets may be given by the buccal or sublingual routes. Except for the point at which you give the tablet to the patient, the steps for administering buccal and sublingual drugs are the same as those for drugs administered orally (as outlined in Procedure 38-1). When you administer buccal or sublingual medications, your role usually involves teaching the patient how to administer these medications at home.

For both buccal and sublingual administration, tell the patient not to chew or swallow the tablet. Tell the patient to place a buccal drug, such as hyoscyamine sulfate, between the cheek and gum until it dissolves, as shown in Figure 38-5. Explain that this area has a rich blood supply that promotes rapid drug absorption.

Tell the patient to place a sublingual drug, such as nitroglycerin, under the tongue until it dissolves, as shown in Figure 38-6. Explain that the capillaries in this area promote rapid drug absorption.

Instruct patients not to eat, drink, or smoke until after the tablet completely dissolves. Food and fluids wash the

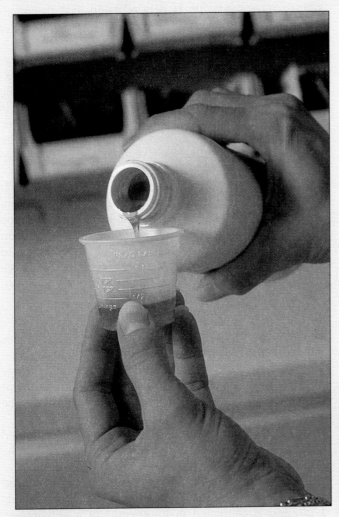

Figure 38-3. Pour a liquid drug into a calibrated medication cup.

9. After pouring the drug, place the cup on a flat surface, and check the drug level again. At eye level the base of the meniscus (the crescent-shaped form at the top of the liquid) should align with the mark that indicates the prescribed dose (Figure 38-4). If you poured out too much, discard it. Do not return it to the container because medicine cups are not sterile.
10. Give the medicine cup to the patient with instructions to drink the liquid. If appropriate, offer a glass of water or juice to wash down the drug.

After You Have Given an Oral Drug

11. Wash your hands.
12. Give the patient an information sheet about the drug. Discuss the information with the patient and answer any questions she may have. If the patient has questions you cannot answer, refer her to the physician.
13. Document the drug administration with date, time, drug name, dosage, route, site, and significant patient reactions in the patient's chart. Also document patient education about the drug.

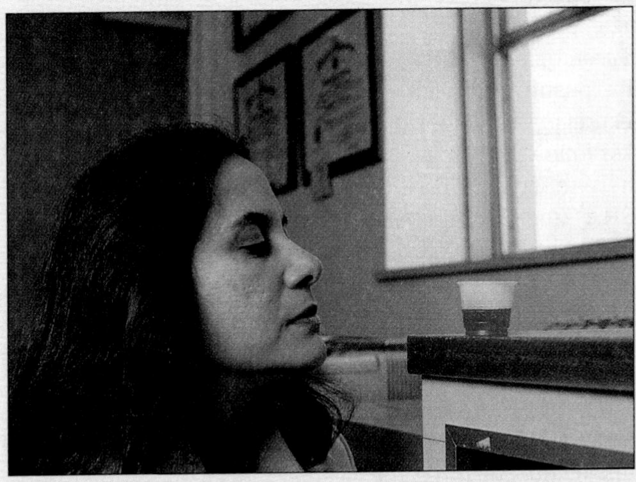

Figure 38-4. Read the measurement at eye level.

drug into the GI tract, slowing absorption or allowing gastric juices to destroy it. Smoking increases salivation, causing impaired absorption of the drug.

Remain with patients until their tablet dissolves to monitor for possible adverse reaction and to ensure that patients have allowed the tablet to dissolve in the mouth instead of chewing or swallowing it. Give patients an information sheet about the drug. Discuss it with them, and answer their questions. If they have questions you cannot answer, refer them to the doctor.

As always, immediately document the drug administration with the date, time, drug name, dose, route, site, and any significant patient reactions. Also document patient education about the drug.

Parenteral Administration

Parenteral administration is the administration of a substance such as a drug by muscle, vein, or any means other than through the GI tract (substances administered through the GI tract are usually given by mouth). It

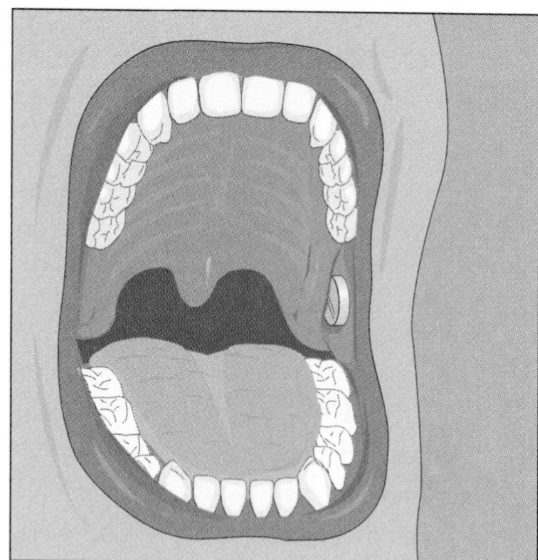

Figure 38-5. Place a buccal drug between the cheek and gum.

generally applies to giving drugs by injection. Although the parenteral route offers the advantage of rapid drug action, it has several potential drawbacks.

Parenteral administration poses more safety risks for the patient than administration by other routes. The reason is that after the drug has been injected, it cannot be retrieved. To reduce the risks, you must administer the drug expertly and observe the "seven rights" meticulously.

Parenteral administration increases your risk of potential exposure to blood-borne pathogens when performing injections and disposing of used needles. To minimize risks, follow Universal Precautions during injections. Also adhere to Occupational Safety and Health Administration (OSHA) and Environmental Protection Agency (EPA) regulations for disposing of contaminated needles and sharp items, as discussed in Chapter 19. Most offices provide a rigid, puncture-proof container for collecting disposable sharp instruments. This container should be self-sealing and have a lock-tight cap and a safety neck.

After using a needle, lancet, or syringe, immediately place it in the sharps container. To avoid puncturing yourself, do not force the needle, lancet, or syringe into the container. If you do accidentally stick yourself, notify the physician at once so you can be treated. OSHA requires medical follow-up for all workers who have been accidentally punctured.

Never let a sharps container become full. When the container is two-thirds full, seal it and follow your office procedure for container disposal.

Needles. When you administer a parenteral drug, you must select the appropriate needle, syringe, and drug form to use on the basis of the type of injection. The following are methods of injection:

- **Intradermal (ID),** or within the upper layers of the skin
- **Subcutaneous (SC),** or beneath the skin
- **Intramuscular (IM),** or within a muscle
- **Intravenous (IV),** or directly into a vein

Needles consist of a hub, hilt, shaft, lumen, point, and bevel (Figure 38-7). The hub of the needle fits onto the syringe. The needle tip is beveled (sloped at the opening). The bevel helps the needle cut through the skin with minimum trauma.

Needles are available in various gauges (inside diameters) and lengths (Figure 38-8). A needle's gauge is expressed with numbers. The smaller the number, the larger the gauge. For example, a 25-gauge needle is smaller than an 18-gauge needle. Use the right gauge for the type of injection and the viscosity (thickness) of the drug to be administered. For example, use a large-gauge needle for a highly viscous drug.

When selecting a needle, also consider its length. It must be long enough to penetrate the appropriate layers of tissue but not so long as to go too deep. Choose the correct needle length on the basis of the type of injection as well as the patient's size, amount of fatty tissue, and injection site. Table 38-6 lists the ranges of needle gauge and length typically used for intradermal, subcutaneous, and intramuscular injections.

Syringes. Syringes have two basic parts: a barrel and a plunger. The barrel is the calibrated cylinder that holds the drug. The plunger forces the drug through the barrel and out the needle, as shown in Figure 38-9. The syringe may be packaged with the needle attached and a guard cap over the needle, or the syringe and needle may be packaged separately.

Syringes come in many sizes and are calibrated according to how the syringe will be used. For example, the common 3-mL syringe is divided into tenths of a milliliter on one side and minims on the other. It is used to measure most drugs. A tuberculin (TB) syringe holds 1 mL and is calibrated in hundredths of a milliliter on one side and minims on the other for small doses of

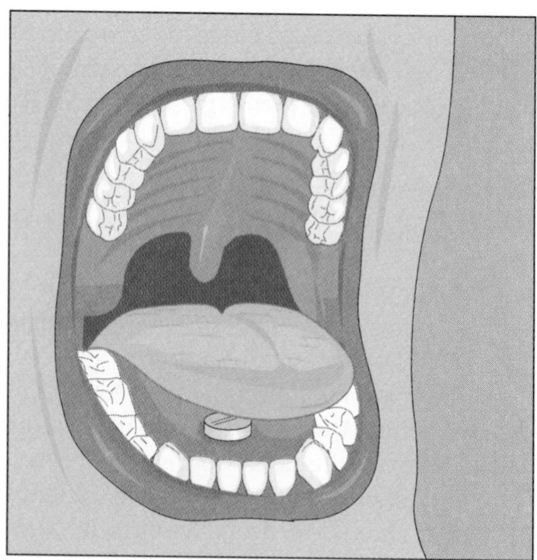

Figure 38-6. Place a sublingual drug under the tongue.

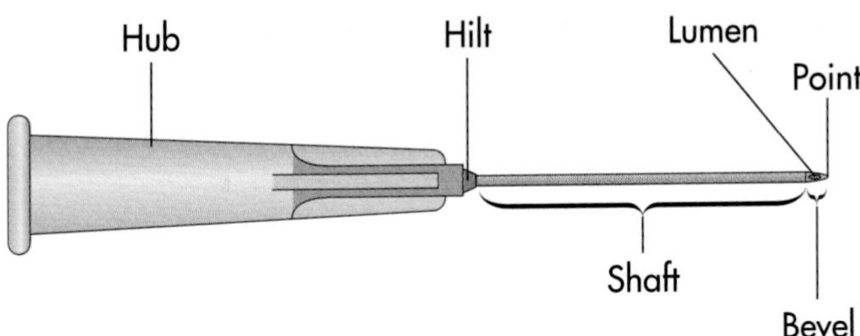

Figure 38-7. Understanding the parts of a needle will help you use it correctly.

drugs (Figure 38-10). Insulin syringes are calibrated in units (U), commonly either 50 U or 100 U (Figure 38-10). Unlike other syringes, insulin syringes have permanently attached needles and no dead space (fluid remaining in the needle or syringe after the plunger is depressed fully). These differences help the patient self-administer the correct amount of insulin.

Forms of Packaging for Parenteral Drugs. Parenteral drugs are supplied in the forms shown in Figure 38-11. They are ampules, cartridges, and vials.

- An ampule is a small glass or plastic container that is sealed to keep its contents sterile. It must be opened and used with care, as described in Procedure 38-2.
- A cartridge is a small barrel prefilled with a sterile drug. It slips into a special, reusable syringe assembly.
- A vial is a small bottle with a rubber diaphragm that can be punctured by needle. A vial contains a liquid or powder, which must first be reconstituted with a **diluent** (liquid used to dissolve and dilute a drug), as described in Procedure 38-3. It may contain a single or multiple dose. This procedure requires two needle and syringe sets—one for inserting the diluent into the vial and another to draw and administer the reconstituted drug—to avoid using a contaminated needle. The first needle is considered contaminated when you set it down to mix the diluent and the drug.

Methods of Injection. Injections are the most common method of drug administration in a medical office. You need to be knowledgeable about all injection methods: intradermal, subcutaneous, intramuscular, and intravenous. You must also become proficient in administering intradermal, subcutaneous, and intramuscular injections, as permitted in your state.

Intradermal. An intradermal injection is administered into the upper layer of skin at an angle almost parallel to the skin, as described in Procedure 38-4, p. 822. Common sites for intradermal injections are the forearm and back. Intradermal injections are usually used to administer a skin test, such as an allergy test or a TB test. When choosing an injection site on patients, avoid scarred, blemished, or hairy areas, because those features interfere with your ability to interpret test results on the skin.

The drug is injected under the top skin layer, and a little bubble or wheal is raised. If the body reacts to the drug, erythema (redness) and induration (hardening) occur. This reaction generally takes place 15 to 20 minutes after an allergy test and from 48 to 72 hours after a TB test.

Subcutaneous. Orally referred to as sub Q by most healthcare professionals, a subcutaneous injection provides a slow, sustained release of a drug and a relatively long duration of action. Generally, 1 mL or less of a drug can be delivered by SC injection (Procedure 38-5, p. 823). Various drugs, such as insulin and heparin, are commonly administered by SC injection.

Common subcutaneous injection sites include an area on the back between the shoulder blades, the outer sides of the upper arms and thighs, and the abdomen (except for a 2-inch area around the umbilicus). To prepare for an SC injection, select a site away from bones and blood vessels. Do not use an area that is edematous (swollen), scarred, or hardened or one that has a large amount of fat, because these areas may not have the capillary network needed for absorption. When patients need regular SC injections, remember to rotate injection sites systematically. Begin the rotation pattern by giving injections in rows in the same area of the body (such as the abdomen). After all those sites have been used once, proceed to the next area on the body (such as the right leg), and follow a similar pattern there. Rotating sites promotes drug absorption and prevents hard subcutaneous lumps from forming.

At the injection site, ensure that you can pinch at least a 1-inch skin fold for the injection. If a patient is frail, dehydrated, or thin, you may need to use a site other than the back or abdomen to provide the necessary fold of skin.

Intramuscular. When a patient requires rapid drug absorption, you may be asked to administer an intramuscular injection, as described in Procedure 38-6, p. 825.

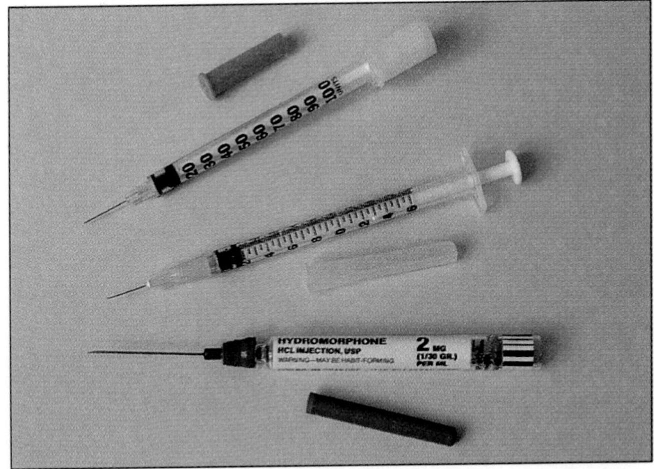

Figure 38-8. Choose a needle with a length, gauge, and bevel appropriate to the type of injection, the drug being injected, and the patient receiving the injection.

Table 38-6

Choosing a Needle

Type of Injection	Gauge of Needle	Length of Needle
Intradermal	25–26 gauge	⅜–½ inch
Subcutaneous	23–27 gauge	½–¾ inch
Intramuscular	18–23 gauge	1–3 inches

An IM injection usually irritates a patient's tissues less than an SC injection and allows administration of a larger amount of drug, usually 3 to 5 mL in an adult.

Common IM injection sites include the dorsogluteal, ventrogluteal, vastus lateralis, and deltoid muscles, illustrated in Figure 38-20, p. 826. Before giving an IM injection, identify the site carefully to prevent injury to blood vessels and nerves in the area. As with SC injections, rotate sites if the patient must receive regular or multiple IM injections.

Take into consideration the patient's layer of fat when choosing an IM injection site. You want the injection to penetrate beyond the fat layer to muscle. If, for example, a patient is heavy in the buttocks and thighs, the deltoid may be the best site for administering an IM injection.

When giving an IM injection to a pediatric patient, use the smallest gauge needle, usually 22 to 25 gauge. Also use the shortest length needle that will allow you to reach muscle, usually 1 inch.

Injection sites vary with age. For an infant or toddler, use the vastus lateralis muscle. For a child who has been walking for about a year, use the ventrogluteal or dorsogluteal site. For an older, well-developed child, use any adult site.

When injecting an IM drug that can irritate subcutaneous tissues, such as iron dextran (Imferon), use the **Z-track method,** illustrated in Figure 38-21, p. 827. To do this, pull the skin and subcutaneous tissue to the side before inserting the needle at the site. After the drug is injected, release the tissue. This technique creates a zigzag path in the tissue layers, which prevents the drug from leaking into the subcutaneous tissue and causing irritation.

Intravenous. Although intravenous injections are not commonly performed in a medical office or by medical assistants, certain drugs may be administered this way. Drugs may also be mixed and dissolved into a **solution** (a homogeneous mixture of a solid, liquid, or gaseous substance in a liquid) and given by IV **infusion** (slow drip) into a vein. Examples of IV drugs include powerful antibiotics, chemotherapeutic drugs, emergency drugs, and electrolytes. Because these drugs are introduced directly into the bloodstream, they produce an almost immediate effect. They also can cause sudden adverse reactions.

Although a doctor or nurse must administer an IV drug, you may assist by laying out supplies and equipment. When assisting with a venipuncture, gather the ordered drug and a tourniquet, bedsaver pad, gloves, iodine and alcohol swabs, venipuncture device, tape, and gauze pad, as ordered. Obtain other supplies and equipment, depending on the specific type of infusion or injection being administered.

Inhalation Therapy

Inhalation therapy can be administered through the mouth or nose. There are a number of disorders for which the physician may order an inhaler or aerosol form of medication. For example, an oral inhaler is frequently

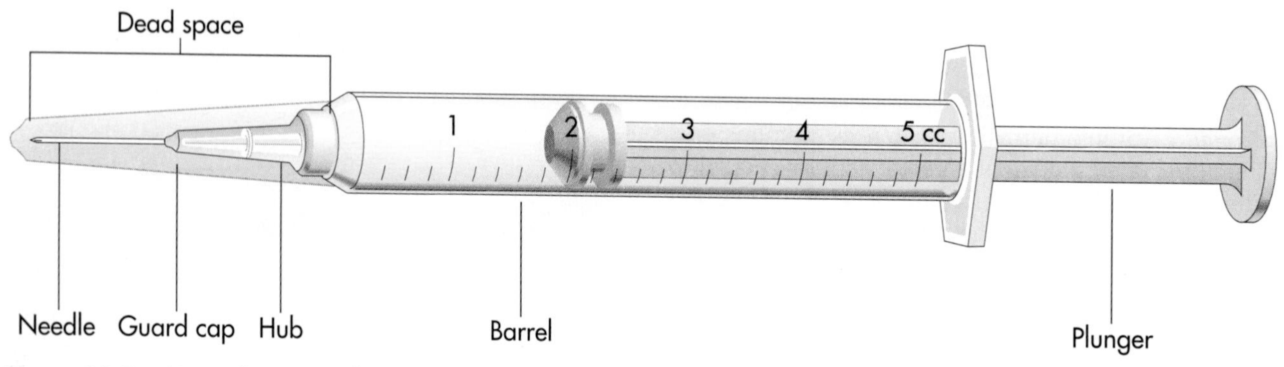

Figure 38-9. Know the parts of a standard syringe.

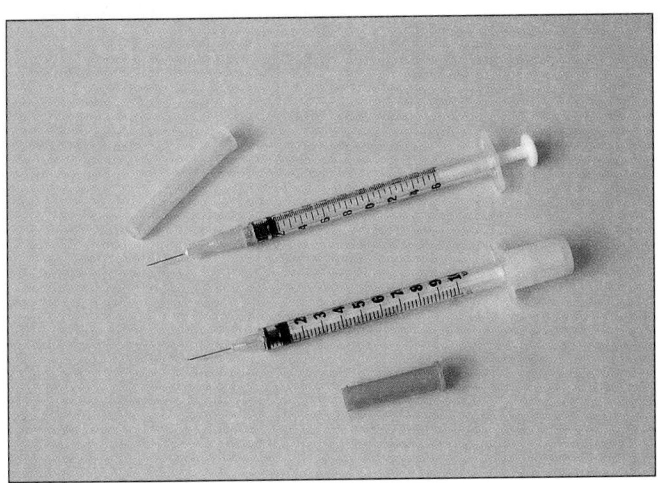

Figure 38-10. You may use the tuberculin syringe (top) to deliver small doses (up to 1.0 mL) of drugs. This insulin syringe (bottom) delivers precisely 100 U of insulin when filled with insulin of the proper concentration (100 U per mL).

used by patients with asthma, whereas a nasal inhaler is frequently used for local treatment of nasal congestion. Nasal inhalers are also used to administer medicines for systemic effect, such as a vasopressin derivative for nocturnal bed-wetting.

Package inserts for inhaled drugs provide detailed descriptions of the correct procedure. If directed by the physician, however, you must teach the patient how to use an inhaler safely and correctly.

As with all drug administrations, check the "seven rights," comparing information against the drug order. Ensure that you have the correct patient, the correct drug, and the correct form (oral or nasal) of inhaler. As you teach the patient, refer to the package insert, and show the patient where to find each step on the instruction sheet, so that he will be familiar with the steps when administering the inhaler at home.

Check the label of the inhaler to determine whether the inhaler must be shaken thoroughly before administration. If shaking the inhaler is indicated, stress this point with the patient. Otherwise, the drug will not be evenly distributed in the inhaler, and its effectiveness will be jeopardized. If indicated, a nasal inhaler must be shaken before administration to each nostril.

Tell patients to follow these steps when administering a nasal inhaler.

1. Wash hands and blow the nose to clear the nostrils as much as possible before using the inhaler.
2. Tilt the head back, and with one hand, place the inhaler tip about ½ inch into the nostril.
3. Point the tip straight up toward the inner corner of the eye. Angling the inhaler downward makes the drug run down the back of the throat, causing a burning sensation.
4. Use the opposite hand to block the other nostril.
5. Inhale gently while quickly and firmly squeezing the inhaler.
6. Remove the inhaler tip and exhale through the mouth.
7. Shake the inhaler and repeat the process in the other nostril.

If indicated in the package insert, instruct patients to keep the head tilted back and not to blow their nose for several minutes. They can then wash their hands while you immediately document the inhaler administration with date, time, drug, dose, route, and any significant patient reactions. Also record your patient education about inhaler use.

Topical Application

Topical application is the direct application of a drug on the skin. Topical drugs can take the form of creams, lotions, **ointments** (salves), tinctures, powders, sprays, and solutions, which are used for their local effects. They include antibacterial and antifungal drugs, as well as corticosteroids.

To apply a cream, lotion, or ointment, use long, even strokes when rubbing it into the skin. Follow the direction of the hair growth to avoid irritating the hair follicles and skin. To apply a powder, shake it on but do not rub it in.

A specialized type of topical administration that produces a systemic effect is the **transdermal** system (or patch). A drug administered through the transdermal patch is absorbed through the skin directly into the bloodstream. The patch slowly and evenly releases a systemic drug, such as scopolamine, nitroglycerin, estrogen, or fentanyl, through the skin. The patient receives a timed-release dose, usually over a day or several days.

Because the release of a drug from a transdermal patch is often crucial to a patient's health, the package inserts with transdermal medications are extremely

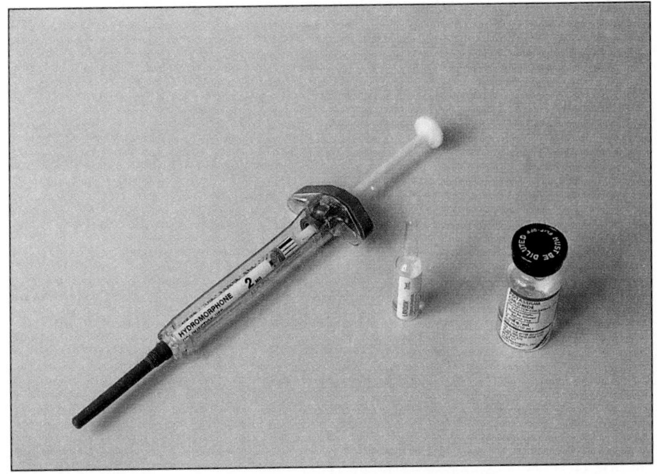

Figure 38-11. Injectable drugs may come in a cartridge (left), an ampule (center), or a vial (right).

PROCEDURE 38-2

Drawing a Drug From an Ampule

Objective: To safely open an ampule and draw a drug, using sterile technique

OSHA Guidelines 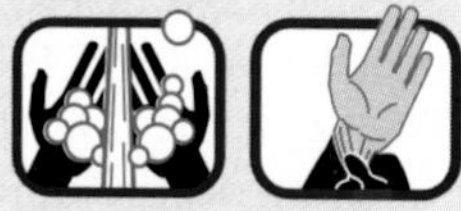

Materials: Ampule of drug, alcohol swab, 2- by 2-inch gauze square, small file (provided by the drug manufacturer), needle and syringe of the appropriate size

Method

1. Wash your hands and put on examination gloves.
2. Gently tap the top of the ampule with your forefinger to settle the liquid to the bottom of the ampule.
3. Wipe the ampule's neck with an alcohol swab.
4. Wrap the 2- by 2-inch gauze square around the ampule's neck. Then snap the neck away from you (Figure 38-12). If it does not snap easily, score the neck with the small file and snap it again.
5. Insert the needle into the ampule without touching the side of the ampule.
6. Pull back on the plunger to aspirate (remove by vacuum or suction) the liquid. The drug is now ready for injection.

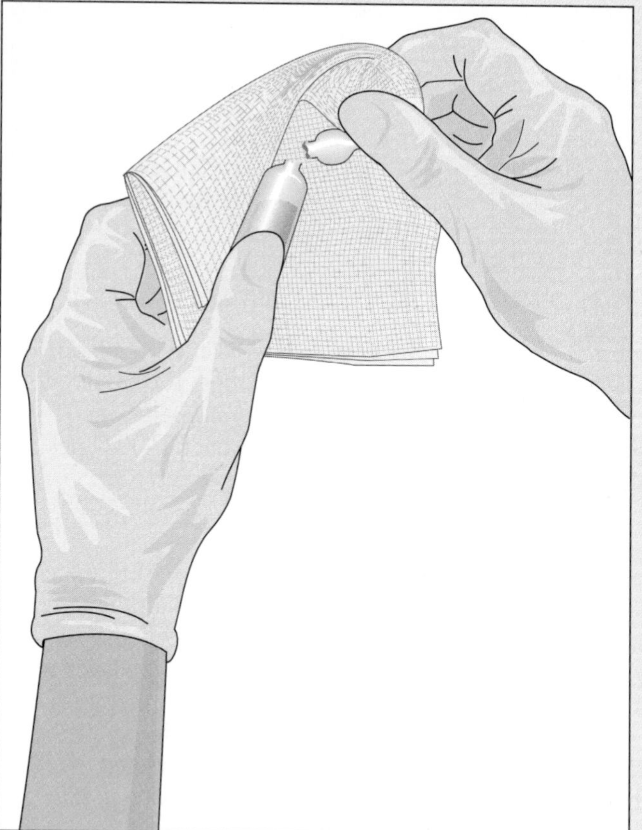

Figure 38-12. You must snap the neck of the ampule before inserting the needle.

detailed. You must instruct the patient to follow the instructions precisely and to be sure to change the patch on the prescribed schedule.

If the doctor directs you to provide some education, your goal is to teach the patient how to apply and remove a transdermal drug unit safely and effectively. Refer to the package insert as you teach, and show the patient where each step is located on the instruction sheet. This identification gives the patient the reference needed for changing the patch at home.

Before showing and administering the patch, check the "seven rights," comparing information against the drug order. Wash your hands and instruct the patient to do the same when preparing for transdermal system application.

Some patches come sealed in a protective pouch. The plastic backing is easily peeled off once the patch is removed from the pouch. The plastic backing on patches without a protective pouch must be manipulated carefully to allow its removal. Show the patient how to bend the sides of the latter type of transdermal unit back and forth until the clear plastic backing snaps down the middle.

For either type of patch, demonstrate how to peel off the clear plastic backing to expose the sticky side of the patch. Then show the patient how to apply the patch to a reasonably hair-free site, such as the abdomen. Figure 38-22, p. 827, shows how to apply both types of patches. Advise the patient to avoid using the extremities below the knee or elbow, skin folds, scar tissue, or burned or irritated areas. Estrogen patches are usually placed on the hip. Wash your hands and instruct the patient to do the same after applying a transdermal system at home.

To remove the patch, instruct the patient to gently lift and slowly peel it back from the skin. Then wash the skin with soap and water, dry the area with a towel, and wash the hands. Explain that the skin may appear red and warm, which is normal. Reassure the patient that the redness will disappear. Instruct the patient to notify the doctor if the redness does not disappear in several days or if a rash develops.

Tell the patient never to apply a new patch to the site just used. It is best to allow each site to rest between applications. Some transdermal systems call for waiting 7

PROCEDURE 38-3

Reconstituting and Drawing a Drug for Injection

Objective: To reconstitute and draw a drug for injection, using sterile technique

OSHA Guidelines

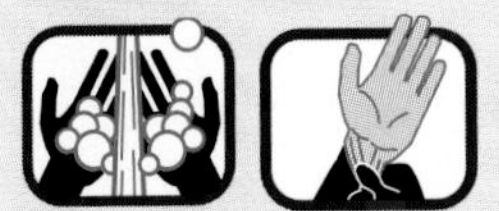
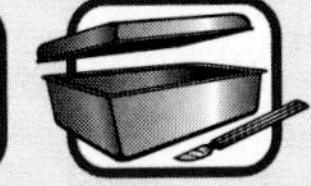

Materials: Vial of drug, vial of diluent, alcohol swabs, two disposable sterile needle and syringe sets of appropriate size

Method

1. Wash your hands and put on examination gloves.
2. Place the drug vial and diluent vial on the countertop. Wipe the rubber diaphragm of each with an alcohol swab.
3. Remove the cap from the needle and the guard from the syringe. Pull the plunger back to the mark that equals the amount of diluent needed to reconstitute the drug ordered. (This action aspirates air into the syringe.)
4. Puncture the diaphragm of the vial of diluent with the needle, and inject the air into the diluent. This action creates positive pressure that lets you draw the diluent easily (Figure 38-13). (If you do not add air, a vacuum forms, making it difficult to draw the diluent.)
5. Invert the vial and aspirate the diluent.
6. Remove the needle from the diluent vial, inject the diluent into the drug vial, and withdraw the needle. Properly dispose of this needle and syringe.
7. Roll the vial between your hands to mix the drug and diluent thoroughly. Do not shake the vial unless so directed on the drug label. When completely mixed, the solution in the vial should have no flakes. The solution will be clear or cloudy when completely mixed (depending on the drug).
8. Remove the cap and guard from the second needle and syringe.
9. Pull back the plunger to the mark that reflects the amount of drug ordered. Inject the air into the drug vial.
10. Invert the vial and aspirate the proper amount of the drug into the syringe (Figure 38-14). The drug is now ready for injection.

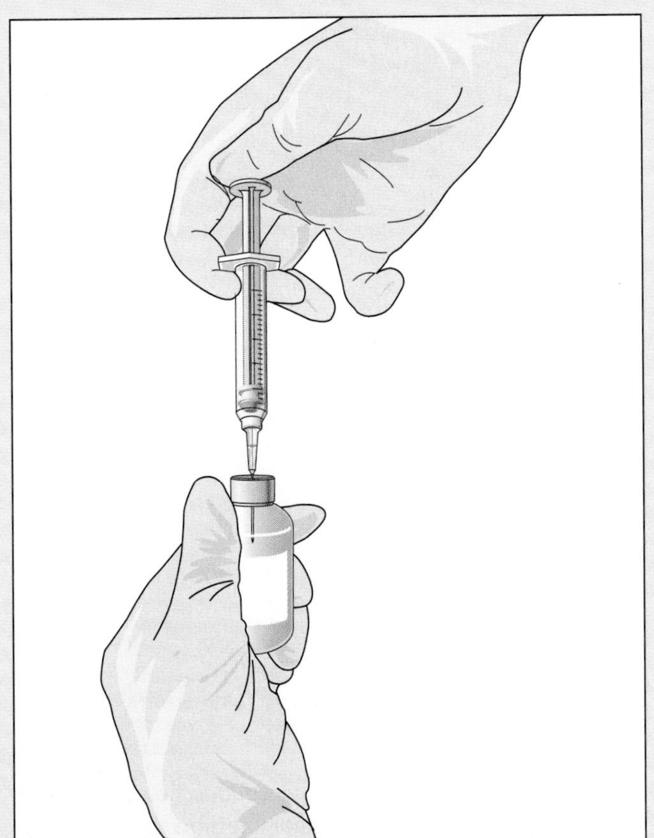

Figure 38-13. Injecting air into the diluent makes it easier to draw.

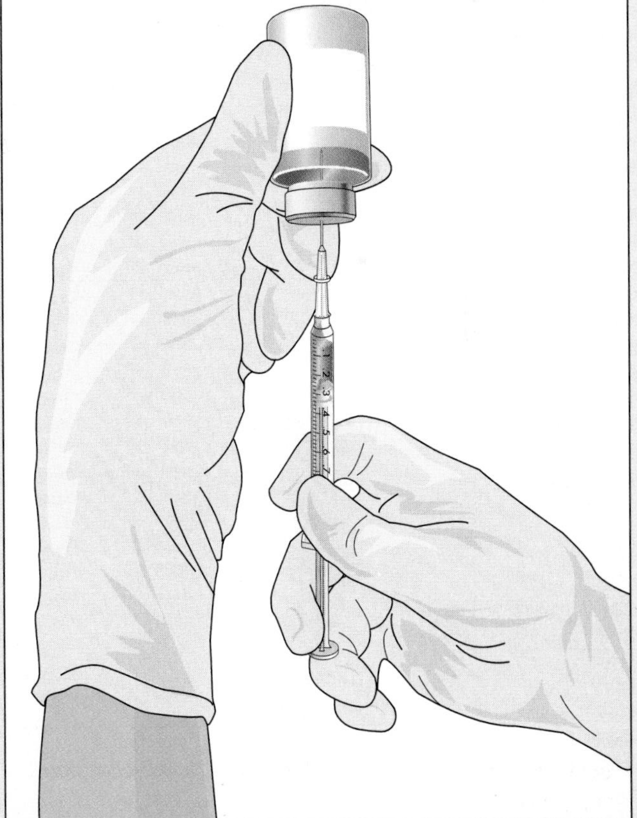

Figure 38-14. Invert the vial and draw the reconstituted drug.

PROCEDURE 38-4

Giving an Intradermal Injection

Objective: To administer an intradermal injection safely and effectively, using sterile technique

OSHA Guidelines

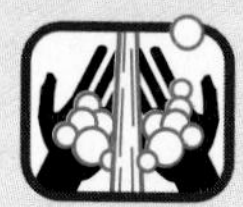
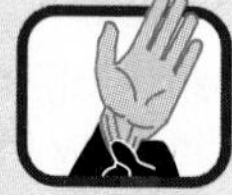

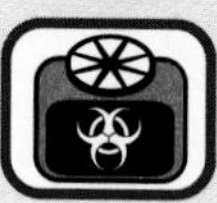
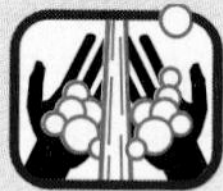

Materials: Drug order (in patient's chart), alcohol swab, disposable needle and syringe of the appropriate size filled with the ordered dose of drug

Method

1. Wash your hands and put on examination gloves.
2. Check the "seven rights," comparing information against the drug order.
3. Identify the injection site on the patient's forearm. To do so, rest the patient's arm on a table with the palm up. Measure 2 to 3 finger-widths below the antecubital space and a hand-width above the wrist. The space between is available for the injection (Figure 38-15).
4. Prepare the skin with the alcohol swab, moving in a circle from the center out.
5. Let the skin dry before giving the injection. Otherwise, you could introduce antiseptic under the skin, which could cause irritation and falsify intradermal test results.
6. Hold the patient's forearm, and stretch the skin taut with one hand.
7. With the other hand, place the needle—bevel up—almost flat against the patient's skin. Press the needle against the skin and insert it.
8. Inject the drug slowly and gently. You should see the needle through the skin and feel resistance. As the drug enters the upper layer of skin, a wheal (raised area of the skin) will form (Figure 38-16).
9. After the full dose of the drug has been injected, withdraw the needle. Properly dispose of used materials and the needle and syringe immediately.
10. Remove the gloves and wash your hands.
11. Stay with the patient to monitor for unexpected reactions.
12. Document the injection with date, time, drug name, dosage, route, site, and significant reactions in the patient's chart.

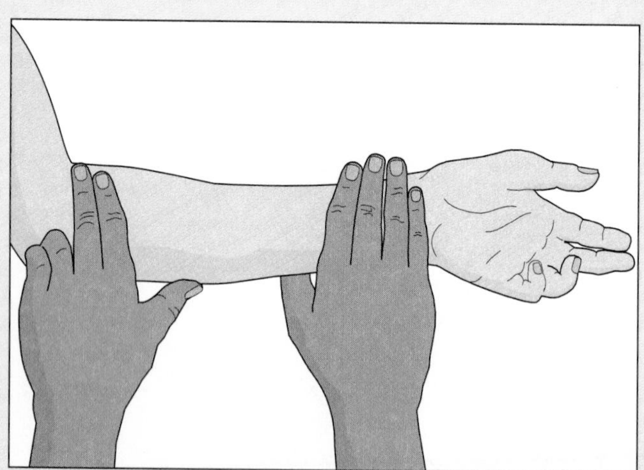

Figure 38-15. This space is available for intradermal injection sites.

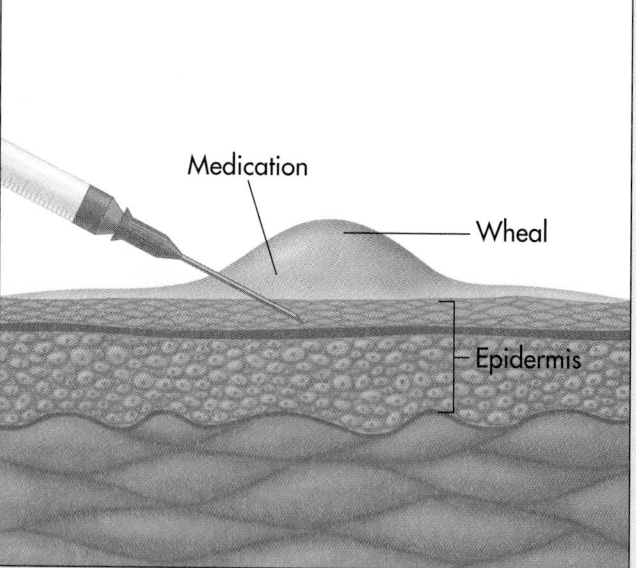

Figure 38-16. Medication collects under the skin, forming a wheal during an intradermal injection.

days before using a site again. Be sure to check the package directions regarding site rotation.

Patients frequently ask whether they can apply lotion or talc to the area after removing the patch. Tell them they may do so if the skin is dry. After answering any other questions, immediately document the drug application with date, time, drug, dose, route, and any significant patient reactions. Also record your patient education about transdermal system application and removal.

Urethral Administration

The urethral route is used when antibiotic and antifungal drugs are needed locally—that is, at the site of infection—for some urinary tract infections. Depending on the nature of the infection and the duration of drug action, the physician or a nurse may instill liquid drugs only one time or several times a day for a week. Urethral administration is used in both men and women.

Urethral drug administration requires passing a small-diameter urinary catheter into the bladder, instilling a drug through it, and clamping the catheter to let the drug bathe the urinary bladder walls. The materials needed for catheterization are included in a urinary catheter kit.

When the physician or nurse administers a urethral drug, you may assist with the following steps as directed.

1. Use sterile technique. Wash your hands and gather the necessary supplies. Depending on the amount of drug to be administered, you will need either a syringe without a needle or tubing and a bag. You will also need a urinary catheter kit, sterile gloves, the prescribed drug, a drape, and a bedsaver pad.

PROCEDURE 38-5

Giving a Subcutaneous Injection

Objective: To administer a subcutaneous injection safely and effectively, using sterile technique

OSHA Guidelines

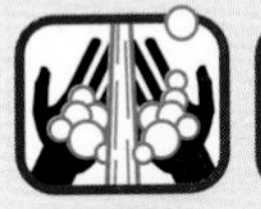
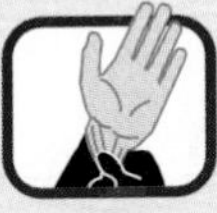

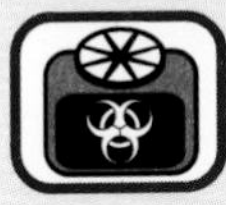
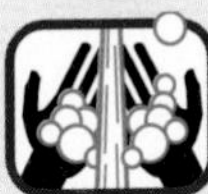

Materials: Drug order (in patient's chart), alcohol swabs, container of the ordered drug, disposable needle and syringe of the appropriate size

Method

1. Wash your hands and put on examination gloves.
2. Check the "seven rights," comparing information against the drug order.
3. Prepare the drug and draw it up to the mark on the syringe that matches the ordered dose. Then pull the plunger back an additional 0.2 to 0.3 mL to create an air bubble. When you inject the drug, the air bubble helps seal the subcutaneous tissue (Figure 38-17).
4. Choose a site (Figure 38-18) and clean it with an alcohol swab, moving in a circle from the center out. Let the area dry.
5. Pinch the skin firmly to lift the subcutaneous tissue.
6. Position the needle—bevel up—at a 45° angle to the skin.
7. Insert the needle in one quick motion. Then release the skin, and aspirate by pulling back slightly on

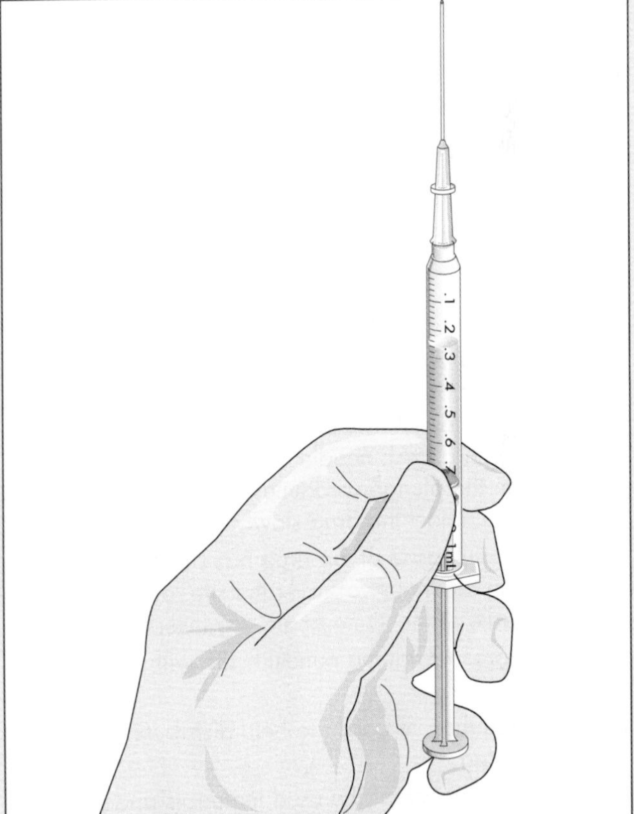

Figure 38-17. Pull back the plunger to create an air bubble in the syringe used in subcutaneous injection.

continued

Giving a Subcutaneous Injection

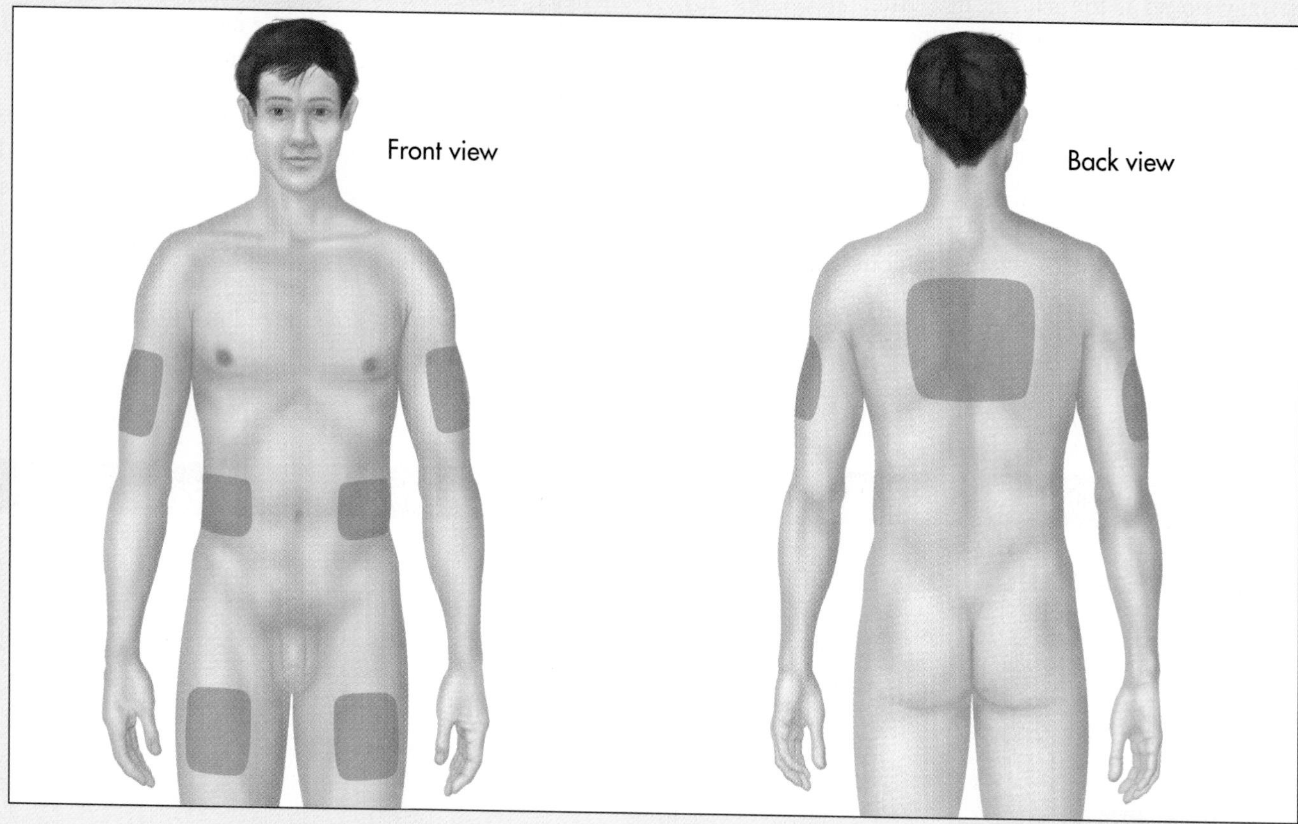

Figure 38-18. Many sites are available for subcutaneous injection.

the plunger to check the needle placement (do not pull back if you are administering insulin or heparin). If pulling back on the plunger produces blood, placement is incorrect and you must begin again with a fresh needle and syringe. If pulling back on the plunger produces no blood, placement is correct. Inject the drug slowly (Figure 38-19).

8. After the full dose of the drug has been injected, place an alcohol swab over the site, and withdraw the needle at the same angle you inserted it.
9. Apply pressure at the puncture site with the alcohol swab.
10. Massage the site gently to help distribute the drug, if indicated.
11. Properly dispose of the used materials and the needle and syringe.
12. Remove the gloves and wash your hands.
13. Stay with the patient to monitor for unexpected reactions.
14. Document the injection with date, time, drug name, dosage, route, site, and significant reactions in the patient's chart.

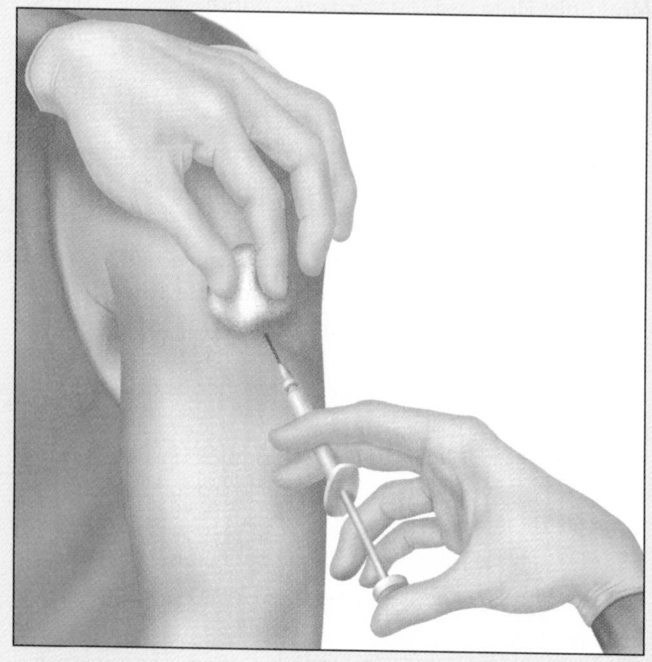

Figure 38-19. Perform a subcutaneous injection.

2. Check the "seven rights," comparing information against the drug order, and explain the procedure and the drug order to the patient.
3. Assist the patient into the lithotomy position, and drape her to preserve her modesty while exposing the vulva.
4. Place a bedsaver pad under the buttocks.
5. Open the catheter kit.
6. Put on sterile gloves.
7. Cleanse the vulva as you would to perform catheterization, using the materials in the kit. As you sweep down with the antiseptic swab, watch for the urethral opening to "wink," which helps you locate it accurately.
8. The physician or nurse will insert the lubricated catheter. Tell the patient that she should feel pressure, not pain, and that the physician or nurse is going to attach the syringe to the catheter and insert the drug (or attach the tubing and bag to the catheter and let the drug run in by gravity).
9. After instilling the drug, the physician or nurse will clamp the catheter and leave the drug in place for the ordered amount of time.
10. Stay with the patient not only to ensure that she remains still but also to reassure her that the full feeling in the bladder is normal. She may also say she feels the need to urinate. Advise her that this feeling, too, is normal and is caused by the catheter.
11. When the time is up, unclamp the catheter, gently remove it, and allow the patient to urinate. Assist the patient as needed.
12. While the patient is dressing, immediately document the drug instillation with date, time, drug, dose, route, and any significant patient reactions.

Vaginal Administration

Physicians usually prescribe vaginal drugs to treat local fungal infections. The drugs may also be used for local bacterial infections. They are usually packaged as suppositories (the most common form), solutions, creams,

PROCEDURE 38-6

Giving an Intramuscular Injection

Objective: To administer an intramuscular injection safely and effectively, using sterile technique

OSHA Guidelines

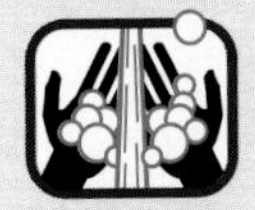
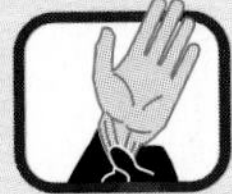

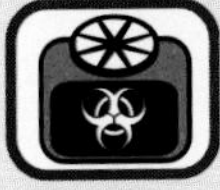
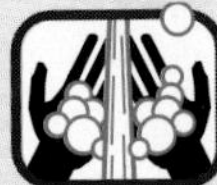

Materials: Drug order (in patient's chart), alcohol swabs, container of the ordered drug, disposable needle and syringe of the appropriate size

Method

1. Wash your hands and put on examination gloves.
2. Check the "seven rights," comparing information against the drug order.
3. Prepare the drug and draw it up to the mark on the syringe that matches the ordered dose. Then pull the plunger back another 0.2 to 0.3 mL to add air. This air clears the drug from the needle and prevents drug seepage.
4. Choose a site (Figure 38-20) and gently tap it. Tapping stimulates the nerve endings and reduces pain caused by the needle insertion.
5. Clean the site with an alcohol swab, moving in a circle from the center out. Let the site dry.
6. Stretch the skin taut over the injection site.
7. Hold the needle and syringe at a 90° angle to the skin. Then insert the needle with a quick, dartlike thrust.
8. Release the skin and aspirate by pulling back slightly on the plunger to check the needle placement. If pulling back on the plunger produces blood, placement is incorrect and you must begin again with a fresh needle and syringe. If pulling back on the plunger produces no blood, placement is correct. Inject the drug slowly.
9. After the full dose of the drug has been injected, place an alcohol swab over the site. Then quickly remove the needle at a 90° angle.
10. Use the alcohol swab to apply pressure to the site and massage it, if indicated.
11. Properly dispose of used materials and the needle and syringe.
12. Remove the gloves and wash your hands.
13. Stay with the patient to monitor for unexpected reactions.
14. Document the injection with date, time, drug name, dosage, route, site, and significant patient reactions in the patient's chart.

continued

Giving an Intramuscular Injection

Iliac crest
Gluteus medius
Gluteus medius
Gluteal fold
Clavicle
Deltoid muscle
Vastus lateralis (mid-portion)

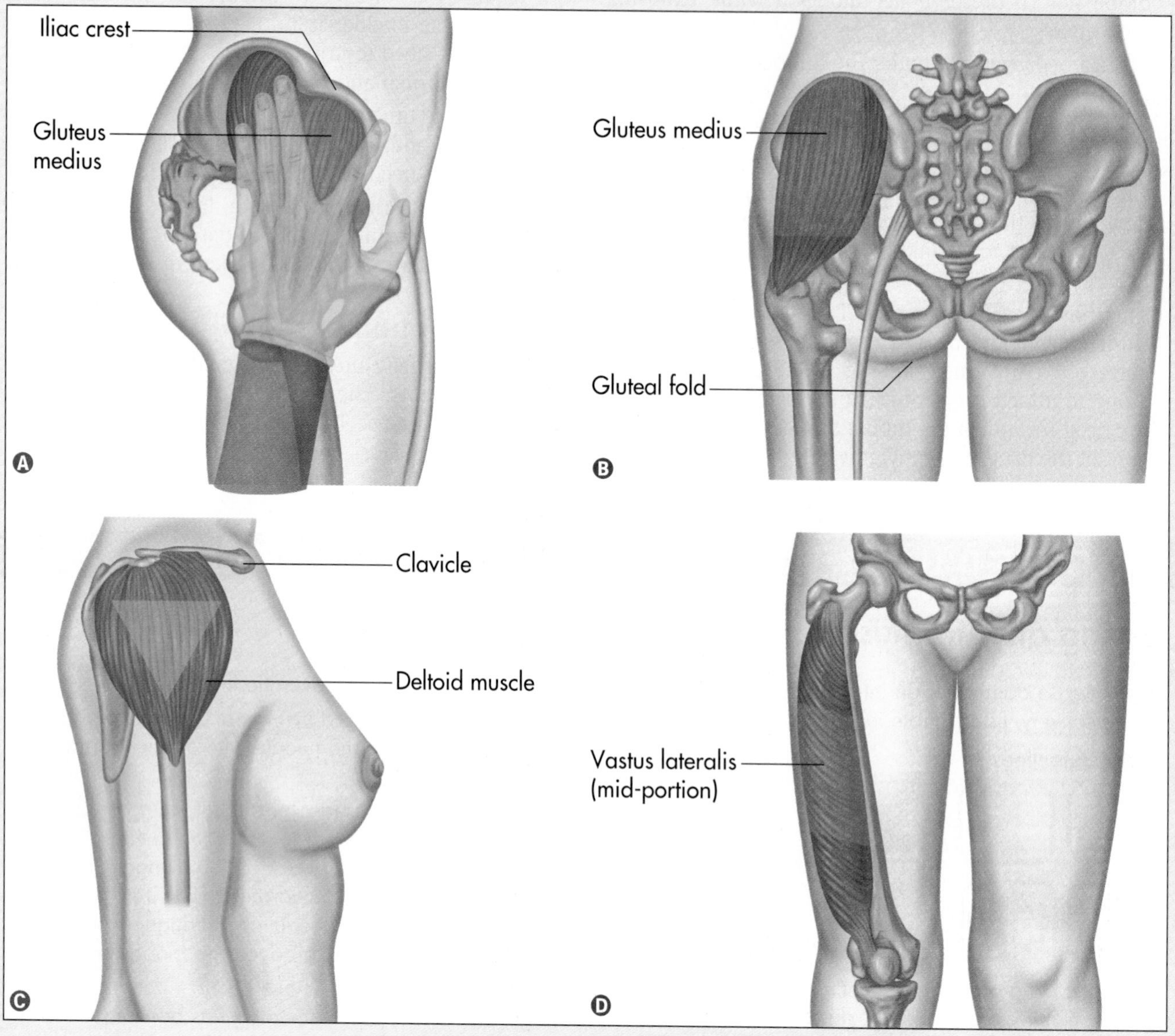

Figure 38-20. For intramuscular injection in an adult, use (a) the ventrogluteal site, (b) the dorsogluteal site, (c) the deltoid site, or (d) the vastus lateralis site.

ointments, and foams. Patients frequently ask about administering vaginal medications, and they usually administer such medications at home. Therefore, you must be prepared to provide detailed patient education for this route of administration. The physician may ask you to administer the first dose as a means of teaching a patient the method to use at home, or you may be asked to administer a one-time-only dose.

To administer a vaginal suppository, follow these steps.

1. Wash your hands and gather the following materials: the prescription or drug order in the patient's chart, a cloth or paper drape, a bedsaver pad, gloves, cotton balls, water-soluble lubricant, and the prescribed drug.
2. Check the "seven rights," comparing information against the drug order, and explain the procedure and the drug order to the patient.
3. Give the patient the opportunity to empty her bladder before beginning.
4. Assist the patient into the lithotomy position, and drape her to preserve her modesty while exposing the vulva.

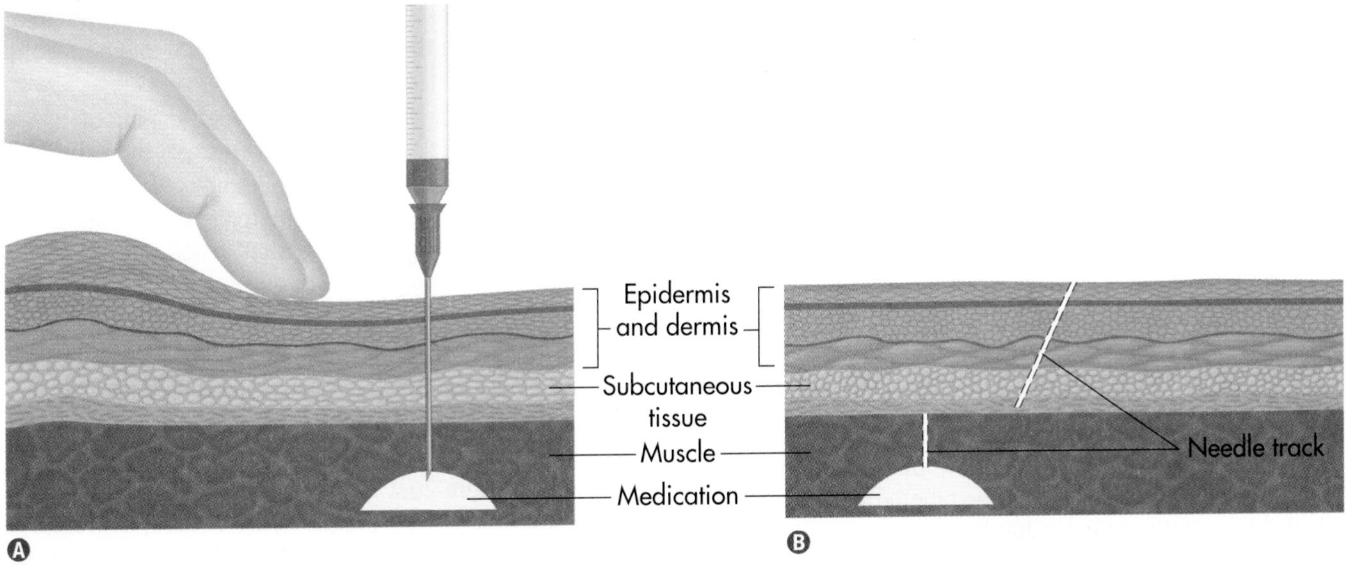

Figure 38-21. Use the Z-track method for IM injection of irritating solutions. **A.** Pull the skin to one side before inserting the needle. **B.** After injecting the drug, release the skin to seal off the needle track.

5. Place a bedsaver pad under the buttocks.
6. Put on sterile gloves.
7. Cleanse the perineum with soap and water, using one cotton ball per stroke, and cleanse the center last, while spreading the labia.
8. Lubricate the vaginal suppository applicator in lubricant spread on a paper towel.
9. While spreading the labia with one hand, insert the applicator with the other (the applicator should be about 2 inches into the vagina and angled toward the sacrum).
10. Release the labia and push the applicator's plunger to release the suppository into the vagina.
11. Remove the applicator, and wipe any excess lubricant off the patient.
12. Help her to a sitting position, and assist with dressing if needed.
13. Document the administration with date, time, drug, dose, route, and any significant patient reactions.

Follow the same steps, using an appropriate applicator, for vaginal drugs in the forms of creams, ointments, gels, and tablets. The liquid form of vaginal medication is administered by performing a **douche** (vaginal irrigation). This process is similar to giving a urethral drug, but it requires a special irrigating nozzle.

Rectal Administration

Certain medications, such as drugs used to treat constipation, nausea, and vomiting, may be administered by the rectal route. These medications may be given in the form of suppositories or enemas and may produce local or systemic effects.

Rectal Suppository. Administering rectal suppositories is rarely done in a doctor's office except on a pediatric patient. The doctor may, however, ask you to give a first suppository to an adult as a means of patient education. To do so, follow these steps.

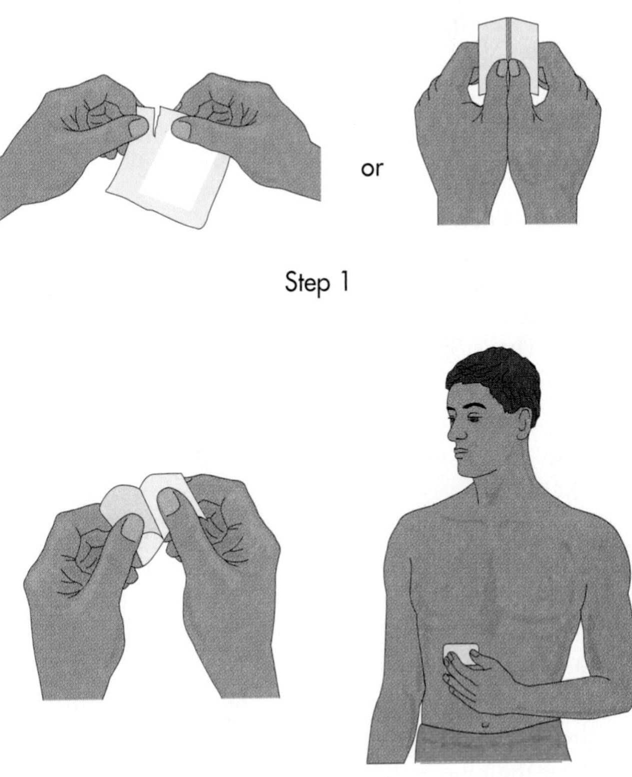

Figure 38-22. To apply a transdermal patch, first either (1) remove it from the pouch, or (1) bend the sides back and forth until the backing snaps; then (2) peel the backing off the patch; and (3) apply the patch, sticky side down, to a clean, relatively hairless site.

1. Check the "seven rights," comparing information against the drug order.
2. Explain the procedure and the drug order to the patient.
3. Give the patient the opportunity to empty the bladder before beginning.
4. Help the patient into Sims' position (shown in Chapter 25, Figure 25-1).
5. Lift the patient's gown to expose the anus.
6. Put on gloves and remove the wrapper from the suppository.
7. Lubricate the tapered end of the suppository with about 1 tsp of lubricant.
8. While spreading the patient's buttocks with one hand, insert the suppository—tapered end first—into the anus with the other hand.
9. Gently advance the suppository past the sphincter with your index finger. Before it passes the sphincter, the suppository may feel as if it is being pushed back out the anus. When it passes the sphincter, it seems to disappear.
10. Use tissues to remove excess lubricant from the area.
11. Remove your gloves and ask the patient to lie quietly and retain the suppository for at least 20 minutes.
12. When the treatment is completed, help the patient to a sitting, then standing, position.
13. Wash your hands and immediately document the drug administration with date, time, drug, dose, route, and any significant patient reactions.

Retention Enema. Retention enemas are usually not administered in a physician's office. You may, however, be asked to perform this procedure in an unusual circumstance, such as for a frail, elderly patient with fecal impaction. The steps for administering a retention enema are as follows.

1. Check the "seven rights."
2. Help the patient lie on the left side and bend the right knee.
3. Put a bedsaver pad under the patient's left hip.
4. Place the tip of a syringe into a rectal tube. Let a little rectal solution flow through the syringe and tube. While holding the tip up, clamp the tubing.
5. Lubricate the end of the tube.
6. Spread the patient's buttocks, and slide the tube into the rectum about 4 inches.
7. After the tube is in place, slowly pour the rectal solution into the syringe, release the clamp, and let gravity move the solution into the patient.
8. When you have administered the ordered amount of solution, clamp the tube, then remove it.
9. Using tissues, apply pressure over the anus for 20 seconds to stifle the patient's urge to defecate.
10. Wipe any excess lubricant or solution from the area, and encourage the patient to retain the enema for the time ordered.
11. When the time has passed, help the patient use a bedpan or direct him to a toilet to expel the solution.
12. Wash your hands and immediately document the drug administration with date, time, drug, dose, route, and any significant patient reactions.

Administering Medications to the Eye or Ear

Doctors commonly administer eye medications to assist patients in eye tests, reduce pressure in the eyes, relieve eye pain, and treat eye infections and inflammation. Refer to Procedure 26-2 in Chapter 26 for instructions on how to administer eye medications. Although most eye medications are administered for local effect, some contain drugs that are absorbed systemically. To prevent systemic absorption, the doctor may request that you apply pressure with one finger just below the inner corner of each eye after instilling medications. Continue applying pressure for 2 to 3 minutes, as directed.

Doctors often administer eardrops to treat patients' ear infections or inflammation, relieve ear pain, or loosen earwax. Like eye medications, eardrops are ordered primarily for their local effects. They are not usually absorbed systemically, nor do they cause systemic effects. Procedure 26-5 in Chapter 26 describes how to administer eardrops.

Educating the Patient About Drug Administration

Educating patients about what drugs do to the body and what the body does to drugs is discussed in detail in Chapter 37. You need to provide additional patient education, however, with regard to routes of administration. This education is extremely important; a patient who does not administer a drug correctly or safely may put health or life at risk.

Reading the Drug Package Label

You must check the *PDR* for information about any drug with which you are not familiar. Likewise, before you teach a patient how to administer a drug, you must review the specific administration instructions for the drug in the *PDR*. An important aspect of this kind of information is teaching the patient how to read a prescription drug label. Instruct the patient to be particularly alert for special instructions and warning labels, such as those shown in Figure 38-23.

Interactions

Drug interactions should not be confused with adverse effects of drugs, discussed in Chapter 37. Patient education with regard to interactions is important. Interactions may

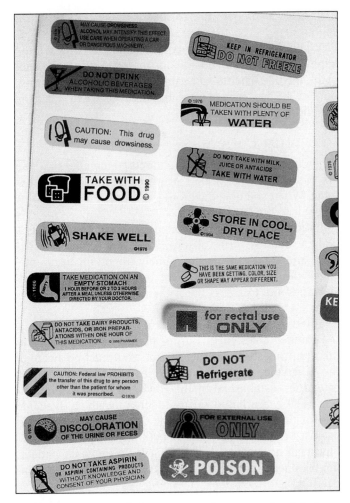

Figure 38-23. Teach the patient to heed warning labels and instructions on drug bottles.

occur between two prescription or nonprescription drugs or between a drug and food and may cause serious effects. Explain that the greater the number of drugs the patient takes, the greater the chance of a drug interaction.

Drug-Drug Interactions. Most drug interactions affect the absorption, distribution, metabolism, or excretion of the drugs. In some cases drug-drug interactions can affect the results of laboratory tests. When two drugs are taken at the same time, there are several possible interactions.

- The effects of both drugs are increased, causing either a toxic or beneficial effect. For example, when alcohol is combined with diazepam (Valium), there is the potential toxic effect of severe central nervous system depression, because one drug intensifies the effect of the other. An example of a beneficial effect is the combination of acetaminophen and codeine, which increases the activity of both drugs, allowing the physician to prescribe a lower dose of each. In fact, this combination of drugs is available in one tablet (Tylenol with codeine).
- The effects of both drugs are decreased, or one drug cancels out the effect of the other. For example, combining propanolol (Inderal) with albuterol (Proventil) causes each drug to lose its effectiveness.
- The effect of one of the drugs is increased by the other. For example, the effect of digoxin (Lanoxin) is increased by the presence of furosemide (Lasix), but the furosemide still works at the same degree of effectiveness as when administered alone.

To help prevent unintentional drug interactions, thoroughly assess the patient's medication use. Be sure to ask about medications prescribed by specialists, as well as over-the-counter (OTC) drugs. Question the patient about past and present use of alcohol and recreational drugs as well as herbal remedies. Update the chart as needed. If you detect a potential for drug interactions, notify the physician.

Also teach patients about possible drug interactions and how to avoid or minimize them. For example, patients may need to take certain drugs at least 2 hours apart. Instruct patients to call the office if they think their drugs are interacting adversely.

Drug-Food Interactions. Interactions between a drug and food can alter a drug's therapeutic effect. For example, taking tetracycline with milk can reduce the drug's effectiveness because of decreased absorption from the GI tract. The drug-food interaction between a monoamine oxidase (MAO) inhibitor (such as Parnate, an antidepressant drug) and aged cheese or meat or other foods containing high levels of tyramine can produce a toxic effect. This interaction can cause a dangerous hypertensive crisis in which the patient's blood pressure rises quickly to dangerous levels, possibly leading to stroke and death.

Some drug-food interactions can affect the body's use of nutrients. For example, the cholesterol-lowering drugs cholestyramine resin and colestipol HCl may reduce the body's absorption of fat-soluble vitamins (A, D, E, and K) from food.

When teaching a patient about drug-food interactions, specify exactly which foods to avoid and when. For example, a patient may drink milk or eat food several hours before or after taking tetracycline, whereas a patient taking an MAO inhibitor must avoid foods that contain high levels of tyramine at all times. Explain what to expect if an interaction occurs, and describe how to deal with it.

Adverse Effects

Adverse effects or reactions associated with a drug and reported in the *PDR* are discussed briefly in the section on toxicology in Chapter 37. These responses are somewhat predictable and range from mild adverse reactions, such as stomach upset, to severe or life-threatening allergic responses. Unpredictable adverse effects can also occur; they are unique to each patient. Always advise the patient to report any change in overall health, because that change could be drug-related.

Elderly patients and patients with liver or kidney disease are more susceptible than others to adverse effects because these conditions affect drug metabolism and excretion. When drugs are not metabolized properly or excreted from the body quickly enough, drugs can reach toxic levels, even with normal doses.

To help prevent adverse effects, teach the patient to take the drug at the right time, in the right amount, and under the right circumstances. For example, the patient may need to take a cephalosporin with food to avoid nausea and diarrhea. Also teach the patient to recognize significant adverse effects and to call the office if any of them occur.

Special Considerations

Pediatric, pregnant, breast-feeding, or elderly patients or patients from different cultures require special considerations. When giving a drug to these patients, you must adjust patient care as needed.

Pediatric Patients

Children pose special challenges in drug administration and use. Their physiology and immature body systems may make drug effects less predictable because drugs are absorbed, distributed, metabolized, and excreted differently in children than in adults. Therefore, plan to observe a pediatric patient closely for adverse effects and interactions.

A child's small size may also increase the risk of overdose and toxicity. These factors may require dosage adjustments and careful measurement of small doses. To help administer drugs safely to pediatric patients, always check your calculations for providing a prescribed dose, and then ask a nurse or the doctor to double-check them.

Remember that administration sites and techniques for a child may differ from those for an adult. For example, fewer IM injection sites can be used for a young child. Also, the technique for eardrop administration varies slightly.

When dealing with an infant or young child, teach the parents—not the patient—about the drug. With an older child, include parents and patient in the teaching session. Be sure to use age-appropriate language when speaking to children.

Pregnant Patients

When dealing with pregnant patients, remember that you are caring for two patients at once: the mother and her fetus. When you give the mother a drug, you may also be giving it to the fetus.

In addition, pregnancy-related changes in the mother's body can affect drug absorption, distribution, metabolism, and excretion. It is extremely important to double-check the drug in the *PDR* for toxicology or pregnancy warnings and to assess the patient carefully for therapeutic and adverse effects of the drug.

Some drugs can cause physical defects in the fetus if the mother takes them during pregnancy (especially in the first trimester). For this reason, you must be aware of the pregnancy drug risk categories (Table 38-7). These categories, established by the Food and Drug Administration (FDA), are based on the degree to which available information has ruled out risk to the fetus, balanced against the drug's potential benefits to the patient. If the physician orders a high-risk drug for a pregnant patient, double-check the order with the physician before administering the drug.

Patients Who Are Breast-Feeding

Some drugs are excreted in breast milk and can thus be ingested by a breast-feeding infant. This ingestion can be dangerous because infants have immature body sys-

Table 38-7

Pregnancy Drug Risk Categories

Category	Meaning
A	Controlled studies in pregnant women have failed to demonstrate risk to the fetus.
B	There is no evidence of risk in humans, either because human findings show no risk or because there are no human findings but animal findings are negative.
C	Human studies are lacking, and animal findings are either positive for fetal risk or lacking as well. However, potential benefits may justify the potential risk.
D	There is positive evidence of risk. Nevertheless, potential benefits may outweigh the potential risk.
X	Fetal risk clearly outweighs any possible benefit to the patient.
NR	No rating is available.

Source: Physicians' Desk Reference, 50th ed. (Montvale, NJ: Medical Economics, 1996), 2888.

tems and cannot metabolize and excrete drugs that are safe for the mother. Some drugs, such as sedatives, diuretics, and hormones, can reduce the mother's flow of breast milk.

Whenever a drug is ordered for a patient who is breast-feeding, check a drug reference work to see whether the drug is contraindicated during lactation. If so, consult the doctor. If not, teach the mother to recognize signs of adverse drug effects in her infant. If a mother must take a drug that affects lactation, advise her to supplement breast-feedings with infant formula.

Elderly Patients

Age-related changes in the body can affect drug absorption, metabolism, distribution, and excretion. These normal changes can be exaggerated by various diseases or disorders. Therefore, as people age, they have an increased risk of drug toxicity, adverse effects, or lack of therapeutic effects. Because of this risk, be especially alert when assessing an elderly patient who is on drug therapy.

Many elderly patients have complex, chronic diseases with unusual symptoms. This situation can make it difficult to tell whether a problem is caused by a drug. Listen closely to elderly patients and their family members; they are more likely to notice subtle changes than you are.

Patient *and family* education is important with elderly patients, particularly if they engage in polypharmacy (take several medications concurrently). Polypharmacy is common in elderly patients, and possible drug-drug interactions can be severe, as described in "Caution: Handle With Care."

If an elderly patient is forgetful or confused, talk to the doctor about simplifying the medication schedule to reduce the risk of drug administration errors or omissions. Suggest the use of pill-organizing devices to help prevent forgotten doses or overdoses. If the patient has vision problems, provide drug instruction sheets in large type. To do this, either type instructions on a word processor in a large type size, enlarge the instructions on a photocopier, or clearly handwrite the instructions in large block letters. You might also contact a local association for the blind or visually impaired for devices and tips.

Patients From Different Cultures

Although cultural background is not likely to affect a drug's action in the body, it can affect a patient's understanding of drug therapy and compliance with it. For example, a patient who speaks little or no English cannot benefit from instructions given in English. To remedy this problem, obtain drug information sheets in the languages that are commonly spoken by patients of the practice. Use simple gestures and drawings to clarify difficult words or concepts. Also try to find a family member of the patient who speaks English.

To improve compliance, ask about the patient's feelings regarding medications and home remedies. Depending on cultural background, the patient may be more likely to use teas, poultices, and other home remedies than prescription or nonprescription drugs. If it appears that home remedies are not likely to affect the prescribed medication, tell the patient that it is all right to continue using the home remedies. Suggest adding the drug to the

CAUTION

HANDLE WITH CARE

Avoiding Unsafe Polypharmacy

Before administering any drug by any route, you must know every drug, both prescription and nonprescription, the patient is taking. Many patients, especially elderly ones, visit several doctors. It is entirely possible that each doctor may prescribe one or more drugs without being aware of other drugs the patient is taking. This practice can result in polypharmacy, which means taking several drugs at once. Polypharmacy can be safe, but if the doctor is unaware of the total drug profile, serious drug interactions can result.

When asking patients to identify *all* other drugs they are taking, including OTC drugs, keep in mind that patients may forget to mention all their medicines or OTC drugs to the doctor. Drugs that patients often forget to mention include antacids (such as Tums or Rolaids), birth control pills (some women do not think of these as medication), and medicines that are used only as needed, such as medicine for migraine headaches.

To help prompt patients about drugs they may have forgotten, ask patients who have seen an orthopedist or cardiologist whether pain medication has been prescribed. Ask women who have seen a gynecologist if they are using a patch or other form of hormone replacement therapy. Ask women of an appropriate age whether there is any chance they are pregnant. Ask a pregnant woman whether she is taking prenatal vitamin and mineral supplements. If a patient has been referred to any other doctor for any reason, ask whether that doctor prescribed medication.

After determining the total drug profile, you should:

- Update the patient's record.
- Consider possible drug interactions, consulting the *PDR* or other drug reference if needed.
- Inform the doctor of your findings.

patient's usual routine to help it work better. Your cultural sensitivity may greatly increase the patient's compliance.

Nonpharmacologic Pain Management

Because of drug interactions, adverse effects, or the risk of dependence, many patients prefer not to take drugs to relieve chronic pain. To meet their needs, some practices now offer nonpharmacologic methods for managing pain, such as biofeedback, guided imagery, and relaxation exercises, in addition to traditional drug therapy. (For other alternative treatments, see Chapter 30.)

Biofeedback requires equipment that measures physical indicators of stress and relaxation, such as the galvanic skin response or pulse rate. This equipment provides feedback to help the patient recognize stress and relaxation responses and, ultimately, to control them. Biofeedback can help a patient learn to evoke relaxation, which helps block pain perception.

Guided imagery helps patients relax by envisioning themselves in a calm, nurturing, wonderful place. Some cancer patients are taught to envision the cancer cells being eaten by healthy cells. Audiotapes and videotapes are available to help lead patients through these mental exercises.

Relaxation exercises involve learning special breathing techniques. Patients also learn how to relax different muscle groups.

Summary

As a medical assistant, you must be prepared to administer drugs safely and effectively. Before you can do so, however, you must be familiar with the metric, apothecaries', and household systems of measurement. You must also be able to convert measures from one system to another and perform calculations to provide a prescribed dose. For both of these skills, you can use the ratio or fraction method.

When preparing to administer a drug, assess the patient for contraindications, and observe the general rules and "seven rights" of drug administration. Depending on the prescription, the drug may be administered by the oral, buccal, sublingual, intradermal, subcutaneous, intramuscular, nasal, topical, transdermal, vaginal, or rectal routes or as eyedrops or eardrops. If directed, assist the physician or nurse with urethral administration and IV drug injection or infusion.

Patient education is an important responsibility related to drug administration. You may need to instruct patients in the proper use of a prescribed drug. In addition, you may have to teach them to prevent or to recognize and report drug interactions and adverse effects.

Some patients require special consideration when receiving drugs. These include pediatric, pregnant, breastfeeding, and elderly patients, as well as patients from different cultures.

Nonpharmacologic methods for managing chronic pain are gaining acceptance. Patients who are interested in learning about such methods should ask the physician for further information.

38 Chapter Review

Discussion Questions

1. What effects may drug interactions produce?
2. Why should you observe the "seven rights" every time you prepare and administer a drug?
3. Compare subcutaneous and intramuscular drug administration in terms of technique and possible dosage levels.

Critical Thinking Questions

1. Mrs. Green, age 78, has been recently widowed. As you assess her, she begins naming all the drugs she takes, including some of her late husband's. What do you need to consider in making your assessment?
2. A patient in her first trimester of pregnancy calls the office saying she has acid indigestion. She says that before her pregnancy, she used to take Tagamet for acid indigestion and wants to know if it is safe to take it now. How can you find this information, and what should you do once you find it?
3. Mr. Lance, age 29, visits the office for his regular IM injection. As you are making a routine assessment, he tells you that the last time the drug was administered, he had a bad reaction to it. What should you do?

Application Activities

1. Perform the necessary calculations for the following conversions. Use a table of equivalents, if needed.
   a. 350 mL = ____ L
   b. 0.17 g = ____ mg

continued →

c. 3 tbsp = ____ tsp

d. ½ tsp = ____ gtt

e. 2 fl dr = ____ mL

2. Using the ratio or fraction method, calculate the following to provide a prescribed drug dose.

a. The doctor orders 60 mg of acetaminophen with codeine, but each tablet contains only 15 mg. How many tablets should the patient take?

b. The doctor orders 300 mg of theophylline anhydrous, but each tablet contains only 100 mg. How many tablets should the patient take?

c. The doctor orders 5 mg of glyburide, but each tablet contains only 1.25 mg. How many tablets should the patient take?

3. In the laboratory, reconstitute a powdered drug for injection.

Further Readings

Baer, Charold L., and Bradley R. Williams. *Clinical Pharmacology in Nursing.* 3d ed. Springhouse, PA: Springhouse, 1996.

Davis, Renée A. *Math and Dosage Calculations for Health Occupations.* Westerville, OH: Glencoe, 1993.

"Elders and Drugs: Trouble in the Mix?" *American Journal of Nursing,* April 1994, 11.

Gerlach, Mary Jo. *Nursing Pharmacology: Concepts and Activities.* Springhouse, PA: Springhouse, 1994.

Harvey, R., et al., eds. *Lippincott's Illustrated Reviews: Pharmacology.* Philadelphia: J. B. Lippincott, 1992.

LaFlash, Elizabeth A. "Self-Care: The New Trend in Asthma Treatment." *The Professional Medical Assistant* 29, no. 5 (September/October 1996): 5–6.

"Metered-Dose Inhaler Misuse." *American Journal of Nursing,* August 1994, 53.

PDR Family Guide to Prescription Drugs. Oradell, NJ: Medical Economics, 1993.

Solomon, J. "Be Sure to Read Medication Orders Carefully." *RN,* August 1992, 71.

"Unraveling Drug Problems in the Elderly." *American Journal of Nursing,* April 1995, 53.

Electrocardiography and Pulmonary Function Testing

CHAPTER OUTLINE

- The Medical Assistant's Role in Electrocardiography and Pulmonary Function Testing
- Anatomy and Physiology of the Heart
- The Conduction System of the Heart
- The Electrocardiograph
- Preparing to Administer an ECG
- Applying the Electrodes and the Connecting Wires
- Operating the Electrocardiograph
- Troubleshooting: Artifacts and Other Problems
- Completing the Procedure
- Interpreting the ECG
- Exercise Electrocardiography (Stress Testing)
- Ambulatory Electrocardiography (Holter Monitoring)
- Anatomy and Physiology of the Respiratory System
- Pulmonary Function Testing
- Spirometry
- Performing Spirometry

OBJECTIVES

After completing Chapter 39, you will be able to:

- Describe the anatomy and physiology of the heart.
- Explain the conduction system of the heart.
- Describe the basic patterns of an electrocardiogram (ECG).
- Identify the components of an electrocardiograph and what each does.
- Explain how to position the limb and precordial electrodes correctly.
- Describe in detail how to obtain an ECG.
- Identify the various types of artifacts and potential equipment problems and how to correct them.
- Discuss how the ECG is interpreted.
- Define exercise electrocardiography.
- Explain the procedure of Holter monitoring.
- Describe the anatomy and physiology of the lungs.
- Describe various types of spirometers.
- Describe the procedure of performing spirometry.

Key Terms

arrhythmia
artifact
atrioventricular (AV) node
calibration syringe
cardiac cycle
deflection
depolarization
electrocardiogram (ECG)
electrocardiograph
electrocardiography
electrode
forced vital capacity
Holter monitor
lead
myocardial infarction
polarity
pulmonary function test
repolarization
sinoatrial (SA) node
spirometer
spirometry
stylus

AREAS OF COMPETENCE
1997 ROLE DELINEATION STUDY

CLINICAL

Fundamental Principles

- Apply principles of aseptic technique and infection control

Diagnostic Orders

- Perform diagnostic tests

Patient Care

- Prepare patient for examinations, procedures, and treatments

The Medical Assistant's Role in Electrocardiography and Pulmonary Function Testing

Electrocardiography and pulmonary function testing are two procedures you may be required to perform in a medical office. **Electrocardiography** is the process by which a graphic pattern is created from the electrical impulses generated within the heart as it pumps. It is often performed to evaluate symptoms of heart disease, to detect abnormal heart rhythms, to evaluate a patient's progress after a heart attack, or to check the effectiveness or side effects of certain medications. Electrocardiography is sometimes performed as part of a general examination.

Pulmonary function tests (PFTs) measure and evaluate a patient's lung capacity and volume. Such tests are commonly performed when a person suffers from shortness of breath, but they may also be performed as part of a general examination. Pulmonary function tests can help detect and diagnose pulmonary problems. They are also used to monitor certain respiratory disorders and to evaluate the effectiveness of treatment.

Anatomy and Physiology of the Heart

A description of the anatomy and physiology of the heart will help you better understand electrocardiography. It will also help you make sense of the electrical activity that electrocardiography records.

Anatomy of the Heart

The heart is a muscular pump that circulates blood throughout the body, carrying oxygen and nutrients to the tissues and removing waste products. The pumping action begins in the muscle tissue of the heart, called the myocardium.

The heart is actually a double pump. The right side of the heart receives blood from the body by way of the superior vena cava and the inferior vena cava. From there, the pulmonary arteries deliver blood to the lungs, where the blood exchanges carbon dioxide for oxygen. Oxygenated blood flows into the left side of the heart through the pulmonary veins. Once in the heart, blood is pumped into the aorta, which pumps oxygenated blood to all parts of the body.

The heart has four sections or chambers: two upper receiving chambers, the atria (singular, atrium), and two lower pumping chambers, the ventricles (Figure 39-1). Valves between each atrium and ventricle prevent blood from regurgitating (backing up) into the atrium while the ventricle contracts. Similar valves between the ventricles and the arteries into which they pump (the aorta and the pulmonary arteries) prevent blood from regurgitating into the ventricles when they relax. A partition, the septum, divides the heart into right and left sides.

Physiology of the Heart

The heart is divided into separate chambers that work as a single unit. Contraction of the atria, followed by contraction of the ventricles, moves the blood. This contraction phase is called systole. Systole is followed by a relaxation phase, called diastole. When you take someone's blood pressure, you are measuring the pressure during the contraction (systolic) and relaxation (diastolic) phases. This sequence of contraction and relaxation makes up a complete heartbeat, known as the **cardiac cycle.** Each cycle lasts an average of 0.8 second.

All the fibers in the cardiac muscle are interconnected and act as one muscle. Consequently, when one fiber is stimulated to contract, the entire group of fibers contracts. This property plays an important role in the conduction system of the heart.

The Conduction System of the Heart

The cardiac cycle is regulated by specialized tissues in the heart wall, shown in Figure 39-1, that transmit electrical impulses. These electrical impulses cause the heart muscle to contract and relax.

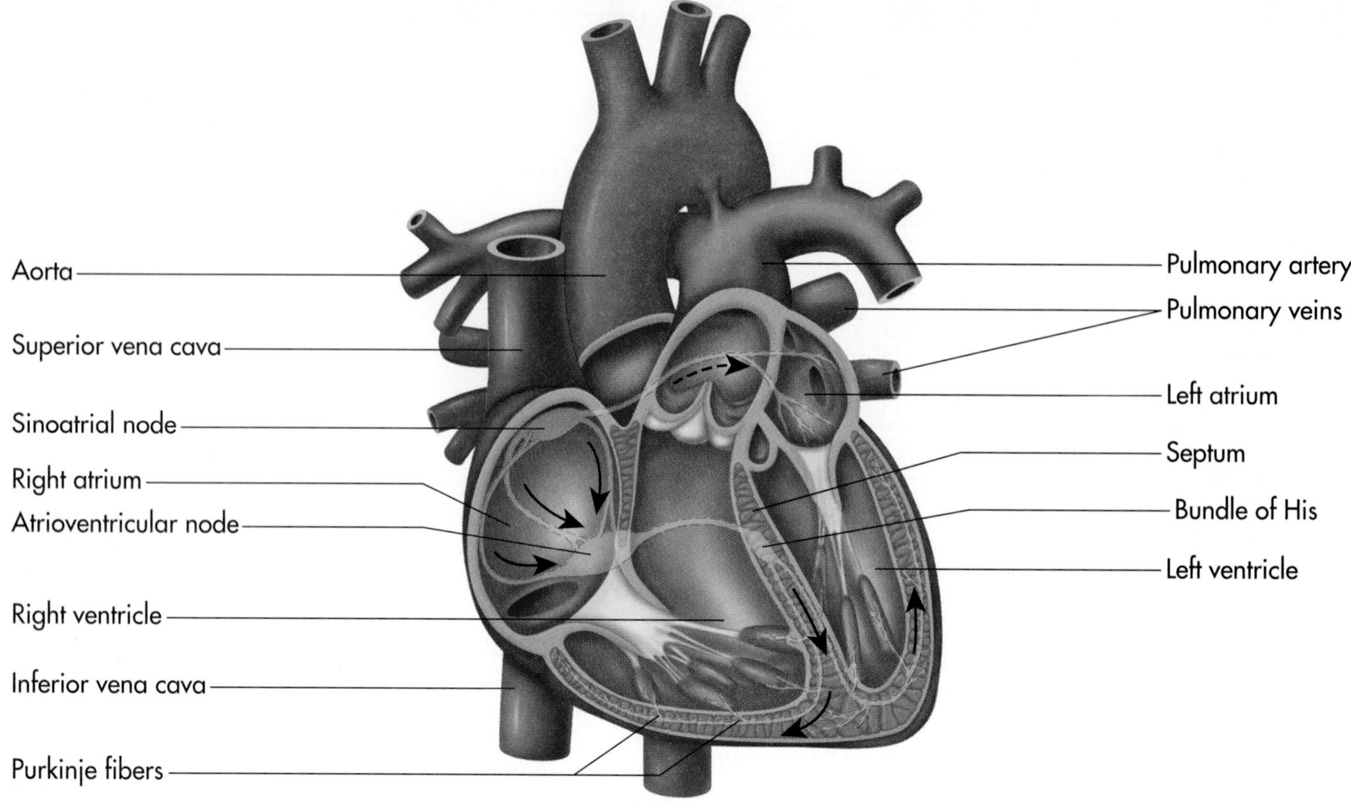

Figure 39-1. Electrical impulses control the cardiac conduction system. Each impulse begins in the sinoatrial node, progresses to the atrioventricular node, and then travels through the bundle of His, the right and left bundle branches, and the Purkinje fibers.

Transmission of electrical impulses in the heart begins in the **sinoatrial (SA) node,** also called the sinus node or the pacemaker of the heart. The sinoatrial node is a small bundle of heart muscle tissue in the superior wall of the right atrium that specializes in producing electrical impulses. The sinoatrial node sets the rhythm (or pattern) of the heart's contractions.

When the electrical impulse for muscle contraction is generated, it travels throughout the muscle of each atrium, causing atrial contraction. The impulse then travels to the **atrioventricular (AV) node,** another mass of specialized conducting cells, similar to those of the SA node. The AV node is located at the bottom of the right atrium, near the junction of the ventricles (the septum), where transmission of the impulse is slightly delayed. This delay gives the atria time to completely contract and fill the ventricles with blood.

The atrioventricular node then passes the impulse to the bundle of His (named after the Swiss physician Wilhelm His, Jr. [1863–1934]), located in the septum between the ventricles. The bundle of His acts as a relay station, sending the impulse through a series of bundle branches to a network of cardiac conducting muscle fibers. These specialized muscle fibers, called Purkinje fibers (named after the Czech physiologist Jan Evangelista Purkinje [1787–1869]), are located in the ventricle walls. When the impulse reaches the Purkinje fibers, the ventricles contract.

Conduction and Electrocardiography

Electrocardiography records the transmission, magnitude, and duration of the various electrical impulses of the heart. Before you can understand how electrocardiography works, you must understand **polarity,** the condition of having two separate poles, one of which is positive and the other negative. A resting cardiac cell is polarized; that is, there is a negative charge inside and a positive charge outside. When the cardiac cell loses its polarity (a natural occurrence), depolarization occurs. **Depolarization** is the electrical impulse that initiates a chain reaction resulting in contraction. This wave of depolarization flows from the SA node to the ventricles and can be detected by **electrodes,** or electrical impulse sensors, that are placed on specific areas on the surface of the body. During electrocardiography, electrodes detect and record the electrical activity of the heart, including disturbances or disruptions in its rhythm.

Depolarization is always followed by a period of electrical recovery called **repolarization,** when polarity is restored. Following repolarization, the heart returns to a resting, polarized state. The electrical cycle is then repeated, leading to another cardiac cycle.

The Basic Pattern of the Electrocardiogram

The waves of electrical impulses responsible for the cardiac cycle produce a series of waves and lines on an **electrocardiogram** (abbreviated **ECG** or EKG), which is the tracing made by an **electrocardiograph,** an instrument that measures and displays these impulses (Figure 39-2). These peaks and valleys, called waves or **deflections,** are labeled with the letters P, Q, R, S, T, and U. Each letter represents a specific part of the pattern, as explained in Table 39-1. The recognition of abnormalities in the size of the waves or the various time intervals can aid in the diagnosis of certain types of heart problems.

The Electrocardiograph

Each type of electrocardiograph works in the same way. The electrical impulses produced by the heart can be detected through the skin; these impulses are measured, amplified, and recorded on the ECG. Detection begins with electrodes that conduct and transmit the electrical impulses to the electrocardiograph through insulated wires. An amplifier increases the signal, making the heartbeat visible. The **stylus,** a penlike instrument, records this movement on the ECG paper. The impulses received through various combinations of electrodes constitute different **leads,** or views of the electrical activity of the heart, that are recorded on the ECG.

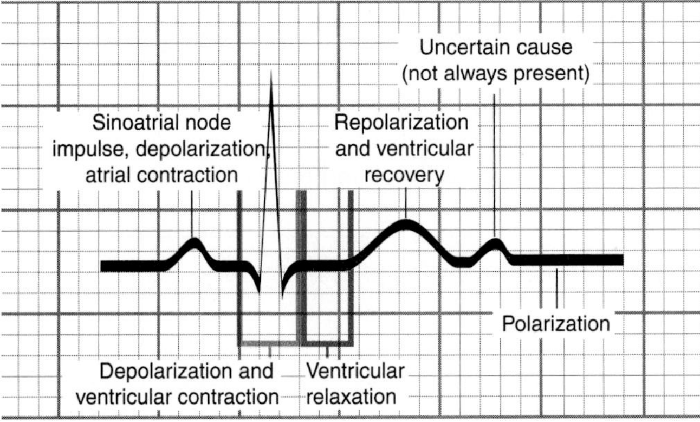

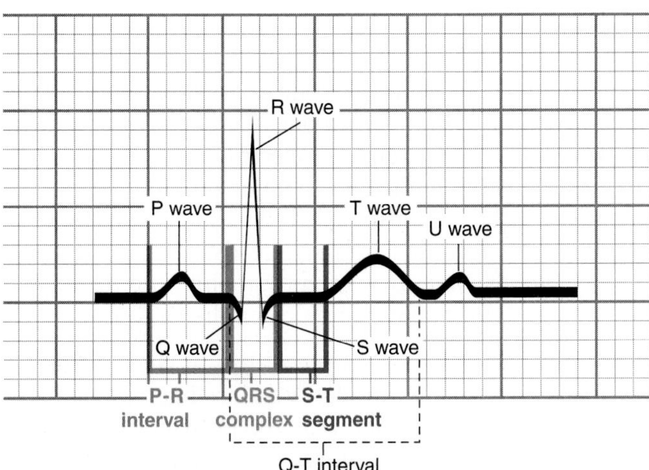

Figure 39-2. This ECG tracing shows the pattern of one cardiac cycle in a normal heart. These specific electrical impulses (top) represent the cycle of cardiac contraction and relaxation. The waves and lines (bottom) represent specific parts of the pattern.

Types of Electrocardiographs

Several different types of electrocardiographs are in use today. Two types are shown in Figure 39-3. The standard machine is a 12-lead electrocardiograph, which simultaneously records the electrical activity of the heart from 12 different views. A single-channel electrocardiograph records the electrical activity of one lead, and consequently, one view of the heart's electrical activity at a time. The record is printed on a long, thin strip of ECG paper. The most common single-channel units allow you to attach all electrodes at the same time and obtain a manual or automatic printout of individual leads. Some older units use fewer electrodes, requiring you to systematically attach, remove, and reposition the electrodes to obtain recordings from different leads.

The newer multichannel units record more than one lead at a time. These machines use wider paper and more than one stylus to record the leads.

Electrodes and Electrolyte Products

Electrodes are attached to the patient's skin during electrocardiography. There are several types of electrodes, including metal plate, suction bulb, and disposable electrodes. Disposable electrodes (Figure 39-4) are the most widely used.

The skin does not conduct electricity well. Consequently, an electrolyte (a substance that enhances transmission of electric current) is needed with each electrode. Disposable electrodes come with an electrolyte preparation in place, but you must apply an electrolyte to reusable electrodes. Electrolytes are available in the form of gels, lotions, and solutions and disposable pads impregnated with electrolyte (Figure 39-5).

When performing routine electrocardiography, you place electrodes on ten areas of the body: one each on the right arm (RA), left arm (LA), right leg (RL), and left leg (LL) and six on specific locations on the chest wall. If the electrocardiograph has only five electrodes, you will position one electrode on each arm and each leg. You will move the fifth electrode to six different positions on the chest for successive readings. Evaluating different leads, that is the electrical activity measured through various combinations of electrodes, enables the physician to pinpoint the origin of certain problems.

Leads

Each lead provides an image of the electrical activity of the heart from a different angle. Together, the images give the doctor a full picture of electrical activity moving

Table 39-1

Parts of the ECG

Name	Appearance	Represents
P wave	Small upward curve	Sinoatrial node impulse, wave of depolarization through atria, and resultant contraction
QRS complex	Includes Q, R, and S waves	Contraction (following depolarization) of ventricles; QRS complex is larger than P wave because ventricles are larger than atria
Q wave	Downward deflection	Impulse traveling down septum toward Purkinje fibers
R wave	Large upward spike	Impulse going through left ventricle
S wave	Downward deflection	Impulse going through both ventricles
T wave	Upward curve	Recovery (repolarization) of ventricles; repolarization of atria is not obvious because it occurs while ventricles are contracting and producing QRS complex
U wave	Small upward curve sometimes found after T wave	May be seen in normal individuals, when there is slow recovery of Purkinje fibers, or in patients who have low potassium levels or other metabolic disturbances
P-R interval	Includes P wave and straight line connecting it to QRS complex	Time it takes for electrical impulse to travel from SA node to AV node
Q-T interval	Includes QRS complex, S-T segment, and T wave	Time it takes for ventricles to contract and recover, or repolarize
S-T segment	Connects end of QRS complex with beginning of T wave	Time between contraction of ventricles and recovery

up and down, left and right, and forward and backward through the heart. Monitoring the electrodes on the arms and legs in two different ways produces six leads that record electrical impulses that move up and down and left and right. The electrodes that are placed on the chest provide six more leads, showing electrical activity moving forward and backward (from the front of the body toward the back and vice versa).

Each lead is given a specific designation and code. The 12 leads are usually marked automatically on the ECG. Some electrocardiographs, however, may require you to clearly mark the codes on each lead manually.

Limb Leads. Of the six leads that directly monitor electrodes on the arms and legs, three are standard leads and three are augmented leads. The standard leads each monitor two limb electrodes, recording electrical activity between them. These leads are also called bipolar leads, because they monitor two electrodes. The augmented leads monitor one limb electrode and a point midway between two other limb electrodes, recording electrical activity between the monitored electrode and the midway point. Because they directly monitor only one electrode, augmented leads are also called unipolar leads. The electrical activity recorded by these leads is very slight, requiring the machine to augment (amplify) the tracings to produce readable waves and lines on the ECG paper.

Precordial Leads. The six precordial, or chest, leads are unipolar leads. The electrodes are placed across the chest in a specific pattern (Figure 39-6). Each precordial lead monitors one electrode and a point within the heart. The precordial leads are each designated by a letter and a number. The designations for the 12 leads of a routine ECG are shown in Table 39-2. The table also indicates which electrodes and points are monitored by each lead. A common system of marking codes completes the information in the table. Other coding systems are in use; be

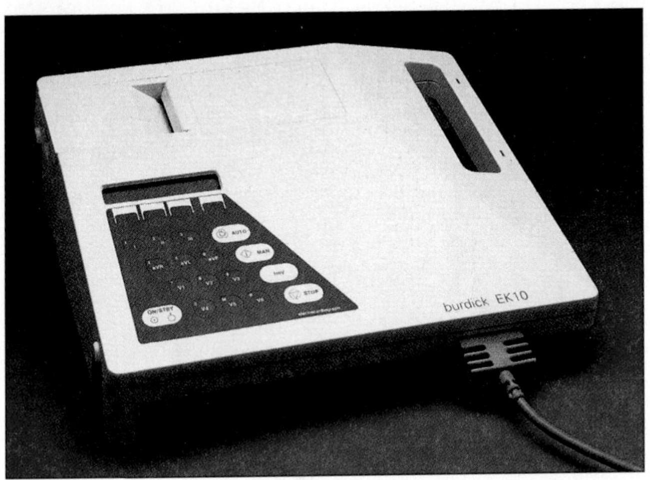

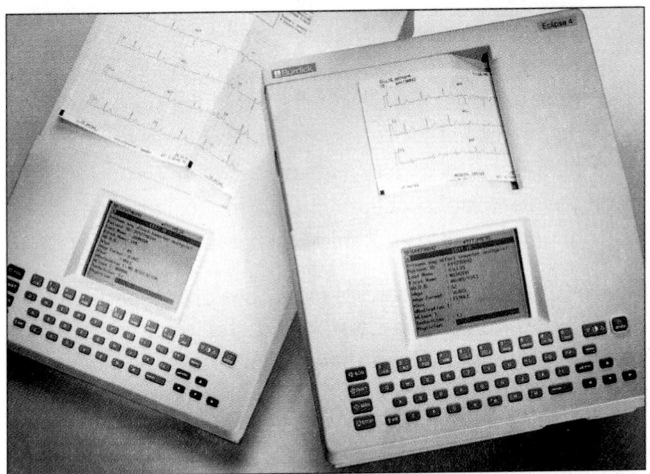

Figure 39-3. Single-channel (top) and multichannel (bottom) electrocardiographs are used to obtain an ECG.

sure to follow office policy or the doctor's preference when you code an ECG.

ECG Paper

ECG paper is provided in a long, continuous roll. If the paper is designed for use with a single-channel electrocardiograph, it is just wide enough for a single trace. Other ECG papers can accommodate several traces at once; these papers are used with multichannel electrocardiography. ECG paper consists of two layers and is both heat- and pressure-sensitive. The heated stylus on the electrocardiograph serves as a "pen" that records the ECG pattern on the paper.

ECG paper (Figure 39-7) is marked with light and dark lines or with dots and lines. The pattern is standardized to permit uniform interpretation by any physician. Each small square, or square area delineated by dots, measures 1 mm by 1 mm. Each large square measures 5 mm by 5 mm.

The vertical, or short, axis of the paper records the voltage, or strength of the impulse; the horizontal axis measures time. Normally the paper moves through the machine at a speed of 25 mm per second. This means that the distance across 1 small square represents 0.04 second. The distance across 1 large square represents 0.2 second. The distance across 5 large squares represents 1.0 second. In 1 minute (60 seconds), the paper advances 300 large squares or 1500 mm (150 cm).

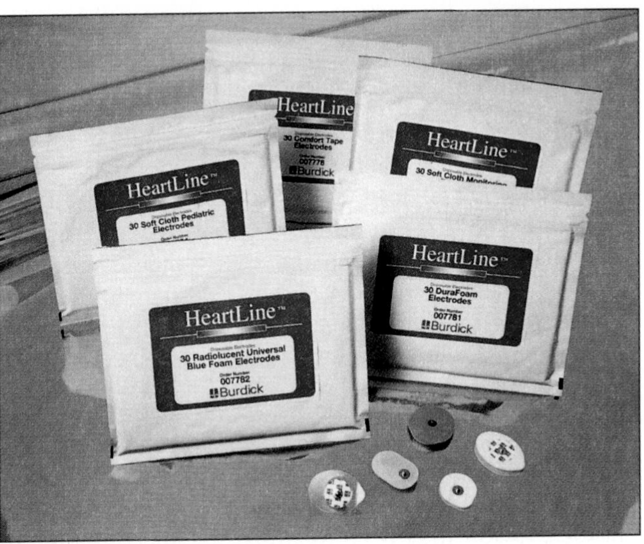

Figure 39-4. Disposable electrodes are available in several varieties.

Each electrocardiograph is standardized before use so that one small square represents 0.1 millivolt (mV). One large square represents 0.5 mV, and two large squares represent 1.0 mV.

Electrocardiograph Controls

The location of certain knobs and buttons on an electrocardiograph may vary from model to model. Certain features, however, are common to most machines. These

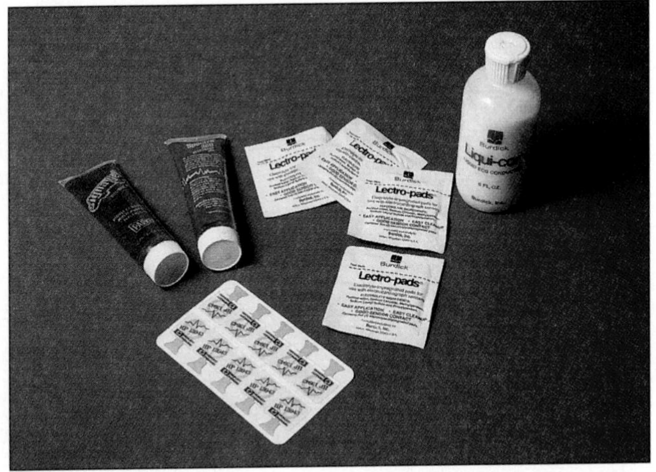

Figure 39-5. An electrolyte (in the form of gel, lotion, solution, or impregnated pad) must be applied to each electrode.

include the standardization control, speed selector, sensitivity control, lead selector, centering control, stylus temperature control, marker control, and on/off switch.

Standardization Control. Before you obtain an ECG, you must correctly standardize the machine. The standardization control uses a 1-mV impulse to produce a standardization mark on the ECG paper. When you press the standardization control, the stylus should move up ten small squares, or 10 mm (1 cm) and remain there for 0.08 second (two small squares, or 2 mm). If it does not, the instrument must be adjusted before you use it.

Speed Selector. The paper is normally set to run at 25 mm per second for adults. When you run an ECG on infants and children or on adults with a rapid heartbeat, the deflections may appear too close together. In these cases you may need to adjust the speed to 50 mm per second to separate the peaks and create a tracing that is easier to read. If you must set the speed at 50 mm per second, note it on the strip. Otherwise, a speed of 25 mm per second is assumed. In any case do not change the speed selection unless the doctor directs you to do so.

Sensitivity Control. The sensitivity control adjusts the height of the standardization mark and the tracing. It is normally set on 1. When the height of an ECG tracing is too high to fit completely on the paper, however, adjust this control to ½ to reduce the size of both the

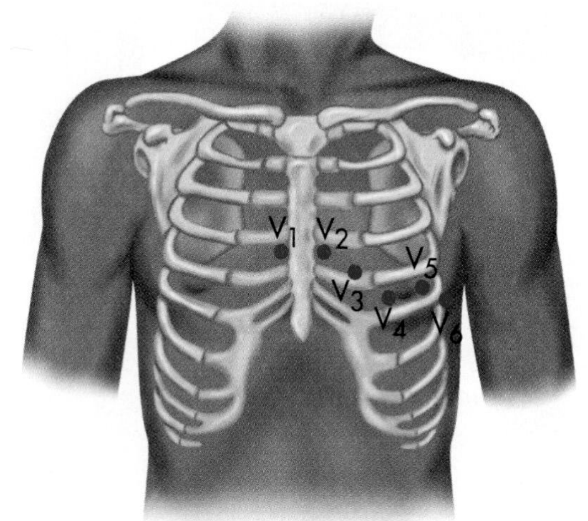

V_1 Fourth intercostal space (between the ribs), to the right of the sternum (breastbone)
V_2 Fourth intercostal space, to the left of the sternum
V_4 Fifth intercostal space, on the left midclavicular line
V_3 Fifth intercostal space, midway between V_2 and V_4
V_6 Fifth intercostal space, on the left midaxillary line
V_5 Fifth intercostal space, midway between V_4 and V_6

Figure 39-6. Six precordial electrodes are arranged in specific positions on the chest. Notice that electrode V_4 must be positioned before V_3 and V_6 before V_5.

Table 39-2

ECG Lead Designations and Marking Codes

Lead	Electrodes and Points Monitored	Marking Codes
Standard limb		
I	RA and LA	•
II	RA and LL	••
III	LA and LL	•••
Augmented limb		
aVR	RA and (LA-LL)	-
aVL	LA and (RA-LL)	--
aVF	LL and (RA-LA)	---
Precordial		
V_1	V_1 and (LA-RA-LL)*	-•
V_2	V_2 and (LA-RA-LL)*	-••
V_3	V_3 and (LA-RA-LL)*	-•••
V_4	V_4 and (LA-RA-LL)*	-••••
V_5	V_5 and (LA-RA-LL)*	-•••••
V_6	V_6 and (LA-RA-LL)*	-••••••

*The point within the heart is identified by averaging the readings from the electrodes.

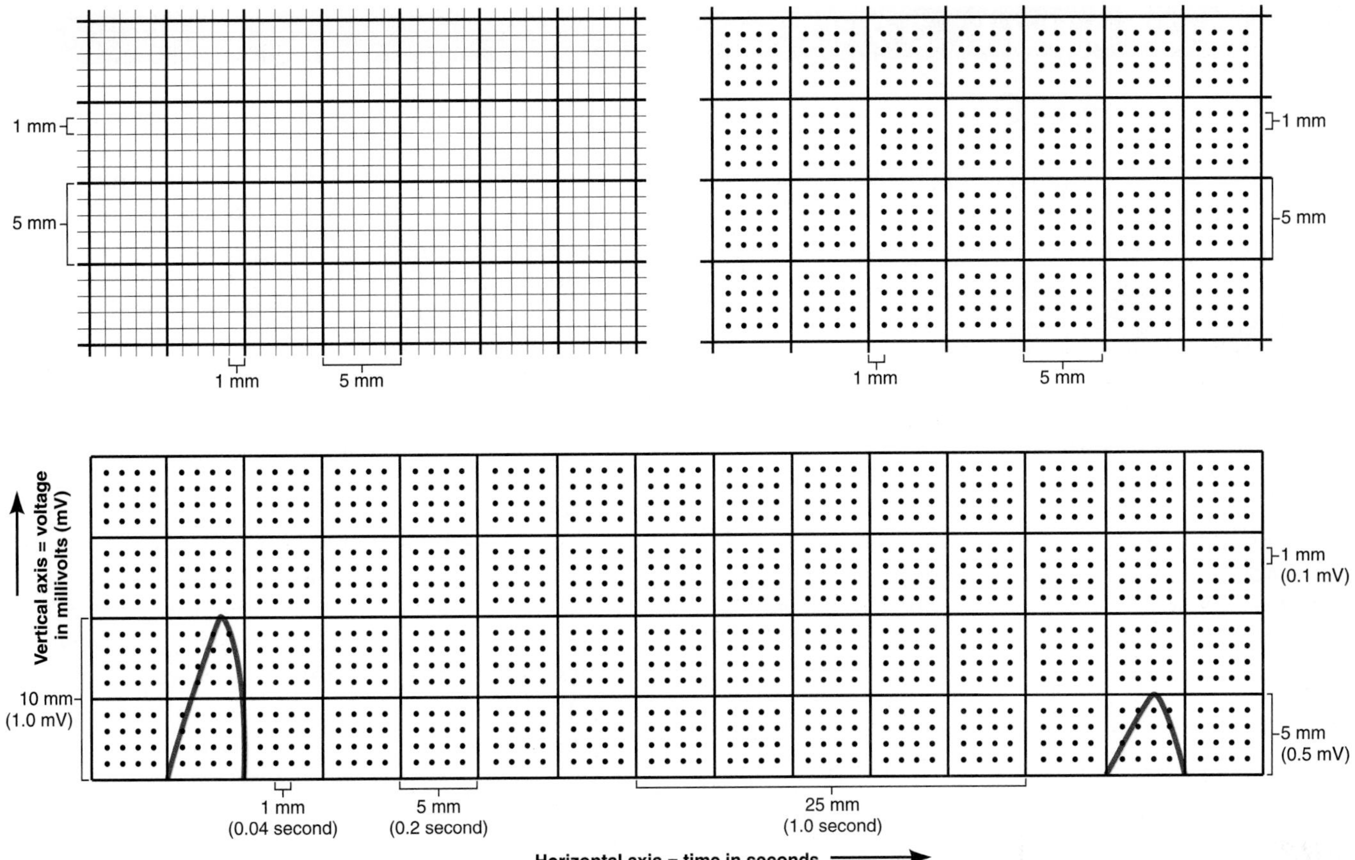

Figure 39-7. The pattern and spacing of lines or lines and dots on ECG paper are standardized and represent specific units of voltage and time.

standardization mark and the tracing by one-half. For tracings that have very low peaks, set this control on 2 to double the standardization mark and the height of the tracing. Note this change on the strip.

Lead Selector. Most newer electrocardiographs have a setting that enables a standard 12-lead tracing to run automatically. All machines, however, have a lead selector that allows you to run each lead individually, in case you need to repeat a strip containing **artifacts** (erroneous marks or defects) during a run.

Centering Control. The centering control allows you to adjust the position of the stylus, which must be centered on the paper. (Centering the stylus simplifies the process of measuring wave heights for the person who interprets the ECG.)

Stylus Temperature Control. Another control allows you to adjust the temperature of the stylus. A higher temperature results in a heavier line, whereas a lower temperature results in a lighter, thinner line. The line should be clear without being so dark that it bleeds or smears on the ECG paper.

Marker Control. Most older machines have a marker control that allows you to place marking codes (see Table 39-2) on the ECG paper to identify the lead during each run. Many newer machines do this automatically.

On/Off Switch. The on/off switch turns the machine on and off. Most machines have an indicator light that signals when the power is on.

Preparing to Administer an ECG

You must obtain a good-quality tracing when performing electrocardiography. To do so, you must be able to recognize an artifact or a generally defective ECG tracing when you see one. Proper technique is also essential to help you obtain the best-quality tracing. The following sections guide you through the process. The steps in obtaining a standard 12-lead ECG using a single-channel electrocardiograph are listed in Procedure 39-1.

Preparing the Room and Equipment

Be sure the room and equipment are properly set up before you begin to administer electrocardiography. The accuracy of an ECG can sometimes be affected by electric currents emitted from nearby machines. Although some

PROCEDURE 39-1

Obtaining an ECG

Objective: To obtain a graphic representation of the electrical activity of a patient's heart

OSHA Guidelines

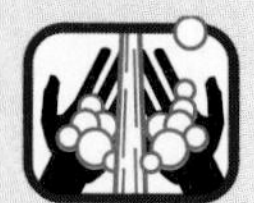

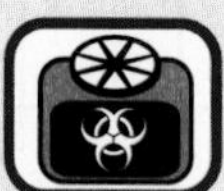
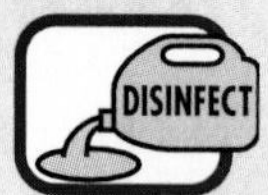

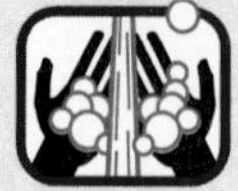

Materials: Electrocardiograph, ECG paper, electrodes, electrolyte preparation, wires, patient gown, drape, blanket, pillows, gauze pads, alcohol, moist towel, disposable shaving supplies (if needed)

Method

1. Turn on the electrocardiograph, and allow the stylus to heat up according to the manufacturer's instructions.
2. Identify the patient, introduce yourself, and explain the procedure.
3. Wash your hands.
4. Ask the patient to disrobe from the waist up and remove jewelry, socks or stockings, and shoes. Have the patient roll up pant legs for placement of electrodes. Provide a gown if the patient is female, and instruct her to wear the gown with the opening in front.
5. Assist the patient onto the table and into a supine position. Cover the patient with a drape (and a blanket if the room is cool). If the patient experiences difficulty breathing or cannot tolerate lying flat, use a Fowler's or semi-Fowler's position, adjusting with pillows under the head and knees for comfort if needed.
6. Tell the patient to rest quietly and breathe normally. Explain the importance of lying still to prevent false readings.
7. Wash the patient's skin, using gauze pads moistened with alcohol. Then rub it vigorously with dry gauze pads to promote better contact of the electrodes.
8. If the patient's leg or chest hair is dense, put on examination gloves, and shave the areas where you will attach the electrodes. Properly dispose of the razor and gloves.
9. Apply electrodes to fleshy portions of the limbs, making sure that the electrodes on one arm and leg are placed similarly to those on the other arm and leg (Figure 39-8). The direction that the tabs (where the wires are fastened) are facing will vary.
   a. If using reusable electrodes, place equal amounts of electrolyte gel, lotion, or solution on each electrode, and secure the electrodes with rubber straps or bulbs.
   b. If using disposable electrodes, peel off the backings, and press them into place.
10. Apply the precordial electrodes at specified locations on the chest.
11. Attach wires and cables, making sure all wire tips follow the patient's body contours.
12. Check all electrodes and wires for proper placement and connection; drape wires over the patient to avoid creating tension on the electrodes that could result in artifacts (Figure 39-9).
13. Set the paper speed to 25 mm per second or as instructed.
14. Set the sensitivity setting to 1 or as instructed.
15. Turn the lead selector to standardization mode.
16. Adjust the stylus so the baseline is centered.

electrocardiographs have filters to minimize outside electrical interference, it is always a good idea to perform electrocardiography in a room where all other electrical equipment is turned off. This equipment includes air conditioners, refrigerators, and fans, as well as laboratory and diagnostic equipment.

The room should be in a quiet location, protected from interruptions. Because the patient must partially disrobe, adjust the room temperature to a comfortable level.

The examining table should be sturdy and comfortable. If the table is made of metal, it must be padded so the patient does not come in contact with any metal parts during the procedure.

Before using the electrocardiograph, check the date of its last inspection. Each machine should be periodically inspected and certified safe to use for a specific period of time. Using a machine only within this time period helps ensure your safety and that of the patient. Be sure to turn the machine on ahead of time to allow the stylus to warm up.

17. Press the on, run, or record button.
18. Press the standardization button. The stylus should move upward above the baseline 10 mm (two large squares).
19. Run the strip.
    a. If the machine has an automatic feature, set the lead selector to automatic.
    b. For manual tracings, turn the lead selector to standby mode. Select the first lead (I), and record the tracing. Switch the machine to standby, and then repeat the procedure for all 12 leads.
20. Check tracings for artifacts.
21. Correct problems and repeat any tracings that are not clear.
22. Disconnect the patient from the machine.
23. Remove the tracing from the machine, and label it with the patient's name, the date, and your initials.
24. Disconnect the wires from the electrodes, and remove the electrodes from the patient.
25. Clean the patient's skin with a moist towel.
26. Assist the patient into a sitting position.
27. Allow a moment for rest, and then assist the patient from the table.
28. Assist the patient in dressing if necessary, or allow the patient privacy to dress.
29. Wash your hands.
30. Record the procedure in the patient's chart.
31. Properly dispose of used materials and disposable electrodes.
32. Clean reusable electrodes and straps with a mild detergent; polish electrodes and dry them thoroughly.
33. Clean and disinfect the equipment and the room according to OSHA guidelines.

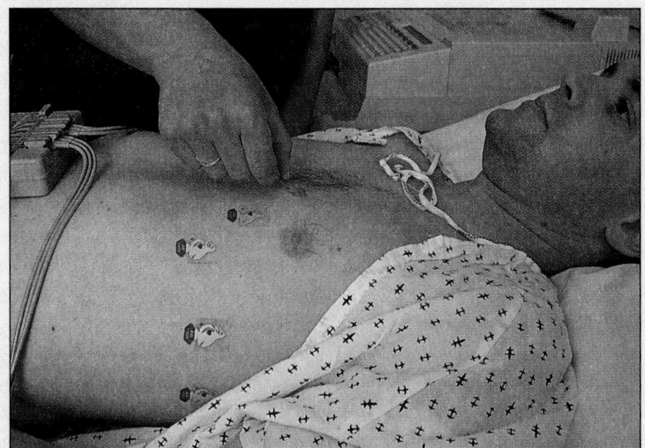

Figure 39-8. Place electrodes at the specified locations on the chest, arms, and legs.

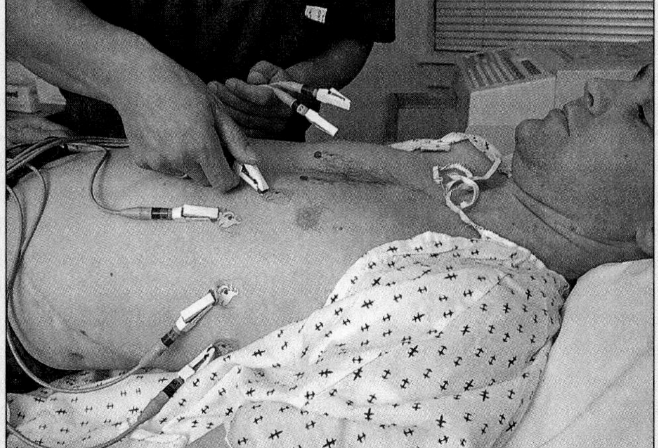

Figure 39-9. Attach wires and cables, draping wires over the patient to avoid tension that can result in artifacts.

Preparing the Patient

Introduce yourself to the patient, explain the procedure, and answer any questions the patient has. Follow the steps described in Procedure 39-1 as you prepare the patient for electrocardiography. Keep in mind that some patients are apprehensive about undergoing electrocardiography. Anxiety often stems from the fear of receiving an electric shock from the machine. See "Caution: Handle With Care" for ways to allay a patient's anxiety about having an ECG.

Applying the Electrodes and the Connecting Wires

You must prepare the patient's skin before applying the electrodes. Proper contact between an electrode and the skin allows for proper conduction of the impulses. Follow the steps described in Procedure 39-1 as you prepare the patient's skin. Depending on your office policy, you may be required to shave chest or leg hair if it is dense to

CAUTION HANDLE WITH CARE

Allaying Patient Anxiety About Having Electrocardiography

The most common reason for a patient's anxiety is not knowing what to expect from electrocardiography. The patient may be fearful of being hooked up to an electrical device and worried about receiving an electric shock.

Calmly and simply explain the procedure in detail, both before you begin and while you prepare the patient for the test. Assure her that it is a safe procedure that will last about 10 to 15 minutes. Explain that the machine measures the electrical activity of the heart and that no outside electricity will pass through the body. It is also helpful to explain why the doctor has ordered the procedure, without giving any diagnosis or prognosis.

Above all, talk to and listen to the patient. Encourage her to express her concerns and ask questions. Respond to the patient's concerns and questions calmly, fully, and respectfully.

Ensuring Patient Comfort

Ensuring that the patient is comfortable will help her feel more at ease. It will also result in less body movement and a more accurate ECG.

Each patient is an individual. You will need to find out from the patient what is and is not comfortable for her. First make sure the room temperature is right for the patient. If she says the room feels too cool, provide an extra blanket to prevent chills. Being chilly can make a patient shiver and increase her anxiety. If the patient says she feels too warm, do not provide a blanket.

Next ensure that the patient is comfortable on the examining table. Placing a small pillow under the head can help. Make sure, however, that the pillow does not touch the shoulders or raise them off the table. For most patients, placing a pillow under the knees helps relax the abdomen and lower extremities and prevents lower-back pain. Try this arrangement and let the patient decide whether it contributes to or detracts from her comfort. If the patient has trouble breathing, shift her into a Fowler's or semi-Fowler's position. Ask the patient which position is more comfortable, and use the position she chooses. If the patient chooses a position other than supine, be sure to note the position in her chart.

ensure proper contact. Because you may be exposed to blood or broken skin when shaving a patient, observe Universal Precautions and wear gloves to prevent contact with potentially contaminated body fluids.

Types of Electrodes

There are three main types of electrodes. It is important to know how to apply each type.

Metal Plates. Metal plate electrodes are secured to the body with a rubber strap. Electrolyte gel, lotion, or solution or a disposable electrolyte pad is placed on the electrode before it is positioned on the skin. If a gel, lotion, or solution is used, the same amount should be used on each electrode to maintain consistency of contact and to lessen the chance of artifacts. Using the electrode, rub the electrolyte on the surface of the skin to provide good contact. Wrap the rubber strap around the patient's arm or leg until a hole on the strap meets the tab on the electrode, then stretch the strap one hole tighter. If the strap is too tight or too loose, the tracing may be inaccurate.

Suction Bulbs. With suction bulb electrodes, first rub electrolyte gel, lotion, or solution onto the patient's skin where the electrode is to be placed. Then squeeze the bulb to create suction, place the electrode on the skin, and holding the electrode in place, release the bulb.

Disposable Electrodes. Disposable electrodes come with an electrolyte product already applied. Simply remove the adhesive backing, and press the electrode firmly into place on the skin.

Positioning the Electrodes

You must position electrodes at ten locations on the body (Figure 39-10). Remember, if the electrocardiograph has only five electrodes, you will need to move the fifth electrode to six different positions on the patient's chest to obtain the necessary tracings.

Limb Electrodes. Placement of limb electrodes need not be exact. Limb electrodes are most commonly placed on the inside of the fleshy part of the calf muscle and on the outside of the upper arm, but they are sometimes placed on the thigh and above the wrist. It is generally better to place arm electrodes on the upper arm because this reduces the amount of artifact caused by arm movement. Attach the electrodes to a smooth and fleshy part of each limb to ensure optimal conduction of impulses. Limb electrodes must always be placed at the same level on both arms and on both legs. If a patient has had a leg amputated, both leg electrodes should be placed on the thighs.

Precordial Electrodes. Unlike the limb electrodes, the precordial electrodes must be placed at specific locations on the chest to obtain accurate readings. These locations

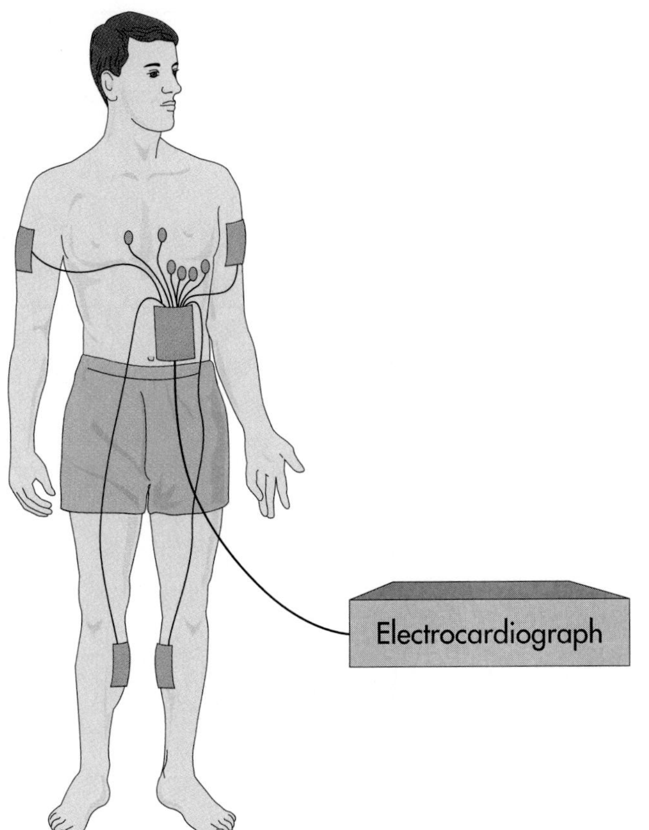

Figure 39-10. There are ten electrode positions for electrocardiography.

specify intercostal spaces, the spaces between the ribs. Intercostal spaces are numbered from top to bottom. Refer to Figure 39-6 for the exact description of each location.

Determine the position for the first precordial electrode (V_1) by counting to the fourth intercostal space to the right of the sternum (breastbone). The V_1 electrode should be placed over this space, directly adjacent to the sternum. After you have this electrode in place, use it as a guide to position the other electrodes.

Place the V_2 electrode in the fourth intercostal space to the left of the sternum in the same manner. Note that the V_1 and V_2 positions may not line up exactly; one may be higher than the other. Perfect symmetry is rare in the human body.

Next place the V_4 electrode in the fifth intercostal space, where it intersects an imaginary line drawn straight down from the middle of the clavicle (midclavicular line). When the V_4 electrode is in place, place the V_3 electrode midway between V_2 and V_4 in the fifth intercostal space.

Place the V_6 electrode in the fifth intercostal space, directly below the middle of the armpit (midaxillary line). Place the last electrode (V_5) in the fifth intercostal space, midway between V_4 and V_6.

You may be using a type of electrocardiograph that has only one chest electrode rather than six separate electrodes. If this is the case, place the chest electrode at position V_1, secure it with a chest strap, and run the ECG. Following this, stop the machine and move the electrode to the next position. You must make separate tracings at each location.

Attaching the Wires

After placing the electrodes, attach the wires that connect the electrodes to the electrocardiograph. Numbers and letters on the wires correspond to numbers and letters for the electrodes. For example, RA stands for right arm, LL stands for left leg, and so on. The precordial electrode wires are labeled V_1 through V_6. Connect the limb wires first, then the precordial wires, in the sequence already described. Some wires are also color-coded.

Depending on the type of electrodes you use, connect the wires to the electrodes by snapping, clipping, or screwing the wire tips tightly in place. Wires should follow the patient's body contours and lie flat against the body. Drape the wires over the patient to avoid putting tension on the electrodes, which could cause interference. You may also bundle the wires together to form a single cable.

Operating the Electrocardiograph

Before running the ECG, remind the patient to remain as still as possible and not to talk. Be sure the patient is comfortable. A comfortable patient is less likely to move around and cause artifacts on the ECG tracing.

Standardizing the Electrocardiograph

Follow the steps described in Procedure 39-1 as you standardize the electrocardiograph. The stylus should move upward above the baseline 10 mm (two large squares) when you press the standardization button. If it does not, you must see to it that the instrument is adjusted before continuing.

Running the ECG

You can now run the ECG. On most newer machines, turning the lead selector to the automatic mode produces a standard 12-lead strip. Because each lead provides a specific view of the heart's electrical activity, each of the 12 leads has a characteristic tracing (Figure 39-11).

Manual ECGs. If your office has a machine without an automatic setting, you must manually run the ECG for each of the 12 leads. You may also be required to repeat certain leads manually if artifacts are detected.

To run a manual ECG, standardize the machine as outlined above. Then turn the lead selector to standby

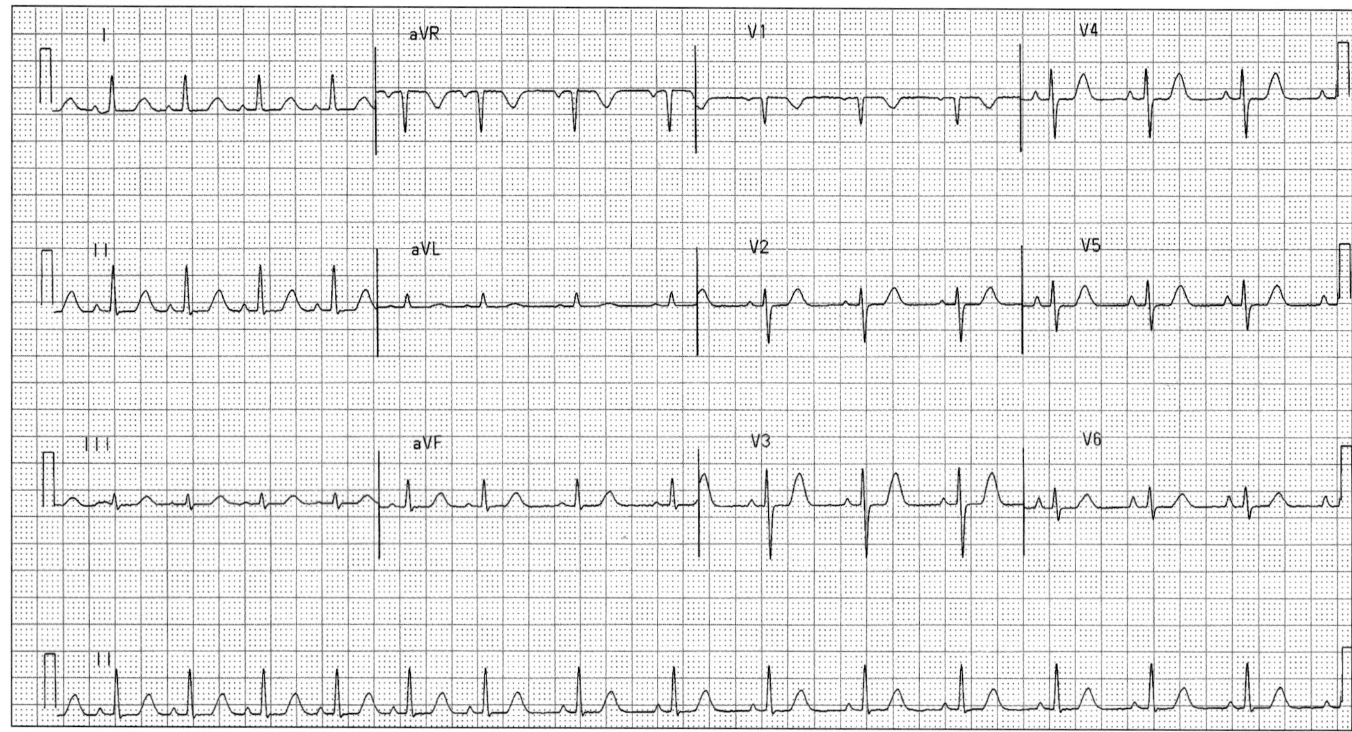

Figure 39-11. The tracing from each lead will differ. The long tracing of a single lead along the bottom is the rhythm strip. (Courtesy of Burdick, Inc., Milton, Wisconsin)

mode. Some older machines may require you to stop the paper before selecting the first lead (I) using the lead selector. Push the marking button on the machine to indicate the lead if the machine does not do this automatically. Allow the strip to run for four to five cardiac cycles, taking about 3 to 5 seconds. Turn the machine back to the standby mode; stop the paper if necessary, and repeat the procedure for leads II and III, the augmented leads, and the precordial leads. Remember to standardize the machine before running each lead for consistency.

Many physicians request another strip on lead II to assess for rhythm. Some physicians choose a different lead for the rhythm strip. Run the rhythm strip on the requested lead to produce a strip that is at least 2 ft long so rhythmic abnormalities can be easily recognized.

Multiple-Channel Electrocardiographs. Some electrocardiographs have multiple channels that can record three, four, or six leads simultaneously (Figure 39-12). Electrode placement is the same for these types of electrocardiographs.

Checking the ECG Tracing

After running the 12 leads and before disconnecting the patient from the machine, check all tracings to make sure they are clear and free of artifacts. If any of the leads do not appear on a tracing, it may mean that a wire has come loose. In this case reconnect the wire, and repeat the tracing. Repeat any tracings that are not clear.

Also check that all tracings are contained within the boundaries of the paper and that no waves peak above the edges of the paper. If this happens, recenter the stylus if it is positioned too high, or set the sensitivity selector to ½ before repeating the tracing. In the reverse situation—where very low peaks appear—set the sensitivity selector to 2 to increase the height of the peaks.

If the peaks in a tracing are too close together, increase the paper speed to 50 mm per second. Increasing the speed separates the peaks and makes the tracing easier to read.

Make a note on the ECG tracing whenever it is necessary to adjust sensitivity or speed settings. This information is vital to the interpretation of the test.

Troubleshooting: Artifacts and Other Problems

To ensure high-quality tracings, it is essential to recognize artifacts and identify sources of interference. You must also know how to correct them.

Artifacts

Artifacts are caused by improper technique, poor conduction, outside interference, or improper handling of a tracing. If artifacts are present on an ECG tracing, the doctor may not be able to make an accurate diagnosis of the patient's condition. Recognizing the presence of an artifact in the baseline during setup allows you to correct the problem before the tracing is recorded.

There are several types of artifacts. Among the common ones you may see are a wandering baseline or a flat line. You may also see marks that are not characteristic of a tracing; large, erratic spikes; or uniform, small spikes. Table 39-3 outlines these artifacts and summarizes possible causes and solutions.

Wandering Baseline. A wandering baseline, shown in Figure 39-13, is identified by a shift in the baseline from the center position for that lead. Causes include somatic interference and a variety of mechanical problems. Mechanical problems may be an inadequately warmed stylus, improper application of electrodes (too loose or incorrectly placed), dirty or corroded electrodes, tension on electrodes caused by a dangling wire, inadequate or unevenly applied electrolyte products, inadequate skin preparation, or the presence of creams or lotions on the skin.

Having the patient lie still can reduce somatic interference. Proper skin preparation and electrode placement are also essential. When the appointment for electrocardiography is made, instruct the patient to use no creams or lotions, deodorant, perfume, or powder. Be sure to include specific instructions in patient education materials, and ask the patient whether any of these substances were used before the procedure. If so, clean each area of electrode placement thoroughly with alcohol to avoid conduction disturbances.

Flat Line. A flat line on the tracing of one of the leads (Figure 39-14) is typically caused by a loose or disconnected wire. If flat lines occur on more than one lead, two of the wires may have been switched. If flat lines occur on all leads, the patient cable may be loose or disconnected, or there may be a break (short) somewhere in the unit. On the other hand, a flat line on all leads can be an indication of cardiac arrest. Always assess the patient's pulse and respiration first when flat lines occur on all leads.

Extraneous Marks. Because ECG graph paper is sensitive to heat and pressure, it can easily be damaged. Any marks on the paper that are not part of the tracing are referred to as extraneous marks. These marks can be

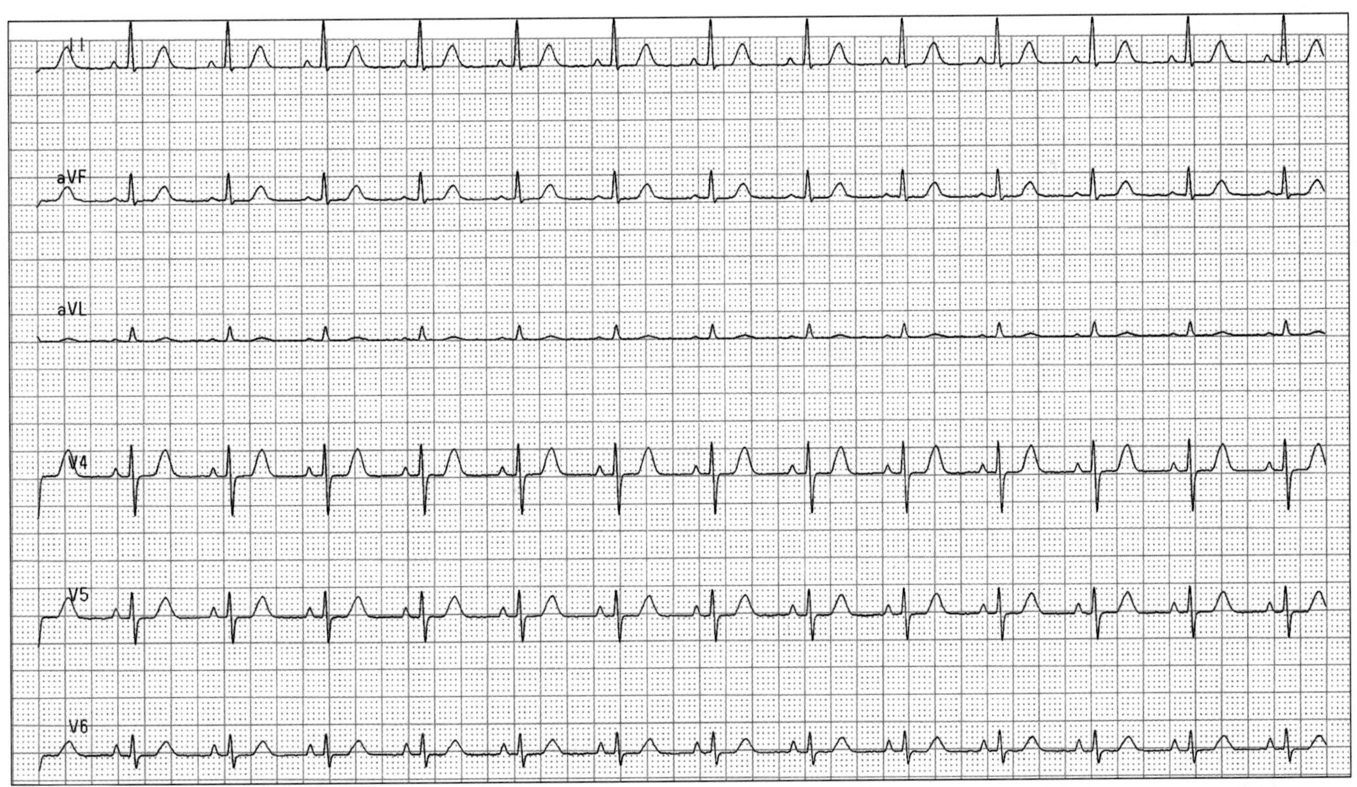

Figure 39-12. Some electrocardiographs allow you to run six leads at the same time. (Courtesy of Burdick, Inc.)

Table 39-3

Correcting ECG Artifacts

Problem	Possible Causes	Solutions
Wandering baseline	Inadequately warmed stylus	Allow electrocardiograph to warm up
	Poor skin preparation	Repeat skin preparation and electrode placement
	Loose electrode	Reapply electrode
	Improper electrode placement	Reapply electrode
	Dirty or corroded electrode	Clean and reapply electrode/replace electrode
	Somatic interference	Help patient relax and be comfortable
	Picking up breathing movement	Reposition electrode
	Tension on electrode	Drape wires over patient
Flat line	Detached/loose wire or cable	Reattach wires/cable
	Wrong selector switch setting	Check/change selector switch setting
	Crossed wires	Check/switch wires
	Short circuit in wires	Check/replace broken equipment
	Cardiac arrest	Check pulse/respiration; begin CPR
Marks not part of tracing	Careless handling	Handle carefully
	Use of paper clips	Use a rubber band
	Wet hands	Ensure hands are dry
	Improper mounting	Mount properly
Uniform, small spikes	AC interference	Turn off/unplug other electrical equipment; remove patient's watch
	Improper electrode placement	Reapply electrode
	Inadequate grounding	Check grounding
	Dirty electrode	Clean and reapply electrode
Large, erratic spikes	Somatic interference	Help patient relax and be comfortable
	Loose/dry electrode	Reapply electrode
	Electrode placed over bone	Reposition electrode

caused by careless handling, such as using paper clips to hold the tracing together or handling the tracing with wet hands.

Causes of Artifacts

You can use the line of the tracing to identify the cause of artifacts. Then you can take steps to eliminate the particular type of interference involved.

Alternating Current (AC) Interference. AC interference occurs when the electrocardiograph picks up a small amount of electric current given off by another piece of electrical equipment. The line of the tracing will be jagged, consisting of a series of uniform, small spikes (Figure 39-15). Many of the newer electrocardiographs have filters to reduce or eliminate most of this interference.

AC interference can often be eliminated by turning off or unplugging other appliances in the room. It is also helpful to keep the examining table away from the wall, because wiring in the wall can contribute to AC interference. If these remedies do not work, check to see whether the electrodes are dirty or attached improperly or whether the machine is incorrectly grounded.

Somatic Interference. Somatic interference is caused by muscle movement. Tensing of voluntary muscles,

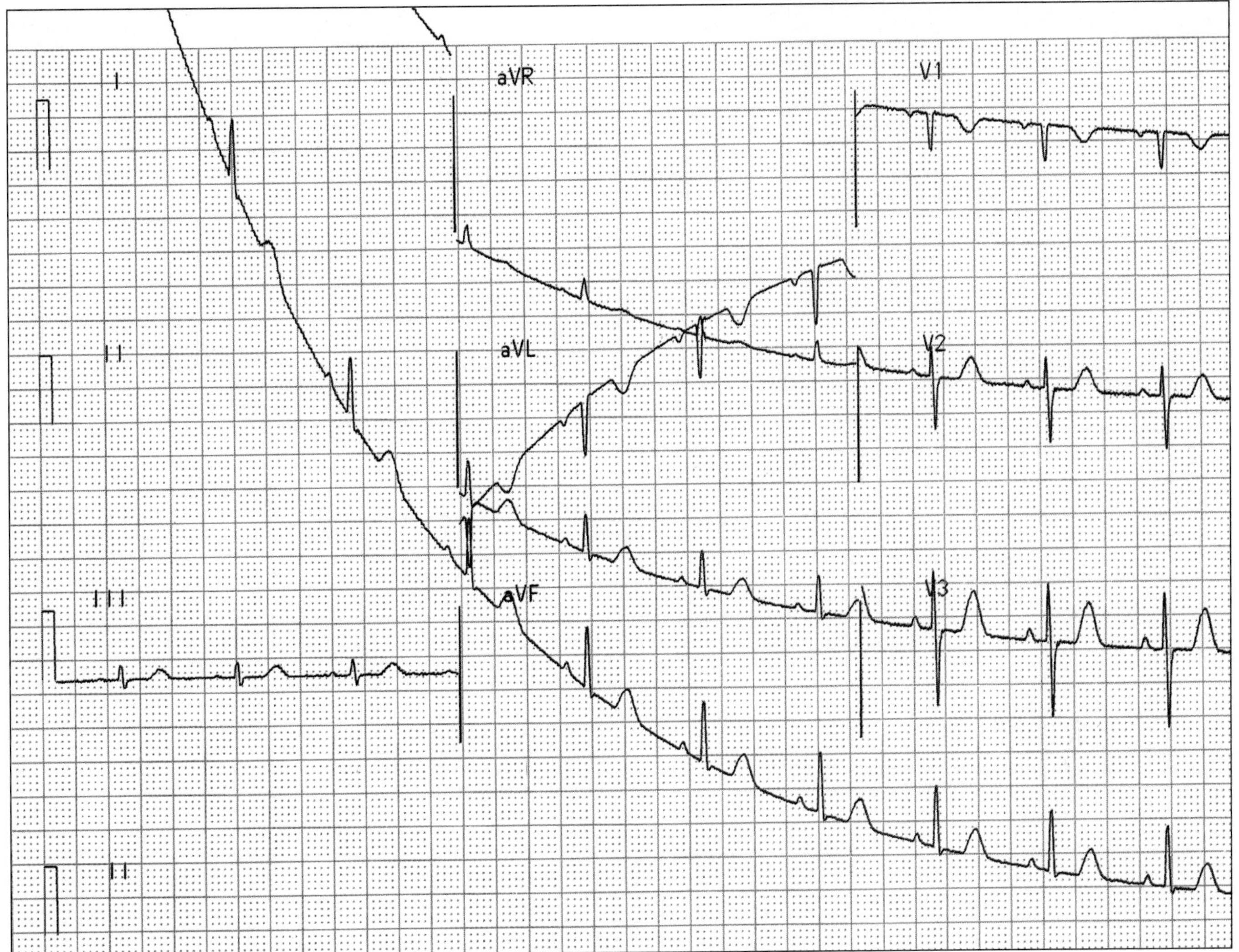

Figure 39-13. A wandering baseline may be caused by somatic interference or a mechanical problem. (Courtesy of Burdick, Inc.)

shifting of body position, tremors, or even talking requires muscular contractions that generate electrical impulses.

A sensitive electrocardiograph detects these impulses. The result is erratic movement of the stylus during the tracing, leading to large, erratic spikes and a shifting baseline (Figure 39-16).

Eliminate this type of interference by reminding the patient to remain still and to refrain from talking. To reduce the chance of shivering, be sure the room temperature is comfortable. Make the patient comfortable to reduce shifting and moving.

Placing the limb electrodes closer to the trunk of the body—on the upper arms, close to the shoulder, and on the upper thighs—can reduce interference. Reducing patient anxiety by explaining the procedure can also help reduce somatic interference. The physician might give an extremely anxious patient a sedative before the procedure.

Certain nervous system disorders, such as Parkinson's disease, cause patients to experience involuntary movements that can cause interference. Placing the limb electrodes closer to the trunk of the body is often helpful; however, it may be necessary to interrupt the tracing until the tremors subside.

Identifying the Source of Interference

The source of interference on an ECG can often be identified by checking the tracings obtained on leads I, II, and III. If there is a problem with a particular limb electrode, the interference will be prominent in two leads. For prominent interference in the following pairs of leads, check the limb electrode indicated:

- Leads I and II, right arm electrode
- Leads I and III, left arm electrode
- Leads II and III, left leg electrode

If the cause of the artifact or the source of interference cannot be determined, stop the machine and notify your supervisor or the physician of the problem. Do not disconnect the patient from the electrocardiograph.

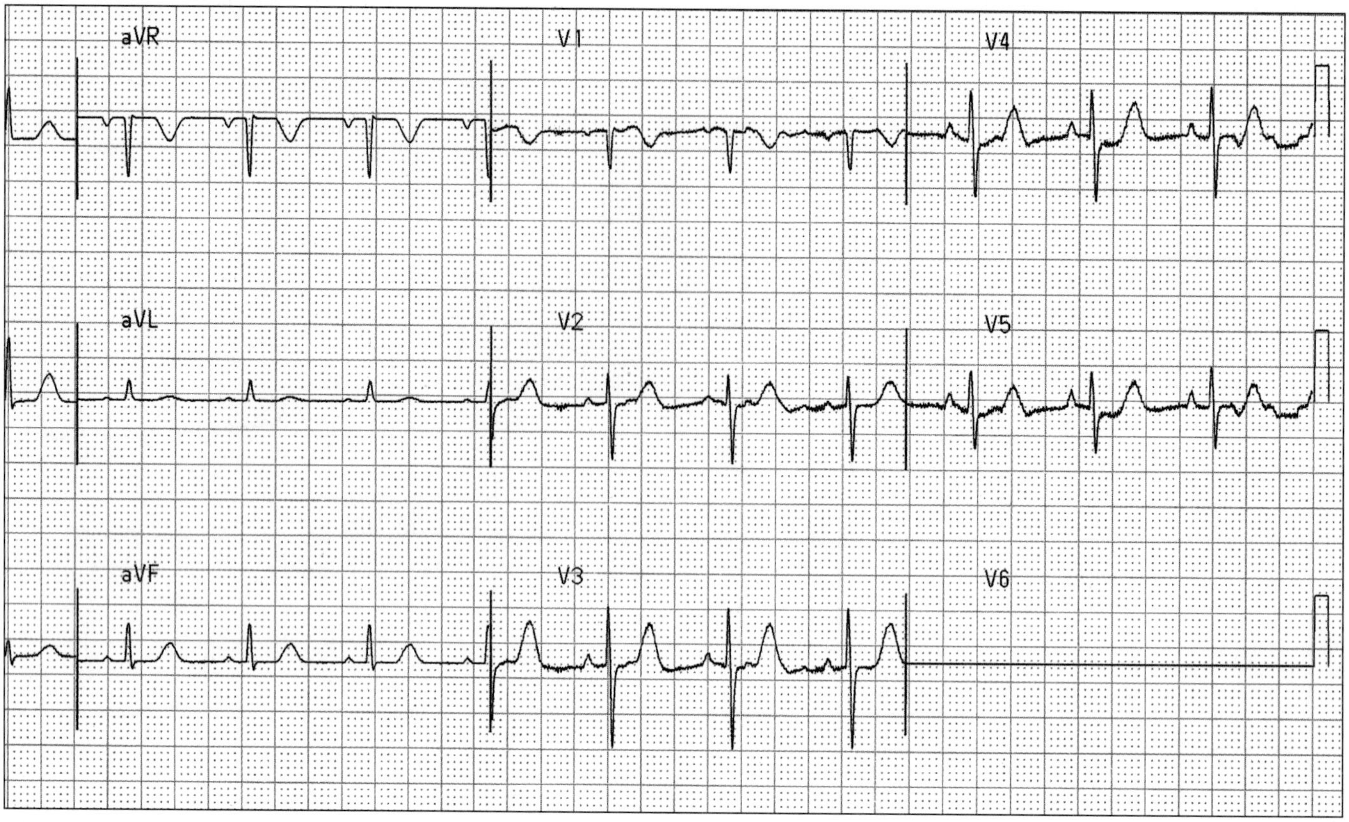

Figure 39-14. A flat line on one of the leads is caused by a loose or disconnected wire. (Courtesy of Burdick, Inc.)

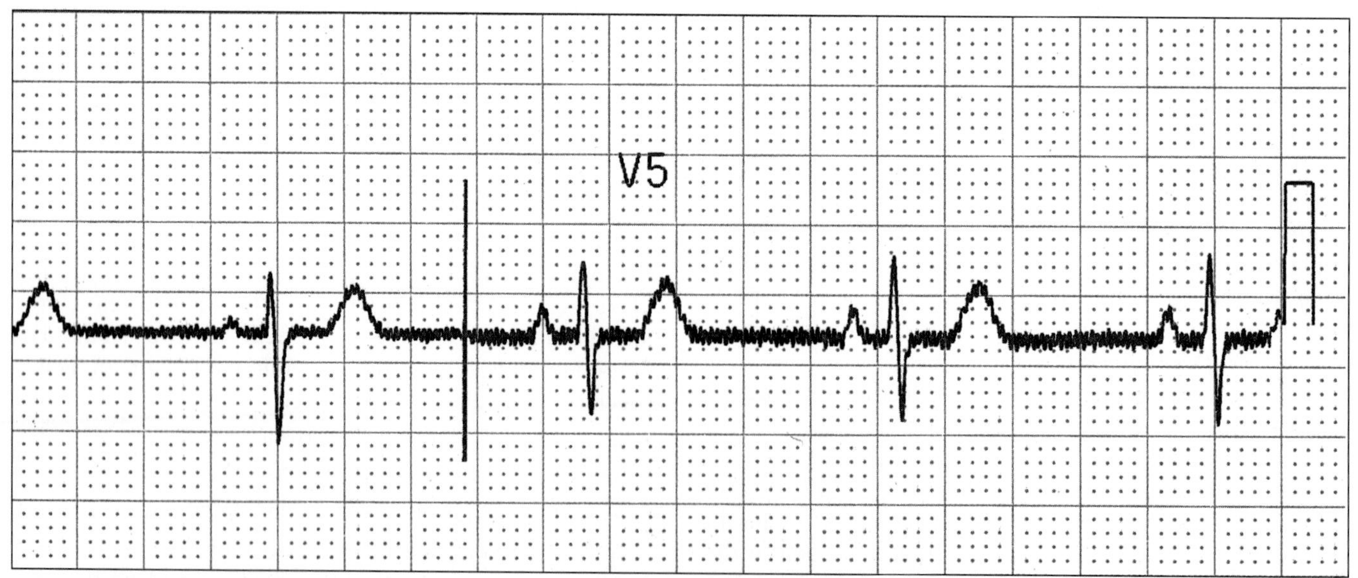

Figure 39-15. This type of artifact is caused by AC interference. (Courtesy of Burdick, Inc.)

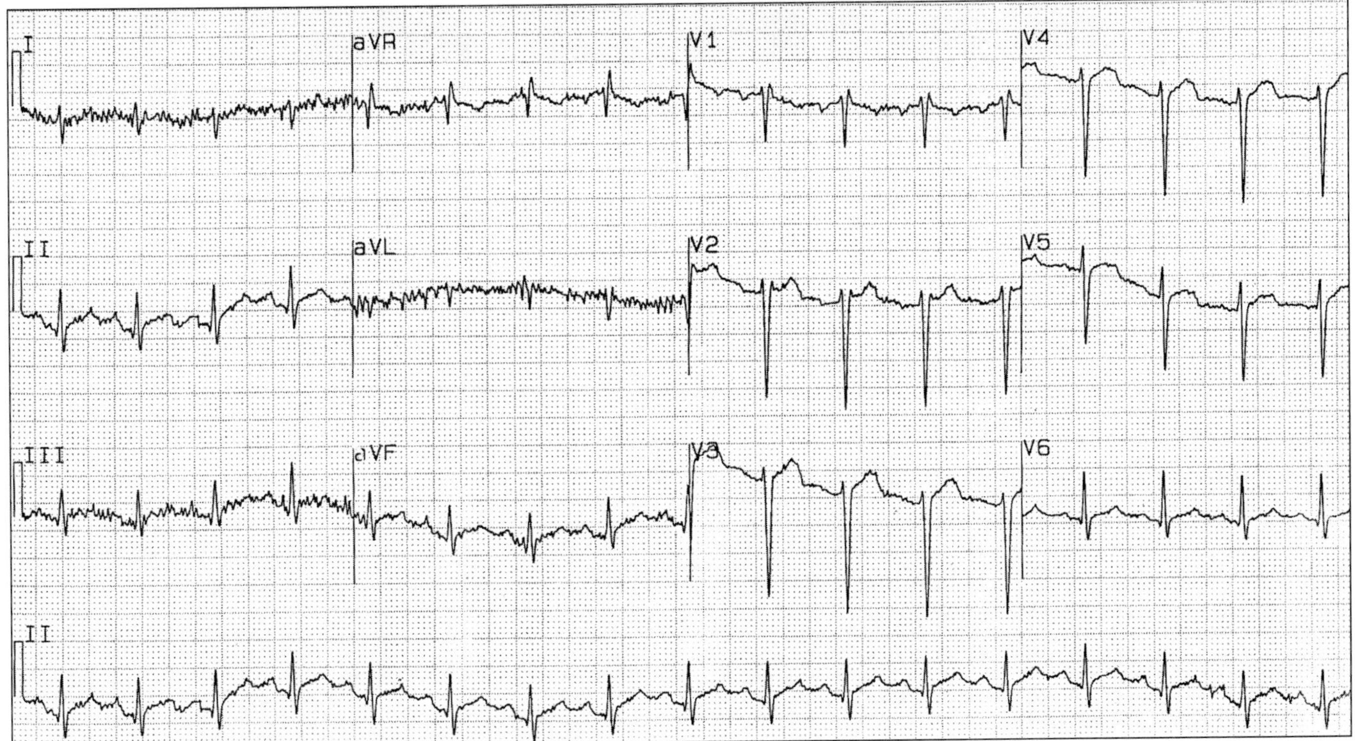

Figure 39-16. The somatic interference in this ECG was caused by patient tremors. (Courtesy of Burdick, Inc.)

Completing the Procedure

When you are sure the quality of all ECG tracings is acceptable, disconnect the patient from the machine. First remove the tracing from the machine, and label it with the patient's name, the date, and your initials. Loosely roll long tapes from single-channel machines with the printed side facing in, and secure them with a rubber band. Do not use paper clips because they can cause extraneous marks on the tracing.

Next disconnect the wires from the electrodes, and remove the electrodes from the patient. Wipe excess electrolyte from the patient's skin with a moist towel. Assist the patient to a sitting position, allowing a moment's rest before assisting the patient from the table. Help the patient dress if necessary, or allow the patient privacy to dress. Remove disposable paper covers from the table and pillows, clean surfaces according to OSHA guidelines, and discard all disposable materials in a biohazardous waste container.

Equipment Maintenance

If your machine has reusable electrodes, wipe off the electrolyte product, and wash the electrodes and rubber straps with a mild detergent. Metal plate electrodes must be polished with a fine grade of scouring powder. Do not use steel wool or metal-base polish because they will cause artifacts. Rinse the electrodes well, and dry them thoroughly before storing.

Mounting the Tracing

There are many types of ECG mounts or holders for single-channel ECG tracings. These mounts form a permanent record of the ECG and allow the doctor to read tracings from all 12 leads at once. Mounts are not typically necessary for multiple-channel ECG tracings because these are compact records of several leads. Several types of mounts are available, including slotted folders and folders with self-adhesive surfaces.

Mounting the ECG tracing involves selecting and cutting representative sections of each of the 12 lead tracings. The procedure used for mounting a tracing depends on the type of mount and the doctor's preference. The steps involved in mounting an ECG tracing are explained in Procedure 39-2.

Interpreting the ECG

As a medical assistant, you are not responsible for interpreting an ECG. Knowing something about how ECGs are interpreted, however, may allow you to recognize a problem that requires immediate attention. Some of the features that are assessed by means of an ECG include

PROCEDURE 39-2

Mounting the ECG Tracing

Objective: To mount an ECG tracing as a permanent record on which tracings from all 12 leads are accurately represented and easy to read

OSHA Guidelines: This procedure does not involve exposure to blood, body fluids, or tissues.

Materials: ECG tracing strip, mount, scissors, tape (if applicable)

Method

1. Gather necessary materials on a flat, uncluttered surface.
2. Label the mount with the following information: patient name, age, sex, the date, and any medications the patient is taking.
3. Indicate any variations from the standard procedure or situations that may have affected the tracing, including:
   a. Paper speed other than 25 mm per second.
   b. Sensitivity setting other than 1.
   c. A position other than supine.
   d. Alternate electrode placements.
   e. An anxious, nervous, or fidgety patient.
   f. A patient who smoked immediately before arriving for the test.
4. Unroll the ECG strip and locate lead I.
5. Locate the standardization mark if applicable.
6. Use scissors to trim the tracing according to office procedure. Include the standardization mark if applicable and four or five complexes in each strip.
7. Mount as required. Be sure that:
   a. The entire tracing is visible in the mount, including all peaks and the standardization mark.
   b. The tracing is right side up.
   c. The tracing is mounted in the correct location on the form.
8. Repeat steps 4 through 7 for each lead.
9. Check the entire mount. Be sure that:
   a. All leads are included and marked properly.
   b. Standardization marks are included.
   c. All patient information is complete.
   d. The mount is neat.
10. Put away all supplies.
11. Place the mounted ECG tracing in the patient's file.

heart rhythm, heart rate, the length and position of intervals and segments, and wave changes. A series of ECGs are often taken before a physician makes a diagnosis. The tracings are compared for changes in a patient's condition, progress, or response to a specific medication.

Heart Rhythm

The ECG is the best way to assess heart rhythm—the regularity of the heartbeat. A normal heart rhythm is indicated on the ECG by regularly spaced complexes. In a regularly spaced complex, the distance between one P wave and the next P wave—or one R wave and the next R wave—is consistent. The physician assesses the patient's rhythm by viewing the rhythm strip you obtain from lead II.

Irregularities in heart rhythm are called **arrhythmias.** Some arrhythmias do not cause problems, but many of them can be dangerous. It is important, therefore, to detect these irregularities with an ECG.

Heart Rate

The heart rate can easily be determined by counting the number of QRS complexes in a 6-second strip of the tracing (30 large squares at 25 mm per second) and multiplying by 10. Irregularities in heart rate may result from conduction abnormalities or reactions to certain drugs.

Intervals and Segments

Variations in the length and position of the intervals and segments can indicate many heart conditions, including conduction disturbances and **myocardial infarction,** or heart attack. For example, following a heart attack, the S-T segment will be elevated in the tracing for a period of time. Thus, the ECG can be used to determine not only the occurrence of a heart attack but also the approximate time it occurred. Electrolyte disturbances in the blood and drug reactions can also affect intervals and segments.

Wave Changes

The direction of certain waves may vary, depending on which lead is being viewed. Normally each wave should have a similar appearance in each of the leads. Changes in the height, width, or direction of a wave may indicate a problem. During the early stages of a heart attack, for example, the T wave forms a large peak. Not long afterward the T wave inverts and appears below the baseline.

Exercise Electrocardiography (Stress Testing)

The resting ECG does not always provide a doctor with enough information to diagnose a problem. Exercise electrocardiography, more commonly known as a stress test, assesses the heart's conduction system during exercise, when the demand for oxygen increases. This test measures a patient's response to a constant or increasing workload.

A stress test may be performed on a patient who has had surgery or a heart attack to determine how the heart is functioning. It is sometimes used to screen a patient for heart disease and to determine a patient's ability to undertake an exercise program.

During the procedure the patient is required to walk on a treadmill, pedal a stationary bicycle, or walk on a stair-stepping ergonometer while ECG readings are taken (Figure 39-17). An ergonometer measures work performed. You are responsible for preparing the patient for electrocardiography and monitoring blood pressure throughout the procedure. The test continues until the patient reaches a target heart rate, experiences chest pain or fatigue, or develops complications, such as tachycardia or dysrhythmia.

A patient who undergoes stress testing is often suspected of having a heart problem or is recovering from a heart attack or surgery. Consequently, there may be a risk of cardiac distress, heart attack, or cardiac arrest during testing. Because of the risks, the patient must be monitored by a physician throughout the test. Emergency medication and equipment, such as a defibrillator, must always be present in the room. The patient must sign an informed consent form before the procedure.

Because of the potential risk, patients may be apprehensive about the test. As a medical assistant, you can be instrumental in helping them feel comfortable about undergoing the procedure and in making the procedure as safe as possible for them. See "Caution: Handle With Care" for ways to help a patient safely undergo stress testing.

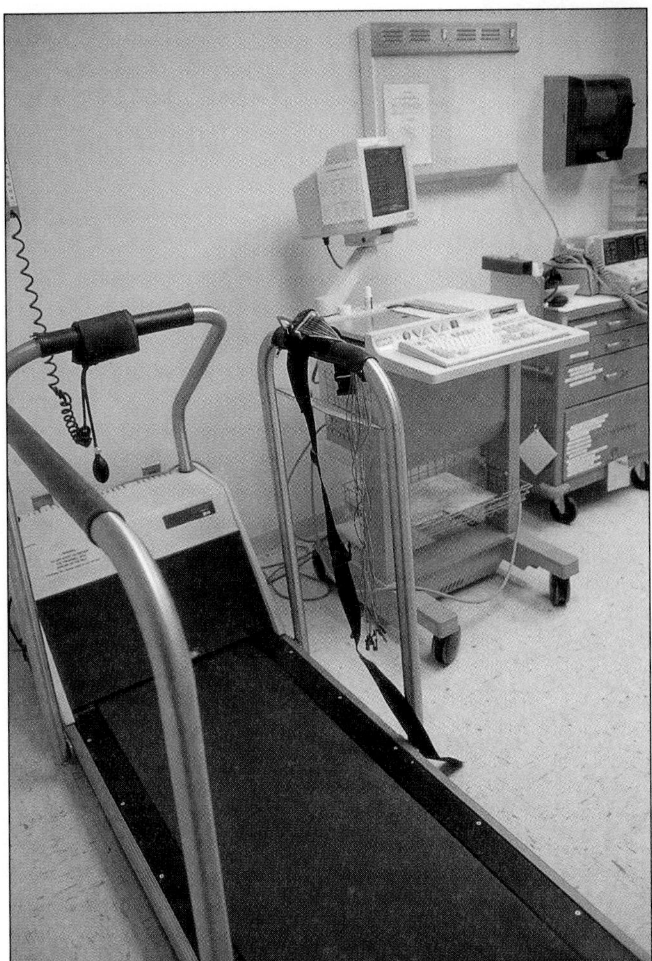

Figure 39-17. During a stress test, the patient exercises on special equipment to see how well the heart handles increased physical demands.

Ambulatory Electrocardiography (Holter Monitoring)

Patients who experience intermittent chest pain or discomfort may have a normal resting ECG and a normal stress test. When this is the case, the electrical activity of the patient's heart can be monitored over a 24-hour period of normal activity to help diagnose the problem. A special monitor, the Holter monitor, is used for this purpose.

Function of the Holter Monitor

The **Holter monitor** is an electrocardiography device that includes a small cassette recorder worn around a patient's waist or on a shoulder strap to record the heart's electrical activity. The monitor is connected to electrodes on the patient's chest (Figure 39-18). During the testing period, the patient is asked to perform usual

CAUTION HANDLE WITH CARE

Ensuring Patient Safety During Stress Testing

Some risk is involved in exercise electrocardiography, because patients who most commonly undergo the test may either already have cardiac problems or be suspected of having them. The risk of having a heart attack during a stress test, however, is less than 1 in 500, and the risk of death is less than 1 in 10,000 (*Illustrated Guide to Diagnostic Tests,* 1994, p. 905). Still, some patients may be apprehensive about the procedure because of the risks.

You can help educate and prepare patients for stress tests and assist them during the procedure. One way to help is to ask patients to wear comfortable shoes and clothes. In addition, there are several ways to help these patients be less fearful of the procedure, while helping to ensure their safety.

A patient who has recently suffered a heart attack may be particularly afraid to undergo stress testing. A stress test may, however, be the only way the physician can accurately determine the functional ability of the patient's heart and assess his physical limitations. This information is vital to preventing future heart attacks.

Informing the patient of how he can expect to feel during the test—fatigued, slightly breathless, increased heart rate, and increased perspiration—will help him better cope with the test. Make clear that he will be given advance warnings of adjustments in the procedure, such as an increased workload.

Assure the patient that the procedure has few risks and that he may stop the test if he experiences chest pain or extreme fatigue. Knowing that he can control the procedure will help him relax and follow instructions.

Tell the patient that both you and the physician will be monitoring him during and after the procedure and that all safety precautions will be taken. Explain the presence of the safety equipment (the crash cart with medication, equipment, and supplies).

During the test, remember to talk to and listen to the patient. Encourage him to report his feelings, even those not related to cardiac symptoms. Observe the patient for signs of distress, and inform the physician immediately if such signs appear.

daily activities and to keep a written log of activities undertaken and of stress or symptoms experienced. Some monitors allow patients to press an event button to mark the area on the recording whenever symptoms appear to aid in the diagnosis.

The patient returns to the office at the end of the 24-hour test period to have the monitor and electrodes removed. The tape is analyzed by a microcomputer in the office or at a reference laboratory, and a printout of the results is prepared. When the tracing has been evaluated, the doctor can correlate cardiac irregularities, such as arrhythmias or S-T segment changes, with the activities and symptoms listed in the patient's diary.

In addition to its role as a diagnostic tool, Holter monitoring can be used to evaluate the status of a patient who is recovering from a heart attack. It can indicate progress or the need to change therapy or modify the rehabilitation plan.

Patient Education

It is absolutely essential that the patient continue normal activities during Holter monitoring. Give the patient the following additional instructions.

- Record all activities, emotional upsets, physical symptoms, and medications taken.
- Wear loose-fitting clothing that opens in the front while wearing the monitor.
- Avoid going near magnets, metal detectors, and high-voltage areas, and avoid using electric blankets during the monitoring period. These devices and areas can interfere with the recording.
- Avoid getting the monitor wet. Do not take a bath or shower. A sponge bath is permissible.

Show the patient how to check the monitor to make sure it is working properly. This step is particularly important if any of the electrodes seem loose. Instruct the patient to inform the office if there are any problems.

Connecting the Patient

Holter monitors have either three or five electrodes, depending on the unit. As with a resting ECG, correct placement of the electrodes is necessary for accurate readings. Because the electrodes must stay in place for 24 hours, you may need to shave the areas where the are attached to permit optimum adherence. The wires may be connected to the electrodes before they are attached to minimize patient discomfort.

After the electrodes and wires are attached and the monitor is in place, tape the wires to the patient's chest to eliminate tension on the wires or electrodes (Figure 39-19). Be sure that the unit has a fresh battery, a cassette tape has been inserted, and the unit is turned on. The steps in performing Holter monitoring are outlined in Procedure 39-3.

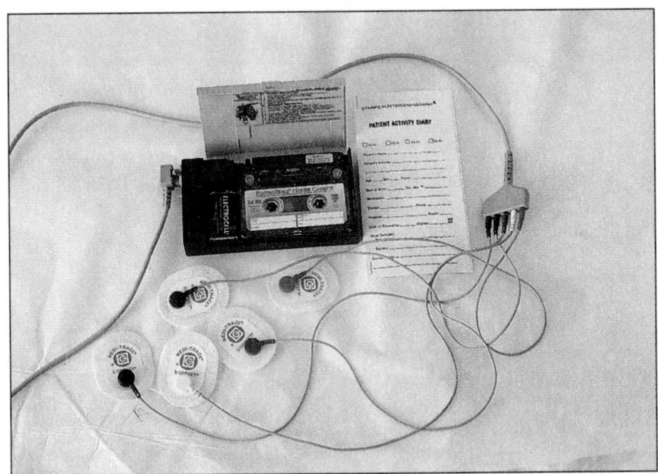

Figure 39-18. The Holter monitor is used to determine electrical activity of a patient's heart over a 24-hour period.

Anatomy and Physiology of the Respiratory System

Pulmonary function tests are used to evaluate a patient's lung volume and capacity. A description of the anatomy and physiology of the respiratory system will help clarify pulmonary function testing and the problems it is used to diagnose.

Anatomy of the Respiratory System

The respiratory system is composed of the nose, pharynx, larynx, trachea, two bronchi, and the lungs. The bronchi branch into bronchioles and eventually into alveoli. In the alveoli, external respiration—the exchange of gases between the air and the blood—occurs. Figure 39-23, p. 859 shows the lungs, bronchi, and alveoli in detail.

Physiology of the Respiratory System

There are two levels of respiration: external and internal. External respiration involves two processes: ventilation and diffusion. Ventilation is the movement of air in and out of the lungs. It results from the contraction and relaxation of the respiratory muscles. The major respiratory muscle is the diaphragm. Other respiratory muscles, including the intercostal muscles (between the ribs), are found in the walls of the chest and back.

Inspiration, or breathing in, results when the respiratory muscles contract. The diaphragm pushes down toward the abdomen when it contracts, while the other respiratory muscles help expand the chest outward and upward. Both actions serve to decrease the pressure within the alveoli so that it is less than the atmospheric pressure. The result is the flow of air into the lungs.

Expiration, or breathing out, results from relaxation of the respiratory muscles and a consequent increase in pressure within the alveoli. As a result, air flows out of the lungs. Expiration is normally a passive process. During fast, hard breathing, however, the abdominal muscles push the diaphragm upward, and certain chest and back muscles pull the ribs downward and inward to decrease the size of the chest cavity and help force the air out.

Diffusion is a passive process wherein oxygen and carbon dioxide cross the capillary and alveolar membranes to enter the capillaries or alveoli. Oxygen diffuses from the alveolar air into the blood, because there is a higher concentration in the alveoli than in the blood. Carbon dioxide, at a higher concentration in the blood, diffuses across the membranes into the alveoli.

Perfusion, or internal respiration, is the exchange of oxygen in the blood for carbon dioxide in the cells of body tissues and organs. Perfusion, diffusion, and ventilation occur simultaneously, as the circulatory system moves the blood from the lungs to the body cells and back.

Pulmonary Function Testing

Pulmonary function tests (PFTs) evaluate lung volume and capacity. These tests are commonly used to evaluate shortness of breath and can help detect and classify pulmonary disorders. They may also be performed as part of a general examination. PFTs are used to monitor conditions such as asthma, certain allergies, cystic fibrosis,

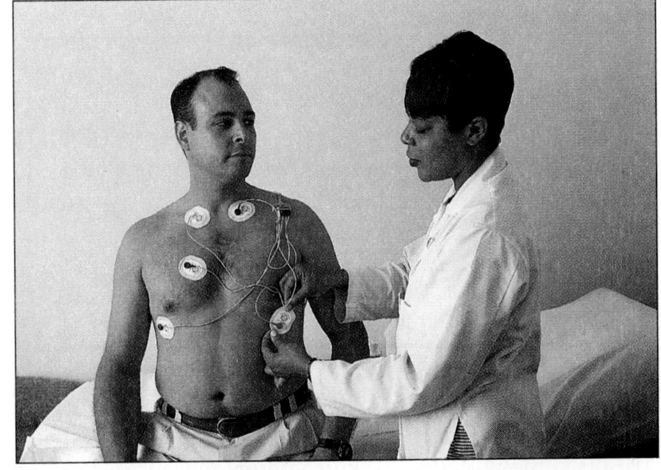

Figure 39-19. Taping the wires to the patient's chest reduces the chance that tension on a wire or electrode will produce artifacts on the ECG.

PROCEDURE 39-3

Holter Monitoring

Objective: To monitor the electrical activity of a patient's heart over a 24-hour period to detect cardiac abnormalities that may go undetected during routine electrocardiography or stress testing

OSHA Guidelines

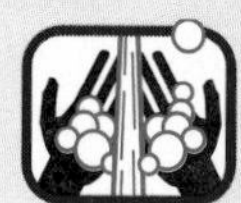 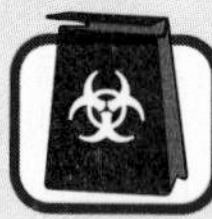 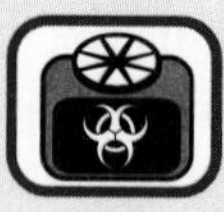 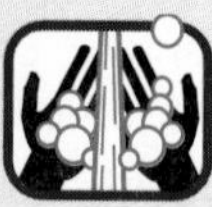

Materials: Holter monitor, battery, cassette tape, patient diary or log, alcohol, gauze pads, disposable shaving supplies, disposable electrodes, hypoallergenic tape, drape, electrocardiograph

Method

1. Identify the patient, introduce yourself, and explain the procedure.
2. Ask the patient to remove clothing from the waist up; provide a drape if necessary.
3. Wash your hands and assemble the equipment.
4. Assist the patient into a comfortable position (sitting or supine).
5. If the patient's body hair is particularly dense, put on examination gloves and shave the areas where the electrodes will be attached. Properly dispose of the razor and the gloves.
6. Clean the electrode sites with alcohol and gauze.
7. Rub each electrode site vigorously with a dry gauze square to help electrodes adhere to the skin.
8. Attach wires to the electrodes, and peel off the paper backing on the electrodes. Apply as indicated (see Figure 39-20), pressing firmly to ensure that each electrode is securely attached, making good contact with the skin.
9. Attach the patient cable.
10. Insert a fresh battery, and position the unit (Figure 39-21).
11. Tape wires, cable, and electrodes as necessary to avoid tension on the wires as the patient moves.

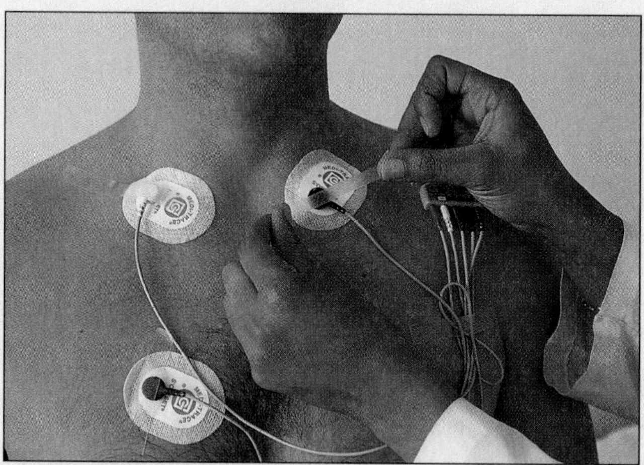

Figure 39-20. Correctly connecting the patient to the Holter monitor is essential.

and chronic obstructive pulmonary disease (COPD), a chronic lung disorder. The tests are also used to evaluate the effectiveness of particular treatments on a patient's lung function.

Spirometry

Spirometry is a test used to measure breathing capacity. An instrument called a **spirometer** measures the air taken in by and expelled from the lungs. Several different measurements related to lung volume and capacity can be made with a spirometer (Table 39-4). Some of these measurements are made directly by the spirometer; others are calculated.

Forced Vital Capacity

Many measurements can be obtained during one particular maneuver—obtaining the **forced vital capacity** (FVC), the greatest volume of air that can be expelled when a person performs rapid, forced expiration. To obtain the FVC, ask the patient to take as deep a breath as possible and to exhale into the spirometer as quickly and completely as possible. You can determine the lung's ability to function by taking into account the volume of air expelled and the time it takes to perform this maneuver.

12. Insert the cassette tape, and turn on the unit.
13. Confirm that the cassette tape is actually running (Figure 39-22). Indicate the start time in the patient's chart.
14. Instruct the patient on proper use of the monitor and how to enter information in the diary. Caution the patient not to alter any diary entries; it is crucial to know what the patient is doing at all times.
15. Schedule the patient's return visit for the same time on the following day.
16. On the following day remove the electrodes, discard them, and clean the electrode sites.
17. Wash your hands.
18. Remove the cassette and obtain a printout of the tracing according to office procedure.

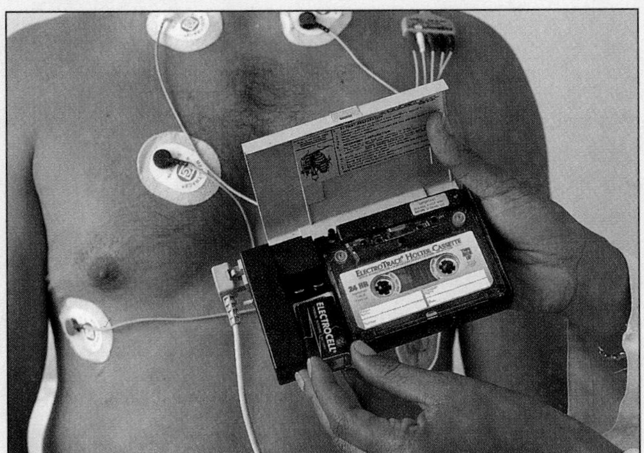

Figure 39-21. Make sure the monitor has a fresh battery and cassette tape.

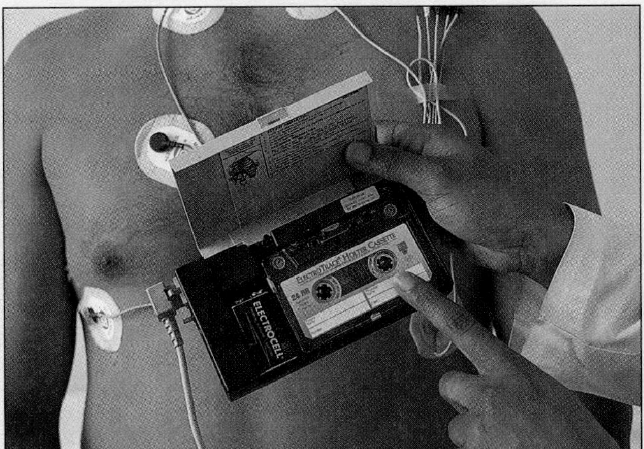

Figure 39-22. Observe the cassette to make sure the tape is moving through the recording unit.

Types of Spirometers

Many types of spirometers are used in physicians' offices. Each consists of a mouthpiece or a mouthpiece and a tube to carry air to the machine, a mechanism to measure the volume or flow of air, and a means of calculating and printing the results.

Computerized spirometers are available that can measure air volume and airflow, perform various calculations, and print a graphic representation of the information. Figure 39-24 shows a computerized spirometer.

Mechanical spirometers directly measure either the air volume displaced or airflow. Spirometers that directly measure airflow calculate air volume using flow rate and time values. The flow-sensing spirometer illustrated in Figure 39-25 calculates airflow by counting the rotations of a turbine.

Performing Spirometry

The technique for performing pulmonary function testing is similar for all types of spirometers. Successful spirometry depends on proper patient preparation and consistent technique in performing the procedure and analyzing the results. The steps involved in measuring forced vital capacity using a spirometer are described in detail here and outlined in Procedure 39-4.

MULTISKILL FOCUS

Respiratory Therapist

To gain medical assistant credentials, you must fulfill the requirements of either the American Association of Medical Assistants (for a Certified Medical Assistant) or the American Medical Technologists (for a Registered Medical Assistant). After obtaining your medical assistant certification or registration, you may wish to acquire additional skills in specialty areas through course work or on-the-job training. Although this course work or training may not lead to an additional certification or degree, it will enable you to expand your role in the medical office and advance your career as the demand for multiskilled health professionals increases.

Skills and Duties

A respiratory therapist diagnoses, treats, and cares for people who have difficulty breathing. Some of his patients are people with chronic lung problems, such as asthma, bronchitis, emphysema, and chronic obstructive pulmonary disease. Others may have difficulty breathing as the result of complications caused by a heart attack, an accident, cystic fibrosis, lung cancer, or acquired immunodeficiency syndrome (AIDS). Some infants who are born prematurely have difficulty breathing and may need respiratory therapy, which may include the use of apnea monitors and oxygen tents.

A respiratory therapist works under the supervision of a physician. Duties include both diagnostic and therapeutic tasks. For example, to diagnose a breathing problem, the therapist analyzes samples of a patient's breath or blood for levels of oxygen, carbon dioxide, and other gases. He also measures the capacity of a patient's lungs to determine whether they are working properly and performs stress tests and other studies of the cardiopulmonary system.

Once a problem is diagnosed, the respiratory therapist may use a variety of treatment options. He may use equipment such as oxygen respirators and oxygen tents to administer oxygen to help the patient breathe. He may administer medication in aerosol form to treat breathing disorders. The respiratory therapist may also set up and maintain mechanical ventilation, such as artificial airways, for patients who cannot breathe on their own.

In addition to diagnosis and treatment of breathing disorders, the respiratory therapist may be responsible for patient education to promote healthy breathing. Education duties may include:

- Teaching smoking cessation programs to help prevent breathing problems associated with smoking.
- Conducting rehabilitation activities, such as low-impact aerobics, to help patients increase their lung capacity.

The respiratory therapist is also often responsible for testing equipment to make sure it is operating effectively.

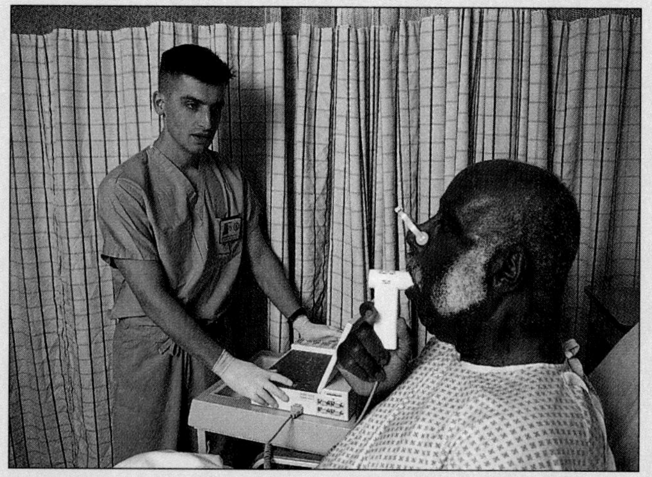

He may make minor repairs to faulty respiratory equipment or arrange for major repair work.

Workplace Settings

Most respiratory therapists work in hospitals. Sometimes, in emergency situations, they also work in ambulances. Increasing numbers of respiratory therapists, however, work in locations outside the hospital. These locations include nursing homes, physicians' offices, home health-care agencies, rehabilitation centers, clinics, medical equipment supply companies, and patients' homes.

Education

Approximately 400 colleges and universities in the United States offer respiratory care programs. To qualify for a program, you must be a high school graduate with a background in math and science.

The National Board for Respiratory Therapists has established two levels of respiratory care practitioners. A Certified Respiratory Therapy Technician (CRTT) has graduated from an approved program (usually 12 to 18 months), has 1 year of work experience, and has passed a voluntary written examination. A Registered Respiratory Therapist (RRT) has completed either a 2-year or 4-year approved program, has 1 year of work experience, and has passed a written and practical examination.

Where to Go for More Information

American Association for Respiratory Care
11030 Ables Lane
Dallas, TX 75229
(214) 243-2272

American Lung Association
1740 Broadway
New York, NY 10019
(212) 315-8700

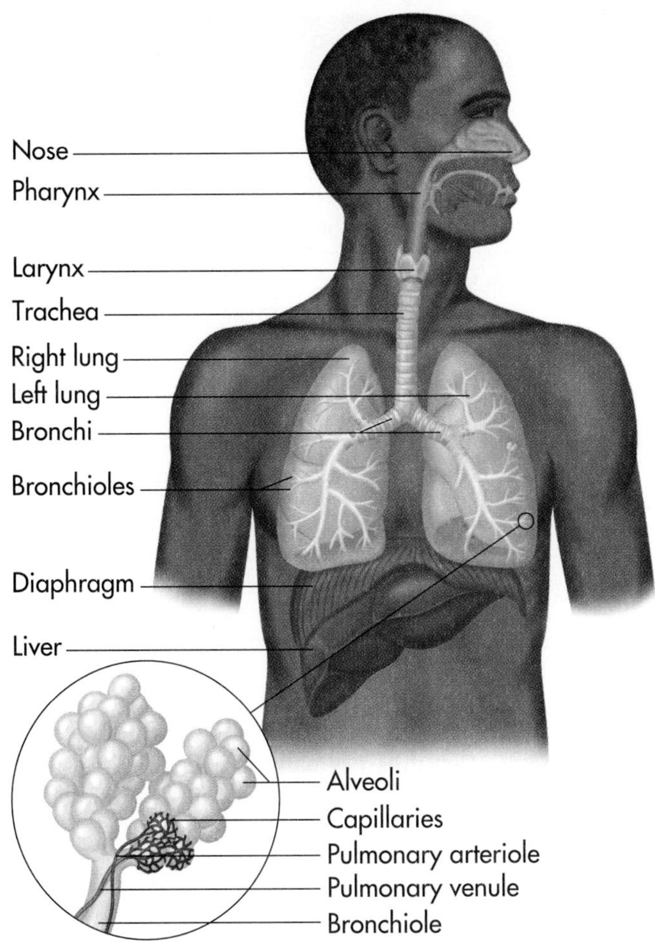

Figure 39-23. Knowing how the respiratory system works will help you understand the application of spirometry.

Patient Preparation

When patients are scheduled for pulmonary function tests, inform them that the following conditions and activities may affect the test's accuracy:

- Viral infection or acute illness within the previous 2 to 3 weeks
- Serious medical condition, such as a recent heart attack
- Recent use of a prescribed medication if test order calls for spirometry before and after prescribed medication
- Use of a sedative or opioid substance before the test
- Smoking or eating a heavy meal within 1 hour of taking the test

Review the conditions and activities with patients again on the day of the test to ensure that none apply. If there are no contraindications, weigh and measure patients. Use simple terms to explain the procedure and its purpose. Have them loosen tight clothing so they will be comfortable and their breathing will not be restricted in any way. The procedure can be performed with patients sitting down or standing up; allow them to choose the more comfortable position. If they choose to sit, make sure their legs are not crossed and that both feet are flat on the floor.

Explain that they need to wear a nose clip or hold the nose tightly closed to be sure that they will inhale and exhale through the mouth. The mouthpiece of the unit

Table 39-4

Pulmonary Function Tests

Lung Capacity Tests	Definition
Vital capacity (VC)	Total volume of air that can be exhaled after maximum inspiration
Inspiratory capacity (IC)	Amount of air that can be inhaled after normal expiration
Functional residual capacity (FRC)	Amount of air remaining in lungs after normal expiration
Total lung capacity (TLC)	Total volume of lungs when maximally inflated
Forced vital capacity (FVC)	Greatest volume of air that can be expelled when person performs rapid, forced expiratory maneuver
Forced expiratory volume (FEV)	Volume of air expelled in first, second, or third second of FVC maneuver
Peak expiratory flow rate (PEFR)	Greatest rate of flow during forced expiration
Forced expiratory flow (FEF)	Average rate of flow during middle half of FVC
Maximal voluntary ventilation (MVV)	Greatest volume of air breathed per unit of time

continued

Table 39-4 continued

Pulmonary Function Tests

Lung Volume Tests	Definition
Tidal volume (T_V)	Amount of air inhaled or exhaled during normal breathing
Minute volume (MV)	Total amount of air expired per minute
Inspiratory reserve volume (IRV)	Amount of air inspired over above-normal inspiration
Expiratory reserve volume (ERV)	Amount of air exhaled after normal expiration
Residual volume (RV)	Amount of air remaining in lungs after forced expiration

Adapted from *Illustrated Guide to Diagnostic Tests,* Student Version (Springhouse, PA: Springhouse, 1994).

may be a disposable cardboard tube or a reusable rubber one that can be disinfected after use. If disposable mouthpieces are used, instruct patients to avoid biting down on them, because that will obstruct the flow of air.

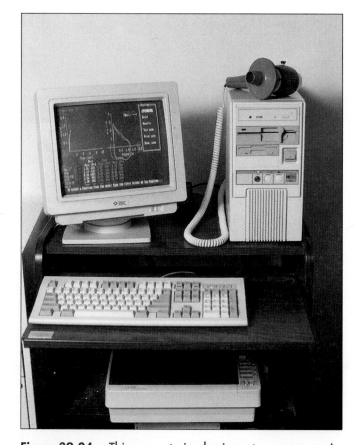

Figure 39-24. This computerized spirometer measures air volume and airflow.

Be sure patients form a tight seal around the mouthpiece with their lips. Dentures normally help maintain a tight seal; however, they should be removed if they hinder the process.

Proper Positioning. Instruct patients to keep their chin and neck in the correct position during the procedure. The chin should be slightly elevated and the neck slightly extended. Bending the chin to the chest tends to restrict the flow of air and should be avoided (Figure 39-26). Some bending at the waist is acceptable.

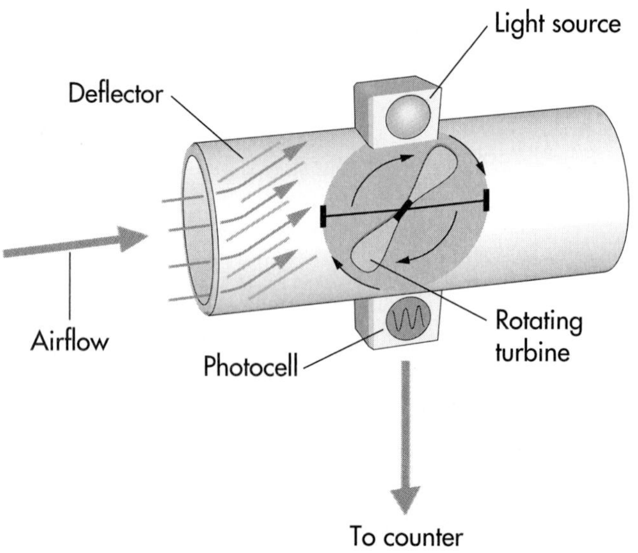

Figure 39-25. One type of flow-sensing spirometer uses a turbine to measure airflow directly from the lungs.

PROCEDURE 39-4

Measuring Forced Vital Capacity Using Spirometry

Objective: To determine a patient's forced vital capacity using a volume-displacing spirometer

OSHA Guidelines

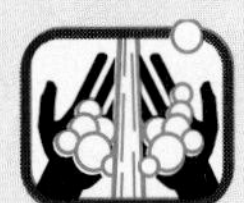
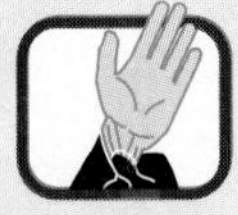

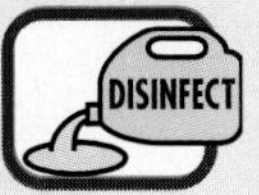

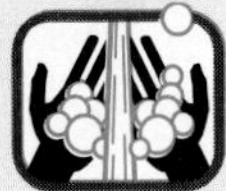

Materials: Adult scale with height bar, spirometer, patient tubing (tubing that runs from the mouthpiece to the machine), mouthpiece, nose clip, disinfectant

Method

1. Prepare the equipment. Ensure that the paper supply in the machine is adequate.
2. Calibrate the machine as necessary.
3. Identify the patient and introduce yourself.
4. Check the patient's chart to see whether there are special instructions to follow.
5. Ask whether the patient has followed instructions.
6. Wash your hands and put on examination gloves.
7. Measure and record the patient's height and weight.
8. Explain the proper positioning.
9. Explain the procedure.
10. Demonstrate the procedure.
11. Turn on the spirometer, and enter applicable patient data and the number of tests to be performed.
12. Ensure that the patient has loosened any tight clothing, is comfortable, and is in the proper position. Apply the nose clip.
13. Have the patient perform the first maneuver, coaching when necessary.
14. Determine whether the maneuver is acceptable.
15. Offer feedback to the patient and recommendations for improvement if necessary.
16. Have the patient perform additional maneuvers until three acceptable maneuvers are obtained.
17. Record the procedure in the patient's chart, and place the chart and the test results on the physician's desk for interpretation.
18. Ask the patient to remain until the physician reviews the results.
19. Properly dispose of used materials and disposable instruments.
20. Sanitize and disinfect patient tubing and reusable mouthpiece and nose clip.
21. Clean and disinfect the equipment and room according to OSHA guidelines.

Explaining and Demonstrating the Procedure. Tell patients to take the deepest breath possible, insert the mouthpiece into the mouth, form a tight seal, and then blow into the mouthpiece as hard and as fast as possible to completely exhale. Tell them to exhale as long as they can to force air from the lungs. Remind them that the initial force of their exhalation must be strong to get a valid reading. Demonstrate the procedure to show how the test is done correctly.

Performing the Maneuver

You can improve patients' performance during the maneuver by actively and forcefully coaching them. Urge patients to blow hard and to continue blowing. After a maneuver, give them feedback on their performance, and indicate corrective actions they can take to improve the next maneuver.

Some spirometers indicate whether a particular maneuver was of adequate force and duration to be measured. Adequate force does not, however, indicate that the maneuver was acceptable. An acceptable maneuver must have the following five features:

1. No coughing, particularly during the first second
2. A quick and forceful start
3. An adequate length of time (a minimum of 6 seconds)
4. A consistent and fast flow with no variability
5. Consistency with other maneuvers

Spirometry tracings plot volume and time. You will need to obtain three acceptable maneuvers, which may require more than three attempts. Observe the patient for signs of breathing difficulty, dizziness, light-headedness, or changes in pulse and blood pressure. If necessary, allow the patient to rest briefly before continuing. Notify the physician immediately if symptoms are severe.

Determining the Effectiveness of Medication. Spirometry is often used to determine the effectiveness of

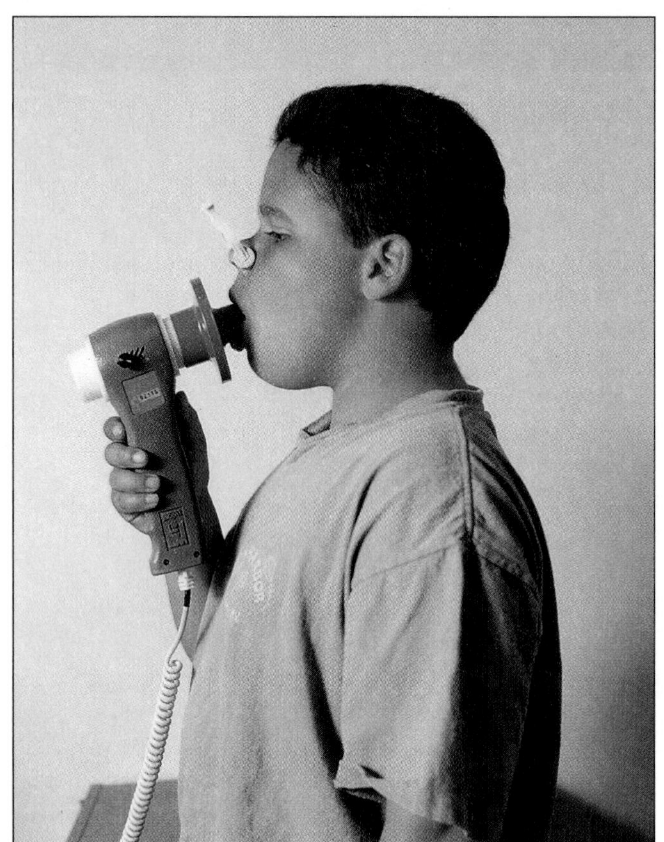

A

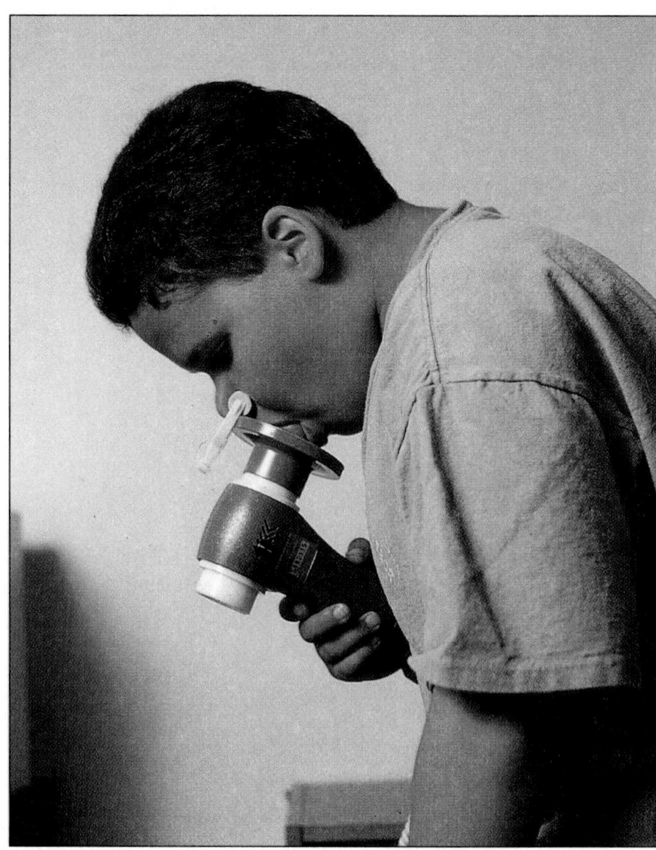

B

Figure 39-26. The patient must maintain the proper position during a pulmonary function test. **A.** The chin should be slightly elevated and the neck slightly extended. **B.** The neck should not approach the chest.

certain medications a patient is taking. You will perform two sets of maneuvers if this determination is required. Instruct the patient to refrain from taking the prescribed medication on the day of the test. Before performing the test, confirm that the patient has followed this instruction. Conduct the first set of maneuvers, ensuring that they are acceptable. After obtaining the results, instruct the patient to take the prescribed medication. Allow the medication to take effect, and then perform a second set of maneuvers. Comparing the two sets of readings shows whether the medication has effectively improved the patient's lung function. Some computerized spirometers can graph both sets of readings together to simplify the comparison (Figure 39-27).

Special Considerations. On occasion you may have to deal with an uncooperative patient, one who cannot understand or follow directions, or one who cannot perform the procedure. In these situations patience and skill are essential to obtaining an acceptable spirometry tracing.

The doctor may be able to convince an uncooperative patient to perform the maneuver. You can help by taking a no-nonsense approach, perhaps stating that the doctor needs these test results to help the patient. Patients who cannot understand or follow directions—the very young, the very old, those who have limited proficiency in English, or those with a hearing impairment—may need extra attention and patience to obtain acceptable results. Explain the procedure in simple terms, and repeat instructions as necessary. If, after eight attempts, the patient is unable to perform the procedure, stop and report the situation to the doctor.

The Importance of Calibration

Spirometers should be calibrated each day they are used to ensure accurate readings. You may be required to perform this procedure. Calibration of a spirometer requires the use of a standardized measuring instrument called a **calibration syringe** (Figure 39-28). When the plunger is pulled back, this syringe contains a fixed volume of air. Connect the syringe to the patient tubing (the tubing that runs from the mouthpiece to the machine), and depress the plunger to inject the entire volume of air. The reading on the spirometer should be within ±3% of the stated volume. It is important to keep a calibration logbook for each spirometer.

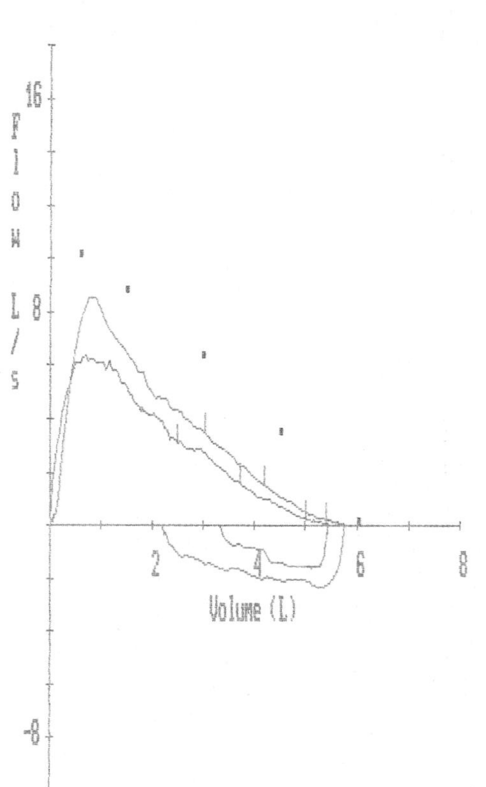

Figure 39-27. These spirometry tracings show air volume per second before and after use of a medication.

While calibrating the spirometer, you can detect leaks by checking the volume/time graph. The volume should remain at a steady reading. If the volume declines with time, there is a leak somewhere in the system.

Infection Control

After a patient completes the pulmonary function test, you must clean the spirometer thoroughly to prevent transmission of microorganisms. If disposable mouthpieces and nose clips are used, discard them in a biohazardous waste container. If reusable mouthpieces and nose clips are used, clean and disinfect them between patients. Also change patient tubing between patients. Thoroughly clean and disinfect patient tubing before reusing it. Most important, wash your hands thoroughly before and after performing a pulmonary function test.

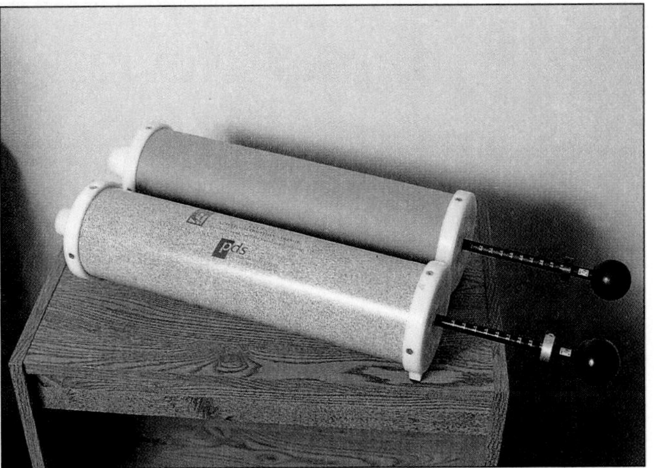

Figure 39-28. A calibration syringe delivers a fixed volume of air.

What the Results Reveal

Pulmonary function tests help the doctor evaluate ventilatory function of the lungs and chest wall. They are good screening tools for pulmonary disorders, such as pulmonary edema, chronic obstructive pulmonary disease, and asthma. These tests also help the doctor determine the nature of a patient's disorder, such as narrowing or obstruction of the airways. Pulmonary function tests can determine the severity of a patient's problem and response to therapy or medication.

Summary

Electrocardiography and pulmonary function testing play a vital role in the diagnosis and treatment of cardiac and pulmonary disease. As a medical assistant, you may be required to perform these procedures in the medical office.

To understand electrocardiography, you need to know the basics of the conduction system of the heart and the components of an electrocardiograph. To obtain accurate electrocardiogram readings, you must properly place the electrodes and be able to recognize artifacts and correct them.

Likewise, to provide accurate assessments of pulmonary function, you must use proper technique and recognize the acceptability of a spirometric maneuver. Because patient compliance is crucial to accurate results, effective patient education is vital to the process.

39 Chapter Review

Discussion Questions

1. Explain the pathway of electrical conduction in the heart.
2. Name and define the waves that can be found in a normal ECG pattern.
3. Explain the importance of nose clips in performing spirometry.

Critical Thinking Questions

1. For each of the ECG artifacts listed, indicate two possible causes and corrective actions that can be taken.
   a. Large, erratic spikes
   b. Wandering baseline
   c. Flat line
2. An elderly woman is in the office today for an ECG. She is anxious about the procedure. How might you allay her fears? What can you do to help her feel more comfortable during the procedure?
3. The physician has ordered pulmonary function testing on a patient who is an ex-smoker and is suffering from shortness of breath. He has had difficulty performing the first two maneuvers. What steps can you take to help him achieve an acceptable maneuver?

Application Activities

1. Practice locating the areas for placement of precordial ECG electrodes on your chest.
2. Explain to another student how to use and care for a Holter monitor.
3. Practice explaining and demonstrating the procedure of obtaining a forced vital capacity to someone who is not familiar with the procedure.

Further Readings

Dracup, Kathleen, et al. "Task Force 3: Partnerships in Delivery of Cardiovascular Care." *Journal of the American College of Cardiology,* August 1994, 296–304.

Illustrated Guide to Diagnostic Tests. Student Version. Springhouse, PA: Springhouse, 1994.

Ruppel, Gregg E. *Manual of Pulmonary Function Testing.* 6th ed. St. Louis, MO: Mosby–Year Book, 1994.

Swearingen, Pamela L. *Photo Atlas of Nursing Procedures.* 2d ed. Redwood City, CA: Addison-Wesley Nursing, 1991.

Thaler, Malcolm S. *The Only EKG Book You'll Ever Need.* 2d ed. Philadelphia: J. B. Lippincott, 1995.

Van Wynsberghe, Donna, Charles R. Noback, and Robert Carola. *Human Anatomy & Physiology.* 3d ed. New York: McGraw-Hill, 1994.

Wanger, Jack. *Pulmonary Function Testing: A Practical Approach.* Baltimore: Williams & Wilkins, 1992.

X-Rays and Diagnostic Radiology

CHAPTER OUTLINE

- Brief History of the X-Ray
- Diagnostic Radiology
- The Medical Assistant's Role in Diagnostic Radiology
- Common Diagnostic Radiologic Tests
- Common Therapeutic Uses of Radiation
- Radiation Safety and Dose
- Storing and Filing X-Rays
- Electronic Medicine

OBJECTIVES

After completing Chapter 40, you will be able to:

- Define x-rays and explain how they are used for diagnostic and therapeutic purposes.
- Compare invasive and noninvasive diagnostic procedures.
- Discuss the medical assistant's role in x-ray and diagnostic radiology testing.
- Describe the imaging process and uses of the various types of x-rays.
- Discuss the medical assistant's duties in preparing a patient for an x-ray.
- Explain the risks and safety precautions associated with radiology work.
- Describe proper procedures for filing and maintaining x-ray films and records.

AREAS OF COMPETENCE

1997 ROLE DELINEATION STUDY

CLINICAL

Patient Care

- Prepare patient for examinations, procedures, and treatments

GENERAL (Transdisciplinary)

Legal Concepts

- Prepare and maintain medical records
- Comply with established risk management and safety procedures

Key Terms

arthrography
barium enema
barium swallow
brachytherapy
cholangiography
contrast medium
diagnostic radiology
intravenous pyelography (IVP)
invasive
KUB radiography
mammography
MUGA scan
myelography
noninvasive
nuclear medicine
PET
radiation therapy
retrograde pyelography
SPECT
stereoscopy
teletherapy
thermography
ultrasound
xeroradiography

Brief History of the X-Ray

In 1895 Wilhelm Konrad Roentgen (1845–1923) discovered the x-ray, or roentgen ray, a type of electromagnetic wave. It has a high energy level, traveling at the speed of light (186,000 miles per second), and an extremely short wavelength (one-billionth of an inch) that can penetrate solid objects. X-rays react with photographic film to produce a permanent record (x-ray, or radiograph). The x-ray image is lightest where the film is struck by the most x-ray energy. Differences in tissue densities produce the x-ray image, with the least dense being lightest and the most dense being darkest on the film.

Today there are both diagnostic and therapeutic uses for x-rays and radioactive substances. Radiologic technologists are trained medical personnel who are certified to perform certain radiologic procedures upon completion of a radiology curriculum lasting 2 to 4 years. Some radiologic technologists receive further training in radiology subspecialties, such as ultrasound, mammography, magnetic resonance imaging, and nuclear medicine. Radiographers, sonographers, radiation therapists, and nuclear medicine technologists are all radiologic technologists. Invasive radiologic procedures or procedures requiring a high degree of expertise are nearly always performed by a radiologist, a physician who specializes in radiology. A radiologist is also the physician who interprets the films for other physicians. Other specialists who perform radiologic procedures, either alone or with the assistance of a radiologist, include cardiologists, orthopedists, obstetricians, and oncologists.

Diagnostic Radiology

Diagnostic radiology is the use of x-ray technology for diagnostic purposes. Radiologic tests sometimes use contrast media, as well as special techniques or instruments for viewing internal body structures and functions. A **contrast medium** is a substance that makes internal organs denser and blocks the passage of x-rays to the photographic film. Introducing contrast media into certain structures or areas of the body can provide a clearer image of organs and tissues and indications of how well they are functioning. Contrast media include gases (air, oxygen, or carbon dioxide), heavy metal salts (barium sulfate or bismuth carbonate), and iodine compounds. They can be administered orally, parenterally (for example, intravenously), or by routes that introduce them into an organ or body cavity (for example, by insertion). Types of diagnostic imaging include x-rays, computed tomography (CT), nuclear medicine, magnetic resonance imaging (MRI), and ultrasound.

Invasive Procedures

Diagnostic tests can be invasive or noninvasive. An **invasive** procedure (such as angiography) requires a radiologist to insert a catheter, wire, or other testing device into a patient's blood vessel or organ through the skin or a body orifice. All invasive tests require surgical aseptic technique. Some procedures, including angiography, are performed in a hospital or same-day surgical facility. The patient may need general anesthesia for some procedures. The anesthetist must closely monitor the patient who is under anesthesia during and after the test for life-threatening complications, such as anaphylaxis.

Noninvasive Procedures

Noninvasive procedures, such as standard x-rays or ultrasound, use other technologies to view internal structures. They do not require inserting devices, breaking the skin, or the degree of monitoring needed with invasive procedures.

The most familiar equipment used for diagnostic imaging is the conventional x-ray machine, as shown in Figure 40-1. This machine consists of a table, an x-ray tube, a control panel, and a high-voltage generator. Other equipment used for diagnostic radiology includes instruments specifically designed for the test. Examples are a mammography unit, a scanner for CT, and a transducer for ultrasound.

The Medical Assistant's Role in Diagnostic Radiology

You may deal with diagnostic radiology in a radiology facility or in a medical office. Your duties in a radiology facility will include assisting a radiologic technologist or a radiologist in performing diagnostic radiologic procedures. Depending on the scope of practice in your state, you may be allowed to learn how to operate certain x-ray

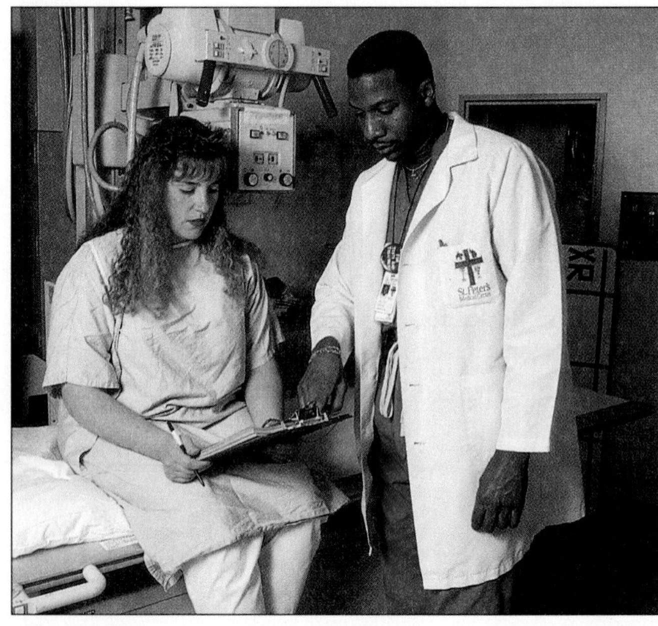

Figure 40-1. A standard x-ray is one of the most frequently performed radiologic tests.

equipment. Even if you are not allowed to assist with an x-ray procedure or to operate x-ray equipment, you will probably provide preprocedure and postprocedure care of the patient.

Your duties in a medical facility, such as an orthopedic office, may include assisting a radiologic technologist in performing x-ray procedures. In an obstetric practice, you might assist a physician in performing an ultrasound examination of a pregnant woman. Even if you work in a medical office that does no radiologic testing, you must still provide a certain amount of preprocedure care. To properly explain a test to a patient and to assist a radiologic technologist or radiologist in performing a test, you must have a basic understanding of x-ray technology. You may also need in-service training to ensure accuracy and patient safety for some procedures.

Preprocedure Care

Preprocedure care varies somewhat, depending on the test. In general, however, you may do the following:

- Schedule the patient's appointment, if necessary. Inform the patient of the location, date, and time of the procedure.
- Provide preparation instructions. Advise the patient about diet restrictions or requirements (such as fasting or drinking liquids), as well as medication requirements (such as taking a laxative). Always check with the radiology facility for specific requirements, and be sure the patient receives this information.
- Explain the procedure to the patient briefly and clearly. Use proper terminology and nontechnical language, but do not talk down to the patient. Reinforce the doctor's reason for requesting the procedure, and provide any available written information about the test. Inform the patient about the length of the examination, about possible side effects or safety precautions and warnings, and about injections or uncomfortable steps.
- Ask pertinent questions. Obtain a medication history from the patient (current medications could interfere with some procedures). If the patient is a woman of childbearing age, ask whether she is pregnant or whether there is any chance she could be pregnant. Report the answers to the physician in a medical office or to the radiologic technologist in a radiology facility.
- Ask about insurance coverage and policy information and answer any questions the patient may have, such as how much the procedure costs and what portion of the cost is covered by insurance (if you have that information).

Care During and After the Procedure

If you work in a radiology facility, your responsibilities include preparing the patient and guiding him through the procedure. You may also assist the radiologic technologist or the radiologist in performing the procedure by placing, removing, and developing film in the x-ray machine. Procedure 40-1 describes the general process of assisting with a radiologic procedure.

You may care for a patient and assist the radiologic technologist or radiologist during a wide variety of x-ray and other diagnostic imaging tests. Although requirements vary depending on the procedure, you will probably be asked to perform many of the duties described in Procedure 40-1. Although you are unlikely to position the patient, you should know that the position relative to the x-ray source determines the path of the x-rays and the sorts of images that result. Figure 40-2 illustrates common x-ray pathways and the images produced.

Common Diagnostic Radiologic Tests

A variety of radiologic imaging tests are available. Table 40-1 identifies some of the most frequently ordered tests and the disorders they are used to diagnose.

Contrast Media in Diagnostic Tests

Various procedures involve the use of contrast media to visualize body structures and observe their function. These procedures include angiography, arthrography, barium enema, barium swallow, cholangiography, cholecystography, fluoroscopy, intravenous pyelography, magnetic resonance imaging (sometimes), myelography, nuclear medicine studies, and retrograde pyelography.

As mentioned, contrast media can be administered by mouth, by needle or catheter into a blood vessel, or by a route that introduces the medium into an organ or body cavity (for example, into the colon). A contrast medium can cause adverse effects in some patients. Common adverse effects with oral agents include mild and transient abdominal cramping, constipation, nausea, vomiting, diarrhea, skin rashes, itching, heartburn, dizziness, and headache. Intravenous agents cause some of the same adverse effects, as well as localized injection-site reactions and more serious reactions such as anaphylaxis. Because many contrast media contain iodine, a common allergen, patients should be questioned about known allergies to iodine or shellfish, which contain iodine, before procedures involving the use of contrast media. All patients should be observed during such procedures for signs of allergic reaction.

Fluoroscopy

X-rays can cause certain chemicals to fluoresce, or emit visible light. When x-rays penetrate a body structure and are directed onto a fluorescent screen, they produce an image the radiologist can view either directly or through special glasses. Usually, fluoroscopic procedures are performed by a radiologist rather than by a radiology technician or a medical assistant.

PROCEDURE 40-1

Assisting With an X-Ray Examination

Objective: To assist with a radiologic procedure under the supervision of a radiologic technologist

OSHA Guidelines: This procedure does not involve exposure to blood, body fluids, or tissue. You must wear a radiation exposure badge (dosimeter), however, and will be required to wear a garment containing a lead shield if you remain in the room during the operation of x-ray equipment

Materials: X-ray examination order, x-ray machine, x-ray film and holder, x-ray film developer, drape, patient shield

Method

1. Check the x-ray examination order and equipment needed.
2. Identify the patient and introduce yourself.
3. Determine whether the patient has complied with the preprocedure instructions.
4. Explain the procedure and the purpose of the examination to the patient.
5. Instruct the patient to remove clothing and all metals (including jewelry) as needed, according to body area to be examined, and to put on a gown. Explain that metals may interfere with the image. Ask whether the patient has any surgical metal or a pacemaker, and report this information to the radiologic technologist. Leave the room to ensure patient privacy.

Note: Steps 6 through 11 are nearly always performed by a radiologic technologist.

6. Position the patient according to the x-ray view ordered.
7. Drape the patient and place the patient shield appropriately.
8. Instruct the patient about the need to remain still and to hold his breath when requested.
9. Leave the room or stand behind a lead shield during the exposure.
10. Ask the patient to assume a comfortable position while the films are developed. Explain that x-rays sometimes must be repeated.
11. Develop the films.
12. If the x-ray films are satisfactory, instruct the patient to dress and tell him when to contact his physician's office for the results.
13. Label the dry, finished x-ray films, place them in a properly labeled envelope, and file them according to the policies of your office.
14. Record the x-ray examination, along with the final written findings, in the patient's chart.

Many diagnostic procedures involve fluoroscopy, which allows viewing of internal organ movement or the movement of a contrast medium, such as barium sulfate, while the contrast medium travels through the alimentary canal. Fluoroscopy also guides the radiologist in locating a precise internal area that needs to be recorded on film.

Fluoroscopic images are sometimes photographed for further study. Photofluorography is a series of these photographs that records the body's internal movements over time. Cinefluorography is a motion picture of the images.

Angiography

Angiography requires a physician (usually a radiologist) to insert a catheter into the patient's vein (venography) or artery (arteriography). The test may be performed jointly by a radiologist and a vascular surgeon or other specialist. Typically, the femoral, brachial, or carotid artery is evaluated. The physician guides the catheter tip to the vessel being examined. Then the physician injects a contrast medium through the catheter and takes a series of x-rays to assess the vessel's blood flow and condition.

Because this procedure requires insertion of a catheter into a blood vessel and the use of local anesthesia, the patient is admitted to a hospital or same-day surgical facility. The physician who performs the examination provides the patient with instructions immediately before the procedure. You will, however, schedule the procedure, and you can encourage the patient to ask questions. Radiology facilities usually have information sheets for each procedure. If the patient has questions you cannot answer or if you have any doubt about preprocedure instructions, check with your supervisor.

Arthrography

Arthrography is performed by a radiologist, who uses a contrast medium and fluoroscopy to help diagnose abnormalities or injuries in the cartilage, tendons, or ligaments of the joints—usually the knee or shoulder. When preparing patients for arthrography or assisting with the procedure, follow these guidelines.

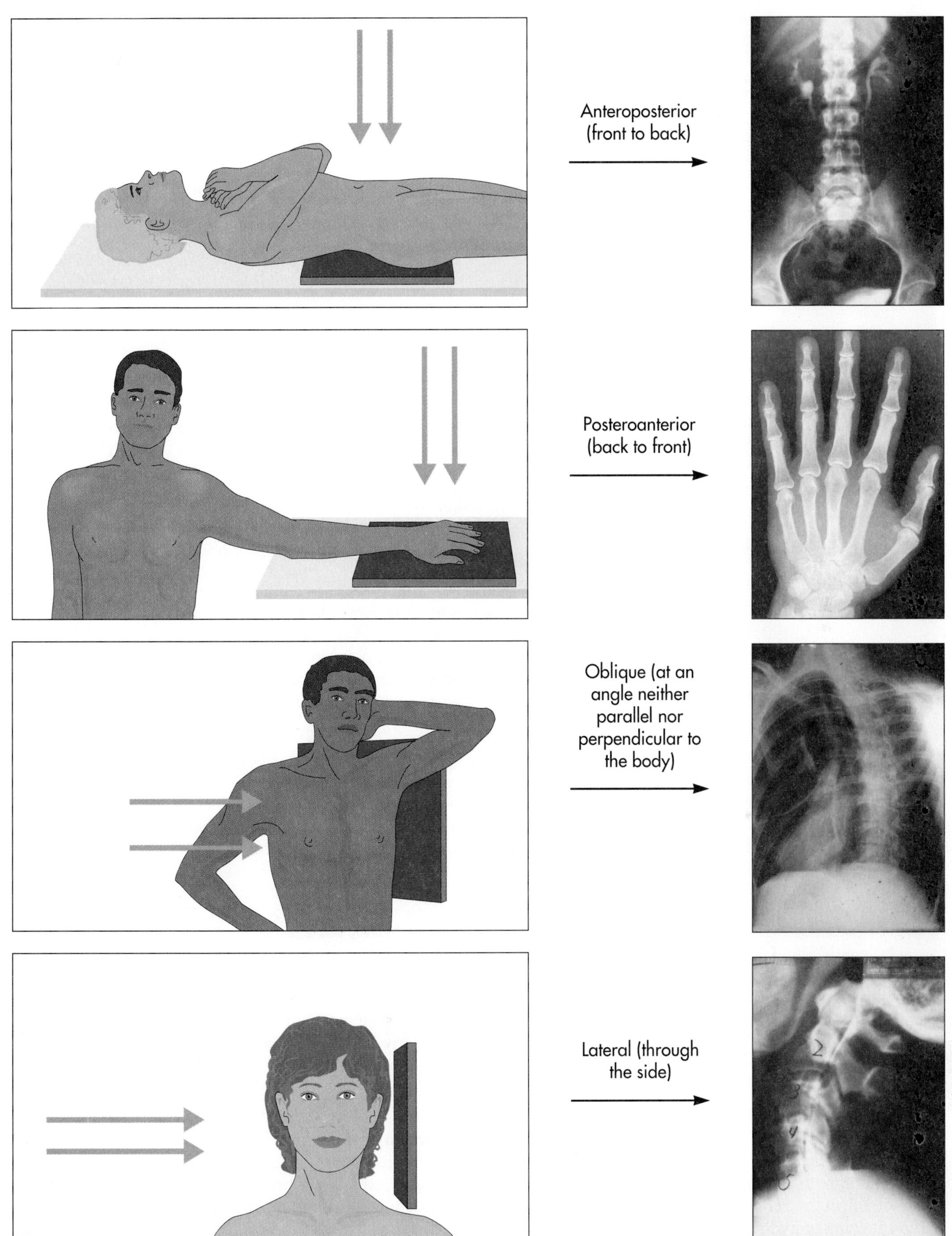

Figure 40-2. These are the x-ray pathways and resulting projections for the most common types of x-rays.

Table 40-1

Common Radiologic Tests and Disorders Diagnosed

Test	Disorders Diagnosed/Treated
Angiography	
Cardiovascular	Status of blood flow, collateral circulation, malformed vessels, aneurysm, narrowing or blockages of vessels, presence of hemorrhage
Cerebral	Aneurysm, hemorrhage, evidence of cerebrovascular accident, arteriosclerosis
Gastrointestinal (GI)	Upper gastrointestinal bleeding
Pulmonary	Pulmonary emboli (especially when lung scan is inconclusive), evaluation of pulmonary circulation in some heart conditions before surgery
Renal	Abnormalities of blood vessels in urinary system
Arthrography	Joint conditions
Barium enema (lower GI series)	Obstructions, ulcers, polyps, diverticulosis, tumor, and motility problems of colon or rectum
Barium swallow (upper GI series)	Obstructions, ulcers, polyps, diverticulosis, tumor, and motility problems of esophagus, stomach, duodenum, and small intestine
Cholangiography, cholecystography	Gallstones, gallbladder or common bile duct stones or obstructions; ability of gallbladder to concentrate and store dye
Computed tomography (CT)	Aortic and heart aneurysms, disorders of liver and biliary systems, renal and pulmonary tumors, brain abnormalities (tumors, blood clots, evidence of cerebrovascular accident, outlines of brain ventricles), GI tract lesions, GI disorders (acute pseudocyst of pancreas, abdominal abscesses, biliary obstruction), breast diseases and disorders, spinal disorders; to guide biopsy procedures
Fluoroscopy	Structure, process, and function of organs in motion to detect abnormalities
Intravenous pyelography (IVP) (excretory urography)	Urinary system abnormalities, including renal pelvis, ureters, and bladder (for example, kidney stones); abnormal size, shape, or structure of kidneys, ureters, or bladder; space-occupying lesions; pyelonephrosis; hydronephrosis; trauma to the urinary system

continued

- Describe the procedure to patients, and inform them that the examination will take about 1 hour. Ask patients about possible allergies to contrast media, iodine, or shellfish. If they have any of these allergies, inform the radiologist immediately.
- Explain to patients that no special preprocedure preparations are necessary.
- Tell patients the doctor will first inject a local anesthetic to numb the area being examined. Then the doctor will inject the contrast medium (dye, air, or both) into the joint and will use a fluoroscope to evaluate the joint's function. Inform patients who are having a knee examined that the doctor may ask them to walk a few steps to spread the contrast medium.
- After the test is completed, advise patients that for 1 or 2 days they may experience some pain or swelling, particularly if the joint is exercised. Tell them to rest and avoid putting strain on the joint.

Barium Enema (Lower GI Series)

A **barium enema** is performed by a radiologist, who instills barium sulfate through the anus into the rectum and then into the colon, to help diagnose and evaluate obstructions, ulcers, polyps, diverticulosis, tumors, or motility problems of the colon or rectum. This procedure is called a lower GI (gastrointestinal) series, a series of x-rays of the colon and rectum. The two types of barium enema techniques are single-contrast, in which only bar-

Table 40-1 continued

Common Radiologic Tests and Disorders Diagnosed

Test	Disorders Diagnosed/Treated
KUB (kidneys, ureters, bladder) radiography	Size, shape, and position of urinary organs; urinary system diseases or disorders; kidney stones
Magnetic resonance imaging (MRI)	Cancerous tissue, atherosclerotic tissue, blood clots, tumors, and deformities, particularly of the heart valves, brain, spine, and joints
Mammography	Breast tumors and lesions
Myelography	Irregularities or compression of spinal cord
Nuclear medicine (radionuclide imaging)	Abnormal function (defects), lesions, or disorders of bone, brain, lungs, kidneys, liver, pancreas, thyroid, and spleen
Radiation therapy	Treatment of cancer
Retrograde pyelogram	Obstruction of ureters, bladder, or urethra (including tumors, stones, strictures, or blood clots); perinephritic abscess
Stereoscopy	Fractures, dense areas that indicate a tumor or increased pressure within the skull
Thermography	Breast tumors, breast abscesses, fibrocystic breast disease
Ultrasound	Abnormalities of gallbladder, liver, spleen, heart, kidneys, gonads, blood vessels, and lymph system; fetal conditions (including number of fetuses, age and sex of fetus, fetal development, position, and deformities)
Xeroradiography	Breast cancer, abscesses, lesions, calcifications

ium is instilled into the colon, and double-contrast, in which air is forced into the colon to distend the tissue. The air may be added while the barium is present, after it has been expelled, or both. The double-contrast technique makes structures more visible by fluoroscopy and allows identification of small lesions. The digestive tract must be totally empty, requiring the patient to thoroughly cleanse the tract with a series of preparatory steps and to have nothing by mouth for 8 hours before the test, except for 1 c of liquid on the morning of the test. In most facilities a nurse assists with a barium enema, but you may assist the patient before and after the procedure. If you do assist with a barium enema, you will have various responsibilities before, during, and after the procedure.

Before the Procedure. Include the following steps when you instruct a patient about the preparation for a barium enema.

- Schedule the patient's appointment in the morning so he can sleep through most of the period during which his digestive tract must be empty and thus avoid experiencing hunger unnecessarily.
- Describe the procedure to the patient, and tell him the examination will take 1 to 2 hours. Ask about possible allergies to contrast media, iodine, or shellfish, and report such allergies to the radiologist.
- Explain to the patient the importance of following the preparation instructions so the colon and rectum are free of residual material. (Residual material in the

colon or rectum could cause blockages or shadows, resulting in an inaccurate test.) Preprocedure preparation on the day before the examination includes following an all-liquid diet beginning in the morning (coffee, tea, carbonated beverages, sherbet, clear gelatin, strained fruit juice, bouillon, clear broths, or tomato juice; milk is not permitted) and taking prescribed amounts of electrolyte solution or other laxative preparations and fluids on a specified schedule. Tell the patient he may have one cup of coffee, tea, or water on the morning of the examination.

During the Procedure. Follow these steps when assisting during a barium enema.

- Have the patient undress and put on a gown.
- Tell the patient to expect some discomfort during the examination, as well as frequent side-to-side turning.
- Have the patient lie on his side. The radiologist inserts the enema tip, which is designed to help the patient hold the liquid, into the rectum and instills the barium sulfate into the colon. If the patient experiences cramping or the urge to defecate during instillation of the barium, instruct him to relax the abdominal muscles by breathing slowly and deeply through the mouth.
- Instruct the patient to remain still and hold his breath when x-rays are taken. Using a fluoroscope, the doctor observes the barium as it flows through the lower bowel and periodically takes x-rays while the patient is placed in various positions. You may be asked to assist with placing the patient in these positions.
- Tell the patient if a double-contrast study is being performed. Explain that air will be introduced into the colon to expand the colon tissue. Also tell the patient that the combination of air and barium provides a clearer view of structures than only one contrast medium would provide and allows possible identification of small lesions if they are present.
- Tell the patient that when the doctor has completed the barium portion of the examination, including x-rays with both barium and air, the patient should use the toilet and expel as much barium as possible. Explain that if enough barium is expelled, the doctor may take a final x-ray of the empty colon.
- Have the patient wait to dress until the doctor tells you that no additional x-rays are needed.

After the Procedure. After the radiologist has completed the barium enema, instruct the patient in postprocedure care. Tell the patient the following.

- He may now have a regular meal.
- The residual barium may make his stools appear whitish or lighter than usual, but this is normal.
- The barium may cause constipation, so he should drink extra water to help relieve constipation and to eliminate remaining barium sulfate. The physician may order a laxative to be taken if constipation is not relieved within 1 or 2 days.

Barium Swallow (Upper GI Series)

A **barium swallow** involves oral administration of a barium sulfate drink to help diagnose and evaluate obstructions, ulcers, polyps, diverticulosis, tumors, or motility problems of the esophagus, stomach, duodenum, and small intestine. This test is called an upper GI series. In preparation for this test, the patient can have nothing by mouth for at least 8 hours before the test. You will have various responsibilities before, during, and after the procedure.

Before the Procedure. When instructing a patient about the preparation for an upper GI series (see Figure 40-3), include the following steps.

- Schedule the patient's appointment in the morning so she can sleep through most of the period during which her digestive tract is empty and thus avoid experiencing hunger unnecessarily.
- Describe the procedure to the patient, and tell her the examination will take about 1 hour. If x-rays of the small bowel are needed, the test may take several hours. Ask about possible allergies to contrast media, iodine, or shellfish, and report such allergies to the radiologist.
- Explain to the patient the importance of following the preparation instructions so that the stomach is empty. Preprocedure requirements include having nothing by mouth (food or liquids) after midnight the night before the examination and no breakfast the morning of the examination. If the patient's small bowel is to be evaluated, also tell her to take the prescribed laxative preparation between 2:00 and 4:00 P.M. the day before the examination.
- Instruct the patient not to swallow water when brushing her teeth or rinsing her mouth and, if applicable,

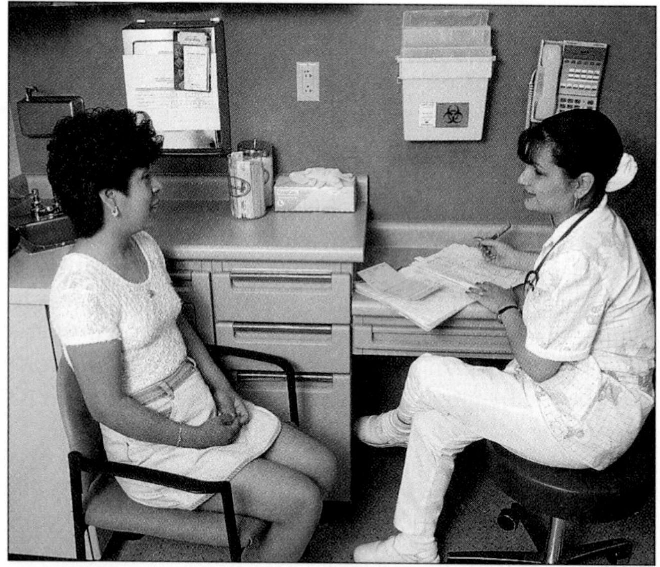

Figure 40-3. Preprocedure instruction is essential to a successful barium swallow procedure.

MULTISKILL FOCUS

Radiographer/Sonographer

To gain medical assistant credentials, you must fulfill the requirements of either the American Association of Medical Assistants (for a Certified Medical Assistant) or the American Medical Technologists (for a Registered Medical Assistant). After obtaining your medical assistant certification or registration, you may wish to acquire additional skills in specialty areas through course work or on-the-job training. Although this course work or training may not lead to an additional certification or degree, it will enable you to expand your role in the medical office and advance your career as the demand for multiskilled health professionals increases.

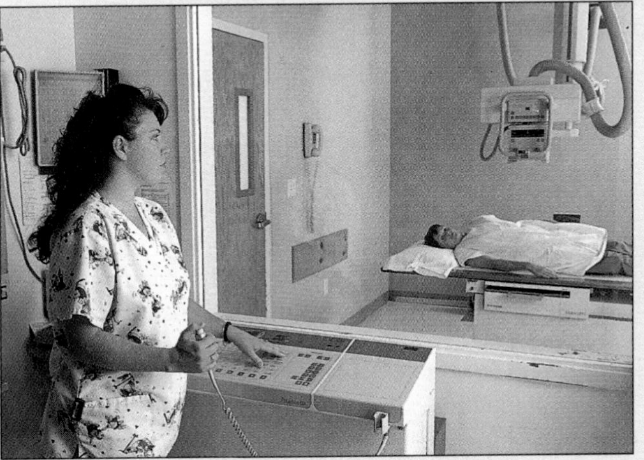

Skills and Duties

Radiographers and sonographers obtain images of internal organs, tissues, bones, and blood vessels. Physicians use these images to diagnose disease or to monitor health status.

A radiographer uses x-rays to produce the images. The radiographer positions the patient for imaging, covering parts of the body that are not to be x-rayed with a lead drape to protect them from the radiation. She then positions the x-ray machine, sets the controls, and makes the requested number of exposures.

The resulting black-and-white images can reveal whether a patient has a broken bone, tumor, ulcer, or other condition. Sometimes the radiographer or a physician administers a special material before the imaging process to make organs and blood vessels more visible on the x-ray film. The physician, usually a radiologist, examines the film and makes a diagnosis.

Sonographers use ultrasound machines that rely on sound waves rather than electromagnetic radiation to produce the images. The images are displayed on a television screen and can be videotaped or printed on film for further review by the physician.

The sonographer prepares the patient by applying a sound-enhancing gel. She then strokes the machine's handheld pad across the gel to create the image. She must be well-versed in anatomy to determine which parts of the image are important as she records measurements and data from the examination. Again, the physician uses the image to make a diagnosis and prescribe treatment if needed.

Sonographers can specialize in a variety of fields. Because sound waves are considered safe, sonography is frequently used in obstetrics and gynecology to take pictures of a fetus in the womb. Sonographers may also specialize in echocardiography, where they focus on heart problems.

Workplace Settings

Radiographers and sonographers most often work in hospitals. Some are employed in clinics, physicians' offices, and imaging centers. Radiographers may also work in dentists' offices, in mobile units, or in private industry. People in this field generally work 40-hour weeks, including some nights, weekends, and holidays.

Education

To become a radiographer or sonographer, you must complete an accredited 2- to 4-year program in radiography/sonography from an accredited vocational school, college, or university. (For those who are already employed in health care, a 1-year certificate program may be available.) Typically, such a program provides instruction in physics, biology, anatomy, medical terminology, radiation safety, and imaging techniques. The program may also include brief courses in nuclear medicine, computed tomography, magnetic resonance imaging, and radiation therapy—each of which can be further studied as a specialty.

After completing the program, you may take a national registry examination from the American Registry of Radiologic Technologists. The disciplines of sonography, nuclear medicine, and radiation therapy require a national registration examination for entry-level work. Radiographers must also have a license from the state to practice.

Where to Go for More Information

American Society of Radiologic Technologists
15000 Central Avenue SE
Albuquerque, NM 87123
(505) 298-4500

Society of Diagnostic Medical Sonographers
12770 Coit Road, Suite 508
Dallas, TX 75251
(214) 239-7367

to stop smoking, because nicotine stimulates gastric secretions and can affect the test results.

During the Procedure. When assisting during an upper GI series, take the following steps.

- Have the patient undress and put on a gown.
- Explain to the patient that she will be drinking a barium sulfate drink that tastes chalky and resembles a milk shake.
- Have the patient stand and drink part of the barium. The radiologist will use a fluoroscope to observe the flow of the barium and to assess the functioning of the esophagus, stomach, duodenum, and small intestine as the barium passes through the structures. (The doctor will then direct the patient to drink additional barium and continue to observe the function of the various structures.)
- Place the patient on the x-ray table, and move her to different positions (if medical assistants are permitted to do so in your state) as instructed by the doctor, to allow x-rays to be taken of the upper digestive tract. Instruct the patient to remain still and hold her breath when x-rays are taken.

After the Procedure. After the physician completes the upper GI series, instruct the patient in postprocedure care. Give the patient the following information.

- She may now have a regular meal.
- Her stools may appear whitish or lighter than usual as the barium is eliminated, but this is normal.
- Sometimes another examination may be required after 24 hours to determine whether the barium has moved into the large intestine. If this test is indicated, tell the patient to follow a liquid diet (coffee, tea, carbonated beverages, sherbet, clear gelatin, strained fruit juices, bouillon, clear broths, or tomato juice; milk is not permitted) and to return in 24 hours.

Cholecystography and Cholangiography

Two similar tests performed by a radiologist are cholecystography and cholangiography. Both tests involve use of a contrast medium to view parts of the gallbladder.

Cholecystography. A radiologist uses cholecystography to detect gallstones and other abnormalities of the gallbladder. The doctor x-rays the patient's gallbladder after the patient has ingested an oral contrast medium. Cholecystography is usually used when ultrasound does not provide enough information for a diagnosis. You will be responsible for preparing the patient for the procedure and assisting during the procedure.

Before the Procedure. When instructing a patient about preparing for a cholecystography, follow these guidelines.

- Schedule the patient's appointment in the morning so he can sleep through most of the period during which his digestive tract is empty and thus avoid experiencing hunger unnecessarily.
- Describe the procedure to the patient, and explain that the examination will take about 1 to 2 hours. Ask the patient about possible allergies to contrast media, iodine, or shellfish, and report them to the radiologist.
- Explain to the patient the diet restrictions necessary to prepare for the test. Tell the patient to have a fat-free dinner (dry toast, tea, fruit, gelatin dessert) the evening before the examination. He should not smoke or have any food or liquids after midnight, and he should have no breakfast the morning of the examination.
- Instruct the patient to take the oral contrast medium (usually in tablet form) beginning about 2 hours after dinner or as prescribed by the doctor. The tablets should be taken one at a time, 5 minutes apart, with a small amount of water, until six tablets have been taken. Explain to the patient that the contrast agent may cause nausea or diarrhea but that nothing should be taken for these conditions. In the case of severe nausea, the doctor may prescribe an antiemetic; diarrhea is an expected result of the contrast medium used for this test.
- Some doctors also order a laxative for the patient to take the day before the examination.

During and After the Procedure. When assisting during a cholecystography, take the following steps.

- Have the patient undress and put on a gown.
- Have the patient lie on the x-ray table in the supine position (face up).
- Explain that the radiologist will take x-rays of the gallbladder, which will be filled with the contrast medium the patient took the night before. Then the radiologist will use a fluoroscope to study the gallbladder's function. A functioning gallbladder absorbs the contrast agent properly.
- Next give the patient a specially prepared fatty meal, which should stimulate the gallbladder to empty bile into the duodenum. After about 1 hour, the doctor takes more x-rays to study the gallbladder's function. A functioning gallbladder empties the contrast medium properly. A nonfunctioning gallbladder may indicate, for example, the presence of gallstones or obstruction of the bile ducts.
- After the examination advise the patient to return to a normal diet and to drink plenty of fluids to replace those lost with diarrhea.

Cholangiography. Cholangiography is similar to cholecystography and is performed by a radiologist to evaluate the function of the bile ducts. It involves injection of the contrast medium directly into the common bile duct (during gallbladder surgery) or through a T tube (after gallbladder surgery or during radiologic testing). X-rays are taken immediately after injection. Use the guidelines for cholecystography. In addition, follow these steps.

- Describe the procedure to the patient, and tell him the examination will take about 2 to 3 hours. Ask the patient about possible allergies to contrast media, iodine, or shellfish, and report them to the radiologist.
- Explain the preparation instructions to the patient. Tell the patient to eat a light evening meal the night before the examination, to take a laxative (as prescribed by the doctor), and to have no food or liquids after midnight. He should also have no solid food the morning of the examination.

Conventional Tomography and Computed Tomography

Conventional tomography produces tomograms, and computed tomography produces CT scans. These two techniques are frequently confused. Computers are involved in producing both kinds of images, but the computers are different and have different functions.

Conventional tomography uses a computerized x-ray camera that moves back and forth in an arc over the patient to produce a series of views of a body part. The computer sets the angle and layer for each arc; the camera produces one view per arc.

In CT scans produced by computed tomography, the x-ray camera rotates completely around the patient, and the computer compiles one cross-sectional view from each rotation of the camera. The patient is lying on a special table that gradually moves through the doughnut-shaped machine containing the rotating camera. Figure 40-4 compares the two kinds of images (tomogram and CT scan) with those produced by x-ray, magnetic resonance imaging (MRI), and myelography.

The preparation is essentially the same for the two procedures. Reassure the patient that he will not be inserted into an enclosed space, as is the case in magnetic resonance imaging. The patient will be able to see around the room during the test.

Tomograms and CT scans are used to diagnose abnormalities in almost all body structures, including the head, kidneys, heart, chest, liver, biliary tract, pancreas, GI tract, spine, pelvis, bones, and breast. When preparing the patient for a tomogram or a CT scan, use the following guidelines.

- Ask the patient about possible allergies to contrast media, iodine, or shellfish, and report them to the radiologist.
- Tell the patient that he will be placed on a table that moves through the scanner for CT scans or on an x-ray table for tomograms.
- Inform the patient that the procedure will last about 45 to 90 minutes and that he must lie still while the scans are taken. The patient may breathe normally while the CT scans are taken but must hold his breath for each of the tomograms.
- If a contrast medium will be used, advise the patient that it will be injected into a vein in the arm or on the back of the hand (except with a CT scan of the spine) to enhance detail of the structure being evaluated.
- If the patient is having a CT scan of the head or chest, instruct him not to eat anything for 4 hours or drink any liquids for 2 hours before the examination. Explain that he may experience mild nausea after injection of the contrast medium if the stomach is too full.
- If the patient is having tomograms or a CT scan of the abdomen or pelvis, tell him to obtain a preparation kit from the office or hospital the day before the examination. This kit includes a special drink the patient must take the night before the examination that helps outline the intestines. Inform the patient that the drink should not produce a laxative effect or any discomfort.
- Tell the patient to remove metallic objects that could interfere with the path of the x-rays. Also, ask if the patient has skin staples or metallic prostheses that could interfere.
- Inform the patient that a written report of the results should be available within 24 hours of the test and that a report will be sent to his primary care physician (or the referring physician).

Heart X-Ray

An x-ray of the heart, using a contrast medium, may be necessary to show the configuration of the heart and to reveal cardiac enlargement and aortic dilation. Angiography of the heart is called angiocardiography, in which a contrast medium is injected into a major blood vessel. X-rays are taken while the medium flows through the heart, lungs, and major vessels. Coronary arteriography uses a dye inserted through a catheter that has been passed through an artery to the heart. Both procedures require hospital admission, usually in a day surgery or ambulatory surgery unit.

Intravenous Pyelography

Also known as excretory urography, **intravenous pyelography (IVP)** is performed by a radiologist who injects a contrast medium into a vein. The doctor then takes a series of x-rays as the contrast medium travels through the kidneys, ureters, and bladder. IVP is used to evaluate urinary system abnormalities or trauma to the urinary system. In most facilities a nurse assists with IVP, but you may assist the patient before the procedure. If you assist with IVP, you will have several responsibilities both before and during the procedure.

Before the Procedure. When instructing a patient about the preparation for an IVP, include the following steps.

- Schedule the patient's appointment in the morning so she can sleep through most of the period during which her digestive tract is empty and thus avoid experiencing hunger unnecessarily.
- Describe the procedure to the patient, and tell her that the examination will take about 1½ hours. Ask about

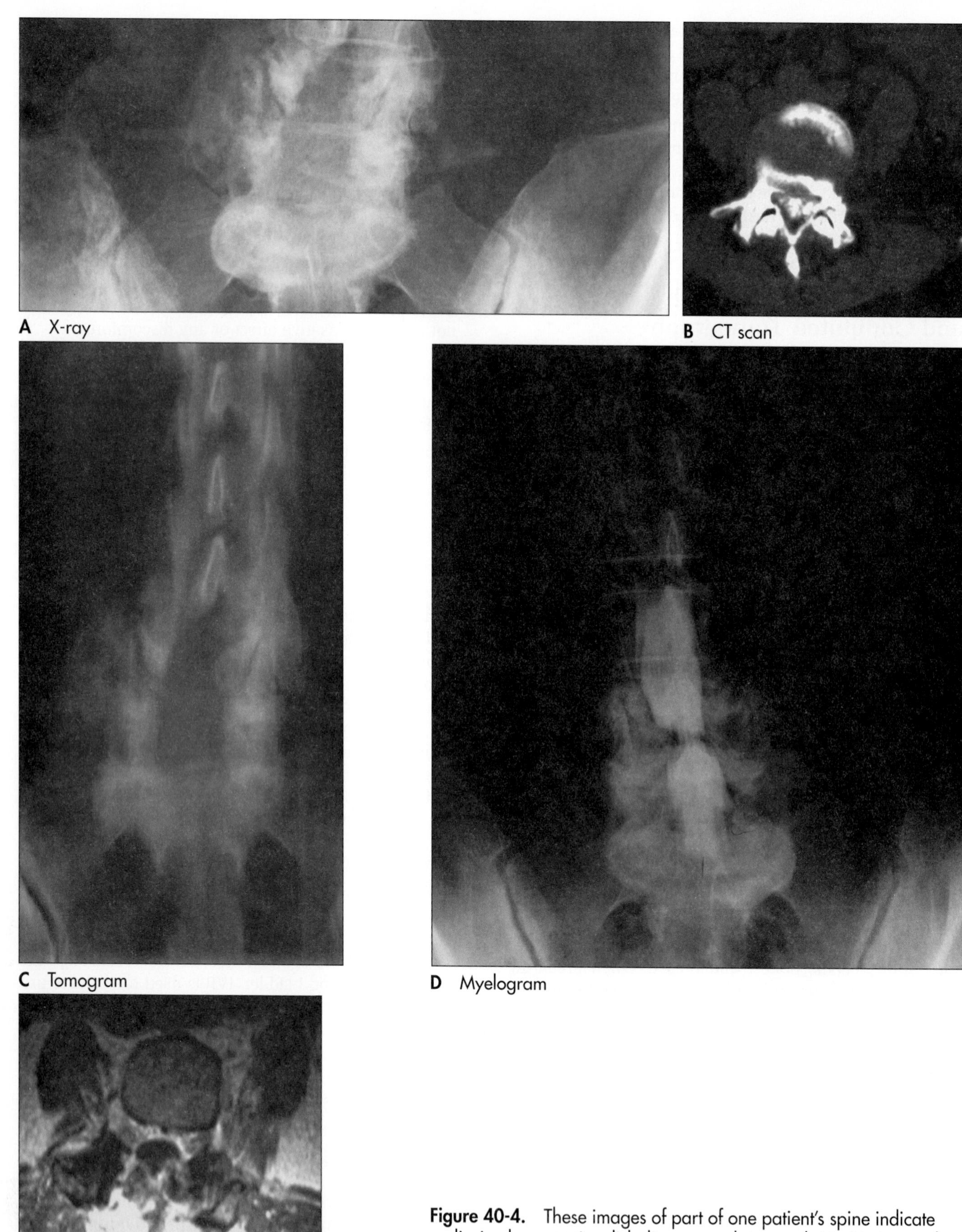

Figure 40-4. These images of part of one patient's spine indicate scoliosis, degenerative disk disease, and osteoarthritis. Various techniques and x-ray pathways were involved: (a) x-ray, anteroposterior; (b) CT scan, full rotation; (c) tomogram, anteroposterior arc; (d) myelogram, posteroanterior; and (e) MRI, full rotation.

possible allergies to contrast media, iodine, or shellfish, and report such allergies to the radiologist.

- Explain the importance of adhering to the preparation instructions, so that the bowel is free of any material that could obstruct the view of the urinary organs. Tell the patient to follow a liquid diet (coffee, tea, carbonated beverages, sherbet, clear gelatin, strained fruit juice, bouillon, clear broths, or tomato juice, but no milk) the day before the examination. The patient should take the prescribed amount of electrolyte solution or other laxative preparation as specified the night before the examination and have no food or liquids after midnight and no breakfast the morning of the examination. Some physicians also order an enema to be taken about 2 hours before the examination.

During and After the Procedure. When assisting during an IVP, you will generally proceed in this manner.

- Have the patient undress and put on a gown.
- Explain that a contrast medium will be injected into her vein (usually in the arm). Instruct her to inform the physician if she notices shortness of breath or itching after injection of the dye. This type of symptom can indicate an allergic reaction.
- Have the patient lie on the x-ray table, and move her to different positions as instructed by the physician, to allow x-rays to be taken of the urinary tract as the contrast medium is excreted. Instruct the patient to remain still and hold her breath when x-rays are taken.
- Note that some physicians place a compression device on the abdomen, which helps hold the contrast medium in the kidneys and ureters by exerting moderate pressure.
- After the physician takes the series of x-rays to evaluate urinary system function, ask the patient to urinate, and explain that a final x-ray will be taken.
- Inform the patient that she may resume a normal diet after the test and that the contrast medium will be eliminated in the urine.

Retrograde Pyelography

Retrograde pyelography is similar to the IVP, except that the doctor injects the contrast medium through a urethral catheter. This procedure, which evaluates function of the ureters, bladder, and urethra, is often used for patients with poor kidney function. Follow the same preparation and assistance instructions as for the IVP.

KUB (Kidneys, Ureters, and Bladder) Radiography

Also called a flat plate of the abdomen, **KUB radiography** is an x-ray of the abdomen used to assess the size, shape, and position of the urinary organs; to evaluate urinary system diseases or disorders; and to determine the presence of kidney stones. It can also be helpful in determining the position of an intrauterine device (IUD) or in locating foreign bodies in the digestive tract. No patient preparation is required. A KUB x-ray is taken by a radiologic technologist; thus, you follow the guidelines you would use for a patient having any type of standard, noninvasive x-ray.

Magnetic Resonance Imaging (MRI)

Nonionizing radiation and a strong magnetic field are combined in magnetic resonance imaging to allow the physician to examine internal structures and soft tissues of any area of the body. The combination of nonionizing radiation and magnetic field, which allows the MRI scanner to produce images based primarily on the water content of tissues, appears to have no harmful effects on the patient. The test may be performed without or with contrast. You will be responsible for preparing the patient for an MRI and assisting with the procedure.

Before the Procedure. When instructing a patient about preparing for an MRI, include the following steps.

- If a contrast medium is going to be used, ask the patient and inform the radiologist about possible allergies to contrast media, iodine, or shellfish.
- Screen the patient to determine whether any internal metallic materials are present. (This is especially important because a magnetic field is involved in creating the image.) Ask about a pacemaker, brain or aneurysm clips, brain or heart surgery, shunts and heart valves, other surgeries, and shrapnel or metal fragments (particularly in an eye).
- Ask the patient whether he is or has been a metalworker. If so, he may carry metal slivers, chips, or filings under his nails or skin.
- Describe the procedure to the patient, and tell him the examination will take between 45 minutes and 2 hours.
- Tell the patient he does not need to fast before the examination or follow any preprocedure diet, unless he is having an MRI of the pelvis. In that case instruct him to have no solid food for 6 hours and no liquids for 4 hours before the examination. Inform the patient that he may take prescription medications.
- Explain that he will not be required to drink an oral contrast preparation but that he should avoid caffeine for 4 hours before the examination. (Instruct women not to wear eye makeup the day of the examination, because eye makeup often contains metallic ingredients.)
- Tell the patient that he will probably have no side effects from the examination but that some nausea may occur as a result of the contrast medium.

During and After the Procedure. When assisting during an MRI, you will need to follow these specific steps.

- Inform the patient that he may wear street clothing, unless it has metallic thread, metal stays or grippers, or thick elastic. Tell the patient that he will probably be asked to undress, however, and put on a gown.

- Have the patient lie on the padded table.
- Explain that the table will be placed inside a long, narrow tube about 22 inches in diameter and that he will hear a loud knocking noise as the machine scans. Warn the patient to remain still to avoid blurring the image and the consequent need for a retake. Note that physicians commonly order sedation for patients who are claustrophobic or cannot lie still for a long period (Figure 40-5).
- Advise the patient that although the technician will not be in the scanning room during the examination, she will maintain contact with a camera and a microphone. The patient may speak to the technician at any time in case of a problem, but he is encouraged to be still for each series.
- Inform the patient that his primary care physician or referring doctor should have a preliminary report of test results within about 24 hours.

Mammography

Mammography, the x-ray examination of the internal breast tissues, helps in diagnosing breast abnormalities (see Figure 40-6). A specially trained radiologic technologist takes mammograms. Types of mammography include film-screen, thermography, diaphanography, and ultrasonography (ultrasound). Diaphanography is produced by directing a high-intensity light through the breast or soft tissue; images are then produced on a screen (a process called transillumination). Unlike other forms of mammography, diaphanography does not require ionizing radiation.

You will have several responsibilities during both setup and patient care before and after mammography. A medical assistant does not assist during mammography in most states. Instead, you will prepare the patient for the procedure and ease her fears. "Educating the Patient" provides information on this topic.

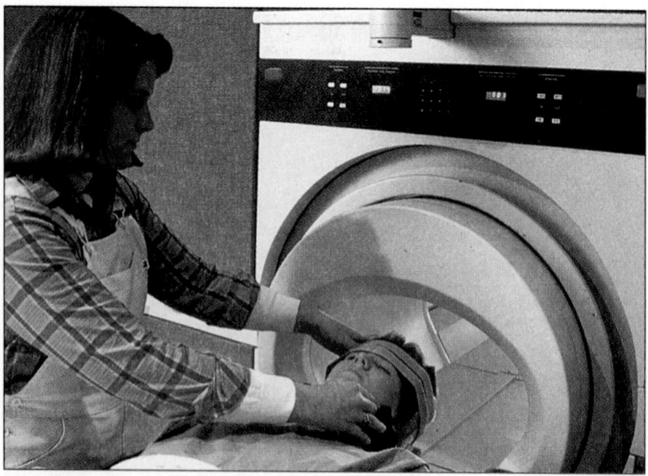

Figure 40-5. A patient who is claustrophobic or unable to lie still may require sedation during an MRI.

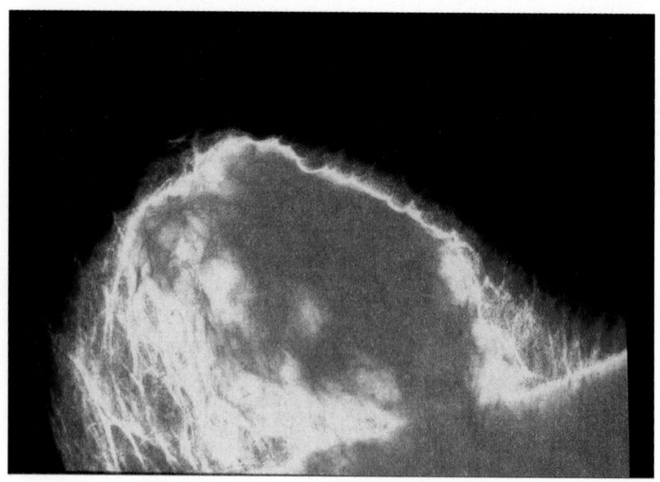

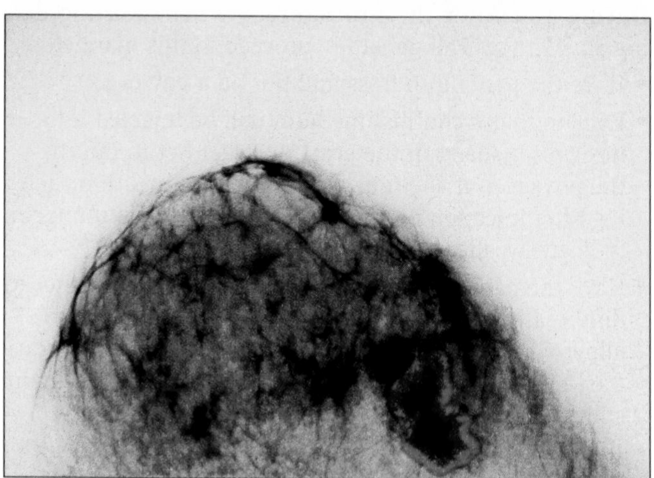

Figure 40-6. Mammograms can reveal the presence of tumors that are not detected by other means. The upper mammogram indicates normal breast tissue, whereas the lower suggests a malignancy.

Myelography

Myelography is a kind of fluoroscopy of the spinal cord. The physician performs a lumbar puncture, removes some cerebrospinal fluid (CSF), and instills a contrast medium to evaluate spinal abnormalities, such as compression of the spinal cord. Sometimes the physician performs pneumoencephalography, which involves instilling air after removal of the CSF to allow visualization of the cerebral cavities.

The physician who performs myelography or pneumoencephalography must be skilled in performing lumbar puncture—most likely a radiologist, neurologist, neurosurgeon, or anesthetist. A radiologic technologist is typically the only other person present for the test. Although myelography is not used as frequently as it was before the invention of CT and MRI, it is still performed when these newer techniques do not provide enough information about the spinal canal. Myelography may be reserved for cases in which the clinical findings are unusual or the scanning results uncertain.

EDUCATING THE PATIENT

Preprocedure Care for Mammography

A patient who is scheduled for mammography must know the guidelines to follow before the examination. You can help educate the patient by instructing her in the following preprocedure care.

- The mammography should be scheduled for the first week after the patient's menstrual cycle. This timing helps minimize discomfort from compression of the breasts and ensures that the breasts are in their most normal state.
- No special preprocedure diet or medication requirements are necessary, but the patient should consider avoiding caffeine for 7 to 10 days before the examination (in some patients caffeine may cause swelling and soreness that would heighten discomfort during the procedure). Have the patient decrease caffeine intake gradually, however, to avoid getting headaches.
- The patient should shower or bathe as close as possible to the time of the mammography and wear loose clothing that is easy to remove. A blouse and pants or skirt work best to allow undressing only to the waist.
- The patient should not use deodorants, powders, or perfumes on the breasts or underarm areas before the examination, because these products could produce a false result on the x-ray.

In addition to providing these instructions, you may need to reassure a patient who is fearful about mammography. Explain that although mammography is uncomfortable, it is usually not painful. Describing how the procedure is performed may alleviate the patient's fears. Provide the patient with the following information.

- The procedure usually takes 15 to 20 minutes.
- A lead apron will be placed on the patient's abdominal area to protect her from unnecessary radiation exposure.
- The patient will be positioned in front of the machine. The technician will compress the left breast between the machine plates and take two x-rays—one horizontal view and one vertical view—of the left breast.
- The technician will then position and compress the right breast between the machine plates. Two x-rays will be taken of the right breast.
- If needed, the physician may order a mild pain reliever after the procedure to alleviate discomfort or aching.

Nuclear Medicine

Also known as radionuclide imaging, **nuclear medicine** involves use of radionuclides, or radioisotopes (radioactive elements or their compounds). The radionuclides are administered orally, intravenously, or through routes that introduce them into organs or body cavities. The purpose is to evaluate the bone, brain, lungs, kidneys, liver, pancreas, thyroid, or spleen. Sometimes the entire body is scanned for "hot spots," or places where the radioisotope is concentrated.

For common nuclear medicine scans, the technician uses a scanner called a gamma camera. This scanner detects radiation from the radioisotope and converts it into an image (called a scintiscan or scintigram) to be photographed or displayed on a screen (see Figure 40-7). Some images are produced immediately, whereas others may take up to several days. Radionuclide imaging exposes patients to lower doses of radiation than some radiologic techniques, because the amount of ionizing radiation in the isotope is less than that emitted from x-ray cameras.

Other nuclear medicine procedures include single photon emission computed tomography (SPECT), positron emission tomography (PET), and MUGA (multiple gated acquisition) scan.

- **SPECT** is often used to locate and determine the extent of brain damage from a stroke. The gamma camera detects signals induced by gamma radiation, and a computer converts these signals into either two- or three-dimensional images that are displayed on a screen.
- **PET** entails injecting isotopes combined with other substances involved in metabolic activity, such as glucose. These special isotopes emit positrons, which a computer processes and displays on a screen. PET is especially useful for diagnosing brain-related conditions, such as epilepsy, mental illnesses, and Parkinson's disease.
- The **MUGA scan** evaluates the condition of the heart's myocardium. It can be done while the patient is at rest or in stress (exercise) and involves the injection of radioisotopes that concentrate in the myocardium. The gamma camera allows the physician to measure ventricular contractions to evaluate the patient's heart wall.

When preparing a patient for a nuclear medicine procedure, describe the procedure and tell her how long the examination will take. Explain any preparation requirements and other special instructions, and tell the patient she will need to wait the required length of time for the uptake of the radioisotope. Length of examination and requirements for common scans are as follows.

- Bone scan lasts about 1 hour; it is done 2 to 3 hours after a 15-minute injection; the patient drinks 1 qt of liquid between the injection and the scan; a normal diet is permitted.

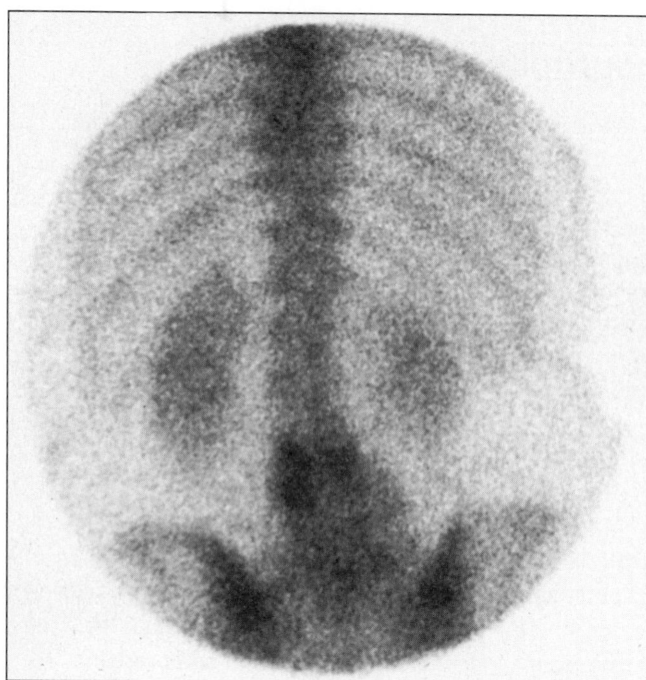

Figure 40-7. This bone scan of the spine (same patient as in Figure 40-4) shows the uptake of the radioactive contrast medium, which is darkest in the areas of inflammation.

- Liver/spleen or lung scan lasts approximately 1 hour; there are no diet restrictions.
- Kidney scan lasts about 2 hours; there are no diet restrictions.
- Thyroid uptake and scan test usually requires 2 days; the patient takes a capsule of contrast medium in the morning and has the scan on the first day; the patient returns 24 hours later for the second scan; there are no diet restrictions, except that the patient must have no fish because of its natural iodine content.

Stereoscopy

Used primarily to study the skull, **stereoscopy** is an x-ray procedure that uses a specially designed microscope (stereoscopic, or Greenough, microscope) with double eyepieces and objectives to take films at different angles. Stereoscopy identifies fractures and dense areas to produce three-dimensional images. The images, which have depth as well as height and width, can indicate a tumor or increased pressure within the skull. No special preparation is required. Follow the guidelines you would use with any other noninvasive x-ray.

Thermography

Thermography is performed to diagnose breast tumors, breast abscesses, and fibrocystic breast disease. The procedure uses an infrared camera to take photographs that record variations in skin temperature as dark (cool areas), light (warm areas), or shades of gray (areas with temperatures between cool and warm). Tumors or inflammations produce more heat than healthy tissues and therefore show up lighter on these photographs; areas with lack of circulation are cooler than tissues with adequate circulation and show up as dark. Because no preparation requirements are necessary for this test, you need only to schedule the procedure and to assist as needed with reassurance during the examination.

Ultrasound

Ultrasound directs high-frequency sound waves through the skin over the area of the body being examined and produces an image based on the echoes. A radiologist or an ultrasound radiologic technologist coats the body area with a special gel and passes a transducer (instrument similar to a microphone) over the area. As the transducer passes back and forth over the area, it picks up echoes from the sound waves, which a computer converts into an image on a screen. Ultrasound is used to detect abnormalities in the gallbladder, liver, spleen, heart, and kidneys. It is also safe to use in obstetrics to evaluate the developing fetus or to detect multiple fetuses, because it does not expose the patient (or the fetus) to radiation (Figure 40-8). In this case the obstetrician may perform the test in the office.

One form of ultrasound is called Doppler echocardiography, which involves sound waves that echo against the flow of blood through vessels. Doppler echocardiography is usually performed by a cardiologist to determine whether blood flow is laminar (normal) or turbulent (disturbed).

When preparing the patient for an ultrasound or assisting with the examination, follow these guidelines.

- Describe the procedure to the patient and inform her that the examination will take about ½ to 2 hours, depending on the type of ultrasound. For example, a cardiac ultrasound takes about 1½ hours; pelvic, 1 to 2 hours; and abdominal, ½ to 1 hour.
- Explain the preparation requirements, which vary according to the type of ultrasound. Tell a patient who is

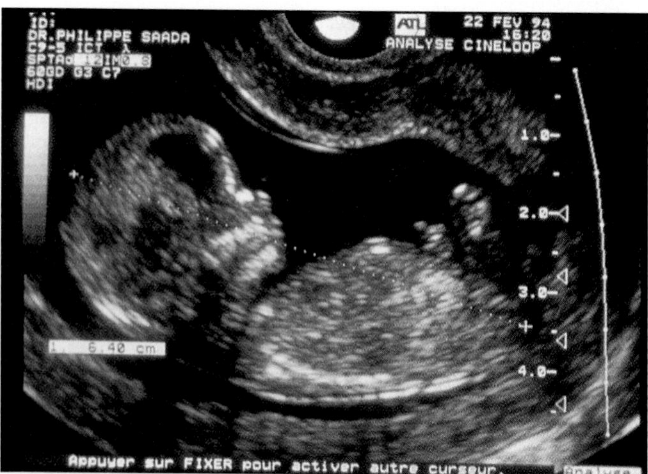

Figure 40-8. Ultrasound is commonly used to evaluate the health of a developing fetus.

having a gallbladder or liver ultrasound not to eat for several hours before the test. Tell a pregnant patient to drink the prescribed amount of water 1 hour before the examination and not to void. Advise a patient having a pelvic ultrasound to take the prescribed laxative (if indicated), drink three to four glasses of water within 1 hour, and not to void within 1 hour of the test. If the patient is having an abdominal ultrasound, instruct her to take a laxative the night before the examination and not to have any food or fluids for 8 hours before the test.

- Advise the patient to wear loose clothing that is easy to remove.

Xeroradiography

Xeroradiography is used to diagnose breast cancer, abscesses, lesions, and calcifications. The xeroradiographic x-rays are developed with a powder toner, similar to the toner in photocopiers, and the image is processed on specially treated xerographic paper. Xeroradiography uses lower exposure times and less radiation than standard x-rays.

Common Therapeutic Uses of Radiation

Used therapeutically, radiology is called **radiation therapy.** Radiation therapy is used to treat cancer by preventing cellular reproduction. The two types of radiation therapy are teletherapy and brachytherapy. **Teletherapy** allows deep penetration and is used primarily for deep tumors; it is done on an outpatient basis. The patient experiences minimal side effects, and superficial tissues are not damaged.

Localized cancers are treated with **brachytherapy.** In this technique the radiologist places temporary radioactive implants close to or directly into cancerous tissue. Both the staff and patient are subject to radiation exposure. Therefore, radiation safety precautions must be closely followed. When preparing the patient for radiation therapy, follow these guidelines.

- Describe the procedure to the patient, and tell him how long the procedure will take, as determined by the radiologist and oncologist according to the diagnosis and the condition of the patient.
- Inform the patient that the radiologist or oncologist will explain the possible side effects of the treatment. Common side effects include nausea, vomiting, hair loss, ulceration of mucous membranes, weakness, and malaise. Other possible effects include localized burns on tissue and damage to organs in the path of treatment. Encourage the patient to discuss with the doctor (or the oncology nurse specialist) measures to relieve or minimize stress and discomfort.
- Advise the patient to immediately report any other symptoms to the doctor.

Radiation Safety and Dose

For many years after the discovery of the x-ray, the seriousness of radiation hazards was not addressed. In the 1920s the government of Great Britain took the first steps to limit x-ray exposure. Since World War II, studies have been performed, mostly on the effects of high-dose radiation. Other studies on the effects of background radiation and nonradiologic versus radiologic (x-ray–related) risks have enabled scientists to assess the risks of diagnostic x-rays. Results from these studies show the risk of excess radiation from routine x-rays to be minimal.

Reducing Patient Exposure

Advances in diagnostic imaging technology, as well as limits to radiation exposure, have helped reduce the dose of radiation to which a patient is exposed during a diagnostic procedure. Another way to reduce the risk of excessive radiation exposure lies with the physician, who must assess the benefit-to-risk ratio when recommending a diagnostic radiology procedure. Because radiation has a cumulative effect, the physician must have valid medical reasons for ordering the test, particularly if the patient has recently had other x-rays. Some types of x-rays, such as mammograms, should be repeated regularly, however, because of their potential to prevent or promote treatment of life-threatening disorders.

According to a National Council on Radiation Protection and Measurements (NCRP) report, *Limitation of Exposure to Ionizing Radiation* (1993), one of the earliest pieces of legislation in the United States to limit occupational radiation exposure was enacted as early as the 1930s. The first legislation to limit public exposure, however, was not enacted until the 1950s. The NCRP report of 1993 set guidelines for protection from radiation in and out of the workplace. The two primary objectives outlined in the report are to prevent serious general tissue damage from radiation by limiting radiation dose to levels below known thresholds for such damage and to reduce the risk of cancer and genetic effects to a level that is balanced by potential benefits to the individual and society.

Because exposure to radiation always poses some degree of risk, the NCRP recommends that any activity involving radiation exposure be justified, or balanced against the expected benefits to society. Furthermore, the NCRP recommends that the cost, or detriment, to society from such activities be kept *as low as reasonably achievable* (ALARA) and that individual dose limits be applied to ensure that justification and ALARA principles do not result in unacceptable levels of risk for individuals or groups.

The NCRP has developed detailed lists on radiation doses to achieve the primary objectives stated in the report. There are separate specific limits for occupational exposure and public exposure.

Safety Precautions

Understanding and following standard safety precautions are crucial for protection from radiation exposure. These precautions are essential to the health and safety of both medical personnel and patients.

Personnel Safety. If you work in a medical facility that performs radiologic tests, you are at risk for excessive radiation exposure. To protect yourself from radiation exposure, you must adhere to the following specific guidelines.

- You (and other members of the medical staff) must always wear a radiation exposure badge, or dosimeter, which is a sensitized piece of film in a holder (see Figure 40-9). You must have the badge checked regularly by specially qualified personnel, who measure the degree of radiation uptake on the film to determine the amount of radiation to which you have been exposed.
- Make sure that all equipment is in good working order and is checked routinely for radiation leakage and any other problems.
- Be aware that the technician and any other staff members present when equipment is operating should always wear a garment that contains a lead shield.

Patient Safety. You must follow all rules governing patient safety from radiation exposure. "Educating the Patient" explains safety measures and information that help protect a patient from exposure to unnecessary radiation.

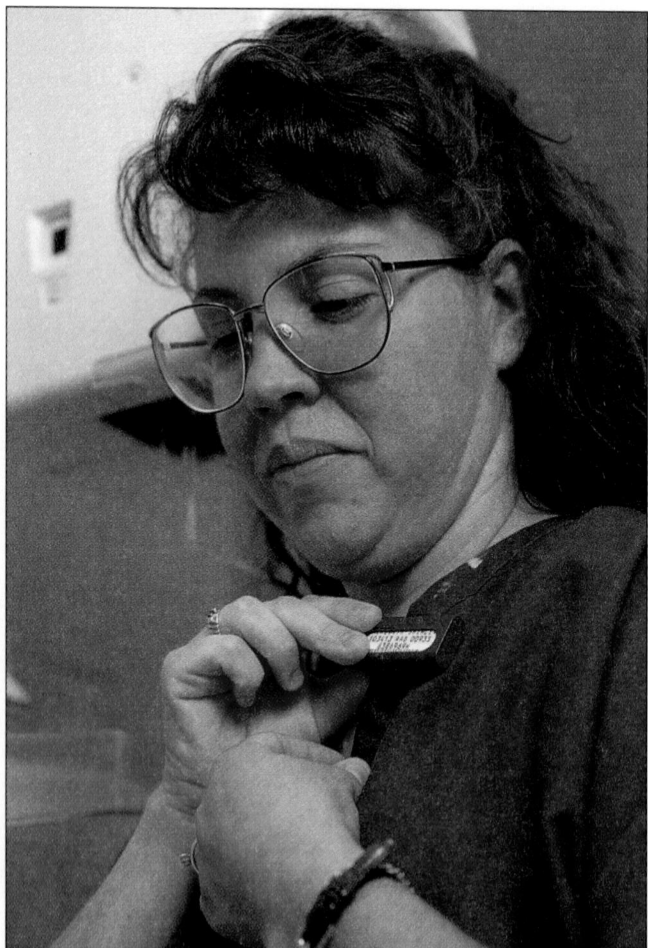

Figure 40-9. A radiation exposure badge contains a film that registers the levels of radiation to which a medical staff member is exposed at work.

Storing and Filing X-Rays

You will be responsible for storing x-ray films if you work in a radiology facility. Follow these guidelines for proper storage of x-rays.

- Keep fresh film on hand at all times.
- Maintain new and exposed films in as good a condition as possible by keeping them at a temperature between 50° and 70°F (between 10° and 20° C) and a relative humidity between 30% and 50%. Radiology facilities usually have one or more special rooms for films.
- Prevent pressure marks and keep expiration dates visible by storing packages on end; do not stack them on top of each other. Use a first-in, first-out method for using film (that is, use the oldest film first).
- Open film packages or boxes only in the darkroom.
- Do not store film near acid or ammonia vapors.

You will also be responsible for providing accurate record keeping of x-rays. See Procedure 40-2 for guidelines on documentation and filing techniques.

Remember that x-ray films are the property of the radiology facility or the doctor's office where they are taken. Although the films may be sent (or taken by the patient) to a hospital or another doctor for consultation, they should be returned to the original facility (for example, the radiologist's office). In some facilities, the images are stored on a specialized computer disk, and the patient receives a copy of films to take to another doctor or medical facility. The information, however, is the property of the patient. Thus, the patient need not return reports.

Electronic Medicine

Recent major advances in telemedicine technology, including rapid video and computer-based communications of medical information, enable physicians to "examine" a patient in another city, view highly detailed medical images, consult with specialists in other cities, and supervise complex medical procedures. In addition, health-care personnel, including medical assistants, can participate in interactive teaching conferences by means of closed-circuit television.

EDUCATING THE PATIENT

Safety With X-Rays

You are responsible for teaching the patient about x-ray safety. You will need to obtain pertinent patient history data, answer questions, and provide basic information on x-rays, possible side effects, and other important guidelines. Consider the points below when teaching the patient about x-ray safety.

Patient History

- Ask the patient about x-rays received in the past, including how many and what type, and about the possibility of exposure to radiation in the home, school, or workplace. Explain that the effects of radiation exposure are cumulative; that is, the effects are related to total exposure over the lifetime as well as to exposure from each procedure.
- Ask a female patient about the possibility of pregnancy. Use the 10-day rule—take an x-ray only within 10 days of the last menstrual period to avoid taking an x-ray of a patient who is unknowingly pregnant. If the patient knows that she is pregnant, do not schedule an x-ray unless approved by the radiologist.
- Inform the patient about possible side effects of radiation exposure. These effects include fetal abnormality or genetic mutation in a fetus (when a patient is pregnant) and the depression of bone marrow activity, which decreases the production of red blood cells and white blood cells.

Patient Questions

- Always answer questions in simple, easy-to-understand language; make explanations brief and clear. Do not use complex medical terms; however, do include proper terminology. Offer written information about the test, if available.
- Answer fully any questions about examinations, including descriptions of procedures; the doctor's reason for ordering them; their length, side effects, injections or other uncomfortable aspects; preprocedure requirements; cost and insurance issues; and availability of test results.
- Help the patient reduce fear or anxiety surrounding the scheduled test and feel comfortable and informed about the procedure.

General X-Ray Information

- Be aware of the most current guidelines established by the American College of Radiology. Always keep up with new studies on the risks of radiation exposure.
- Encourage the patient to ask questions about the need for x-rays ordered by the doctor and risks associated with those x-rays.
- If the patient's employer requires annual x-rays or a potential employer asks for preemployment x-rays, advise the patient to question the necessity of these tests. Suggest that the patient find out whether the doctor has x-rays on file that could be submitted.
- Advise the patient to discuss testing options with the doctor. For instance, if the doctor orders fluoroscopy, the patient might ask whether standard x-rays can be taken instead, because fluoroscopy often represents a higher risk for exposure to radiation than standard x-rays. (Mobile x-ray examinations often pose a higher exposure risk as well.)
- Advise the patient to ask questions about x-ray safety standards in the office or hospital in which the tests are to take place.
- Tell the patient to avoid dental x-rays that are performed with wide-beamed plastic cones; narrow-beamed cones are more exact and less dangerous. In addition, educate the patient about the opinions of the American Dental Association and the National Conference of Dental Radiology, both of which believe that x-rays should not be performed solely for insurance claim purposes.
- Advise the patient to always ask for a lead apron over organs not being studied.
- Tell the patient to avoid retakes of x-rays because of blurriness or shadows (which are caused by movements or breathing) by remaining still when instructed to do so during x-ray examinations.
- Explain to the patient the importance of x-rays in proper diagnosis of disorders. Inform the patient about the constant improvements in equipment and x-ray procedures and the much lower doses of radiation now used in these procedures.
- Advise the patient to keep a family record of x-ray examinations.
- Educate a female patient without breast disease on the correct schedule for mammography examinations. The patient should have the following:
  - —A baseline mammogram between ages 35 and 40
  - —A mammogram every 1 to 2 years between ages 40 and 49
  - —An annual mammogram after age 50
- Also tell the patient to see a doctor immediately if she notices a breast mass, lump, or nipple discharge.

PROCEDURE 40-2

Documentation and Filing Techniques for X-Rays

Objective: To document x-ray information and file x-ray films properly

OSHA Guidelines: This procedure does not involve exposure to blood, body fluids, or tissues.

Materials: X-ray film(s), patient x-ray record card or book, label, film-filing envelopes, film-filing cabinet, inserts, marking pen

X-RAY EXAMINATIONS RECORD

Patient	Date	Type X-Ray	No. Taken	Referring Doctor	Comments
Jill Cabot	2/16	Chest	4	Wapnir	
M. C. Gaines	2/16	Right knee	8	Wright	
J. Hale	2/19	Right wrist	6	McCarthy	
L. Becker	2/23	Left hip	4	Wright	
R. Bell	2/24	Chest	4	Wapnir	
Donna Lin	2/24	Sinuses	6	Harris	
Jon Carey	2/26	Right hand	2	Cohen	

Figure 40-10. Keeping accurate records of patient x-ray information is an important duty of the medical assistant.

In some cities emergency medical technicians (EMTs) are able to transmit an electrocardiogram (ECG) electronically to an emergency room physician to obtain lifesaving directives from the physician. These directives may involve administration of drugs or other measures the EMTs otherwise would not be permitted to perform without a physician's order. Similarly, some patients are monitored by cardiologists by the transmission of daily ECGs through telephone lines to the cardiologist's office.

Another new technology is stereotaxis, a magnetic neurosurgery procedure that allows surgeons to treat or remove brain tissue safely while being guided by a computer screen. Traditionally, neurosurgeons risked causing severe damage while gaining access to an affected area of a patient's brain. With stereotaxis, however, the computer screen shows a view of the brain containing a surgically implanted magnetic pellet in a safe area of the brain. The neurosurgeon then uses magnetic resonance imaging to guide the pellet, which is the size of a grain of rice, toward a critical area. Using this technique, the surgeon can avoid critical neurons and deliver treatment to the high-risk area. The pellet can be used to move a catheter, probe, or other implement into place to remove

Method

1. Document the patient's x-ray information on the patient record card or in the record book (see Figure 40-10). Include the patient's name, the date, the type of x-ray, and the number of x-rays taken.
2. Verify that the film is properly labeled with the referring doctor's name, the date, and the patient's name. To note corrections or unusual positions or to identify a film that does not include labeling, attach the appropriate label and complete the necessary information (see Figure 40-11). Some facilities also record the name of the radiologist who interpreted the x-ray.
3. Place the processed film in a film-filing envelope. File the envelope alphabetically or chronologically (or according to your office's protocol) in the filing cabinet.
4. If you remove an envelope for any reason, put an insert or an "out card" in its place until it is returned to the cabinet.

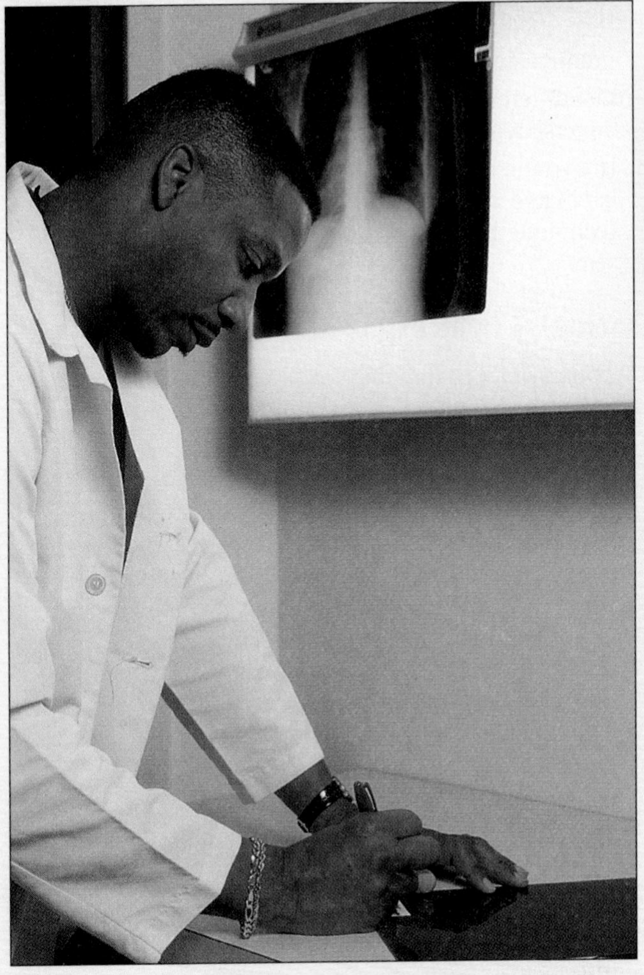

Figure 40-11. You may need to provide labeling information on an x-ray film before you file it.

tissue or deliver a drug. Researchers hope to expand this technology to other parts of the body, such as the liver or blood vessels.

Summary

Diagnostic tests are an important part of medical care because they help doctors diagnose a variety of diseases and disorders. As a medical assistant, you will be asked to assist with patient care before, and sometimes during and after, diagnostic radiology procedures. Your responsibilities include providing instructions and explanations to patients, preparing patients for various tests, and assisting the doctor or technician with the procedures. Your duties may also include storing and filing x-rays.

Safety is a vital concern with radiologic tests. Understanding and following safety precautions will help you ensure your patients' health and well-being as well as your own.

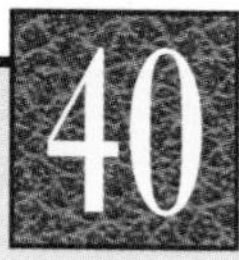

Chapter Review

Discussion Questions

1. Describe the differences between invasive and noninvasive diagnostic procedures.
2. List different types of contrast media and possible adverse reactions the patient may experience.
3. If a young child has a condition that can be evaluated by either CT scan or MRI, would either technique have an advantage over the other, and why?

Critical Thinking Questions

1. Upon arrival at the office for a lower GI series, a patient tells you he did not follow the preparation instructions he was given. Although he was supposed to follow an all-liquid diet the day before, he ate some solid food. What would you do?
2. A 40-year-old patient, scheduled for her first mammography, calls the office to cancel her appointment. You ask when she can come in for the procedure, and she says she does not want to reschedule. She sounds uneasy and you suspect she is afraid the examination will be painful. What would you say to this patient?
3. A patient who is scheduled for a series of x-rays tells you he is concerned about the amount of radiation he will be receiving. What would you say to ease this patient's fears?

Application Activities

1. Write a list of instructions to give to a patient who is going to have an upper GI series. Exchange lists with a classmate, and evaluate each other's work.
2. With another student, role-play a situation in which a medical assistant is preparing a patient for an MRI of the pelvis. Then switch roles and critique each other's technique.
3. With another student, role-play a situation in which a medical assistant is training a new coworker in how to document and file x-rays. Have your classmate evaluate the thoroughness of your instructions.

Further Readings

Diagnostic Tests, Nurse's Ready Reference. Springhouse, PA: Springhouse, 1990.

Fallon, Carol. "The Use of Ultrasound in Ophthalmology." *The Professional Medical Assistant,* November/December 1996, 6.

Fischback, F. T. *A Manual of Laboratory and Diagnostic Tests.* 4th ed. Philadelphia: J. B. Lippincott, 1992.

Gurley, LaVerne T., and William J. Callaway, eds. *Introduction to Radiologic Technology.* 4th ed. St. Louis, MO: Mosby–Year Book, 1996.

Health & Medical Horizons. New York: Macmillan Educational Company, 1991.

Limitation of Exposure to Ionizing Radiation. Bethesda, MD: National Council on Radiation Protection and Measurements, 1993.

"Screening for Gynecologic Malignancies in Primary Care." *Emergency Medicine,* March 1993, 113–124.

Appendixes

Appendix I
Medical Assistant Role Delineation Chart

ADMINISTRATIVE

Administrative Procedures

- Perform basic clerical functions
- Schedule, coordinate, and monitor appointments
- Schedule inpatient/outpatient admissions and procedures
- Understand and apply third-party guidelines
- Obtain reimbursement through accurate claims submission
- Monitor third-party reimbursement
- Perform medical transcription
- Understand and adhere to managed care policies and procedures
- * *Negotiate managed care contracts (adv)*

Practice Finances

- Perform procedural and diagnostic coding
- Apply bookkeeping principles
- Document and maintain accounting and banking records
- Manage accounts receivable
- Manage accounts payable
- Process payroll
- * *Develop and maintain fee schedules (adv)*
- * *Manage renewals of business and professional insurance policies (adv)*
- * *Manage personnel benefits and maintain records (adv)*

CLINICAL

Fundamental Principles

- Apply principles of aseptic technique and infection control
- Comply with quality assurance practices
- Screen and follow up patient test results

Diagnostic Orders

- Collect and process specimens
- Perform diagnostic tests

Patient Care

- Adhere to established triage procedures
- Obtain patient history and vital signs
- Prepare and maintain examination and treatment areas
- Prepare patient for examinations, procedures, and treatments
- Assist with examinations, procedures, and treatments
- Prepare and administer medications and immunizations
- Maintain medication and immunization records
- Recognize and respond to emergencies
- Coordinate patient care information with other health care providers

* Denotes advanced skills.

Medical Assistant Role Delineation Chart

GENERAL (Transdisciplinary)

Professionalism

- Project a professional manner and image
- Adhere to ethical principles
- Demonstrate initiative and responsibility
- Work as a team member
- Manage time effectively
- Prioritize and perform multiple tasks
- Adapt to change
- Promote the CMA credential
- Enhance skills through continuing education

Communication Skills

- Treat all patients with compassion and empathy
- Recognize and respect cultural diversity
- Adapt communications to individual's ability to understand
- Use professional telephone technique
- Use effective and correct verbal and written communications
- Recognize and respond to verbal and nonverbal communications
- Use medical terminology appropriately
- Receive, organize, prioritize, and transmit information
- Serve as liaison
- Promote the practice through positive public relations

Legal Concepts

- Maintain confidentiality
- Practice within the scope of education, training, and personal capabilities
- Prepare and maintain medical records
- Document accurately
- Use appropriate guidelines when releasing information
- Follow employer's established policies dealing with the health care contract
- Follow federal, state, and local legal guidelines
- Maintain awareness of federal and state health care legislation and regulations
- Maintain and dispose of regulated substances in compliance with government guidelines
- Comply with established risk management and safety procedures
- Recognize professional credentialing criteria
- Participate in the development and maintenance of personnel, policy, and procedure manuals

* *Develop and maintain personnel, policy, and procedure manuals (adv)*

Instruction

- Instruct individuals according to their needs
- Explain office policies and procedures
- Teach methods of health promotion and disease prevention
- Locate community resources and disseminate information

* *Orient and train personnel (adv)*

* *Develop educational materials (adv)*

* *Conduct continuing education activities (adv)*

Operational Functions

- Maintain supply inventory
- Evaluate and recommend equipment and supplies
- Apply computer techniques to support office operations

* *Supervise personnel (adv)*

* *Interview and recommend job applicants (adv)*

* *Negotiate leases and prices for equipment and supply contracts (adv)*

Source: This chart is part of the "AAMA Role Delineation Study: Occupational Analysis of the Medical Assisting Profession," released by the American Association of Medical Assistants in May 1997.

Appendix II
Prefixes and Suffixes Commonly Used in Medical Terms

a-, an- without, not
ab- from, away
ad-, -ad to, toward
adeno- gland, glandular
aero- air
-aesthesia sensation
-al characterized by
-algia pain
ambi-, amph-, amphi- both, on both sides, around
andr-, andro- man, male
angio- blood vessel
ano- anus
ante- before
antero- in front of
anti- against, opposing
arterio- artery
arthro- joint
-ase enzyme
auto- self
bi- twice, double
bili- bile
bio- life
blasto-, -blast developing stage, bud
brachy- short
brady- slow
broncho- bronchial (windpipe)
cardio- heart
cata- down, lower, under
-cele swelling, tumor
-centesis puncture, tapping
centi- hundred
cephal-, cephalo- head
cerebr-, cerebro- brain
chol-, chole-, cholo- gall
chondro- cartilage
chromo- color
-cide causing death
circum- around
-cise cut
co-, com-, con- together, with
-coele cavity
colo- colon
colp-, colpo- vagina
contra- against
cost-, costo- rib
crani-, cranio- skull
cryo- cold
cysto-, -cyst bladder, bag
-cyte, cyto- cell, cellular
dacry-, dacryo- tears, lacrimal apparatus
dactyl-, dactylo- finger, toe
de- down, from
deca- ten
deci- tenth
demi- half
dent-, denti-, dento- teeth
derma-, dermat-, dermato-, -derm skin
dextro- to the right
di- double, twice
dia- through, apart, between
dipla-, diplo- double, twin
dis- apart, away from
dorsi-, dorso- back
dys- difficult, painful, bad, abnormal
e-, ec-, ecto- away, from, without, outside
-ectomy cutting out, surgical removal
em-, en- in, into
-emesis vomiting
-emia blood
encephalo- brain
endo- within
entero- intestine
ento- within, inner
epi- on, above
erythro- red
esthesio-, -esthesia sensation
eu- good, true, normal
ex-, exo- outside of, beyond, without
extra- outside of, beyond, in addition
fibro- connective tissue
fore- before, in front of
-form shape
-fuge driving away
galact-, galacto- milk
gastr-, gastro- stomach
-gene, -genic, -genetic, -genous arising from, origin, formation
glosso- tongue
gluco-, glyco- sugar, sweet
-gram recorded information
-graph instrument for recording
-graphy the process of recording
gyn-, gyno-, gyne-, gyneco- woman, female
haemo-, hemato-, hem-, hemo- blood
hemi- half
hepa-, hepar-, hepato- liver
herni- rupture
hetero- other, unlike
histo- tissue
homeo, homo- same, like
hydra-, hydro- water
hyper- above, over, increased
hypo- below, under, decreased
hyster-, hystero- uterus
-iasis condition of
-ic, -ical pertaining to
ictero- jaundice
idio- personal, self-produced
ileo- ileum
im-, in-, ir- not
in- in, into
infra- beneath
inter- between, among
intra-, intro- into, within, during
-ism condition, process, theory
-itis inflammation of
-ize to cause to be, to become, to treat by special method
juxta- near, nearby
karyo- nucleus, nut
kata-, kath- down, lower, under
kera-, kerato- horn, hardness, cornea
kineto-, -kinesis, -kinetic motion
lact- milk
laparo- abdomen
latero- side
-lepsis, -lepsy seizure, convulsion
leuco-, leuko- white
levo- to the left
lipo- fat
lith-, -lith stone

Appendix II
Prefixes and Suffixes Commonly Used in Medical Terms

-logy science of, study of
-lysis setting free, disintegration, decomposition
macro- large, long
mal- bad
-malacia abnormal softening
-mania insanity, abnormal desire
mast-, masto- breast
med-, medi- middle
mega-, megalo- large, great
meio- contraction
melan-, melano- black
meno- month
mes-, meso- middle
meta- beyond
-meter measure
metro-, metra- uterus
micro- small
mio- smaller, less
mono- single, one
multi- many
my-, myo- muscle
myel-, myelo- marrow
narco- sleep
nas-, naso- nose
necro- dead
neo- new
nephr-, nephro- kidney
neu-, neuro- nerve
niter-, nitro- nitrogen
non-, not- no
nucleo- nucleus
ob- against
oculo- eye
odont- tooth
-odynia pain
-oid resembling
olig-, oligo- few, less than normal
-oma tumor
onco- tumor
oo- ovum, egg
oophor- ovary
ophthalmo- eye
-opia vision
orchid- testicle
ortho- straight
os- mouth, bone
-osis disease, condition of
oste-, osteo- bone
-ostomy to make a mouth, opening
oto- ear
-otomy incision, surgical cutting
-ous having
oxy- sharp, acid
pachy- thick
paedo, pedo- child
pan- all, every
para- alongside of, with
path-, patho-, -pathy disease, suffering
ped-, pedi-, pedo- foot
-penia too few, lack
per- through, excessive
peri- around
phag-, phago-, -phage eating, consuming
pharyng- throat, pharynx
phlebo- vein
-phobia fear
-phylaxis protection
-plastic molded
-plasty operation to reconstruct
-plegia paralysis
pleuro- side, rib
pluri- more, several
pneo-, -pnea breathing
pneumo- air, lungs
poly- many, much
post- after, behind
pre-, pro- before, in front of
presby-, presbyo- old age
procto- rectum
proto- first
pseudo- false
psych- the mind
pulmon-, pulmono- lung
pyelo- pelvis (renal)
pyo- pus
pyro- fever, heat
quadri- four
re- back, again
reni-, reno- kidney
retro- backward, behind
rhino- nose
-rrhage, -rrhagia abnormal or excessive discharge, hemorrhage, flow
-rrhaphy suture of
-rrhea flow
sacchar- sugar
sacro- sacrum
salpingo- tube, fallopian tube
sarco- flesh
sclero- hard, sclera
-sclerosis hardening
-scopy examining
semi- half
septi-, septic-, septico- poison, infection
-stasis stoppage
steno- contracted, narrow
stereo- firm, solid, three-dimensional
stomato- mouth
-stomy opening
sub- under
super-, supra- above, upon
sym-, syn- with, together
tachy- fast
tele- distant, far
teno-, tenoto- tendon
tetra- four
-therapy treatment
thermo-, -thermy heat
thio- sulfur
thoraco- chest
thrombo- blood clot
thyro- thyroid gland
tomo-, -tomy incision, section
trans- across
tri- three
tropho-, -trophy nutrition, growth
-tropy turning, tendency
ultra- beyond, excess
uni- one
-uria urine
urino-, uro- urine, urinary organs
utero- uterus, uterine
vaso- vessel
ventri-, ventro- abdomen
xanth- yellow

Appendix III
Latin and Greek Equivalents Commonly Used in Medical Terms

abdomen venter
adhesion adhaesio
and et
arm brachium; brachion (Gr*)
artery arteria
back dorsum
backbone spina
backward retro; opistho (Gr)
bend flexus
bile bilis; chole (Gr)
bladder vesica, cystus
blister vesicula
blood sanguis; haima (Gr)
body corpus; soma (Gr)
bone os, ossis; osteon (Gr)
brain encephalon
break ruptura
breast mamma; mastos (Gr)
buttock gloutos (Gr)
cartilage cartilago; chondros (Gr)
cavity cavum
chest pectoris, pectus; thorax (Gr)
child puer, puerilis
choke strangulo
corn clavus
cornea kerat (Gr)
cough tussis
deadly lethalis
death mors
dental dentalis
digestive pepticos
disease morbus
dislocation luxatio
doctor medicus
dose dosis (Gr)
ear auris; ous (Gr)
egg ovum
erotic erotikos (Gr)
exhalation exhalatio, expiro
external externus
extract extractum
eye oculus; ophthalmos (Gr)
eyelid palpebra
face facies
fat adeps; lipos (Gr)
female femella
fever febris
finger (or toe) digitus
flesh carnis, caro
foot pes
forehead frons
gum gingiva
hair capillus, pilus; thrix (Gr)
hand manus; cheir (Gr)
harelip labrum fissum; cheiloschisis (Gr)
head caput; kephale (Gr)
health sanitas
hear audire
heart cor; kardia (Gr)
heat calor; therme (Gr)
heel calx, talus
hysterics hysteria
infant infans
infectious contagiosus
injection injectio
intellect intellectus
internal internus
intestine intestinum; enteron (Gr)
itching pruritis
jawbone maxilla
joint vertebra; arthron (Gr)
kidney ren, renis; nephros (Gr)
knee genu
kneecap patella
lacerate lacerare
larynx guttur
lateral lateralis
limb membrum
lip labium, labrum; cheilos (Gr)
listen auscultare
liver jecur; hepar (Gr)
loin lapara
looseness laxativus
lung pulmo; pneumon (Gr)
male masculinus
malignant malignons
milk lac
moisture humiditas
month mensis
monthly menstruus
mouth oris, os; stoma, stomato (Gr)
nail unguis; onyx (Gr)
navel umbilicus; omphalos (Gr)
neck cervix; trachelos (Gr)
nerve nervus; neuron (Gr)
nipple papilla; thele (Gr)
no, none nullus
nose nasus; rhis (Gr)
nostril naris
nourishment alimentum
ointment unguentum
pain dolor; algia
patient patiens
pectoral pectoralis
pimple pustula
poison venenum
powder pulvis
pregnant praegnans, gravida
pubic bone os pubis
pupil pupilla
rash exanthema (Gr)
recover convalescere
redness rubor
rib costa
ringing tinnitus
scaly squamosus
sciatica sciaticus; ischiadikos (Gr)
seed semen
senile senilis
sheath vagina; theke (Gr)
short brevis; brachys (Gr)
shoulder omos (Gr)
shoulder blade scapula
side latus
skin cutis; derma (Gr)
skull cranium; kranion (Gr)
sleep somnus
solution solutio
spinal spinalis
stomach stomachus; gaster (Gr)
stone calculus
sugar saccharum
swallow glutio
tail cauda
taste gustatio
tear lacrima
testicle testis; orchis (Gr)
thigh femur
throat fauces; pharynx (Gr)
tongue lingua; glossa (Gr)
tooth dens; odontos (Gr)
touch tactus
tremor tremere
twin gemellus
ulcer ulcus
urine urina; ouran (Gr)
uterus hystera (Gr)
vagina vagina; kolpos (Gr)
vein vena; phlebos, phleps (Gr)
vertebra spondylos (Gr)
vessel vas
wash diluere
water aqua
wax cera
weak debilis
windpipe arteria aspera
wrist carpus; karpos (Gr)

* Parenthetical "Gr" means the preceding term is Greek. Other terms in the column are Latin.

Appendix IV
Abbreviations Commonly Used in Medical Notations

a before
a.c. before meals
ADL activities of daily living
ad lib as desired
ADT admission, discharge, transfer
AIDS acquired immunodeficiency syndrome
a.m.a. against medical advice
amp. ampule
amt amount
aq., AQ water; aqueous
ausc. auscultation
ax axis
Bib, bib drink
b.i.d., bid, BID twice a day
BM bowel movement
BP, B/P blood pressure
c., c̄ with
cap, caps capsules
CBC complete blood (cell) count
cc cubic centimeter
C.C., CC chief complaint
CDC Centers for Disease Control and Prevention
CHF congestive heart failure
chr chronic
CNS central nervous system
Comp, comp compound
COPD chronic obstructive pulmonary disease
CPE complete physical examination
CPR cardiopulmonary resuscitation
CSF cerebrospinal fluid
CV cardiovascular
d day
d/c, D/C discontinue
D & C dilation and curettage
Dil, dil dilute
DTP diptheria-tetanus-pertussis vaccine
Dr. doctor
DTs delirium tremens
D/W dextrose in water
Dx, dx diagnosis
ECG, EKG electrocardiogram
EEG electroencephalogram
EENT eyes, ears, nose, and throat
ER emergency room
ESR erythrocyte sedimentation rate
FBS fasting blood sugar
FDA Food and Drug Administration
FH family history
Fl, fl, fld fluid
F/u follow-up
Fx fracture
GBS gallbladder series
GI gastrointestinal
gt, gtt drops
GU genitourinary
GYN gynecology
HB, Hgb hemoglobin
HEENT head, ears, eyes, nose, throat
HIV human immunodeficiency virus
h.s., hs, HS hour of sleep/at bed-time
Hx history
ICU intensive care unit
I & D incision and drainage
IM intramuscular
inf. infusion; inferior
inj injection
IT inhalation therapy
IUD intrauterine device
IV intravenous
lab laboratory
liq liquid
LMP last menstrual period
MI myocardial infarction
MM mucous membrane
NB newborn
NED no evidence of disease
no. number
noc, noct night
npo, NPO nothing by mouth
NS normal saline
NTP normal temperature and pressure
N & V nausea and vomiting
NYD not yet diagnosed
OB obstetrics
OC oral contraceptive
o.d. once a day
OD overdose
O.D., OD right eye
oint ointment
OOB out of bed
OPD outpatient department
OR operating room
O.S., OS left eye
OTC over-the-counter
O.U., OU both eyes
p.c., pc after meals
PE physical examination
PH past history
PID pelvic inflammatory disease
p/o postoperative
POMR problem-oriented medical record
p.r.n., prn, PRN whenever necessary
Pt patient
PT physical therapy
PTA prior to admission
pulv powder
q. every
q2, q2h every 2 hours
q.a.m., qam every morning
q.d., qd every day
q.h., qh every hour
qhs every night, at bedtime
q.i.d., QID four times a day
qns, QNS quantity not sufficient
qod every other day
qs, QS quantity sufficient
RBC red blood cells; red blood (cell) count
REM rapid eye movement
R/O rule out
ROM range of motion
ROS/SR review of systems/systems review
Rx prescription, take
SAD seasonal affective disorder
s.c., SC, SQ, subq, SubQ subcuta-neously
SIDS sudden infant death syndrome
Sig directions
SOAP subjective, objective, assess-ment, plan

Appendix IV continued
Abbreviations Commonly Used in Medical Notations

SOB shortness of breath
sol solution
S/R suture removal
ss, $\overline{ss}$ one-half
Staph staphylococcus
stat, STAT immediately
STD sexually transmitted disease
Strep streptococcus
subling, SL sublingual
S/W saline in water
T & A tonsillectomy and adenoidectomy
tab tablet
TB tuberculosis
t.i.d., tid, TID three times a day
tinc, tinct, tr tincture
top topically
TPR temperature, pulse, and respiration
Tx treatment
U unit
UA urinalysis
UCHD usual childhood diseases
ung, ungt ointment
URI upper respiratory infection
u/s ultrasound
UTI urinary tract infection
VA visual acuity
VD venereal disease
Vf visual field
VS vital signs
WBC white blood cells; white blood (cell) count
WNL within normal limits
wt weight
y/o year old

Appendix V
Symbols Commonly Used in Medical Notations

Apothecaries' Weights and Measures
♏ minim
℈ scruple
ʒ dram
fʒ fluidram
℥ ounce
f℥ fluidounce
O pint
℔ pound

Other Weights and Measures
\# pounds
° degrees
′ foot; minute
″ inch; second
μm micrometer
μ micron (former term for micrometer)
mμ millimicron; nanometer
μg microgram
mEq milliequivalent
mL milliliter
dL deciliter
mg% milligrams percent; milligrams per 100 mL

Abbreviations
$\overline{aa}$, $\overline{AA}$ of each
$\bar{c}$ with
M mix (Latin *misce*)
m- meta-
o- ortho-
p- para-
$\bar{p}$ after
$\bar{s}$ without
ss, $\overline{ss}$ one-half (Latin *semis*)

Mathematical Functions and Terms
\# number
\+ plus; positive; acid reaction
\- minus; negative; alkaline reaction
± plus or minus; either positive or negative; indefinite
× multiply; magnification; crossed with, hybrid
÷, / divided by
= equal to
≈ approximately equal to
> greater than; from which is derived
< less than; derived from
≮ not less than
≯ not greater than
≤ equal to or less than
≥ equal to or greater than
≠ not equal to
√ square root
$\sqrt[3]{}$ cube root
∞ infinity
: ratio; "is to"
∴ therefore
% percent
π pi (3.14159)—the ratio of circumference of a circle to its diameter

Chemical Notations
Δ change; heat
⇌ reversible reaction
↑ increase
↓ decrease

Warnings
C-I Schedule I controlled substance
C-II Schedule II controlled substance
C-III Schedule III controlled substance
C-IV Schedule IV controlled substance
C-V Schedule V controlled substance
☠ poison
☢ radiation
☣ biohazard

Others
℞ prescription; take
□, ♂ male
○, ♀ female
$\dot{\text{T}}$ one
$\dot{\text{T}}\dot{\text{T}}$ two
$\dot{\text{T}}\dot{\text{T}}\dot{\text{T}}$ three

Glossary

AAMA Role Delineation Study 1997 occupational analysis of the medical assisting profession by the American Association of Medical Assistants; the areas of competence identified in the study replace DACUM competencies. (1*)

abandonment A situation in which a health-care professional stops caring for a patient without arranging for care by an equally qualified substitute. (3)

ABA number A fraction appearing in the upper right-hand corner of all printed checks that identifies the geographic area and specific bank on which the check is drawn. (16)

ABCs The assessments to make first in a medical emergency—the patient's airway, breathing, and circulation. (31)

abduction Movement away from the body. (23)

abscess A collection of pus (white blood cells, bacteria, and dead skin cells) that forms as a result of infection. (29)

absorption The process by which one substance is absorbed, or taken in and incorporated, into another, as when the body converts food or drugs into a form it can use. (37)

access The way patients enter and exit a medical office. (13)

accessibility The ease with which people can move into and out of a space. (22)

accounts payable Money owed by a business; the practice's expenses. (16)

accounts receivable Income or money owed to a business. (16)

accreditation The documenting of official authorization or approval of a program. (1)

acid-fast stain A staining procedure for identifying bacteria that have a waxy cell wall. (35)

active file A file used on a consistent basis. (10)

active listening Part of two-way communication, such as offering feedback or asking questions; contrast with **passive listening.** (4)

active voice The feature of a verb that indicates the subject of a sentence is performing an action, as in "We sent the report yesterday"; contrast with **passive voice.** (7)

acute Having a rapid onset and progress, as acute appendicitis. (27)

addiction A physical or psychological dependence on a substance, usually involving a pattern of behavior that includes obsessive or compulsive preoccupation with the substance and the security of its supply, as well as a high rate of relapse after withdrawal. (26)

adduction Movement toward the body. (23)

administer To give a drug directly by injection, by mouth, or by any other route that introduces the drug into the body. (37)

advance directive See **living will.** (3)

advance scheduling Booking an appointment several weeks or even months in advance. (12)

aerobes Bacteria that grow best in the presence of oxygen. (35)

afebrile Having a body temperature within one's normal range. (24)

agar A gelatinlike substance derived from seaweed that gives a culture medium its semisolid consistency. (35)

age analysis The process of clarifying and reviewing past due accounts by age from the first date of billing. (17)

agenda The list of topics discussed or presented at a meeting, in order of presentation. (12)

agent (legal) A person who acts on a physician's behalf while performing professional tasks; (clinical) an active principle or entity that produces a certain effect; for example, an infectious agent. (3)

aggressive Imposing one's position on others or trying to manipulate them. (4)

agranular leukocyte See **nongranular leukocyte.** (34)

allergen An antigen that induces an allergic reaction. (28)

allergist A specialist who diagnoses and treats physical reactions to substances including mold, dust, fur, pollen, foods, drugs, and chemicals. (2)

alphabetic filing system A filing system in which the files are arranged in alphabetic order, with the patient's last name first, followed by the first name and middle initial. (10)

alveoli Clusters of air sacs in which the exchange of gases between air and blood takes place; located in the lungs. (23)

ambulate To move from place to place; walk. (25)

American Association of Medical Assistants (AAMA) The professional organization that certifies medical assistants and works to maintain professional standards in the medical assisting profession. (1)

American Medical Technologists (AMT) The national certifying body for laboratory personnel that registers medical assistants who have met AMT educational requirements and passed the AMT certification examination. (1)

Americans With Disabilities Act (ADA) A U.S. civil rights act forbidding discrimination against people because of a physical or mental handicap. (13)

amino acids Natural organic compounds found in plant and animal foods and used by the body to create protein. (36)

anabolism The stage of metabolism in which substances such as nutrients are changed into more complex substances and used to build body tissues. (36)

anaerobe A bacterium that grows best in the absence of oxygen. (35)

anaphylaxis A severe allergic reaction with symptoms that include respiratory distress, difficulty in swallowing, pallor, and a drastic drop in blood pressure that can lead to circulatory collapse. (28)

anergic reaction A lack of response to skin testing that indicates the body's inability to mount a normal response to invasion by a pathogen. (21)

anesthesia A loss of sensation, particularly the feeling of pain. (29)

anesthesiologist A specialist who uses medications to cause patients to lose sensation or feeling during surgery. (2)

anesthetic A medication that causes anesthesia. (29)

angiography An x-ray examination of a blood vessel, performed after the injection of a contrast medium, that evaluates the function and structure of one or more arteries or veins. (28)

annotate To underline or highlight key points of a document or to write reminders, make comments, and suggest actions in the margins. (7)

anorexia nervosa An eating disorder in which people starve themselves because they fear that if they lose control of eating they will become grossly overweight. (36)

antecubital space The inner side or bend of the elbow; the site at which the brachial artery is felt or heard when a pulse or blood pressure is taken. (24)

antibodies Highly specific proteins that attach themselves to foreign substances in an initial step in destroying such substances, as part of the body's defenses. (19)

* Parenthetical numbers indicate the chapter in which the entry is a key term or is first defined in context. Entries not followed by a chapter number are important terms related to material covered but not specifically defined in the text.

anticoagulant A chemical agent that keeps blood from clotting. (20)
antigen A foreign substance that stimulates white blood cells to create antibodies when it enters the body. (19)
antimicrobial An agent that kills microorganisms or suppresses their growth. (35)
antioxidants Chemical agents that fight cell-destroying chemical substances called free radicals. (36)
antiseptic A cleaning product used on human tissue as an anti-infection agent. (20)
anuria The absence of urine production. (33)
anvil See **incus.** (26)
apex The left lower corner of the heart, where the strongest heart sounds can be heard. (24)
apical Located at the apex of the heart. (24)
approximation The process of bringing the edges of a wound together, so the tissue surfaces are close, to protect the area from further contamination and to minimize scar and scab formation. (29)
aqueous humor A liquid produced by the eye's ciliary body that fills the space between the cornea and the lens. (26)
arbitration A process in which opposing sides choose a person or persons outside the court system, often someone with special knowledge in the field, to hear and decide a dispute. (3)
arrhythmia Irregularity in heart rhythm. (39)
arterial blood gases (ABGs) A test that measures the amount of gases, such as oxygen and carbon dioxide, dissolved in arterial blood. (27)
arthrography A radiologic procedure performed by a radiologist, who uses a contrast medium and fluoroscopy to help diagnose abnormalities or injuries in the cartilage, tendons, or ligaments of the joints—usually the knee or shoulder. (40)
arthroscopy A procedure in which an orthopedist examines a joint, usually the knee or shoulder, with a tubular instrument called an arthroscope; also used to guide surgical procedures. (28)
artifact Any irrelevant object or mark observed when examining specimens or graphic records that is not related to the object being examined; for example, a foreign object visible through a microscope or an erroneous mark on an ECG strip. (32)
asepsis The condition in which pathogens are absent or controlled. (19)
assertive Being firm and standing up for oneself while showing respect for others. (4)
asset An item owned by the practice that has a dollar value, such as the medical practice building, office equipment, or accounts receivable. (16)
assignment of benefits An authorization for an insurance carrier to pay a physician or practice directly. (15)
astigmatism A condition in which vision is distorted because the cornea is unevenly curved. (28)
atherosclerosis The accumulation of fatty deposits along the inner walls of arteries. (27)
atrioventricular (AV) node A mass of specialized conducting cells in the heart, located at the bottom of the right atrium, that slightly delays the contraction impulse, then transmits the impulse to another mass of conducting cells called the bundle of His. (39)
atrium An upper, receiving chamber of the heart. (23)
audiologist A health-care specialist who focuses on evaluating and correcting hearing problems. (26)
audiometer An electronic device that measures hearing acuity by producing sounds in specific frequencies and intensities. (26)
auricle The outside part of the ear, made of cartilage and covered with skin. (26)
auscultated blood pressure Blood pressure as measured by listening with a stethoscope. (24)
autoclave A device that uses pressurized steam to sterilize instruments and equipment. (20)
axilla Armpit; one of the four locations for temperature readings. (24)

B lymphocyte A type of nongranular leukocyte that produces antibodies to combat specific pathogens. (34)
bacilli See **bacillus.**
bacillus A rod-shaped bacterium. (35)
bacteria See **bacterium.** (35)
bacterial spore A primitive, thick-walled reproductive body capable of developing into a new individual; resistant to killing through disinfection. (19)
bacterium A single-celled prokaryotic organism that reproduces quickly; bacteria are one of the major causes of disease. (35)
barium enema A radiologic procedure performed by a radiologist who administers barium sulfate through the anus, into the rectum, and then into the colon to help diagnose and evaluate obstructions, ulcers, polyps, diverticulosis, tumors, or motility problems of the colon or rectum; also called a lower GI (gastrointestinal) series. (40)
barium swallow A radiologic procedure that involves oral administration of a barium sulfate drink to help diagnose and evaluate obstructions, ulcers, polyps, diverticulosis, tumors, or motility problems of the esophagus, stomach, duodenum, and small intestine; also called an upper GI (gastrointestinal) series. (40)
basophil A type of granular leukocyte that produces the chemical histamine, which aids the body in controlling allergic reactions and other exaggerated immunologic responses. (34)
behavior modification The altering of personal habits to promote a healthier lifestyle. (36)
benefit A type of employee compensation other than salary, such as paid vacation, paid holidays, or insurance. (16)
bilirubin A bile pigment formed by the breakdown of hemoglobin in the liver. (33)
bilirubinuria The presence of bilirubin in the urine; one of the first signs of liver disease or conditions that involve the liver. (33)
bioethics Principles of right and wrong in issues that arise from medical advances. (3)
biohazardous materials Biological agents that can spread disease to living things. (19)
biohazardous waste container A leakproof, puncture-resistant container, color-coded red or labeled with a special biohazard symbol, that is used to store and dispose of contaminated supplies and equipment. (19)
biohazard symbol A symbol that must appear on all containers used to store waste products, blood, blood products, or other specimens that may be infectious. (32)
biopsy specimen A small amount of tissue removed from the body for examination under a microscope to diagnose an illness. (29)
birthday rule A rule that states that the insurance policy of a policyholder whose birthday comes first in the year is the primary payer for all dependents. (15)
block style See **full-block letter style.** (7)
blood-borne pathogen A disease-causing microorganism carried in a host's blood and transmitted through contact with infected blood, tissue, or body fluids. (21)
body language Nonverbal communication, including facial expressions, eye contact, posture, touch, and attention to personal space. (4)
bone conduction The process by which sound waves pass through the bones of the skull directly to the inner ear, bypassing the outer and middle ears. (26)
bookkeeping The systematic recording of business transactions. (16)
botulism A life-threatening type of food poisoning that results from eating improperly canned or preserved foods that have been contaminated with the bacterium *Clostridium botulinum.* (31)

brachial artery An artery that provides a palpable pulse and audible vascular sounds in the antecubital space (the bend of the elbow). (24)

brachytherapy A radiation therapy technique in which a radiologist places temporary radioactive implants close to or directly into cancerous tissue; used for treating localized cancers. (40)

breach of contract The violation of or failure to live up to a contract's terms. (3)

bronchi The two branches of the trachea that enter the lungs. (23)

buccal Between the cheek and gum. (38)

buffer To neutralize changes in pH (hydrogen ion concentration, which determines the acidic or basic quality of a substance such as a body fluid).

buffy coat The layer between the packed red blood cells and plasma in a centrifuged blood sample; this layer contains the white blood cells and platelets. (34)

bulimia An eating disorder in which people eat a large quantity of food in a short period of time (bingeing) and then attempt to counter the effects of bingeing by self-induced vomiting, use of laxatives or diuretics, and/or excessive exercise. (36)

bundle of His An area located in the septum of the heart between the ventricles that acts as a relay station, sending the electrical impulse for muscle contraction through a series of bundle branches to the Purkinje fibers. (39)

burn An injury to tissue that can occur from heat, chemicals, electricity, or radiation. (31)

calibration syringe A standardized measuring instrument used to check and adjust the volume indicator on a spirometer. (39)

calorie (kilocalorie) A unit used to measure the amount of energy food produces; the amount of energy needed to raise the temperature of 1 kg of water by 1°C. (36)

capillary puncture A blood-drawing technique that requires a superficial puncture of the skin with a sharp point. (34)

capitation A payment structure in which a health maintenance organization prepays an annual set fee per patient to a physician. (15)

cardiac catheterization A diagnostic method in which a catheter is inserted into a vein or artery in the arm or leg and passed through blood vessels into the heart. (28)

cardiac cycle The sequence of contraction and relaxation that makes up a complete heartbeat. (39)

cardiologist A specialist who diagnoses and treats diseases of the heart and blood vessels (cardiovascular diseases). (2)

cardiomyopathy Disease of the heart muscle causing fatigue and breathing problems and possibly leading to heart failure. (28)

cardiopulmonary resuscitation (CPR) A basic life-support technique consisting of a prescribed sequence of steps designed to provide ventilation and blood circulation for a patient who is not breathing and has no pulse. (31)

carrier A reservoir host who is unaware of the presence of a pathogen and so spreads the disease while exhibiting no symptoms of infection; (insurance) an insurance provider. (19)

cash flow statement A statement that shows the cash on hand at the beginning of a period, the income and disbursements made during the period, and the new amount of cash on hand at the end of the period. (18)

cashier's check A bank check issued by a bank on bank paper and signed by a bank representative; usually purchased by individuals who do not have checking accounts. (16)

cast A rigid, external dressing, usually made of plaster or fiberglass, that is molded to the contours of the body part to which it is applied; used to immobilize a fractured or dislocated bone. (31)

casts Cylinder-shaped elements with flat or rounded ends, differing in composition and size, that form when protein from the breakdown of cells accumulates and precipitates in the kidney tubules and is washed into the urine. (33)

catabolism The stage of metabolism in which complex substances, including nutrients and body tissues, are broken down into simpler substances and converted into energy. (36)

catheter A slender, sterile tube inserted into a vessel, an organ, or a body cavity for diagnostic or therapeutic purposes.

catheterization The procedure during which a catheter is inserted into a vessel, an organ, or a body cavity. (33)

CAT scan See **computed tomography.** (28)

CD-ROM A compact disc that contains software programs; an abbreviation for "compact disc—read-only memory." (6)

Celsius (centigrade) One of two common scales for measuring temperature; measured in degrees Celsius, or °C. (24)

Centers for Disease Control and Prevention (CDC) A division of the Department of Health and Human Services that sets guidelines for the control of infectious diseases. (19)

central processing unit (CPU) A microprocessor, the primary computer chip responsible for interpreting and executing programs. (6)

Certificate of Waiver tests Laboratory tests that pose an insignificant risk to the patient if they are performed or interpreted incorrectly, are simple and accurate to such a degree that the risk of obtaining incorrect results is minimal, and have been approved by the Food and Drug Administration for use by patients at home; laboratories performing only Certificate of Waiver tests must meet less stringent standards than laboratories that perform tests in other categories. (32)

certified check A payer's check written and signed by the payer, which is stamped "certified" by the bank. The bank has already drawn money from the payer's account to guarantee that the check will be paid. (16)

Certified Medical Assistant (CMA) A medical assistant whose knowledge about the skills of medical assistants, as summarized by the 1997 AAMA Role Delineation Study areas of competence, has been certified by the Certifying Board of the American Association of Medical Assistants (AAMA). (1)

centrifuge A device used to spin a specimen at high speed until it separates into its component parts. (32)

cerumen A waxlike substance produced by glands in the ear canal; also called earwax. (26)

chain of custody A procedure for ensuring that a specimen is obtained from a specified individual, is correctly identified, is under the uninterrupted control of authorized personnel, and has not been altered or replaced. (31)

chancre A painless ulcer that may appear on the tongue, the lips, the genitalia, the rectum, or elsewhere. (21)

charge slip The original record of services performed for a patient and the charges for those services. (16)

check A bank draft or order written by a payer that directs the bank to pay a sum of money on demand to the payee. (16)

chiropractic A holistic approach to health that involves adjustment of the spine to aid the body's natural defenses and healing processes. (30)

cholangiography A test that evaluates the function of the bile ducts by injection of a contrast medium directly into the common bile duct (during gallbladder surgery) or through a T-tube (after gallbladder surgery or during radiologic testing) and taking an x-ray. (40)

cholecystography A gallbladder function test performed by x-ray after the patient ingests an oral contrast agent; used to detect gallstones and bile duct obstruction. (28)

cholesterol A fat-related substance the body produces in the liver and obtains from dietary sources; needed in small amounts to carry out several vital functions. High levels of cholesterol in the blood increase the risk of heart and artery disease. (36)

choroid The middle layer of the eye, which contains the iris, the ciliary body, and most of the eye's blood vessels. (26)

chromosome A threadlike structure in the nucleus of a cell, made of deoxyribonucleic acid (DNA), that directs all cell activities and allows the cell to reproduce. (23)

chronic Lasting a long time or recurring frequently, as in chronic osteoarthritis. (27)

ciliary body A wedge-shaped thickening in the middle layer of the eyeball that contains the muscles that control the shape of the lens. (26)

Civilian Health and Medical Program of the Veterans Administration (CHAMPVA) A program that covers the expenses of the dependents of veterans with total, permanent, service-connected disabilities, as well as surviving spouses and dependent children of veterans who died in the line of duty or as a result of service-related disabilities. (15)

clarity Clearness in writing or stating a message. (7)

class-action lawsuit A lawsuit in which one or more people sue a company or other legal entity that allegedly wronged all of them in the same way. (17)

clean-catch midstream urine specimen A type of urine specimen that requires special cleansing of the external genitalia to avoid contamination by organisms residing near the external opening of the urethra and is used to identify the number and types of pathogens present in urine; sometimes referred to as midvoid. (33)

clean technique See **medical asepsis.** (29)

clinical diagnosis A diagnosis based on the signs and symptoms of a disease or condition. (25)

clinical drug trial An internationally recognized research protocol designed to evaluate the efficacy or safety of drugs and to produce scientifically valid results. (21)

Clinical Laboratory Improvement Amendments (CLIA '88) A law enacted by Congress in 1988 that placed all laboratory facilities that conduct tests for diagnosing, preventing, or treating human disease or for assessing human health under federal regulations administered by the Health Care Financing Administration (HCFA) and the Centers for Disease Control and Prevention (CDC). (32)

clinical pharmacology See **pharmacotherapeutics.** (37)

closed file A file for a patient who has died, moved away, or for some other reason no longer consults the office for medical expertise. (10)

closed posture A position that conveys the feeling of not being totally receptive to what is being said; arms are often rigid or folded across the chest. (4)

cluster scheduling The scheduling of similar appointments together at a certain time of the day or week. (12)

coagulation The process by which a clot forms in blood. (34)

cocci See **coccus.**

coccus A spherical, round, or ovoid bacterium. (35)

cochlea A spiral-shaped canal in the inner ear that contains the hearing receptors. (26)

coinsurance A fixed percentage of covered charges paid by the insured person after a deductible has been met. (15)

collection percentage The total amount of payments received by the practice compared to the total amount of charges assessed for the year. (17)

colonoscopy A procedure used to determine the cause of diarrhea, constipation, bleeding, or lower abdominal pain by inserting a scope through the anus to provide direct visualization of the large intestine. (28)

colony A distinct group of microorganisms, visible with the naked eye, on the surface of a culture medium. (35)

color family A group of colors that share certain characteristics, such as warmth or coolness, allowing them to blend well together. (13)

colposcopy The examination of the vagina and cervix with an instrument called a colposcope to identify abnormal tissue, such as cancerous or precancerous cells. (27)

comorbidity A preexisting condition unrelated to the condition for which the patient is currently being treated. (15)

compactible file Files kept on rolling shelves that slide along permanent tracks in the floor and are stored close together or stacked when not in use. (10)

complete proteins Proteins that contain all nine essential amino acids. (36)

complex carbohydrates Long chains of sugar units; also known as polysaccharides. (36)

compound microscope A microscope that uses two lenses to magnify the image created by condensed light focused through the object being examined. (32)

computed tomography (CAT scan) A radiographic examination that produces a three-dimensional, cross-sectional view of an area of the body; may be performed with or without a contrast medium. (28)

conciseness Brevity; the use of no unnecessary words. (7)

concussion A jarring injury to the brain; the most common type of head injury. (31)

conductive hearing loss A type of hearing loss caused by an interruption in the transmission of sound waves to the inner ear. (26)

cones Light-sensing nerve cells in the eye, at the posterior of the retina, that are sensitive to color, provide sharp images, and function only in bright light. (26)

conflict An opposition of opinions or ideas. (4)

conjunctiva The protective membrane that lines the eyelid and covers the anterior of the sclera, or the white of the eye. (26)

consumable Able to be emptied or used up, as with supplies. (22)

consumer education The process by which the average person learns to make informed decisions about goods and services, including health care. (14)

contagious Having a disease that can easily be transmitted to others. (13)

contaminated Soiled or stained, particularly through contact with potentially infectious substances; no longer clean or sterile. (1)

contraindication A symptom that renders use of a remedy or procedure inadvisable, usually because of risk. (20)

contrast medium A substance that makes internal organs denser and blocks the passage of x-rays to photographic film. Introducing a contrast medium into certain structures or areas of the body can provide a clear image of organs and tissues and highlight indications of how well they are functioning. (40)

controlled substance A drug or drug product that is categorized as potentially dangerous and addictive and is strictly regulated by federal laws. (37)

control sample A specimen that has a known value; used as a comparison for test results on a patient sample. (32)

contusion A closed wound, or bruise. (31)

convulsion See **seizure.** (31)

coordination of benefits A legal principle that limits payment by insurance companies to 100% of the cost of covered expenses. (15)

co-payment A small fee paid by the insured at the time of a medical service rather than by the insurance company. (15)

cornea A transparent area on the front of the outer layer of the eye that acts as a window to let light into the eye. (26)

counter check A special bank check that allows a depositor to draw funds from his own account only, as when he has forgotten his checkbook. (18)

courtesy title A title used before a person's name, such as Dr., Mr., or Ms. (7)

cover sheet A form sent with a fax that provides details about the transmission. (5)

craniosacral therapy An alternative therapy in which the bones of the skull are manipulated through rhythmic motions that shift the pressure of the cerebrospinal fluid. (30)

crash cart A rolling cart of emergency supplies and equipment. (31)

credit An extension of time to pay for services, which are provided on trust. (17)

credit bureau A company that provides information about the creditworthiness of a person seeking credit. (17)

cross-referenced Filed in two or more places, with each place noted in each file; the exact contents of the file may be duplicated, or a cross-reference form can be created, listing all the places to find the file. (10)

cryosurgery The use of extreme cold to destroy unwanted tissue, such as skin lesions. (29)

cryotherapy The application of cold to a patient's body for therapeutic reasons. (30)

crystals Naturally produced solids of definite form; commonly seen in urine specimens, especially those permitted to cool. (33)

CT scan See **computed tomography.** (28)

culture In the sociological sense, a pattern of assumptions, beliefs, and practices that shape the way people think and act. (25)

culture To place a sample of a specimen in or on a substance that allows microorganisms to grow in order to identify the microorganisms present. (35)

culture and sensitivity (C & S) A procedure that involves culturing a specimen and then testing the isolated bacteria's susceptibility (sensitivity) to certain antibiotics to determine which antibiotics would be most effective in treating an infection. (35)

culture medium A substance containing all the nutrients a particular type of microorganism needs to grow. (35)

curriculum vitae A concise summary of one's education, skills, and experience; see also **résumé.** (1)

cursor A blinking line or cube on a computer screen that shows where the next character that is keyed will appear. (6)

cycle billing A system that sends invoices to groups of patients every few days, spreading the work of billing all patients over the month while billing each patient only once. (17)

DACUM (Developing A CurriculUM) A process developed by the AAMA to analyze the medical assisting profession and outline the duties and competencies that an effective medical assistant must have. (1)

damages Money paid as compensation for violating legal rights. (17)

database A collection of records created and stored on a computer. (6)

dateline The line at the top of a letter that contains the month, day, and year. (7)

debridement The removal of debris or dead tissue from a wound to expose healthy tissue. (29)

decibel A unit for measuring the relative intensity of sounds on a scale from 0 to 130. (26)

deductible A fixed dollar amount that must be paid by the insured before additional expenses are covered by an insurer. (15)

defibrillator An electrical device that shocks the heart to restore normal beating; normally found in a crash cart. (31)

deflection A peak or valley on an electrocardiogram. (39)

dehydration The condition that results from a lack of adequate water in the body. (31)

dependent A person who depends on another person for financial support. (18)

depolarization The loss of polarity, or opposite charges inside and outside; the electrical impulse that initiates a chain reaction resulting in contraction. (39)

dermatologist A specialist who diagnoses and treats diseases of the skin, hair, and nails. (2)

dermis The middle layer of the skin, which contains connective tissue, nerve endings, hair follicles, sweat glands, and oil glands. (23)

diabetes mellitus Any of several related endocrine disorders characterized by an elevated level of glucose in the blood, caused by a deficiency of insulin or insulin resistance at the cellular level. (28)

diagnosis-related group (DRG) A group of procedures or tests that is related directly to a given diagnosis and constitutes a reasonable set of procedures to be covered by an insurer. (15)

diagnostic radiology The use of x-ray technology to determine the cause of a patient's symptoms. (40)

diastolic pressure The blood pressure measured when the heart relaxes. (24)

diathermy A type of heat therapy in which a machine produces high-frequency waves that achieve deep heat penetration in muscle tissue. (30)

differential diagnosis The process of determining the correct diagnosis when two or more diagnoses are possible. (25)

differently abled Having a condition that limits or changes a person's abilities and may require special accommodations. (13)

digital examination Part of a physical examination in which the physician inserts one or two fingers of one hand into the opening of a body canal such as the vagina or the rectum; used to palpate canal and related structures. (25)

diluent A liquid used to dissolve and dilute another substance, such as a drug. (38)

disability insurance Insurance that provides a monthly, prearranged payment to an individual who cannot work as the result of an injury or disability. (15)

disbursement Any payment of funds made by the physician's office for goods and services. (8)

disclosure statement A written description of agreed terms of payment; also called a federal Truth in Lending statement. (17)

disease A disturbed or abnormal state of the body. (23)

disinfectant A cleaning product applied to instruments and equipment to reduce or eliminate infectious organisms; not used on human tissue. (20)

disinfection The destruction of infectious agents on an object or surface by direct application of chemical or physical means. (19)

dislocation The displacement of a bone end from a joint. (31)

dispense To distribute a drug, in a properly labeled container, to a patient who is to use it. (37)

distribution The biochemical process of transporting a drug from its administration site in the body to its site of action. (37)

doctor of osteopathy A doctor who focuses special attention on the musculoskeletal system and uses hands and eyes to identify and adjust structural problems, supporting the body's natural tendency toward health and self-healing. (2)

documentation The recording of information in a patient's medical record; includes detailed notes about each contact with the patient and about the treatment plan, patient progress, and treatment outcomes. (9)

dosage The size, frequency, and number of doses. (37)

dose The amount of a drug given or taken at one time. (37)

dot matrix printer An impact printer that creates characters by placing a series of tiny dots next to one another. (6)

double-booking system A system of scheduling where two or more patients are booked for the same appointment slot, assuming both patients will be seen by the doctor within the scheduled period. (12)

douche Vaginal irrigation, which can be used to administer vaginal medication in liquid form. (38)

drainage catheter A type of catheter used to withdraw fluids. (33)

dressings Sterile materials used to cover a surgical or other wound. (29)

durable item A piece of equipment that is used repeatedly, such as a telephone, computer, or examination table; contrast with **expendable item.** (8)

durable power of attorney A document naming the person who will make decisions regarding medical care on behalf of another person if that person becomes unable to do so. (3)

dyspnea Difficult or painful breathing. (24)

eardrum See **tympanic membrane.** (26)

echocardiography A procedure that tests the structure and function of the heart through the use of reflected sound waves, or echoes. (28)

edema An excessive buildup of fluid in body tissue. (30)

editing The process of ensuring that a document is accurate, clear, and complete; free of grammatical errors; organized logically; and written in the appropriate style. (7)

efficacy The therapeutic value of a procedure or therapy, such as a drug. (37)

efficiency The ability to produce a desired result with the least effort, expense, and waste. (8)

eggs See **ova.** (23)

electrical stimulation The delivery of controlled amounts of low-voltage electric current to motor and sensory nerves to stimulate muscles. (30)

electrocardiogram (ECG or **EKG)** The tracing made by an electrocardiograph. (39)

electrocardiograph An instrument that measures and displays the waves of electrical impulses responsible for the cardiac cycle. (39)

electrocardiography The process by which a graphic pattern is created to reflect the electrical impulses generated by the heart as it pumps. (39)

electrocauterization The use of a needle, probe, or loop heated by electric current to remove growths such as warts, to stop bleeding, and to control nosebleeds that either will not subside or continually recur. (29)

electrodes Sensors that detect electrical activity. (39)

electroencephalography A procedure that records the electrical activity of the brain as a tracing called an electroencephalogram, or EEG, on a strip of graph paper. (28)

electrolyte A compound that separates into positively and negatively charged parts (ions) when it dissolves. In the diet, electrolytes are essential to fluid balance, muscle contraction, nerve conduction, and other body functions; they also enhance transmission of electric current. (23)

electromyography A procedure in which needle electrodes are inserted into some of the skeletal muscles and a monitor records the nerve impulses and measures conduction time; used to detect neuromuscular disorders or nerve damage. (28)

electronic mail A method of sending and receiving messages through a computer network; commonly known as E-mail. (6)

electron microscope A microscope that uses a beam of electrons instead of a beam of light; can magnify an image several million times. (32)

eligibility The status of a person's qualification for coverage by an insurance plan. (15)

embolism An obstruction in a blood vessel. (27)

emergency medical services (EMS) system A network of qualified emergency personnel who use community resources and equipment to provide emergency care to victims of injury or sudden illness. (31)

empathy Identification with or sensitivity to another person's feelings and problems. (4)

employment contract A written agreement of employment terms between employer and employee that describes the employee's duties and the considerations (money, benefits, and so on) to be given by the employer in exchange. (18)

endocrinologist A specialist who diagnoses and treats disorders of the endocrine system, which regulates many body functions by circulating hormones that are secreted by glands throughout the body. (2)

endogenous infection An infection in which an abnormality or malfunction in routine body processes causes normally beneficial or harmless microorganisms to become pathogenic. (19)

endorse To sign or stamp the back of a check with the proper identification of the person or organization to whom the check is made out, to prevent the check from being cashed if it is stolen or lost. (16)

endoscopy Any procedure in which a scope is used to visually inspect a canal or cavity within the body. (28)

enunciation Clear and distinct speaking. (11)

enzyme A protein that speeds up chemical processes necessary for life. (23)

enzyme-linked immunosorbent assay (ELISA) test A blood test that confirms the presence of antibodies developed by the body's immune system in response to an initial HIV infection. (21)

eosinophil A type of granular leukocyte that captures invading bacteria and antigen-antibody complexes through phagocytosis. (34)

epidermis The outermost layer of the skin, consisting entirely of epithelial cells. (23)

epistaxis Nosebleed. (31)

erythema Redness of the skin. (30)

erythrocytes Red blood cells. (34)

erythrocyte sedimentation rate (ESR) The rate at which red blood cells, the heaviest blood component, settle to the bottom of a blood sample. (34)

estrogen A female sex hormone; when produced during ovulation, estrogen causes a buildup of the lining of the uterus (womb) to prepare it for a possible pregnancy. (23)

ethics General principles of right and wrong, as opposed to requirements of law. (3)

etiologic agent A living microorganism or its toxin that may cause human disease. (35)

etiquette Good manners. (11)

eukaryotic Having a complex cell structure, including a nucleus, cytoplasm, and cytoplasmic organelles. (35)

eustachian tube An opening in the middle ear, leading to the back of the throat, that helps equalize air pressure on both sides of the eardrum. (26)

exclusion An expense that is not covered by a particular insurance policy, such as an eye examination or dental care. (15)

excretion The elimination of waste by a discharge; in drug metabolism, the manner in which a drug is eliminated from the body. (37)

excretory urography See **intravenous pyelography.** (40)

exogenous infection An infection that is caused by the introduction of a pathogen from outside the body. (19)

expendable item An item that is used and must then be restocked; also known collectively as supplies. Contrast with **durable item.** (8)

explanation of benefits (EOB) A form sent by the insurance company to both the subscriber and the medical practice that contains information on a claim, including amount billed and amount covered by the insurance policy, co-payments, and deductibles; the copy sent to the designated recipient for that claim is accompanied by claim payment. (15)

extension An unbending or straightening movement of the two elements of a jointed body part. (23)

externship A period of practical work experience performed by a medical assisting student in a physician's office, hospital, or other health-care facility. (1)

facultative Able to adapt to different conditions; in microbiology, able to grow in environments either with or without oxygen. (35)

Fahrenheit One of two common scales used for measuring temperature; measured in degrees Fahrenheit, or °F. (24)

family practitioner A physician who does not specialize in a branch of medicine but treats all types and ages of patients; also called a general practitioner. (2)

farsightedness See **hyperopia.** (28)

fast To refrain from eating or drinking; required by some procedures and tests. (12)

febrile Having a body temperature above one's normal range. (24)

federal Truth in Lending statement See **disclosure statement.** (17)

feedback Verbal and nonverbal evidence that a message was received and understood. (5)

fee schedule A list of the costs of common services and procedures performed by a physician. (15)

fenestrated drape A drape that has a round or slitlike opening that provides access to the surgical site. (29)

fiber The tough, stringy part of vegetables and grains, which is not absorbed by the body but aids in a variety of bodily functions. (36)

file guide A heavy cardboard or plastic insert used to identify a group of file folders in a file drawer. (10)

first aid The immediate care given to a person who is injured or suddenly becomes ill before complete medical care can be obtained. (31)

first morning urine specimen A urine specimen that is collected after a night's sleep; contains greater concentrations of substances that collect over time than specimens taken during the day. (33)

fixative A chemical spray used to preserve a specimen obtained from the body for pathologic examination. (22)

flexion A bending movement of the two elements of a jointed body part. (23)

floater A nonsterile assistant who is free to move about the room during surgery and attend to unsterile needs. (29)

fluidotherapy A technique for stimulating healing, particularly in the hands and feet, by placing the affected body part in a container of glass beads that are heated and agitated with hot air. (30)

fomite An inanimate object, such as clothing, body fluids, water, or food, that may be contaminated with infectious organisms and thus serve to transmit disease. (19)

food exchange A unit of food in a particular food category that provides the same amounts of protein, fat, and carbohydrates as all other units of food in that category. (36)

forced vital capacity The greatest volume of air that a person is able to expel when performing rapid, forced expiration. (39)

formalin A dilute solution of formaldehyde used to preserve biological specimens. (29)

formed elements Red blood cells, white blood cells, and platelets; comprise 45% of blood volume. (34)

401(k) plan A specific type of pension plan in which the employer deposits part of the employee's paycheck in a trust account. The amount is taken out of the employee's salary before taxes are calculated and not taxed until the money is withdrawn. (16)

fracture Any break in a bone. (28)

frequency The number of complete fluctuations of energy per second in the form of waves. (26)

full-block letter style A letter format in which all lines begin flush left; also called block style. (7)

fungus A eukaryotic organism that has a rigid cell wall at some stage in the life cycle. (35)

gait The way a person walks, consisting of two phases: stance and swing. (30)

gastroenterologist A specialist who diagnoses and treats disorders of the entire gastrointestinal tract, including the stomach, intestines, and associated digestive organs. (2)

general physical examination An examination performed by a physician to confirm a patient's health or to diagnose a medical problem. (22)

general practitioner See **family practitioner.** (2)

generic name A drug's official name. (37)

geriatrics The branch of medicine that deals with the diagnosis and treatment of problems and diseases of the older adult.

gerontologist A specialist who studies the aging process. (2)

glomerular filtration The process by which urine forms in the kidneys as blood moves through a tight ball of capillaries called the glomerulus. (33)

glycosuria The presence of significant levels of glucose in the urine. (33)

goniometer A protractor device that measures range of motion. (30)

gram-negative Referring to bacteria that lose their purple color when a decolorizer has been added during a Gram's stain. (35)

gram-positive Referring to bacteria that retain their purple color after a decolorizer has been added during a Gram's stain. (35)

Gram's stain A method of staining that differentiates bacteria according to the chemical composition of their cell walls. (35)

granular leukocyte A type of leukocyte (white blood cell) with a segmented nucleus and granulated cytoplasm; also known as a polymorphonuclear leukocyte. (34)

gross earnings The total amount an employee earns before deductions. (18)

gynecologist A specialist who performs routine physical care and examinations of the female reproductive system. (2)

hairy leukoplakia A white lesion on the tongue associated with AIDS. (21)

hammer See **malleus.** (26)

hard copy A readable paper copy or printout of information. (6)

hardware The physical components of a computer system, including the monitor, keyboard, and printer. (6)

hazard label A shortened version of the Material Safety Data Sheet; permanently affixed to a hazardous substance container. (32)

health insurance provider The company that covers a portion of a patient's health-care costs. (15)

health maintenance organization (HMO) A health-care organization that provides specific services to individuals and their dependents who are enrolled in the plan. Doctors who enroll in an HMO agree to provide certain services in exchange for a prepaid fee. (15)

helper T-cells White blood cells that are a key component of the body's immune system and that work in coordination with other white blood cells to combat infection. (21)

hematemesis The vomiting of blood. (31)

hematocrit The percentage of the volume of a sample made up of red blood cells after the sample has been spun in a centrifuge. (34)

hematology The study of blood. (34)

hematoma A swelling caused by blood under the skin. (31)

hematuria The presence of blood in the urine. (33)

hemocytometer A special microscope slide that allows blood cells to be counted when a diluted blood sample is examined under the microscope. (34)

hemoglobin A protein that contains iron and bonds with and carries oxygen to cells; the main component of erythrocytes. (34)

hemoglobinuria The presence of free hemoglobin in the urine; a rare condition caused by transfusion reactions, malaria, drug reactions, snake bites, or severe burns. (33)

hemolysis The rupturing of red blood cells, which releases hemoglobin. (34)

Holter monitor An electrocardiography device that includes a small portable cassette recorder worn around a patient's waist or on a shoulder strap to record the heart's electrical activity. (39)

homeopathy The use of natural substances from plants, minerals, and animals to stimulate the body's healing. (30)

homeostasis A balanced, stable state within the body. (23)

hormone A chemical produced within the body that can affect activities such as growth, metabolism, and reproduction. (23)

host A body in which a microorganism can survive, multiply, and thrive. (19)

hydrotherapy The therapeutic use of water to treat physical problems. (30)

hyperglycemia High blood sugar. (31)

hypermetropia See **hyperopia.**

hyperopia A condition in which images come into focus behind the retina, so that faraway objects are seen clearly, but nearby objects are unclear; also called hypermetropia or farsightedness. (28)

hyperpnea Abnormally deep, rapid breathing. (24)

hypertension High blood pressure. (24)

hyperventilation Overly deep breathing that leads to a loss of carbon dioxide in the blood. (25)

hypoglycemia Low blood sugar. (31)

hypotension Low blood pressure. (24)

hypovolemic shock A state of shock resulting from insufficient blood volume in the circulatory system. (31)

icon A pictorial image; on a computer screen, a graphic symbol that identifies a menu choice. (6)

identification line A line at the bottom of a letter containing the letter writer's initials and the typist's initials. (7)

immunity The condition of being resistant or not susceptible to pathogens and the diseases they cause. (19)

immunization The administration of a vaccine or toxoid to protect susceptible individuals from communicable diseases. (20)

immunocompromised Having an impaired or weakened immune system. (21)

immunofluorescent antibody (IFA) test A blood test used to confirm enzyme-linked immunosorbent assay (ELISA) test results for HIV infection. (21)

inactive file A file used infrequently. (10)

incision A surgical wound made by cutting into body tissue. (29)

incomplete proteins Proteins that lack one or more of the essential amino acids. (36)

incus A small bone in the middle ear, located between the malleus and the stapes; also called the anvil. (26)

independent practice association (IPA) An HMO that uses only certain doctors, under contract, to provide procedures and services. IPAs are composed of physicians who practice independently. (15)

indication The purpose or reason for using a drug, as approved by the FDA. (37)

infectious waste Waste that can be dangerous to those who handle it or to the environment; includes human waste, human tissue, and body fluids, as well as potentially hazardous waste, such as used needles, scalpels, and dressings, and cultures of human cells. (13)

infestation An infection caused by a parasite. (35)

informed consent form A form that verifies that a patient understands the offered treatment and its possible outcomes or side effects. (9)

infusion A slow drip, as of an intravenous solution into a vein. (38)

ingestion Swallowing. (22)

inhalation Breathing. (22)

ink-jet printer A nonimpact printer that forms characters by using a series of dots created by tiny drops of ink. (6)

inoculate To place a sample of a specimen on or in a culture medium. (35)

inpatient A patient who is confined to a hospital and receives treatment there. (15)

insulin A hormone that regulates the amount of sugar in the blood by facilitating its entry into the cells. (23)

insured See **subscriber.** (15)

interim room A room off the patient reception area and away from the examination rooms for occasions when patients require privacy. (13)

Internet A global network of computers. (6)

internist A doctor who specializes in diagnosing and treating problems related to the internal organs. (2)

interpersonal skills Attitudes, qualities, and abilities that influence the level of success and satisfaction achieved in interacting with other people. (4)

intradermal Within the upper layers of the skin. (38)

intradermal test An allergy test in which dilute solutions of allergens are introduced into the skin of the inner forearm or upper back with a fine-gauge needle. (28)

intramuscular (IM) Within muscle; an IM injection allows administration of a larger amount of a drug than a subcutaneous injection allows. (38)

intraoperative Taking place during surgery. (29)

intravenous (IV) Injected directly into a vein. (38)

intravenous pyelography (IVP) A radiologic procedure in which the doctor injects a contrast medium into a vein and takes a series of x-rays of the kidneys, ureters, and bladder to evaluate urinary system abnormalities or trauma to the urinary system. Also known as excretory urography. (40)

invasive Referring to a procedure in which a catheter, wire, or other foreign object is introduced into a blood vessel or organ through the skin or a body orifice. Surgical asepsis is required during all invasive tests. (40)

inventory A list of supplies used regularly and the quantities in stock. (8)

invoice A bill for materials or services received by or services performed by the practice. (8)

iris The colored part of the eye, made of muscular tissue that contracts and relaxes, altering the size of the pupil. (26)

itinerary A detailed travel plan listing dates and times for specific transportation arrangements and events, the location of meetings and lodgings, and phone numbers. (12)

jaundice A condition characterized by yellowness of the skin, eyes, mucous membranes, and excretions; occurs during the second stage of hepatitis infection. (21)

journalizing The process of logging charges and receipts in a chronological list each day; used in the single-entry system of bookkeeping. (16)

Kaposi's sarcoma Abnormal tissue occurring in the skin, and sometimes in the lymph nodes and organs, manifested by reddish-purple to dark blue patches or spots on the skin. (21)

keratin A tough, hard protein contained in skin, hair, and nails. (35)

kilocalorie See **calorie.** (36)

KOH mount (potassium hydroxide mount) A type of mount used when a physician suspects a patient has a fungal infection of the skin, nails, or hair and to which potassium hydroxide is added to dissolve the keratin in cell walls. (35)

KUB (kidneys, ureters, and bladder) radiography The process of x-raying the abdomen to help assess the size, shape, and position of the urinary organs; evaluate urinary system diseases or disorders; or determine the presence of kidney stones. It can also be helpful in determining the position of an intrauterine device (IUD) or in locating foreign bodies in the digestive tract. Also called a "flat plate of the abdomen." (40)

labeling Information provided with a drug, including FDA-approved indications and the form of the drug. (37)

labyrinth The inner ear. (26)

laceration A jagged, open wound in the skin that can extend down into the underlying tissue. (29)

lacrimal gland A gland in the eye that produces tears. (26)

lag phase The initial phase of wound healing, in which bleeding is reduced as blood vessels in the affected area constrict. (29)

lancet A small, disposable instrument with a sharp point used to puncture the skin and make a shallow incision; used for capillary puncture. (34)

laser printer A high-resolution printer that uses a technology similar to that of a photocopier. It is the fastest type of computer printer and produces the highest-quality output. (6)

lateral file A horizontal filing cabinet that features doors that flip up and a pull-out drawer, where files are arranged with sides facing out. (10)

law A rule of conduct established and enforced by an authority or governing body, such as the federal government. (3)

law of agency A law stating that an employee is considered to be acting on the physician's behalf while performing professional duties. (3)

lead A view of a specific area of the heart on an electrocardiogram. (39)

lease To rent an item or piece of equipment. (5)

legal custody The court-decreed right to have control over a child's upbringing and to take responsibility for the child's care, including health care. (17)

lens A clear, circular disc located in the eye, just posterior to the iris, that can change shape to help the eye focus images of objects that are near or far away. (26)

letterhead Formal business stationery, with the doctor's (or office's) name and address printed at the top, used for correspondence with patients, colleagues, and vendors. (7)

leukocytes White blood cells. (34)

Level I tests Laboratory tests of moderate complexity; make up approximately 75% of all tests performed in the laboratory and require stricter standards for certification than Certificate of Waiver tests. (32)

Level II tests High-complexity laboratory procedures; require stricter standards for certification than either Certificate of Waiver or Level I tests. (32)

liable Legally responsible. (3)

ligament A tough, fibrous band of tissue that connects bone to bone. (23)

ligature Suture material. (29)

limited check A check that is void after a certain time limit; commonly used for payroll. (18)

lipoproteins Large molecules that are fat-soluble on the inside and water-soluble on the outside and carry lipids such as cholesterol and triglycerides through the bloodstream. (36)

living will A legal document addressed to a patient's family and health-care providers stating what type of treatment the patient wishes or does not wish to receive if he becomes terminally ill, unconscious, or permanently comatose; sometimes called an advance directive. (3)

locum tenens A substitute physician hired to see patients while the regular physician is away from the office. (12)

lower GI (gastrointestinal) series See **barium enema.** (40)

lymph The part of the blood that does not return from body tissue to the capillaries but drains into lymph vessels and is filtered through a series of lymph nodes to remove any foreign material or bacteria. (23)

macrophage A type of phagocytic cell found in the liver, spleen, lungs, bone marrow, and connective tissue. Macrophages play several roles in humoral and cell-mediated immunity, including presenting the antigens to the lymphocytes involved in these defenses. Also known as monocytes while in the bloodstream. (19)

magnetic resonance imaging (MRI) A viewing technique that uses a powerful magnetic field to produce an image of internal body structures. (28)

maintenance contract A contract that specifies when a piece of equipment will be cleaned, checked for worn parts, and repaired. (5)

malleus A small bone in the middle ear that is attached to the eardrum; also called the hammer. (26)

malpractice claim A lawsuit brought by a patient against a physician for errors in diagnosis or treatment. (3)

managed care Health care managed by organizations that negotiate and contract health care to keep costs down. (15)

Material Safety Data Sheet (MSDS) A form that is required for all hazardous chemicals or other substances used in the laboratory and that contains information about the product's name, ingredients, chemical characteristics, physical and health hazards, guidelines for safe handling, and procedures to be followed in the event of exposure. (32)

matrix The basic format of an appointment book, established by blocking off times on the schedule during which the doctor is able to see patients. (12)

maturation phase The third phase of wound healing, in which scar tissue forms. (29)

Mayo stand A movable stainless steel instrument tray on a stand. (29)

Medicaid A federally funded health cost assistance program for low-income, blind, and disabled patients; families receiving aid to dependent children; foster children; and children with birth defects. (15)

medical asepsis Measures taken to reduce the number of microorganisms, such as hand washing and wearing examination gloves, that do not necessarily eliminate microorganisms; also called clean technique. (29)

medical emergency Any situation in which a person suddenly becomes ill or sustains an injury that requires immediate help by a health-care professional. (31)

Medicare A national health insurance program for Americans aged 65 and older. (15)

Medigap Private insurance that Medicare recipients can purchase to reduce the gap in coverage—the amount they would have to pay from their own pockets after receiving Medicare benefits. (15)

meiosis A type of cell division in which each new cell contains only one member of each chromosome pair. (23)

meniscus The curve in the air-to-liquid surface of a liquid specimen in a container. (24)

menstruation The monthly shedding of the lining of the uterus when pregnancy does not occur. (23)

mensuration The measurment of weight and height. (24)

metabolism The overall chemical functioning of the body, including all body processes that build small molecules into large ones (anabolism) and break down large molecules into small ones (catabolism). (24)

metastasis The transfer of abnormal cells to body sites far removed from the original tumor. (28)

microbiology The study of microorganisms. (35)

microfiche Microfilm in rectangular sheets. (5)

microfilm A roll of film stored on a reel and imprinted with information on a reduced scale to minimize storage space requirements. (5)

microorganism A simple form of life, commonly made up of a single cell and so small that it can be seen only with a microscope. (19)

micropipette A small pipette that holds a small, precise volume of fluid; used to collect capillary blood. (34)

minerals Natural, inorganic substances the body needs to help build and maintain body tissues and carry on life functions. (36)

minutes A report of what happened and what was discussed and decided at a meeting. (12)

mitosis A type of cell division that produces ordinary body, or somatic, cells; each new cell receives a complete set of paired chromosomes. (23)

mobility aids Devices that improve one's ability to move from one place to another; also called mobility assistive devices. (30)

mobility assistive devices See **mobility aids.**

modeling The process of teaching the patient a new skill by having the patient observe and imitate it. (14)

modem A device used to transfer information from one computer to another through telephone lines. (6)

modified-block letter style A letter format similar to full-block style, except that the dateline, complimentary closing, signature block, and notations are aligned and begin at the center of the page or slightly to the right of center. (7)

modified-wave scheduling A scheduling system similar to the wave system, with patients arriving at planned intervals during the hour, allowing time to catch up before the next hour begins. (12)

mold Fungi that grow into large, fuzzy, multicelled organisms that produce spores. (35)

money order A certificate of guaranteed payment, which may be purchased from a bank, a post office, or some convenience stores. (16)

monocyte A large white blood cell with an oval or horseshoe-shaped nucleus that defends the body by phagocytosis; develops into a macrophage when it moves from blood into other tissues. (34)

mordant A substance, such as iodine, that can intensify or deepen the response a specimen has to a stain. (35)

morphology The study of the shape or form of objects. (34)

motherboard The main circuit board of a computer that controls the other components in the system. (6)

mucocutaneous exposure Exposure to a pathogen through mucous membranes. (21)

MUGA scan A radiologic procedure that evaluates the condition of the heart's myocardium; involves injection of radioisotopes that concentrate in the myocardium, followed by the use of a gamma camera to measure ventricular contractions to evaluate the patient's heart wall. (40)

multimedia More than one medium, such as in graphics, sound, and text used to convey information. (6)

multitasking Running two or more computer software programs simultaneously. (6)

myelography An x-ray visualization of the spinal cord after the injection of a radioactive contrast medium or air into the spinal subarachnoid space (between the second and innermost of three membranes that cover the spinal cord). This test can reveal tumors, cysts, spinal stenosis, or herniated disks. (28)

myocardial infarction (MI) A heart attack that occurrs when the blood flow to the heart is reduced as a result of blockage in the coronary arteries or their branches. (31)

myoglobinuria The presence of myoglobin in the urine; can be caused by injured or damaged muscle tissue. (33)

myopia A condition in which images come into focus in front of the retina, so that nearby objects are seen clearly but faraway objects are unclear. (28)

narcotic A popular term for an opioid and term of choice in government agencies; see **opioid.** (37)

nasal mucosa The lining of the nose. (25)

naturopathy The treatment of conditions through diet, herbs, and preventive techniques that rely on the body's natural mechanisms of healing. (30)

needle biopsy A procedure in which a needle and syringe are used to aspirate (withdraw by suction) fluid or tissue cells. (29)

negligence A medical professional's failure to perform an essential action or his performance of an improper action that directly results in the harm of a patient. (3)

negotiable Legally transferable from one person to another. (16)

nephrologist A specialist who studies, diagnoses, and manages diseases of the kidney. (2)

nephron The functional unit of the kidneys that filters water and waste products from the blood. (23)

net earnings Take-home pay, calculated by subtracting total deductions from gross earnings. (18)

network A system that links several computers together. (6)

neurologist A specialist who diagnoses and treats disorders and diseases of the nervous system, including the brain, spinal cord, and nerves. (2)

neuron A nerve cell, which carries nerve impulses between the brain or spinal cord and other parts of the body. (23)

neutrophil A type of granular leukocyte that aids in phagocytosis by attacking bacterial invaders; also responsible for the release of pyrogens. (34)

nocturia Excessive nighttime urination. (33)

nongranular leukocyte A type of leukocyte (white blood cell) with a solid nucleus and clear cytoplasm; includes lymphocytes and monocytes; also called agranular leukocyte. (34)

noninvasive Referring to procedures that do not require inserting devices, breaking the skin, or monitoring to the degree needed with invasive procedures. (40)

normal flora Beneficial bacteria found in the body that create a barrier against pathogens by producing substances that may harm invaders and using up the resources pathogens need to live. (19)

no-show A patient who does not call to cancel and does not come to an appointment. (12)

nosocomial infection An infection contracted in a hospital. (20)

nuclear medicine The use of radionuclides, or radioisotopes (radioactive elements or their compounds), to evaluate the bone, brain, lungs, kidneys, liver, pancreas, thyroid, and spleen; also known as radionuclide imaging. (40)

nucleus The control center of a cell; contains the chromosomes that direct cellular processes. (23)

numeric filing system A filing system that organizes files by numbers instead of names. Each patient is assigned a number in the order in which she joins the practice. (10)

O and P specimen An ova and parasites specimen, or a stool sample, that is examined for the presence of certain forms of protozoans or parasites, including their eggs (ova). (35)

objectives The set of magnifying lenses contained in the nosepiece of a compound microscope. (32)

occult blood Blood contained in some other substance, not visible to the naked eye. (22)

ocular An eyepiece of a microscope. (32)

oil-immersion objective A microscope objective that is designed to be lowered into a drop of immersion oil placed directly above the prepared specimen under examination, eliminating the air space between the microscope slide and the objective and producing a much sharper, brighter image. (32)

ointment A form of topical drug; also known as a salve. (38)

Older Americans Act of 1965 A U.S. law that guarantees certain benefits to elderly citizens, including health care, retirement income, and protection against abuse. (13)

oliguria Insufficient production (or volume) of urine. (33)

oncologist A specialist who identifies tumors and treats patients who have cancer. (2)

onychectomy The removal of a fingernail or toenail. (29)

open-book account An account that is open to charges made occasionally as needed. (17)

open hours scheduling A system of scheduling where patients arrive at the doctor's office at their convenience and are seen on a first-come, first-served basis. (12)

open posture A position that conveys a feeling of receptiveness and friendliness; facing another person with arms comfortably at the sides or in the lap. (4)

ophthalmologist A medical doctor who is an eye specialist. (26)

ophthalmoscope A hand-held instrument with a light; used to view inner eye structures. (28)

opioid A natural or synthetic drug that produces opiumlike effects. (37)

opportunistic infection Infection by microorganisms that can cause disease only when a host's resistance is low. (19)

optical microscope A microscope that uses light, concentrated through a condenser and focused through the object being examined, to project an image. (32)

optometrist A trained and licensed vision specialist who is not a physician. (26)

orbit The eye socket, which forms a protective shell around the eye. (26)

orthopedist A specialist who diagnoses and treats diseases and disorders of the muscles and bones. (2)

osteoporosis An endocrine and metabolic disorder of the musculoskeletal system, more common in women than in men, characterized by hunched-over posture. (27)

otologist A medical doctor who specializes in the health of the ear. (26)

otorhinolaryngologist A specialist who diagnoses and treats diseases of the ear, nose, and throat. (2)

out guide A marker made of stiff material and used as a placeholder when a file is taken out of a filing system. (10)

outpatient A patient who travels to a hospital for care but who is not confined to the hospital. (15)

ova Female reproductive cells; also called eggs. (23)

overbooking Scheduling appointments for more patients than can reasonably be seen in the time allowed. (12)

ovulation The process by which the ovaries release one ovum (egg) approximately every 28 days. (23)

pacemaker See **sinoatrial (SA) node.** (39)

packed red blood cells Red blood cells that collect at the bottom of a centrifuged blood sample. (34)

palpated systolic pressure Systolic blood pressure measured by using the sense of touch. This measurement provides a necessary preliminary approximation of the systolic blood pressure to ensure an adequate level of inflation when the actual auscultatory measurement is made. (24)

palpitations Unusually rapid, strong, or irregular pulsations of the heart. (31)

parasite An organism that lives on or in another organism and relies on it for nourishment or some other advantage to the detriment of the host organism. (35)

parasympathetic nervous system The part of the peripheral autonomic nervous system that responds by returning the body to its normal state after stress has passed. (23)

parenteral nutrition Nutrition obtained when specially prepared nutrients are injected directly into patients' veins rather than taken by mouth. (36)

passive listening Hearing what a person has to say without responding in any way; contrast with **active listening.** (4)

passive voice The feature of a verb that indicates the subject of a sentence is being acted upon, or receiving the action, as in "The report was sent to us yesterday"; contrast with **active voice.** (7)

patch See **transdermal.** (38)

patch test An allergy test in which a gauze patch soaked with a suspected allergen is taped onto the skin with nonallergenic tape; used to discover the cause of contact dermatitis. (28)

pathogen A microorganism capable of causing disease. (19)

pathologist A medical doctor who studies the changes a disease produces in the cells, fluids, and processes of the entire body. (2)

patient compliance Obedience in terms of following a physician's orders. (25)

patient ledger card A card containing information needed for insurance purposes, including the patient's name, address, telephone number, Social Security number, insurance information, employer's name, and any special billing instructions. It also includes the name of the person who is responsible for charges if this is anyone other than the patient. (16)

patient record/chart A compilation of important information about a patient's medical history and present condition. (9)

payee A person who receives a payment. (16)

payer A person who pays a bill or writes a check. (16)

payroll deductions Amounts regularly withheld from a paycheck, such as those for federal, state, and local taxes, as well as those for such options as a 401(k) plan, life insurance, or savings bonds. (16)

pay schedule A list showing how often an employee is paid, such as weekly, biweekly, or monthly. (18)

pediatrician A specialist who diagnoses and treats childhood diseases and teaches parents skills for keeping their children healthy. (2)

peer review organization (PRO) An organization of health-care professionals who check hospital diagnoses, quality of services, and patient admissions and discharges related to government-funded health care within a state. (15)

pegboard system A bookkeeping system that uses a lightweight board with pegs on which forms can be stacked, allowing each transaction to be entered and recorded on four different bookkeeping forms at once; also called the one-write system. (16)

pension plan A retirement benefit that pays a fixed monthly amount to an employee after retirement. (16)

percutaneous exposure Exposure to a pathogen through a puncture wound or needle stick. (21)

peristalsis The rhythmic muscular contractions that move food through the digestive tract. (23)

personal space A certain area that surrounds an individual and within which another person's physical presence is felt as an intrusion. (4)

PET Positron emission tomography; a radiologic procedure that entails injecting isotopes combined with other substances involved in metabolic activity, such as glucose. These special isotopes emit positrons, which a computer processes and displays on a screen. (40)

petty cash fund Cash kept on hand in the office for small purchases. (18)

pH A standard measure of acidity or alkalinity; pH 7.0 is neutral, lower than 7.0 is acidic, higher than 7.0 is alkaline (or basic).

phagocyte A specialized white blood cell that engulfs and digests pathogens. (19)

phagocytosis The process by which white blood cells defend the body against infection by engulfing invading pathogens. (34)

pharmaceutical Pertaining to medicinal drugs. (37)

pharmacodynamics The study of what drugs do to the body: the mechanism of action, or how they work to produce a therapeutic effect. (37)

pharmacognosy The study of characteristics of natural drugs and their sources. (37)

pharmacokinetics The study of what the body does to drugs: how the body absorbs, metabolizes, distributes, and excretes the drugs. (37)

pharmacology The study of drugs. (37)

pharmacotherapeutics The study of how drugs are used to treat disease; also called clinical pharmacology. (37)

phenylketonuria (PKU) A genetically inherited disorder in which the body cannot properly metabolize the nutrient phenylalanine, resulting in the buildup of phenylketones in the blood and their presence in the urine. The accumulation of phenylketones results in mental retardation. (33)

philosophy The system of values and principles an office has adopted in its everyday practice. (14)

phlebotomy The insertion of a needle or cannula (small tube) into a vein for the purpose of withdrawing blood. (34)

photometer An instrument that measures light intensity. (32)

physiatrist A physical medicine specialist, who diagnoses and treats diseases and disorders with physical therapy. (2)

physical therapy A medical specialty that uses cold, heat, water, exercise, massage, traction, and other physical means to treat musculoskeletal, nervous, and cardiopulmonary disorders. (30)

physician's office laboratory (POL) A laboratory contained in a physician's office; processing tests in the POL produces quick turnaround and eliminates the need for patients to travel to other test locations. (32)

pitch The high or low quality in the sound of a person's speaking voice. (11)

plasma The fluid component of blood, in which formed elements are suspended; makes up 55% of blood volume. (34)

plastic surgeon A specialist who reconstructs, corrects, or improves body structures. (2)

platelets Fragments of cytoplasm in the blood that are crucial to clot formation; also called thrombocytes. (34)

poison Any substance that produces harmful effects if it enters the body. (31)

polarity The condition of having two separate poles, one of which is positive whereas the other is negative. (39)

polymorphonuclear leukocyte See **granular leukocyte.** (34)

POMR The problem-oriented medical record system for keeping patients' charts. Information in a POMR includes the database of information about the patient and the patient's condition, the problem list, the diagnostic and treatment plan, and progress notes. (9)

portfolio A collection of an applicant's résumé, reference letters, and other documents of interest to a potential employer. (1)

postoperative Taking place after a surgical procedure. (29)

posture Body position and alignment. (30)

power of attorney The legal right to act as the attorney or agent of another person, including handling that person's financial matters. (16)

practitioner One who practices a profession. (1)

preferred provider organization (PPO) A type of HMO where physicians agree to accept predetermined fees, often for complex and unusual procedures. (15)

premium The basic annual cost of health-care insurance. (15)

preoperative Taking place prior to surgery. (29)

presbyopia A condition in which aging eyes lose the ability to accommodate or thicken the lens by contracting muscles in the ciliary body, because the lens becomes more rigid. As a result, images come into focus behind the retina, as they do with farsightedness. (28)

prescribe To give a patient a prescription to be filled by a pharmacy. (37)

prescription A physician's written order for medication. (37)

prescription drug A drug that can be legally used only by order of a physician and must be administered or dispensed by a licensed health-care professional. (37)

pressure point An area of the body where major blood vessels can be occluded by direct pressure; used to help control external bleeding. (31)

P-R interval An area on an electrocardiogram that represents the time it takes for an electrical impulse to travel from the SA node to the AV node; includes the P wave and a straight line connecting it to the QRS complex. (39)

proctoscopy An examination of the lower rectum and anal canal with a 3-inch instrument called a proctoscope to detect hemorrhoids, polyps, fissures, fistulas, and abscesses. (27)

proficiency testing program A required set of tests for clinical laboratories; the tests measure the accuracy of the laboratory's test results and adherence to standard operating procedures. (32)

profit-sharing plan A special type of pension plan in which the employer adds an amount to the employee's account each year based on the organization's profits. (15)

prognosis A prediction of the probable course of a disease in an individual and the chances of recovery. (15)

prokaryotic Having a simple cell structure with no nucleus and no organelles in the cytoplasm. (35)

proliferation phase The second phase of wound healing, in which new tissue forms, closing off the wound. (29)

pronunciation The sounding out of words. (11)

proofreading Checking a document for formatting, data, and mechanical errors. (7)

protease inhibitor A drug that blocks the production of a key enzyme, protease, that is required for a host cell to replicate the HIV virus. (21)

proteinuria An excess of protein in the urine. (33)

protozoan A single-celled eukaryotic organism much larger than a bacterium; some protozoans can cause disease in humans. (35)

provider of medical services A doctor. (15)

puberty The period of adolescence when a person begins to develop secondary sexual traits and reproductive functions. (27)

pulmonary function test (PFT) A test that evaluates a patient's lung volume and capacity; used to detect and diagnose pulmonary problems or to monitor certain respiratory disorders and evaluate the effectiveness of treatment. (39)

puncture wound A deep wound caused by a sharp, pointed object. (29)

punitive damages Money paid as punishment for intentionally breaking the law. (17)

pupil The opening at the center of the iris, which grows smaller or larger as the iris contracts or relaxes, respectively; it regulates the amount of light that enters the eye. (26)

purchase order A form that authorizes a purchase for the practice. (8)

purchasing groups Groups of medical offices associated with a nearby hospital that order supplies through the hospital to obtain a quantity discount. (8)

Purkinje fibers A network of cardiac muscle fibers in the ventricle walls that causes the ventricles to contract when the electrical impulse for muscle contraction reaches them. (39)

P wave A small upward curve on an electrocardiogram that represents the wave of depolarization through the atria and the resultant contraction. (39)

pyrogens Fever-producing substances released by neutrophils. (34)

QRS complex An area on an electrocardiogram that represents the contraction (following depolarization) of the ventricles; includes the Q, R, and S waves. (39)

Q-T interval An area on an electrocardiogram that represents the time it takes for the ventricles to contract and recover, or repolarize; includes the QRS complex, S-T segment, and T wave. (39)

quadrants Four equal sections, such as those into which the abdomen is figuratively divided during an examination. (25)

qualitative analysis In microbiology, identification of bacteria present in a specimen by the appearance of colonies grown on a culture plate. (35)

qualitative test response A test result that indicates the substance tested for is either present or absent. (32)

quality assurance program A required program for clinical laboratories designed to monitor the quality of patient care, including quality control, instrument and equipment maintenance, proficiency testing, training and continuing education, and standard operating procedures documentation. (32)

quality control (QC) An ongoing system, required in every physician's office, to evaluate the quality of medical care provided. (35)

quality control program A component of a quality assurance program that focuses on ensuring accuracy in laboratory test results through careful monitoring of test procedures. (32)

quantitative analysis In microbiology, a determination of the number of bacteria present in a specimen by direct count of colonies grown on a culture plate. (35)

quantitative test results The concentration of a test substance in a specimen. (32)

quarterly return The Employer's Quarterly Federal Tax Return, a form submitted to the IRS every 3 months that summarizes the federal income and employment taxes withheld from employees' paychecks. (18)

Q wave A downward deflection on an electrocardiogram that represents the impulse for contraction traveling down the septum toward the Purkinje fibers. (39)

radial artery An artery located in the groove on the thumb side of the inner wrist, where the pulse is taken on adults. (24)

radiation therapy The use of x-rays and radioactive substances to treat cancer. (40)

radiologist A physician who specializes in taking and reading x-rays. (2)

radionuclide imaging See **nuclear medicine.** (40)

random access memory (RAM) The temporary, or programmable, memory in a computer. (6)

random urine specimen A single urine specimen taken at any time of the day; the most common type of sample collected. (33)

range of motion (ROM) The degree to which a joint is able to move. (30)

rapport A harmonious, positive relationship. (4)

read only memory (ROM) A computer's permanent memory, which can be read by the computer but not changed. It provides the computer with the basic operating instructions it needs to function. (6)

reagent A chemical or chemically treated substance used in test procedures and formulated to react in specific ways when exposed under specific conditions. (32)

reconciliation A comparison of the office's financial records with bank records to ensure that they are consistent and accurate; usually done when the monthly checking account statement is received from the bank. (16)

records management system How patient records are created, filed, and maintained. (10)

reference laboratory A laboratory owned and operated by an organization outside the physician's practice. (32)

referral An authorization from a medical practice for a patient to have specialized services performed by another practice; often required for insurance purposes. (15)

refraction examination An eye examination in which the patient looks through a succession of different lenses to find out which ones create the clearest image. (28)

refractometer An optical instrument that measures the refraction, or bending, of light as it passes through a liquid. (33)

Registered Medical Assistant (RMA) A medical assistant who has met the educational requirements and taken and passed the certification examination for medical assisting given by the American Medical Technologists (AMT). (1)

Release of Medical Information form A form signed by a patient granting permission to insurers, physicians, and other qualified personnel to examine the patient's records. (15)

repolarization The restoration of polarity after depolarization. (39)

reputable Having a good reputation. (8)

requisition A formal request from a staff member or doctor for the purchase of equipment or supplies. (8)

reservoir host An animal, insect, or human whose body is susceptible to growth of a pathogen. (19)

respiration The exchange of gases between air and blood and between blood and body cells. (23)

résumé A typewritten document summarizing one's employment and educational history. (1)

retention schedule A schedule that details how long to keep different types of patient records in the office after they have become inactive or closed and how long the records should be stored. (10)

retina The inner layer of the eye; contains light-sensing nerve cells. (26)

retrograde pyelography A radiologic procedure in which the doctor injects a contrast medium through a urethral catheter and takes a series of x-rays to evaluate function of the ureters, bladder, and urethra. (40)

rods Light-sensing nerve cells in the eye, at the posterior of the retina, that function in dim light but do not provide sharp images or detect color. (26)

Role Delineation Study See **AAMA Role Delineation Study.** (1)

route The way a drug is introduced into the body. (38)

R wave A large upward spike on an electrocardiogram that represents the impulse for depolarization traveling through the left ventricle. (39)

salutation A written greeting, such as "Dear," used at the beginning of a letter. (7)

sanitization A reduction of the number of microorganisms on an object or a surface to a fairly safe level. (19)

saturated fats Fats, derived primarily from animal sources, that are usually solid at room temperature and that tend to raise blood cholesterol levels. (36)

scanner An optical device that converts printed matter into a format that can be read by the computer and inputs the converted information. (6)

sclera The tough, outermost layer, or "white," of the eye, through which light cannot pass; covers all except the front of the eye. (26)

scoliosis A lateral curvature of the spine, which is normally straight when viewed from behind. (25)

scratch test An allergy test in which extracts of suspected allergens are applied to the patient's skin and the skin is then scratched to allow the extracts to penetrate. (28)

screening Performing a diagnostic test on a person who is typically free of symptoms. (14)

screen saver A program that automatically changes the monitor display at short intervals or constantly shows moving images to prevent burn-in of images on the computer screen. (6)

seizure A series of violent and involuntary contractions of the muscles; also called a convulsion. (31)

semen Sperm and the various substances that nourish and transport them. (23)

semicircular canals Structures in the inner ear that help a person maintain balance; each of the three canals is positioned at right angles to the other two. (26)

sensorineural hearing loss A type of hearing loss in which sound waves reach the inner ear but the brain does not perceive them as sound. (26)

septic shock A state of shock resulting from massive, widespread infection that affects the blood vessels' ability to circulate blood. (31)

sequential order One after another in a predictable pattern or sequence. (10)

serum The clear, yellow liquid that remains after a blood clot forms; it is separated from the clotted elements by centrifugation. (34)

service contract A contract that covers services for equipment that are not included in a standard maintenance contract. (5)

set point The weight that a body automatically maintains, which may be elevated in people who are obese. (36)

shock A life-threatening state, associated with failure of the cardiovascular system, that prevents adequate blood circulation to the vital organs. (31)

sigmoidoscopy A procedure in which the interior of the sigmoid area of the large intestine, between the descending colon and the rectum, is examined with a sigmoidoscope, a lighted instrument with a magnifying lens. (28)

sign An objective or external factor, such as blood pressure, rash, or swelling, that can be seen or felt by the physician or measured by an instrument. (9)

simplified letter style A modification of the full-block style in which the salutation and complimentary closing are omitted and a subject line typed in all capital letters is placed between the address and the body of the letter. (7)

single-entry account An account that has only one charge, usually for a small amount, for a patient who does not come in regularly. (17)

sinoatrial (SA) node A small bundle of heart muscle tissue in the superior wall of the right atrium that sets the rhythm (or pattern) of the heart's contractions; also called sinus node or pacemaker. (39)

sinus node See **sinoatrial (SA) node.**

skinfold test A method of measuring fat as a percentage of body weight by measuring the thickness of a fold of skin with a caliper. (36)

slit lamp An instrument composed of a magnifying lens combined with a light source; used to provide a minute examination of the eye's anatomy. (28)

smear A specimen spread thinly and unevenly across a slide. (35)

SOAP An approach to medical records documentation that documents information in the following order: S (subjective data), O (objective data), A (assessment), P (plan of action). (9)

software A program, or set of instructions, that tells a computer what to do. (6)

solution A homogeneous mixture of a solid, liquid, or gaseous substance in a liquid, such as a dissolved drug in liquid form. (38)

SPECT Single photon emission computed tomography; a radiologic procedure in which a gamma camera detects signals induced by gamma radiation and a computer converts these signals into two- or three-dimensional images that are displayed on a screen. (40)

speculum An instrument that expands the vaginal opening to permit viewing of the vagina and cervix. (27)

sperm See **spermatozoa.**

spermatozoa Male reproductive cells; also called sperm. (23)

sphygmomanometer An instrument for measuring blood pressure; consists of an inflatable cuff, a pressure bulb used to inflate the cuff, and a device to read the pressure. (24)

spirilla See **spirillum.**

spirillum A spiral-shaped bacterium. (35)

spirometer An instrument that measures the air taken in and expelled from the lungs. (39)

spirometry A test used to measure breathing capacity. (39)

splinting catheter A type of catheter inserted after plastic repair of the ureter; it must remain in place for at least a week after surgery. (33)

sprain An injury characterized by partial tearing of a ligament that supports a joint, such as the ankle. A sprain may also involve injuries to tendons, muscles, and local blood vessels and contusions of the surrounding soft tissue. (31)

stain In microbiology, a solution of a dye or group of dyes that impart a color to microorganisms. (35)

standard A specimen for which test values are already known; used to calibrate test equipment. (32)

Standard Precautions A combination of Universal Precautions and Body Substance Isolation guidelines; used in hospitals for the care of all patients. (19)

stapes A small bone in the middle ear that is attached to the inner ear; also called the stirrup. (26)

statement A form similar to an invoice; contains a courteous reminder to the patient that payment is due. (17)

statute of limitations A state law that sets a time limit on when a collection suit on a past-due account can legally be filed. (17)

stereoscopy An x-ray procedure that uses a specially designed microscope (stereoscopic, or Greenough, microscope) with double eyepieces and objectives to take films at different angles and produce three-dimensional images; used primarily to study the skull. (40)

sterile field An area free of microorganisms used as a work area during a surgical procedure. (29)

sterile scrub assistant An assistant who handles sterile equipment during a surgical procedure. (29)

sterile technique See **surgical asepsis.** (29)

sterilization The destruction of all microorganisms, including bacterial spores, by specific means. (19)

sterilization indicator A tag, insert, tape, tube, or strip that confirms that the items in an autoclave have been exposed to the correct volume of steam at the correct temperature for the correct amount of time. (20)

stethoscope An instrument that amplifies body sounds. (24)

stirrup See **stapes.** (26)

strain A muscle injury that results from overexertion or overstretching. (31)

stress test A procedure that involves recording an electrocardiogram while the patient is exercising on a stationary bicycle, treadmill, or stair-stepping ergometer, which measures work performed. (28)

S-T segment An area on an electrocardiogram that represents the time between contraction of the ventricles and their recovery; connects the end of the QRS complex with the beginning of the T wave. (39)

stylus A penlike instrument that records electrical impulses on ECG paper. (39)

subclinical case An infection in which the host experiences only some of the symptoms of the infection or milder symptoms than in a full case. (19)

subcutaneous (SC) Under the skin. (38)

sublingual Under the tongue. (38)

subpoena A written court order that is addressed to a specific person and requires that person's presence in court on a specific date at a specific time. (3)

subscriber The person in whose name an insurance policy is carried; also called the insured. (15)

subscriber liability The amount for which a subscriber is responsible, whether deductible, co-payment, coinsurance, or some combination of these. (15)

substance abuse The use of a substance in a way that is not medically approved, such as using diet pills to stay awake or consuming large quantities of cough syrup that contains codeine. Substance abusers are not necessarily addicts. (24)

superbill A form that combines the charges for services rendered, an invoice for payment or insurance co-payment, and all the information for submitting an insurance claim. (17)

supernatant The liquid portion of a substance from which solids have settled to the bottom, as with a urine specimen after centrifugation. (33)

surgeon A physician who uses hands and medical instruments to diagnose and correct deformities and treat external and internal injuries or disease. (2)

surgical asepsis The elimination of all microorganisms from objects or working areas; also called sterile technique. (29)

susceptible host An individual who has little or no immunity to infection by a particular organism. (19)

suture A surgical stitch made to close a wound. (29)

S wave A downward deflection on an electrocardiogram that represents the impulse for depolarization traveling through both ventricles. (39)

symmetry The degree to which one side of the body is the same as the other. (25)

sympathetic nervous system The part of the peripheral autonomic nervous system that responds to body stress. (23)

symptom A subjective, or internal, condition felt by a patient, such as pain, headache, or nausea, or another indication that generally cannot be seen or felt by the doctor or measured by instruments. (9)

systolic pressure The blood pressure measured when the left ventricle of the heart contracts. (24)

tab A tapered rectangular or rounded extension at the top of a file folder. (10)

tachycardia Rapid heart rate, generally in excess of 100 beats per minute. (31)

tachypnea Abnormally rapid breathing. (24)

tax liability Money withheld from employees' paychecks and held in a separate account that must be used to pay taxes to appropriate government agencies. (18)

telephone triage A process of determining the level of urgency of each incoming telephone call and how it should be handled. (11)

teletherapy A radiation therapy technique that allows deeper penetration than brachytherapy; used primarily for deep tumors. (40)

tendon A cordlike fibrous tissue that connects muscle to bone. (23)

10× lens A magnifying lens in the ocular of a microscope that magnifies an image ten times. (32)

terminal Fatal. (21)

testosterone A hormone produced by the testes that maintains the male reproductive structures and male characteristics such as deep voice, body hair, and muscle mass. (23)

therapeutic team A group of physicians, nurses, medical assistants, and other specialists who work with patients dealing with chronic illness or recovery from major injuries. (30)

thermography A radiologic procedure in which an infrared camera is used to take photographs that record variations in skin temperature as dark (cool areas), light (warm areas), or shades of gray (areas with temperatures between cool and warm); used to diagnose breast tumors, breast abscesses, and fibrocystic breast disease. (40)

thermotherapy The application of heat to the body to treat a disorder or injury. (30)

third-party check A check made out to one recipient and given in payment to another, as with one made out to a patient rather than the medical practice. (16)

thrombocytes See **platelets.** (34)

thrombus A blood clot. (27)

tickler file A reminder file for keeping track of time-sensitive obligations. (10)

time-specified scheduling A system of scheduling where patients arrive at regular, specified intervals, assuring the practice a steady stream of patients throughout the day. (12)

timed urine specimen A specimen of a patient's urine collected over a specific time period. (33)

T lymphocyte A type of nongranular leukocyte that regulates immunologic response; includes helper T cells and suppressor T cells. (34)

topical Applied to the skin. (29)

tort In civil law, a breach of some obligation that causes harm or injury to someone. (3)

tower case A vertical housing for the system unit of a personal computer. (6)

toxicology The study of poisons or poisonous effects of drugs. (37)

tracking (financial) Watching for changes in spending so as to help control expenses. (18)

traction The pulling or stretching of the musculoskeletal system to treat dislocated joints, joints afflicted by arthritis or other diseases, and fractured bones. (30)

trade name A drug's brand or proprietary name. (37)

transcription The transforming of spoken notes into accurate written form. (9)

transcutaneous absorption Entry (as of a pathogen) through a cut or crack in the skin. (22)

transdermal A type of topical drug administration that slowly and evenly releases a systemic drug through the skin directly into the bloodstream; a transdermal unit is also called a patch. (38)

transfer To give something, such as information, to another party outside the doctor's office. (9)

traveler's check A check purchased and signed at a bank and later signed over to a payee. (18)

triage To assess the urgency and types of conditions patients present, as well as their immediate medical needs. (2)

trial balance A preliminary check performed on calculations in a disbursements journal. (18)

triglycerides Simple lipids consisting of glycerol (an alcohol) and three fatty acids. (36)

troubleshooting Trying to determine and correct a problem without having to call a service supplier. (5)

tutorial A small program included in a software package designed to give users an overall picture of the product and its functions. (6)

T wave An upward curve on an electrocardiogram that represents recovery (repolarization) of the ventricles. (39)

24-hour urine specimen A urine specimen collected over a 24-hour period and used to complete a quantitative and qualitative analysis of one or more substances, such as sodium, chloride, and calcium. (33)

tympanic membrane A fibrous partition located at the inner end of the ear canal and separating the outer ear from the middle ear; also called the eardrum. (26)

tympanic thermometer A type of electronic thermometer that measures infrared energy emitted from the tympanic membrane. (24)

ultrasonic cleaning A method of sanitization that involves placing instruments in a cleaning solution in a special receptacle that generates sound waves through the cleaning solution, loosening contaminants. Ultrasonic cleaning is safe for even very fragile instruments. (20)

underbooking Leaving large, unused gaps in the doctor's schedule; this approach does not make the best use of the doctor's time. (12)

Uniform Donor Card A legal document that states a person's wish to make a gift upon death of one or more organs for medical research, organ transplants, or placement in a tissue bank. (3)

unit price The total price of a package divided by the number of items that comprise the package. (8)

Universal Precautions Specific precautions required by the Department of Health and Human Services' Centers for Disease Control and Prevention (CDC) to prevent health-care workers from exposing themselves and others to infection by blood-borne pathogens. (19)

unsaturated fats Fats, including most vegetable oils, that are usually liquid at room temperature and tend to lower blood cholesterol. (36)

upper GI series See **barium swallow.** (40)

urinalysis The physical, chemical, and microscopic evaluation of urine to obtain information about body health and disease. (33)

urinary catheter A sterile plastic tube inserted to provide urinary drainage. (33)
urinary pH A measure of the degree of acidity or alkalinity of urine. (33)
urine specific gravity A measure of the concentration or amount (total weight) of substances dissolved in urine. (33)
urinometer A sealed glass float with a calibrated scale on the stem; used to measure urine specific gravity. (33)
urobilinogen A colorless compound formed by the breakdown of hemoglobin in the intestines. Elevated levels in urine may indicate increased red blood cell destruction or liver disease, whereas lack of urobilinogen in the urine may suggest total bile duct obstruction. (33)
urologist A specialist who diagnoses and treats diseases of the kidney, bladder, and urinary system. (2)
U wave A small upward curve sometimes found on an electrocardiogram after a T wave. (39)

vaccine A special preparation made from microorganisms and administered to a person to produce reduced sensitivity to, or increased immunity to, an infectious disease. (37)
vasectomy A male sterilization procedure in which a section of each of the vas deferens is removed. (28)
vector A living organism, such as an insect, that carries microorganisms from an infected person to another person. (19)
venipuncture The puncture of a vein, usually with a needle, for the purpose of drawing blood. (34)
ventricle A lower, pumping chamber of the heart. (23)
vertical file A filing cabinet featuring pull-out drawers that usually contain a metal frame or bar equipped to handle letter- or legal-sized documents in hanging file folders. (10)
vesting Giving a person the legal right to the money in an account. (16)
vial A small glass bottle with a self-sealing rubber stopper. (29)
vibrio A comma-shaped bacterium. (35)
vibrios See **vibrio.**
virulence A microorganism's disease-producing power. (19)
virus One of the smallest known infectious agents, consisting only of nucleic acid surrounded by a protein coat; can live and grow only within the living cells of other organisms. (35)
vital signs Primary indicators of a patient's condition: temperature, pulse, respiration, and blood pressure. (24)
vitamins Organic substances that are essential for normal body growth and maintenance and resistance to infection. (36)
vitreous humor A jellylike substance that fills the part of the eye behind the lens and helps the eye keep its shape. (26)
voice mail An advanced form of answering machine that allows a caller to leave a message when the phone line is busy. (5)
volume The amount of space an object, such as a drug, occupies. (38)
voucher check A business check with an attached stub, which is kept as a receipt. (18)

walk-in A patient who arrives without an appointment. (12)
warranty A contract that specifies free service and replacement of parts for a piece of equipment during a certain period, usually a year. (5)
wave scheduling A system of scheduling where the number of patients seen each hour is determined by dividing the hour by the length of the average visit and then giving that number of patients appointments with the doctor at the beginning of each hour. (12)
Western blot test A blood test used to confirm enzyme-linked immunosorbent assay (ELISA) test results for HIV infection. (21)
wet mount A preparation of a specimen in a liquid that allows the organisms to remain alive and mobile while they are being identified. (35)
whole-body skin examination An examination of the visible top layer of the entire surface of the skin, including the scalp, genital area, and areas between the toes, to look for lesions, especially suspicious moles or precancerous growths. (28)
whole blood The total volume of plasma and formed elements, or blood in which the elements have not been separated by coagulation or centrifugation. (34)
Wood's light examination A type of dermatologic examination in which a physician inspects the patient's skin under an ultraviolet lamp in a darkened room. (28)
wound An injury in which the skin or tissues under the skin are damaged. (29)
written-contract account An agreement between the physician and patient stating that the patient will pay a bill in more than four installments. (17)

xeroradiography A radiologic procedure in which x-rays are developed with a powder toner, similar to the toner in photocopiers, and the x-ray image is processed on specially treated xerographic paper; used to diagnose breast cancer, abscesses, lesions, or calcifications. (40)
xiphoid process The lower extension of the breastbone. (31)

yeast A fungus that grows mainly as a single-celled organism and reproduces by budding. (35)

Z-track method A technique used when injecting an intramuscular (IM) drug that can irritate subcutaneous tissue; involves pulling the skin and subcutaneous tissue to the side before inserting the needle at the site, creating a zigzag path in the tissue layers that prevents the drug from leaking into the subcutaneous tissue and causing irritation. (38)

Index

Index

Page numbers in **boldface** indicate figures. Page numbers followed by (t) indicate tables, by (p) procedures, and by (b) other boxed material.

Natasha
Marie
Valenzuela
4-10-97

Natalie
Miranda
2-11-78

Margarita
Miranda

Mar
Maritza

Natalie Miranda

Natalie Miranda

Natalie Miranda

Maritza Miranda

Natasha Marie Valenzuela

Emanuel Miranda

Jose Miranda

Na

N

Aida Miranda

Natalie

Natalie

Natalie Miranda

Maritza Miranda